A TEXTBOOK O

CLINICAL
PHARMACOL

A TEXTBOOK OF
CLINICAL PHARMACOLOGY

Second Edition

H. C. Gillies, BSc, MB, BS, MRCP
Lecturer in Clinical Pharmacology

H. J. Rogers, MA, MB, BChir, PhD, FRCP
Professor of Clinical Pharmacology

R. G. Spector, MD, PhD, FRCP, FRCPath,
Professor of Applied Pharmacology

J. R. Trounce, MD, FRCP
Professor Emeritus of Clinical Pharmacology,
United Medical and Dental Schools,
Guy's Hospital, London

HODDER AND STOUGHTON
LONDON SYDNEY AUCKLAND TORONTO

British Library Cataloguing in Publication Data

A Textbook of clinical pharmacology.—
2nd ed.
1. Chemotherapy
I. Gillies, H. C. II. Rogers, H. J.
615.5′8 RM262

ISBN 0 340 37674 0

First published 1981
Reprinted 1982, 1983, 1984
Second edition 1986

Typeset by Macmillan India Ltd., Bangalore 25.

Printed and bound in Great Britain
For Hodder and Stoughton Educational,
a division of Hodder and Stoughton Ltd.,
Mill Road, Dunton Green, Sevenoaks, Kent
by Page Bros (Norwich) Ltd.

PREFACE

The last thirty years have seen an unprecedented increase in the number and in the range of activity of drugs used in the treatment of human disease. Although their use goes back far into antiquity, it has only been relatively recently that mythology and empiricism have given way to systematic and scientific study. In parallel with the drug explosion, clinical pharmacology has emerged as a distinct discipline, one of the chief reasons for this being the realisation that the use of drugs in man posed special problems which were not necessarily solved by animal models. An important catalyst was the thalidomide disaster which highlighted the casual and often uninformed way in which drugs were introduced and used.

Clinical pharmacology is not merely a link between pharmacology and clinical medicine. It is a rapidly developing and evolving subject with its own methods and techniques. Although animal pharmacology provides much of the essential background to the development and use of drugs, it gives only part of the story. This is because the handling and toxicity of drugs often show considerable species difference, and also because many disease states appear to be unique to man and can therefore only be studied in the human context. In this book we portray clinical pharmacology as a subject in its own right, not as an appendage to either pharmacology or medicine. We have tried to indicate how an understanding of the subject is essential for the rational use of drugs as therapeutic agents. In a world where drugs are so widely prescribed and where many of them have so great a potential to do harm or good, the training of a doctor should include a thorough grounding in clinical pharmacology.

The importance attached to clinical pharmacology and therapeutics in the education of doctors is emphasised by the fact that in most universities in the United Kingdom it is accorded equal status with medicine, surgery and gynaecology and obstetrics in the final qualifying examination. Our objectives in this book are therefore to encourage an understanding of how drugs act and may best be used in the clinic. It is also hoped that readers will be encouraged to evaluate critically both their own clinical decisions and therapeutic innovations. In some areas we have not hesitated to introduce both complexity and controversy since clinical pharmacology is presently a rapidly changing subject. Although some of the pharmacokinetic equations are, at first sight, fearsome to many doctors of our generation it is unlikely that they will intimidate many of our students who nowadays enter our medical schools with sufficient grasp of mathematics to comprehend them with ease.

The first part of the book deals with general aspects of the subject. This section not only considers pharmacokinetics and the various factors which may modify drug disposition, but also reviews the problems of toxicity, monitoring of adverse effects and the introduction of new drugs: topics which are important, not only to the practising doctor, but also to those concerned with drugs in industry and in government.

The second part is devoted to a systematic review of the disposition and action of drugs together with their therapeutic use. Particular emphasis is laid on side effects and interactions and where it is relevant the underlying disease processes are described.

A number of appendices which may be useful to the reader have been included. As this is not a comprehensive reference book but essentially a book for study and learning it is not fully referenced but further reading is suggested in one of the appendices. Throughout the text every effort has been made to indicate the growing points of the subject so that it is seen not as a static body of knowledge but as an expanding and developing branch of medicine.

Although it is little more than four years since the first edition of this book appeared, the advances in the subject have been so great that considerable sections have had to be entirely rewritten and an extensive revision of the text has been necessary. The rapid introduction of effective new drugs with widely differing pharmacological actions makes the task of the student and practising doctor increasingly difficult. We have tried to define not only the pharmacology of these drugs in man, but also where they fit into the therapeutic scene, for pharmacology without reference to therapeutic application is of little use to the clinician. We have been pleased to share this task of revision with Dr Helen Gillies who assisted with the previous edition and now joins the team of authors.

We would emphasise that learning Clinical Pharmacology can only be effective if accompanied by clinical experience for, perhaps despite initial impressions, this is a practical subject and, just like clinical medicine, the patient is the best teacher. We make no apology for the size of the book. As different drugs are used for the same purpose in different hospitals we advise the student to select those parts which relate to the practice of his own institution. We recommend our own students to review each drug or treatment as it is encountered for the first time in practice. By this means it is possible to achieve a secure background in therapeutics very quickly. It is our experience that attempts to learn the subject in isolation from clinical work usually fail.

We would like to thank numerous colleagues who have helped us with advice and criticism and in particular Dr Glyn Volans and Dr John Henry of the National Poisons Centre, Dr J G Lewis, Dr Lionel Lewis, Dr Laurence Youlton, Dr Peter Harper, Dr William Van't Hoff, and the Drug Information Unit, Guy's Hospital. We would also like to thank the Southwark and North Lewisham Formulary Committee for permission to publish their guide to the use of antibiotics in modified form. Special thanks are due to Christine Wier and Lorraine White who typed the revisions and to Stuart Gillies who assisted with the Index.

United Medical and Dental Schools
Guy's Hospital Campus
LONDON
SE1 9RT

Helen Gillies
Howard Rogers
Roy Spector
John Trounce

CONTENTS

A. General Principles

Chapter 1

INTRODUCTION TO PHARMACOKINETICS

Pharmacokinetics may be defined as the study of the time course of absorption, distribution, metabolism and excretion of drugs and the corresponding pharmacological response. The use of mathematical models to describe these processes allows predictions to be made about such matters as drug concentration in various parts of the body, design of dosage regimes and adjustment of dosage in diseases affecting absorption, metabolism or elimination. In view of the complexity of the human body it is not surprising that pharmacokinetic formulations may be complex and require mathematical methods which can make pharmacokinetic literature and concepts unintelligible to many clinicians. In this chapter a brief synopsis of the field is given, sufficient to allow comprehension of the increasing number of publications appearing in clinical journals which make use of pharmacokinetic methods.

SINGLE-COMPARTMENT MODELS AND FIRST ORDER KINETICS

A common approach to the study of pharmacokinetic behaviour is to consider the body as a series of well-stirred compartments. These compartments have no physiological or anatomical meaning but are mathematical concepts from which a model may be built. The simplest model (Fig. 1.1) considers the body as a single compartment (a 'black box') into which the administered drug simultaneously distributes and equilibrates. This model often adequately describes the changes with time of plasma concentration or urinary excretion for drugs which rapidly distribute between plasma and tissue after administration. To assume a one-compartment model does not necessarily imply that plasma and tissue concentrations are the same, i.e. uniformity within the

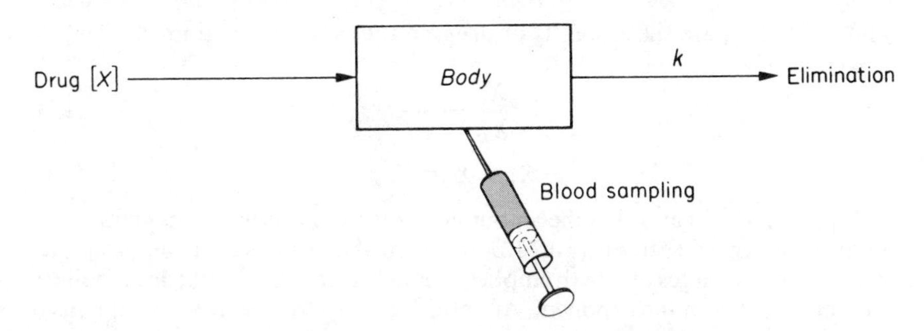

Fig. 1.1 A one-compartment model.

compartment is not necessary, but it is essential that changes occurring in the plasma quantitatively reflect changes in tissue drug levels, i.e. a constant relationship exists between these variables. Thus, if the concentration of a drug in fat at time t after a dose X is one third of the plasma concentration, then at time t after a dose $2X$ the fat concentration is still one third of the plasma concentration.

Elimination from the compartment is often assumed to follow so-called *first-order kinetics*, i.e. the rate of a given process is proportional to the amount of drug present. To describe this it is convenient to use the methods of differential and integral calculus. Thus, the rate of change ($\mathrm{d}X/\mathrm{d}t$) in the amount of drug present in the body (X) is expressed in this notation by

$$-\frac{\mathrm{d}X}{\mathrm{d}t} \propto X \quad \text{so} \quad \frac{\mathrm{d}X}{\mathrm{d}t} = -kX, \tag{1.1}$$

where k is a proportionality constant otherwise known as the *first-order elimination rate constant* (its units are of time^{-1}). The negative sign in eq. (1.1) indicates drug is being lost from the body. Differential equations of this type are known as linear (the dependent variable X appears only in its first power) and homogeneous (X appears only once in every term). *First-order processes therefore give rise to so-called linear kinetics.* An important consequence of a linear system in kinetics is that the total area under the plasma concentration–time curve (AUC) following intravenous administration is a linear function of the administered dose. Thus doubling the dose will, other factors being equal, double the AUC. By analogy, building bricks could be considered to form a linear system in the sense that two bricks placed one on top of the other stand twice as high as a single brick. Equation (1.1) may be solved to give an expression which will allow us to obtain values of X at any time t by integration between the limits of zero time and t. Thus

$$\int_{X_0}^{X_t} \frac{\mathrm{d}X}{X} = -\int_0^t k\,\mathrm{d}t \tag{1.2}$$

which gives $\ln X_t - \ln X_0 = -kt$, where ln is the notation for logarithms (natural logarithms) taken to the base e, i.e. $\log_e$ (where e is defined as

$$e = \lim_{n \to \infty} \left(1 + \frac{1}{n}\right)^n = 2.71828\ldots)$$

and X_0 and X_t are the amounts of drug present at time 0 and time t. This is solved as

$$\ln \frac{X_t}{X_0} = -kt \tag{1.3}$$

so

$$X_t = X_0 e^{-kt}. \tag{1.4}$$

Equation (1.4) states that the amount of drug in the body declines with time in an exponential fashion (Fig. 1.2) in much the same way as an electrical condenser discharges or a bath empties. It is called an exponential decline since the variable, t, is in the exponent. An intuitive grasp for the meaning of k may be gained by considering that:

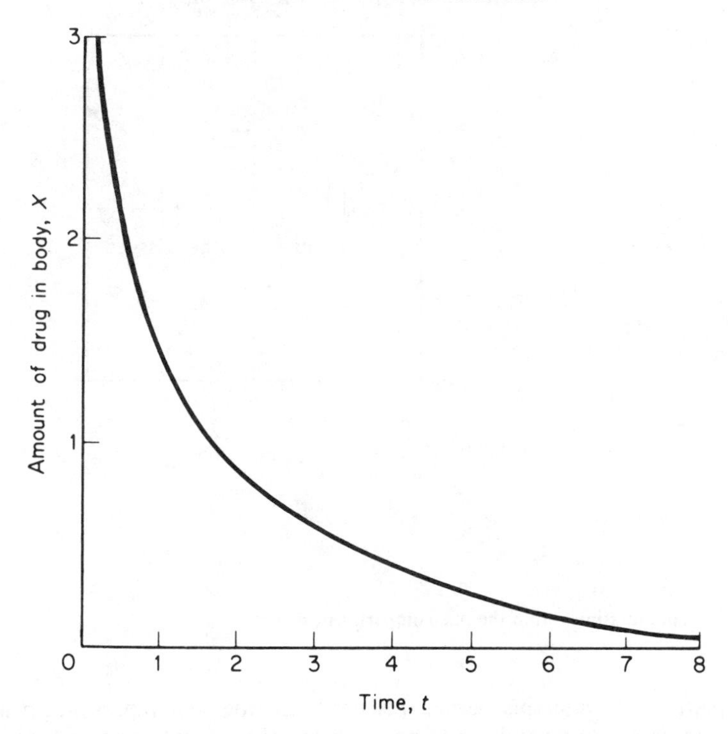

Fig. 1.2 Decline in amount of drug in body with time according to $X_t = X_0 e^{-kt}$ plotted on linear (Cartesian) coordinates.

Amount of drug eliminated in time t is

$$X_0 - X_t = X_0 - X_0 e^{-kt} = X_0(1 - e^{-kt}) \tag{1.5}$$

If a table of k in arbitrary units is prepared we have

k (*time*$^{-1}$)	0.001	0.01	0.1	0.2	0.3
Fraction of drug lost in unit time $(1 - e^{-k})$	0.000 999	0.009 95	0.095 2	0.181	0.259

Thus k and $(1 - e^{-k})$ are approximately equal for values of k below 0.2 and it is roughly true to say that if $k = 0.01$ hours^{-1} then 1% of the drug in the body is eliminated per hour.

Even if the data will fit a one-compartment model obviously the drug levels in liver, heart, fat, etc, are not equal to that in plasma. The one-compartment model assumes, however, that a constant relationship exists between the drug concentration in the plasma and the amount of drug in the body (see Fig. 1.3), that is

$$X = V_d C, \tag{1.6}$$

where C is the plasma concentration and V_d is a proportionality constant which has the units of volume and is, rather confusingly, called the *volume of*

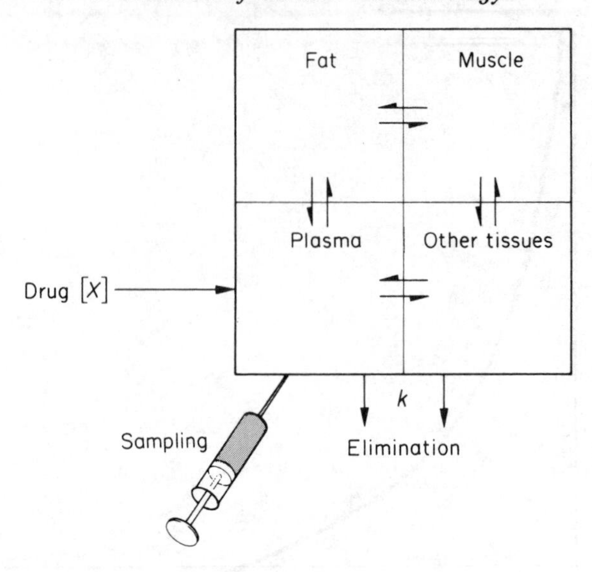

Fig. 1.3 Equilibration within the one-compartment model.

distribution. Despite this name, this constant does *not* represent an actual physiological volume and for some drugs may be several hundred litres in an adult. The size of the V_d is related partly to the characteristics of the drug, e.g. lipid solubility, and partly to patient characteristics such as body size, plasma protein concentration, degree of protein and tissue binding of the drug, body water and fat content. In general, drugs which are highly protein bound exhibit small V_d values, whilst highly lipid soluble compounds able to penetrate into cells and fatty tissues possess a large V_d. The V_d should be regarded as a multiplying factor relating the amount of drug in the whole body to the plasma concentration.

Example: for gentamicin the V_d is 0.25 l/kg; thus to calculate a dose of gentamicin for an 80 kg man in whom the maximum serum concentration is not to exceed 8 μg/ml, we substitute in (1.6) and

$$X = 0.25 \times 80 \times 8 = 160 \text{ mg.}$$

Use of eq. (1.6) allows eqs. (1.1)–(1.4) to be rewritten in terms of concentration. For example,

$$C_t = C_0 e^{-kt}. \tag{1.7}$$

Equation (1.7) may be rewritten as

$$\ln C = \ln C_0 - kt \tag{1.8}$$

and converted into common logarithms (i.e. logarithms to the base 10) by dividing by 2.303:

$$\log C = \log C_0 - \frac{kt}{2.303}. \tag{1.9}$$

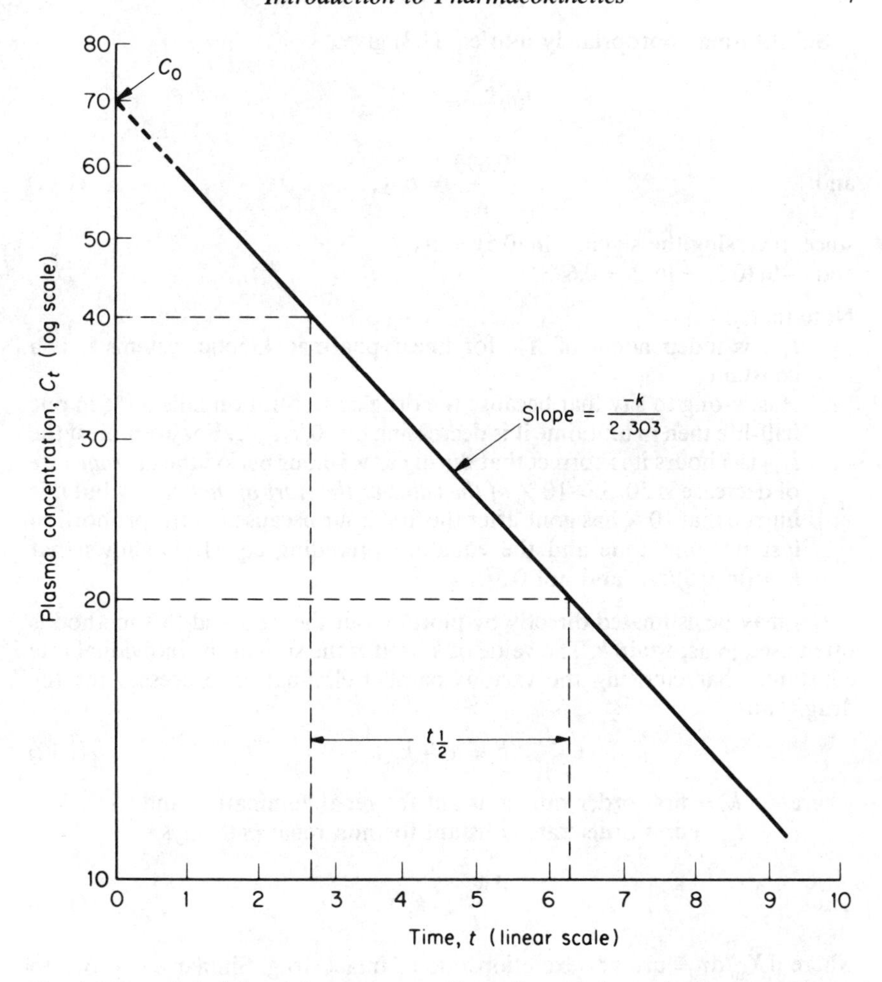

Fig. 1.4 Hypothetical plot of plasma concentration decline with time on log-linear coordinates.

Thus plotting $\log C$ against t yields a straight line and C_0 may be obtained by extrapolation of the line to zero time (Fig. 1.4). The slope of the line is $-k/2.303$. Straight lines are mathematically much easier to handle than exponential curves and so log concentration–time plots frequently occur in pharmacokinetics. Since X_0 is the dose of drug administered, eq. (1.10) may be used to find V_d from

$$V_d = \frac{X_0}{C_0}. \tag{1.10}$$

Half life and clearance

A commonly used constant to characterise first-order processes is the *half-life*, *i.e. the time taken for the drug concentration to decline by* 50%.

Substituting appropriately into eq. (1.3) gives

$$\ln\frac{0.5}{1} = -kt_{1/2},$$

and
$$\frac{0.693}{k} = t_{1/2}, \tag{1.11}$$

since, reversing the signs $-\ln(0.5) = kt_{1/2}$
and $-\ln(0.5) = \ln 2 = 0.693$.

Note that:

1. $t_{1/2}$ is independent of X_0: for linear pharmacokinetic systems it is a constant
2. It is wrong to say that because the drug concentration falls 50% in one half-life then in unit time it is decreasing by $50/t_{1/2}$ %. For example if the $t_{1/2}$ is 5 hours it is correct that during any 5-hour period the *average* rate of decrease is 50/5 = 10% *of the value at the start of that period* but it is untrue that 10% has gone after the first hour because k is the proportion lost per unit time and the equation preceding eq. (1.11) shows that $k = (\ln 0.5)/t_{1/2}$ and not $0.5/t_{1/2}$.

$t_{1/2}$ may be estimated directly by plotting out the data and this method is often used to ascertain k. The value of k itself is the sum of the individual rate constants characterising the various parallel elimination processes for the drug. Thus

$$k = k_r + k_{nr}, \tag{1.12}$$

where k_r = first-order rate constant for renal elimination and
k_{nr} = first order rate constant for non-renal pathways.

Thus
$$\frac{dX_u}{dt} = k_r X, \tag{1.13}$$

where dX_u/dt = urinary excretion rate of intact drug. Similar equations to those for the decline in plasma drug concentrations may be written for urinary excretion and a log/linear plot of urinary excretion rate of unchanged drug versus time may be used to determine k (cf. Fig. 1.4).

The $t_{1/2}$ is often regarded as a direct measure of the efficiency of drug elimination. This is incorrect since $t_{1/2}$ is dependent upon two independent variables, the volume of distribution and the total clearance of the drug (Cl):

$$t_{1/2} = \frac{0.693\,V_d}{Cl}. \tag{1.14}$$

Clearance is a more accurate measure of the efficiency with which the eliminating organs remove a drug since it is defined as the fraction of the apparent volume of distribution cleared of drug by the body in unit time. *Clearance is a physiologically meaningful parameter* having units of flow. It is *independent of the model used*. Clearance is constant for drugs excreted by first-order kinetics: in any time interval a constant fraction of the drug is eliminated.

Drugs not eliminated by first order kinetics (see below) will have changing clearance values with time as the total amount of drug in the body declines. Total body clearance is assessed by several methods including eq. (1.15)

$$Cl = \frac{X_0}{\int_0^\infty C\,\mathrm{d}t} = \frac{X_0}{\mathrm{AUC}} \tag{1.15}$$

$$= kV_\mathrm{d}. \tag{1.16}$$

The area under the plasma concentration–time curve (AUC) is symbolically expressed as

$$\mathrm{AUC} = \int_0^t C\,\mathrm{d}t \quad \text{for an area up to time } t$$

or $$\mathrm{AUC} = \int_0^\infty C\,\mathrm{d}t \quad \text{for an area extrapolated to infinite time.}$$

Practically this may be assessed by measuring the area with a planimeter or cutting out the curve and weighing it with reference to a standard area cut from the same piece of graph paper, or most usually by a numerical approximation such as the trapezoidal rule. If the curve is fitted to a particular pharmacokinetic model, then the exact solution of the integral for that model may be used after substituting the appropriate variables derived from the data. Thus for the one-compartment model the exact solution to the integral is

$$\int_0^\infty C\,\mathrm{d}t = \int_0^\infty C_0 e^{-kt}\,\mathrm{d}t = \frac{C_0}{k}. \tag{1.17}$$

Thus the total body clearance for a one-compartment model is also given by substituting (1.17) into (1.15):

$$Cl = \frac{X_0 k}{C_0}. \tag{1.18}$$

In passing we may note that therefore

$$C_0 = k\int_0^\infty C\,\mathrm{d}t \tag{1.19}$$

and this may be substituted into (1.10) to give a method for calculating the apparent volume of distribution which, because it utilises the area, is model independent:

$$V_\mathrm{d} = \frac{X_0}{k\int_0^\infty C\,\mathrm{d}t} = \frac{X_0}{k(\mathrm{AUC})} \tag{1.20}$$

Clearances are additive and total body clearance is the sum of clearance by each eliminating organ: for example,

total body clearance = renal clearance + metabolic clearance.

The maximum body clearance is determined by the blood flow through these organs and is approximately 3 l/min.

Renal clearance Cl_r is defined as the urinary drug excretion rate divided by the plasma concentration

$$Cl_r = \frac{dX_u/dt}{C}. \tag{1.21}$$

substituting from (1.13) gives

$$Cl_r = \frac{k_r X}{C}. \tag{1.22}$$

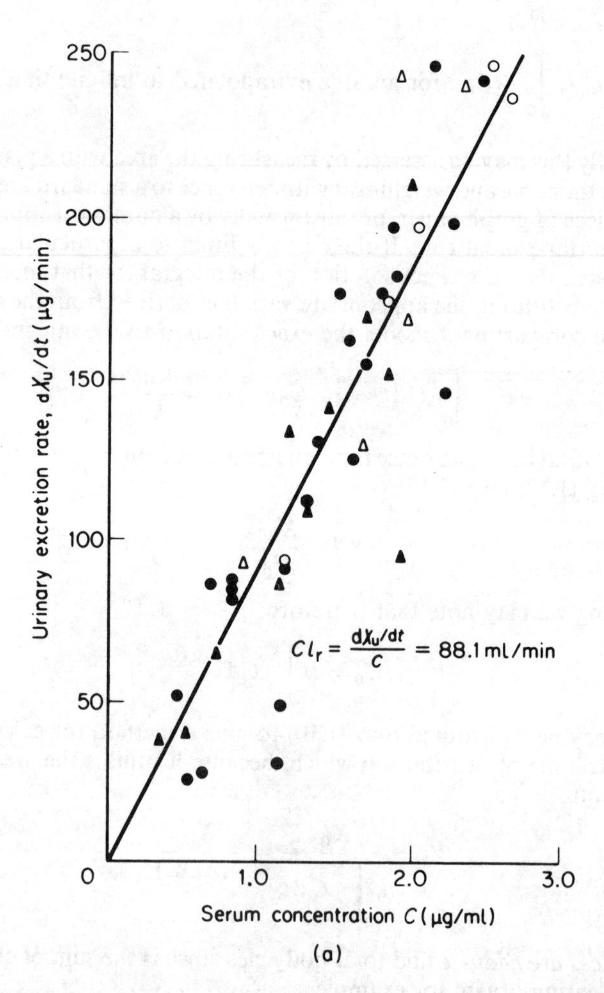

Fig. 1.5 Use of eqs (1.21) and (1.24) to determine renal clearance of tetracycline: (a) plot of mean urinary excretion rates versus serum tetracycline concentration. (b) *See facing page.*

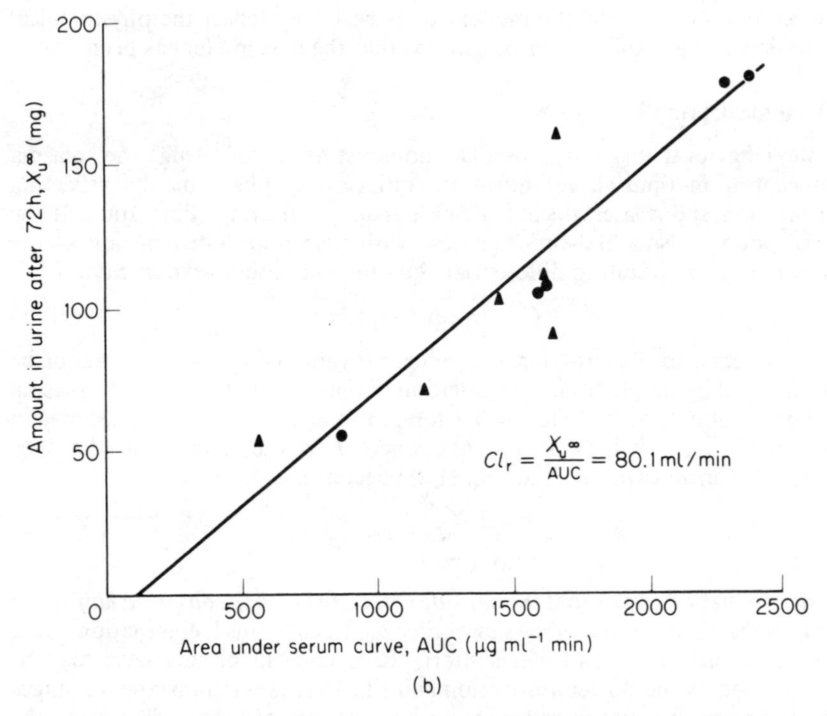

Fig. 1.5(b) Plot of cumulative tetracycline excretion in urine at 72 hours versus AUC following oral administration of 250 mg tetracycline hydrochloride. In each case the slope of the line represents renal clearance. (From W. H. Barr *et al*, *Clin. Pharmacol. Ther.*, **13**, 97 (1972).)

Since $X/C = V_d$ from (1.10), eq. (1.22) may also be written

$$Cl_r = k_r V_d \tag{1.23}$$

Substitution from (1.23) for Cl_r into (1.21) followed by integration from time zero to infinity and rearrangement of the equation yields an expression for average renal clearance:

$$Cl_r = k_r V_d = \frac{X_u^\infty}{\int_0^\infty C\,dt} \tag{1.24}$$

where X_u^∞ = total amount of free drug excreted in the urine (see Fig. 1.5).

Complementary changes in half-life and volume of distribution can be consistent with the same clearance. Thus an increased half-life with aging has been found for diazepam but the clearance remains constant at all ages because of a compensatory increase in volume of distribution.

It should be noted that pharmacokinetic 'constants' are not constants in the mathematical sense. They are fitted model parameters and subject to errors in their estimation which may vary with the concentrations obtained, analytical techniques and methods of data handling. These constants result from the operation of various physiological processes and although the model used may be reasonably accurate, the model can at best only reflect the physiological situation and it should never be claimed that the true model has been found.

Drug absorption kinetics

Following oral or intramuscular administration of drug the plasma concentration–time curve shows an initial rising phase mainly reflecting absorption and a later, declining phase mainly reflecting elimination. If the absorption is also a first-order process, with absorption rate constant k_a, the solution of the resulting differential equation is a double exponential:

$$C = C_0(e^{-kt} - e^{-k_a t}). \quad (1.25)$$

In contrast to the situation following intravenous injection C_0 cannot be determined by simple back-extrapolation of the declining phase of the plasma concentration–time curve to $t = 0$ (c.f. Fig. 1.4) since the intercept as shown in eq. (1.26) is $\log(k_a F X_0 / V_d(k_a - k))$, where F is the fraction of the dose available for absorption. Thus eq. (1.25) becomes

$$C = \frac{k_a F X_0}{V_d(k_a - k)}(e^{-kt} - e^{-k_a t}). \quad (1.26)$$

This equation shows that *the half-life associated with the observed half-life of drug in the plasma is that of the slower process.* Usually this is elimination but, if the true elimination half-life is short, the decline in plasma level may be determined by the slower absorption half-life. In these circumstances changes in absorption kinetics produce changes in the rate of loss of drug from the body. Because of this variable determination of the rate of decline in plasma concentration this type of equation is sometimes called a 'flip-flop'.

The transposed equation

$$F X_0 = \frac{C V_d (k_a - k)}{k_a(e^{-kt} - e^{-k_a t})} \quad (1.27)$$

is useful to calculate dosage regimes. Thus suppose it is desired to find the intramuscular dose of gentamicin for a normal 70 kg man to achieve a serum concentration of not greater than 8 mg/l at 1 hour. From volunteer studies, k_a for intramuscular injection is 2.47 h^{-1}, from Table 5.4 k is 0.30 h^{-1} and the $V_d = 0.25$ l/kg. Thus assuming $F = 1$ (i.e. complete absorption) we have

$$X_0 = \frac{8 \times 0.25 \times 70(2.47 - 0.30)}{2.47(e^{-0.30} - e^{-2.47})} = 187 \text{ mg}.$$

The time at which the maximum plasma concentration is reached is given by

$$t_{max} = \frac{2.303}{k_a - k} \log \frac{k_a}{k}, \quad (1.28)$$

and the actual maximum concentration is as would be expected from (1.4).

$$C_{max} = \frac{F X_0}{V_d} e^{-kt_{max}} \quad (1.29)$$

For the above example t_{max} is 0.97 hours and C_{max} is 7.99 μg/ml.

THE TWO-COMPARTMENT MODEL

Although useful for many purposes the one-compartment model is too simple to account accurately for the plasma level–time curves resulting from the administration of many drugs. For these a more complex two-compartment model may be suitable (Fig. 1.6). This resolves the body into a smaller central compartment and a larger peripheral compartment. Again, these compartments have no physiological or anatomical reality, although we assume the central compartment comprises blood (from which samples are taken for analysis) with the extracellular spaces of some well-perfused tissues such as heart, lungs, liver and kidneys. The peripheral compartment comprises less well-perfused tissues such as muscle, skin and fat into which drug permeates more slowly. Reversible transfer of drug occurs between these two compartments depending upon such factors as blood flow, affinity of tissues for the drug and the drug's partition coefficients. When a drug is instantaneously introduced into the central compartment (i.e. by intravenous or intra-arterial injection) the blood level of drug falls in a biphasic fashion. The initial rapid fall reflects mainly drug distribution from central to peripheral compartments, although elimination will be occurring from the moment the drug enters the body. At some point in time a *pseudodistribution equilibrium* is attained between the central and peripheral compartments when the ratio of drug in each compartment approaches a constant value which is maintained during the second slower phase of decline in blood concentration, which reflects largely elimination. A theoretical plot of these events is shown in Fig. 1.7. During this second phase, loss of drug from the body is described by a monoexponential process indicative of the kinetic homogeneity with respect to drug levels in all fluids and tissues of the body (see Fig. 1.8). At this stage the model may be said to have 'collapsed' into a one-compartment form. For a two-compartment model the net rate of change of drug concentration C_1 in the

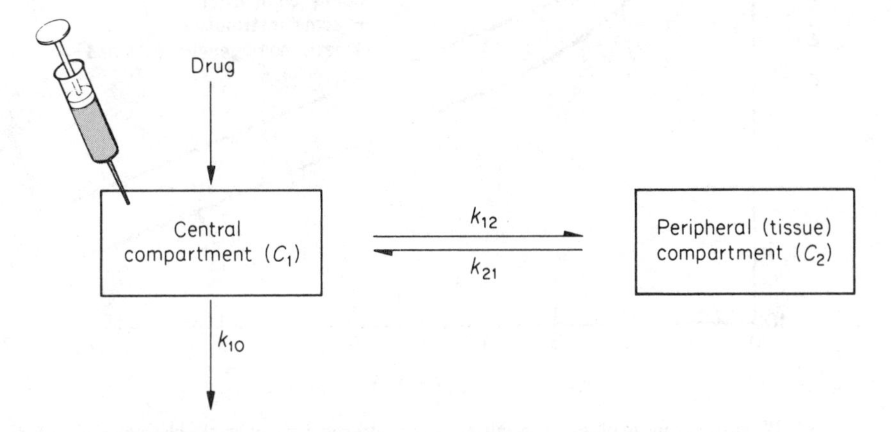

Fig. 1.6 Schematic representation of a two-compartment model.

central compartment is given by

$$\frac{dC_1}{dt} = -(k_{12}+k_{10})C_1 + k_{21}C_2, \tag{1.30}$$

where C_2 is the concentration in the peripheral compartment. This is a linear, homogeneous equation with constant coefficients and like all such equations has a solution which is the sum of exponential terms each of which may be multiplied by a constant. Thus the solution of the differential equations describing an instantaneous drug input into the central compartment is

$$C_1 = Ae^{-\alpha t} + Be^{-\beta t}, \tag{1.31}$$

where α is the rate constant of the distributive phase and the distribution half-life is

$$t_{1/2,\alpha} = \frac{0.693}{\alpha}, \tag{1.32}$$

while β is the rate constant of the elimination or β-phase and is sometimes called the disposition rate constant. β may be estimated from the slope of the

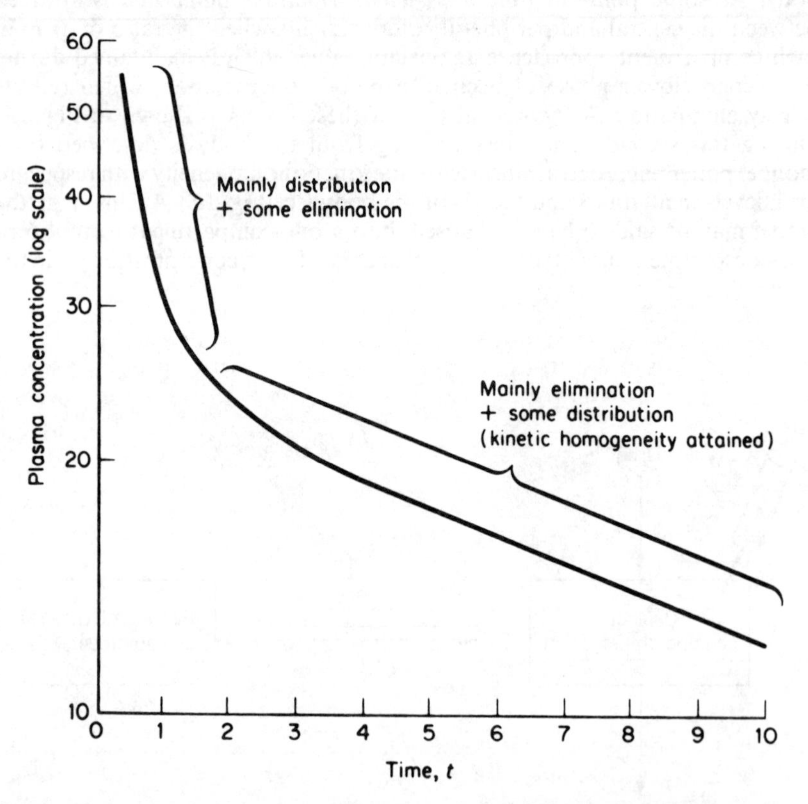

Fig. 1.7 Biphasic decline in plasma concentration for a drug which confers the characteristics of a two-compartment system on the body.

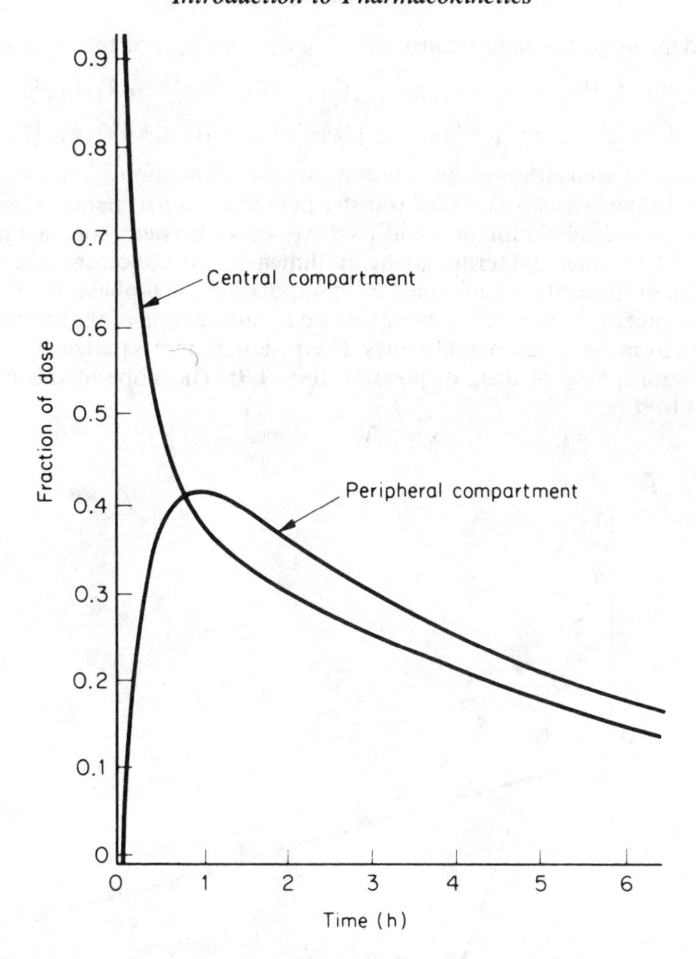

Fig. 1.8 Time course of hypothetical drug distribution in central and peripheral compartments following rapid intravenous injection. Note the parallel curves during the elimination (β-) phase.

elimination (second) phase of the log plasma concentration–time plot according to the equation

$$\beta = 2.303 \times \text{slope} \tag{1.33}$$

or from $t_{1/2,\beta}$, the elimination half-life (which is the half-life most usually and properly quoted), using

$$t_{1/2,\beta} = \frac{0.693}{\beta} \tag{1.34}$$

α and β have units of time^{-1} but neither correspond to the elimination rate constant k of the one-compartment model. They are both hybrid coefficients dependent upon the micro-constants (k_{12}, k_{21} and k_{10}) of the model, thus

$$\alpha = \tfrac{1}{2}\{(k_{12}+k_{21}+k_{10})+\sqrt{[(k_{12}+k_{21}+k_{10})^2-4k_{21}k_{10}]}\} \quad (1.35)$$

and $$\beta = \tfrac{1}{2}\{(k_{12}+k_{21}+k_{10})-\sqrt{[(k_{12}+k_{21}+k_{10})^2-4k_{21}k_{10}]}\} \quad (1.36)$$

and as can be seen although the rate constant for elimination k_{10} determines β, so also do the rate constants for transfer between compartments. β therefore reflects both drug elimination and its distribution between compartments.

A and B are intercept terms having the dimensions of concentration. B is the intercept on the ordinate obtained by extrapolating the β-phase to $t = 0$, A is the intercept of the secondary curve formed by subtraction of the extrapolated β-phase from the experimental values. This residual curve is that describing the distribution phase of drug disposition (Fig. 1.9). The slope of this curve is related to α by

$$\alpha = 2.303 \times \text{slope}. \quad (1.37)$$

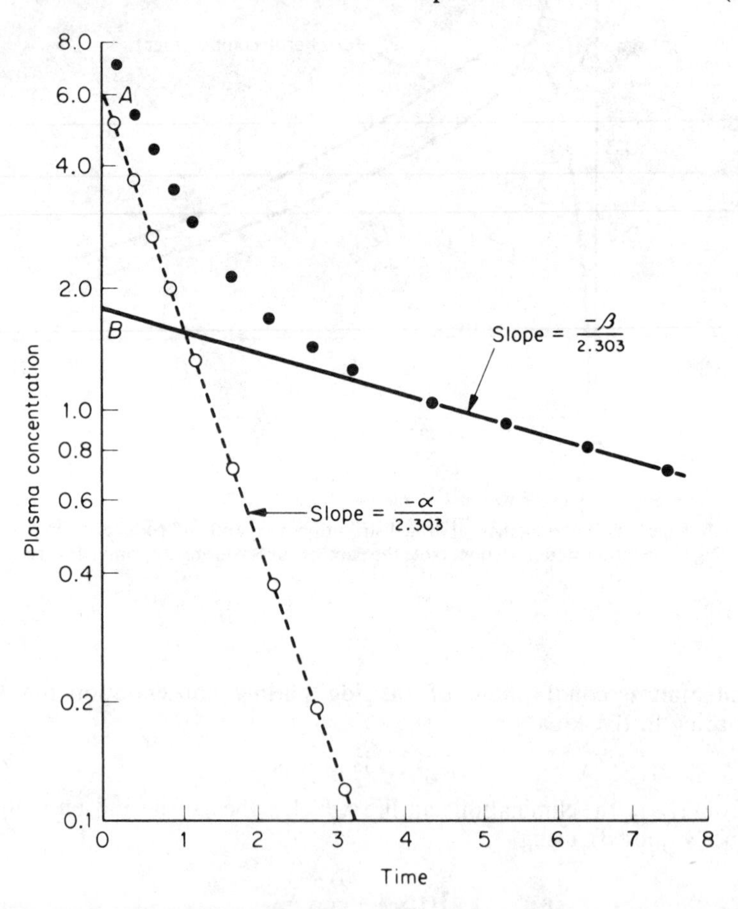

Fig. 1.9 Determination of A, B, α and β from experimental data (●) by method of residuals. A line of best fit is constructed through the terminal monoexponential (β) phase. Subtraction of this line from the remaining data points yields a second series of points (O) through which the residual line may be fitted to yield A and α.

A and B correspond to C_0 in a one compartment model. The micro-constants of the model may be found from the following:

$$k_{10} = \frac{A+B}{(A/\alpha)+(B/\beta)} = \frac{\alpha\beta}{k_{21}}, \tag{1.38}$$

$$k_{12} = \frac{AB}{(A+B)^2} \frac{(\beta-\alpha)^2}{k_{21}}, \tag{1.39}$$

$$k_{21} = \frac{A\beta + B\alpha}{A+B}. \tag{1.40}$$

There are a number of different volumes of distribution for a two-compartment model illustrating the point that these apparent volumes are not to be regarded as physical spaces but as multiplying factors. The volume of the central compartment V_1 is calculated by a method analogous to that for the one-compartment model:

$$V_1 = \frac{X_0}{A+B}. \tag{1.41}$$

The volume of distribution of the peripheral compartment

$$V_2 = V_1 \frac{k_{12}}{k_{21}}. \tag{1.42}$$

It is the more useful distribution volumes which describe the whole model that cause confusion. Using the usual definition of volume of distribution as the total drug in the body divided by the concentration at equilibrium in the reference (central) compartment at steady state, this is given by

$$V_{d(ss)} = V_1 + V_2 \tag{1.43}$$

$$= V_1\left(1 + \frac{k_{12}}{k_{21}}\right). \tag{1.44}$$

This is the apparent V_d at steady state and due to the requirement for equilibrium between compartments to be attained has a physiological meaning only when the drug is either not eliminated or is being infused at the same rate at which it is being eliminated. During a single dose it gives the correct relationship between the amount of drug in the body and the plasma concentration only when the net transfer of drug from central to peripheral compartment is zero. This obtains only at that single point in time when the peripheral compartment drug concentration has reached a maximum. A more useful estimate of the apparent volume of distribution is that which relates drug concentration in the plasma to the total amount of drug in the body at all times during the β-phase. This is $V_{d(\beta)}$ sometimes called $V_{d(area)}$ because of the mode of its calculation.

$$V_{d(\beta)} = \frac{X_0}{\beta\left(\int_0^\infty C\,dt\right)} \tag{1.45}$$

$$= \frac{X_0}{\beta(\text{AUC})}, \tag{1.46}$$

and since AUC for a two compartment model is given by

$$\int_0^\infty C\,\mathrm{d}t = \frac{A}{\alpha} + \frac{B}{\beta}, \text{ (c.f. (1.17))} \tag{1.47}$$

then

$$V_{\mathrm{d}(\beta)} = \frac{X_0}{\beta[(A/\alpha)+(B/\beta)]}. \tag{1.48}$$

Clearance is calculated using

$$Cl = V_1 k_{10} \tag{1.49}$$

or

$$Cl = \beta V_{\mathrm{d}(\beta)}, \tag{1.50}$$

which from (1.46) gives

$$Cl = \frac{X_0}{\mathrm{AUC}}. \tag{1.51}$$

It is seen that clearance depends upon k_{10} and V_1 and so changes in clearance may involve alterations in V_1 apart from altered elimination. Similarly $t_{1/2,\beta}$ depends not only on k_{10} but also upon k_{12} and k_{21}; thus conclusions about altered elimination cannot be based solely upon changes in $t_{1/2}$. Clearance is inversely proportional to $t_{1/2,\beta}$ and directly proportional to $V_{\mathrm{d}(\beta)}$ and changes in $V_{\mathrm{d}(\beta)}$ can change the $t_{1/2,\beta}$ in the presence of a constant total body clearance.

For a first-order input rate which is usually assumed for oral or intramuscular drug administration into a two-compartment system, eq. (1.31) becomes

$$C = A'e^{-\alpha t} + B'e^{-\beta t} - (A'+B')e^{-k_a t}. \tag{1.52}$$

A' and B' are not identical with A and B since they are influenced by the rate and extent of absorption. Their derivation lies outside the scope of this text. If k_a is approximately equal to α, a distributive α-phase is not observed after first-order input and the plasma concentration–time curve appears biexponential rather than triexponential. Thus the drug in question appears to confer single rather than two-compartment characteristics upon the body. Even rigorous analysis of data may fail to obtain α, β and k_a from oral absorption experiments and estimation of these constants may be impossible without an additional intravenous experiment.

CONSTANT INTRAVENOUS INFUSION

Many drugs are given by a constant rate (sometimes called zero-order—see below) infusion. At steady state the amount in the body

$$X_{ss} = C_{ss} V_d \text{ (from (1.6))}, \tag{1.53}$$

where C_{ss} is the steady-state plasma concentration. When the plasma level is at steady state the rate of infusion k_0 will equal the rate of elimination, which for a one-compartment model gives

$$k_0 = C_{ss} V_d k. \tag{1.54}$$

Similar reasoning applies to a two-compartment model,

thus
$$C_{ss} = \frac{k_0}{V_d k} = \frac{\text{infusion rate}}{\text{clearance}} \tag{1.55}$$

or
$$C_{ss} = \frac{k_0}{\beta V_{d(\beta)}} \tag{1.56}$$

Thus C_{ss} is high when $t_{1/2}$ is long, that is when β is small or if $V_{d(\beta)}$ is small. At steady state $V_{d(ss)}$ as discussed above is more applicable, but the use of $V_{d(\beta)}$ is accompanied by little error.

An appropriate infusion rate may be calculated from (1.56). Thus to determine the rate of intravenous infusion to produce a therapeutic (2 mg/l) level of lignocaine in a 70 kg man it is necessary to know that $V_d = 1.7$ l/kg and to find $\beta = 0.39\ \text{h}^{-1}$ from Table 5.4. Then

$$k_0 = 2 \times 1.7 \times 70 \times 0.39 = 92.8\ \text{mg/h} = 1.5\ \text{mg/min}.$$

Theoretically the concentration C at any time t is given by

$$C = C_{ss}(1 - e^{-kt}). \tag{1.57}$$

The rate at which C_{ss} is attained is independent of dose, V_d, C_{ss} itself or the route of administration but is dependent on $t_{1/2}$. During drug elimination a single dose is nearly eliminated when five half-lives have elapsed (since at this time $(\frac{1}{2})^5$ or $\frac{1}{32}$ of the dose is present in the body, i.e. 97 % has been eliminated). *During the accumulation of drug in the body the plateau is likewise reached in about five half-lives.*

Thus the elimination half-life which is related to k (or β) by eq. (1.34) solely determines the time to reach the plateau. Thus for lignocaine, for which $\beta = 0.39$ h,

$$t_{1/2} = \frac{0.693}{\beta} = \frac{0.693}{0.39} = 1.78\ \text{h}$$

and the plateau will not be reached for about 5 × 1.78 h or 8.9 h. Clearly this may be too long for clinical purposes, and under such circumstances an instantaneous bolus injection may be required to achieve the therapeutic level more rapidly. Similarly any change in a steady infusion rate will not reach the new plateau level for $5 \times t_{1/2}$, and so a bolus may be also required under these circumstances. The loading dose required to obtain C_{ss} is $C_{ss} \cdot V_d$ (i.e. 238 mg lignocaine in the above example). It may be noted that from eq. (1.54) we also have

$$\text{loading dose} = \frac{k_0}{k}.\quad \text{or} \quad \frac{k_0}{\beta} \tag{1.58}$$

(which in the above example gives 92.8/0.39 = 238 mg).

MULTIPLE-DOSE KINETICS

Few drugs are used in a single dose: the majority are repetitively administered at a specific dosage interval (T). Under these circumstances, just as with an infusion which is a limiting case of multiple-dose kinetics where T is zero, drug accumulation occurs. Unlike the infusion, the plasma drug concentration fluctuates between a minimum (C_{min}) immediately before the next dose to a maximum (C_{max}) just after a dose. The time to reach the plateau concentration, when the amount of drug administered in a dosage interval equals the amount of drug eliminated during the dose interval, is again approximately $5 \times t_{1/2}$. When the plateau is reached

$$C_{max} - C_{min} = \text{dose}/V_d \tag{1.59}$$

and

$$\frac{C_{max}}{C_{min}} = 2^{(T/t_{1/2})}, \tag{1.60}$$

e.g. if doses are given every three half lives as for 6 hourly dosing with ampicillin ($t_{1/2}$ about 2 h)

$$\frac{C_{max}}{C_{min}} = 2^{6/2} = 2^3 = 8$$

i.e. C_{max} is 8 times C_{min}. Thus it is possible to calculate this ratio easily knowing only the $t_{1/2}$ of the drug and the dosing interval.

Extremely complex equations describe the plasma concentration occurring at any time in a linear multicompartment system with oral or intramuscular absorption. For the simplest case of repetitive intravenous injections, such as may be used for antibiotics, for a one-compartment system,

$$C_{ss}^t = \frac{X_0}{V_d}\left(\frac{1}{1-e^{-kT}}\right)e^{-kt}, \tag{1.61}$$

where C_{ss}^t is the concentration at any time t during a dosage interval T after plateau conditions are attained.

$$C_{max} = \frac{X_0}{V_d}\left(\frac{1}{1-e^{-kT}}\right) \tag{1.62}$$

and

$$C_{min} = \frac{X_0}{V_d}\left(\frac{1}{1-e^{-kT}}\right)e^{-kT} \tag{1.63}$$

A useful concept in multiple dosing is the average plasma drug concentration at steady state, $\bar{C}$. This is defined as

$$\bar{C} = \frac{\int_0^T C_\infty \, dt}{T}, \tag{1.64}$$

i.e. it is neither the arithmetic nor the geometric mean of C_{min} and C_{max} but is the plasma concentration which when multiplied by T equals the area ($\int_0^T C_\infty \, dt$) under the plasma concentration–time curve during a dosage interval. Integration of (1.61) from zero to T, i.e. during a dosage interval, gives

$$\int_0^T C_\infty \, dt = \frac{X_0}{V_d k}, \tag{1.65}$$

and substitution of (1.65) into (1.64) yields

$$\bar{C} = \frac{X_0}{V_d k T}. \tag{1.66}$$

Since $k = \dfrac{0.693}{t_{1/2}}$ this may also be written

$$\bar{C} = \frac{1.44 X_0 t_{1/2}}{V_d T}, \tag{1.67}$$

as 1/0.693 = 1.44. An additional factor, F, may be required to account for the variable drug availability due to oral administration (see Chapter 2).

So $$\bar{C} = 1.44\, F X_0 t_{1/2} / V_d T. \tag{1.68}$$

Equation (1.68) is equivalent to

$$\bar{C} = \frac{F X_0}{T} \frac{1}{\text{Clearance}} \tag{1.69}$$

(see Figure 9.5) and the appropriate expression for a two-compartment model is

$$\bar{C} = \frac{F X_0}{T} \frac{1}{V_{d(\beta)} \beta}. \tag{1.70}$$

These equations are formally independent of the route of administration and assume no particular pharmacokinetic model although first-order kinetics must apply. An approximation is that drug will accumulate in the body if it is given at intervals of less than 1.4 times the $t_{1/2}$. This can also be expressed as an accumulation ratio R, where

$$R = \frac{1}{1 - e^{-kT}} = \frac{\text{average plasma drug concentration at steady state}}{\text{average plasma drug concentration during single dose}}$$

$$= \frac{\bar{C}}{\bar{C}_1} \tag{1.71}$$

Also:

$$R = \frac{(C)_{\max}}{(C_1)_{\max}} = \frac{\text{maximum plasma drug concentration at steady state}}{\text{maximum plasma drug concentration after single dose}}. \tag{1.72}$$

To exemplify the use of eq. (1.68) consider the calculation of $\bar{C}$ for 12 hourly oral dosage of 250 μg digoxin as Lanoxin (for which $F = 0.6$, see Chapter 12) to a 70 kg man with normal renal function. V_d for digoxin is 7.3 l/kg lean body mass. Table 5.4 gives $\beta = 0.45$ days^{-1} so that $t_{1/2} = 24 \times (0.693)/0.45 = 37$ h. Thus substituting in (1.68) gives

$$\bar{C} = \frac{1.44 \times 0.6 \times 250 \times 37}{7.3 \times 70 \times 12}$$

$$= 1.3\ \mu\text{g/l} \quad \text{(which is within the therapeutic range).}$$

We have seen from eq. (1.17) that

$$\int_0^\infty C\,dt = \frac{C_0}{k}.$$

Therefore from (1.10)
$$\int_0^\infty C\,dt = \frac{X_0}{V_d k} \tag{1.73}$$

and from (1.65)
$$\int_0^\infty C\,dt = \int_0^T C\,dt, \tag{1.74}$$

i.e. the AUC at steady state during one dosing interval T is the same as the AUC after an equal dose given on a single occasion.

Therefore $\bar{C}$ at steady state can be predicted from a single dose study using

$$\bar{C} = \frac{\int_0^\infty C\,dt}{T}, \tag{1.75}$$

which does not require knowledge of k or V_d.

A loading dose (L) is sometimes required during oral therapy and may be calculated from the maintenance dose (this applies to oral, intramuscular and intravenous administration). As can be seen from Fig. 1.10, at the end of the dosing interval T the amount of drug left from the loading dose L will be Le^{-kT} (or $Le^{-\beta T}$). To this will be added the maintenance dose X_0, which must replace the amount of the loading dose which has been eliminated during T so as to keep the plasma levels within the therapeutic range. Therefore

$$L = Le^{-kT} + X_0, \tag{1.76}$$

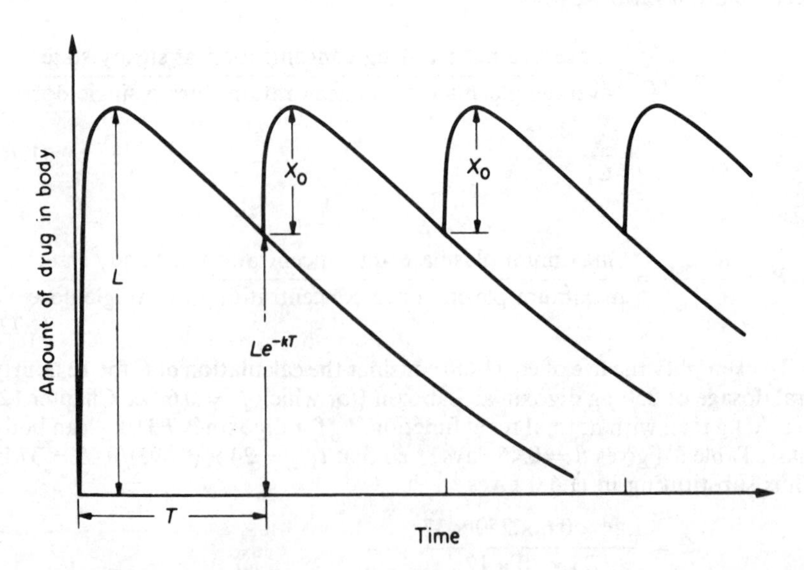

Fig. 1.10 Amount of drug in body resulting from administration of loading dose L followed by repeated maintenance doses X_0 at dosing interval T.

so that

$$X_0 = L(1 - e^{-kT}) \tag{1.77}$$

and

$$L = \frac{X_0}{1 - e^{kT}} = \frac{X_0}{1 - e^{-\beta T}}. \tag{1.78}$$

Thus for digoxin for which $\beta = 0.019\ \text{h}^{-1}$ the loading dose for the patient with normal renal function if the maintenance dose is 250 μg 12 hourly is

$$L = 250 \frac{1}{1 - e^{-(0.019 \times 12)}} = 1226\ \mu\text{g} \quad \text{(i.e. 1.25 mg approximately)}$$

The advantages of using a loading dose for digoxin are illustrated by Fig. 1.11.

The effects on the plasma concentration–time profile when dose or dosage interval are varied can be calculated and is illustrated in Figs. 1.12 and 1.13 for a drug with a $t_{1/2}$ of 3.5 h. Figure 1.12 shows the effect of giving 0.75 g, 0.5 g or 0.25 g every 3 h. Obviously, the higher the dose the higher the steady-state plasma level, but also note that with a high dose the fluctuation between maximum and minimum concentration is greater. Figure 1.13 shows the effect

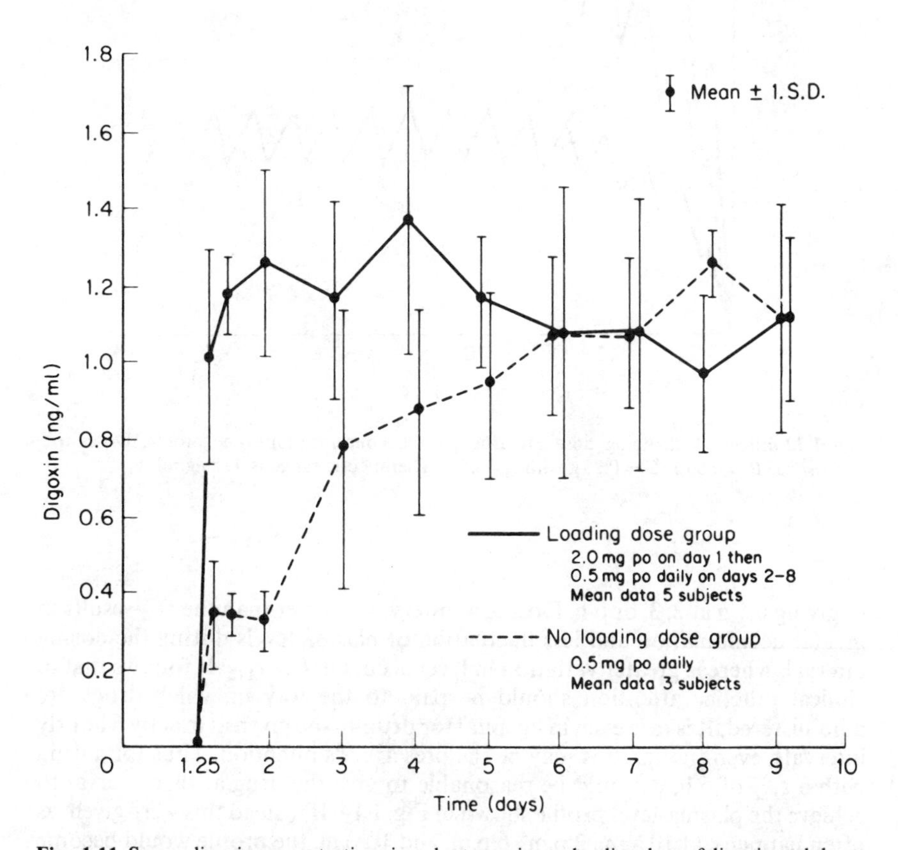

Fig. 1.11 Serum digoxin concentrations in volunteers given a loading dose of digoxin and those in whom a loading dose was omitted (From F. Marcus *et al*, *Circulation*, **34**, 865 (1966). By permission of the American Heart Association Inc.).

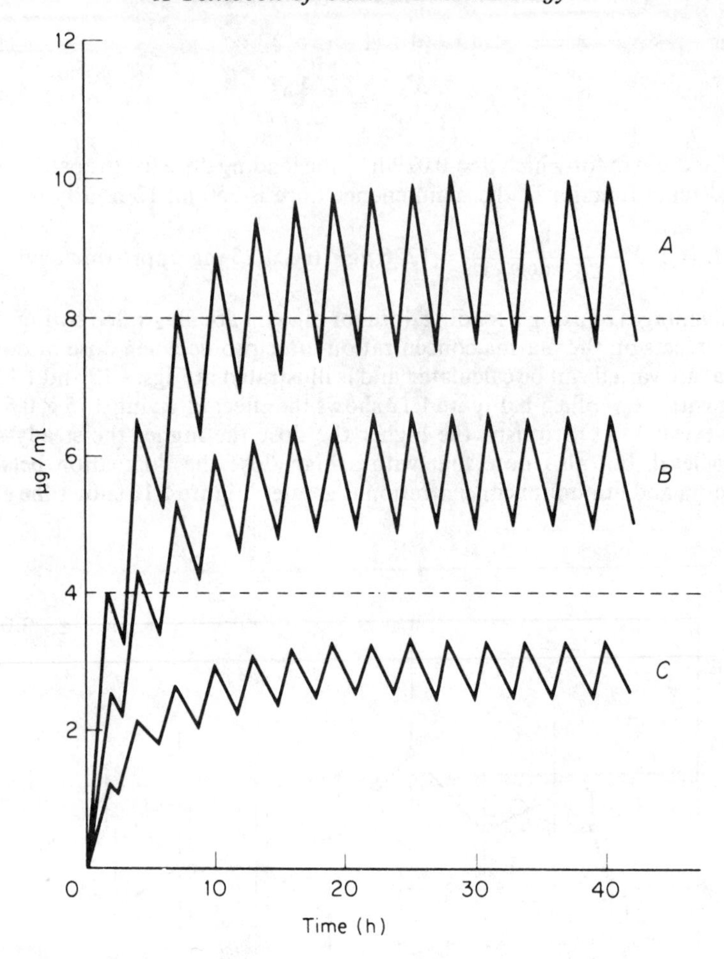

Fig. 1.12 Effect of changing dose on drug plasma concentration–time profile. Doses are $A = 0.75$ g; $B = 0.50$ g; $C = 0.25$ g with $t_{1/2}$ 3.5 h. Therapeutic range is 4–8 μg/ml.

of giving 0.5 g at 2, 3, or 6 h. Dosing at intervals shorter than the $t_{1/2}$ results in greater accumulation and less fluctuation of plasma levels during the dosing interval, whereas greater variation in level occurs if $T > t_{1/2}$. It follows that in clinical practice attention should be paid to the way in which drugs are administered. It is rare even in hospital for drugs to be given at exactly 6 hourly intervals, even though this may be the prescriber's intention. Thus for a drug with a $t_{1/2}$ of 6 h, it would be reasonable to give the drug at this interval to achieve the plasma-level profile shown in Fig. 1.14. If instead this were given, as often happens, at 10 a.m., 2 p.m., 6 p.m. and 10 p.m. the profile would become as shown in Fig. 1.15, which may produce both ineffective and toxic levels daily.

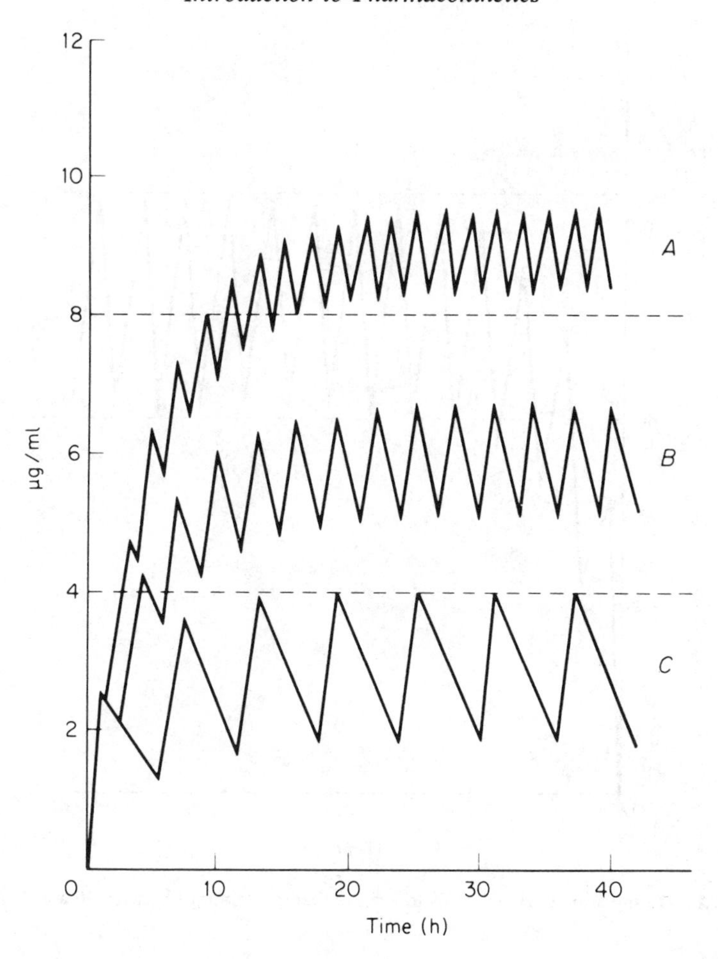

Fig. 1.13 Effect of altered dosing interval: A, $T = 2$h; B, $T = 3$h and C, $T = 6$h.

CHOICE OF APPROPRIATE PHARMACOKINETIC MODEL

In the case of some drugs even the two-compartment model is insufficient to predict the behaviour of the drug in the body. More complex models, such as a three-compartment model with central and 'shallow' and 'deep' peripheral compartments have been postulated to explain the triphasic decline in the log plasma concentration, time curves of diazepam, chlordiazepoxide, lignocaine, digoxin and many other drugs. The assignment of a particular model is determined by a consideration of the number of exponential terms required to best fit the plasma concentration–time curve. Linear kinetic models may be summarised as the polyexponential equation

$$C = \sum_{i=1}^{n} C_i e^{-\lambda_i t}, \tag{1.79}$$

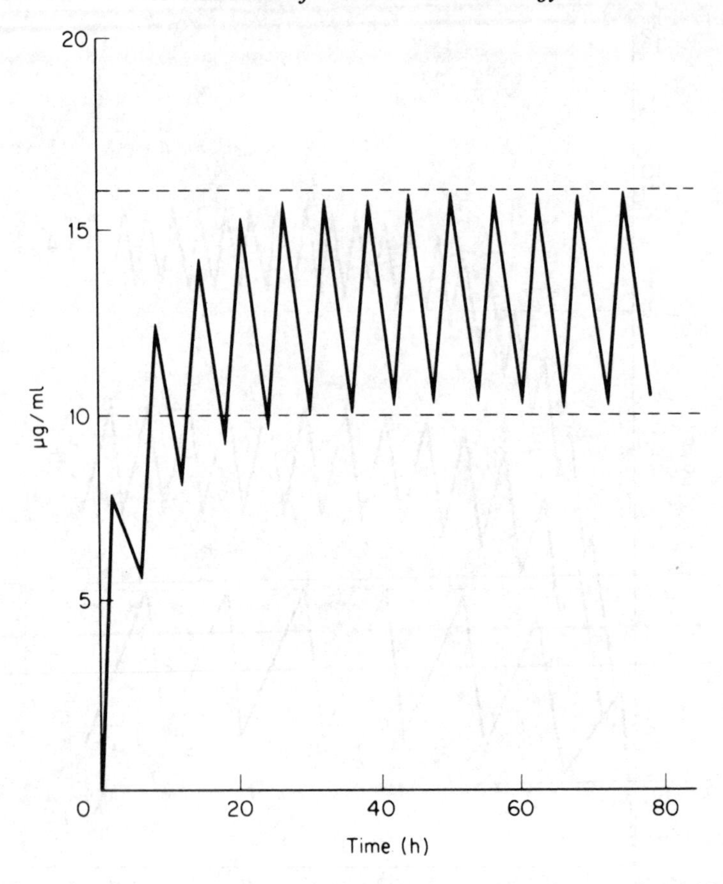

Fig. 1.14 Dosing at 6 hourly intervals to achieve therapeutic range between 10 and 16 μg/ml.

where n is the number of compartments. Expanded forms of eq. (1.79) corresponding to one and two-compartment models are eqs. (1.80) and (1.81)

$$C = C_1 e^{-\lambda_1 t}, \tag{1.80}$$

$$C = C_1 e^{-\lambda_1 t} + C_2 e^{-\lambda_2 t}, \tag{1.81}$$

where C_1, C_2 are the coefficients (corresponding to A, B) and λ_1, λ_2 are the exponents (corresponding to α, β for the two-compartment model). The number of exponential terms equals the number of compartments required in the disposition model. Thus an equation such as (1.81) suggests a two-compartment model is necessary. However the situation is more complex than this. Firstly it has been known for some time that the same drug might be described by different compartmental models in different subjects or even in the same subject on different occasions. Secondly, the mathematical analysis of the experimental data does not suggest which of several alternative models is applicable. Thus the model of Fig. 1.6 is only one of three possible two-

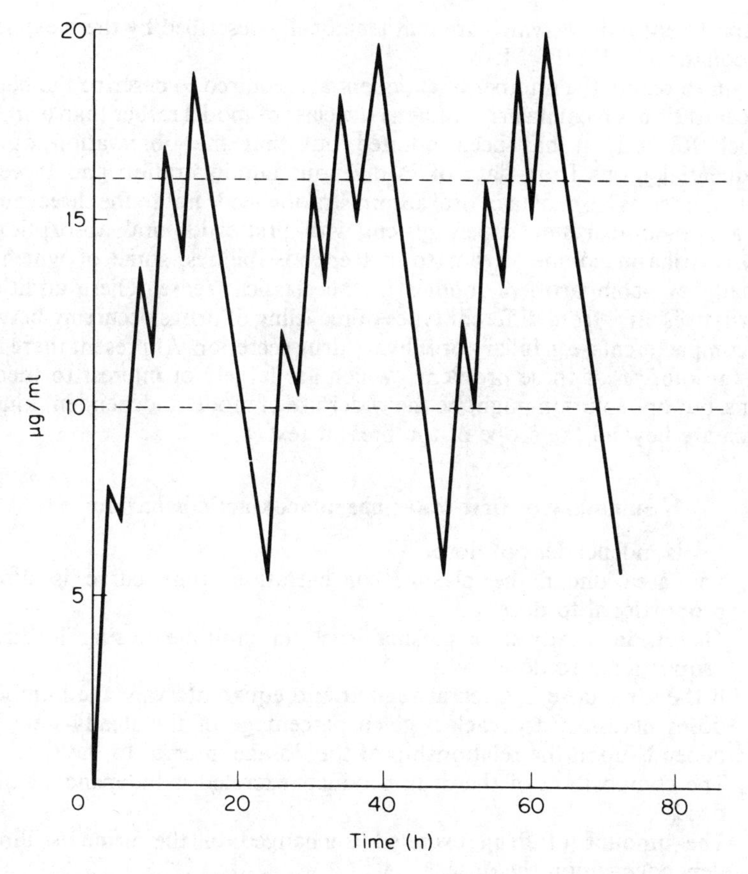

Fig. 1.15 Dosing at 10 a.m., 2 p.m., 6 p.m. and 10 p.m. instead of at strict 6 hourly intervals may produce both toxicity and lack of therapeutic effect.

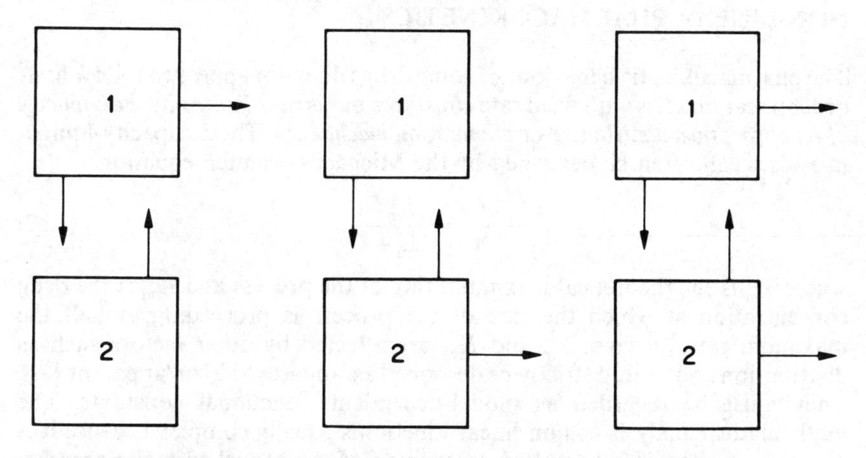

Fig. 1.16 The three possible two-compartment open models. In each, compartment 1 is assumed to include the compartment from which sampling for drug analysis occurs, e.g. plasma.

compartment models which are mathematically described by the biexponential equation (1.31) (Fig. 1.16).

Thus in reality the number of exponentials required to describe the plasma concentration, time data array assigns the class of model rather than a specific model. Recently it has been pointed out that the observation of two exponential terms from data of intravenous administration and three exponential terms from data of oral administration leads not to the three models for a two-compartment open system with first-order oral absorption of classical pharmacokinetics but to sixteen possibilities, some of which are actually one-compartment models in the classical sense. These additional alternatives arise from different types of recycling of drugs occurring between the compartments, e.g. biliary or salivary drug secretion. At present there is no clear resolution of these problems, which are largely of interest to theoreticians, but one solution might be the wider use of model-independent kinetics which are beyond the scope of the present text.

Summary of first-order pharmacokinetic behaviour

1. $t_{1/2}$ is independent of dose.
2. The area under the plasma concentration, time curve is directly proportional to dose.
3. The mean steady-state plasma level on multiple dosing is directly proportional to dose and $t_{1/2}$.
4. If the same dose is given at regular and equal intervals, the number of doses necessary to reach a given percentage of the steady-state level depends upon the relationship of the dosage interval to the $t_{1/2}$.
5. The composition of the drug products excreted is independent of the dose.
6. The amount of drug excreted unchanged in the urine is directly dependent upon the dose.

NON-LINEAR PHARMACOKINETICS

The pharmacokinetic behaviour of some drugs does not appear to follow first-order linear kinetics with fixed rate constants but is *rate-limited by the capacity of an absorptive, distributive or elimination mechanism.* These capacity-limited processes can often be described by the Michaelis–Menten equation

$$-\frac{\mathrm{d}C}{\mathrm{d}t}=\frac{V_{\mathrm{m}}C}{K_{\mathrm{m}}+C}, \qquad (1.82)$$

where V_{m} is the theoretical maximum rate of the process and K_{m} is the drug concentration at which the rate of the process is proceeding at half the maximum rate. In vivo, V_{m} and K_{m} are affected by other factors such as distribution and should strictly be described as 'apparent V_{m}' or 'apparent K_{m}'. They must be regarded as model-dependent, functional constants. The mathematical analysis of non-linear kinetics is usually complex because it is necessary to obtain a complete description of the model to make accurate predictions.

There are two limiting cases of eq. (1.82). When $K_m \gg C$, (1.82) reduces to

$$-\frac{dC}{dt} = \frac{V_m}{K_m} C = \text{constant} \times C, \tag{1.83}$$

indicating that when the drug concentration resulting from the usual therapeutic regime is far below the K_m of the processes involved in the disposition of the drug, then first-order kinetics apply (see Fig. 1.17). Alternatively when $C \gg K_m$, eq. (1.82) becomes

$$-\frac{dC}{dt} = V_m, \tag{1.84}$$

i.e. the decline in drug concentration is independent of the drug concentration and proceeds at a fixed rate. Because it does not depend on the concentration of any of the reactants this type of process is called zero order.

Capacity-limited processes include biotransformation mediated by enzymes, specialised intestinal and renal transport mechanisms and binding by plasma protein. A number of drugs including salicylate, phenytoin and ethanol obey non-linear kinetics in the therapeutic range. Some drugs in toxic doses such as barbiturates also show non-linearity. The implications of such behaviour include the following:

(a) The decline of drug levels in the body is not exponential but is described by the integrated Michaelis–Menten equation

$$V_m(t - t_0) = C_0 - C + K_m \ln \frac{C_0}{C}, \tag{1.85}$$

where $(t - t_0)$ is the time elapsed for C_0 to fall to C. On Cartesian coordinates a 'hockey-stick' shaped curve is described (Fig. 1.17). For zero-order kinetics the situation is simpler: integration of (1.84) yields

$$C = C_0 - V_m t \tag{1.86}$$

A plot of plasma concentration against time is therefore linear with slope of $-V_m$ and ordinate intercept C_0 (Fig. 1.18).

(b) The times required to eliminate 50% of a dose increase with increasing dose and the concept of a constant half-life is meaningless since the fractional elimination rate is dose-dependent.

(c) Kinetic linearity has been defined as direct proportionality of transfer rates to concentrations or concentration differences as expressed by for example the first equation in this chapter. In practice this means that the area under the plasma level–time curve is proportional to the dose. Thus doubling the dose of say, penicillin doubles the amount of drug in the body and hence doubles the plasma concentration. This is not the case for drugs exhibiting non-linear kinetics (Figs. 1.19 and 9.10). We have seen (eq. (1.15), reproduced for convenience as (1.87)) that for a one-compartment model

$$\int_0^\infty C\,dt = \frac{X_0}{V_d k}, \tag{1.87}$$

i.e.

$$\int_0^\infty C\,dt = \text{constant} \times X_0 \propto X_0. \tag{1.88}$$

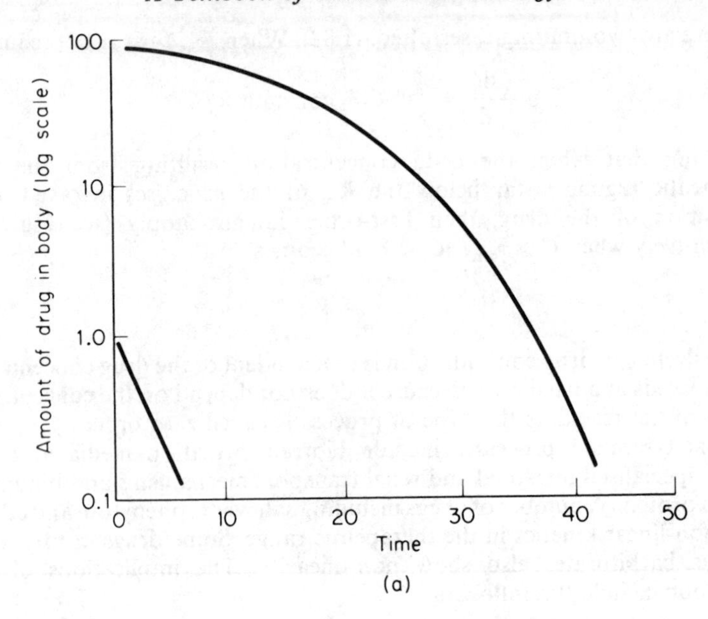

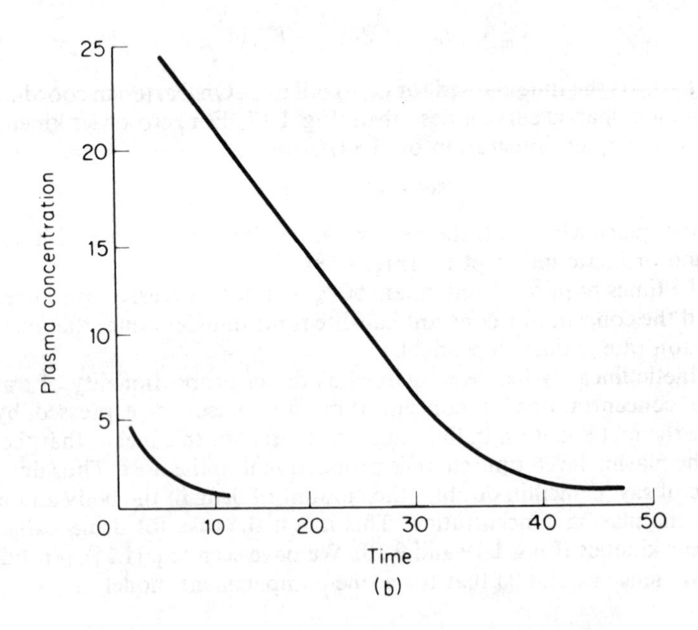

Fig. 1.17 Time course of a hypothetical drug obeying Michaelis–Menten elimination kinetics: (a) the lower curve shows that if the dose is small compared to K_m the kinetics are apparently linear; (b) on linear coordinates large doses are initially described by a linear segment (apparent zero-order kinetics) and as the concentration falls the curve takes on a 'hockey stick' shape.

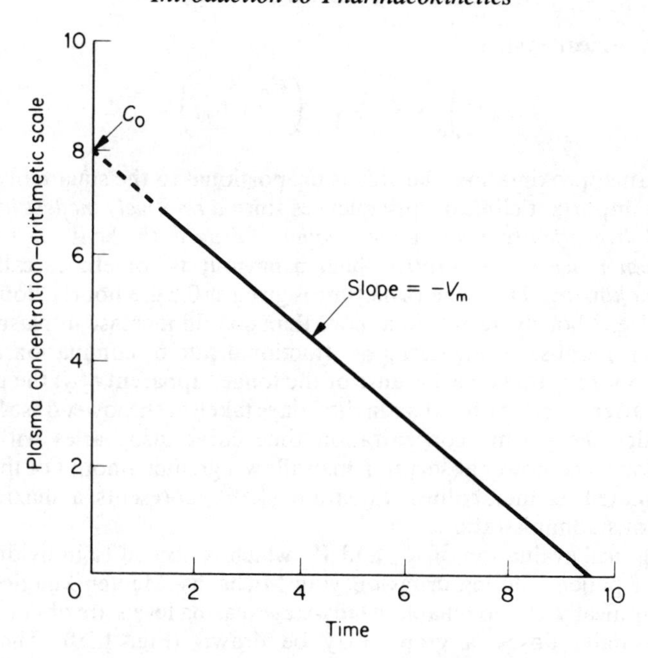

Fig. 1.18 Time course of hypothetical drug demonstrating apparent zero-order kinetics.

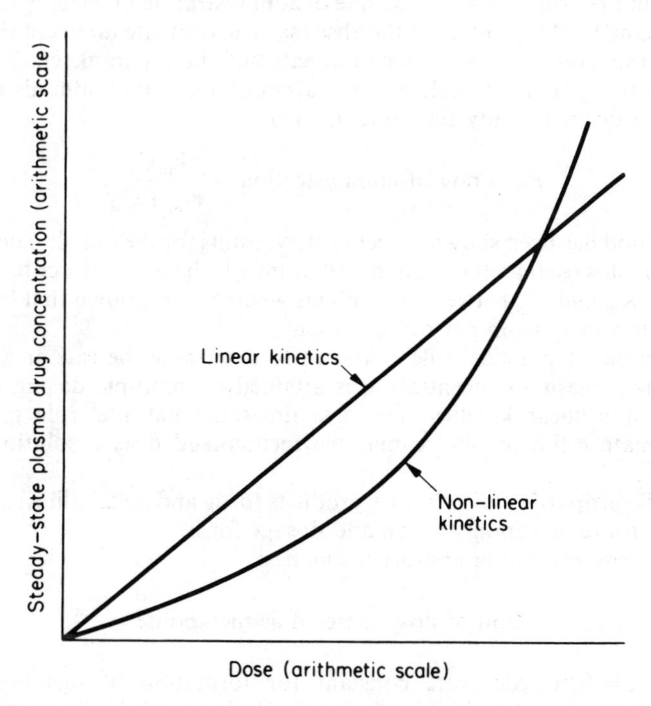

Fig. 1.19 Effect of increase in dose on steady-state plasma concentration (and AUC) for drugs obeying linear and non-linear kinetics.

For a non-linear system

$$\int_0^\infty C\,dt = \frac{C_0}{V_m}\left(\frac{C_0}{2} + K_m\right) \tag{1.89}$$

thus, as an approximation, the area is proportional to the square of the dose. This has important clinical consequences since *a relatively modest increase in dose will dramatically increase the amount of drug in the body once the drug-elimination process is saturated.* Such behaviour is sometimes called *dose-dependent kinetics.* Thus when salicylate is given as 0.5 g, 8 hourly, doubling the dose to 1 g, 8 hourly, results in a more than sixfold increase in plasma levels. Moreover, because of the decreased fractional rate of elimination at higher plasma concentrations (i.e. because of the longer apparent $t_{1/2}$) the plateau is attained after 1 week rather than in the 2 days taken at the lower dose level. The area under the plasma concentration–time curve also varies with rate of absorption since slower absorption may allow a greater amount of the drug to be eliminated as metabolites. Equation (1.89) represents a maximum for intravenous administration.

The clinical evaluation of K_m and V_m which is needed to individualise the dosing of patients taking drugs obeying Michaelis–Menten kinetics may be done graphically. If two reliable steady-state plasma levels are obtained at two different daily doses, a graph may be drawn (Fig. 1.20). The rate of administration which at steady state equals the rate of drug elimination is plotted on the ordinate whilst the rate of administration divided by the steady state plasma level is plotted on the abscissa. The ordinate intercept then gives V_m and the slope is $-K_m$. Once estimates of these parameters have been obtained it is possible to calculate the appropriate rate of administration to produce a desired steady-state level C_{ss} from

$$R_0 = \text{rate of administration} = \frac{V_m C_{ss}}{K_m + C_{ss}}. \tag{1.90}$$

This method has been shown to yield better results for the individualisation of phenytoin dosage than the use of nomograms which have perforce to assume a constant K_m and V_m between individuals whereas it is known that these may vary quite widely from person to person.

No simple or practical rule is known to determine the rate at which the steady-state plasma concentration is attained on multiple dosing of drugs obeying non-linear kinetics. The 'five times the half-life' rule gives only approximate estimates and cannot be recommended as a solution to the problem.

(d) The proportion of excretory products (drug and metabolites) is affected by dose, route of administration and dosage form.

For a drug exhibiting first-order kinetics:

$$\text{Fraction of dose excreted as metabolite} = \frac{k_m}{k} \tag{1.91}$$

where k_m = first-order rate constant for formation of metabolite. For capacity-limited metabolite formation the fraction of the dose excreted as metabolite will obviously fall with an increase in dose once metabolite

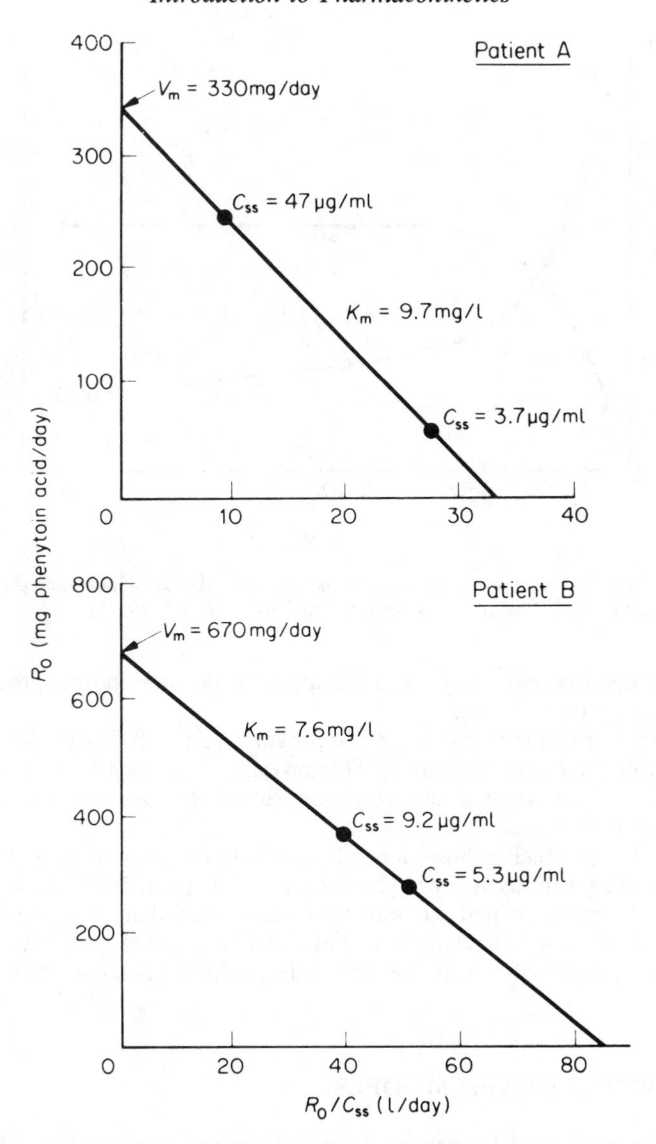

Fig. 1.20 Graphical estimation of V_m and K_m values for phenytoin in two patients (From T. M. Ludden *et al.*, *Clin. Pharm. Ther.*, **21**, 287 (1977).)

formation has attained its maximum, i.e. it is dose-dependent. Figure 1.21 demonstrates these points with respect to the formation of salicylamide sulphate and glucuronide from salicylamide in man. Administration of salicylamide in the form of slowly dissolving pellets increases the amount of salicylamide sulphate excreted since slower absorption results in much lower drug levels in the body and the sulphation pathway does not become saturated.

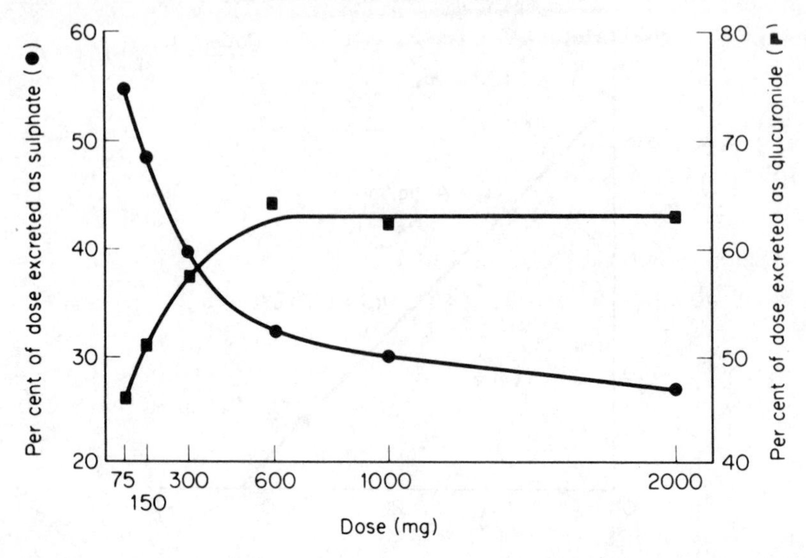

Fig. 1.21 Effect of dose of salicylamide on formation of salicylamide sulphate and glucuronide. (From G. Levy and T. Matsuzawa, *J. Pharm. exp Ther.*, **156**, 285 (1967).)

(e) Competitive effects by drugs sharing the same rate-limiting process may produce drug interactions.

(f) Some drug metabolites, e.g. 5-(*p*-hydroxyphenyl)-5-phenylhydantoin, may inhibit their own formation. This process of product inhibition causes larger doses to be excreted relatively more slowly than small doses and hence dose-dependent effects.

(g) Drugs producing dose-dependent effects on physiological functions affecting drug elimination or disposition, e.g. hepatic blood flow, cardiac output, urinary pH, will also demonstrate dose-dependent pharmacokinetics.

Some drugs, e.g. salicylate, may have several parallel pathways of drug elimination, some of which are first-order, others Michaelis–Menten (see p. 286).

FLOW RATE-LIMITED MODELS

Compartmental models such as discussed above are usually developed in practice by fitting curves of plasma concentration versus time to multiexponential or Michaelis–Menten equations by appropriate non-linear least-squares computer programs. The limitations of this approach usually mean that no representation more complex than a two, or at the most three, compartment open model is justified to describe the time course of drug concentrations in the plasma. In most cases the derived parameters of the system such as compartment volumes or transfer constants have no anatomical or physiological reality. Moreover these models are very species dependent and although such classical pharmacokinetic models have many clinical uses, the amount of basic information is limited, this being especially true for the prediction of tissue levels. Compartmental models do not directly take account of drug–protein binding, although the shape and height of a plasma level–time curve are altered by protein binding and compartmental analysis yields constants which are sensitive to protein binding. New types of models which are anatomically and physiologically realistic are being developed. These are based upon actual organ blood flows and volumes and take into account both bound and unbound drug in blood and tissues. Naturally such models involve many compartments (Fig. 1.22) and require a firm and extensive data base to be useful. They may also be mathematically complex. In principle such models permit the prediction of drug concentrations in any tissue at any time and drug distribution in pathological states may be predicted by altering estimates of organ blood flow. Using concepts developed in chemical engineering in which a laboratory-developed process may be 'scaled up' in size for commercial production in a factory-sized chemical plant, physiological models could be scaled to apply to several species. Thus the large amount of information required to develop a physiological pharmacokinetic model may be collected in a laboratory animal and then scaled to apply to man. This approach has

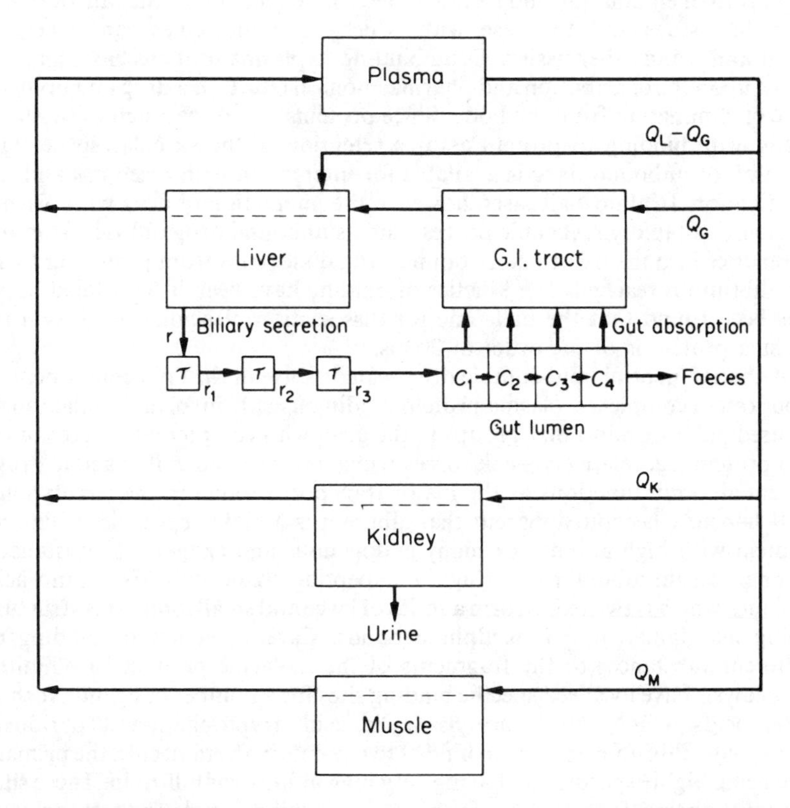

Fig. 1.22 Physiologically based pharmacokinetic multicompartmental model for methotrexate kinetics (From K. B. Bischoff *et al.*, *J. Pharm. Sci.*, **60**, 1128 (1971) Reproduced with permission of the copyright owner.)

been explored for a few drugs, which include methotrexate, 6-mercaptopurine, cytarabine, salicylate, lignocaine, cephalosporins and digoxin, and is at present in its infancy. There are several problems associated with this concept which include the difficulties of assessing some of the important variables characterising biological processes such as enterohepatic recirculation and gastrointestinal absorption and the high cost of the great amounts of computer time required to numerically integrate the differential equations involved. Nevertheless, this remains a bold and innovative approach to pharmacokinetic modelling and in the future may prove a viable alternative to classical pharmacokinetic models firmly based on anatomical, physiological and physico-chemical reality.

DRUG DISTRIBUTION, ELIMINATION AND PLASMA PROTEIN BINDING

Upon entering the circulation most drugs are simultaneously distributed throughout the body and eliminated. Distribution usually occurs much more rapidly than elimination and its rate is determined mainly by the rate of blood flow to tissues and the ease with which drug molecules can penetrate membranes and other tissues. Drug binding to plasma proteins has a marked effect upon the distribution and pharmacological effects of a drug and upon its rate of elimination from the body. Since proteins do not pass across capillary walls drug binding to protein assures retention in the vascular space. The fraction of unbound drug is available for interaction with receptors and for elimination. In almost all cases, however, the interaction of drug with plasma protein is a rapidly reversible process and as unbound drug diffuses from the capillaries into the tissues more bound drug dissociates from protein until an equilibrium is reached. The kinetics of binding have been little studied but it has been found that the half-time for dissociation of acidic azo dyes from plasma protein is of the order of 20 ms.

Although neutral lipid-soluble drugs can dissolve in the lipid component of lipoprotein complexes, plasma protein binding usually involves interaction of ionised polar or non-polar groups in the drug with corresponding groups on the protein, i.e. relatively weak forces which are reversible. For acidic drugs serum albumin functions as the major transport protein in the circulation.

It has now become apparent that albumin is a highly specialised binding protein with high affinity for many endogenous and exogenous substances. Human serum albumin is a single polypeptide chain with 584 amino acid residues which is twisted to form a series of large and small loops, this structure being maintained by 17 disulphide bonds. Careful studies of binding of different substances to the fragments of the molecule produced by limited proteolysis have localised specific binding sites for a number of ligands such as fatty acids, Cu^{2+}, Ni^{2+}, acetylsalicylic acid, tryptophan and pyridoxal phosphate. Bilirubin appears to bind at two points in the molecule, the primary site being highly specific and having very high affinity for bilirubin. These sites are quite distinct from the sites for binding of sulphonamide and fatty acids. A great variety of drugs, however, have been shown to bind to the same two sites on the albumin molecule. Site 1 is the primary binding site for sulphonamides, sulphonylureas, coumarin anticoagulants and some radio-contrast agents. Site 2 binds ibuprofen and substances containing a phenylalkanoic structure, although in the presence of high (2 : 1) ratios of fatty acid these molecules may be displaced to bind to the less specific coumarin binding site (site 1). Some sites, e.g. for bilirubin, are so highly specific and have such high affinity that competition for binding by other ligands is virtually impossible. Other sites, e.g. for benzodiazepines, have strongly stereospecific properties and yet are able to bind a number of ligands of diverse structure. Changes in albumin conformation resulting from ligand binding may occur since the binding sites, although structurally and spatially distinct, are not independent. Thus the affinity, specificity and number of binding sites for a given ligand may alter in the presence of a second ligand binding to a separate site.

Basic drugs may bind to a number of other proteins which are distinct from albumin. Thus quinidine binds to albumin, lipoproteins and α_1-acid glycoprotein. This latter component also avidly binds imipramine, chlorpromazine, dipyridamole, propranolol and alprenolol. This protein is an acute phase reactant and its serum concentration rises markedly (3–4 times) when the ESR is elevated by inflammatory disease. The total plasma propranolol level has been shown to be elevated by 3–4 times in inflammatory disease although its half-life is unaltered. The increased binding may, however, change the apparent volume of distribution. The clinical relevance of such effects has yet to be established.

There also exist a number of other specific carrier proteins in the plasma, e.g. corticosteroid binding globulin (transcortin) which binds steroids and also carrier proteins for vitamin B_{12} and thyroxine. The binding of individual drugs to plasma protein varies from very little to almost complete binding of all the drug in the blood. The interaction of drug and protein is affected by their relative concentrations and is best defined in terms of the association constant, K_a, which may be derived from the mass–action expression for the equilibrium:

$$\text{free drug} + \text{protein} \underset{k_2}{\overset{k_1}{\rightleftharpoons}} \text{drug–protein complex},$$

where
$$K_a = \frac{k_1}{k_2} = \frac{(\text{drug–protein complex})}{(\text{free drug})(\text{protein})} \qquad (1.92)$$

The dissociation constant $K_d = 1/K_a$ and is the free-drug concentration at which half the drug binding sites on the protein are saturated. For most drugs the number of binding sites per protein molecule is one or two although secondary, less specific sites may also be present.

Since the protein concentration of most extravascular fluids is considerably less than in plasma the total drug concentration in plasma is usually higher than in lymph, cerebrospinal fluid, saliva or synovial fluid. The total drug concentration in these fluids is often approximated by the free-drug concentration in plasma. Thus the percentages of phenytoin and phenobarbitone unbound in plasma are 10 % and 45 % and the CSF/plasma ratios for these drugs are 0.1 and 0.43 respectively. The penetration of drugs into the CSF is of therapeutic importance for the treatment of meningitis: in the presence of inflamed meninges the penetration of antibiotics is increased. Normal synovial fluid contains about 10 g/l albumin (cf. 40 g/l in plasma). However, albumin levels may be elevated several fold in synovial inflammation or degenerative joint disease and drug concentrations within the joint may be likewise increased.

Only free drug is available for glomerular filtration and elimination. *Saturation of plasma protein binding may introduce non-linearities into the kinetic behaviour of a drug.* Thus it has been shown that when single doses of naproxen are given, although at low doses the area under the plasma concentration–time curve increases proportionately to dose (linear behaviour) when doses of 0.5, 1, 2, 3 or 4 g are given (up to 8 times the clinically effective dose in rheumatoid arthritis) the area-to-dose ratio flattens out and shows only small increases. This non-linear behaviour is accompanied by an increase in urinary naproxen excretion rate and is thought to result from saturation of plasma protein binding and consequent increased urinary elimination rate of the free drug. Similar considerations apply to the protein binding of prednisolone, phenylbutazone (see Fig. 10.5) and clofibrate (see Fig. 16.1).

A pharmacokinetic consequence of decreased protein binding is an increase in the apparent volume of distribution of a drug compared to normal. The apparent volume of distribution is related to plasma and tissue binding by

$$V_d = V_b + V_t\left(\frac{f_b}{f_t}\right), \tag{1.93}$$

where V_b and V_t are the actual volumes of water in the blood and tissues respectively (i.e. $V_b + V_t$ = total body water) and f_b and f_t are the fractions of free drug in blood and tissues respectively. Thus changes in the unbound fraction of drug in plasma without commensurate change in tissue binding alter the apparent volume of distribution. For example in normal patients phenytoin is about 88% bound and has a mean apparent volume of distribution of 0.64 l/kg. In uraemia the plasma protein binding is reduced to 74%, and the apparent volume of distribution increases to 1.4 l/kg. This results in an increased total body clearance and a decreased half-life, and a given dose of phenytoin will produce a lower plasma level in a uraemic patient. These problems are further discussed in Chapter 5.

The free-drug concentration in the plasma is a critical determinant of drug effect because only free drug can reach the receptor and exert a pharmacological effect. Binding to protein decreases the maximum intensity of action of a single dose of a drug since it lowers the peak concentration attained at the receptor. Conversely decreased binding increases the intensity of drug action. Because binding slows drug elimination by glomerular filtration or diffusion into hepatocytes prior to metabolism it increases the duration of action of the drug. Thus the duration of action of sulphonamides, tetracyclines and thiazide diuretics is correlated with their degree of protein binding. The relationship between plasma protein binding and hepatic drug elimination is more complex and there are circumstances in which increased plasma protein binding may enhance drug elimination. The rate of intravenous injection of highly protein-bound drugs may be important for the intensity of their action. During rapid intravenous injection the binding capacity of plasma protein in the limited volume of blood with which the drug mixes may be exceeded. This produces higher concentrations of free drug at the sites of action in highly perfused tissues. A more intense action has been observed after rapid injections of thiopentone and diazoxide as compared to slow injections of the same amount.

Competition for protein binding

Highly protein-bound drugs may compete for binding or else one drug may bind and alter the tertiary structure of the protein thus altering the affinity of the protein for another drug. Aspirin alters drug binding to albumin by permanent acetylation of a lysine residue of the albumin molecule. This modifies the binding of some acidic drugs like phenylbutazone and flufenamic acid. Such mechanisms result in an increased free fraction of the displaced drug. Thus displacement from protein binding of 1 % of a drug which is 99 % bound will double the percentage of free drug. This will not necessarily double the free-drug concentration in the plasma since this free drug is available for distribution throughout the body and may bind in the tissues. The amount by which the plasma free-drug level rises is therefore dependent upon the apparent volume of distribution. If this is small, as in the case of warfarin or tolbutamide, the changed level of free drug may produce pharmacodynamic effects. If the apparent volume of distribution is large, e.g. tricyclic antidepressants, there is unlikely to be any clinical consequence of the displacement. Increased pharmacological activity is not the only consequence of this type of interaction. The increased concentration of free drug in the plasma makes more drug available for glomerular filtration or diffusion into hepatocytes which results in a higher rate of elimination. This is reflected in a shortened plasma half-life and the steady-state level of total drug attained by a given dosage declines to a new steady state. At this new steady state the free drug in plasma returns to the same concentration as obtained before the displacement and the half-life of the drug returns to normal (see Fig. 1.23). Thus the potentiation of pharmacological action tends to be greatest shortly after therapy with the displacing drug is initiated, but if dosage is continued the pharmacological effects will return to their initial intensity. Clinically this may take too long for an expectant attitude to be adopted. For example, catastrophic haemorrhage or hypoglycaemia may ensue when phenylbutazone is initially added to warfarin or tolbutamide therapy and therefore it is prudent to reduce dosage with these agents or better still to avoid the combination altogether. Although the mechanism of drug displacement from protein binding by another drug is often proposed as underlying a drug interaction (see Chapter 8) there are few cases in which this mechanism has been rigorously and quantitatively proven. Thus in the case of the warfarin/phenylbutazone interaction an alternative explanation which is equally plausible has been proposed which involves alterations in drug metabolism (see p. 596).

Competition for binding sites occurs not only between drugs but also between drugs and endogenous ligands. Displacement of hormones from their carrier proteins is of no clinical importance because of the attainment of a new equilibrium as outlined above. Thus phenytoin, although lowering the protein-bound iodine, does not produce hypothyroidism or alter the uptake of radioiodine by the thyroid. Several anti-inflammatory drugs, e.g. salicylates, indomethacin, phenylbutazone, displace cortisol from transcortin without any effect. The displacement of bilirubin from protein binding in the neonate by

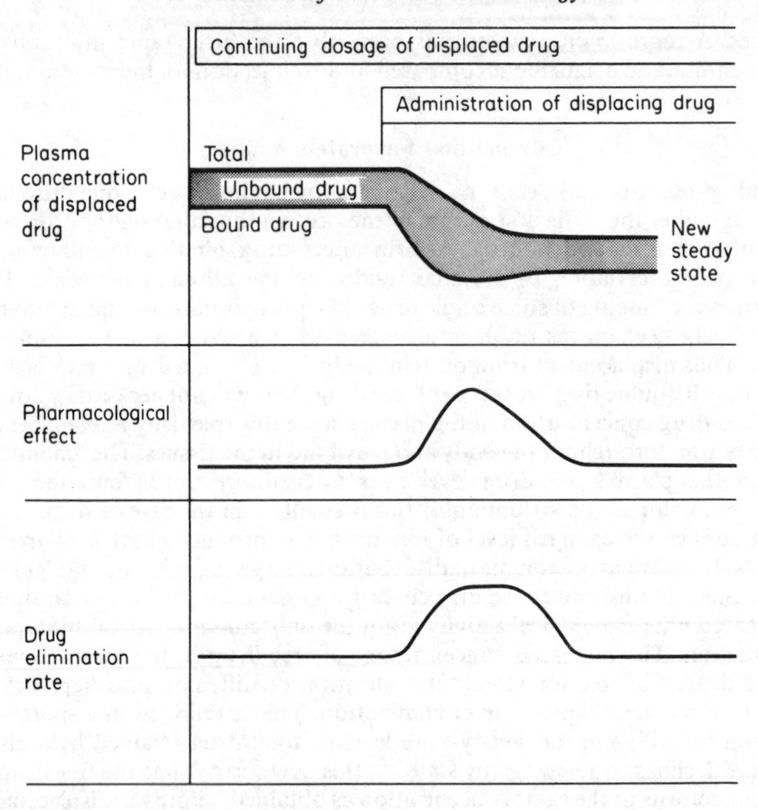

Fig. 1.23 Diagrammatic representation of effects of displacement of a drug from plasma protein binding by a concurrently administered drug.

the administration of sulphonamides is of clinical importance since the resultant high levels of unbound bilirubin are able to cross the immature blood–brain barrier to produce kernicterus and brain damage. As mentioned above the specificity and affinity of bilirubin for its binding site on albumin is such that its displacement by another drug is unlikely. It has been shown, however, that the specific bilirubin-binding capacity of albumin is decreased by a stress such as infection in neonates, and thus more bilirubin is bound to the non-specific drug binding site (site 1) on the molecule where it is available for displacement by sulphonamide. There is some evidence from animal studies that the converse action, i.e. displacement of bound drug by an endogenous molecule, can also occur, for high levels of triglycerides occurring in stress can displace clofibrate from protein binding thereby shortening its half-life.

Intersubject differences in protein binding

This may contribute significantly to the variable clinical response to drugs. Thus the free fraction of imipramine in the plasma of depressed patients varies from 5.4 to 21.0%. This may explain some of the difficulties in correlating the plasma levels of antidepressants with clinical response. The interindividual differences are partly under genetic control (Chapter 4) and may also be affected by disease (Chapter 5) and age (Chapter 6).

Renal excretion of drugs

The kidneys are involved to some degree in the elimination of virtually every drug or drug metabolite in man. The kidneys receive 20% of the cardiac output and about 130 ml/minute of protein-free filtrate is formed at the glomeruli, although only 1–2 ml of this filtrate finally appears in the urine. The renal elimination of a drug may be a rather complex phenomenon since a number of processes occur in the renal tubule which may alter its concentration in the tubular fluid. Depending upon which of these processes predominates, the renal clearance of a drug may be either an important or a trivial component in its overall elimination.

1. *Glomerular filtration*: The ultrafiltrate has a composition similar to that of plasma water and contains the same concentration of solutes as plasma but molecules with a molecular weight of 66 000 or above (which includes plasma proteins and drug–protein complexes) do not pass the glomerulus. Accordingly only free drug passes into the filtrate.

2. *Proximal tubular secretion*: Mechanisms for active secretion of both acids and bases exist in this segment. These are relatively non-specific in their structural requirements and share many of the characteristics of the transport systems in the intestine. The organic acid transport mechanism excretes hippuric acid, endogenous phenols, sulphates and glucuronides as well as acidic drugs such as probenecid, penicillin and some sulphonamides. For many acidic drugs like benzylpenicillin this tubular secretion is so efficient that virtually all of the drug is excreted by this mechanism. The organic base transport mechanism contributes little to the elimination of basic drugs from the body: quinine, procaine and tetraethyl ammonium are examples of drugs which are secreted by this system.

Each mechanism is characterised by a maximal rate of transport for a given drug so that the process is theoretically saturable although this maximum is rarely reached in practice. Competitive effects can occur between drugs carried on these systems. Thus probenecid, a weak acid, competitively inhibits the tubular secretion of the penicillins and methotrexate whilst cimetidine competes with procainamide for the basic drug transport system.

3. *Passive distal tubular reabsorption*: The renal tubule behaves like a lipid barrier separating the high drug concentration (further increased by tubular reabsorption of water) in the tubular lumen and the lower concentration in the interstitial fluid and plasma. Reabsorption of drug down its concentration gradient therefore occurs by passive diffusion. To traverse the lipid membrane of the tubule the drug should be lipid soluble, so that for highly lipid soluble drugs such as griseofulvin, reabsorption is so effective that its renal clearance is virtually zero. Conversely polar substances, such as mannitol, are too water soluble to be absorbed and are eliminated virtually without reabsorption.

The reabsorption of drugs that are weak acids or bases depends upon the pH of the tubular fluids, and for acidic drugs, the more alkaline the urine, the greater the renal clearance and vice versa for basic drugs. The extent to which urinary pH affects renal excretion of such compounds depends upon the pK_a of the drug, since the Henderson–Hasselbalch equations state:

$$pH = pK_a + \log \frac{(\text{unionised})}{(\text{ionised})} \quad \text{for a base} \qquad (1.94)$$

and

$$pH = pK_a + \log \frac{(\text{ionised})}{(\text{unionised})} \quad \text{for an acid.} \qquad (1.95)$$

The pK_a determines the ratio of ionised to unionised at any given pH. Thus relatively strong acids or bases are virtually ionised (and therefore lipid insoluble) over the entire range of physiological urine pH values, and so undergo little reabsorption. The critical range of pK_a values for pH-dependent excretion is about 3.0–6.5 for acids and 7.5–10.5 for bases. Figure 1.24 gives some representative pK_a values for weak acids or bases. At any pH the pK_a determines the ratio of ionised to unionised drug. For strong acids ($pK_a < 3$) the concentration of unionised drug will be very low regardless of the plasma pH and the renal clearance will be high (because little reabsorption occurs) and unaffected by pH. Weak acids, however, ($pK_a > 7.5$) are less ionised at physiological urinary pHs and a high gradient for reabsorption exists which is again insensitive to pH changes. Only between these pK_a ranges is renal clearance sensitive to pH changes. Similar arguments apply to bases. Thus if urine pH is decreased to pH 5.5 by administration of ammonium chloride the elimination of amphetamine (pK_a 9.8) is increased some seven times as compared to its elimination from subjects with uncontrolled urinary pH.

Urinary pH may also influence the fraction of the total dose which is excreted unchanged. Thus about 57% of a dose of amphetamine is excreted unchanged in acid urine (pH 4.5–5.6) as compared to about 7% in subjects with alkaline urine (pH 7.1–8.0). Administration of amphetamines with sodium bicarbonate has sometimes been used illicitly by athletes to enhance the pharmacological effects of the drug on performance as well as to make its detection by urinary screening tests more difficult. The extent to which urinary pH changes alter the rate of drug elimination naturally depends upon the contribution that renal clearance makes to the total drug clearance from the body. Manipulation of urinary pH may play an important role in the management of some drug overdoses (see Chapter 22).

Tubular reabsorption may also be influenced by urinary flow rate. Diuresis may increase the renal clearance of drugs that are passively reabsorbed since the concentration gradient is reduced. Figure 1.25 exemplifies this. Diuresis may be used to increase drug elimination during overdose.

4. Active tubular reabsorption is a relatively unusual process. Uric acid is reabsorbed by an active transport system which may be inhibited by uricosuric drugs. Lithium, riboflavine and fluoride also appear to undergo active tubular reabsorption.

Monitoring plasma drug levels

The large variability in the responses to drugs by patients may result from two main sources:

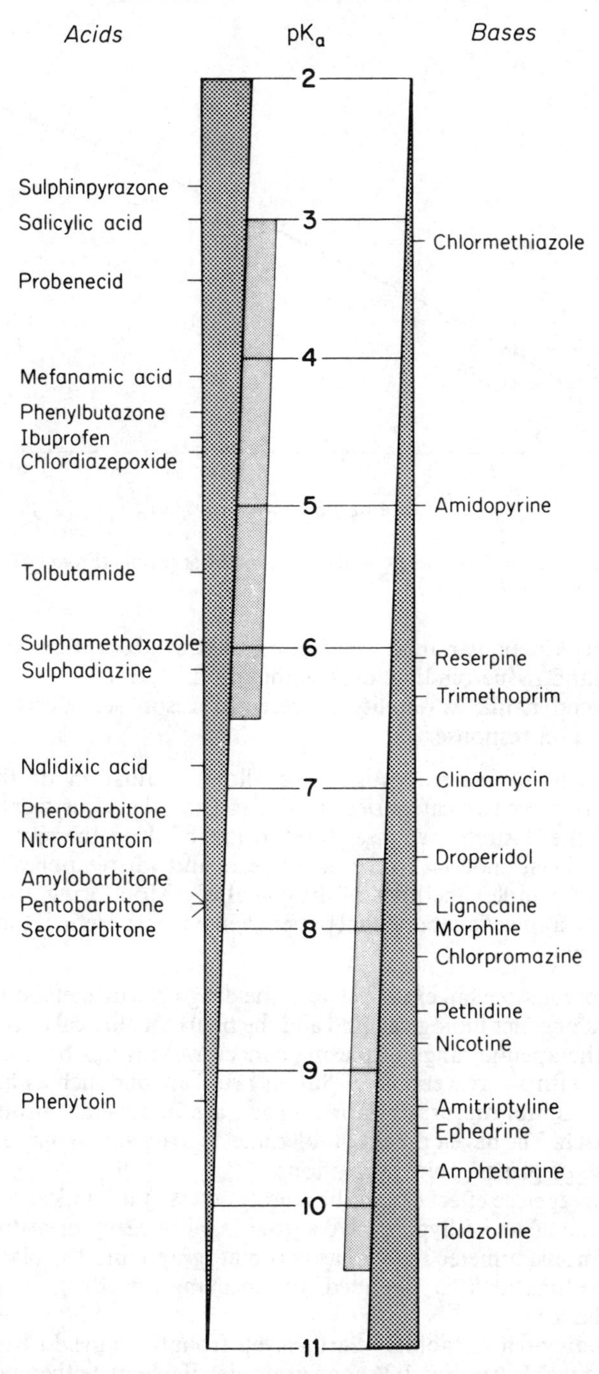

Fig. 1.24 pK_a of various drugs that are weak acids or bases. Width of wedge indicates increasing strength of acid (or base). Drugs with pK_a within shaded range may have their excretion influenced by urinary pH change.

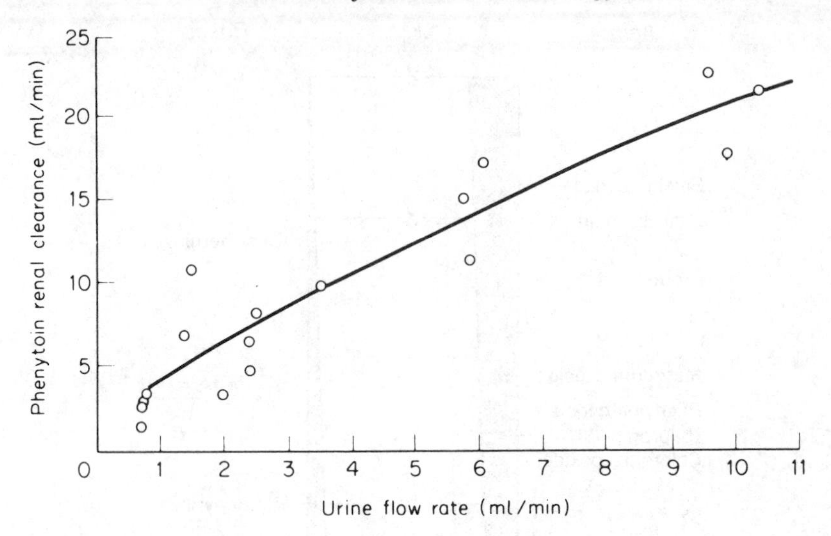

Fig. 1.25 Effect of urine flow rate on renal elimination of phenytoin (From F. Bochner *et al.*, *Clin. Pharm. Ther.*, **14**, 791 (1973).)

(a) Pharmacokinetic variability in factors such as absorption, metabolism, plasma and tissue binding, drug elimination.
(b) Pharmacodynamic variability in receptor response, effects of disease processes on response.

Measurement of plasma drug levels allows evaluation of the relative importance of these two categories of variation and the adjustment of dosage to produce the desired response. Monitoring of drug therapy by clinical response has been undertaken for many years and where applicable is more valuable than complex methods of drug analysis. Monitoring drug levels to assist in the therapy of an individual patient will be most useful if the following criteria are met:

1. A direct relationship exists between the drug or drug metabolite levels in plasma or other biological fluid and the pharmocological or toxic effects, i.e. a therapeutic range of plasma concentrations has been established. Drugs with an irreversible or 'hit and run' actions such as monoamine oxidase inhibitors or alkylating agents are in general unsuited to this approach. The development of tolerance to drug action may also restrict the use of plasma level estimations.
2. The therapeutic effect cannot be readily assessed by clinical observation. Thus the effect of hypotensive agents is more easily measured using a sphygmomanometer than a gas chromatograph and the place of drug-level estimations is confined to checking on drug resistance or compliance.
3. Interindividual variability in drug levels from the same dose is large and unpredictable (see Fig. 1.26 as an example). If adequate therapeutic levels can be reached in all patients by administration of a standard dose there is clearly no place for estimation of drug levels.

4. A low therapeutic ratio. Such drugs are particularly suitable for plasma level monitoring as they put the patient at risk. Similarly drug-level estimations may help when several drugs are being given and serious interactions may be anticipated.

Kinetic factors may influence the relationship between plasma level and response:

(a) Rate of change of plasma level has been found to determine the response to barbiturates, alcohol, amphetamine and indomethacin. Thus for amphetamine there is a close relationship between both its side-effects and the effects on systolic blood pressure and the initial rate of entry of the drug into the circulation, but not the peak plasma level or the area under the concentration–time curve.

(b) Time course of drug distribution and formation of active metabolites may affect the relationship as may binding to tissues and alterations of physiological homeostatic mechanisms. It should be recalled that only during the β-phase is there a constant tissue/plasma drug-concentration ratio. Thus studies should allow time for equilibrium to occur and preferably use steady-state conditions to define the relationship between plasma and tissue concentrations and effect.

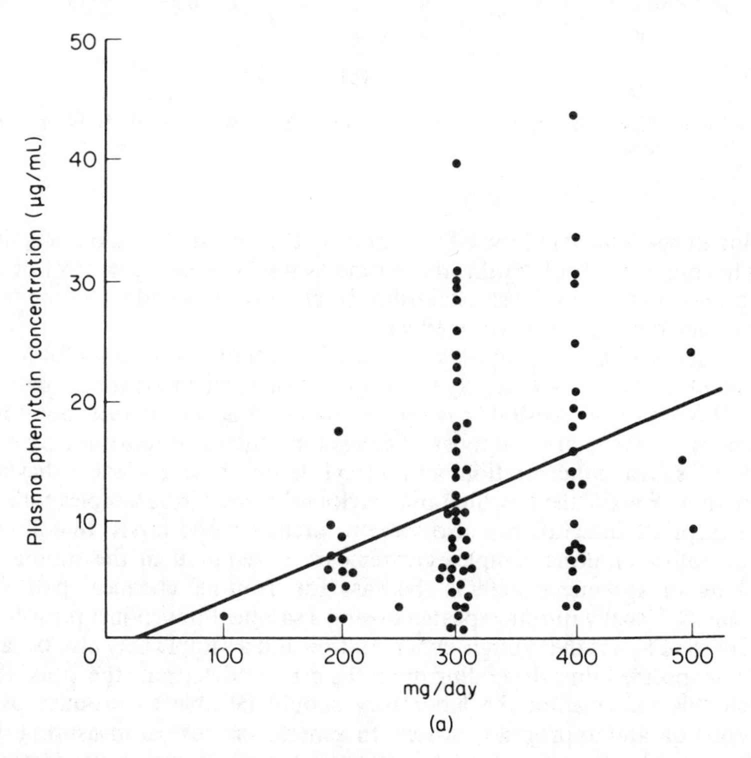

Fig. 1.26 Plasma phenytoin level at steady state expressed as total daily dose in (a) and as daily dose on a body weight basis in (b), *See next page.*

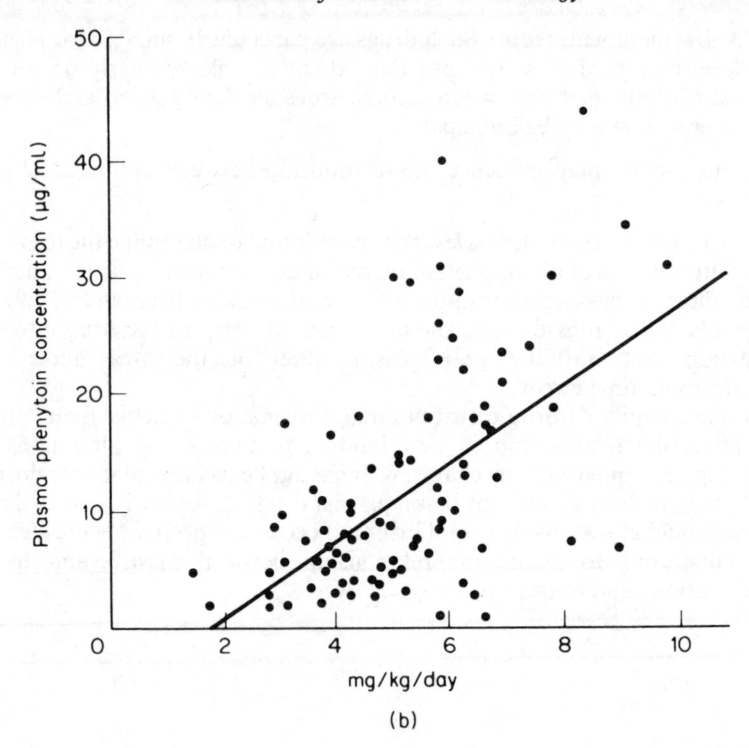

Fig. 1.26 (b) Data derived from 97 adults taking only phenytoin. (From W. D. Hooper *et al.*, *Aust. N. Z. J. Med.*, **4**, 449 (1974).)

Not all assessments of the efficacy of drug therapy are based on drug-level monitoring: the use of prothrombin time estimations in the control of oral anticoagulant therapy is well established by clinical usage and is an example of laboratory monitoring of drug effect.

In order to obtain appropriate kinetic information it is often useful to take several blood samples. This may be inconvenient, particularly for outpatients, and a hopeful new possibility is the use of saliva as an indirect monitor of blood levels. There are a number of drugs for which a proportionality exists between saliva concentration and blood level: these include salicylates, phenytoin, digoxin, theophylline and amylobarbitone. Urine samples collected at appropriate intervals can also serve to predict blood levels. In collecting blood, saliva or urine samples greater care is required in the timing and labelling of specimens than is the case for 'routine' chemical pathology specimens. Usually during repeated dosing a sample is taken just prior to the next dose to assess the 'trough' concentration and a sample may also be taken at some specified time depending upon the drug to determine the 'peak' level. Given this information the laboratory should be able to produce useful information and appropriate advice. In general the cost of measuring drug levels is greater than for clinical chemical estimations and to use expensive facilities to produce 'numbers' resulting from analysis of samples taken at random from patients described only by name or number may be meaningless and even misleading, as well as being a waste of money. Analytical techniques should estimate the appropriate substances in a specific manner: several of the older spectrophotometric methods for drugs such as theophylline estimate inactive metabolites. It should also be remembered that co-administered drugs may interfere with assays, e.g. many laboratories assay antibiotics by a microbiological assay, and if the patient is given a second antibiotic concurrently the results will be meaningless. As with all laboratory reports the clinician should realise that they may be in error. Experience with quality control monitoring of anticonvulsant analyses performed by laboratories both in the UK and in the USA reveals that analysis of a reference sample can produce some startlingly different results. *Plasma drug levels must always be interpreted in a clinical context.*

It must be admitted that few prospective studies of the effects of using plasma-monitoring services on the quality of patient care have been carried out. However, the same applies to more established procedures such as the use of prothrombin times in the control of warfarin therapy. A retrospective survey carried out at the Massachusetts General Hospital showed that whilst prior to the use of digoxin monitoring 13.9 % of all patients receiving this drug showed evidence of intoxication, following introduction of monitoring this fell to 5.9 %.

Drugs for which the case for monitoring seems clearest are:

1. Digoxin, digitoxin and other cardiac glycosides
2. Lithium
3. Aminoglycoside antibiotics: gentamicin, kanamycin, amikacin, tobramycin
4. Salicylates in rheumatic fever
5. Phenytoin.
6. Methotrexate
7. Theophylline.

Drugs for which the case may become better established over the next few years:

1. Some other anticonvulsants especially sodium valproate, clonazepam and carbamazepine.
2. Tricyclic antidepressants
3. Antiarrhythmic drugs: mexiletine, procainamide, quinidine, lignocaine and amiodarone.

COMPUTERS AND PHARMACOKINETICS

The availability of high-speed digital computers and of programs for simulation of drug kinetics in model systems has considerably increased the scope of pharmacokinetics. Computer programs may be designed to calculate drug-dosage regimes for individual patients when given appropriate patient data. They are based on three main modes of operation:

(a) A fixed pharmacokinetic model, usually of the one-compartment type, in which some of the model dimensions are calculated from patient data, e.g.

weight determines the volume of distribution, but the remainder of which are not easily assessed for a given patient, e.g. k_a for oral or intramuscular absorption will be determined from previous experiments. Such simulations allow compensation for some changes in the condition of patients, e.g. creatinine clearance, but in practice have been rather disappointing.

(b) Adaptive pharmacokinetic models also utilise a kinetic model but incorporate a facility whereby the program modifies the model according to the response of the patient to the suggested drug dosage. This adjusted model is then used to predict the next dose and is modified again according to the response. Such a program may accumulate experience based on many patients and incorporate this experience for future predictions.

(c) Model-independent programs do not utilise a formal pharmacokinetic model, which, provided a large enough group of patients is studied using an adaptive type of program, is not strictly necessary. The information provided by the panel of patients studied is used to predict the required dosage empirically. One simple approach is to find a linear regression between patient characteristics and individual maintenance doses of drug. Thus for gentamicin the creatinine clearance accounts for more than 80% of the variation in daily dose requirement and a simple regression equation of the form:

$$\text{daily dose} = a(\text{creatinine clearance}) + b$$

can be found, where a and b are constants (see p. 124).

A simple substitution in the formula is all that is then required to determine the correct dose. More complex multiple linear regressions may be devised, e.g. for digoxin the creatinine clearance, serum albumin, age, body size and liver function tests, may be taken into account although the prediction of appropriate dosage is only marginally improved by this complication. Such equations can, in the case of digoxin, account for about 70% of the variance observed in patients.

In several trials the performance of computer programs in predicting the required drug dosage has been somewhat better than that of clinicians. A reduction in the frequency of adverse reactions to cardiac glycosides from 35% to 12% has been demonstrated in one group of patients and to 4% in another group by the use of computer-generated dosage regimes. There remains, however, a group of patients (10–20%) in most clinical studies carried out with several types of drug in whom as yet drug dosage cannot be accurately predicted from the usually selected patient characteristics.

Chapter 2
DRUG ABSORPTION AND BIOAVAILABILITY

DRUG ABSORPTION

Regardless of route of administration a drug traverses a number of biological membranes to reach its site of action. The ease of penetration of such membranes thus determines the routes by which a drug may be absorbed and also the duration and intensity of its action. Although the architecture of membranes is still a matter of dispute, most membranes allow penetration of lipid-soluble substances and low molecular weight lipid-insoluble molecules whilst obstructing larger lipid-insoluble ones. A simple model would be to consider the membrane as a lipid barrier containing small aqueous channels. The best-understood absorption processes are those occurring in the alimentary tract and these will be considered in some detail.

1. Absorption from the alimentary tract

There are three main mechanisms for drug absorption by the gut:

(a) *Active transport* which requires a specific, carrier-mediated, energy-consuming mechanism. This is utilised by some naturally occurring substrates such as sugars, amino acids and some vitamins. Drugs related to such molecules may compete with these natural substrates and enter on the carrier. Examples include dopamine, methyldopa, some antimetabolites (such as methotrexate, 5-fluorouracil), lithium, iodine.

(b) *Pore filtration* through aqueous channels is limited to drugs with molecular weights less than 100 and to ions. The contribution of this route is likely to be negligible.

(c) *Passive diffusion* is undoubtedly the most important mechanism. Unlike active transport no energy is consumed and there is no competition between structurally related compounds for transport. The rate of transport of a drug across the membrane is described by Fick's law:

$$\frac{\mathrm{d}X}{\mathrm{d}t} = -\frac{DRA\Delta x}{M}, \qquad (2.1)$$

where $\mathrm{d}X/\mathrm{d}t$ is the diffusion rate, D is the diffusion coefficient (number of moles of drug diffusing across a unit area of membrane in unit time with a concentration gradient Δx of unity) A is the area of the membrane, R is the partition of drug between membrane and surrounding medium, and M is the thickness of the membrane.

The incorporation of R in the equation demonstrates the importance of lipid solubility in the process. Usually a simplified equation is written replacing the constants D, R and M by P, the permeability coefficient:

$$\frac{dX}{dt} = -PA(x_1 - x_2), \tag{2.2}$$

where x_1 and x_2 are the concentrations of drug on either side of the membrane, so that the rate of diffusion is proportional to this concentration difference. Therefore, it might be expected that no further transmembrane movement would occur once the drug attained equal concentration on either side of the membrane. However, because only uncharged drug molecules are able to partition into the membrane and because most drugs are weak electrolytes, the lipid–water solubility properties of which will vary with pH, it is possible for a considerable disparity of concentration to arise.

The Henderson–Hasselbalch equation states:

$$\text{pH} = \text{pK}_a + \log\frac{(\text{base})}{(\text{acid})} \tag{2.3}$$

(N.B. when pH = pK_a, the drug is 50% ionised, so that acids are more highly ionised when the pH exceeds the pK_a), so that salicyclic acid ($\text{pK}_a = 3.4$) distributes:

Stomach (pH 1.4)	Plasma (pH 7.4)
$\log\frac{(A^-)}{(HA)} = \text{pH} - \text{pK}_a$	$\log\frac{(A^-)}{(HA)} = \text{pH} - \text{pK}_a$
$= 1.4 - 3.4$	$= 7.4 - 3.4$
$\therefore \frac{(A^-)}{(HA)} = 10^{-2}$	$\therefore \frac{(A^-)}{(HA)} = 10^{4}$
$= \frac{0.01}{1}$	$= \frac{10\,000}{1}$

Thus there is 10 000 times more drug in the plasma than the stomach and the drug is thus well absorbed from the stomach when given orally. Conversely the absorption of aspirin is diminished in conditions associated with achlorhydria. In addition, this ion-trapping mechanism can result in strongly basic drugs, like quinine or levorphanol, passing into the stomach from the plasma. Furthermore, some drugs, such as aminoglycosides, are so completely ionised at any pH that they are not absorbed.

(a) Gastric pH Conflicting evidence exists for the effects of achlorhydria on the absorption of drugs. This may possibly be explained by the considerable variation found in gastric emptying in achlorhydric patients.

Antacids are widely consumed, sometimes without the knowledge or prescription of a physician. By altering gastric pH they may interfere with drug absorption in a number of ways:

1. Altered drug ionisation, e.g. carbenoxolone absorption is completely inhibited above pH 2 and therefore it should not be given with antacids; cimetidine (and food)-induced elevation of gastric pH reduces the absorption of ketoconazole.

2. Alteration of gastric emptying (the stomach empties more rapidly when the pH increases). This may partly explain the rapid absorption of buffered aspirin which is quickly exposed to the larger surface area of the small intestine from which it is rapidly absorbed. Trivalent aluminium ion also has the pharmacological effect of depressing gastric motility whilst magnesium ion has the reverse effect. Isoniazid absorption is depressed by aluminium but not magnesium-containing antacids, whilst sodium bicarbonate appears to enhance indomethacin absorption and aluminium hydroxide reduces it. Cimetidine in clinically employed dosage does not appear to alter gastric emptying rate.
3. Drug dissolution may be affected by pH changes. Thus sodium bicarbonate decreases tetracycline absorption probably by impeding dissolution of the solid. This is in contrast to the interference with tetracycline absorption produced by magnesium, aluminium, calcium and iron salts due to chelation of the cation by tetracycline.

(b) Gastric emptying and intestinal motility This may be changed by disease states but little is known about the influence of this on drug absorption. It has been shown that during a migraine headache there is delayed gastric emptying which reduces the absorption of orally administered aspirin. This may be countered by co-administration of metoclopramide with relief of headache (see Fig. 9.11). Presumably gastrointestinal hurry seen in anxiety or thyrotoxicosis may decrease drug absorption because of failure of adequate tablet dissolution during its passage through the small intestine where most drug absorption occurs. This is probably of most importance for those drugs with slow dissolution e.g. digoxin, or in enteric or delayed release formulations.

Table 2.1 Altered drug absorption resulting from drug-induced changes in gastric emptying and intestinal motility

Drug altering absorption	*Effect on absorption*	*Drugs whose absorption altered*
Anticholinergic drugs (atropine, propantheline)	Decreased	Lignocaine, paracetamol, lithium (slow release preparations), pivampicillin, tetracycline, sulphamethoxazole, phenylbutazone.
	Increased	Digoxin
Diphenhydramine (antihistamine with anti-cholinergic properties)	Decreased	Para-aminosalicylic acid
Narcotic analgesics (morphine, pethidine)	Decreased	Mexiletine, paracetamol, ethanol.
Tricyclic antidepressants (with anticholinergic properties, e.g. nortriptyline, amitriptyline)	Decreased	Phenylbutazone
	Increased	Para-aminosalicylic acid
Metoclopramide	Decreased	Digoxin
	Increased	Aspirin, levodopa, lithium (slow release preparations), paracetamol, pivampicillin, tetracycline, ethanol.

Surgical interference with gastric emptying by gastrectomy reduces the absorption of digoxin, levodopa, sulphonamides, ethambutol, ethionamide, iron and folic acid.

Drugs affecting gastric emptying alter the absorption patterns of many drugs. The effects of these drugs are not always easily predicted (see Table 2.1). Thus metoclopramide which coordinates gastric activity and improves emptying accelerates absorption of some drugs like paracetamol but conversely reduces digoxin absorption (see Fig. 12.5), perhaps by reducing the length of time that digoxin remains at the optimum site of absorption in the most favourably disaggregated state. As a general rule it is thus wise to avoid giving any drug which could potentially alter gastric emptying or gut motility when several drugs are given orally simultaneously.

(c) Presence of food or other substances in the gut These may act by dilution of the drug or by adsorbing or otherwise complexing with it. Food may also influence the rate and/or extent of absorption by altering gastric emptying. Table 2.2 gives some examples of the effects of food on drug absorption. In most cases the underlying mechanism is not understood. For amoxycillin, ampicillin and cephalexin it appears that the effect depends upon the presence of solid food in the stomach since a liquid isocaloric meal does not impair drug absorption like solid food. Enhanced absorption might be explained by delayed gastric emptying and transit time which allows more complete dissolution or a prolonged exposure to a specific intestinal absorption site. For drugs with a significant hepatic first-pass metabolism (see p. 89) transient increases in hepatic portal blood flow such as often occur after a meal may result in greater availability of drug if the drug is eliminated by capacity limited metabolism. The kinetics of such drugs are highly dependent upon hepatic blood flow and a sustained increase in hepatic blood flow increases systemic availability by reducing the extent of first-pass metabolism. Thus propranolol and metoprolol plasma levels are considerably higher when the drugs are given with food.

Any change in blood flow through mucosal capillaries may influence drug absorption. The degree of change in splanchnic blood flow varies with different foods, e.g. after a high-protein liquid meal, splanchnic blood flow increases but it is decreased by a liquid carbohydrate meal.

A high protein diet reduces levodopa absorption. Taking a diet with less than 10 g protein/day almost doubles the plasma concentration. This effect probably has two causes: delayed gastric emptying retains levodopa in the stomach where it is degraded, also digestion liberates amino acids from the protein which compete with levodopa for active uptake in the small intestine.

Ion-exchange resins such as cholestyramine will bind a number of acid drugs including warfarin, aspirin, phenylbutazone, digoxin, clindamycin, trimethoprim, tetracycline and cephalexin. Such resins should not therefore be given with these drugs and are best taken with meals to maximise their bile-binding properties. Activated charcoal binds a number of drugs including occasionally tricyclic antidepressants and this is occasionally useful in the management of overdose.

The timing of drug administration in relation to food can influence the effects of the drug. In general oral antibiotics should be given on an empty

Table 2.2 Effect of food on drug absorption

Reduced absorption	*Increased absorption*	*Unchanged absorption*	*Delayed absorption*
Aspirin	Hydralazine	Chlorpropamide	Cephalexin
Isoniazid	Nitrofurantoin	Metronidazole	Digoxin
Tetracyclines	Dextropropoxyphene	Oxazepam	Frusemide
(doxycycline least affected)	Lithium citrate	Nitrazepam	Paracetamol
Benzylpenicillin	Griseofulvin	Propylthiouracil	Sulphadiazine
Amoxycillin	(fat specifically enhances)	Prednisone	Glibenclamide
Ampicillin	Riboflavin	Theophylline	
Cephalexin	Carbamazepine	Phenoxymethylpenicillin	
Rifampicin	Metoprolol		
Levodopa	Propranolol		
	Spironolactone		

stomach to avoid impairment of absorption by food. Anthelmintics should also be taken similarly to improve contact with parasites. On the other hand, indomethacin, levodopa, iron preparations, phenylbutazone and other drugs likely to cause indigestion when given on an empty stomach should be taken with food.

(d) Absorptive area in the small intestine, especially the jejunum, is large and many natural substances are absorbed there, although some, such as bile salts and vitamin B_{12}, are known to be mainly absorbed in the terminal ileum. Little is known about the absorption site of drugs but by analogy it is believed that the upper small intestine is probably most important for passive absorption of drugs. The absorptive capacity of the bowel may be diminished by malabsorption syndromes and inflammatory bowel disease (see Chapter 5). The effects of these diseases, however, are unpredictable and may result in decreased or conversely increased drug absorption for no clearly defined reason. A single case of isolated malabsorption of phenytoin has been reported in which absorption of several other drugs was normal. Whether this type of phenomenon extends to other drugs is unknown.

(e) Gastro-intestinal blood flow is important only for those drugs in which absorption is perfusion-limited. For most polar drugs it is absorption which is the rate-limiting process and therefore blood flow does not affect absorption. Salicylamide, a lipid soluble analgesic, shows perfusion-limited absorption but its more polar glucuronide formed within the gut epithelial cells does not. Changes in blood flow to the gut brought about by stress might affect this process. Procainamide, which is usually rapidly and well absorbed, is more slowly and incompletely absorbed by patients with acute myocardial infarction. Blood flow to the gut is greater in supine compared to ambulant patients (although intestinal motility is decreased) but tetracycline absorption is decreased by bed rest although the responsible factors are undetermined.

(f) Metabolism by intestinal microflora may affect drug absorption. Studies of the metabolism of levodopa and sulphasalazine (salicylazosulphapyridine) in normal and germ-free rats indicate that some metabolic transformations of these drugs are due exclusively to the activity of the intestinal microflora. Similar effects are believed to occur in man. The breakdown of sulphasalazine into its constituent sulphapyridine and 5-aminosalicylate occurs at its presumed site of action in the colon. These metabolites are responsible for the effectiveness of the drug and the intestinal microflora govern its efficacy since suppression of the flora by neomycin diminishes sulphasalazine splitting. Apart from drugs, other substances such as cyclamate are transformed by the intestinal microflora and the activity of these bacteria may influence factors such as weight gain, resistance to infection or production of carcinogens.

2. Rectal absorption

The following advantages are claimed for this route:

(a) the acidity and enzymes of the gastric juice are avoided
(b) the portal circulation is bypassed to a variable extent, thus reducing first-pass metabolism (q.v.)

(c) it can be used in patients unable to swallow
(d) the duration of action may be prolonged.

In practice the rectal route is occasionally useful for nocturnal absorption of drugs, e.g. theophylline for asthma, indomethacin for the morning stiffness of rheumatoid arthritis or when the drug is poorly absorbed orally, e.g. ergotamine during a migraine attack.

The absorption of naproxen appears to be approximately equivalent by either oral or rectal administration, but little has been published regarding other anti-inflammatory analgesics. Unfortunately even when administered rectally these compounds may produce gastric irritation. It might be anticipated that more rapid absorption of substances which delay gastric emptying might be achieved by rectal administration. Such an advantage has not been shown for pentazocine but meptazinol gives more rapid and higher peak blood levels when given by suppository which could be of clinical benefit. A similar result has been shown for rectal aminophylline which produces earlier therapeutic levels and effects than tablets.

3. Buccal and sublingual absorption

This is used infrequently but has distinct advantages over oral administration for some drugs with pronounced first-pass hepatic metabolism, since by this route rapid systemic absorption occurs bypassing the liver. Thus for methyltestosterone a 40–50% increase in the amount of drug absorbed is seen after sub-lingual administration as compared to oral administration. Glyceryl trinitrate, isosorbide dinitrate and buprenorphine are also given by this route for similar reasons. As in the rectum the absorption rate is related to the degree of ionisation and the lipid to water partition coefficient of the compound.

4. Absorption from intramuscular injection

Lipid-soluble drugs can directly diffuse through capillary walls and are rapidly absorbed by this route. Drugs which are water soluble but completely lipid insoluble can also be taken up rapidly, providing that they have a molecular weight low enough to pass through the pores in the capillary membrane. Lipid-insoluble drugs of high molecular weight are only slowly taken up because removal from the injection site depends upon the relatively slow process of lymphatic absorption. The drug must be sufficiently water soluble at physiological pH to remain in solution at the injection site until absorption occurs: this does not appear to occur for some drugs such as phenytoin, diazepam or digoxin and crystallization and/or poor absorption occurs when they are given by intramuscular injection. The rate of absorption is also governed by the total surface area available for diffusion and the rate is increased when the solution is distributed throughout a large volume of muscle. Spreading of the solution is enhanced by massage of the injection site or by the use of high-pressure 'jet' injector devices. Transport away from the injection site is governed by muscle blood flow and this varies from site to site. Thus the speed of absorption of a number of drugs is increased by nearly 20% following injections into the deltoid compared to gluteal injection, injections into the vastus lateralis occupying an intermediate position. Females appear to absorb less cephradine when given into any of these sites, presumably due to increased fatty tissue and lower perfusion rates. Blood flow to muscle is increased by exercise and absorption rates are increased in all sites after exercise and conversely shock, heart failure or other conditions reducing muscular blood flow may be expected to reduce absorption. Slow absorption may be deliberately promoted to produce clinically effective drug blood levels for prolonged periods. This may be used to ensure compliance in psychiatric patients. One technique uses viscous injection vehicles such as oils, glycerine or polyethylene glycol, e.g. hydroxyprogesterone injection B.P. Alternatively a fatty acid ester of the drug may be injected which is slowly hydrolysed to release active free drug, e.g. fluphenazine decanoate.

Apart from complications associated with reduced and possibly unexpected availability a number of complications are associated with intramuscular injection:

(a) Pain: muscle is poorly innervated with pain fibres compared to skin but distension with large volumes (over 4 ml) is painful and injected volumes should be small. Solutions of abnormal pH or toxicity, e.g. phenytoin injection which has pH 10.5, are painful. Local anaesthetics are sometimes added in intramuscular injections but it is not established whether this is effective.
(b) Sciatic-nerve palsy following injection into the buttock is avoided by injecting into the upper outer gluteal quadrant.
(c) Sterile abscess may occur with some drugs: digoxin and paraldehyde have a reported propensity to cause this.
(d) Elevated serum creatine phosphokinase levels due to enzyme release from muscle cells may obscure diagnosis in suspected myocardial infarction.

The intramuscular route is somewhat more hazardous than an intravenous injection because if some adverse effect of the drug develops shortly after injection there is no way of stopping absorption of the drug, whereas a slow intravenous injection can be immediately discontinued. The intramuscular route is not always more effective or rapid than the oral route, e.g. for diazepam or chlordiazepoxide oral administration requires a lower dose of drug and produces a given level of sedation more rapidly than intramuscular injection.

5. Intravenous injection

This has the following advantages:

(a) Rapid action
(b) Complete availability of drug to the body since first-pass metabolism (q.v.) of the drug is avoided by direct introduction into the central compartment.
(c) It can be used for drugs which are not absorbed by mouth, e.g. kanamycin, or which are too painful to be given intramuscularly, e.g. nitrogen mustard. These latter drugs must not, however, be allowed to leak from the vein.

(d) It is easily controlled, which may be essential for some relatively toxic drugs where titration of drug levels to a therapeutic plateau is required.

The chief drawbacks of this route are:

(a) Drugs once injected cannot easily be recalled (orally administered drugs may be removed by gastric lavage).
(b) Very high drug levels may result if the drug is given too rapidly, one circulation time is optimal.
(c) Embolism of foreign particles or air, sepsis or thrombosis are all possible. Probably the greatest hazard is sepsis occurring via intravenous catheters in immunosuppressed or debilitated patients.
(d) Inadvertent intra-arterial injection may cause arterial spasm and possible peripheral gangrene.
(e) Inadvertant extravascular injection or leakage of toxic drugs, e.g. doxorubicin, vincristine, may produce severe local tissue necrosis.

6. Absorption from subcutaneous injections

This is influenced by identical factors to those affecting intramuscular injections. Cutaneous blood flow is slower than in muscle and therefore absorption is slower. If the skin of a limb is injected drug absorption may be increased by exercise, which may be one factor in exercise-induced hypoglycaemia in insulin-dependent diabetics (see Fig. 2.1). Absorption is retarded by immobilisation, reduction of blood flow by a tourniquet and local cooling, all of these measures being used to reduce absorption in wasp stings and snake bites. Adrenaline incorporated into an injection will reduce absorption rate by promoting vasoconstriction, conversely hyaluronidase will increase it by spreading the injection more widely within the subcutaneous tissues.

Sustained effects may be obtained from the subcutaneous injections by using oily suspensions of drug or by implanting a compressed pellet of drug subcutaneously. Such implants should resist disintegration and are optimally coin-shaped, which gives a constant (zero-order) absorption rate since the surface area hardly alters as the disc becomes thinner. Cylindrical pellets give a slightly different absorption pattern (see Fig. 2.2). Spherical particles have a reduced surface area to volume ratio with increasing diameter and therefore absorption rate from such particles is controlled by altering their diameter. Ultralente insulin zinc is a suspension of uniform (30 μm) crystals of insulin which provide reproducible absorption over about 36 h, which is much slower than Semilente (amorphous) insulin with a duration of action of 16 h. A 3:7 mixture of semilente and ultralente is known as lente insulin and has a duration of action of about 30 h.

7. Absorption through the skin

The skin has evolved as an impermeable integument so that the problems of getting drugs through the skin are completely different from transport through an absorptive surface such as the gut. There are three potential routes of absorption through the stratum corneum:

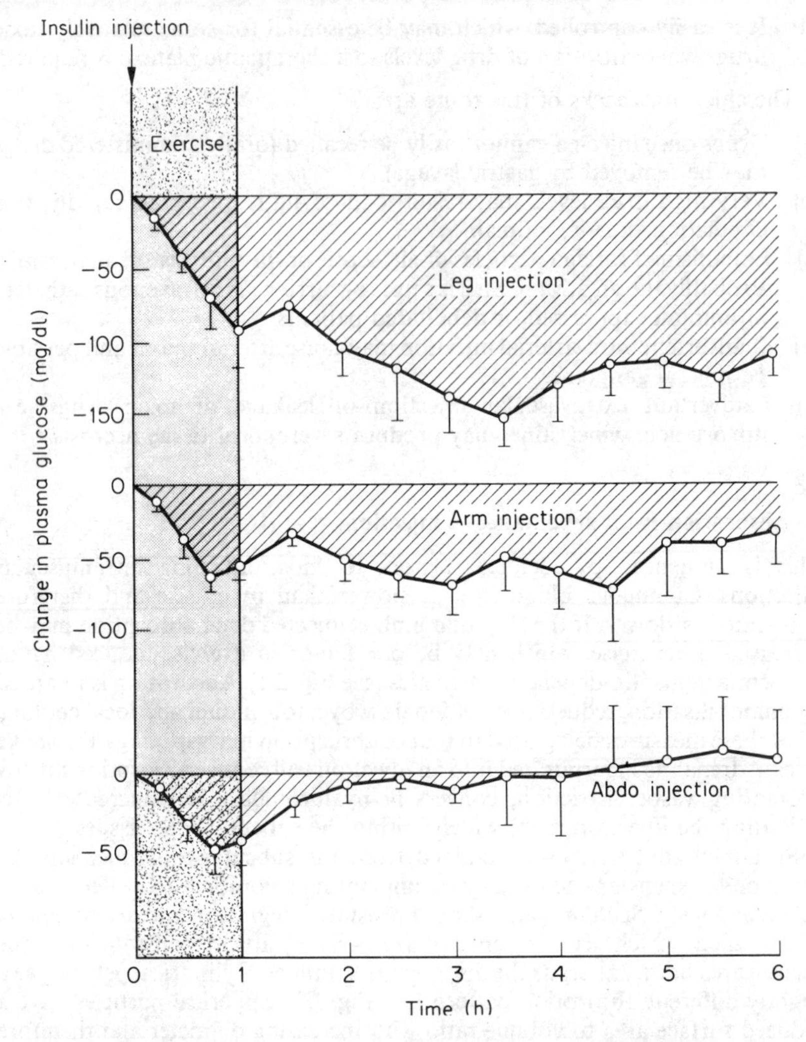

Fig. 2.1 Influence of injection site on plasma glucose response to subcutaneous insulin injection. The area above the curve for leg injection (thigh) is significantly greater than that for arm or abdominal sites: use of these latter sites reduces exercise-induced hypoglycaemia (From V. A. Koivisto and P. Felig, *New Eng. J. Med.*, **298**, 79 (1978).)

(a) sweat ducts (0.04 % of the surface);
(b) hair follicles (0.2 % of the surface);
(c) unbroken stratum corneum.

Sweat ducts play little part in drug penetration but for most drugs the other two routes play a varying role. Early penetration probably takes place via the follicles and is followed by steady-state transport directly through the cells. For some drugs such as steroids, which move very slowly through the stratum corneum, the follicles may at all times be the major route of percutaneous

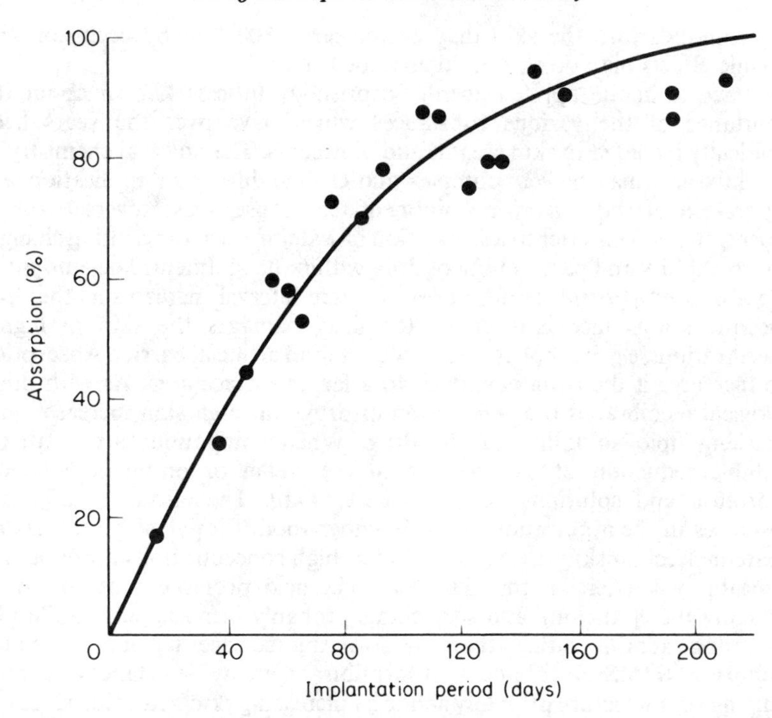

Fig. 2.2 Change in weight of testosterone pellets (cylinders diameter 2.5 mm, thickness 4.6 mm) after subcutaneous implantation in man. Curve is calculated from an arbitrary rate constant for absorption and assumes that absorption is proportional to surface area (From P. M. F. Bishop and S. J. Folley, *Lancet*, **1**, 434 (1944).)

absorption. A depot within the skin may exist for at least some topically applied drugs, explaining why drugs applied to the skin are excreted from the body more slowly than when injected intradermally. Factors affecting percutaneous drug absorption include:

1. Skin condition: injury and disease affecting the stratum corneum result in artificial shunts across the horny layer allowing greater penetration. The penetration of isotopically labelled hydrocortisone increases from 1–2% to 78–90% after removal of the stratum corneum by repeated stripping with cellophane tape.

2. Skin age: infant skin is more permeable than adult skin and steroids penetrate more completely.

3. Regional skin sites differ in permeability. In order of increasing permeability: plantar, anterior forearm, instep, scalp, scrotum, posterior auricular skin.

4. Hydration of the stratum corneum is one of the most important factors which increases the passage of all substances that penetrate skin. Under plastic-film occlusion as employed by dermatologists the stratum corneum changes from a tissue normally containing very little (10%) water to one containing up to 50% water with increased permeability. Thus penetration of

corticosteroids into the skin may be increased 100 fold by occlusion and systemic effects may occur due to absorbed steroid.

5. Factors in the applied agent. Surprisingly little is known about the importance of the various substances which have over the years been empirically included in skin creams and ointments. The physical chemistry of these mixtures may be very complex and change during an application, e.g. evaporation of water from an ointment may cause phase reversal from a suspension of oil in water to a suspension of water in oil with resulting changes in the solubility and partitioning of drug within the ointment. The amount of drug absorbed per unit surface area per time interval increases as the drug concentration is increased unless the drug damages the skin in higher concentrations, e.g. phenol, thereby producing an artificial barrier. Absorption also increases if the drug is applied to a larger surface area. As with other biological membranes the penetration of drugs through skin increases with increasing lipid solubility of the drug. When compounds are relatively insoluble reduction of particle size in the cream or ointment enhances absorption and solutions penetrate best of all. The effects of adjuvant substances in the application are little understood. Propylene glycol has no apparent effect on skin permeability but at high concentrations decreases the permeability barriers in the skin. Salicyclic acid promotes absorption by damaging the epithelium and surfactants probably increase permeability by denaturing keratin rather than by lowering surface tension. Dimethyl sulphoxide (DMSO) enhances absorption of many substances without changing skin structure probably acting by increasing skin hydration since it is a very hygroscopic substance.

Despite the low permeability of skin, recent interest has centred upon the possibility of using the skin as a site for administration of drugs with a large hepatic first-pass metabolism. Absorption into the systemic circulation via the skin bypasses this first-pass effect. New techniques now make transdermal drug administration reproducible and reliable. This is exemplified by percutaneous administration of glyceryl trinitrate in the form of a medicated plaster. This transdermal system (Fig. 2.3) consists of a nitroglycerine reservoir sandwiched between an impermeable backing and a membrane which controls the flow rate of drug to provide a uniform rate over 24 hours. This membrane

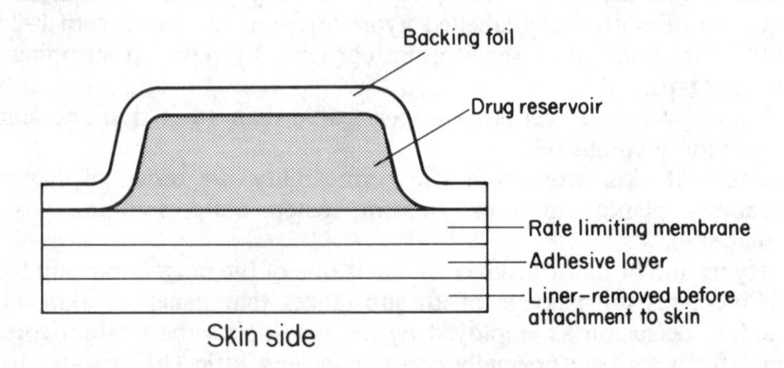

Fig. 2.3 Device for percutaneous drug administration.

is made of ethylene vinyl copolymer and the drug passes through it by diffusion. The plaster is stuck to the skin after removal of the liner and remains in place for 24 hours delivering approximately 25 μg glyceryl trinitrate cm^{-2} h^{-1} producing plasma concentrations of about 150 pg/ml (c.f. the transient levels of 2000–3000 pg/ml after sublingual tablets). These levels are adequate for angina prophylaxis without producing adverse effects and the system can be worn for swimming or other physical activities. Other systems are available in the USA, e.g. scopolamine–used for such diverse purposes as controlling excess salivation in orchestral horn players or motion sickness. One advantage of transdermal systems is that drug effects may be terminated simply by removing the device from the skin.

8. Absorption through the lungs

The lungs are ideally suited for drug absorption since the total respiratory surface area is about 60 m^2 through which only 60 ml of blood is percolating in the capillaries, thus presenting an enormous surface area for absorption. Drugs (or toxic environmental compounds) may be administered as gases, aerosols or particles for absorption through the lungs although the former usage in general anaesthesia is obviously the commonest.

Table 2.3 Some constants relevant to uptake of gaseous anaesthetics

Anaesthetic	*Ostwald solubility coefficient (blood/gas) at 37°*	*Partition coefficient (oil/water)*	*Concentration (mg/ml blood) at Stage III anaesthesia*
Diethyl ether	12.1	3.2	1.5
Chloroform	10.3	100	0.21
Halothane	2.3	220	0.21
Cyclopropane	0.42	34	0.17
Nitrous oxide	0.46	3.2	1.3

The amount of an anaesthetic gas entering the alveoli depends upon the partial pressure at which it is inspired and the alveolar ventilation. Initially the gas is diluted in the anatomical dead space but the partial pressure in the alveoli rises rapidly and this is followed by rapid diffusion into the blood. Equilibrium between the inspired and alveolar partial pressures of anaesthetic gas is not complete, since the gas is carried away from the lungs by the blood to the tissues. The rate at which equilibrium is attained is dependent upon the solubility of the anaesthetic in blood. This is defined as the Ostwald solubility coefficient (concentration of gas in blood/concentration in the gaseous phase at body temperature at equilibrium). The more soluble a gas is in blood, the greater the amount that must be dissolved in the blood volume to reach equilibrium and therefore the longer it takes for the equilibrium to be reached. Thus the blood represents a reservoir which must be filled before attainment of equilibrium. The larger the reservoir, the longer it takes to be filled and the longer it takes to induce anaesthesia with the gas. The rate of attainment of equilibrium therefore varies with the agent and is longest for the most soluble

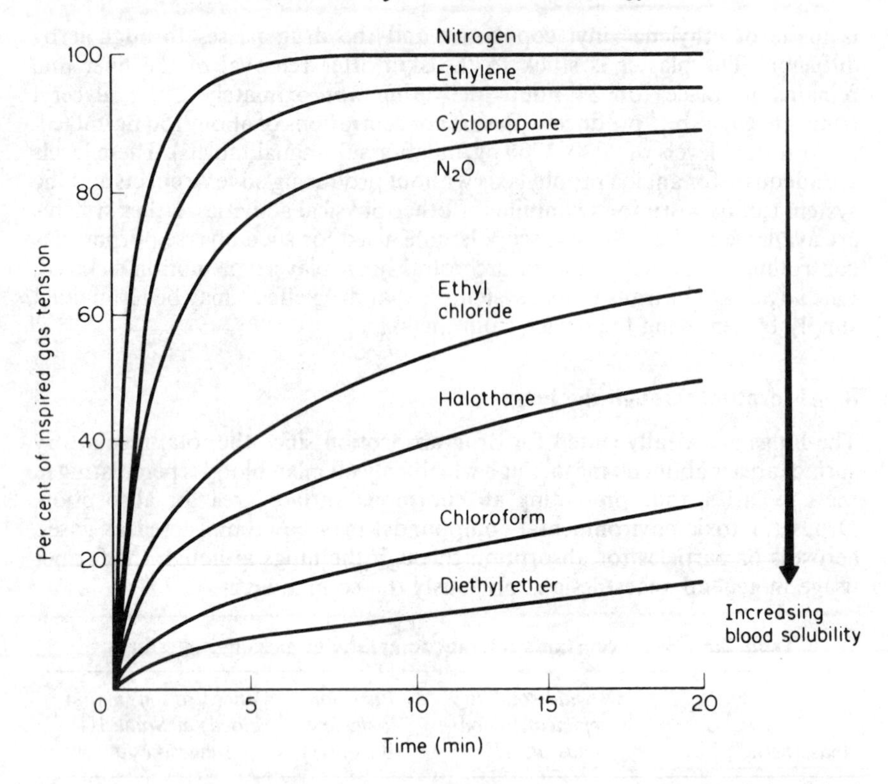

Fig. 2.4 Rate of attainment of equilibrium between arterial blood and inspired gas is determined by the blood solubility of the gas.

(Fig. 2.4). In practice equilibrium is rarely attained since anaesthetics are sufficiently selective upon the brain so as to produce anaesthesia before this happens. However, for highly soluble agents like ether, the time required to induce anaesthesia would be impractically long and therefore an initial 'loading' dose is given (using concentrations of 20–25% v/v) which is reduced to a maintenance dose (say 3–5% v/v) once the patient is asleep.

Anaesthetic gases rapidly distribute throughout the body thus the volume of distribution exceeds the blood volume so lengthening the process of equilibrium. Furthermore, attainment of equilibrium is slowed by a progressively decreasing difference in the pulmonary arteriovenous anaesthetic concentration as blood returning to the lungs contains increasing amounts of anaesthetic. Since the rate of diffusion across the alveolar membrane is proportional to this arteriovenous difference, the volume of gas transferred in unit time gradually falls. The rate of uptake of sparingly soluble gases (e.g. nitrous oxide, cyclopropane) is perfusion-limited, i.e. increasing the cardiac output will reduce the induction/equilibration time but this is unaltered by increased alveolar ventilation since the blood is carrying the maximum amount of gas possible. Conversely, with agents of high solubility such as chloroform or ether the alveolar concentration is rapidly reduced before the next breath

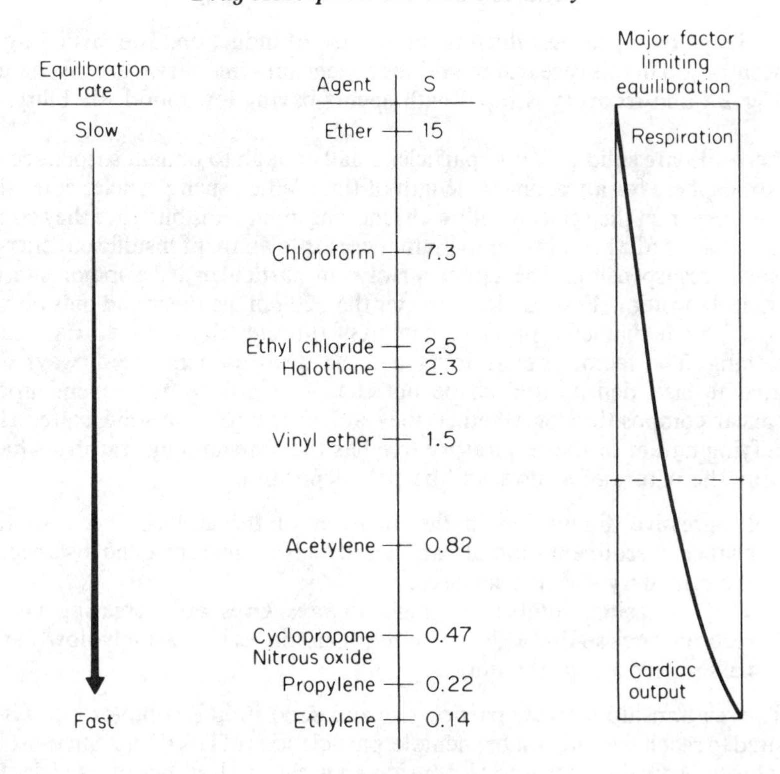

Fig. 2.5 Relation of anaesthetic solubility of equilibration rate and its relative limitation by respiration and cardiac output (From A. Goldstein *et al.*, *Principles of Drug Action*, Wiley, 1974).

and equilibration may be hastened by increasing the respiratory minute volume. Gases with intermediate solubilities like halothane have their uptake affected by both cardiac output and respiration (Fig. 2.5).

The fat/blood partition coefficient (roughly paralleled by the oil/water coefficient) is relevant to penetration into the CNS and anaesthetic potency. The rapidity with which a patient loses consciousness is directly related to this factor. It might be imagined that because anaesthetics are lipid soluble, body fat might absorb much of the administered drug. In practice this does not happen partly because true equilibrium is not always attained under clinical circumstances and partly because although adipose tissue comprises at least 15% of body weight it receives only 3% of the cardiac output (cf. 15% for the brain).

At equilibrium a predictable relationship exists between the anaesthetic concentration in blood and alveoli which is defined by the solubility of the gas. Therefore the concentration of anaesthetic in alveolar air to produce a given level of anaesthesia is fixed and is equivalent to the dose of a drug administered by tablet or injection.

Recovery rapidly follows stopping the anaesthetic and because most anaesthetics undergo relatively little metabolism the main route of elimination is the lungs by a process which is the reverse of induction. The inspired-gas concentration in this case is zero and so the tension–time curves are inversions of Fig. 2.4 and recovery is rapid with agents having low blood solubility.

Aerosols are solid or liquid particles small enough to remain suspended in an atmosphere for a reasonable length of time. When such particles enter the respiratory tract they closely follow the moving airstreams but once they come into contact with the lining epithelium these airflows are of insufficient energy to cause resuspension. The upper airways in particular are a major site of particle deposition. Few particles greater than 20 μm diameter and only about 50% of 5 μm diameter particles can pass through the nose during quiet breathing. The factors determining particle deposition in the airways are related to size, density and shape but the process does not depend upon chemical composition or whether they are in a liquid or solid state. The ramifying nature of the respiratory tree has two outstanding features which modify the nature of airflow and particle deposition:

(a) Progressive diminution in the diameter of the airways increases the chance of sedimentation of particles in a given time since the distance to the boundary wall is decreased.
(b) The increasing number of small airways gives an increasing cross-sectional area so that a given volume of air moves increasingly slowly as it passes deeper into the lung.

The relationship between particle size and deposition is complex but if it is desired to reach the smallest bronchiole, particle sizes of less than 2 μm must be employed. A further factor to be considered is ciliary clearance of particles by the ciliated epithelium which lines the respiratory tract right down to the terminal bronchioles. These cilia sweep particles back up the bronchi until they reach the pharynx. This remarkably efficient process can remove particles within 30 min, so a solid must dissolve and be absorbed more rapidly than this. Fortunately drugs may be absorbed rapidly by this route.

Aerosol inhalation has largely, but not exclusively, been used in the therapy of obstructive airways disease. Certainly a local action may be important for some of these drugs (Chapter 13). Although there is little firm evidence that different effects are obtained using different size particles it is best that inhalation is via the mouth and so absorption whilst still largely occurring in the pharynx can occur in smaller bronchioles. Pressurised aerosol nebulisers are convenient and meter the dose relatively accurately. The most usual problem with them is the failure of the patient to obey the instructions and careful explanation and guidance by the doctor is essential if patients are to obtain maximum benefit.

Disodium cromoglycate (p. 478) is prescribed as a dry powder for inhalation via a 'Spinhaler' without initial solution in liquids. The drug is delivered from special 20 mg capsules which are punctured within the 'spinhaler' to release a dust with about 50% of the particles of diameter 2–6 μm. However, aggregation of particles occurs readily and probably only 10% of the particles are within the range on inhalation. Much of the drug is therefore deposited at a high level in the respiratory tract. The plasma concentration of cromoglycate rises to a peak within 10 min of inhalation and falls to undetectable levels within an hour. This drug is almost unabsorbed by the gut but by inhalation about 8% is absorbed (possibly by some form of pinocytosis).

BIOAVAILABILITY

In order that a drug can exert a pharmacological effect it must reach the general circulation in an active form. It has until recently been assumed that this is assured once the drug preparation has been administered. A recent major advance in clinical pharmacology has been the demonstration of the incomplete and variable availability of drugs and a partial understanding of the causes of this variation. *Bioavailability may be defined as the extent to which and the rate at which the active substance in a drug product is taken up by the body in a form which is physiologically active.* The rate at which the drug enters the body controls the onset, intensity and sometimes the duration of pharmacological effect. It is therefore as important as the extent of drug availability. A number of processes determine bioavailability and are summarised in Table 2.4. Some of these are described in this and subsequent chapters.

Table 2.4 Factors affecting bioavailability of a drug from its dosage form

Dosage form factors	*Physiological factors*
1. Physical properties of drug Lipid solubility Water solubility pK_a 2. Properties of dosage form Disintegration time Dissolution rate Manufacturing variables e.g. compression pressure, lubricant concentration, ageing of product	1. Effect of luminal fluids pH Mucus Presence of bile salts Complexing components 2. G.I. transit time Gastric emptying Food Bed rest and exercise Enterohepatic cycling Drugs 3. Absorptive site Surface area Local blood flow 4. Metabolism of drug (first-pass effect) by gut wall, liver, skin, bronchial mucosa and all factors affecting this. 5. Pharmacogenetic factors determining rate of hepatic metabolism. 6. Disease states, e.g. malabsorption, thyrotoxicosis, achlorhydria. 7. Gut flora

There is now overwhelming evidence that the bioavailability of different drug products may vary significantly (Fig. 2.6) and the list of drugs for which this has been demonstrated grows longer each year. It is important to distinguish between *bioinequivalence*, a statistically significant difference in

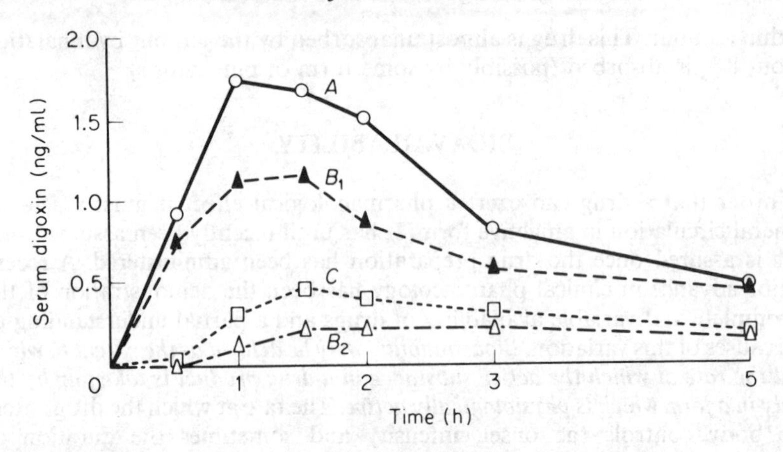

Fig. 2.6 Mean absorption curves following oral administration of four digoxin products A, B_1, B_2, C to healthy volunteers. B_1 and B_2 represent lots from the same manufacturer (From J. Lindenbaum *et al.*, *New Eng. J. Med.*, **285**, 1344 (1971).)

bioavailability, and *therapeutic inequivalence*, a clinically significant difference in bioavailability. The frequency of bioinequivalence is unknown but it is likely to be common. Therapeutic inequivalence is clearly less common and the degree of difference in bioavailability which must occur before therapeutic consequences occur will vary with the drug. Major differences in bioavailability will always be of significance. Small differences are likely to be of consequence for drugs with a steep dose–response curve or a small therapeutic ratio. Dose-dependent pharmacokinetics will magnify any changes in bioavailability. Fortunately most drugs have relatively flat dose—response curves, making it likely that only marked bioinequivalence will produce therapeutic inequivalence. A couple of examples will suffice to demonstrate the clinical significance of bioinequivalence.

In 1968–9 a number of reports were made of an epidemic of anticonvulsant intoxication in Australian epileptics. This was investigated in Brisbane where all affected patients were found to be taking one brand of phenytoin, and in these patients reduction of the dosage relieved the symptoms. It was shown that the excipient in the responsible phenytoin capsules was changed from calcium sulphate to lactose several months before the outbreak and that this change can result in altered bioavailability of the drug (Fig. 2.7) and consequent toxicity.

In 1971 Finnish workers showed that the blood levels resulting from continuous dosing with two commercially available digoxin preparations were markedly different, the disparity being sufficient to intoxicate some patients supposedly receiving an amount of the more bioavailable preparation equivalent to a previously satisfactory maintenance dose. At about the same time an apparently minor change in the manufacturing process of Lanoxin (a digoxin preparation made in Britain by Wellcome) resulted in reduced potency due to poor bioavailability, making this comparable with the potency of most other brands. Restoration of the potency by alteration of manufacturing conditions in 1972 led to some confusion and considerable variation occurred

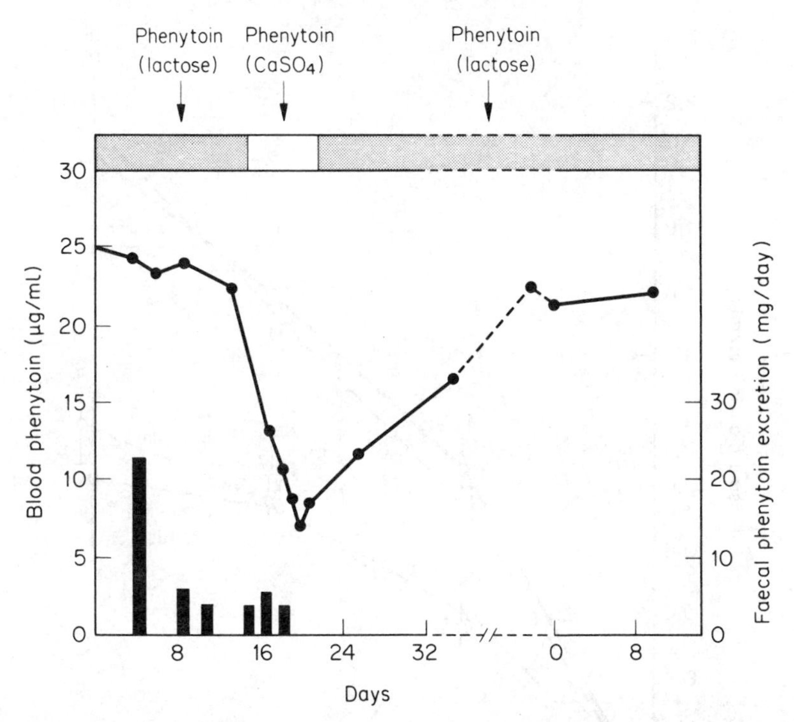

Fig. 2.7 Blood phenytoin concentrations in a patient taking phenytoin (400 mg/day), with excipients as shown (lactose; calcium sulphate). Vertical columns represent daily faecal phenytoin excretion (From J. H. Tyrer *et al.*, *Brit. Med. J.*, **4**, 271 (1970). Reproduced by permission of the Editor.)

in the blood levels recorded in patients who changed from 'old' to 'new' Lanoxin (although in fact the bioavailability had been restored to pre-1969 levels, see Fig. 2.8). These happenings drew attention to the non-equivalence of digoxin tablets available in the UK and alerted physicians to the potential for toxicity under treatment with different digoxin formulations. The clinical situation was complicated by the marked differences in digoxin absorption noted in patients changed from slowly dissolving to quickly dissolving tablets. It is now known that brands of digoxin vary markedly from one to another and even from batch to batch of the same manufacture. It may be that improvements in the B.P. dissolution standard for digoxin tablets will result in more uniformity but the difficulties are compounded by biological variation between individuals, some of whom are more affected by changes in brand than others.

An often cited example of therapeutic non-equivalence followed the testing of 16 different brands of oxytetracycline in the USA in 1969 which showed that only one met standard regulations and resulted in the discontinuation of licences for distribution of the other 15 products. These and other examples raise the question of whether in prescribing a drug the doctor should do so by *generic* name or by *proprietary or brand name.* It is difficult to give a dogmatic

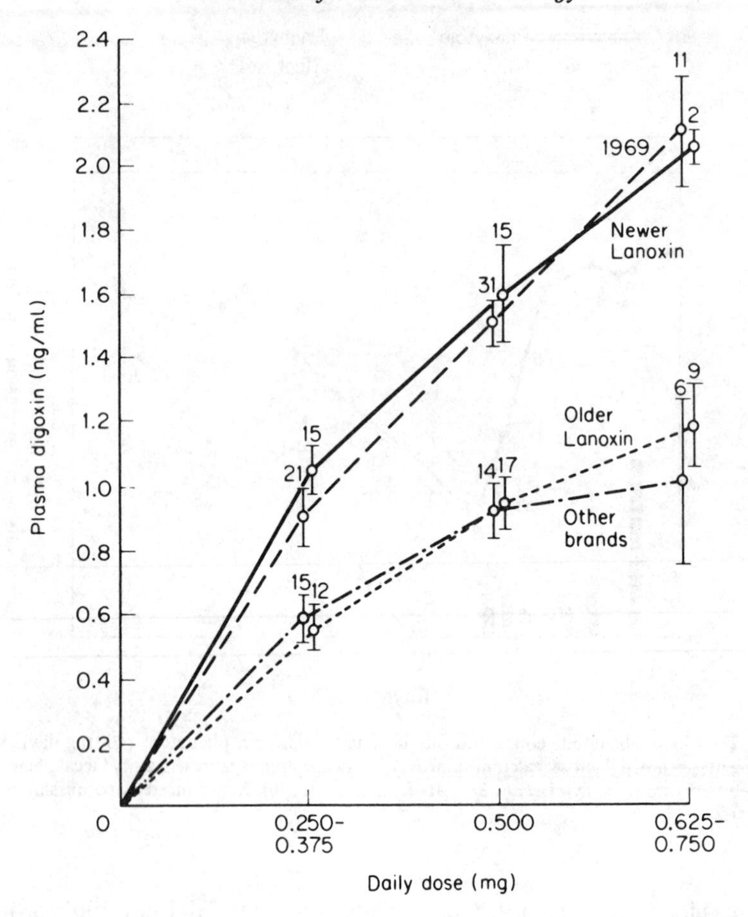

Fig. 2.8 Steady-state plasma digoxin levels (mean + standard error) resulting from use of pre-1969 Lanoxin, post-1972 Lanoxin ('newer'), 1969–72 Lanoxin ('older') and miscellaneous other brands. Numbers refer to total patients in each group (From T. R. D. Shaw *et al.*, *Brit. Heart J.*, **36**, 85 (1974).)

answer to this problem. Certainly in many cases substitution of a generic product will not result in demonstrable therapeutic inequivalence and such preparations are generally cheaper than branded products. It may also be added that brand names introduce confusion into therapeutics by creating a dual, parallel nomenclature to the approved name and often the brand name does not reveal the pharmacological nature or relationships of a drug. In a study of prescribing in a hospital group it was found that currently just over half of some 7000 prescriptions were by brand name. Since brand names are not generally taught in courses in therapeutics, this presumably reflects other sources of drug information, which include the activities of the pharmaceutical companies which rely upon sales of proprietary drugs to fund their research programmes and for profits.

Determination of bioavailability

This requires specific and sensitive methods for the estimation of drug concentrations in body fluids. In a few cases, e.g. anticoagulants, anticholinergic drugs, it is possible to determine bioavailability by the relative magnitude of therapeutic or pharmacological responses. In general this is not possible and a study of plasma levels following a single (or occasionally multiple) dose of the drug is necessary. If possible reference is made to the plasma levels resulting from intravenous administration of the drug since this route has 100% bioavailability. If this is not technically possible the reference preparation may be a drug solution or a formulation of recognised efficacy. Bioequivalence data usually consider three measurements:

1. *Peak plasma concentration* which depends upon
   (a) completeness of absorption;
   (b) rate of absorption;
   (c) "rate of elimination" (because elimination begins as soon as the drug enters the body).

   Taken alone therefore this measurement can be misleading.
2. *Time to peak plasma concentration* depends mainly on absorption rate and is reached when the rate of drug entry into the circulation is exceeded by the rates of drug elimination and distribution, absorption cannot therefore be considered to have been completed at this stage.
3. *Area under the plasma concentration–time curve* (*AUC*) which represents the amount of drug absorbed. For drugs administered chronically this is more critical than the absorption rate.

Since $\text{AUC} = \int_0^\infty C\,\mathrm{d}t$ it is essential for the plasma levels to be measured over at least three elimination half-lives because the error in estimation of AUC is reduced the nearer the integral approaches its limit of $t = \infty$. If this is not done AUC will be influenced by absorption rate as well as its completeness.

$$\text{Apparent bioavailability} = F = \frac{\left(\int_0^\infty C\,\mathrm{d}t\right)_0}{\left(\int_0^\infty C\,\mathrm{d}t\right)_{\text{i.v.}}} \tag{2.4}$$

$$= \frac{(\text{AUC})_{\text{oral}}}{(\text{AUC})_{\text{i.v.}}}. \tag{2.5}$$

F is the product of a bioavailability factor for completeness of absorption of the dose and a bioavailability factor describing any first-pass metabolism (q.v.), that is

$$F = F_{(\text{absorption})} \times F_{(\text{first-pass})}. \tag{2.6}$$

If absorption is complete, then eq. (2.4) estimates the first-pass effect. Similar expressions to eq. (2.5) may be written for comparison of intramuscular and intravenous administration or with reference to a secondary standard oral preparation.

These expressions are valid only if the apparent volume of distribution (V_d) and elimination rate constant (k) of the drug are independent of the route and the duration of administration since for the simplest, one-compartment case

$$\left(\int_0^\infty C\,dt\right)_{i.v.} = \left(\frac{X_0}{V_d k}\right)_{i.v.} \quad \text{and} \quad \left(\int_0^\infty C\,dt\right)_0 = \left(\frac{X_0}{V_d k}\right)_0 F$$

and similar arguments hold for more complex models. The error may be reduced by determining the half-life for each route of administration and correcting for any difference between them by using

$$F = \frac{(\text{AUC})_0 \ (t_{1/2})_{i.v.}}{(\text{AUC})_{i.v.} \ (t_{1/2})_0} \tag{2.7}$$

There are some circumstances which make single-dose bioavailability estimations difficult:

(a) Long $t_{1/2}$ may require blood sampling to be carried out for impossibly long times.
(b) Assay methods may be inadequate to detect plasma levels after a single dose.
(c) Availability estimates may need to be carried out in patients from whom therapy cannot be withdrawn.

It is possible to carry out bioavailability estimates employing steady-state plasma levels. The AUC during a dosing interval T, at steady state after first-order absorption for a drug which confers upon the body the characteristics of a one-compartment model, is

$$(\text{AUC})_0 = \left(\int_0^T C_{ss}\,dt\right)_0 = \left\{\frac{FX_0}{V_d k}\right\}_0 \quad \text{for both preparations.} \tag{2.8}$$

Thus,

$$\text{Apparent availability} = F = \frac{\left(\int_0^T C_{ss}\,dt\right)_0}{\left(\int_0^T C_{ss}\,dt\right)_{0,\ \text{reference}}}. \tag{2.9}$$

Hence the bioavailability of a drug can be estimated by comparison of the AUCs during a single dosage interval at steady state. This approach is valid for drugs which confer multicompartment characteristics to the body. As with single-dose studies a correction for variable $t_{1/2}$ can be applied.

It is not necessary to consider only plasma drug concentrations and methods exist for the assessment of bioavailability from a study of drug levels in the urine or of drug metabolites.

A good deal of space is taken in textbooks of pharmacokinetics concerning the estimation of absorption-rate constants. This is complex for drugs which are described by a multicompartment model. In fact, although data can sometimes be made to fit a single-compartment model, a true single compartment is unusual, and, since the absorption rate constant is a model-dependent parameter, errors may arise if the wrong model is adopted. For this and other technical reasons the determination of the absorption-rate constant experimentally seldom yields a value which gives quantitative insight into the kinetics of absorption or the performance of a dosage form. The measurements detailed above will allow statements to be made about bioavailability. The question of how these measurements can be interpreted in practical terms is not completely settled. Clearly a 10% difference in any or all of the measurements would probably be of little concern whilst differences of 50% between preparations are likely to be clinically significant. Differences in the range of 10–50% require consideration of the effects of the drug and the steepness of the dose–response curve to be taken into account. For antibiotics a value of 20% difference in bioavailability between preparations has been proposed as being an appropriate one for legislative action by drug-regulation authorities.

Pharmaceutical factors determining bioavailability

To be bioavailable a drug must be at the absorption site in a form capable of being absorbed. Figure 2.9 represents the processes taking place when a solid dosage form undergoes dissolution. Many factors involved in the manufacture of the dosage form cause marked changes in the rates of disintegration and dispersion of the granules and these processes govern the rate at which surfaces become available for dissolution. Therefore pharmaceutical factors are extremely important in the control of drug availability. The average tablet or capsule is a complex product often containing as many as 20 different ingredients, for in addition to the drug substance there are excipients, disintegrating agents, binders, diluents, lubricants and dyes, all of which may contribute to the performance of the dosage form as a drug delivery system. The active drug substances may comprise less than 10% of the total tablet weight. Under conditions of fast disintegration the dissolution rate of the particles themselves will limit the appearance of drug in the blood. Noyes and Whitney (1897) propounded a law which characterises the dissolution rate:

$$\frac{\mathrm{d}W}{\mathrm{d}t} = KS(C_s - C) \tag{2.10}$$

where $\mathrm{d}W/\mathrm{d}t$ = dissolution rate, K is a rate constant, S = surface area of dissolving solid, C = concentration of drug in dissolution medium and C_s = concentration of a saturated drug solution. This simplifies to (2.11) if $C_s \gg C$:

$$\frac{\mathrm{d}W}{\mathrm{d}t} \propto SC_s. \tag{2.11}$$

The dissolution rate may therefore be controlled by manipulation of the surface area of the drug particles or solubility.

(a) Alteration in surface area by control of particle size. Figure 2.10 shows that the amount of griseofulvin absorbed increases linearly with the logarithm of the surface area. 0.5g of microcrystalline griseofulvin produces higher levels than 1g powdered griseofulvin and this is now the form used clinically. Nitrofurantoin when given in microcrystalline form may produce nausea and vomiting, possibly due to overshoot of the toxic plasma level. When given as

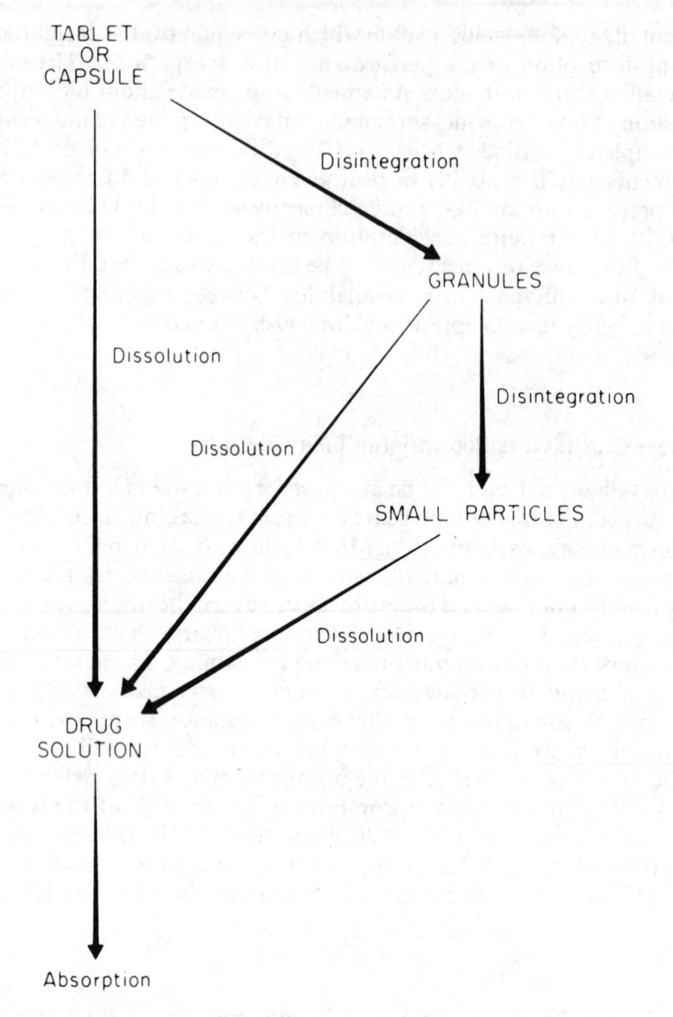

Fig. 2.9 Schematic representation of disintegration and dissolution processes occurring before absorption from a dosage form.

macrocrystals of the appropriate size the toxic level is not reached but the amount absorbed (area under the curve) is the same for both preparations and clinically the cure rate for urinary tract infection is maintained.

(b) Drug solubility may be altered in a number of ways. As shown above, a weak base is freely soluble at the low pH of the stomach but a weak acid is less soluble. Thus by controlling the pH of the microenvironment of the drug particles the solubility is altered. Some preparations of buffered aspirin contain aluminium or magnesium hydroxide and although the pH of the stomach contents is unchanged the rate of aspirin absorption is increased (Fig. 2.11). Alternatively the salt of a weak acid may be employed. When a weak acid

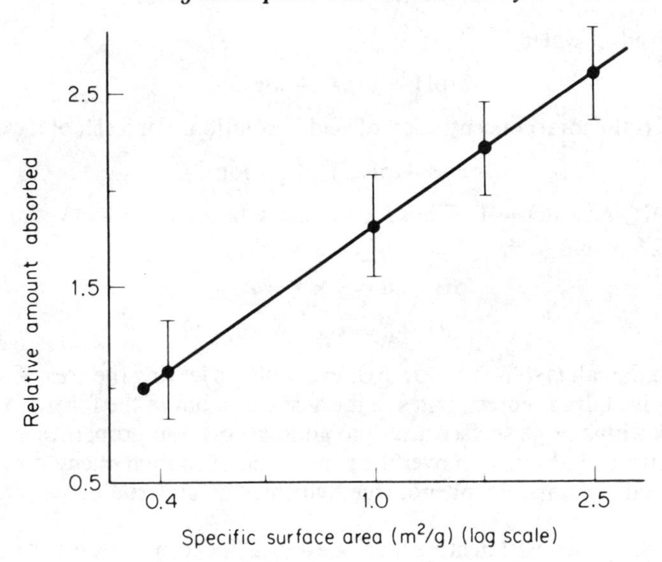

Fig. 2.10 Effect of surface area of particles on absorption of griseofulvin in man (From R. M. Atkinson *et al.*, *Nature*, **193**, 588 (1962).)

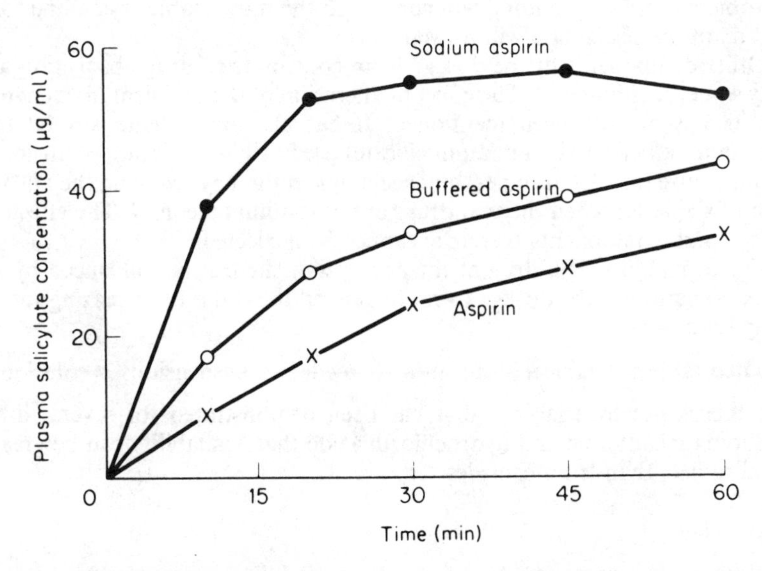

Fig. 2.11 Mean plasma salicylate concentrations in normal volunteers following administration of different aspirin preparations in doses equivalent to 640 mg (From J. R. Leonards, *Clin. Pharm. Ther.*, 4,476 (1963).)

is dissolved in water

$$\mathrm{pH} \simeq \tfrac{1}{2}(\mathrm{pK_a} - \log C), \tag{2.12}$$

where C is the total concentration of acid in solution. For a salt of a weak acid

$$\mathrm{pH} \simeq \tfrac{1}{2}(\mathrm{pK_w} + \mathrm{pK_a} + \log C), \tag{2.13}$$

where $\mathrm{pK_w}$ for water = 14. Thus for a molar solution of an acid with $\mathrm{pK_a} = 4$, since $\log C = \log 1 = 0$,

$$\mathrm{pH\ acid} \simeq \tfrac{1}{2} \times 4 = 2$$

and

$$\mathrm{pH\ salt} \simeq \tfrac{1}{2} \times (14 + 4) = 9.$$

Hence the salt is soluble at low pH. Probably on leaving the area of the solid the dissolved drug reprecipitates in the acid form, but in the form of very fine particles with a large surface area and good absorption properties. Examples are the superior absorption over the parent acid of sodium phenytoin, sodium tolbutamide, potassium phenoxymethylpenicillin and sodium aspirin (Fig. 2.11).

Some drugs can exist in more than one crystalline form, e.g. cortisone acetate exists in five different forms differing in dissolution rate. The most unstable polymorph has the most rapid dissolution rate, thus the metastable form of methylprednisolone is some 50% more available when administered as a subcutaneous pellet. The anhydrous form of ampicillin is 20% more soluble than the trihydrate and thus is more rapidly available. The optimum metastable form can usually be prepared by careful adjustment of manufacturing conditions but may require additional stabilisation to prolong shelf-life. Thus novobiocin in the amorphous state is ten times more soluble than crystalline novobiocin, but on standing will convert to the more stable crystalline form and addition of alginate will prevent this.

Other components of the dosage form contribute to drug absorption and may sometimes hinder it. The effect of alteration of the excipient in phenytoin tablets has already been mentioned. It has also been demonstrated that bentonite (a hydrated aluminium silicate) used as a granulating agent in the manufacture of PAS granules, binds rifampicin thereby reducing the absorption of the latter when the two drugs are used simultaneously. The effects of these 'inert' components therefore cannot be neglected.

The availability of a drug at the absorption site can be influenced by the physical nature of the dosage form. In general the order of increasing rate of drug release is

coated tablets < tablets < capsules < powders < suspensions < solutions,

but this is not invariable and it has been demonstrated for several drugs including triamterine and hydrochlorthiazide that availability can be greater from tablets than from capsules.

Pro-Drugs

A different approach to improving bioavailability is to modify the drug molecule chemically to a better absorbed compound which will liberate the active drug *in vivo* after absorption has been accomplished. Such modified drugs are termed *pro-drugs*. For example, carbenicillin is poorly absorbed by mouth but the esters indanyl carbenicillin and carfecillin are much better absorbed. Once absorbed they are hydrolysed to carbenicillin and cannot be found free in the circulation. These esters, unlike carbenicillin, are not active antibiotics. Some other examples are shown in Table 2.5.

Table 2.5 Pro-drugs and their final products released into the circulation

Prodrug	*Product*
Pivampicillin	Ampicillin
Talampicillin	Ampicillin
Pivmecillinam	Mecillinam
Benorylate	Aspirin + paracetamol
Ibuterol	Terbutaline
Prazepam	Desmethyldiazepam
Clorazepate	Desmethyldiazepam

Sustained release preparations

An alternative type of drug formulation is the sustained-release preparation which releases drug slowly into the gut for sustained absorption and effect. Such formulations are suitable if the half-life is short so that the drug would otherwise have to be taken very frequently. However, they cannot reliably prolong a dosage interval from 12 to 24 hours because the transit time through the small intestine where most drugs are absorbed is only about 6 hours. Because absorption is influenced by transit time, the presence of food, disease, drugs changing gut motility, immobility and constipation may alter the amount of drug absorbed. This may be particularly important in the old who have prolonged transit times and hence increased drug absorption. If the gut lumen is narrowed there is also a danger that the formulation will become impacted and release high concentrations of drug locally thus causing mucosal damage. Preparations with a soluble matrix or which produce small particles are less likely to produce this problem. Another problem is that overdose with sustained release preparations may be difficult to treat because large amounts of the drug may continue to be absorbed several hours after the tablets have left the stomach. They are not suitable for potent drugs (when variations in drug release may exceed the safety margin), poorly absorbed drugs or those absorbed by zero-order processes or when the drug effect is unrelated to blood levels. A slow-release formulation may improve patient compliance and theoretically, by maintaining a continuous blood level, should prevent symptom breakthrough. In the case of some drugs, e.g. quinidine, adverse effects due to high peak plasma concentrations may be avoided and it should be possible to avoid rapid delivery of an irritant drug to localised areas of the gut wall. A number of mechanisms are used to produce sustained release of drug:

(a) Tablets with an outer immediately absorbed dose enclosing a slowly released core of drug bound to resin or in a wax matrix.

(b) Capsules containing pellets of drug. One group of pellets are uncoated and constitute the immediately absorbed portion, the other pellets are coated with variable amounts of a retarding coat which controls the rate of dissolution by its thickness and nature.

(c) Tablets of a plastic matrix so that drug is leached from within its interstices and the spent matrix is shed in the faeces. The dose is controlled by the geometry of the tablet and the rate at which channels are opened up into its material to allow drug dissolution.

(d) Tablets or capsules containing drug bound to ion exchange resin, e.g. as a salt with a polystyrine sulphonic acid resin. The release of drug depends upon the exchange of ions such as sodium and potassium from the digestive juices for ionised drug from the resin.

(e) Osmotic pump systems: These are tablets comprising a strong, rigid semipermeable coating containing the drug and an osmotically active 'driver' substance (usually an electrolyte). An accurately bored hole is made into the coat using a laser. In the gut water is attracted osmotically into the core, dissolving the contents and generating a pressure of several atmospheres. The resulting solution of drug is then squirted out of the hole to relieve the pressure. By adjustment of the size of the hole and the concentrations in the core a constant rate of drug release from the system is provided. Although several experimental preparations are under trial the only example of this formulation on the UK market (Osmosin – a preparation of indomethacin) was withdrawn following reports of small bowel ulceration. It seems likely that Osmosin tablets became stuck in the bowel so increasing local indomethacin concentrations and causing bleeding and ulceration.

Sustained release preparations tend to be expensive and have their own complications and problems so the decision to use them must be carefully considered. Patients should be warned not to cut or chew the tablets or capsules and to take them after food with water. They should also be told not to worry if the unabsorbed remnants of the tablet or capsule appear in the stool.

Local delivery systems

Systems have been developed to apply drugs locally using rate-controlling membranes. One of these is presently available as the pilocarpine Ocusert system for glaucoma. This is a flat flexible elliptical-shaped device consisting of a drug reservoir core containing pilocarpine enclosed in two outer plastic polymer membranes. These membranes give a zero-order release rate of pilocarpine, i.e. the release is at a constant rate and does not decrease as the reservoir empties. The device is small enough to insert comfortably into the lower conjunctival sac and can remain there releasing drug for several days. This device might be expected to improve compliance since the alternative is using pilocarpine drops several times daily. It also provides smoother control of intraocular pressure with a reduced total pilocarpine dosage.

Slow release formulations may however reduce flexibility for dosage adjustment since it may not be possible to divide the capsule or tablet to reduce dosage. Sometimes, it can be more appropriate to substitute a different drug with similar properties but longer half-life, e.g. isosorbide mononitrate for isosorbide dinitrate, piroxicam for ketoprofen, rather than to use a sustained release preparation.

Chapter 3

DRUG METABOLISM

METABOLIC PATHWAYS

Biochemical modification of drugs alters their pharmacological activity and rate of excretion. Although activity is often reduced or abolished (as in oxidation of barbiturates, phenytoin and alcohol), it may sometimes be increased (as in the conversion of chloral hydrate to trichlorethanol). The formation of polar metabolites which have reduced lipid solubility results in reduced reabsorption from the renal tubules and therefore an increased rate of drug excretion. Some metabolic transformations however result in compounds with a slower rate of elimination than the parent substance (e.g. desmethyldiazepam has a plasma half-life of 100 h compared with a half-life of 20–50 h for diazepam).

Drug metabolism in man may involve two phases. *Phase I* is a metabolic modification of the drug: oxidation, reduction and hydrolysis. *Phase II* is a synthetic reaction called conjugation. This may affect the parent drug or one of its metabolites. Conjugation involves combination with another molecule or group such as glucuronic acid, glycine, glutamine, sulphate or acetate. Synthesis of a thiocyanate or mercapturic acid is also possible.

Conjugate formation may occur with the original drug, as for example with isoprenaline, as shown in Fig. 3.1. Characteristically conjugate formation occurs with the product of phase I metabolism. This sequence can in general terms be expressed as shown in Fig. 3.2.

PHASE I METABOLISM

The most important site of drug metabolism is the liver. The endoplasmic reticulum, cytosol and mitochondria are all concerned in various metabolic pathways in drug degradation.

(a) Endoplasmic reticulum

The smooth endoplasmic reticulum is a membrane system which contains enzymic protein with the ability to metabolise exogenous substances. Cellular homogenates yield the endoplasmic reticulum membrane (microsomes) by centrifugation at 100 000 g for $\frac{1}{2}-1$ h. Microsomes ('small bodies') are artifacts of homogenisation and centrifugation and contain, amongst other cell-derived structures, the enzymes of the endoplasmic reticulum trapped within membranes which coalesce.

(i) *Oxidation* Microsomal oxidation may result in aromatic and aliphatic hydroxylation, deamination, dealkylation and S-oxidation. These are all primarily a hydroxylation reaction involving reduced NADP, atmospheric oxygen, mixed function oxidase and a haemoprotein (or probably a group of

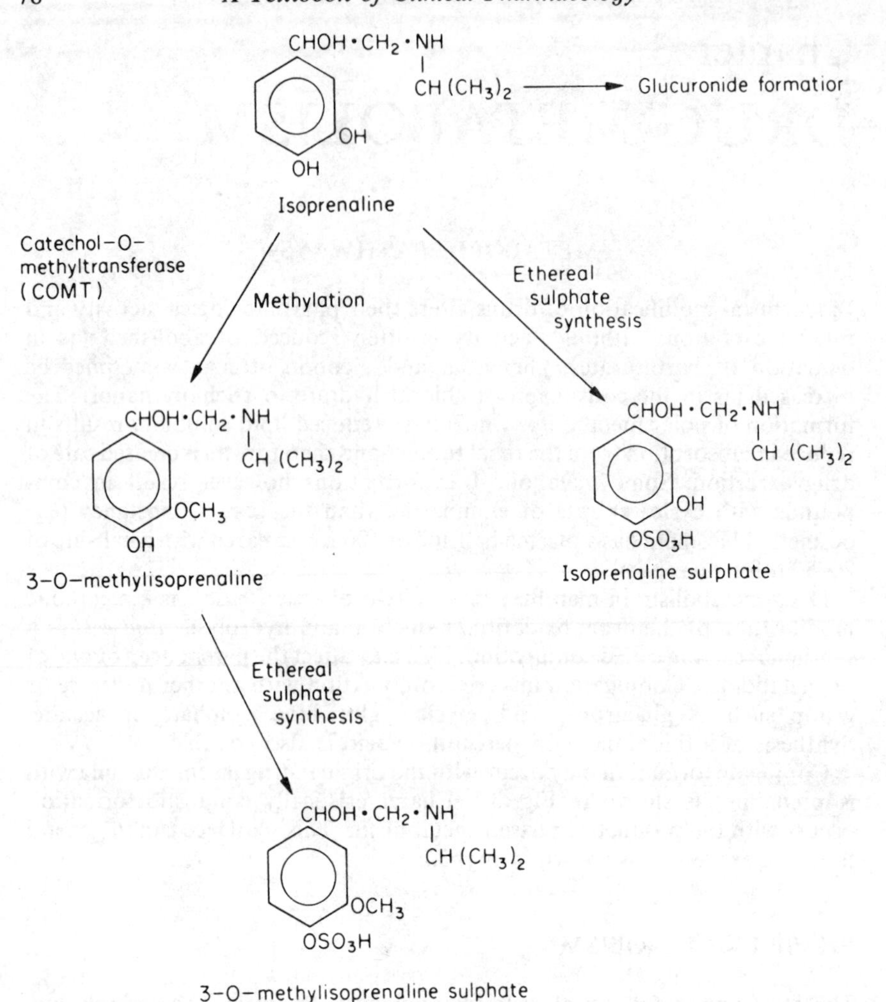

Fig. 3.1 The metabolic fate of isoprenaline.

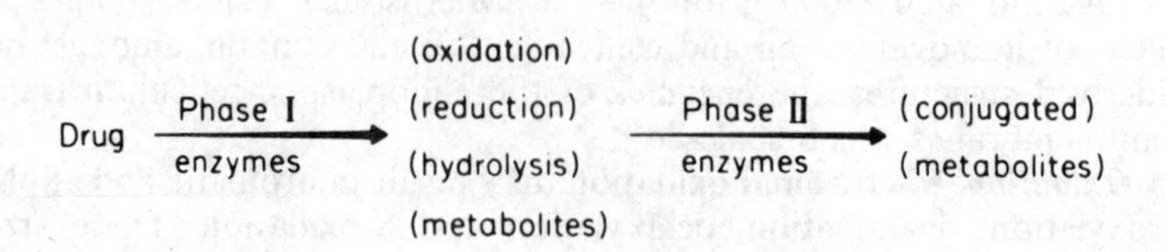

Fig. 3.2 Phase I and II of drug metabolism.

closely related haemoproteins) called cytochrome P_{450}. This acts as a terminal oxidase in the oxidation reaction and is so called because the reduced form can react with carbon monoxide to yield a complex with an absorption peak at 450 nm. A simplified scheme for the oxidation pathway is shown in Fig. 3.3.

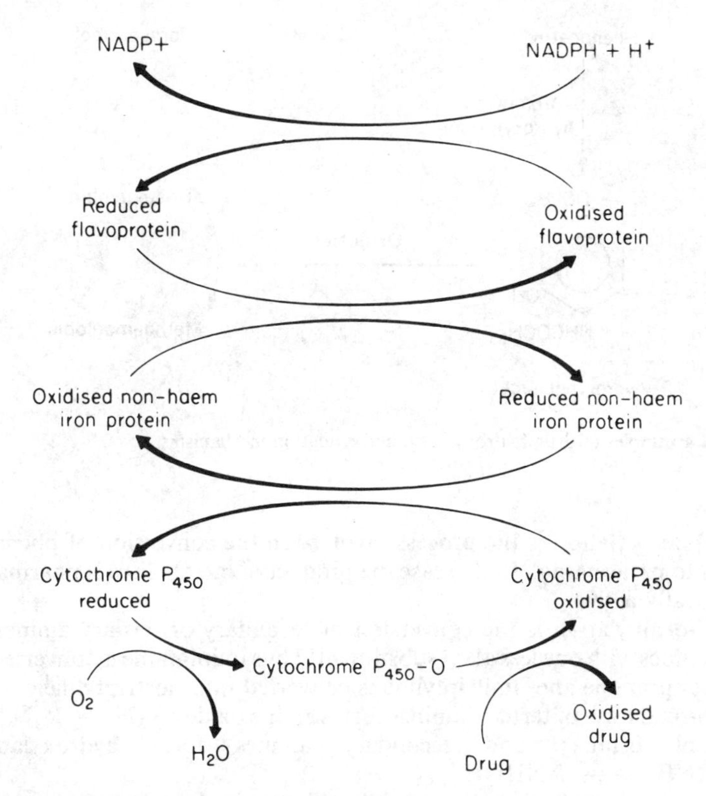

Fig. 3.3 Simplified scheme for the oxidation pathway.

Cytochrome P_{450} also occurs in adrenal cortex, kidney and intestinal mucosa which are also sites of drug metabolism.

Typical examples of drug oxidation mechanisms are:

1. Aromatic hydroxylation to form phenols, e.g. the conversion of phenacetin into 2-hydroxyphenacetin. Normally much of a dose of phenacetin is converted into paracetamol by dealkylation. In patients with a genetic inability to carry out this reaction, large amounts of the 2-hydroxy derivative are formed instead. This oxidises haemoglobin and methaemoglobinaemia can result, as shown in Fig. 3.4.
2. Aliphatic hydroxylation occurs in the side chains of barbiturates (at carbon 5 of the ring) and this results in complete loss of pharmacological activity.

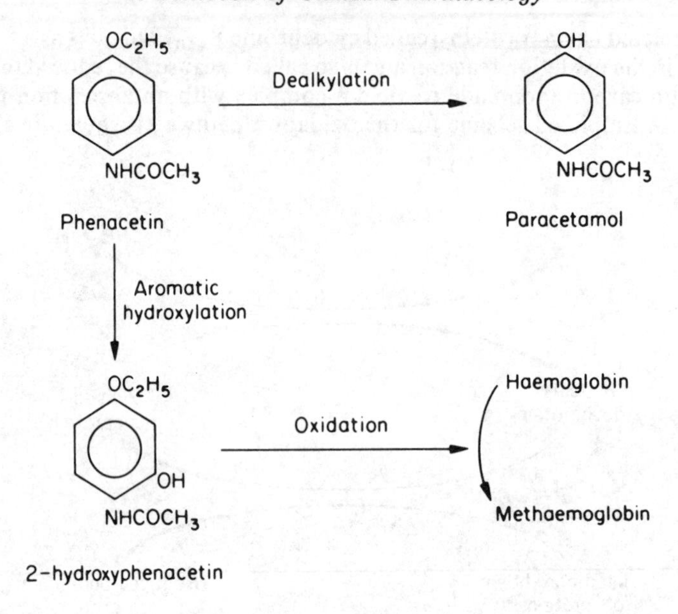

Fig. 3.4 Examples of drug hydroxylation and oxidation mechanisms.

3. O-dealkylation is the process involved in the conversion of phenacetin into paracetamol. In this case the product of metabolism is pharmacologically active.
4. N-dealkylation is the conversion of secondary or tertiary amines into amines with one less alkyl substituent. Thus imipramine is converted into desipramine and amitriptyline is converted into nortriptyline.
5. N-oxidation of tertiary amines forms amine oxides: R_3N — R_3N^+—O′ and primary and secondary amines form hydroxylamines: RNH_2 —— RNHOH.
6. S-oxidation of sulphides to sulphoxides, as in the metabolic conversion of chlorpromazine into chlorpromazine sulphoxide.

(ii) *Microsomal reduction* requires reduced NADP-cytochrome c reductase or reduced NAD-cytochrome b_5 reductase. Chloramphenicol is reduced by NADH and a nitroreductase in the liver by this mechanism.

(iii) *Microsomal hydrolysis* Pethidine is de-esterified to meperidinic acid by hepatic membrane-bound esterase activity.

(b) Non-endoplasmic reticulum drug metabolism

(i) *Oxidation* of alcohol to acetaldehyde and chloral to trichlorethanol is catalysed by a cytosol enzyme whose substrates also include vitamin A and the aldehyde retinene. Diamine oxidase (DAO) and monoamine oxidase (MAO) are both membrane-bound mitochondrial enzymes which oxidatively deaminate primary amines to aldehydes (which can be further oxidised to carboxylic acids) or ketones. MAO occurs in liver, kidney, intestine and nervous tissue and its substrates include catecholamines (dopamine, noradrenaline, adrenaline), tyramine, phenylephrine and tryptophan derivatives (5-hydroxytryptamine and tryptamine). DAO has a substrate specificity overlapping that of MAO and is involved in histamine metabolism.

(ii) Non microsomal *reduction* reactions are involved in enzymic reduction of double bonds.

(iii) Soluble *esterases* catalyse hydrolytic reactions including the cleavage of suxamethonium to form inactive products, a mechanism with pharmacogenetic variation (see Chapter 4). Not all esters undergo hydrolysis in the body. Atropine, whilst hydrolysed extensively by some strains of rabbits, in which species this plasma esterase demonstrates pharmacogenetic variation, is hydrolysed to an insignificant extent by man.

(iv) *Purine oxidation by xanthine oxidase* is non-microsomal; 6-mercaptopurine is transformed to inactive 6-thiouric acid by this mechanism. Thus concurrent administration of allopurinol, a xanthine oxidase inhibitor, results in 6-mercaptopurine toxicity.

(c) **Metabolism of drugs by intestinal organisms** (see p. 54).

This is important for drugs undergoing enterohepatic circulation. Thus carbenoxolone, for example, which is excreted in the bile as a glucuronide conjugate, loses glucuronic acid by microbial activity and so the free drug is available for reabsorption via the terminal ileum.

PHASE II METABOLISM (CONJUGATION REACTIONS)

(a) *Glucuronidation* O-glucuronides are formed by linking glucuronic acid to a hydroxyl or carboxyl group in the drug molecule. N-glucuronides result from linking glucuronic acid to an amino group. When linking is to mercapto or dithiocarboxyl groups, S-glucuronides are formed. In all cases the C_1 hydroxyl of glucuronic acid is the group involved in the conjugation. The cytosol of liver cells contains enzymes which synthesise uridine diphosphate–glucuronic acid from glucose-1-phosphate and uridine triphosphate. This serves as the glucuronic acid donor in reactions mediated by microsomal transferase enzymes. Conjugations between glucuronic acid and carboxyl groups are involved for example in the metabolism of bilirubin, salicylate, nicotinic acid and probenecid. In patients with an inherited deficiency of glucuronide formation (which presents clinically as a non-haemolytic jaundice due to excess unconjugated bilirubin) as in the Crigler—Najjar syndrome, the administration of drugs which are normally conjugated in this way may aggravate the jaundice.

The formation of O-glucuronides by reaction with a hydroxyl group of the drug results in the formation of an ether glucuronide. It occurs with trichloroethanol, morphine, paracetamol, phenacetin and chloramphenicol. The ether glucuronides are stable in alkaline urine, whereas ester glucuronides are unstable and thus if the classical cupric ion reduction test (e.g. Benedict's solution, Clinitest) is used, the ester glucuronide will give a positive test for sugar in the urine.

(b) *The amino acids chiefly involved in conjugation reactions in man are glycine and glutamine.* The use of these amino acids is not general throughout the animal kingdom but apes and monkeys share these pathways with man. Thus studies of drug metabolism or kinetics in lower animals may be invalid if this pathway is important for the drug under consideration. Glycine forms conjugates with nicotinic acid, salicylate and benzoic acid whilst glutamine conjugates *p*-aminosalicylate. Hepatocellular damage may deplete the intracellular pool of these amino acids, thus restricting the use of this pathway which may also be reduced in the newborn.

(c) *Acetate can also act as a conjugating agent.* The active donor is acetyl coenzyme-A which reacts with an amino group on the drug to form an acetyl amide. Drugs which are acetylated include isoniazid, hydralazine, procainamide, sulphonamides (see Chapter 4 regarding pharmacogenetic variation in this pathway), histamine and *p*-aminosalicylate. Acetylating activity resides in the cytosol and is widely distributed, occurring in leucocytes and gastrointestinal cells as well as the liver. In the liver it is the reticuloendothelial cells rather than parenchymal cells which perform acetylation.

(d) *Methylation* proceeds by a pathway involving S-adenosyl methionine as methyl donor to drugs with free amino, hydroxyl or thiol groups. Catechol O-methyltransferase, a cytosol enzyme, is an example of such a methylating enzyme. It catalyses the transfer of a methyl group to a phenolic hydroxyl of catecholamines and is involved in the physiological inactivation of neurotransmitter. Other enzymes methylate histamine, mercaptoethanol and thiouracil. An important methylation is that controlled by phenylethanolamine N-methyltransferase which methylates the terminal-NH_2 of noradrenaline to form adrenaline but which also acts upon phenylethanolamine, phenylephrine, norephedrine and octopamine.

(e) *Sulphation of a hydroxyl (alcoholic or phenolic) or amine group*, via an active sulphate compound, 3′-phosphoadenosine 5′-phosphosulphate (PAPS) can occur in the cytosol. The system is normally concerned in formation of sulphates such as heparin and chondroitin sulphate but sulphatransferases can also produce ethereal sulphates from dihydroandrosterone, oestrone, 3-hydroxycoumarin, 3-hydroxysteroids, hydroxyacetanilide and chloramphenicol. There are a number of transferases in liver, each specific for different receptor molecules. Ethanol is conjugated with sulphate by a minor pathway, the route being more important for some other alcohols. The sulphate pool is easily exhausted so that glucuronide formation predominates over sulphate conjugation (see Fig. 1.21).

(f) *Mercapturic acid formation* via reaction with cysteine in glutathione is a relatively unusual pathway: naphthalene and some sulphonamides form these conjugates.

ENZYME INDUCTION

Enzyme induction is a process in which there is an enhancement of enzymic activity because of an increase in the synthesis or decrease in the destruction of the enzyme. This increased enzyme activity may be accompanied by hypertrophy of the endoplasmic reticulum as the anatomical counterpart of increased activity. There is a rise in cytochrome P_{450} content and increased cytochrome P_{450} reductase activity. The size of the liver itself increases and in association with this liver blood flow increases. Thus in one study the blood flow increased from a mean of 565 to 825 ml/min after two weeks treatment with 1 g of antipyrine orally per day. The effect of enzyme inducers may therefore not only be solely on enzyme activity but also on the rate of presentation of drug to the functioning liver mass which may be important for drugs exhibiting flow-dependent metabolism (see p. 92).

Other tissues apart from the liver may demonstrate enzyme induction. Thus fibroblasts in culture develop increased proteolytic and collagenolytic activity when exposed to a number of anti-inflammatory drugs and aryl hydrocarbon hydroxylase induction may be demonstrated in lymphocytes and fibroblasts.

In a wider biological sense enzyme induction is a model of variable expression of a constant genetic constitution. Medical aspects of this process mainly are involved in variations in the rate of drug metabolism; however, other aspects may also be important:

Adaptation to extrauterine life

This is in part a series of biochemical changes. Delay in such events may be hazardous to the infant. Many of the mediators are hormones, such as glucocorticoids, thyroxine and glucagon. Immature neonates may be unable to form glucuronide conjugates because of immaturity of hepatic glucuronyl transferase. Not only will chloramphenicol conjugation (and hence excretion) be impaired, but bilirubin will not be conjugated. The administration of glucocorticoids or phenobarbitone to the mother before delivery may induce the early appearance of glucuronyl transferase.

Another important consequence of immature enzyme systems in prematurely born infants is a low level of synthesis of lung surfactant (surface-active lecithin). The appearance of this substance is necessary for expansion of the lungs. The early secretion of surfactant can be stimulated by the administration of glucocorticoids to the mother.

Enzyme synthesis in adult life

This is constantly varying due to changes in hormone secretion. Despite such fine physiological control, this opportunity for therapeutic manipulation has not yet been exploited to any significant extent. The jaundice due to an inherited deficiency of glucuronyl transferase (Gilbert's disease) can be improved by the administration of inducing agents such as barbiturates or antipyrine. Similarly phenytoin has been tried to stimulate steroid metabolism in Cushing's disease and glycogen breakdown in glycogenoses. Patients with galactosaemia treated with progesterone show enhanced galactose metabolism and in glycogen storage disease the activity of hepatic glucose-6-phosphate can be stimulated with steroids. The therapeutic benefit of such induction therapy in these severely disabling metabolic diseases has yet to be demonstrated.

Induction by exogenous substances

There is no apparent relationship between the chemical structure or pharmacological actions of substances which act as inducing agents. As with any drug some degree of lipid solubility at physiological pH is necessary for absorption and tissue penetration, but for barbiturates at least there is a poor correlation between inducing ability and lipid solubility. There exists a good deal of interindividual variability between the degree of induction produced by a given agent. Part of this may be inherited. Often the greatest change in $t_{1/2}$ of a marker substance is seen in those individuals with an initially long $t_{1/2}$. There is no correlation between the rate of elimination of an inducing agent and the degree of induction produced.

Studies of induction indicate selectivity, e.g. the degree of induction of phenacetin oxidation relative to that of antipyrine is far greater with hydrocarbons than with rifampicin. In addition, rifampicin and pentobarbitone selectively increase the N-demethylation of antipyrine relative to its 4-hydroxylation and 3-methylhydroxylation. This and other evidence suggests multiple forms of cytochrome P_{450} proteins. Studies in animals have shown at least six distinct classes of mono-oxygenase inducers. Although representatives of most of these classes have been administered to man there is little information available on specificity of induction although some, e.g. barbiturates, induce many pathways whilst others such as polycyclic hydrocarbons (e.g. 3,4-benzo(a) pyrine) have more limited inducing properties. At least eight varieties of cytochrome P_{450} have been isolated from rodent liver and following induction a single form may increase from less than 10% of the total to almost 80%. Analogous information for man has not yet been obtained although by analogy with immunoglobulins the possibility exists that any individual mammal may have the capacity to produce hundreds or even thousands of unique P_{450} proteins.

Exogenous inducing agents include not only drugs but also halogenated insecticides (particularly DDT and gamma benzene hexachloride), herbicides, polycyclic aromatic hydrocarbons, dyes, food preservatives, nicotine and alcohol. A practical consequence of enzyme induction is that if two or more drugs are given simultaneously, then one substance which is an inducing agent can accelerate the rate of metabolism of other drugs (Table 3.1). In addition to drugs, substrates can include pollutants, carcinogens and normal body constituents (e.g. steroids, bilirubin, thyroxine and fat-soluble vitamins).

Table 3.1 lists some known drug interactions due to enzyme induction. Clinically important interactions include:

(a) Decreased efficacy of oral anticoagulants.
(b) Osteomalacia following anti-epileptics or prolonged barbiturate hypnotic treatment.
(c) Increased requirements of analgesics and benzodiazepines in smokers.
(d) Decreased efficacy of oral contraceptive pill.
(e) Decreased efficacy of antiepileptic drugs.
(f) Failure of doxycycline treatment due to depression of plasma levels out of bacteriostatic range.
(g) Decreased digitoxin levels.
(h) Decreased tricyclic antidepressant levels.

Table 3.1 Effects of enzyme-inducing substances on metabolism of endogenous and exogenous chemicals

Enzyme inducing agent	*Substances whose metabolism is enhanced*
Barbiturates	Barbiturates, coumarins, phenytoin, digitoxin, chlorpromazine, phenylbutazone, cortisol, testosterone, bilirubin, vitamin D_3, tricyclic antidepressants, contraceptive pill
Glutethimide	Glutethimide, warfarin, vitamin D_3
Meprobamate	Meprobamate
Phenylbutazone	Digitoxin, cortisol, aminopyrine
Phenytoin	Digitoxin, dexamethasone, cortisol, thyroxine, DDT, tricyclic antidepressants, contraceptive pill, vitamin D_3
Ethanol	Ethanol, warfarin, phenytoin, barbiturates, meprobamate, tolbutamide, bilirubin
Cigarette smoking	Benzpyrine, nicotine, phenacetin, propoxyphene, pentazocine
DDT, gamma benzene hexachloride (Lindane)	Cortisol, phenylbutazone, bilirubin, phenazone
Phenothiazines	Phenothiazines
Aldrin, Dieldrin, Endrin	Widespread acceleration of drug metabolism
Phenazone	Bilirubin, warfarin, cortisol
Griseofulvin	Warfarin
Rifampicin	Steroids including contraceptive steroids

Although Table 3.1 shows the effects on the metabolism of exogenous and endogenous chemicals due to administration of enzyme inducing agents, in practice some of these interactions are complicated by other pharmacokinetic factors. Thus chronic administration of alcohol may reduce the effects of barbiturates by accelerating their destruction. However, a single large dose of ethyl alcohol enhances barbiturate effects due to inhibition of hepatic metabolism of these drugs. Further chronic administration of sedatives may reduce the responsiveness of the brain to cerebral depressants, whilst the simultaneous administration of alcohol and a hypnotic result in profound additive effects on the brain. Tolerance to narcotic action appears to be mainly a central effect and enzyme induction is not a significant feature.

Induction of aryl hydrocarbon hydroxylase (AHH) AHH is a membrane-bound multicomponent hydroxylase which uses NADH, NADPH, and oxygen involved in the metabolism of a number of polycyclic hydrocarbons. Phenols and other hydroxy derivatives are formed. Some polycyclic hydrocarbons are carcinogenic and the action of AHH may include their conversion to products which are weakly or non-carcinogenic. However, some foreign compounds may be converted by AHH into carcinogenic or other toxic substances. AHH is highly inducible by benzo(a) anthracene and there is evidence from animal studies that inducibility of the enzyme may be under genetic control. This may be of relevance to cancer in man. Cigarette smoke contains benzo(a) pyrene which induces AHH in lung macrophages. About one half of the population have lung macrophages with low induction potential for their AHH. One study has suggested that only 4% of patients with bronchial carcinoma have this macrophage type. This could be interpreted as a genetic predisposition to bronchial cancer which is characterised as lung macrophages whose AHH is highly inducible by benzo(a) pyrene, and which in this stimulated state can more readily convert procarcinogens in the cigarette smoke into active carcinogens within the lung. Other studies have failed to confirm this work: the disagreement may be due to a variety of technical subtleties related to isolation and culture of the cells, and further clarification is awaited.

Induction and drug toxicity Another example of metabolism increasing the toxicity of exogenous compounds is the conversion by the liver of unstable toxic epoxides from chemically stable halogenated hydrocarbons. Thus phenobarbitone can enhance the toxicity of halothane by increasing the formation of epoxides which react covalently with nucleophilic groups in proteins and nucleic acids. A similar mechanism involving formation of intermediate toxic metabolites which are increased by inducing agents underlies the hepatotoxicity of paracetamol (see p. 868).

Tests for induction The level of induction of liver enzymes can be assessed by administering a single test dose of antipyrine and plotting plasma levels in order to determine the $t_{1/2}$ which is reduced as hepatic enzymes are induced. An alternative method is measurement of the urinary excretion of compounds which are normally formed by hepatic microsomal activity. Urinary d-glucaric acid excretion has been proposed, but since it is formed by enzymes distinct from those concerned with drug metabolism it is used mainly as a screening test for populations. Plasma levels of γ-glutamyl transpeptidase and the urinary concentration of 6-β-hydroxycortisol have also been used but suffer from the same drawbacks. The use of marker drugs such as phenylbutazone and amylobarbitone has also been explored, but no one test is entirely satisfactory or completely predictive of the handling of other drugs by an individual. It is unlikely that a single test will ever be reliable, since the mixed function oxidase system is extremely complex and at any given time the activity of some enzymes may be increased and others minimal.

ENZYME INHIBITION

Inhibition of drug metabolism by a concurrently administered drug can lead to drug accumulation and toxicity. This effect is relatively unusual compared to the commoner enzyme induction phenomenon. A number of drugs such as monoamine oxidase inhibitors, allopurinol, methotrexate rely upon enzyme inhibition to exert their therapeutic effect. Drugs interacting at an enzyme site may do so competitively or non-competitively.

The specificity of enzyme inhibition is sometimes incomplete, e.g. disulfiram, which inhibits acetaldehyde oxidation following administration of ethanol, also prolongs antipyrine half-life and raises the steady-state plasma levels of warfarin and phenytoin. The mechanism of these last two interactions is unknown but presumably results from inhibition of microsomal metabolism. Diazepam and phenytoin both undergo hydroxylation and occasionally interact causing phenytoin intoxication, presumably due to a competitive action at the microsomes. Dicoumarol and phenytoin also act competitively with elevation of plasma steady-state levels of both drugs. Chloramphenicol on the other hand is a non-competitive inhibitor of microsomal enzymes in animals and inhibits phenytoin, tolbutamide and chlorpropamide metabolism without elevation of chloramphenicol levels. Conventional oral-contraceptive therapy also inhibits metabolism of other compounds: that of antipyrine is reduced by 21% despite an increased liver size. They are perhaps the most commonly administered enzyme inhibitors and prolongation of the $t_{1/2}$ of compounds as different as caffeine, chlordiazepoxide, pethidine and phenylbutazone has been reported. This is probably due to the oestrogen component which *in vitro* competitively inhibits metabolism of barbiturates, benzpyrine and some other compounds. Whether these effects are of clinical importance has yet to be determined.

Many of the adverse drug interactions occurring with MAOIs (see p. 237) and cimetidine (see p. 523) result from inhibition of drug metabolism by these agents.

FURTHER FACTORS INFLUENCING DRUG METABOLISM

1. Species differences. Even within mammals there are wide differences in drug metabolism by different species although the basis of this is not clear. Rates of metabolism may differ although the amounts of hepatic cytochrome P_{450} and NADPH-cytochrome reductase are relatively constant in various mammalian species. Different mammals may also have entirely different pathways for dealing with the same drug. These differences make the interpretation of pharmacological effects in animals and their extrapolation to man very difficult. Thus the $t_{1/2}$ of phenylbutazone in the rabbit is 3 h, in the rat, dog, and guinea pig 6 h, yet in man the $t_{1/2}$ is 3 days. Similarly for hexobarbitone the $t_{1/2}$ varies from 19 min (mice), through 60 min (rabbits), 260 min (dogs) to 360 min (man). It is problematical how many compounds have been discarded on the basis of an unsatisfactory pharmacological profile in animals, but would have been very suitable for human use. There exist racial differences in human drug metabolism (see Chapter 4) but this aspect has not been investigated extensively.

2. Temporal variations. Circadian rhythms in drug effectiveness and toxicity have been well established for animals. Thus the lethal dose to kill 50% of a group of mice (LD50) has been found to show diurnal rhythmicity for drugs such as acetylcholine, nikethimide, metyrapone and aurothioglucose. These effects can clearly be of clinical importance.

The effectiveness of an anabolic steroid, oxymetholone, in preventing skeletal demineralisation in immobilised paraplegics demonstrates circadian fluctuations in efficacy. Calcium loss occurs mainly during a few hours in the middle of the day and administration of oxymetholone at 6 a.m. reduces this urinary calcium loss although a similar dose at other times of the day is not significantly effective. The cause of this diurnal variation in efficacy has not been determined. Temporal variations in microsomal enzyme activity also occur in animals. In man the $t_{1/2}$ of antipyrine has been shown to alter diurnally, in some cases the changes being almost two-fold. There does not appear to be a consistent time of day between individuals at which this process is maximal. The hepatic cytosol enzyme alcohol dehydrogenase also shows diurnal swings in activity which coincide with diurnal variations in ethanol elimination in rats. A similar chronopharmacokinetic pattern for ethanol with the fastest elimination in the early morning has been demonstrated in man. Circadian changes in plasma proteins may also affect drug elimination. Healthy young adults have a large-amplitude (20%) swing in plasma proteins with a peak at 16.00 h and a trough at 04.00 h. It has been shown for example that transcortin, which carries corticosteroids in the plasma, shows a similar diurnal variation and this may underline the shorter $t_{1/2}$ of hydrocortisone when it is administered at 16.00 h as compared to 08.00 h.

Diurnal changes in drug disposition have now been demonstrated for many drugs, e.g. indomethacin, theophylline, propranolol, erythromycin but in most cases the underlying mechanism is unknown although rhythmic changes in drug absorption or more likely metabolism or excretion must be responsible.

3. Nutritional status. The nutritional status of the individual may affect drug metabolism. Malnutrition may lead to changes in the activity of mixed function oxidases in animals and frank malnutrition among adult Indians has been reported to shorten antipyrine half-life, possibly the stress of malnutrition results in enzyme induction. On the other hand, patients with severe protein-calorie nutrition and nutritional oedema may show a prolonged half-life, possibly reflecting a decreased hepatic capacity for drug metabolism. Although starvation in animals may alter drug elimination, a study of the disposition of antipyrine and tolbutamide (microsomal metabolism), sulphisoxazole and isoniazid (acetylation) and procaine (pseudocholinesterase) were found to be unchanged by fasting in obese subjects. Extrapolation from species to species concerning the effects of fasting on drug metabolism may therefore lead to erroneous conclusions.

The nature of the diet is important in animals and this may apply in man too. Asian vegetarians living in London have significantly longer antipyrine half-lives than Caucasian non-vegetarians. Changing normal volunteers' diets to a low-carbohydrate–high-protein mixture substantially reduces antipyrine and tolbutamide half-lives and reversion to the original high-carbohydrate diet reverses this trend. Feeding charcoal-broiled beef to volunteers has been shown to reduce phenacetin half-life, an effect attributed not to the increased protein intake but to the polycyclic hydrocarbons in the beef after charcoal cooking which produce hepatic enzyme induction. This demonstrates the complex interaction between both composition and nature of diet and effects on drug handling. At present the implications of these studies are not clear but patients who are malnourished, debilitated or receiving prolonged intravenous feeding may have an altered capacity to metabolise drugs.

4. Sex. Despite differences in body composition, e.g. the differing relative proportions of fat and muscle which could influence volume of distribution and drug clearance and the changes in hormone, water and electrolyte balance occurring during the menstrual cycle, sex has only a minor or no influence on the metabolism of most of the drugs studied, e.g. cimetidine, propranolol, metoprolol. Whilst the half life of diazepam, demethyldiazepam, chlordiazepoxide, oxazepam and temazepam is longer in women there is no difference for nitrazepam or lorazepam. The situation is more complicated than this however since the weight-normalised clearance of unbound drug in men was lower for diazepam and demethyldiazepam but higher for the other three benzodiazepines. The metabolic clearance of methaqualone varies during the menstrual cycle being highest at mid-cycle. Similar changes may occur in the case of paracetamol and antipyrine but for some other drugs, e.g. phenytoin, carbamazepine, salicylate, no effect of the menstrual cycle has been demonstrated.

Other factors influencing drug metabolism include:

age (Chapter 6);
disease states (Chapter 5);
genetic factors (Chapter 4).

THE FIRST-PASS EFFECT (PRE-SYSTEMIC ELIMINATION)

The metabolism of some drugs may be markedly dependent upon the route of administration. Orally administered drugs gain access to the systemic circulation almost exclusively via the hepatic portal system which first presents the drug to the liver. Thus the entire absorbed dose of drug is exposed to the liver during the first pass through the body. A considerably smaller fraction of the absorbed dose goes through the liver in subsequent passes because of distribution to other tissues and elimination of drug by other routes. If a drug is subject to a high hepatic clearance (i.e. it is rapidly metabolised by the liver) a substantial fraction of the drug may be extracted from the portal blood and metabolised before it reaches the systemic circulation. This is known as the first-pass effect and may contribute to a significant reduction in bioavailability. For example, despite complete absorption only 30–80% of an orally administered dose of imipramine enters the systemic circulation intact.

The route of administration and consequent first-pass effect may also influence the pattern of drug metabolism. Thus when salbutamol is given to asthmatic subjects the ratio of unchanged drug to metabolite excreted in the urine is 2 : 1 after intravenous administration but 1 : 2 after an oral dose. Again, when lignocaine is given orally the levels of the major primary metabolite monoethyl glycine xylidide (MEGX) are comparable to those of lignocaine itself, whereas after a single intravenous dose, MEGX levels are about 15–20% of those of lignocaine. The metabolic fate of a drug can also change according to route of administration. Thus when propranolol is given orally, pharmacologically active quantities of 4-hydroxypropranolol are formed although this metabolite is produced in very small amounts after intravenous administration. This may be because the high concentration of propranolol passing through the liver saturates the usual metabolic pathway to naphthoxylacetic acid and some drug is therefore metabolised by a lower affinity alternative pathway to 4-hydroxypropranolol. Propranolol undergoes a large hepatic first-pass effect and small doses given orally are completely metabolised before reaching the systematic circulation. After intravenous administration the area

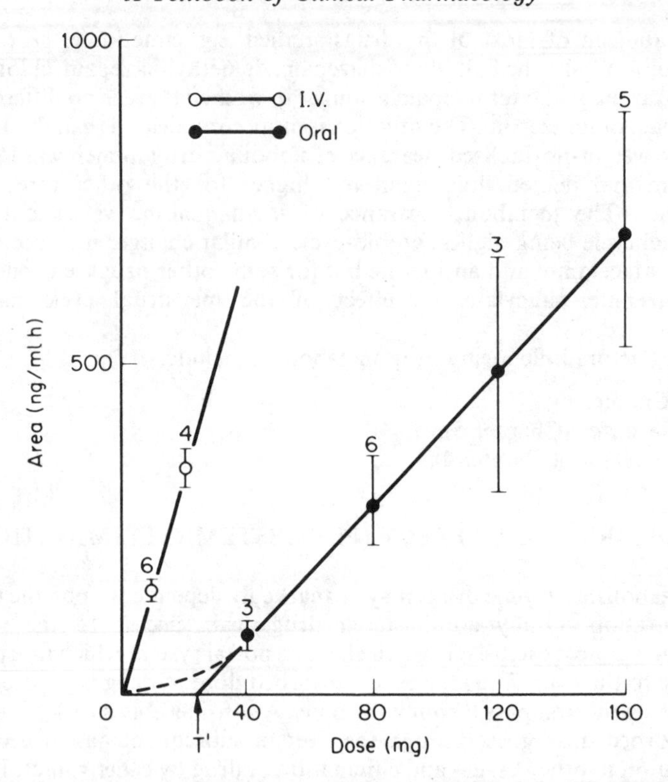

Fig. 3.5 Area under blood concentration–time curve after oral (●) and intravenous (O) administration of propranolol to man in various doses. T′ is the apparent threshold for propranolol following oral administration. (From D. G. Shand and R. E. Rangno, *Pharmacology*, 7, 159 (1972). Reproduced by permission of S. Karger AG, Basle.)

under the plasma concentration–time curve is proportional to the dose administered and passes through the origin (Fig. 3.5). After oral administration, although linear, the relationship does not pass through the origin and an apparent dose threshold is seen below which measurable levels of propranolol are not produced in the plasma. Administration of propranolol to a patient with a portocaval anastomosis which bypassed the liver showed that the drug was fully available and no threshold was observed.

The pharmacokinetic models of Chapter 1 assumed that the central compartment is directly accessible to administered drug regardless of route of administration. Clearly this assumption does not hold for drugs undergoing first-pass effects and an alternative scheme is required. The essential feature of such models (Fig. 3.6) is that elimination occurs, at least in part, from a compartment other than the central one and that drug may be given directly into this eliminating compartment, which in this case lies within the hepatic portal system.

Mathematical analysis of this model shows that, assuming complete absorption from the gut, and defining the systemic availability $\underline{F}$ as the ratio of

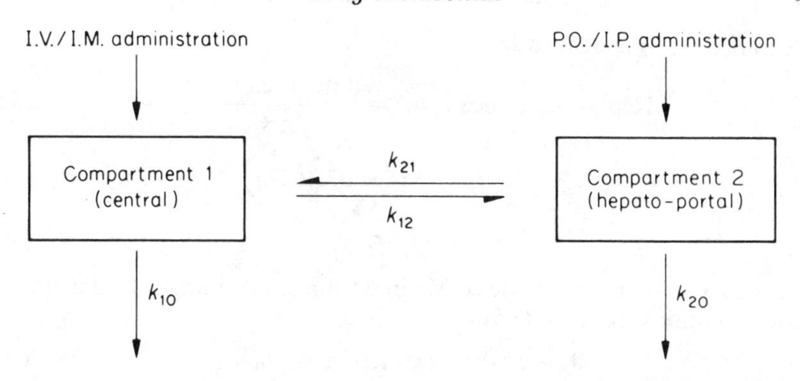

Fig. 3.6 First-pass pharmacokinetic model (k_{10} and k_{20} are rate constants characterising renal and hepatic drug elimination respectively).

areas under the plasma concentration–time curve, then:

$$\underline{F} = \frac{(\text{AUC})_{\text{oral}}}{(\text{AUC})_{\text{i.v.}}} = \frac{k_{21}}{k_{21} + k_{20}}. \tag{3.1}$$

Equation (3.1) shows that theoretically the area under the curve following oral administration will always be less than that observed after intravenous administration. Whether this is significant depends upon the magnitudes of k_{21} and k_{20} for a given drug. If $k_{21} \gg k_{20}$, then no first-pass effect is evident; if $k_{21} \ll k_{20}$, then virtually all of the administered dose will be metabolised by the liver before reaching the systemic circulation. If $k_{21} \simeq k_{20}$ then the first-pass effect may range from modest to substantial. Equation (3.1) cannot be solved since in practice the critical pharmcokinetic constants k_{20}, k_{21} and k_{12} cannot be experimentally ascertained in man.

When the liver is the only site of drug elimination

$$\begin{aligned} \underline{F} &= 1 - \text{hepatic extraction ratio} \\ &= 1 - \text{E} \end{aligned} \tag{3.2}$$

The hepatic extraction ratio is the fraction of drug entering the liver that is eliminated by the organ.

i.e.

$$E = \frac{C_a - C_v}{C_a} \tag{3.3}$$

where C_a is the mixed portal venous and hepatic arterial and C_v the hepatic venous blood drug concentrations. For example, propranolol has a hepatic extraction ratio of 0.8 and therefore its oral bioavailability is only 20%.

The rate of presentation of drug to the liver = $Q_L . C_a$ where Q_L is the combined hepatic blood flow via the portal vein (about 1050 ml/min in adults) and artery (300 ml/min). The rate at which the drug leaves the liver will be $Q_L . C_v$. Therefore:

$$\text{Rate of drug elimination} = Q_L(C_a - C_v) \tag{3.4}$$

Clearance (p. 8) is defined by

$$\text{Hepatic clearance } (Cl_H) = \frac{\text{Rate of elimination}}{C_a} \tag{3.5}$$

Thus

$$Cl_H = \frac{Q_L(C_a - C_v)}{C_a} \tag{3.6}$$

i.e.

$$Cl_H = Q_L . E \tag{3.7}$$

The extraction ratio may be considered from another angle. Under steady-state conditions from eq. (3.5).

$$\text{Rate of drug extraction} = Cl_H . C_a \tag{3.8}$$

which equals

$$\text{Rate of presentation of drug to liver} = Q_L . C_a \tag{3.6}$$

Consequently, by definition

$$E = \frac{Cl_H . C_a}{Q_L . C_a}$$

$$= \frac{Cl_H}{Q_L} \tag{3.7}$$

Thus subsitituting (3.7) in (3.2)

$$\underline{F} = 1 - \frac{Cl_H}{Q_L} \tag{3.8}$$

Thus hepatic clearance is a function of liver blood flow and the ability of the liver to extract the drug as it passes through the hepatic capillaries. This latter is a function of the overall activity of the hepatic drug-metabolising enzymes. A quantitative approach to the removal process is obtained by considering the total intrinsic clearance (Cl_{int}) of the liver to be the maximal ability of the liver to remove drug irreversibly by all pathways in the absence of all flow restrictions. Cl_{int} is a distinctive characteristic of a drug in a given situation; in terms of enzyme kinetics

$$Cl_{int} = \frac{V_{max}}{K_m} \tag{3.9}$$

where V_{max} is the maximum velocity of the reaction and K_m the Michaelis constant for the enzyme. Some progress has been made in the prediction of Cl_{int} values *in vivo* from *in vitro* studies of drug metabolism by liver slices.

As hepatic blood flow increases, actual drug clearance increases to a plateau value, the height of this plateau and the flow at which it is attained being dependent upon Cl_{int}. This process is described by eq. (3.10) and illustrated by Fig. 3.7

$$Cl_H = Q_L\left(\frac{Cl_{int}}{Q_L + Cl_{int}}\right) \tag{3.10}$$

Physiological restrictions on hepatic blood determine which part of the curve in Fig. 3.7 is operative for any given drug. When $Cl_{int} \gg Q_L$, then

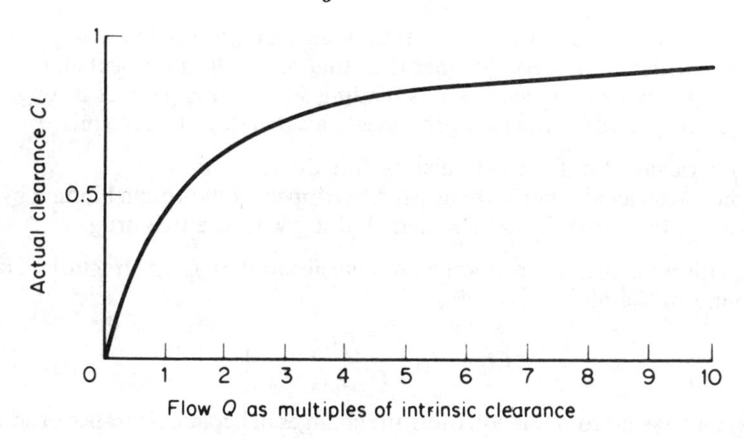

Fig. 3.7 Theoretical relationship between liver blood flow and actual drug clearance (From R. A. Branch *et al.*, *Drug Metab. Disp.*, **1**, 687 (1973).)

eq. (3.10) simplifies to

$$Cl_H = Q_L \tag{3.11}$$

and the plateau is not attained *in vivo*. Thus drug elimination varies with liver blood flow and is said to be *flow-dependent* and the drug is removed by the liver almost as rapidly as it is presented. Examples are lignocaine, propranolol, glyceryl trinitrate. Elimination falls if blood flow declines: propranolol for example diminishes its own clearance and that of lignocaine by reducing liver blood flow by decreasing cardiac output. Similarly the reduced hepatic perfusion following myocardial infarction reduces lignocaine metabolism (see p. 405). The lower the extraction ratio the less effect does blood flow exert on drug clearance. In such cases, e.g. theophylline, procainamide, warfarin $Q \gg Cl_{int}$ and drug clearance is more affected by the intrinsic activity of hepatic enzymes.

Enzyme-inducing agents increase the functional hepatic parenchymal mass by elevating the hepatic enzyme concentration, and increase hepatic blood flow. The increased clearance of propranolol after phenobarbitone treatment in monkeys has been apportioned as being 57 % due to increased hepatic blood flow and 43 % due to enhanced enzyme activity. Antipyrine, on the other hand, which has a low intrinsic hepatic clearance initially, shows a 300 % increase in intrinsic clearance after phenobarbitone but the additional effect due to increased hepatic blood flow is trivial. Thus the effects of any given degree of enzyme induction will be smaller the higher the initial intrinsic clearance of the drug in contrast to the effects of flow changes which will be higher the greater the initial intrinsic clearance.

It should be noted that eqs (3.3) to (3.11) are based upon drug concentrations in whole blood: plasma flow and plasma drug concentrations cannot be substituted unless the drug is confined to plasma, when a correction based upon haematocrit may be applied. Usually the blood to plasma concentration ratio must be known.

Many drugs are bound to plasma protein and circulate through the liver as bound and free drug. It is usually assumed that only free drug is available for hepatic extraction but this is not totally correct since if the avidity of the hepatic extraction process is higher than that of the drug for protein binding, then drug may be removed from its binding sites during passage through the liver. Two types of extraction processes may therefore be recognised:

(a) restricted—limited to circulating free drug;
(b) non-restricted—bound drug can be stripped from protein binding by the extraction process and eliminated along with the free drug.

Equation (3.10) may be modified to take account of f_B, the fraction of drug unbound in the blood

$$Cl_H = Q_L\left(\frac{f_B\,Cl_{int}}{Q_L + f_B\,Cl_{int}}\right). \tag{3.12}$$

As can be seen from this equation, the changes in hepatic clearance produced by alterations in protein binding are likely to be complex. Paradoxically there may be occasions when for drugs with non-restricted binding increased protein binding increases the hepatic clearance. Thus the $t_{1/2}$ of propranolol is reduced by higher protein binding which delivers more drug in unit time to the avid hepatic elimination mechanisms. Conversely drugs with restricted binding such as warfarin show a longer $t_{1/2}$ when protein binding is increased, since protein-bound drug is inaccessible for elimination.

The number of drugs in which first-pass hepatic metabolism is suspected is large; some of them are listed in Table 3.2,

Table 3.2 Drugs in which first-pass hepatic metabolism is significant

Propranolol	Lignocaine	Imipramine	Pethidine	Aspirin
Alprenolol	Aldosterone	Nortriptyline	Morphine	Propoxyphene
Reserpine	Verapamil	Hydralazine	Pentazocine	Cortisone
Oxyphenbutazone	Dopamine	Tryptophan	Organic Nitrates	Chlorpromazine

First-pass metabolism is not limited to the liver since the gastrointestinal mucosa may also metabolise drugs such as isoprenaline, dopamine, chlorpromazine before they enter the hepatic portal blood. Drugs administered by inhalation also may be exposed to a first-pass pulmonary metabolism. Thus inhaled isoprenaline must pass through bronchial mucosa containing high levels of catechol-O-methyltransferase before entering the pulmonary circulation. A greater proportion of inhaled isoprenaline appears in the urine as the methylated metabolite when it is inhaled as compared to when it is given intravenously. Nicotine from tobacco smoke also undergoes some pulmonary first-pass metabolism.

Clinical consequences of first-pass metabolism

Pronounced first-pass metabolism by either the gastrointestinal mucosa or flora, e.g. isoprenaline, levodopa, or liver, e.g. glyceryl trinitrate, naloxone, may preclude the use of these drugs by the oral route or require very high doses to be effective. Alternative routes of drug delivery such as rectal, buccal, sublingual, aerosol or transdermal may bypass the presystemic elimination processes and permit the attainment of effective plasma levels.

Drugs that undergo extensive first-pass metabolism exhibit pronounced interindividual variability in drug disposition. This can result in highly variable responses to therapy and is one of the major difficulties in their clinical use. This variability in first-pass metabolism results from:

(a) Genetic variation, e.g. the bioavailability of hydralazine is about doubled in slow acetylators as compared to fast acetylators (see p. 100). Similarly the first-pass elimination of debrisoquine, metoprolol and encainide has been shown to depend upon a genetic polymorphism (see p. 109).

(b) Enzyme induction and inhibition may profoundly affect bioavailability, e.g. although phenobarbitone did not alter the clearance of intravenously injected alprenolol the mean oral bioavailability fell from 28% to 7%.

(c) Food may increase liver blood flow and increase the availability of highly extracted drugs such as propranolol, metoprolol, hydralazine (see p. 52).

(d) Drugs which change liver blood flow may have similar effects, e.g. hydralazine may increase propranolol bioavailability by one third without altering its elimination half-life.

(e) Non-linear first-pass kinetics have been observed for several drugs, e.g. hydralazine, propranolol, 5-fluorouracil, so that increasing the dose produces a disproportionate increase in bioavailability. Other drugs show time-dependent non-linearity, i.e. their bioavailability increases when they are given repeatedly. This occurs for example with repeated oral doses of propranolol, verapamil, dextropropoxyphene but is not seen if multiple intravenous doses are given. This is most probably due to saturation of metabolism at the higher plasma drug concentrations achieved during multiple dosing than after a single dose.

(f) Liver disease may increase the bioavailability of some drugs suffering extensive first-pass extraction, e.g. chlormethiazole, labetalol, propranolol, pethidine (see p. 136).

CYCLING PROCESSES

Many drugs undergo cyclical processes involving secretion and reabsorption back into the blood. A drug involved in such a cycle persists in the body for longer and thus has a longer half-life than would otherwise occur. Some drugs show a remarkable persistence as a result of this. The formerly used radio-opaque medium iophenoxic acid persists in man with a plasma $t_{1/2}$ of $2\frac{1}{2}$ years and enterohepatic circulation probably contributes to the persistence of other compounds such as polychlorinated hydrocarbon pesticides, carcinogenic hydrocarbons and the antitrypanosomal agents ethidium and prothidium. The influence of the enterohepatic cycle may be demonstrated if the cycle can be interrupted, e.g. by giving an ion-exchange resin to bind the drug in the gut and so interrupt the enterohepatic cycle. It has also been suggested that cycling processes may result in increases in drug concentrations in the plasma in the post-absorptive phase ('secondary peaks'). This must be rare since the volumes of the secretions concerned are relatively small and the kinetics of absorption exert a smoothing effect on the entry of drug into the plasma. Thus a secondary increment in plasma levels due to absorption of a recycled bolus of drug is unlikely. The existence of recycling processes, which may in themselves obey saturation kinetics, limits, at least in theory, the applicability of the simple one- and two-compartment models thus far described.

Examples of cycling processes include:

(a) *Salivary secretion* of drugs occurs only occasionally by active secretion (e.g. lithium, iodide) and is most usually by a passive diffusion process. Lipid solubility and the degree of ionisation are thus important determinants of the saliva/plasma ratio. For an acidic compound

$$R_{S/P} = \frac{1 + 10^{(pH_s - pK_a)}}{1 + 10^{(pH_p - pK_a)}}, \tag{3.13}$$

where pH_s is salivary pH, pH_p is plasma pH and the pK_a is that of the compound in question. If, as is usual, the total drug concentration in plasma (bound and unbound) is measured, then this ratio is multiplied by f_b/f_s, where

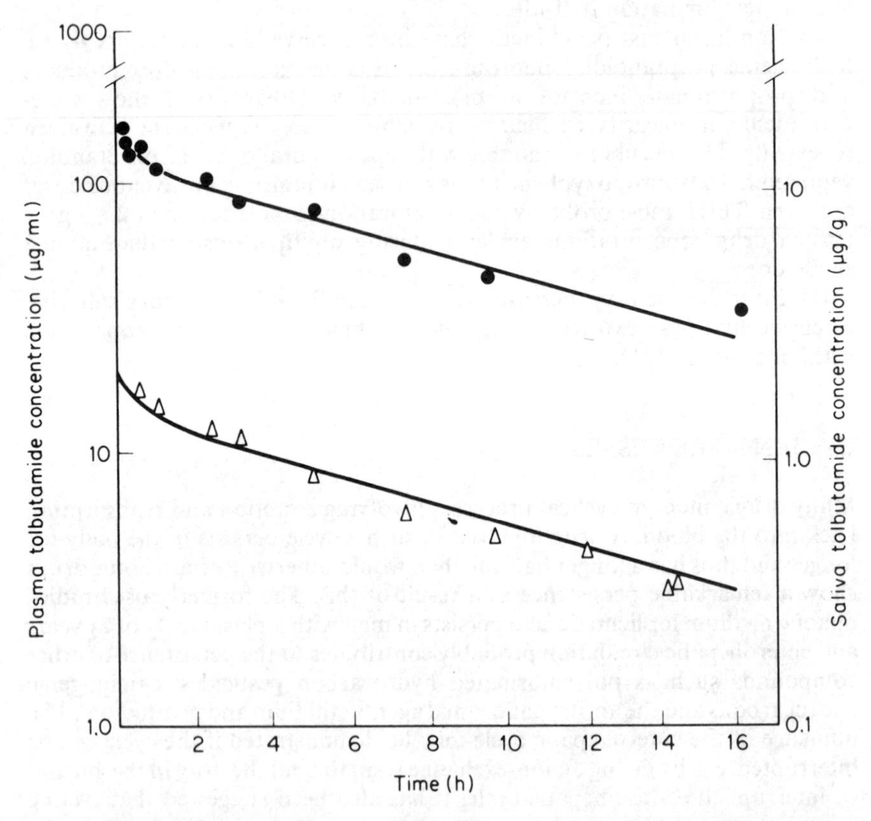

Fig. 3.8 Plasma (●) and salivary (△) concentrations of tolbutamide following 1 g given intravenously to a single subject. For tolbutamide $f_p = 0.093$. (From S. B. Matin *et al.*, *Clin. Pharm. Ther.*, **16**, 1052 (1974).)

f_b is the unbound fraction of drug in plasma and f_s is the unbound fraction in saliva.

For a basic compound this becomes

$$R_{S/P} = \frac{1 + 10^{-(pH_s - pK_a)}}{1 + 10^{-(pH_p - pK_a)}} \times \frac{f_b}{f_s}. \tag{3.14}$$

It has been shown for some drugs that their concentration in saliva equals the free drug in plasma (Fig. 3.8) and this may offer advantages for therapeutic monitoring of drug levels where the assay available for plasma levels measures both free and bound drug. If saliva is to be used for therapeutic monitoring or pharmacokinetic purposes it is important that $R_{S/P}$ is constant. This may not always be so, and time-dependent variations have been shown for some drugs such as procainamide and theophylline, suggesting that active or non-linear processes may be operating in these cases. Examples of drugs undergoing salivary secretion include caffeine, cyclophosphamide, amylobarbitone, clonidine, phenytoin, phenobarbitone, ethosuximide, carbamazepine, digoxin, sulphonamides, tolbutamide and amitriptyline.

(b) *Gastric secretion.* Basic drugs such as quinine and pethidine may undergo appreciable secretion into the stomach followed by reabsorption from the intestine. The pharmacological significance of this cycle has not been quantitated.

(c) *Enterohepatic cycling* in which the drug, following absorption, is excreted into the bile, absorbed from the intestine and returned via the portal system to the liver from where it is recycled once more through the bile (Fig. 3.9). Drug may be lost from the cycle either by excretion with the faeces or

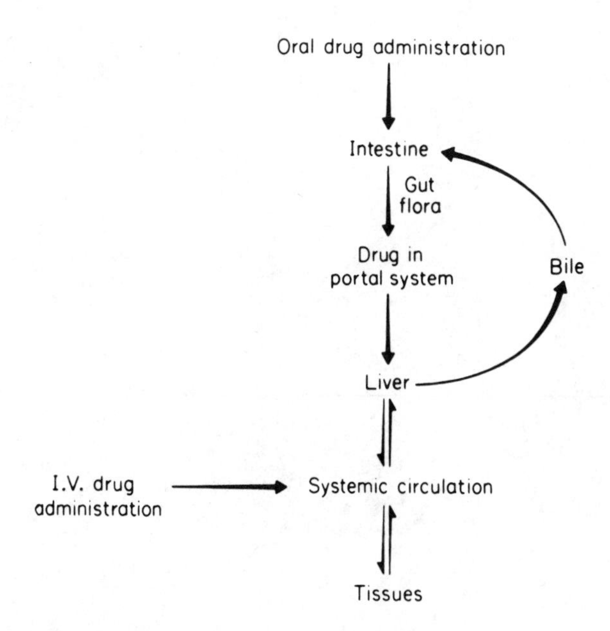

Fig. 3.9 Enterohepatic cycling of drug.

via renal elimination. The classical example of enterohepatic circulation is seen with the bile salts. In man it has been calculated that two circulations of the complete bile-salt pool occur with each meal. The cycle was probably evolved to conserve and reutilise the physiologically important bile acids. Other endogenous compounds undergoing enterohepatic cycling are oestrogens, progestogens, thyroxine and vitamin A. Drugs involved in this process include stilboestrol, phenytoin, rifampicin and digitoxin. Drug excretion in bile is commonly in the form of water-soluble drug metabolites such as glucuronides which are not reabsorbed as such from the intestine. Enterohepatic circulation involves hydrolysis of these conjugates by intestinal enzymes and microflora. Marked differences occur in enterohepatic circulation between species, rodents being particularly active in secreting compounds into the bile as compared to man. Thus whilst chloramphenicol and morphine undergo prolonged enterohepatic cycling in the rat they do not do so in man. This again stresses the difficulties of extrapolating from animal data to man.

Chapter 4
PHARMACOGENETICS

The individual response to drugs shows great variation. Administration of a drug in the same dose to a group of individuals may result in a range of effects varying in a continuous or discontinuous manner. Such differences may be due to environmental and genetic effects on drug absorption, distribution, metabolism, excretion and receptor sensitivity. The study of variations in drug responses under hereditary control is called pharmacogenetics. Pharmacogenetic variation may exist due to the actions of a single mutant gene (as in genetic polymorphism or discontinuous variation) or result from polygenic influences (Fig. 4.1).

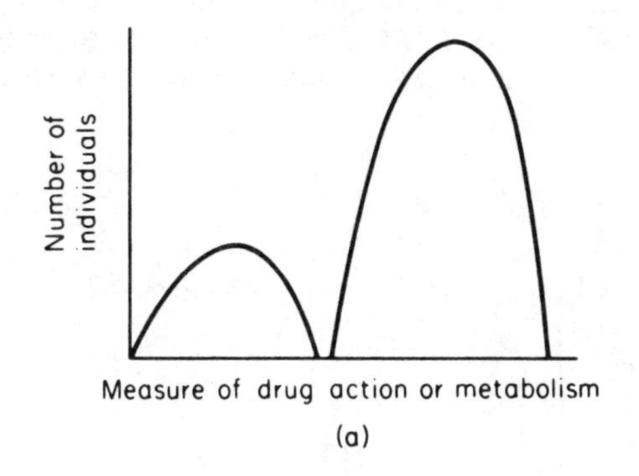

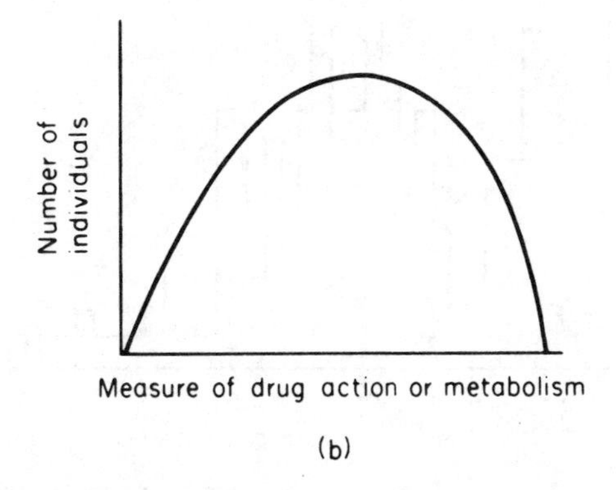

Fig. 4.1 Frequency distributions of (a) discontinuous and (b) continuous variation observed when a population of individuals are given a standard dose of drug.

GENETIC POLYMORPHISM

Genetic polymorphism is the type of variation in which individuals with sharply distinct characteristics co-exist as normal members of a population. Such differences may affect drug metabolism and drug responses. Tables 4.1 and 4.2 show examples of each type.

Acetylator Status

The administration of *isoniazid* (INH) to patients in identical doses per kg weight reveals great variation in blood levels attained. A distribution histogram of blood levels shows two distinct groups of individuals (Fig. 4.2). INH is metabolised in the liver by acetylation and the patients with lower INH blood levels acetylate the drug more rapidly because of larger amounts of hepatic enzyme compared with the slow acetylators who have higher INH levels.

Slow and rapid acetylator status are inherited in a simple Mendelian manner.

Heterozygotes as well as homozygotes are rapid acetylators because rapid metabolism is an autosomal dominant. Thus, if the rapid metabolism homozygote has a genotype E^aE^a, then E^ae^a the heterozygote is also a rapid metaboliser and e^ae^a, the recessive homozygote is a slow metaboliser. 55–

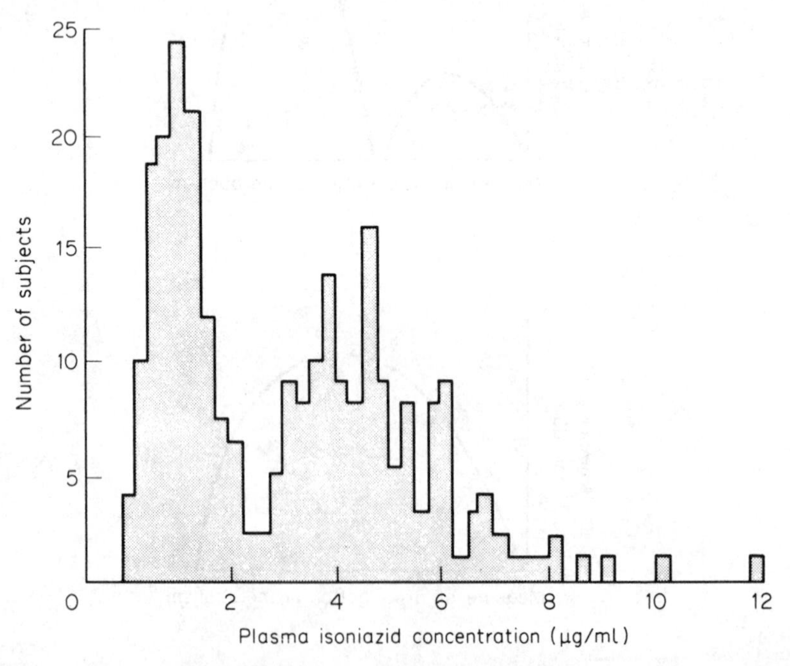

Fig. 4.2 Plasma isoniazid concentrations in 483 subjects 6 h after oral isoniazid (9.8 mg/kg). Acetylator polymorphism produces a bimodal distribution into fast and slow acetylators. (From D. A. P. Evans *et al.*, *Brit. Med. J.*, **2**, 485 (1960). Reproduced by permission of the Editor.)

Table 4.1 Variations in Drug Metabolism due to Genetic Polymorphism

Pharmacogenetic variation	*Mechanism*	*Inheritance*	*Occurrence*	*Drugs involved*
Acatalasia	Lack of RBC catalase	Autosomal recessive	Up to 1 % of some Japanese populations	Hydrogen peroxide
Rapid acetylator status	Increased hepatic N-acetyltransferase	Autosomal dominant	40 % whites	Isoniazid; Hydralazine; some Sulphonamides; Phenelzine; Dapsone Procainamide.
Suxamethonium sensitivity	Several types of abnormal plasma pseudocholinesterase	Autosomal recessive	Most common form 1 : 2500	Suxamethonium
Suxamethonium resistance	Increased amount of normal cholinesterase e.g. Cynthiana variant	Autosomal autonomous	? 1 : 1000	Suxamethonium
Phenacetin-induced methaemoglobinaemia	Deficiency of mixed function hepatic de-ethylating microsomal enzyme	Autosomal recessive	Rare	Phenacetin
Slow inactivation of tolbutamide	Decreased activity of microsomal oxidation to hydroxytolbutamide	Autosomal	Unknown	Tolbutamide
Defective alicyclic hydroxylation of debrisoquine	Functionally defective cytochrome P_{450} ? Two cytochromes involved	? Autosomal recessive	8 % Britons; 1 % Saudi Arabians; 30 % Chinese	Debrisoquine; Phenformin Guanoxan; Perhexiline; Phenacetin; Nortriptyline

Table 4.1 (*Continued*)

Pharmacogenetic variation	*Mechanism*	*Inheritance*	*Occurrence*	*Drugs involved*
Inherited failure of glucuronidation	Deficiency of UDP glucuronyl transferase	Different forms: e.g. Gilbert's autosomal dominant	Uncertain. Mild forms are common	Paracetamol, chloral tolbutamide
Defective metabolism of phenytoin	Abnormal cytochrome P_{450} mixed function oxidase	Autosomal dominant	Rare	Phenytoin ? related to defective debrisoquine metabolism
Defective metabolism of dicoumarol	Poor hydroxylation of dicoumarol due to abnormal cytochrome P_{450} mixed function oxidase	Unknown	Rare	Warfarin: bishydroxycoumarin
Ethanol sensitivity	Relatively low rate of alcohol metabolism	Usual in some ethnic groups	Eskimos and Orientals	Alcohol
Increased elimination of ethanol	Atypical enzyme on alcohol DH_2 locus	Autosomal autonomous	4–20% of Western Europeans	Alcohol
Deficient N-glucosidation of amylobarbitone	Unknown	Autosomal recessive	2% Canadian whites	Amylobarbitone

Table 4.2 Variations in Drug Response due to Genetic Polymorphism

Pharmacogenetic variation	*Mechanism*	*Inheritance*	*Occurrence*	*Drugs involved*
G6PD deficiency, favism, drug-induced haemolytic anaemia	80 distinct forms of G6PD	X-linked incomplete codominant	10 000 000 affected in the world	Many—including 8-aminoquinolines, antimicrobials and minor analgesics (see text)
Steroid-induced raised intraocular pressure	Unknown	Autosomal recessive (heterozygotes show some response)	5 % white population	Glucocorticosteroids
Warfarin resistance	Insensitive variant of vitamin K oxide reducing enzyme	Autosomal dominant	Rare	Warfarin
Haemoglobin Zurich: Sulphonamide-induced haemolysis	Arginine substituted for histidine at 63rd position of β chain of haemoglobin	Autosomal dominant	Rare	Sulphonamides
Haemoglobin H: drug-induced haemolysis	Haemoglobin composed of four β chains	Autosomal recessive	1 : 300 births in Bangkok	Same drugs as for G6PD deficiency
Methaemoglobinaemia: drug-induced haemolysis	Methaemoglobinaemia reductase deficiency	Autosomal recessive (heterozygotes show some response)	1 : 100 are heterozygotes	Same drugs as for G6PD deficiency

Table 4.2 (*Continued*)

Pharmacogenetic variation	*Mechanism*	*Inheritance*	*Occurrence*	*Drugs involved*
Malignant hyperthermia with muscular rigidity	Unknown	Autosomal dominant	1 : 20 000 of population	Some anaesthetics especially halothane. Suxamethonium
Inability to taste phenythiourea or phenylthiocarbamide	Unknown	Autosomal recessive	1 : 3 of whites	Drugs containing the N–C = S group such as thiouracils
Acute intermittent porphyria: exacerbation induced by drugs	Increased activity of ˆ-amino levulinic acid synthetase secondary to defective porphyrin synthesis	Autosomal dominant	Acute intermittent type 15 : 1 000 000 in Sweden; Porphyria cutanea tarda 1 : 100 in Afrikaaners	Barbiturates, chloral, chloroquine, ethanol, sulphonamides, phenytoin, griseofulvin.

60% of the European population are slow acetylators and 40–45% are rapid acetylators. The rapid acetylator phenotype is most common in Eskimos and Japanese (95%) and is lowest among some Mediterranean Jews (20%).

In the treatment of tuberculosis with INH, toxicity (in the form of peripheral neuropathy) occurs most commonly in slow acetylators, whilst slower response and relapse of the infection is more frequent in rapid acetylators, particularly when the drug is not given daily, but twice weekly. Experimental slow-release matrix preparations of INH have been produced to attain sustained blood concentrations similar to those produced by ordinary INH formulations in slow acetylators during intermittent chemotherapy. In addition, slow acetylators are more likely to show phenytoin toxicity when this drug is given with INH, probably because the accumulated INH inhibits hepatic microsomal hydroxylation of phenytoin resulting in increased blood levels of phenytoin.

Isoniazid hepatitis may be commoner among rapid acetylators and the greater liberation of acetylhydrazine, a hepatotoxic isoniazid metabolite, could be responsible. However, this metabolite is itself polymorphically acetylated and therefore would be more rapidly detoxicated to diacetylhydrazine in rapid acetylators. Further studies are required to define the exact risk to fast acetylators of taking isoniazid.

Acetylator status affects other drugs which are inactivated by acetylation. *Procainamide* is one such drug and about 40% of patients treated with this drug for six months develop antinuclear antibodies. Slow acetylators are more likely to develop such antibodies than rapid acetylators (Fig. 4.3), and more

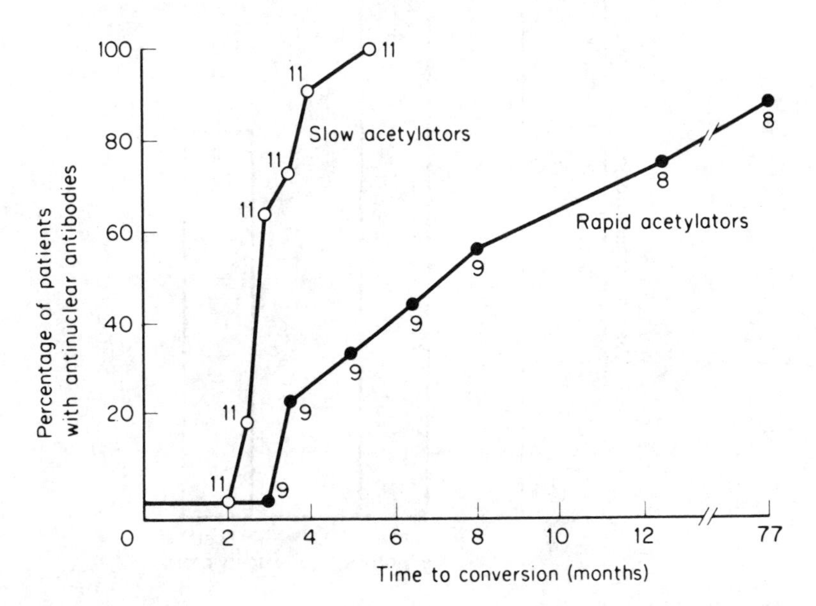

Fig. 4.3 Development of procainamide-induced antinuclear antibody in slow acetylators (open circles) and rapid acetylators (closed circles) with time. Number of patients shown at each point (From R. L. Woosley *et al.* Reprinted by permission from the *New Eng. J. Med.*, **298**, 1157 (1978).)

slow acetylators go on to develop procainamide-induced lupus erythematosus (see p. 410). There is also a correlation between acetylator status and procainamide plasma levels which are associated with clinical response. Slow acetylators develop higher plasma levels and show more rapid control of arrhythmias. Similarly, hypertension may be controlled by lower doses of *hydralazine* in slow acetylators (Fig. 4.4), and in these individuals higher doses (above 200 mg/day) are much more likely to lead to the production of antinuclear antibodies, and the disseminated lupus erythematosus and rheumatoid syndromes. Slow acetylators are also more likely to experience toxic effects from the monoamine oxidase inhibitor *phenelzine* but the antidepressant effect in these patients is significantly greater. *Sulphonamides* are metabolised by acetylation and acetylator status affects the hepatic metabolism of *some* of this group as well. Thus sulphamethazine and the sulphapyridine released by metabolism of sulphasalazine show polymorphic acetylation. With sulphasalazine, red-cell damage and mild haemolysis in patients receiving the drug for ulcerative colitis may be associated with

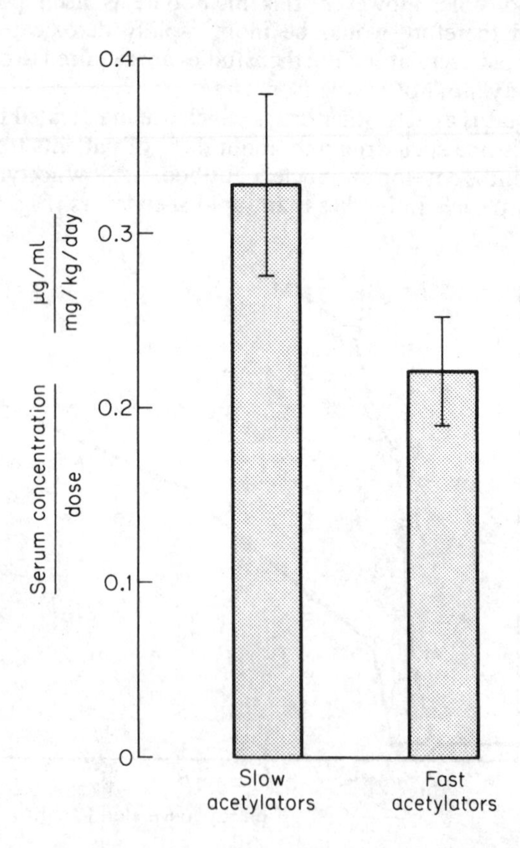

Fig. 4.4 Relationship between acetylator status and dose-normalised serum hydralazine concentration (i.e. serum level corrected for variable daily dose). Serum concentrations were measured 1–2 h after oral hydralazine doses of 25–100 mg in 24 slow and 11 fast acetylators. (From J. Koch-Weser, *Med. Clin. N. Amer.*, **58**, 1027 (1974).)

slow acetylator status. Sulphanilamide, para-aminobenzoic acid and para-aminosalicylic acid are also acetylated, but monomorphically, which suggests that more than one N-acetyltransferase may exist. Evidence for this is provided by *in vitro* studies showing that hepatic sulphamethazine N-acetyltransferase activity reflects the isoniazid acetylator phenotype whilst the enzyme in blood does not reflect acetylator status.

Dapsone, aminoglutethimide and metabolites of caffeine and clonazepam also show polymorphic acetylation although this does not have apparent clinical significance.

It has recently been observed that there is a significantly higher proportion of fast acetylators among diabetics with symptomatic peripheral neuropathy as compared with diabetics without neuropathy or in the normal population. The reasons for this are not understood but possibly this inherited metabolic trait in some way modifies the manifestations of the diabetic diathesis.

Acetylation may also detoxicate carcinogens: the incidence of bladder cancer in men exposed to arylamines whilst employed in the dyestuffs industry is higher in slow acetylators although there is no clear association with sporadic bladder cancer.

Suxamethonium sensitivity

The usual response to a single intravenous dose of suxamethonium is muscular paralysis for about 6 min. This shortness of effect is because suxamethonium is rapidly hydrolysed by plasma pseudocholinesterase. Occasional individuals show a much more prolonged response and may remain paralysed and require artificial ventilation for two or more hours. This results from the presence of an aberrant form of plasma cholinesterase. The usual genotype is designated $E_1^u E_1^u$ and is present in 94% of the population. The commonest variant which causes suxamethonium sensitivity is $E_1^a E_1^a$ and occurs at a frequency of 1 in 2500. Heterozygotes $E_1^u E_1^a$ are unaffected carriers and comprise about 4% of the population.

$E_1^u E_1^u$ individuals may show increased sensitivity to suxamethonium, particularly in the presence of liver disease, malnutrition, body cooling and the effects of drugs (including general anaesthetics).

Measurement of pseudocholinesterase activity in groups containing suxamethonium-sensitive individuals and their unaffected relatives may not show two distinct populations with low and with normal enzyme levels, but an almost continuous variation. However, if butyrylcholine is used as the substrate and the effect of adding dibucaine is observed, three distinct phenotypes are discovered, corresponding to $E_1^u E_1^u$, $E_1^u E_1^a$ and $E_1^a E_1^a$. Under arbitrarily standardised conditions, using benzoylcholine as a substrate, 10^{-5} M dibucaine inhibits normal plasma pseudocholinesterase by 80% but atypical cholinesterase is less affected. The percentage inhibition which dibucaine produces under these conditions is known as the dibucaine number (see Fig. 4.5). Fluoride also reveals a polymorphism in pseudocholinesterase activity but the individuals revealed are not those diagnosed by dibucaine resistance. In this way another enzyme variant was discovered. Heterozygotes ($E_1^a E_1^f$) show a milder degree of suxamethonium sensitivity compared with $E_1^a E_1^a$ patients. A silent gene has been found on the E_1 locus and is the $E_1{}^s$

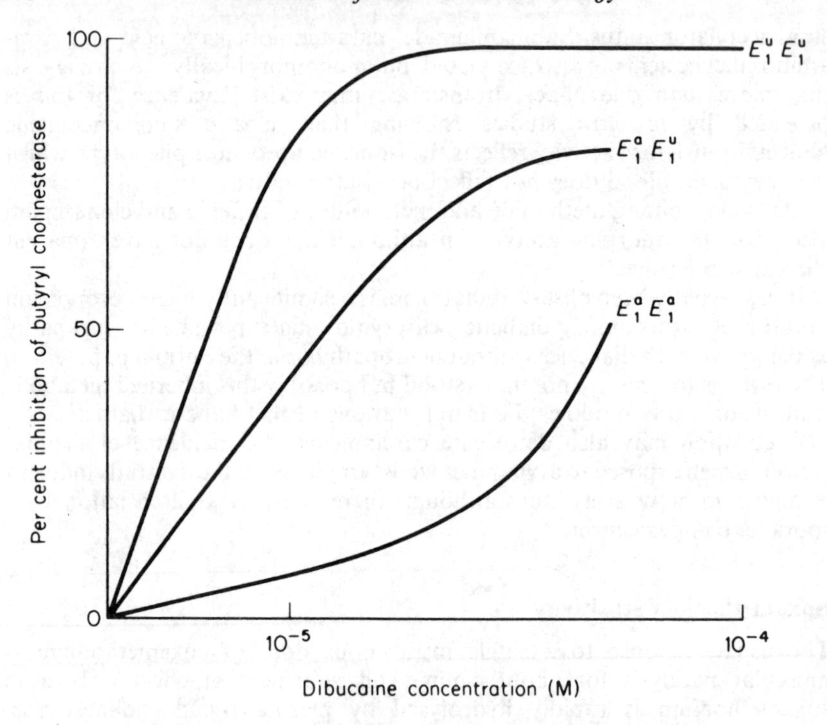

Fig. 4.5 Effects of dibucaine on hydrolysis of a choline ester *in vitro* by different cholinesterase variants.

allele. This variant has a high incidence in Eskimos. In one form (type 1) there is a total lack of functioning enzyme. In type 2 there is about 2% of the usual enzyme concentration. Table 4.3 is a summary of some of the genotypes which have been described.

A high activity cholinesterase, designated E_{cyn}, produces suxamethonium resistance.

Methaemoglobinaemia may arise because of an inherited failure to convert phenacetin to paracetamol. Thus relatively large amounts of the drug are available to enter other metabolic pathways and form hydroxyphenacetin and hydroxyphenetidin. These are potent methaemoglobin-forming agents. By this mechanism, ingestion of phenacetin over a prolonged period can produce methaemoglobinaemia in such patients.

There are several other compounds which oxidise haemoglobin to methaemoglobin. These include nitrates, nitrites, chlorates, sulphonamides, sulphones, nitrobenzenes, nitrotoluenes and anilines. In certain haemoglobin variants (e.g. HbM; HbH) the oxidised (methaemoglobin) form is not readily converted back into reduced, functioning haemoglobin and thus exposure to the above substances can lead to methaemoglobinaemia cyanosis. In a similar way administration of nitrites, chlorates, dapsone and primaquine can cause cyanosis in patients with a deficiency of NADH-methaemoglobin reductase.

Table 4.3 Some genotypes of cholinesterase

Genotype	*Phenotype*	*Prevalence*	*Response to suxamethonium*
$E_1^u E_1^u$	Usual type of esterase	94%	Normal
$E_1^a E_1^a$	Atypical esterase. Dibucaine resistant	1:2500	Grossly prolonged
$E_1^f E_1^f$	Atypical esterase. Fluoride resistant	1:300 000	Prolonged
$E_1^s E_1^s$	Silent. Little or no esterase activity	1:140 000	Grossly prolonged
$E_1^u E_1^a$	Heterozygote pattern	1:25	Normal or almost normal
$E_1^u E_1^f$	Heterozygote pattern	1:280	Normal or almost normal
$E_1^a E_1^f$	Heterozygote pattern	1:29 000	Prolonged
$E_1^u E_1^s$	Heterozygote pattern	1:200	Normal or almost normal
$E_1^a E_1^s$	Heterozygote pattern	1:20 000	Grossly prolonged
$E_{cynthiana}$	2–3 × normal esterase	1:10 in UK	Resistance

Defective alicyclic hydroxylation of debrisoquine 4-Hydroxylation of the antihypertensive drug debrisoquine is deficient in about 8% of the British population (see Table 4.1). A similar defect in oxidation of sparteine (an antiarrhythmic drug with uterine-stimulating effects unavailable in the UK) was found in about 5% of Germans. Although initially it was believed that these effects were identical it is now known that the two do not co-incide in about 3% of subjects. This could reflect linkage disequilibrium, i.e. two different cytochromes governed by two different genes with deficient and non-deficient forms plus some natural selective process which favours association of the two deficient and the two non-deficient forms. Alternatively there could be multiple alleles which produce several varieties of a functionally deficient cytochrome. Family studies show that poor metabolisers are homozygous for an autosomal recessive gene.

Debrisoquine is often used to phenotype individuals using the metabolic ratio:

$$\frac{\%\text{ of dose as debrisoquine}}{\%\text{ of dose as 4-hydroxydebrisoquine}}$$

excreted in the urine collected in the 8 hours following an oral dose of 10 mg debrisoquine. Poor metabolisers are defined as having a log metabolic ratio > 1.1.

This polymorphism explains several clinical phenomena:

Drug	*Effect in poor metaboliser*
Debrisoquine	Excessive hypotension
Sparteine	Fetal distress due to excessive uterine contraction
Perhexiline	Neuropathy and hepatotoxicity more common

Phenformin	Lactic acidosis more likely
Encainide	Reduced antiarrhythmic action (less active metabolite)
Nortriptyline	Headache, confusion

Several other drugs, e.g. metoprolol, propranolol, timolol, dextromethorphan and phenacetin also exhibit oxidation polymorphism associated with debrisoquine-linked defective metabolism. As yet the clinical importance of this defect in these cases is not established. It is also possible that oxidation phenotype determines susceptibility to cancer, thus there is an over-representation of extensive metabolisers in West African patients with primary liver cancer. One (unproven) hypothesis is that such individuals activate natural carcinogens like aflatoxin more extensively than poor metabolisers. Similarly a study of smokers has shown that poor oxidisers enjoy a 4 to 5-fold lower incidence of lung cancer.

There is preliminary evidence for at least two other oxidation polymorphisms (for nifedipine and mephenytoin respectively) which are distinct from the debrisoquine/sparteine systems.

Polymorphic sulphoxidation Sulphoxidation shows polymorphism analogous to that of nitrogen. There is a nearly hundred-fold difference between individuals with respect to the amount of sulphoxide metabolites in the urine following carbocysteine (Mucodyne). Preliminary data indicate that sulphoxidation capacity is inherited autosomally and is incompletely recessive. It is apparently independent of the nitrogen oxidation ('debrisoquine') system. As yet it is not known whether this genotype controls oxidation of other sulphur-containing drugs like phenothiazines but an association has been demonstrated between impaired sulphoxidation and an increased incidence of adverse reactions to penicillamine therapy for rheumatoid arthritis.

Alcohol dehydrogenase polymorphism Not all enzyme variants produce distinct clinical syndromes. Alcohol dehydrogenase in human liver exists as an atypical variant form with a specific activity about five times higher than the normal enzyme. It occurs in 20% of subjects studied in London. In spite of the high specific activity of the atypical enzyme the alcohol oxidation rate is no higher in individuals possessing this variant.

Slow metabolism of tolbutamide This pharmacogenetic variant has recently been described following the finding of a ninefold variation in the rate of tolbutamide elimination. Preliminary investigations suggest autosomal transmission of rapid and slow inactivation of tolbutamide which is apparently almost entirely under genetic control. It is believed that the primary site of genetic control is at the level of microsomal oxidation of the drug to hydroxytolbutamide. The clinical implication of this finding is that a fixed dose regime cannot be applied to all diabetics.

Deficiency of glucose-6-phosphate dehydrogenase (G6PD)

This defect is determined by a sex-linked gene carried on the X chromosome, which is of irregular dominance. The gene is present in a high proportion of Sephardic Jews, Africans and their descendants, the population of the Indian Continent, throughout the Mediterranean countries and in the Far East. The condition consists of an abnormal form of G6PD with reduced enzymic activity resulting in acute haemolysis when the red cells are exposed to oxidising substances, including the broad bean (*Vicia fava*) or its pollen, hibiscus flower, naphthalene derivatives and some drugs. G6PD catalyses the formation of NADPH, which maintains glutathione in its reduced form. This reaction converts methaemoglobin (i.e. oxidised) into haemoglobin (see Fig. 4.6). Lack of the dehydrogenase is associated with increased concentrations of red-cell methaemoglobin, Heinz body formation and haemolysis on exposure to oxidants.

Over 80 distinct variants of the G6PD molecule have been identified but not all are associated with drug-induced haemolysis. Only those in which dehydrogenase activity is reduced to less than 30% of normal produce haemolytic reactions. There are at least 15 varieties of clinically significant G6PD deficiency and these occur in different races. Two main types, A and B, are distinguished on the basis of their differing electrophoretic mobilities. Africans usually have either phenotypes A or B whilst white races have only type B. Thus the deficiency is found to be less severe in affected Africans whose

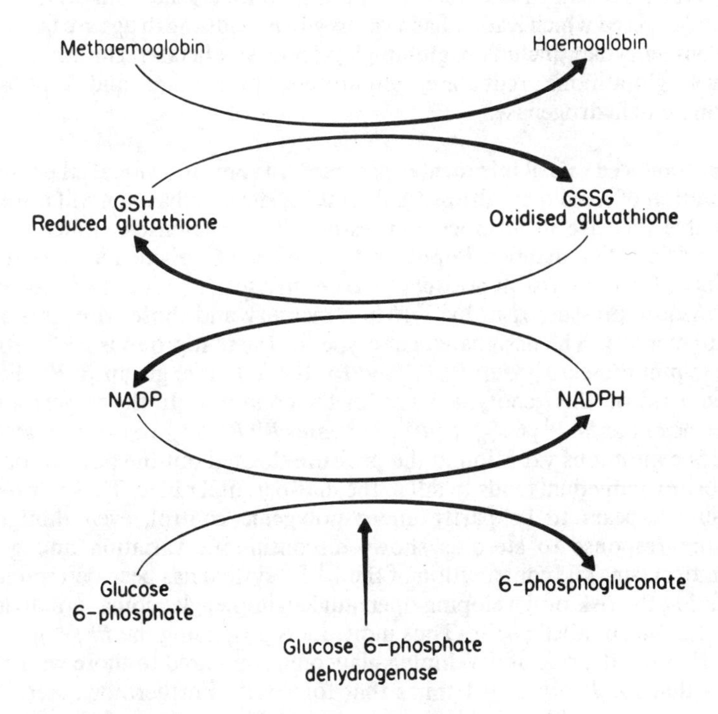

Fig. 4.6 Site of glucose 6-phosphate dehydrogenase deficiency.

red cells contain about 10% of normal activity, whilst in deficient whites only 1–3% of normal activity remains. The latter suffer from favism (sensitivity to broad beans) whilst Africans do not. In patients with G6PD deficiency the following drugs can produce haemolysis:

analgesics	*aspirin, phenacetin, acetanilid, antipyrine, aminopyrine.*
antimalarials	*primaquine, pamaquine, pentaquine, quinacrine, quinine.*
antibacterials	*sulphonamides, sulphones, nitrofurantoin, chloramphenicol, PAS*
miscellaneous	*quinidine, probenecid, BAL, vitamin K, naphthalene.*

Treatment should consist of preventing this drug reaction. Patients treated with an 8-aminoquinoline, e.g. primaquine, should spend at least the first few days in hospital under supervision. If this treatment does produce acute haemolysis the drug should be withdrawn and blood transfusion may be necessary. 100–200 mg of cortisol is given intravenously and the urine should be made alkaline to reduce the chance of deposition of acid haematin in the renal tubules.

The high incidence of the condition in some areas is attributed to a protective effect of the enzyme deficiency against falciparum malaria. In regions of Sardinia there is a positive correlation between genes for both thalassaemia and G6PD deficiency and previous malarial endemicity. The resistance may arise because parasites survive less well in enzyme-deficient cells because they are more rapidly removed from the circulation.

Several other enzymic defects in the glutathione-generating system have been discovered which lead to haemolysis when oxidising drugs are taken. The deficient enzymes include γ-glutamylcysteine synthetase, glutathione synthetase, glutathione reductase, glutathione peroxidase and 6-phosphogluconate dehydrogenase.

Steroid-induced raised intraocular pressure In some individuals the repeated application of steroid eye drops (such as 0.1% dexamethasone) will result in a reversible increase in intraocular pressure. This response is inherited in a simple Mendelian manner. Populations tested can be divided into those who produce little or no rise in pressure (maximum rise in pressure 5 mm mercury), those whose pressure rises by 5–15 mm mercury and those with rises above 15 mm mercury. The designated genotype for the first group is $P^L P^L$, for the over 15 mm pressure group $P^H P^H$ and for the 5–15 mm group $P^L P^H$. Family studies confirm this genotypic basis for the condition. In the population the frequencies are $P^L P^L$, 66%; $P^L P^H$, 29% and $P^H P^H$ 5%. In the untreated eye there is continuous variation in the pressure throughout the population, and that of any individual tends to fall in the mid-parental range. Thus intraocular pressure appears to be partly under polygenic control, even though the pressure response to steroids shows discontinuous variation and genetic polymorphism. The contribution of the $P^H P^L$ system has been determined by observing the risk of developing open angle (simple) glaucoma in individuals with the various allelic pairs. Thus individuals possessing the $P^L P^H$ genotype have 18 times the risk of developing glaucoma compared to those with $P^L P^L$, whilst that for $P^H P^H$ is 101 times that for $P^L P^L$. Furthermore, steroid eye drops in some $P^H P^H$ individuals can precipitate an attack of glaucoma.

Warfarin resistance has been observed in only two pedigrees in man, but has become very common in rats.

In man the condition was originally observed in a male whose prothrombin time was not affected by even large doses of warfarin. Vitamin K is necessary for the activation of factors II, VII, IX and X and is itself oxidised in the process. The enzyme which reactivates vitamin K (by reduction) is inhibited by warfarin. Patients resistant to warfarin appear to have a reducing enzyme insensitive to the action of warfarin.

Haemoglobin variants Hb Zurich may lead to acute haemolytic reactions when sulphonamides are administered. Even without drug therapy, red-cell survival time is shortened. Heterozygotes may also suffer spontaneous mild episodes of haemolytic jaundice.

Hb H is a relatively common variant in the East, and in Bangkok has been detected once every 300 births. Oxidants can cause acute haemolysis in homozygotes, in the same way as in patients with G6PD deficiency.

Methaemoglobinaemia due to lack of methaemoglobin reductase also leads to a drug sensitivity similar to that seen with G6PD deficiency.

Malignant hyperthermia (malignant hyperpyrexia) This is a rare but potentially fatal complication of general anaesthesia. The causative agents are usually halothane or suxamethonium. The sufferers exhibit a rapid rise in temperature and (usually) increasing muscular rigidity. In addition there is tachycardia, sweating, cyanosis and rapid respiration. There appear to be several forms of this condition, one of the more common (in which there is halothane induced rigidity) is inherited as a Mendelian dominant. The frequency of the phenotype is 1:20000. A number of different underlying muscle diseases may predispose. These include myopathies, myotonia congenita and central core disease. The serum creatine phosphokinase level is often elevated in susceptible individuals but a more accurate prediction of susceptibility may be made from muscle biopsy. Affected individuals' muscle has heightened sensitivity to caffeine *in vitro* and responds by a strong contraction, and it responds in a similar way to halothane or suxamethonium. It has been suggested that the essential abnormality lies in the muscle-cell membrane which shows impaired binding of calcium ion which can therefore be easily displaced by caffeine or halothane, producing contraction and the clinical features of the syndrome. The management of malignant hyperthermia is considered on p. 364.

Tasting polymorphisms for phenylthiocarbamide, prophylthiouracil and thiopentone

The ability of different people to taste these three drugs varies greatly: some individuals can taste them as bitter at great dilutions, others can only taste them when the crystals are placed on the tongue. The ability to taste these drugs is dominantly inherited. A high incidence of non-tasters is found among patients with adenomatous goitre and athyreotic cretinism whilst there are greater numbers of tasters among patients with toxic diffuse goitre. The efficacy of the thiouracils as antithyroid drugs suggests that there may be some pathological linkage between these observations but its nature has not been determined at present.

Acute porphyria

This group of diseases comprises acute intermittent porphyria, variegate porphyria and hereditary coproporphyria. In all three varieties acute illness can be precipitated by drugs because of inherited enzyme deficiencies in the pathway of haem synthesis (Fig. 4.7).

In variegate porphyria and hereditary coproporphyria skin lesions are present as well. In porphyria cutanea tarda, a non-acute porphyria, there are skin lesions but drugs do not precipitate acute attacks, although the condition may be aggravated by alcohol, oestrogens, iron and polychlorinated aromatic compounds. All the drugs which precipitate acute exacerbations of porphyria (neurological, psychiatric, cardiovascular and gastrointestinal disturbances which are occasionally fatal) are accompanied by increased urinary excretion of 5-ALA and porphobilinogen. These are not all enzyme inducers but all raise ALA synthetase levels in the liver. These drugs include:

hypnosedatives	*barbiturates, glutethimide, dichloralphenazone, meprobamate and chlordiazepoxide*
anticonvulsants	*phenytoin, succinimides*
oral hypoglycaemics	*sulphonylureas*
miscellaneous	*ethanol, griseofulvin, sulphonamides, sex hormones, methyldopa, imipramine, pentazocine, ergot, theophylline, rifampicin, pyrazinamide, chloramphenicol*

Often a single dose of one drug of this type can precipitate an acute episode, but in some patients, repeated doses are necessary to provoke a reaction.

CONTINUOUS VARIABILITY IN DRUG RESPONSE

The above are examples of discontinuous variation in drug response. This is usually due to the effects of variations in a single allele. The response to most drugs in a population demonstrates continuous variation and is the result of multiple genetic and environmental factors. Twin studies have been used to investigate the role of genetic influences acting in this type of distribution. With the drugs ethanol, bishydroxycoumarin, phenylbutazone, antipyrine, phenytoin, halothane and nortriptyline there is much greater similarity between identical than between fraternal twins (see Fig. 4.8). Family studies have confirmed this type of inheritance despite complications arising from differences in drug disposition according to age, sex, disease and exposure to chemicals in the environment. Thus, like intelligence, blood pressure and height, which are under polygenic control, the patterns of drug metabolism of these drugs in offspring tend to lie between those of the two parents. An estimate of the relative contributions of genetic and environmental factors in the control of drug metabolism may be made by estimating the mean variance of measurements, e.g. drug half-life, within the sets of identical and fraternal

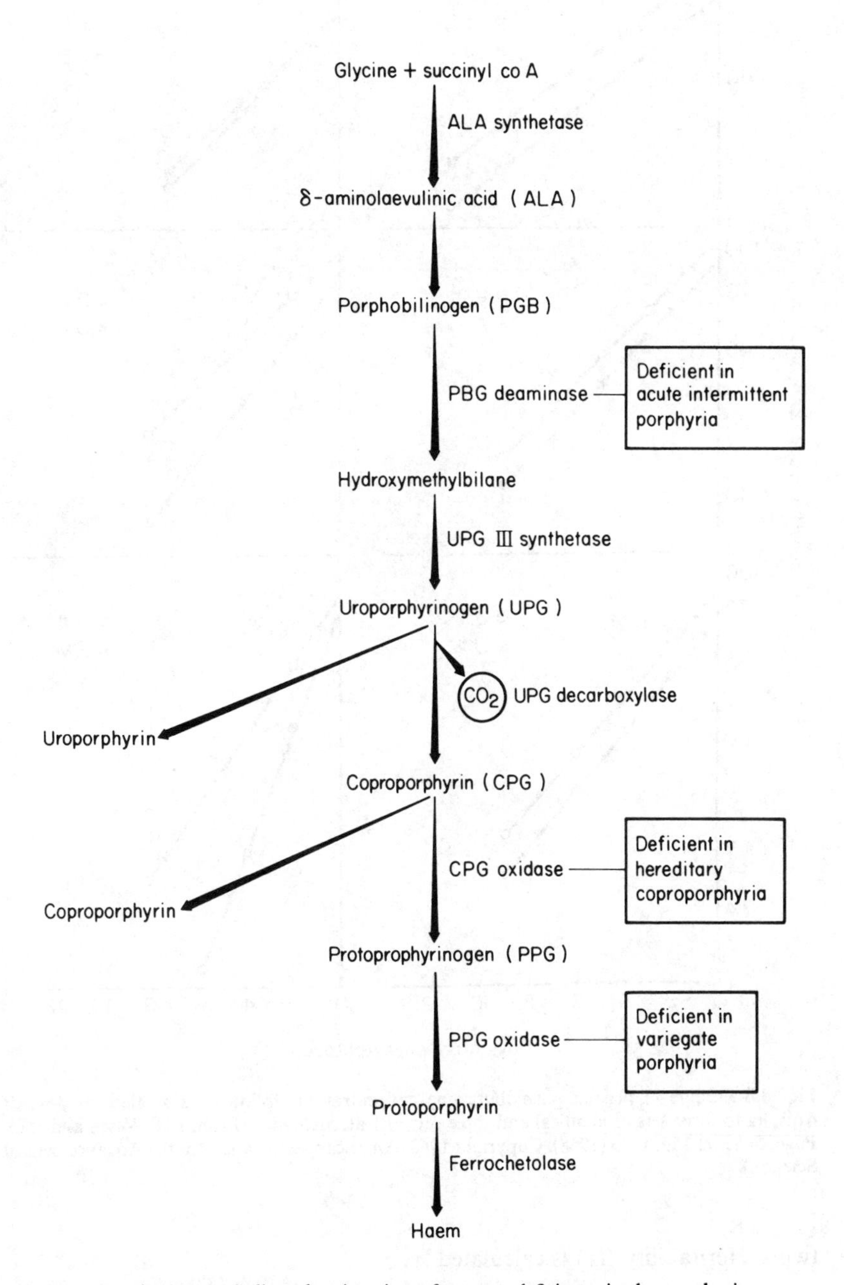

Fig. 4.7 Porphyrin metabolism showing sites of enzyme deficiency in the porphyrins.

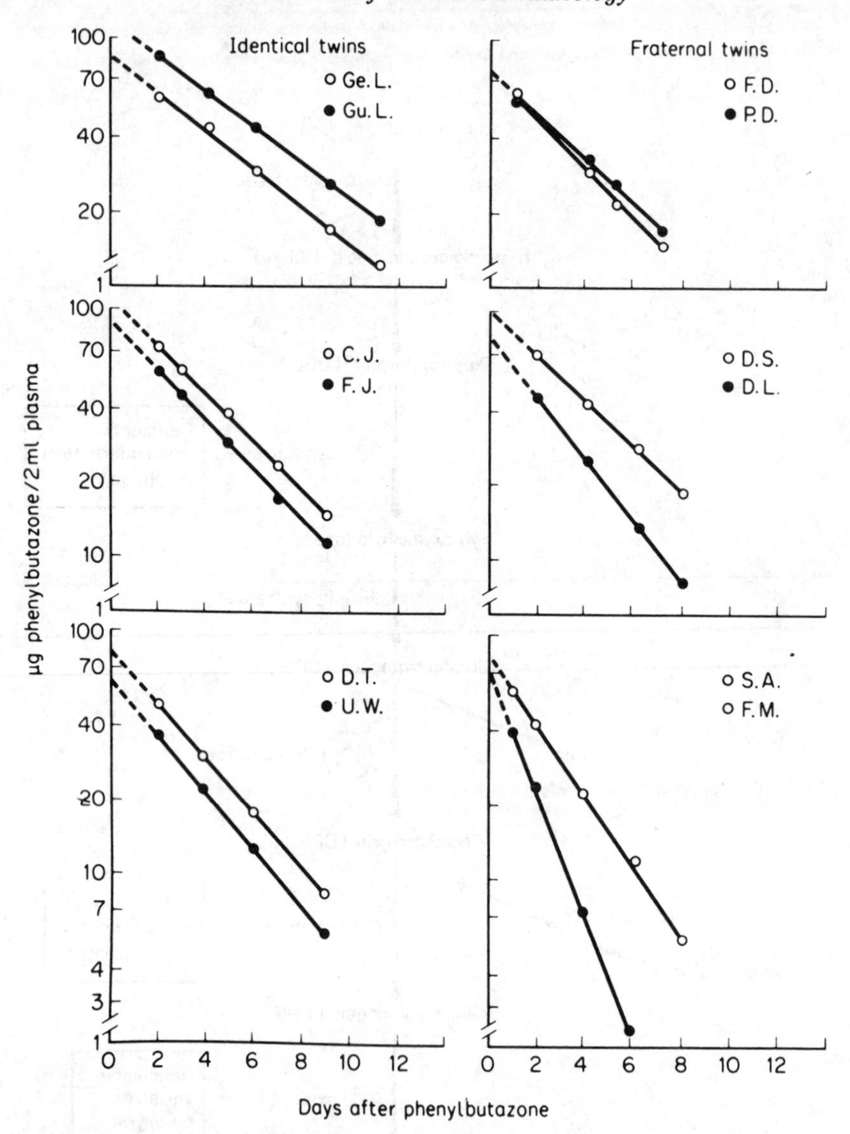

Fig. 4.8 Decline in plasma phenylbutazone concentrations following a single oral dose of 6 mg/kg to three sets of identical and three sets of fraternal twins (From E. S. Vesell and J. G. Page, *Science*, **159**, 1479 (1968). Copyright 1968. American Association for the Advancement of Science.)

twins. Heritability (H) is calculated from

$$H = \frac{\begin{pmatrix}\text{variance within pairs}\\ \text{of fraternal twins}\end{pmatrix} - \begin{pmatrix}\text{variance within pairs}\\ \text{of identical twins}\end{pmatrix}}{(\text{variance within pairs of fraternal twins})}.$$

Negligible hereditary control gives $H = 0$, whereas complete control is indicated by $H = 1$. Estimates of heritability for antipyrine, bishydroxy-coumarin and ethanol metabolism have been put as high as 0.98, 0.97 and 0.99 respectively for identical twins and 0.47, 0.66 and 0.38 for fraternal twins. Clearly for these drugs, large interindividual differences in the rates of elimination are remarkably free from environmental influences, since the expected values for fraternal twins who have approximately half their genes in common is 0.5 and for identical twins with identical genotypes H should be 1. Since antipyrine and ethanol exhibit little protein binding these effects are likely to result from genetic differences in elimination rather than drug distribution.

Progress is being made into the nature of genetic influences on pharmaco-kinetic parameters. In a study of amylobarbitone metabolism in twins it has been found that genetic control is exerted on kinetic parameters determining the rate of drug elimination and therefore its rate of metabolism. In the case of warfarin, the study of monozygotic and dizygotic twins showed that mainly genetic factors control the large intersubject variations in both the association constants for warfarin binding and the number of warfarin binding sites per albumin molecule. This appears to be associated with different albumin variants since charcoal treatment to remove endogenous ligands (i.e. sub-stances produced by the individual which could bind to albumin and so displace warfarin) did not alter the binding characteristics. Albumins from monozygotic twins exhibit greater structural similarities than do those from dizygotic twins. Genetic factors account for some 85% of this similarity.

Even drugs whose metabolism is mainly influenced by variations in a single gene (i.e. exhibit genetic polymorphism) may show additional variation due to superimposed polygenic effects. Isoniazid is an example of this state of affairs: there is continuous variation within each of the two populations of rapid and slow acetylators.

GENETIC DISORDERS WITH ALTERED DRUG SENSITIVITY

1. Children with *Down's syndrome*, show excessive sensitivity to anti-cholinergic drugs of the atropine type.
2. *Gout* is commonly the result of an inherited abnormality in purine metabolism. The disease can be aggravated by:

   (a) Ethanol. This is metabolised by oxidation and simultaneous forma-tion of NADH from NAD^+. NADH favours the conversion of pyruvate to lactate which impairs the renal excretion of urate.
   (b) Diuretics such as thiazide, ethacrynic acid, frusemide and bume-tanide. These impair renal excretion of uric acid.
   (c) Allopurinol normally reduces the frequency of acute gouty attacks by inhibiting xanthine oxidase and thus blocks the conversion of xanthine and hypoxanthine to uric acid. Allopurinol also inhibits total synthesis of purines. In some patients (0.5%) with reduced hypoxanthine–guanine phosphoribosyltransferase (HGPRT) activity, this second action of allopurinol does not operate and thus the drug can cause xanthine renal

stones to form. Complete absence of HGPRT is the cause of the very rare Lesch–Nyhan syndrome which is associated with hyperuricaemia and presents in infancy with choreoathetosis, spasticity, mental retardation and compulsive self-mutilation.

3. For the purine antimetabolites 6-mercaptopurine and azathioprine to become activated in the body HGPRT must operate. In patients lacking this enzyme, the therapeutic effects of these drugs may not be attained.
4. *Gilbert's disease* is a chronic form of hyperbilirubinaemia due to an inherited lack of a hepatic conjugating enzyme—glucuronyl transferase. Drugs such as cholecystographic agents and oestrogens may impair bilirubin uptake and aggravate the jaundice in this syndrome.
5. *Transketolase deficiency* It has been suggested recently that some individuals inherit an abnormal form of transketolase with reduced avidity for its cofactor, thiamine pyrophosphate. If the dietary intake of thiamine is reduced because of chronic alcoholism the activity of transketolase becomes compromised. This may explain why only some alcoholics develop Wernicke–Korsakov syndrome (see p. 852) whereas many others with the same degree of malnutrition are unaffected.

Chapter 5

EFFECTS OF DISEASE ON DRUG KINETICS

GASTROINTESTINAL DISEASE

It is obvious that gastrointestinal disease may alter the absorption of orally administered drugs.

(a) *Gastric emptying* is an important determinant of the rate and sometimes extent of drug absorption (Chapter 2). A number of pathological factors apart from drugs are known to alter gastric emptying (Table 5.1).

Table 5.1 Pathological factors influencing the rate of gastric emptying

Decreased	*Increased*
Trauma	Duodenal ulcer
Pain (including myocardial infarction, acute abdomen)	Gastroenterostomy
Labour	Coeliac disease
Migraine	
Myxoedema	
Raised intracranial pressure	
Intestinal obstruction	
Gastric ulcer	

There is relatively little information about the effect of these diseases on drug absorption. The absorption of effervescent aspirin is delayed in a migraine attack and this delay correlates with the severity of symptoms. More rapid relief is gained by increasing the gastric emptying rate and thus aspirin absorption by administering aspirin with metoclopramide. Pyloric stenosis results in impaired paracetamol absorption and it may be anticipated that effects on absorption of other drugs will occur with such conditions. Rarely however has a clinically significant effect been demonstrated.

(b) *Small intestinal disease* alters gastric emptying but the most significant changes occur in the gut mucosa. In coeliac disease destruction of the villi and microvilli reduces the area available for drug absorption, alters intraluminal pH, decreases the amount of mucosal enzyme present and thus alters enterohepatic cycling. There appears to be no consistent pattern in the effects on drug absorption, thus whilst ampicillin is unaffected, amoxycillin and pivampicillin show decreased absorption and cephalexin, clindamycin, fusidic acid, sulphamethoxazole and trimethoprim exhibit an increased absorption.

Crohn's disease primarily affects the terminal ileum (cf. coeliac disease which affects the jejunum) but may involve any part of the small intestine and the colon. It has been shown that the absorption of clindamycin and sulphamethoxazole increases in this disease, the peak concentration of the latter being three times that occurring in normal controls. The absorption of trimethoprim is slightly reduced and hypothetically this change in the ratio of the two components of cotrimoxazole could allow development of bacterial resistance. Although the absorption of a water-soluble drug like practolol is delayed and peak levels of the lipid-soluble propranolol are increased, there is little evidence that this is a general rule for altered drug absorption in coeliacs.

(c) *Pancreatic disease* can produce steatorrhoea and this may reduce the absorption of highly lipophilic molecules. Significant reduction in absorption of clindamycin and cephalexin have been demonstrated in mucoviscidosis. On the other hand, the low plasma levels after oral dicloxacillin are apparently not due to malabsorption but result from unusually high renal clearance of this drug. Increased doses of the antibiotic in such patients are therefore necessary.

CARDIAC FAILURE

Cardiac failure and the consequent pathophysiological changes produce a number of alterations in drug pharmacokinetics, although their clinical importance has yet to be established. The following factors must be considered:

(a) *Alterations in drug absorption* Malabsorption of orally administered fat occurs in cardiac failure and improves after diuretic therapy. This has been attributed to mucosal oedema and drug absorption could be affected similarly.

In addition to structural changes, altered gastro-intestinal blood flow subsequent to reduced cardiac output may reduce drug absorption since gastrointestinal blood flow may be the rate-limiting step in the absorption of some drugs. Furthermore, redistribution of cardiac output during failure produces splanchnic vasoconstriction. Other secondary changes in gastrointestinal motility, secretion, altered pH etc. may also adversely affect drug absorption.

Only limited information is yet available concerning the effect of cardiac failure on drug absorption. The absorption of two diuretics, metolazone and hydrochlorothiazide, is reduced by 30–40%. Frusemide absorption is delayed in heart failure, probably due to delayed gastric emptying, but the overall absorption is no more erratic than normal. Although procainamide is well absorbed by healthy volunteers with peak concentrations achieved at 1 h, after acute myocardial infarction there may be a lag time of up to 2 h before drug is detected in the blood, and the peak occurs at around 5 h. Occasionally the bioavailability is reduced by more than 50% and therapeutic concentrations cannot be reached with usual oral regimes. There is also a clinical impression that oral absorption of digoxin is erratic in heart failure. Whilst some patients seem to show marked changes (Fig. 5.1) overall the objective evidence is at present less impressive and suggests great inter-patient variability may be more important.

(b) *Drug distribution* changes during cardiac failure. Thus after oral administration of quinidine, the apparent volume of distribution in patients with congestive cardiac failure is approximately one third of normal. This

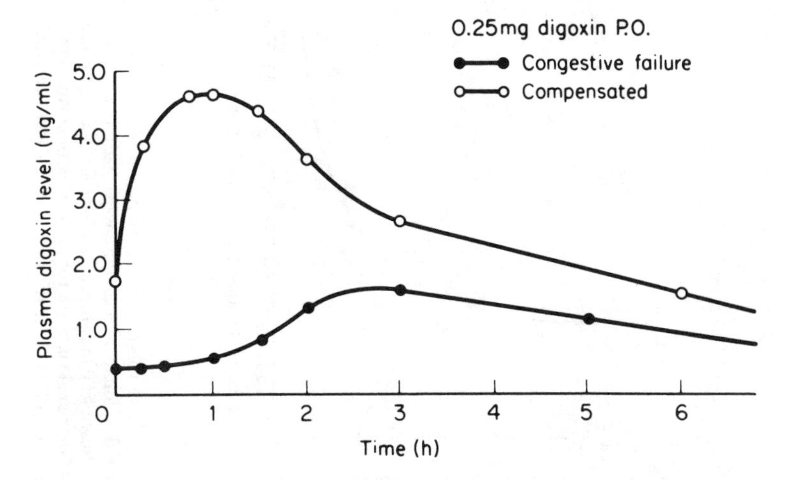

Fig. 5.1 Plasma digoxin levels following 0.25 mg orally during and after clearing of cardiac failure (From G. C. Oliver *et al.*, in Symposium on digitalis (Editor: O. Storstein), *Gyldenal Norsk Forlag*, Oslo (1973).)

results in elevated plasma levels and under these circumstances the heart and brain, which retain high perfusion rates even during cardiac failure, could receive excessively high amounts of quinidine, producing toxicity. The half-life of quinidine is unaltered by cardiac failure. The volume of distribution of procainamide is reduced by 25% in heart failure and that of lignocaine is similarly reduced with an increase in plasma levels. The decreased distribution volume in patients with heart failure may be related to decreased tissue perfusion and perhaps by alteration in the partition of lignocaine between blood and tissue components. Frusemide, a drug largely confined to the vascular compartment with a low apparent volume of distribution, has an unchanged distribution volume in heart failure.

Tissue injury following myocardial infarction results in a rise in ESR and the concentration of acute phase reactant proteins in the blood rises. These latter include α_1-acid glycoprotein which binds many basic drugs (see p. 37). Thus acute myocardial infarction is associated with increased binding and hence it may be supposed reduced efficacy of such drugs. A decrease of approximately 50% in free disopyramide concentration has been documented over the first five days following an infarct and similar but less-marked changes have been reported for lignocaine and flecainide. The clinical significance of such changes has yet to be determined.

(c) *Drug elimination* by the liver or kidneys may diminish in heart failure. Decreased hepatic perfusion accompanies the reduced cardiac output of heart failure and drugs having an extraction ratio $> 70\%$ show blood-flow-limited clearance. Lignocaine conforms to this criterion and steady-state levels are related to cardiac output and diminished hepatic blood flow (Fig. 5.2). Terminal half-lives of lignocaine and its two pharmacologically active metabolites monoethylglycinexylidide (MEGX) and glycinexylidide (GX) are also prolonged (see Table 5.2) in patients following a myocardial infarct, the prolongation being more pronounced in those with clinically apparent failure.

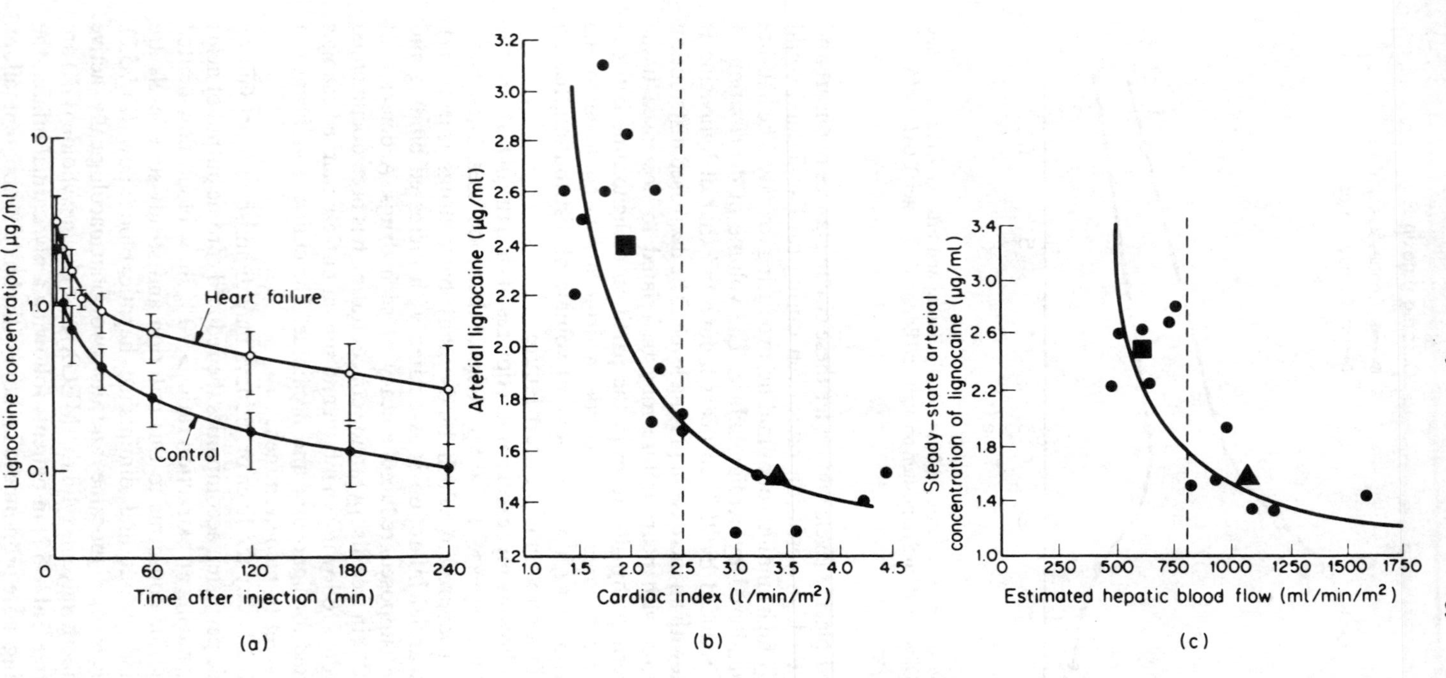

Fig. 5.2 (a) Mean (and standard deviations) of plasma lignocaine concentrations in seven heart failure patients and controls following a 50 mg intravenous bolus; (b) relationship of arterial lignocaine level and cardiac index (dotted vertical line is lower limit of normal cardiac index, square is mean for low cardiac index patients, traingle is mean for patients with normal cardiac index); (c) relationship of steady-state arterial lignocaine level following 50 mg bolus and infusion of 40 mg/kg/min (vertical line is lower limit of normal hepatic blood flow, sauare is mean for patients with low hepatic blood flow, triangle is mean for patients with normal flow). (From (a) P. D. Thompson *et al.*, *Amer. Heart J.*, **82**, 417 (1971) (b & c) R. E. Stenson *et al.*, *Circulation*, **43**, 205 (1971). By permission of the American Heart Association Inc.)

Table 5.2 Mean plasma half lives of lignocaine, MEGX and GX (± S.E. of mean) in healthy subjects and in patients with and without clinically apparent cardiac failure following acute myocardial infarction. From Prescott *et al.*, *Brit. Med. J.*, I, 939 (1976).

	Plasma half-life (h)		
	Lignocaine	*MEGX*	*GX*
Healthy subjects	1.4 ± 0.1	2.3 ± 0.1	15
Patients without cardiac failure	4.3 ± 0.8	6.7 ± 1.3	17.3 ± 4.8
Patients with cardiac failure	10.2 ± 2.0	7.8 ± 1.0	40.4

Thus following a prolonged infusion of lignocaine the steady-state levels attained are almost 50 % higher in patients with cardiac failure. In one patient with cardiogenic shock no decline occurred following termination of infusion, suggesting markedly impaired hepatic clearance. The potential for lignocaine intoxication may be increased by the accumulation of MEGX and GX which have cardiodepressant and central stimulant properties. Similar decreases in elimination may be anticipated with other drugs possessing high extraction ratios. The total body clearance of theophylline is decreased and the half-life doubled in patients with cardiac failure and pulmonary oedema, although the inter-patient variability with this drug is wide relative to these kinetic changes. As the apparent volume of distribution of this drug is unchanged, a single dose gives relatively reproducible plasma levels in cardiac failure, but because of the variable plasma clearance of the drug in this situation, plasma concentrations and toxicity would be unpredictable after repeated doses or infusions.

The metabolic capacity of the liver is probably also affected in heart failure either by hypoxia impairing drug oxidation or by hepatocellular damage resulting from hepatic congestion or hypoperfusion. Liver-biopsy samples show reduced drug-metabolising activity under these circumstances. The extraction ratio of antipyrine is approximately 3 % and the half-life of this compound is prolonged in patients after myocardial infarction, particularly if clinically apparent failure is present (Table 5.3).

Heart failure may reduce renal drug elimination by reduction in glomerular filtration rate and by increased tubular reabsorption secondary to redistribution of intrarenal blood flow. Procainamide shows a prolonged half-life and accumulation in heart failure due to reduced renal excretion. In addition,

Table 5.3 Mean plasma antipyrine half lives (± S.E. of mean) in patients after myocardial infarction measured on second hospital day and during convalescence. From Prescott *et al.*, *Brit. Med. J.*, I 939 (1976).

	Plasma antipyrine half-life (h)	
	In hospital	*During convalescence*
Patients without cardiac failure	12.2 ± 0.6	9.9 ± 0.7
Patients with cardiac failure	19.4 ± 1.9	13.2 ± 1.0

accumulation of the pharmacologically active metabolite N-acetyl-procainamide occurs in renal insufficiency and may contribute to drug toxicity.

RENAL DISEASE

Renal excretion is a major route of elimination for many drugs and metabolites. In renal failure drugs eliminated predominantly through the kidneys may accumulate within the body after repeated dosing. Additionally, drug metabolites can also accumulate and exert pharmacological effects, inhibit the metabolism of their parent compound or displace it from protein binding and cause toxic effects. Drugs are cleared by passive glomerular filtration and also by active tubular excretion. Once within the renal tubule compounds may be passively reabsorbed back into the circulation. Glomerular filtration rate is approximated by endogenous creatinine clearance (normally 100–130 ml/min) which is relatively easily determined clinically. Much work has been directed to finding simple clinical measurements which will predict the behaviour of drugs in patients with various degrees of renal impairment. For a drug which distributes in the body according to a linear one-compartment model the apparent first-order elimination rate constant k is the sum of k_r, the rate constant for renal elimination, and k_{nr}, the rate constant for non-renal elimination. That is,

$$k = k_r + k_{nr}. \qquad (5.1)$$

If renal elimination is proportional to the creatinine clearance Cl_{cr}, then

$$k_r = aCl_{cr}, \qquad (5.2)$$

where a is a proportionality constant, and substitution into (5.1) yields

$$k = aCl_{cr} + k_{nr}. \qquad (5.3)$$

This is the equation of a straight line for a plot of k versus creatinine clearance with a slope of a and y-intercept of k_{nr}. According to this relationship, drugs may exhibit three types of behaviour (Fig. 5.3):

Type A Drug elimination is almost entirely via the renal route ($k_{nr} = 0; a > 0$) and the line passes through the origin and shows a marked dependence of drug elimination on renal function.
Type B Drug elimination is almost entirely extrarenal ($k_{nr} > 0; a = 0$) yielding a horizontal line with the ordinate intercept $y = k_{nr}$, i.e. the rate of elimination is independent of renal function.
Type C Drug elimination occurs by renal and non-renal routes ($k_{nr} > 0$; $a > 0$), again the ordinate $y = k_{nr}$ but the line is rising to the right.

For a type A drug if the slope of the line of the plot of k versus creatinine clearance is known, a simple rule can be determined for changes in drug elimination with altered renal function. As an example, for gentamicin the percentage hourly loss $= 0.2 + (0.25 \times Cl_{cr})$ as shown in Fig. 5.4. Therefore the percentage hourly gentamicin loss is approximated by dividing endogenous creatinine clearance by four.

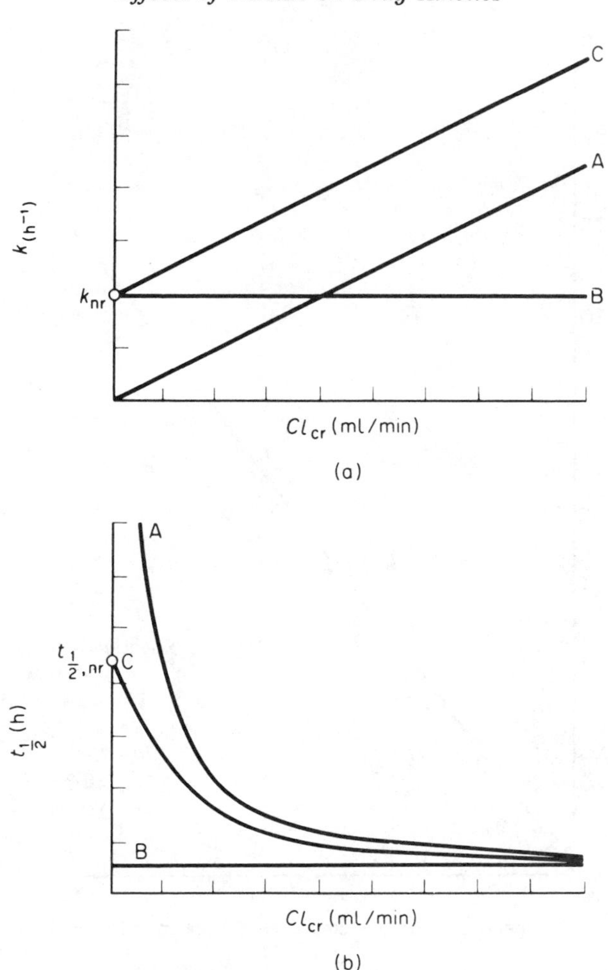

Fig. 5.3 (a) Dependence of elimination rate constant k on the endogenous creatinine clearance Cl_{cr} for drugs of type A, B and C (see text); (b) dependence of the elimination half-life $t_{1/2}$ on creatinine clearance for drugs of type A, B and C.

Equation (5.3) can be expressed in terms of $t_{1/2}$ as follows:

$$t_{1/2} = \frac{0.693}{k} = \frac{0.693}{k_{nr} + aCl_{cr}}. \qquad (5.4)$$

As can be seen from Fig. 5.3, this is a more complex curvilinear function. It is readily apparent that substantial changes in $t_{1/2}$ do not occur until renal function is significantly depressed. Practically, the linear relationship of creatinine clearance with k is more useful than the relationship with $t_{1/2}$. If values of k for normals and for subjects with various degrees of renal impairment or in the limiting case for anephric ($Cl_{cr} = 0$) subjects are obtained, then constructing a straight line between these two points will allow the

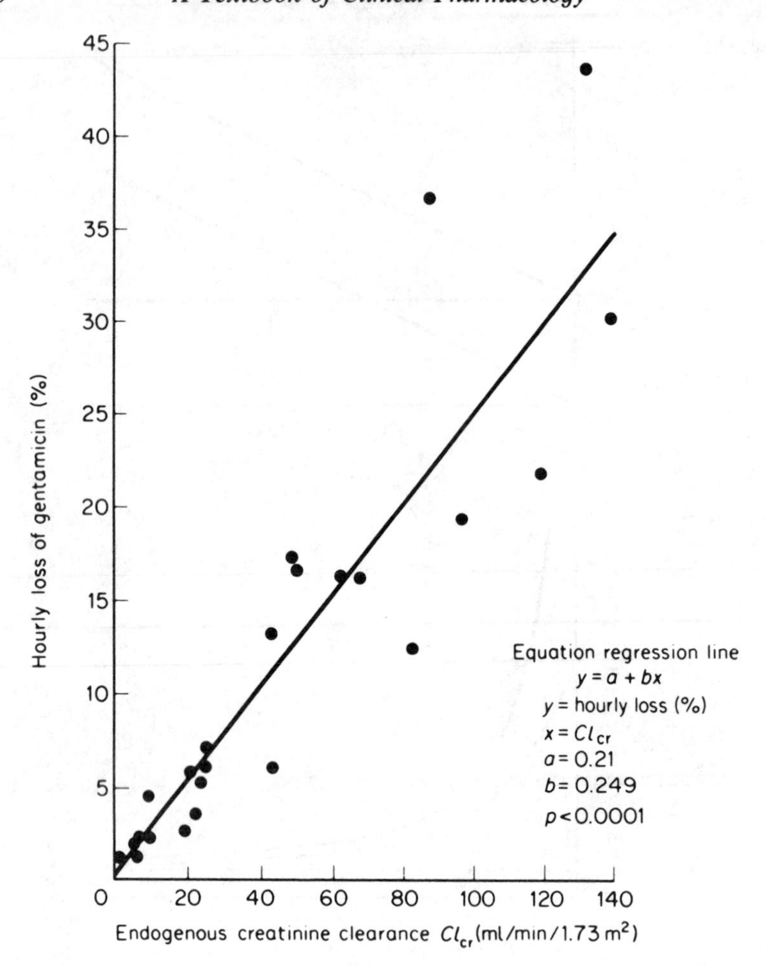

Fig. 5.4 Relationship of per cent hourly loss of gentamicin and creatinine clearance in 24 patients. The slope of the line (b) is 0.25. (From M. C. McHenry *et al.*, *Ann. Int. Med.* **74**, 192 (1971).)

estimation of k for other patients. Table 5.4 is a collection of such values. Thus to determine k for carbenicillin in a patient with a creatinine clearance of 10 ml/min, the table is consulted and a graph drawn as shown in Fig. 5.5.

When k_{nr} from anephric patients is unknown it is possible to calculate an approximate value assuming a simple one-compartment model, since from eqs. (1.11) and (5.1),

$$t_{1/2} = \frac{0.693}{k} = \frac{0.693}{k_r + k_{nr}}. \tag{5.5}$$

The fraction f of the absorbed dose excreted unchanged in the urine is given by

$$f = \frac{k_r}{k_r + k_{nr}}. \tag{5.6}$$

Table 5.4 Reported elimination rate constants (k) for drugs in patients with normal renal function (k_N) and in anephric patients ($k = k_{nr}$). The quotient $k_{nr}/k_N(\%)$ is the relative amount of any drug excreted extrarenally. Normal renal function is defined as a creatinine clearance of 100 ml/minute.

	k_N (h^{-1})	k_{nr} (h^{-1})	$\frac{k_{nr}}{k_N} \times 100\,(\%)$
Rifampicin	0.25	0.25	100.0
Minocycline	0.04	0.04	100.0
Chlortetracycline*	0.1	0.1	100.0
Lignocaine	0.39	0.36	92.3
Doxycycline	0.037	0.031	83.8
Clindamycin	0.16	0.12	75.0
Chloramphenicol*	0.26	0.19	73.1
Propranolol	0.22	0.16	72.8
Erythromycin	0.39	0.28	71.8
Trimethoprim	0.054	0.031	57.4
Isoniazid (fast acetylator)	0.53	0.30	56.6
Isoniazid (slow acetylator)	0.23	0.13	56.5
Sulphamethoxazole	0.084	0.037	44.0
Chlorpropamide	0.020	0.008	40.0
Lincomycin	0.15	0.06	40.0
Tetracycline	0.12	0.033	27.5
Cloxacillin	1.21	0.31	25.6
Oxytetracycline*	0.075	0.014	18.7
Methyldopa	0.17(?)	0.03(?)	17.6
Amoxycillin	0.70	0.10	14.3
Methicillin*	1.4	0.19	13·6
Penicillin G	1.24	0.13	10.5
Ampicillin	0.53	0.05	9.4
Carbenicillin	0.55	0.05	9.1
Cephaloridine*	0.51	0.03	5.9
Cephalothin	1.2	0.06	5.0
Gentamicin	0.30	0.015	5.0
Flucytosine	0.18	0.007	3.9
Kanamycin	0.28	0.01	3.6
Tobramycin	0.32	0.01	3.1
Procainamide*	0.21 (days^{-1})	0.007 (days^{-1})	3.3
Digitoxin	0.1 (days^{-1})	0.07 (days^{-1})	70.0
β-Methyldigoxin	0.38 (days^{-1})	0.17 (days^{-1})	44.7
Digoxin	0.45 (days^{-1})	0.15 (days^{-1})	33.0

* Drugs which should not be administered in renal failure

Equations (5.5) and (5.6) can be solved simultaneously for k_r and k_{nr} if f and $t_{1/2}$ are found from normal subjects.

With declining renal function the concentration of endogenous substances usually cleared by the kidneys increases. Blood urea is relatively useless as an index of renal drug elimination, since it is influenced by protein intake and metabolism, liver function, urine flow and other factors. Plasma creatinine depends upon age, sex and muscle mass but unlike the creatinine clearance

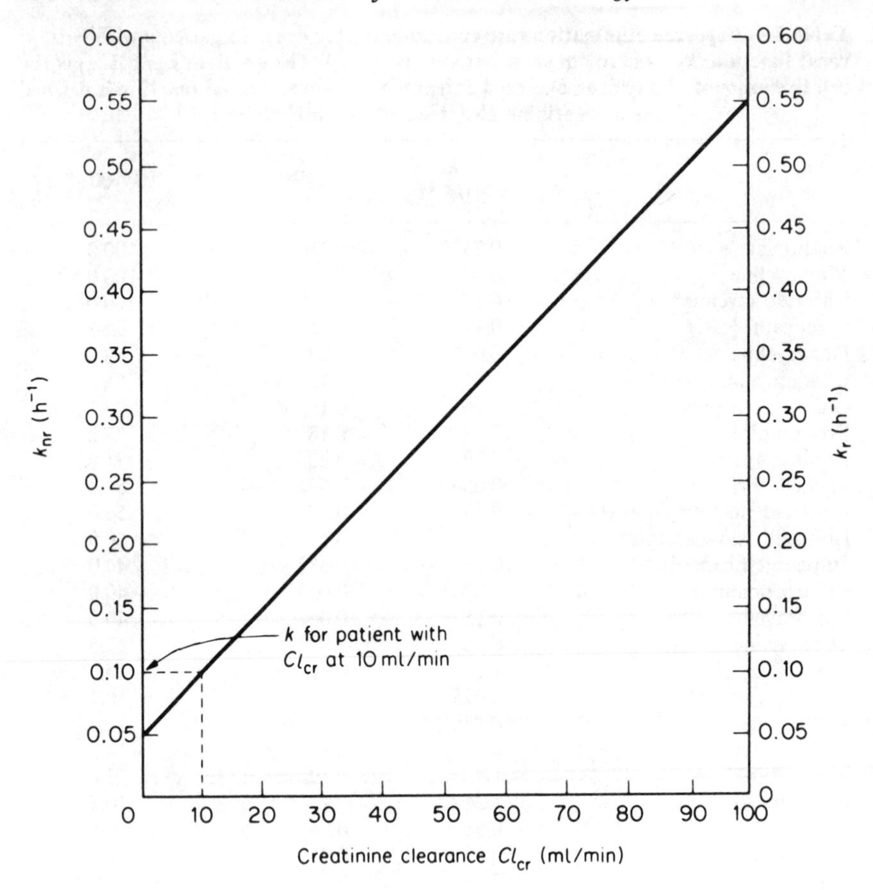

Fig. 5.5 Use of data in Table 5.4 to determine elimination rate constant for carbenicillin in a patient with a creatinine clearance of 10 ml/min.

does not require a urine collection to be made (a procedure which is rarely accurately performed).

By definition the plasma creatinine concentration, C_{cr}, is related to the rate of endogenous creatinine production, K_0, and creatinine clearance by

$$C_{cr} = \frac{K_0}{Cl_{cr}}. \tag{5.7}$$

Solving (5.7) for Cl_{cr} and substituting into eq. (5.3) yields

$$k = \frac{aK_0}{C_{cr}} + k_{nr}. \tag{5.8}$$

Thus a linear relationship exists between k and $1/C_{cr}$ with intercept and slope of k_{nr} and aK_0 respectively. Such a plot could be used to determine k under conditions of renal failure, but requires determination in each patient. The relationship between drug half-life and plasma creatinine may be determined by solving (5.7) for Cl_{cr} and substitution into (5.4), yielding

$$t_{1/2} = \frac{0.693C_{cr}}{aK_0 + k_{nr}C_{cr}}. \tag{5.9}$$

The half-life $t_{1/2}$ is linearly related to C_{cr} only when k_{nr} is very small relative to k; as k_{nr} approaches k the relationship becomes curvilinear and $t_{1/2}$ becomes independent of C_{cr}. Thus only for drugs cleared unchanged solely through the kidneys is the creatinine concentration itself of direct value, an example being gentamicin (Fig. 5.4). An additional problem arises if a drug demonstrates very marked multi compartment characteristics, since under these circumstances the terminal exponential phase of the plasma concentration–time curve has a $t_{1/2}$ which is determined by both drug elimination and distribution (i.e., $t_{1/2} = 0.693/\beta$). Under these circumstances β and hence $t_{1/2}$ are not linearly related to the plasma creatinine concentration. The assumption that creatinine production is constant (K_0) is not necessarily true in the aged where K_0 falls but the plasma concentration remains constant, probably due to a corresponding decrease in creatinine clearance. Consequently dosage-regime adjustments for the elderly should not be based on data employing plasma creatinine measurements obtained in a younger population. Plasma creatinine levels are stable in chronic renal failure, but it should be remembered that they reflect acute fluctuations in renal function with a lag time of several days.

The plasma creatinine level may be employed to estimate the creatinine clearance either by use of the nomogram of Siersbaek–Nielsen *et al.* (Fig. 5.6) or by the approximations:

for males
$$Cl_{cr} = \frac{1.23\,(140 - \text{age (yrs)} \times \text{weight (kg)})}{\text{plasma creatinine } (\mu\text{M})} \tag{5.10}$$

for females
$$Cl_{cr} = \frac{1.04(140 - \text{age (yrs)} \times \text{weight (kg)})}{\text{plasma creatinine } (\mu\text{M})} \tag{5.11}$$

An alternative estimate is gained from

$$Cl_{cr}(\text{male}) = \frac{W(29.3 - 0.203Y)}{14.4\,C_{cr}}, \tag{5.12}$$

$$Cl_{cr}(\text{female}) = 0.8Cl_{cr}\,(\text{male}), \tag{5.13}$$

where W = weight (kg), Y = age (years), C_{cr} = plasma creatinine concn. (mg/100 ml).

The estimated Cl_{cr} may then be used to adjust k for an individual patient.

Adjustment of dosage regimes in renal impairment

Following the administration of multiple doses of a drug at a dosage interval T, the average steady-state concentration $\bar{C}$ can be expressed by a model-independent equation for drugs obeying first-order kinetics (see Chapter 1):

$$\bar{C} = \frac{F}{V_d}\frac{X_0}{kT}, \tag{1.66}$$

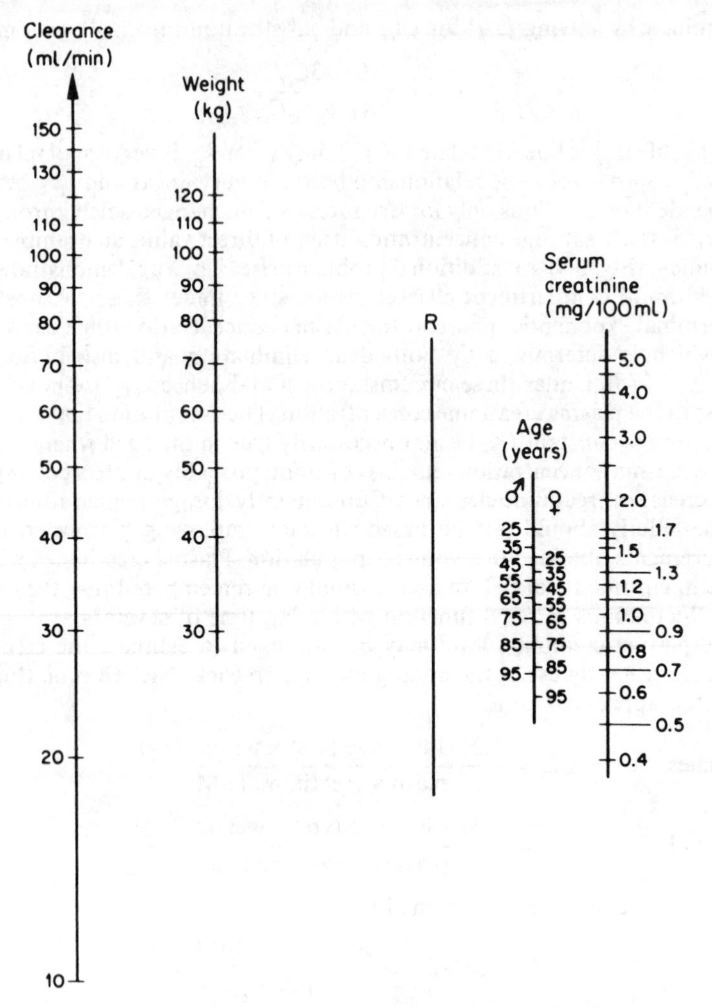

Fig. 5.6 Nomogram for rapid evaluation of endogenous creatinine – with a ruler join weight to age; keep ruler at crossing point on **R**, then move the right-hand side of the ruler to the appropriate serum creatinine value and read off clearance from left-hand scale (From K. Siersbaek – Nielson *et al.*, *Lancet*, **1**, 1133 (1971).)

where V_d is the apparent volume of distribution, F is the fraction of an oral or intramuscular dose X_0 which is absorbed and k is the apparent first-order elimination constant. In a patient with renal impairment it is obviously desirable to achieve the same average steady-state concentration as in patients with normal kidneys; thus, in this circumstance

$$\bar{C} = \frac{\hat{F}\hat{X}_0}{\hat{V}_d \hat{k} \hat{T}}, \tag{5.14}$$

where ^ identifies the characteristics of the patient with renal failure. Thus

$$\frac{FX_0}{V_d kT} = \frac{\hat{F}\hat{X}_0}{\hat{V}_d \hat{k}\hat{T}}. \tag{5.15}$$

Assuming that F and V_d are unaffected by renal failure this simplifies to

$$\frac{X_0}{kT} = \frac{\hat{X}_0}{\hat{k}\hat{T}}. \tag{5.16}$$

Therefore the dosage regime for a patient with renal failure could be adjusted by one of two methods, both of which require the determination of $\hat{k}$, the elimination rate constant, as detailed above.

(i) A lower dose could be used at the same dosing interval, i.e. $T = \hat{T}$, so that (5.16) becomes

$$\frac{X_0}{k} = \frac{\hat{X}_0}{\hat{k}}, \tag{5.17}$$

which is solved for $\hat{X}_0$.

(ii) The same dose could be used but the dosing interval lengthened, i.e. $X_0 = \hat{X}_0$ so that (5.16) becomes

$$\hat{T} = \frac{k}{\hat{k}} T. \tag{5.18}$$

Although there is some disagreement in the literature, it is usually suggested that the loading dose, L, is the same as in patients with normal renal function. Because the desired plasma steady-state concentration is not reached until at least 5 half-lives have elapsed, in patients with renal failure producing an unduly prolonged $t_{1/2}$, a loading dose will be required if an immediate therapeutic effect is desired. This is calculated from

$$\hat{L} = \frac{\hat{X}_0}{1 - e^{-\hat{k}\hat{T}}}. \tag{5.19}$$

Equations (5.17)–(5.19) may be easily solved using a pocket calculator or tables of natural exponential functions.

As an example, consider the dose of gentamicin required for a patient with a creatinine clearance of 10 ml/min. The usual dose of gentamicin for patients with normal kidneys might be 480 mg daily. Table 5.4 gives $k_N = 0.3\ h^{-1}$ and $k_{nr} = 0.015\ h^{-1}$ and construction of a graph similar to Fig. 5.5 yields $\hat{k}$ as $0.035\ h^{-1}$.

Thus $$\hat{X}_0 = \frac{480 \times 0.035}{0.3} = 56\ \text{mg}/24\ \text{h}.$$

The $t_{1/2}$ corresponding to $\hat{k} = 0.035\ h^{-1}$ is 0.693/0.035 h = 19.8 h, so that the plateau will not be reached until some 100 h have elapsed (i.e. $5 \times t_{1/2}$). Thus a loading dose in required:

$$\hat{L} = \frac{56}{1 - e^{-0.035 \times 24}} = 98.5\ \text{mg}.$$

Gentamicin is dispensed in solution for injection as 40 mg/ml, and to minimise errors in administration the drug is usually prescribed in multiples of this, so that a practical regime for the patient would be a loading dose of 80 mg followed by doses of 40 mg at 24 h intervals. There can be no substitute for careful monitoring of gentamicin levels during therapy coupled with acute clinical observation of the patient. Mathematical exactitude should not give a false sense of security since patients do not completely correspond to pharmacokinetic models, which by their simplicity cannot account for some sources of variability. Amongst the factors which undermine the assumptions of the model, the following should be considered:

(a) Metabolism of drugs in renal failure has not been extensively studied but obviously alterations will be of consequence only for drugs eliminated extensively by metabolism. In general, oxidative drug metabolism appears to be normal in uraemia and although antipyrine oxidation is increased in uraemic patients, a state of maximal induction of these enzymes does not appear to occur. Reductive metabolic pathways as exemplified by cortisol reduction are slowed. Acetylation of sulphonamides, but not that of the polymorphic (isoniazid) type, is reduced, whilst glucuronide formation is normal. Hydrolysis of esters such as procaine is prolonged and may be of consequence for drugs such as clindamycin phosphate or erythromycin estolate which require hydrolysis for activity. Renal metabolism may also change in uraemia: the vitamin D metabolite 25-hydroxycholecalciferol is hydroxylated to active 1, 25-dihydroxycholecalciferol in the kidney and uraemic patients require massive doses of calciferol to avoid 'renal rickets'. Alternatively, the metabolic block is bypassed with a synthetic analogue of 1, 25-dihydroxycholecalciferol, 1-α-hydroxycholecalciferol.

(b) Drug distribution is assumed to be unchanged by renal failure but simulations of renal failure using two-compartment pharmacokinetic models suggest that in renal impairment drug may concentrate in the central compartment at the expense of the peripheral compartment. This concept is theoretical, although one piece of evidence in its favour is the fall in the apparent volume of distribution of digoxin at steady state in renal failure from an average of around 500 litres in normals to about 280 litres in patients with renal disease, although there is great variability. However, there may be explanations other than pharmacokinetic ones for these observations, since in animals with experimentally induced uraemia there is widespread inhibition of Na^+K^+ATPase which could decrease digoxin binding. Direct measurement of amounts of digoxin bound to myocardium at post mortem suggests that decreased binding is linearly correlated with ante-mortem creatinine clearance. Every acidic drug, e.g. warfarin, phenytoin, sulphonamide, that binds to albumin shows decreased binding in serum from uraemic patients and an increased volume of distribution. These changes in distribution are associated with decreased plasma protein binding of drugs and predicted by

$$V_d = V_b + V_t\left(\frac{f_b}{f_t}\right), \tag{1.93}$$

where V_b and V_t are the actual volumes of water in the blood and the tissues respectively (i.e. $V_b + V_t$ = total body water) and f_b and f_t are the fractions of free drug in blood and tissues respectively. Thus decreased plasma protein binding (which increases f_b) without comparable changes in tissue binding will increase the apparent volume of distribution and decrease the plasma levels of the drug. The clinical consequences of these effects are difficult to predict. Although a higher fraction of unbound drug may lead to more intense effects and a higher incidence of adverse effects, impaired binding may also increase drug clearance and decrease half-life. A further kinetic factor may contribute to the increased incidence of adverse effects with decreased protein binding, for it can be shown theoretically that the peak concentrations achieved at steady state with decreased binding are higher than those occurring under normal conditions, so that increased pharmacological effects may occur. The theory is supported by the fact that after a single dose the maximum hypotensive effect of diazoxide and the maximum hypoprothrombinaemic effect of phenindione are greater in patients with impaired protein binding.

The precise nature of the changes in binding to protein in uraemia are not clearly understood. Phenytoin binding is clearly correlated with the serum creatinine (see Fig. 5.7). This decreased binding in uraemic serum is greater than can be accounted for by hypoalbuminaemia, which may occur in the

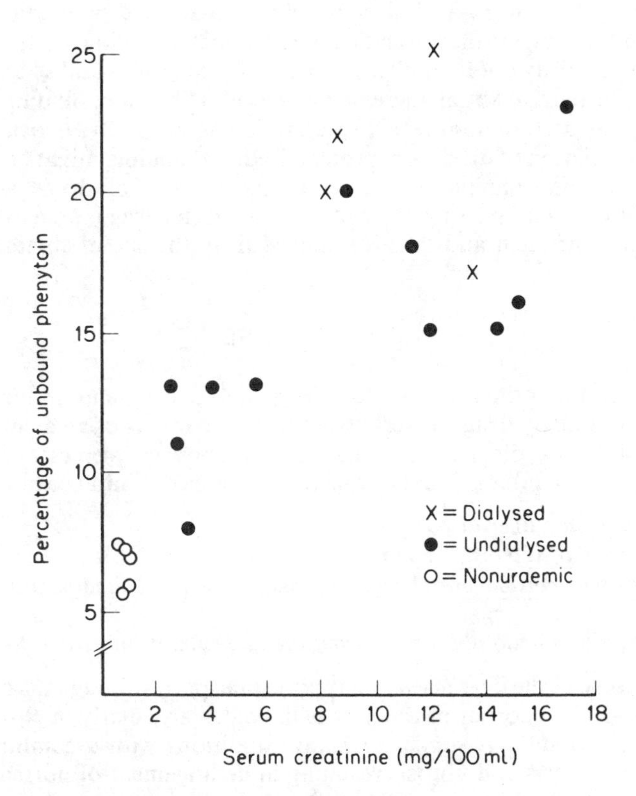

Fig. 5.7 Relationship between unbound phenytoin in plasma of 15 uraemic patients and 5 normal volunteers and serum creatinine ($r = 0.80$) (From M. M. Reidenberg *et al.* Reprinted by permission from the *New Eng. J. Med.*, **285**, 264 (1971).)

nephrotic syndrome. The defective binding cannot be corrected by dialysis but is restored to normal by successful renal transplantation. It appears to reside in the nature of the plasma protein since adding an ultrafiltrate of ureamic serum to normal plasma protein does not alter the binding properties of the protein. Charcoal treatment of uraemic serum may, however, restore normal binding properties and on these grounds it is thought that some endogenous binding inhibitor may compete for binding sites. An alternative line of research has shown differences in amino-acid composition between normal and uraemic plasma albumin, suggesting that altered protein synthesis and structure may also be involved. Since the fraction of unbound drug is associated with pharmacodynamic activity, this implies that in uraemia the total (bound and unbound) phenytoin which is necessary for control of seizures and for producing toxicity is reduced, since in this state lower total levels produce the same concentration of unbound phenytoin. In a similar fashion the hypotensive action of diazoxide is correlated with the plasma urea concentration, which in turn relates to the unbound drug fraction responsible for the vasodilator action of the drug (see Fig. 5.8).

The binding and distribution of basic drugs e.g. dapsone, quinidine, nitrofurantoin, trimethoprim, chloramphenicol and desmethylimipramine, which mainly bind to α_1-acid glycoprotein, is unaffected by uraemia.

Changes in drug–protein binding affect renal handling of drugs since protein-bound drug does not filter through the glomerulus and so an increase in free drug is reflected by an increased glomerular filtration. Binding does not affect tubular secretion since active secretion is normally associated with further dissociation of drug from protein. Reduced binding might be expected to decrease renal elimination indirectly, particularly of drugs which are extensively secreted, since a greater proportion of the drug is able to leave the vascular compartment and thus is removed from the site of elimination.

LIVER DISEASE

The liver is the principal site for drug metabolism and influences the disposition of many drugs. Liver disease in man consists of an assortment of pathophysiological disturbances which do not allow easy prediction of their effects on drug handling. Factors which must be taken into account include:

(a) *nature of the liver disease*;
(b) *alteration of intrinsic hepatic clearance of drug*;
(c) *changes in plasma protein binding and subsequent modification of drug distribution*;
(d) *alteration in drug absorption from the gastrointestinal tract.*

(a) **The nature of the liver disease** may play some part, although the repertoire of pathological responses of the liver is limited. Particularly in chronic liver disease the end stage is similar in many conditions with a combination of hepatocyte necrosis and fibrosis resulting in derangement of normal hepatic architecture. Cells that are uninvolved by fibrosis appear morphologically normal and contain normal amounts of mixed-function oxidase. Nevertheless the delicately balanced perfusion of the sinusoids is disturbed and, with

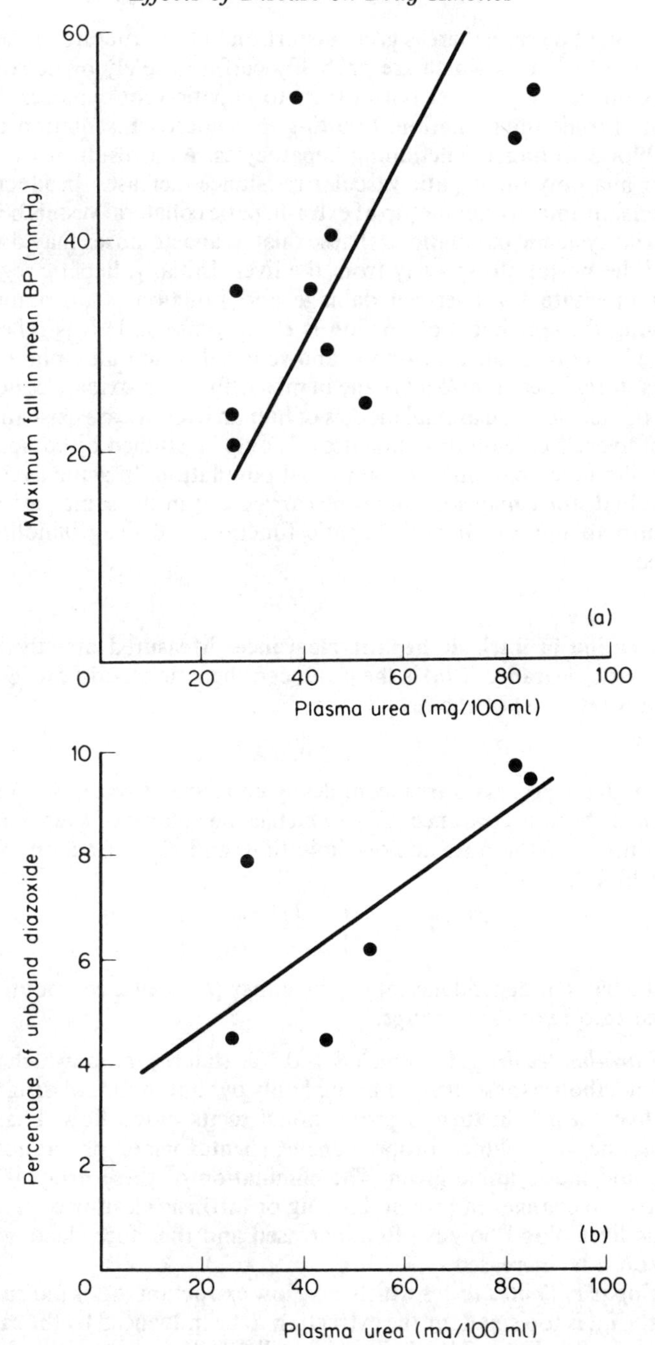

Fig. 5.8 (a) Plasma urea concentration and fall in blood pressure in 10 patients following intravenous injection of diazoxide over 10 s; (b) Plasma urea concentration and unbound diazoxide in plasma from six hypertensives incubated *in vitro* with diazoxide at 250 μg/ml (From R. M. Pearson and A. M. Breckenridge, *Brit. J. Clin. Pharm.*, **3**, 169 (1976).)

progression of disease, there is gross distortion of the structure of the liver and formation of nodules which are probably perfused solely by hepatic arterial blood. Concurrently, direct portal tract to hepatic-vein bypasses develop in areas of chronic inflammation, resulting in reduced presentation of hepatic portal blood to intact functioning hepatocytes. As a result of the distorted vascular anatomy the hepatic vascular resistance increases, producing portal hypertension and an opening-up of extra-hepatic collateral vessels between the portal and systemic circulations. These dilated anastomoses may divert up to 60% of the portal blood away from the liver. Initially, hepatic regeneration may compensate for liver-cell damage and function is maintained. With continuing damage hepatic function is compromised. This is reflected by a decreased rate of protein synthesis and reduced serum albumin and coagulation factors. There is also a decline in mixed-function oxidase concentration in liver tissue. No good animal models of human liver disease exist and thus the effect of liver disease on drug kinetics can only be studied by comparing data from well-studied patients with a normal population. In acute liver disease a longitudinal study may sometimes be carried out in the same patient so that the return to normal in both hepatic function and drug handling can be followed.

(b) **Alteration in intrinsic hepatic clearance**. Measured directly across the liver, hepatic clearance (Cl_H) is the product of hepatic blood flow (Q_L) and the extraction ratio (E) of the drug:

$$Cl_H = Q_L E. \tag{3.7}$$

Although the processes are incompletely understood, one model relates E to the intrinsic hepatic clearance (Cl_{int}) which is the volume of liver water cleared in unit time when there are no flow limitations and f_B the fraction of unbound drug in blood:

$$Cl_H = Q_L \left[\frac{f_B Cl_{int}}{Q_L + f_B Cl_{int}} \right]. \tag{3.12}$$

On the basis of dependence of Cl_H on either Q_L or Cl_{int} compounds may be classified into two main groups:

1. *Flow-limited drugs* for which $E > 0.7$, so that the rate at which the liver is able to metabolise these drugs is limited only by the amount of drug presented to the liver, which in turn is proportional to its blood flow. Examples are nortriptyline, morphine, propoxyphene, pentazocine, propranolol, aldosterone and indocyanine green. The elimination of these drugs is relatively insensitive to changes in protein binding or intrinsic clearance. In acute viral hepatitis liver blood flow is often increased and therefore clearance of such drugs could be increased.
2. *Capacity limited drugs* which have low extraction ratios indicative of the fact that Cl_{int} is too small for the extraction to be influenced by the rate of drug delivery to the liver. These drugs usually follow first order kinetics at therapeutic concentrations and the rate of metabolism is dependent on the concentration of drug at the hepatic enzymes which is dependent upon the plasma free drug concentration. On this basis the group is subdivided into:

(i) Capacity limited, binding sensitive drugs which have a high affinity for plasma protein (usually $> 80\%$ bound) and whose elimination may be affected by altered protein binding, e.g. phenytoin, tolbutamide, diazepam, warfarin, quinidine, digitoxin.

(ii) Capacity limited, binding insensitive drugs which have low plasma protein binding and whose clearance is unaffected by altered binding, e.g. theophylline, amylobarbitone, chloramphenicol, paracetamol, antipyrine.

The relationship between plasma protein binding and extraction ratio is complex but can be summarised by Fig. 5.9.

Equation (3.10) is most successful in predicting the behaviour of flow-limited drugs in states where blood flow may be altered. It has been less successful in anticipating changes in the kinetics of capacity-limited compounds. Thus correlations may be demonstrated between the hepatic clearances of propranolol (high extraction with partial elimination as metabolite) and indocyanine green (high extraction and unchanged elimination) but also, unexpectedly, with antipyrine (low extraction with complete elimination as

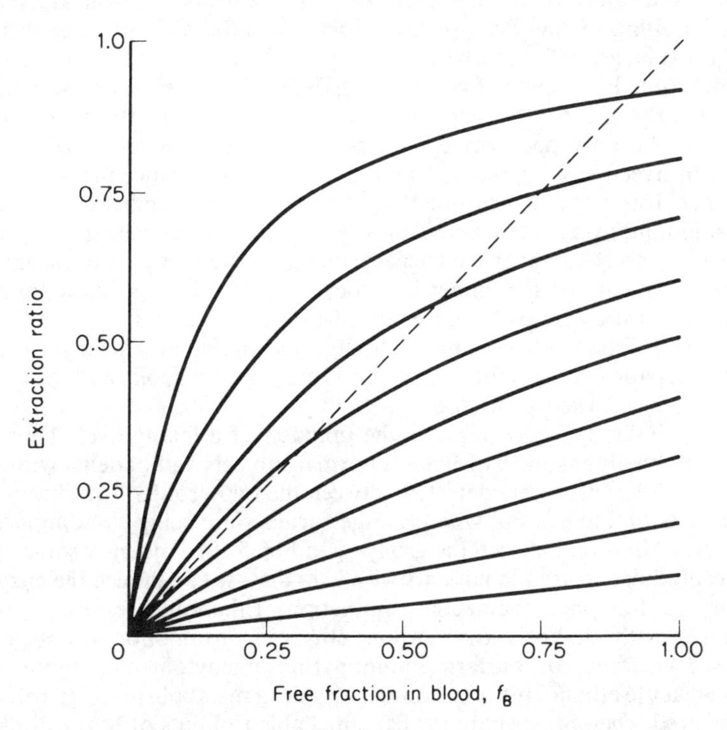

Fig. 5.9 Relationship between extraction ratio and unbound fraction of drug (f_B) according to eq. (3.12). The dashed line indicates when $E = f_B$: below this line extraction is limited to the unbound drug, above the line extraction is non-restrictive. The individual curves represent different values of Cl_{int}/Q_L corresponding to 10% stepwise changes when $f_B = 1$ (From G. R. Wilkinson and D. G. Shand, *Clin. Pharm. Ther.*, **18**, 377 (1975).)

metabolite). Theoretically this correlation might arise if flow and intrinsic hepatic clearance fall in parallel whilst hepatic extraction remains constant. Direct measurement shows this cannot be the case and the reduction in hepatic clearance and extraction ratio implies that intrinsic hepatic clearance falls to a greater extent than blood flow. Two hypotheses have been proposed to explain this parallel reduction in clearance of drugs whose elimination is limited by either flow or enzyme activity.

(i) '*The sick-cell theory*': hepatic damage decreases the intrinsic clearance of both high- and low-clearance drugs. This explains the reduced antipyrine clearance but requires an additional postulation of a proportionately greater effect on the intrinsic clearance of highly extracted drugs.
(ii) '*The intact hepatocyte theory*': disease is associated with a decreased mass of hepatocytes which function approximately normally and have normal perfusion. The reduced extraction of high-extraction drugs is then due to the operation of intrahepatic shunts bypassing these normal cells.

It must be emphasised that liver disease does not impair the metabolism of all drugs to the same extent and it is hazardous to extrapolate from knowledge of the handling of one drug in liver disease to effects on another drug. A possible explanation for this heterogeneity of effect lies in the multiple forms of cytochrome P_{450}, some of which act on different substrates and which may be differently affected by hepatocellular dysfunction. Furthermore, there appears to be only poor correlation between *in vitro* microsomal enzyme activity in liver-biopsy specimens and in vivo drug-clearance measurements. The concentration of cytochrome P_{450} and activity of a number of enzymes is normal in mild liver disease and is only decreased in specimens from patients with very severely compromised hepatic function. These observations may be evidence in favour of the 'intact hepatocyte' theory. Even when a common metabolic pathway is involved, e.g. mixed-function oxidases, some drugs are more affected than others. Thus, although antipyrine and phenytoin both undergo hepatic hydroxylation, in cirrhosis only the metabolism of the former appears to be markedly affected.

Enzyme induction may improve the function of a failing liver. Thus in a study of phenylbutazone half-lives in normal subjects and patients with liver disease no differences were detected between the two-groups. Stratification of the subjects on the basis of whether other drugs were being co-administered gave a clear division between the groups (see Fig. 5.10). Evidently some drugs such as prednisone used in patients with liver disease can induce the enzymes responsible for phenylbutazone elimination. Ethanol ingestion is often associated with cirrhosis and chronic ethanol consumption results in an increased clearance of warfarin, aminopyrine, phenytoin and tolbutamide although acute ethanol intoxication impairs drug metabolism—a factor to be remembered when prescribing for patients liable to bouts of heavy drinking. The activity of alcohol dehydrogenase in cirrhotic liver has been shown to be lowered by about half but other enzymes such as the microsomal ethanol oxidising system show increased activity, possibly in compensation, which accounts for the unchanged ethanol clearance observed in such patients.

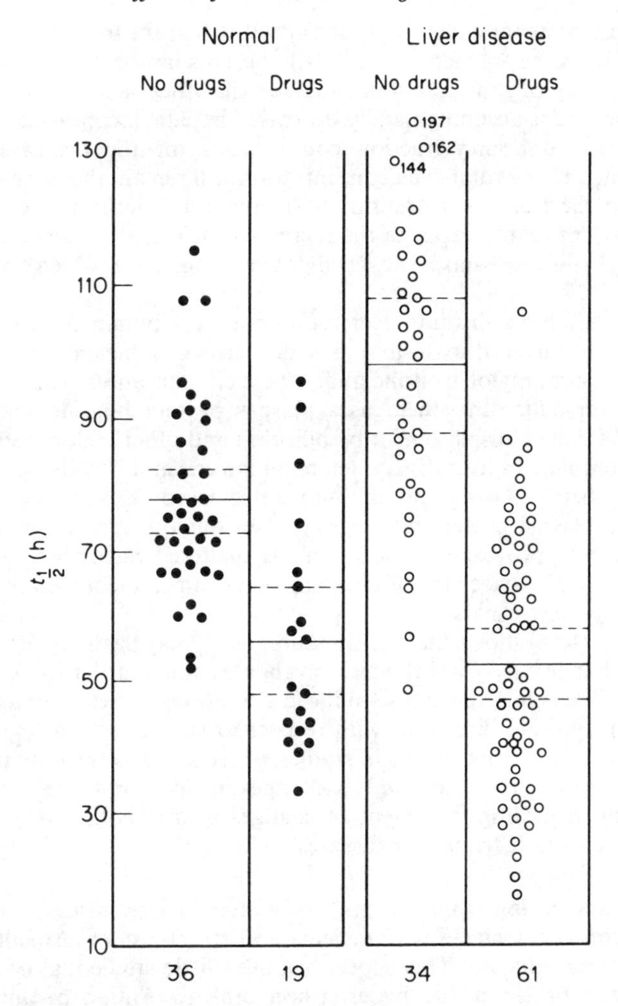

Fig. 5.10 Influence of drug treatment on phenylbutazone half-lives in normal subjects and in patients with liver disease (From A. J. Levi *et al.*, *Lancet*, **1**, 1275 (1968).)

(c) **Plasma protein binding** is often altered in liver disease. Thus the free fraction of tolbutamide is increased by 115 % in cirrhosis and that of phenytoin by up to 40 %. Failure to appreciate the effects of such changes may lead to erroneous conclusions. Decreased binding of flow-limited drugs would not be expected to alter hepatic clearance but would alter the volume of distribution, and from

$$t_{1/2\beta} = \frac{0.693\, V_{\mathrm{d}(\beta)}}{Cl}, \tag{1.14}$$

the $t_{1/2}$ will also change. This effect has been demonstrated for propranolol.

The effect of altered protein binding on the disposition of capacity-limited binding-sensitive drugs is difficult to predict. If protein binding is decreased without loss of hepatic metabolising capacity, then the total drug concentration will fall as the V_d increases (see below). This has been demonstrated for warfarin, phenytoin and tolbutamide. If, on the other hand, decreased plasma protein binding is accompanied by decreased hepatic intrinsic clearance then the increased unbound fraction compensates for the decreased hepatic metabolism and the total drug concentration will remain the same or become higher and the free concentration will increase. Clinically this can result in toxicity and probably explains the increased incidence of adverse reactions with theophylline, prednisolone, phenytoin and diazepam which occur in liver disease.

There is often an absolute decrease in plasma albumin concentrations in severe chronic liver disease and this decrease is sufficient to explain the increased V_d for amylobarbitone under these circumstances. This may also be true for ampicillin. In other cases plasma protein binding may also be influenced by drug displacement by bilirubin and other endogeneous factors which accumulate in liver disease (cf. renal failure) and it is also possible that the affinity between drug and albumin is decreased.

Reduced plasma protein binding increases the apparent volume of distribution (eq. 1.93) providing tissue binding is unaltered. Such observations have been made with diazepam, lorazepam, lignocaine, theophylline and propranolol amongst others.

Equation (1.14) shows that an alteration in V_d may partially or completely explain a change in $t_{1/2}$, a fact which invalidates much earlier work where this fact was not recognised. Disease-induced alterations in clearance and V_d may well act in opposite directions with respect to their effect on $t_{1/2}$, probably accounting for different results in studies where $t_{1/2}$ was the only pharmacokinetic estimate made. Data on $t_{1/2}$ changes in isolation therefore give little information regarding the extent of changes in metabolism or drug distribution which result from liver disease.

(d) **Drug absorption from the gut** may alter in liver disease since portal hypertension is associated with oedema and structural abnormalities of the small intestinal mucosa. This aspect has been little studied, although it has been shown that in portal hypertension oral absorption of antipyrine is delayed, sometimes by several hours.

Portocaval anastomoses allow passage of orally administered drug directly into the systemic circulation preventing hepatic first-pass metabolism from reducing drug bioavailability and suggests a possible hazard if drugs with high clearance and low therapeutic ratio are given orally. This mechanism has been confirmed in man for propranolol. The increased incidence of CNS effects from niridazole in patients with hepatosplenic schistosomiasis in contrast to other forms of this disease, has been attributed to elevated drug levels resulting from shunting of portal blood away from hepatic metabolism. The amount of unmetabolised chlormethiazole reaching the systemic circulation after an oral dose is about ten times higher in patients with advanced cirrhosis than in normal subjects. The low oral bioavailability in healthy people is due to an extensive hepatic first-pass metabolism (see Fig. 5.11). The higher availability in cirrhotics results from both shunting of portal blood past hepatic parenchyma and to reduced metabolic capacity. It is therefore necessary to use

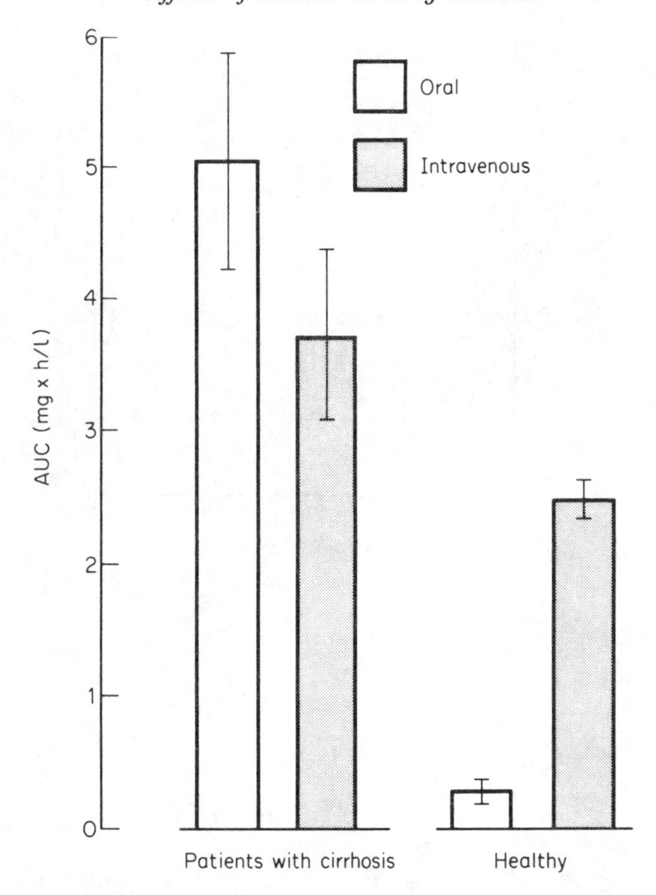

Fig. 5.11 Mean (+ SE) areas under plasma chlormethiazole concentration time curve (AUC) in eight patients with cirrhosis of liver and six healthy volunteers after oral and intravenous doses corresponding to 192 mg chlormethiazole (base) (From P. Pentikainen *et al.*, *Brit. Med. J.*, **2**, 861 (1978). Reproduced by permission of the Editor.)

reduced doses of chlormethiazole when given by mouth to patients with advanced cirrhosis. A similar phenomenon has been described for labetalol, pethidine and pentazocine.

Practical implications of altered pharmacokinetics in liver disease

At the present stage of knowledge it is difficult to discern any clear methods for predicting dosage requirements for a patient with a given degree of liver damage. Attempts to correlate changes in pharmacokinetics of drugs with tests for derangement of liver function have been generally unsuccessful in contrast to the successful use of creatinine clearance in renal impairment. In chronic liver disease, serum albumin is the most useful index of hepatic drug metabolising activity, possibly becasue a low albumin reflects depressed synthesis of hepatic proteins including those involved in drug metabolism (see

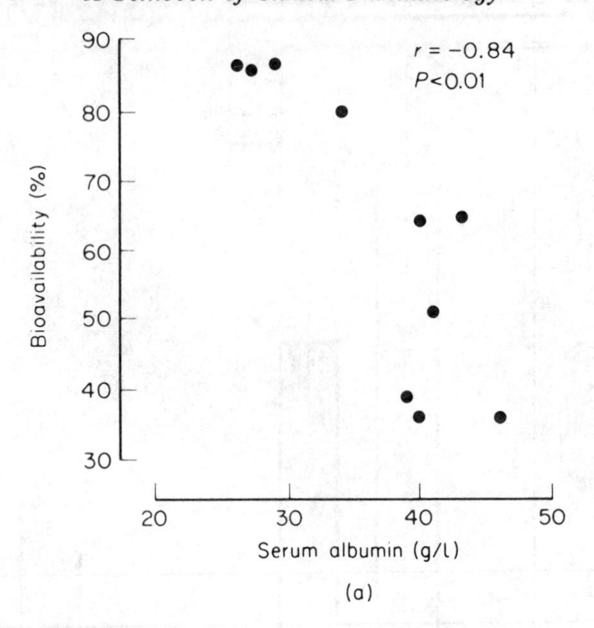

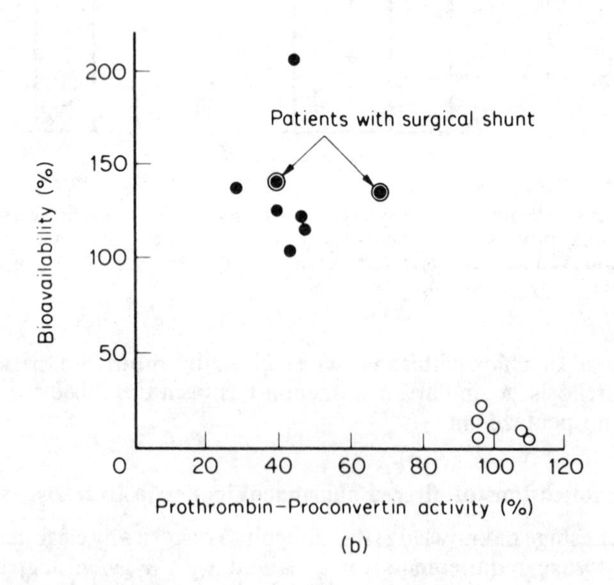

Fig. 5.12 Correlations between (a) serum albumin concentration and systemic bioavailability of labetalol in patients with liver disease (b) bioavailability of chlormethiazole and prothrombin – proconvertin activity in patients (●) and controls (○). (From (a) M. Homeida *et al.*, *Brit. Med. J.*, **2**, 1048 (1978) and (b) P. J. Pentikainen *et al.*, *Brit. Med. J.*, **2**, 861 (1978). Reproduced by permission of the Editor.)

Fig. 5.12). Prothrombin time also shows moderate correlation with drug clearance by the liver (see Fig. 5.12). However, in neither case has a continuous relationship been demonstrated and such indices of hepatic function largely serve to distinguish the severely affected from the milder cases. The use of various drugs such as indocyanine green or antipyrine as markers of hepatic function has also proved of little value, particularly in conditions like acute viral hepatitis which produce complex changes in hepatic drug handling.

Alterations in drug pharmacokinetics due to effects discussed above usually result in no more than two- to three-fold changes in plasma concentration. The significance of such changes in the absence of alterations in receptor sensitivity is questionable, for inter-individual differences of this magnitude in normal subjects are often encountered. It is probable that both the pharmacokinetic and pharmacodynamic alterations are responsible for sedative and analgesic drugs being the second most common precipitant of hepatic coma.

The use of drugs known to cause idiosyncratic liver disease, e.g. imipramine, is not necessarily contraindicated in patients with established liver disease, for there is no evidence of an increased susceptibility to further damage. Predictable hepatotoxins such as cytotoxic drugs should only be used with close biochemical monitoring. Oral contraceptives are not advisable if there is active liver disease or a history of jaundice of pregnancy, but should not be withheld after acute hepatitis if the liver-function tests have returned to normal.

In addition to the effects of liver disease on hepatocellular function the secondary effects of the disorder on other organs impose constraints upon the prescription of drugs (see Table 5.5). Thus in hepatic pre-coma brain metabolism is abnormal and extremely sensitive to a variety of centrally acting drugs, coma being easily precipitated by amounts of drug which in normal people have trivial central effects. Respiratory depressant drugs can also produce coma in patients with moderate hepatic disease because they antagonise the commonly encountered hyperventilation which appears to protect cerebral functioning. Other drugs which may produce hepatic coma are those containing ammonium which may be metabolised by gut micro-organisms to toxic substances which, bypassing the normal protective first-pass hepatic metabolism, enter the CNS. Many of these substances could act as false neurotransmitter amines and drugs which reduce their catabolism such as the monoamine oxidase inhibitors can provoke coma. Kaliuretic drugs such as thiazide diuretics also provoke encephalopathy and potassium-sparing drugs such as amiloride are preferable. Other problems encountered in hepatic disease are fluid overload and ascites which can be exacerbated by drugs causing sodium retention, e.g. phenylbutazone, carbenoxolone, or those containing sodium, e.g. large doses of intravenous penicillins. Changes in the clotting system and not in drug kinetics explain the enhanced anticoagulant response to a dose of warfarin during the acute phase of viral hepatitis.

Presently, therefore, empiricism coupled with an awareness of the possibility of adverse drug effects and plasma-level monitoring of appropriate drugs appear to be the best way to manage the patient with liver disease. Drugs should be used only if absolutely necessary and the risks weighed against any potential advantage. If possible, drugs that are eliminated by routes other than the liver should be employed.

Table 5.5 Drugs to be avoided if possible in liver disease

A.	*Precipitating coma* CNS depressant drugs, e.g. phenobarbitone, phenothiazines Thiazide and loop diuretics Opiates, e.g. pethidine, diphenoxylate (in Lomotil), pentazocine Ammonium-containing compounds Sedative tricyclic antidepressants, e.g. amitriptyline (imipramine or protriptyline which are less sedative are preferable) Monoamine oxidase inhibitors
B.	*Causing sodium retention or overload* Antacid mixtures containing sodium Carbenoxolone Phenylbutazone Large doses of intravenous penicillins, e.g. carbenicillin (contains sodium as cation)
C.	*Increasing risk of gastrointestinal haemorrhage* Liquid paraffin (reduces vitamin K absorption) Cholestyramine (reduces vitamin K absorption) Some non-narcotic analgesics, e.g. salicylates, indomethacin, phenylbutazone Broad-spectrum antibiotics (reduce vitamin K production in gut) Propylthiouracil Alcohol
D.	*Increased effect of drug or toxic effects known to occur* Oral anticoagulants (increased sensitivity) Theophylline (decreased metabolism) Oral hypoglycaemics (risk of hypoglycaemia increased with sulphonylureas; risk of lactic acidosis increased with phenformin) Suxamethonium (reduced level of pseudocholinesterase) Phenytoin (decreased metabolism) Lignocaine (prolonged and increased activity because of decreased rate of metabolism) Azathioprine (impaired metabolism, unchanged drug myelotoxic)

THYROID DISEASE

Thyroid dysfunction may affect drug disposition partly by effects upon the rate of microsomal drug metabolism and partly via changes in renal elimination. At present the existing data refer to only a handful of drugs:

(a) *Digitalis* It has been known for many years that myxoedematous patients are extremely sensitive to digitalis and that conversely larger doses of digitalis are required to control the ventricular rate in thyrotoxic atrial fibrillation. In general, hyperthyroid patients have lower plasma digoxin levels and hypothyroid patients higher plasma levels than euthyroid patients on a similar digoxin dose. No significant difference in half-life exists between these groups and a difference in the apparent volume of distribution has been postulated to explain the alteration of plasma level with thyroid activity. An increased myocardial digoxin concentration has been demonstrated in hyperthyroid dogs and rats, possibly due to an increase in myocardial $Na^+ K^+$ ATPase. Changes in renal function which occur with changes in thyroid status complicate this interpretation. The glomerular filtration rate is increased in thyrotoxicosis and decreased in myxoedema, although there is little information about changes in renal function accompanying heart failure in thyroid disease, i.e. in the patients who usually require digitalis treatment. These changes in renal function will influence elimination and the reduced plasma levels of digoxin correlate well with the increased creatinine clearance in thyrotoxicosis. In addition enhanced biliary clearance, digoxin malabsorption due to intestinal hurry and increased hepatic metabolism have all been postulated as factors in the insensitivity of thyrotoxic patients to cardiac glycosides. At the present time these clinical phenomena are inexplicable solely in terms of altered pharmacokinetics.

(b) *Antipyrine* is cleared more rapidly and has a shorter $t_{1/2}$ in thyrotoxicosis as compared to normal subjects or to the values obtained in the same patients following treatment. In hypothyroidism the plasma $t_{1/2}$ is prolonged, the clearance falls and the volume of distribution increases, these values returning to normal when treatment produces euthyroid status. These effects are believed to reflect the modulating influence of the thyroid upon hepatic metabolism.

(c) *Oral anticoagulants* produce an unduly prolonged prothrombin time in hyperthyroidism which results from increased catabolism of the vitamin K-dependent clotting factors rather than from changes in drug kinetics. The $t_{1/2}$ of both warfarin and discoumarol is unchanged by altered thyroid function.

(d) *Steroids* are metabolised by hepatic mixed-function oxidases which are influenced by thyroid status. Thus in hyperthyroidism there is increased cortisol production and a reduced cortisol half-life, the converse obtaining in myxoedema.

(e) *Thyroid hormones* The normal half-life of thyroxine (6–7 days) is reduced to 3–4 days by hyperthyroidism and prolonged to 9–10 days by hypothyroidism. This may be related to changes in hepatic blood flow and clearance. Studies in animals suggest similar changes occur in the disposition of TSH with altered thyroid status.

(f) *Antithyroid drugs* The $t_{1/2}$ of propylthiouracil and methimazole is prolonged in hypothyroidism and shortened in hyperthyroidism, these values returning to normal on attainment of the euthyroid state. These changes are correlated with similar alterations in antipyrine $t_{1/2}$ and are thought to result from altered hepatic microsomal drug metabolism.

(g) *Propranolol* The clearance of propranolol is increased by hyperthyroidism, this effect being reversed following successful treatment. There is also evidence for an increased apparent volume of distribution which may be related to the decreased plasma protein binding occurring in hyperthyroidism.

(h) *Oxazepam* Clearance is increased three-fold and half-life commensurately shortened in hyperthyroidism suggesting that higher doses or more frequent administration will be needed in such cases.

Chapter 6
DRUGS IN PREGNANCY AND AT THE EXTREMES OF AGE

DRUGS IN PREGNANCY

Drugs which are given to a pregnant woman may affect the fetus in several ways:

(a) They may interfere with some important physiological function in the mother and so indirectly damage the fetus. For instance, if the maternal circulation is sufficiently reduced as a result of drug action, the placental function will be compromised with ultimate fetal death.
(b) Drugs may pass from the mother to the fetus via the placenta. The changes which are occurring rapidly in the fetus make it unduly susceptible to the action of certain drugs which are apparently harmless to the mother.

Little is known about the changes in pharmacokinetics produced by pregnancy in man. Ethical and practical considerations make such studies difficult. There is no evidence however that pregnancy changes pharmacological response and differences in drug effects where they are known are invariably explained by altered pharmacokinetics.

The effects of pregnancy on drug disposition

1. *Absorption* Gastric emptying and small intestinal motility are reduced probably by hormonal factors. This is apparently of little consequence except during labour when the drugs should be given parenterally if rapid action is required.

2. *Distribution* During pregnancy the blood volume increases by a third with the expansion in plasma volume from 2.5 l to 4 l at term being greater than the increase in red cell mass so that the haematocrit falls. There is also an increase in body water due to a larger extravascular volume and the development of organs such as uterus and breasts concerned with pregnancy and the products of conception. Oedema, which at least one third of women experience during pregnancy, may add another 8 l to the volume of extracellular water. For water-soluble drugs (which usually have a relatively small volume of distribution) this increases the apparent volume of distribution and although clearance is unaltered their half-life is prolonged.

During pregnancy plasma protein concentration falls, e.g. plasma albumin decreases by 5–10 g/1 and there is increased competition for binding sites on α_1 acid glycoprotein due to competition by endogenous liquids such as increased hormone levels.

These factors reduce the total amount of drug bound and also expand the apparent volume of distribution. The concentration of free drug however tends to remain unaltered. There are two reasons for this: a greater volume of distribution for free drug accompanied by an increased clearance of free drug. Thus the lower total plasma level of drug is cancelled by the increased free drug fraction so that in practice these changes are rarely of pharmacological significance. They may however cause confusion in monitoring of plasma drug levels since these usually measure only total plasma drug concentration. Thus phenytoin plasma concentration may fall during pregnancy but, because the free fraction increases, there is no need to increase the daily dose. This situation is analogous to that arising in renal failure (p. 133).

3. *Metabolism* of drugs by the pregnant liver is increased, largely due to enzyme induction perhaps by the raised hormone levels in pregnancy. This has been documented for a few drugs such as carbamazepine but the importance of this factor is largely unknown.

4. *Excretion* of drugs via the kidney is increased since during pregnancy the renal plasma flow almost doubles and the glomerular filtration rate increases by two thirds. This has been shown for digoxin, lithium, ampicillin, cephalexin and gentamicin. Most of the alterations are insufficient to be of clinical importance but this may be because no-one has ever looked.

Placental transfer of drugs

In the placenta the maternal blood is separated from the fetal blood by a cellular membrane. The diffusion path is longer in early pregnancy (25 μm) than in late pregnancy (2 μm). Drugs can cross the placenta either by an active transport system or by passive diffusion down the concentration gradient, and it is the latter which is usually involved in drug transfer. Diffusion across the placenta is governed by the same principles which apply when drugs cross cell barriers in other parts of the body. The rate of diffusion depends on:

(a) The concentration of free drug (i.e. not protein bound) on each side of the barrier.
(b) The lipid solubility of the drug.
(c) The degree of ionisation of the drug. Diffusion will only occur if the drug is in the non-ionised state. The degree of ionisation will depend in turn on the pH of the medium in which it is dissolved and on the pKa of the drug.

If a drug can be absorbed from the gut it can usually also cross the placenta into the fetus.

Placental function will also be modified by changes in blood flow which in turn may alter the response to drugs. It is possible that the placenta itself may be able to modify drugs and their actions since the placenta possesses a mixed-function oxidase system, the activity of which is enhanced by smoking. Enzymes are thus present which are capable of drug metabolism but the extent to which this potential is utilised in man is unknown.

Effects of drugs on the fetus

The fetus is liable to be damaged at three main stages in pregnancy:

1. *Implantation* (5–17 days)—interference with the fetus will lead to abortion.
2. *Embryonic stage* (17–57 days)—at this stage the fetus is differentiating to form major organs. Drugs which interfere with this process cause gross structural abnormalities such as absence of limbs, congenital heart lesions etc. Thalidomide produced its defects during this stage of fetal development.
3. *Fetogenic stage*—in this stage the formed fetus undergoes further development and maturation, and although drug damage is less likely it is still possible and the uncontrolled use of drugs is to be discouraged.

Drugs (or other factors) producing deviations or abnormalities in the development of the embryo that are compatible with prenatal life and are observable post-natally are called teratogens. True teratogens cause such anomalies at lower doses than are necessary to cause a toxic effect on the mother or fetus. Table 6.1 shows generally accepted human teratogens. Thalidomide was unusual in the way in which a very small dose of the drug given on only one or two occasions between the 4th and 7th week of pregnancy produced serious malformations. Despite its wide use it was nearly four years before these adverse effects were recognised (cf. other adverse reactions to drugs).

Table 6.1 Drug-induced teratogenesis

A. *Positively implicated as teratogenic*

(i) Thalidomide
(ii) Androgens and some progestogens, e.g. ethisterone
(iii) Oestrogens including diethylstilboestrol
(iv) Many cytotoxic drugs, especially methotrexate, chlorambucil, cyclophosphamide, busulphan
(v) Some anticonvulsants – phenytoin, troxidone, sodium valproate
(vi) Ethanol
(vii) Tetracycline
(viii) Etretinate

B. *Suspected of teratogenic potential*

(i) Oral anticoagulants
(ii) Corticosteroids
(iii) Some cytotoxics including colchicine, vinca alkaloids, actinomycin D, azathioprine
(iv) Anorectics
(v) Carbamazepine
(vi) Phenobarbitone
(vii) Organic solvents
(viii) Gaseous anaesthetics
(ix) Lithium
(x) Anti-tuberculosis drugs: rifampicin, PAS
(xi) Quinine (large doses only)
(xii) High doses vitamin D

Recognition of teratogenic drugs The incidence of serious congenital abnormality is about 2% of all births and probably 1–5% of these are due to drugs.

Two problems face those who try to determine whether a drug is teratogenic when it is used to treat disease in humans:

(a) Many drugs, when given experimentally in large doses to animals, can be shown to produce fetal defects, but this does not necessarily mean that they are teratogenic in man when given in therapeutic doses. Indeed, the metabolism and kinetics of drugs in high doses in other species is so different as to make such studies almost irrelevant.

(b) Fetal defects frequently occur even without drugs. If the incidence of drug-induced abnormalities is low, a very large number of infants will have to be studied to obtain a significant answer. Effects on the fetus may take several years to become clinically manifest, a good example being the high incidence of adenocarcinoma of the vagina which occurred in their late teens in girls whose mothers had been given diethylstilboestrol when they were pregnant. It is therefore best to reduce drug taking to a minimum during the whole pregnancy and whenever possible use only those drugs which have been proved by long usage to be safe.

One interesting problem is why only a proportion of fetuses exposed to a teratogen develop an abnormality. It has been suggested that there are inherited differences in fetal drug metabolising enzymes which may lead in certain cases to the production of a teratogenic metabolite. There is experimental work in animals to support this idea but no clear evidence in man.

Distribution of drugs in the fetus This has been studied in animals by giving radioactively labelled drugs to the mother and comparing distribution in mother and fetus. Generally the distribution is very similar, although there is often a higher uptake by the maternal liver, presumably reflecting the more active metabolism at that site in the adult. Certain drugs are concentrated at particular sites in the fetus, e.g. tetracyline—the skeleton; chlorpromazine—the eye; chloroquine—the eye; thiouracil—the thyroid.

Drug metabolism in the fetus There is evidence that the P_{450} oxidase system is active in the fetal liver within the first three months of pregnancy, and it increases in activity into the second trimester. It is not known whether this is of any practical importance, but drug metabolites have been found in the fetus.

Drug exposure during pregnancy A retrospective study carried out in Scotland in 1972 found that the average number of drugs taken during pregnancy was 4.2, not including drugs given during labour and delivery. The most commonly taken drugs are analgesics, antihistamines, diuretics; bronchodilators and caffeine. It is unfortunate that the signs of pregnancy may be sufficiently delayed that drugs are prescribed to a woman before either she or her doctor realises that she is pregnant, thus exposing the embryo to potential damage. Only a prescribing policy which recognises that any woman of child-bearing age may be pregnant can prevent this risk. During labour and delivery the fetus is exposed to a relatively large number of drugs in a short interval, in one study from the USA the usual number of drugs given was 3, the maximum being 26. The commonly encountered drugs are pethidine, oxytocin, barbiturates, diazepam, caffeine and aspirin. As a result of placental transfer most infants at birth have drugs and drug metabolites stored in their tissues in up to milligram quantities. These are excreted in the first few days after delivery and consequently the urinary drug profile of the neonate is strikingly similar to that of the mother.

SOME INDIVIDUAL DRUGS IN PREGNANCY

Analgesics *Opiates* cross the placenta. This is important in the management of labour as the use of narcotics which will depress the fetal respiratory centre may inhibit the start of normal respiration after birth. If the mother is dependent on opiates the fetus may show distress if the drug is withdrawn and this is liable to occur during childbirth. The infant may also develop withdrawal symptoms after delivery which may be delayed up to three days and can be fatal. In neonates the chief withdrawal symptoms are tremor, irritability, diarrhoea and vomiting. The treatment of withdrawal symptoms in the neonate is chlorpromazine 1.0 mg/kg four hourly, gradually reduced over four to six weeks.

Salicylates given in early pregnancy have been reported to be associated with achondroplasia, hydrocephalus, congenital heart disease and skeletal abnormalities but the case is not proven. They can also produce hypothrombinaemia which can cause bleeding in the neonate. Salicylates are not teratogenic but due to their antiprostaglandin effect, if taken in late pregnancy, they increase post-partum haemorrhage and delay labour (with consequent post-maturity). Large doses could produce kernicterus by displacing bilirubin from protein binding. In the neonate, premature closure of the ductus arteriosus, persistent pulmonary hypertension and haemorrhage due to altered platelet function result from inhibition of prostaglandin synthesis. Paracetamol should replace aspirin in pregnancy when mild analgesia is required.

Indomethacin can cause premature closure of the ductus arteriosus in the fetus leading to pulmonary hypertension in the newborn.

Local anaesthetics (used for regional anaesthesia) readily cross the placenta and may cause fetal methaemoglobinaemia. High doses producing maternal hypotension have caused reduced placental perfusion and fetal distress.

General anaesthetics Neonatal depression has been noted after ether and cyclopropane and depends upon the duration of maternal inhalation.

Although a causal relation is not proved, several studies have shown an increased incidence of spontaneous abortion and perhaps of congenital abnormalities in the infants of women working in operating theatres.

Antibiotics *Tetracyclines* are teratogenic. They also cause depression of bone growth and staining of the teeth with hypoplasia of the enamel from about the eighteenth week of pregnancy until the child is about eight years old, so should be avoided if possible.

Sulphonamides do not appear to be teratogenic, but cotrimoxazole is under some suspicion since trimethoprim is an anti-folate and should not be given during pregnancy. If sulphonamides are used at the end of pregnancy they displace bilirubin from the plasma protein in the neonate and increase the risk of kernicterus. This is especially a risk with long-acting sulphonamides which are highly protein bound and persist in the circulation for several days. Novobiocin has similar effects to sulphonamides.

Streptomycin and other aminoglycosides can damage the eighth cranial nerve of the fetus and cause deafness. They should be avoided unless necessary.

Chloramphenicol is poorly metabolised by the fetus and in neonates can lead to severe toxicity (see below). It should be avoided in pregnancy.

Penicillins appear to be free from ill effects on the fetus.

Antiemetics Nausea is common in the early months of pregnancy. *Meclozine* and *cyclizine* are frequently used to combat this problem. Although they have been suspected from time to time of having some teratogenic effects, this has been widely investigated and never confirmed.

Cytotoxics Although many normal births have been reported in those taking cytotoxic drugs, there are powerful reasons for believing them to increase the risk of fetal abnormality. Anti-folate drugs such as methotrexate are known teratogens in man and produce absence of digits and cranial abnormalities.

Anticonvulsants Here the position is difficult to assess. Fetal abnormalities are approximately twice as common in the children of epileptic mothers. Whether this is due specifically to an anti-epileptic drug or to other factors is not known. *Phenytoin* has been associated with a specific 'hydantoin syndrome' (craniofacial defects, microcephaly, nail and digital hypoplasia, mental deficiency, growth retardation). *Troxidone* may have an even higher potential to produce such effects including cardiac anomalies. A variety of abnormalities, especially spina bifida, have been associated with sodium valproate and carbamazepine has been linked with retardation of fetal head growth. The mechanism of all these effects may involve folate metabolism. There is no definite evidence that phenobarbitone is teratogenic, although it may increase the risks due to other anticonvulsants. No anticonvulsant is definitely free of teratogenic risk but most epileptic mothers have normal babies and the risks do not justify changing the drug regime if the epilepsy is well controlled. Good seizure control should be achieved, if possible, with a single drug at minimum dosage with plasma concentration monitoring. Folate supplements may be advisable and vitamin K should be given in late pregnancy to prevent neonatal coagulation defects (phenytoin and phenobarbitone have been associated with haemorrhagic disease of the newborn).

Carbamazepine may be the favoured anticonvulsant in pregnancy.

Oral anticoagulants Coumarins have been associated with nasal hypoplasia and chondrodysplasia when given in the first trimester and CNS abnormalities after administration in later pregnancy although absolute proof of causation is lacking. Warfarin is associated with a high incidence of haemorrhagic complications towards the end of pregnancy: neonatal haemorrhage is difficult to prevent because of the immature enzymes in fetal liver and low stores of vitamin K. Heparin, which does not cross the placenta, is the anticoagulant of choice in pregnancy although chronic use can cause maternal osteoporosis (see p. 600).

Antidiabetic drugs Sulphonylureas may be associated with fetal abnormalities and prolonged neonatal hypoglycaemia. During pregnancy diabetes is best controlled by insulin.

Hormones *Progestogens*, particularly synthetic ones, can masculinise the female fetus. There is no evidence that this occurs with the small amount of progestogen in the oral contraceptive: the risk applies only to the large doses used to prevent abortion. *Oestrogens* have a similar effect but only if given for a long time: care is needed in prescribing them for vaginal disorders, pruritus or dysmenorrhoea when pregnancy is possible. *Diethylstilboestrol* has caused vaginal adenocarcinoma some 20 years later in the daughters of mothers so treated. Androgens masculinise the fetus.

Corticosteroids These do not appear to give rise to any serious problems. Transient suppression of the fetal hypothalamic-pituitary-adrenal axis has been reported. Rarely cleft palate and congenital cataract have been linked with steroid administration in pregnancy.

Tranquillisers *Barbiturates* may depress the respiration of the neonate as does *diazepam*. These drugs accumulate in the tissues and are slowly eliminated by the neonate, resulting in prolonged hypotonia ('floppy baby'), subnormal temperatures, periodic cessation of respiration and poor sucking. *Chlorpromazine* and other *phenothiazines* given chronically in high doses to the mother may cause retinal damage to the fetus. There is also the fear that future intellectual development could be impaired by exposure of the developing brain to tranquillisers.

Ethanol Excessive ethanol consumption is associated with spontaneous abortion, craniofacial abnormalities, mental retardation, congenital heart disease and impaired growth. Even moderate alcohol intake may adversely affect the baby: the risk of having an abnormal child is about 10% in mothers drinking 30–60 ml ethanol/day rising to 40% in chronic alcoholics.

Lithium may cause fetal goitre and possibly cardiovascular abnormalities.

Iodine and antithyroid drugs Iodine and radio-iodine cross the placenta as does carbimazole and related drugs and can cause hypothyroidism and goitre. The latter drugs should be used in half dosage during the later stages of pregnancy to avoid this.

Antihypertensive agents *Reserpine* may cause fetal bradycardia, neonatal hypothermia and engorgement of the nasal mucous membrane which can cause dangerous respiratory obstruction and imrair feeding. *Thiazides* have allegedly caused thrombocytopenic purpura. *Diazoxide* can interfere with hair growth. *Beta-blockers* are controversial. They have been reported as causing bradycardia and hypoglycaemia but equally oxprenolol has been shown to be satisfactory in the control of maternal blood pressure in hypertensive subjects.

DRUGS IN NEONATES AND CHILDREN

Much less is known about the rational use of drugs in children and knowledge of paediatric pharmacokinetics is rudimentary. This reflects the greater ethical difficulties in performing studies in minors as well as the technical difficulties involved. This has led to these patients being labelled 'therapeutic orphans' in the USA where 78 % of all drugs available in 1976 had not been fully approved as safe and efficacious for use in children according to FDA standards. Children are not miniature adults with respect to their handling of drugs and many differences may be noted.

1. Drug absorption

The anatomy and functions of the gut vary almost continuously from birth until adulthood. The most striking changes occur during the first month of life. The gastric pH at birth is usually 6–8 but within a few hours falls to 2 and then rises again since virtual achlorhydria occurs for several days. As the gastric mucosa develops the acidity increases again until age 3 when adult values are attained. The gastric emptying time is prolonged (up to 8 h) in neonates and approaches adult values only after 6 months. Changes in intestinal microorganisms which may play a part in drug metabolism (see p. 54) also occur.

There is little information about absorption from the gut in the newborn, on the whole it appears to be similar to that found in the adult. Ampicillin and benzylpenicillin are better absorbed by the neonate (60 %) compared with about 30 % in the adult after oral dosage due to the relative achlorhydria. Other drugs which are adequately absorbed and are sometimes used in the neonate include digoxin, sulphonamides, diazepam and trimethoprim. In older children absorption is generally comparable with adults although a few drugs such as imipramine, clonazepam, valproate and phenobarbitone may actually be absorbed more rapidly.

The thinner stratum corneum and higher degree of hydration of the skin of newborns and infants allows drugs to be more easily absorbed through the skin early in life. There have been reports of toxicity from the antiseptic hexachlorophane when applied several times daily to the skin or mucous membranes, particularly in premature babies or when the skin is excoriated.

2. Distribution

The newborn is characterised by a high content of total body water and low body fat. After birth body water falls from about 75 % body weight to adult values (60 %) at about a year. Extracellular water is also high at birth (45 %) and reaches adult values (17 %) at age 10–15. On the contrary, intracellular water is low at birth (33 %) and rises to the adult 40 % at about age 4. Since drugs are distributed between fat and water depending upon their physicochemical characteristics it is clear that these changes will alter the apparent volume of distribution (V_d) of drugs. The majority of drugs have a larger distribution volume during infancy than in adults but for a few drugs, e.g. ethosuximide, clindamycin, the reverse has been found. The pattern for digoxin appears to be unique: the V_d is only slightly larger than adults in early infancy but is as much as three times larger than in adults in the older infant and child.

In the newborn a decreased plasma protein binding for drugs such as imipramine, phenylbutazone, and sulphonamides has been demonstrated, although this reaches normal levels by about 3 months. Despite the presence of plasma albumin in concentrations equivalent to those in adults the total protein level is lower and a number of other factors are operative:

(a) presence of fetal albumin which has low drug binding capacity
(b) presence of competing substances, e.g. bilirubin for binding sites
(c) lower blood pH

Of practical importance is the interaction which occurs between bilirubin and various drugs for binding sites on the plasma albumin. Drugs may displace bilirubin in the plasma and the resulting increase in free bilirubin may cause kernicterus with neurological damage. Drugs which have been implicated and which should be avoided in the first weeks of life include sulphonamides, aspirin, tolbutamide and vitamin K analogues.

3. Drug metabolism

Most studies suggest that drug metabolism is slower in the newborn and probably reaches the adult rate in about one month, although there may be considerable individual variation. Enzyme systems which have been investigated and found deficient are the glucuronidation and N-dealkylation pathways. Neonatal inability to glucuronidate chloramphenicol is responsible for the occurrence of the 'grey baby' syndrome which is cardiovascular shock secondary to high concentrations of unchanged chloramphenicol (p. 724). Thus zero-order kinetics have been demonstrated for aspirin, phenobarbitone and phenytoin in neonates presumably due to inefficiency of the former system. Oxidation and hydroxylation develop relatively early and together with other conjugation mechanisms assume greater importance as a result of the inefficiency of glucuronide formation.

Caffeine provides an illustration of the slowed drug elimination in neonates in that the plasma $t_{1/2}$ in infants is approximately 4 days whereas in adults it is about 4 hours. Since the $t_{1/2}$ of many drugs is prolonged in infants it is important to realise that active drug and metabolites may persist in neonatal tissues for weeks. It is not known whether this is harmful but it is a warning that the minimum number of drugs should be given to mother and newborn.

Among the substances with apparent delay in clearance from the plasma of neonates are:

Nortriptyline	Tolbutamide	Caffeine
Sulphadiazine	Diazepam	Amylobarbitone
Chloramphenicol	Phenytoin	Salicylate

It is possible to induce faster metabolism in the liver by using enzyme inducers, of which phenobarbitone has been the most widely studied. It has been used therapeutically in the treatment of hyperbilirubinaemia of the newborn, in whom phenobarbitone administration increases the amount of glucuronyl transferase and bilirubin binding protein in the liver. The drug is given either to the mother a few days before delivery or to the neonate directly it is born, and it has been shown that it increases the rate of glucuronide formation and causes a rapid decrease in the serum bilirubin level.

Older children may paradoxically appear to metabolise drugs at rates of up to twice those in adults. This has been reported for antipyrine, phenylbutazone, diazoxide, phenobarbitone and clindamycin, which are metabolised primarily by the mixed-function oxidase system dependent upon cytochrome P_{450}. One explanation could be that the ratio of the weight of the liver to body weight may be up to 50% higher than in adults.

4. Renal excretion

Renal function is impaired in the newborn, the GFR being only $20\ ml/1.7\ m^2/min$ and does not reach surface-area-adjusted adult levels until about six months after birth. Decreased elimination of drugs which are excreted via the kidney has been shown after giving various penicillins, aminoglycosides, chloramphenicol and its metabolites, and digoxin. Thus the plasma $t_{1/2}$ for gentamicin has been found to be 18 h in premature infants less than 48 h old, 6 h in premature infants 5–22 days old, 3 h in infants 1–4 weeks old and 2 h in adults.

The effect of diuretics depends upon their concentration in renal tissue. Since the tubular secretion of drugs does not reach adult levels until about six months the maximal diuretic effect in neonates is only achieved by administration of a relatively higher dosage than in adults.

Adverse reactions in the neonate

It is often difficult to pick out the side effects which are clinically important from a mass of theoretical possibilities which rarely, if ever, occur. The list below does not claim to be complete.

Drug	*Syndrome in the neonate*
Chloramphenicol	'Grey' syndrome
Opiates (to the mother during labour)	Respiratory depression
Sulphonamides, etc.	Kernicterus (see p. 39)
Hexachlorophane	Irritability fits, death
Oxygen	Retrolental fibroplasia
Phenacetin	Methaemoglobinaemia

Drugs in breast milk

Essentially the drug has to pass from the capillary in the breast tissue to the lumen of the secreting alveolus. The extent to which this occurs probably depends on various factors.

(1) The concentration of free drug in the plasma.
(2) The degree of ionisation of the drug in the plasma (i.e. pK_a) and thus the amount of unionised drug which could diffuse across lipid membranes.

(3) The lipid solubility of the drug.
(4) Protein binding and lipid solubility of the drug in milk.

In addition, there are factors modifying the volume of milk produced including blood flow to the breast, various hormonal influences, adequate suckling and general nutrition. Information on this subject is still fragmentary.

Table 6.2 lists drugs which should not be given to the nursing mother as they may injure the neonate. There are other drugs which may cause less severe adverse effects.

Table 6.2 Drugs which should not be given to a nursing mother

Chloramphenicol	Oestrogens
Isoniazid	Atropine
Tetracycline	Indomethacin
Nalidixic acid	Phenylbutazone
Phenindione*	Carbimazole
Lithium	Iodides
Cytotoxics	Ergotamine
Senna	Vitamins A and D

* NB Warfarin is safe

Drug doses in children

In general children require smaller doses of drugs than adults and the dose is dependent on size. Several formulae are used to calculate the reduced dose:

1. $$\text{Dose} = \frac{\text{age (years)}}{20} \times \text{adult dose}$$

2. $$\text{Dose} = \frac{\text{patient's weight in kg}}{70} \times \text{adult dose}$$

3. $$\text{Dose} = \frac{\text{patient's body surface area (m}^2\text{)}}{1.7} \times \text{adult dose}$$

All these methods are only approximate and with some drugs do not give a dose which will produce the desired pharmacological effect. The main problem is that dosing by weight is most satisfactory in estimating a loading dose but is less satisfactory for estimating maintenance dose, which is often dependent on the rate of metabolism and therefore more closely related to surface area. Doses related to age nearly always underestimate the required dose, the error becoming greater the younger the child.

Finally, it must be borne in mind that changes in body composition may occur rapidly when the child is ill. If this is extreme it could appreciably affect drug distribution and metabolism.

DRUGS IN OLD AGE

The proportion of elderly people in the population of the UK is increasing steadily. The elderly are subject to a variety of complaints many of which are chronic and incapacitating, and so they receive a great deal of drug treatment. The elderly comprise 12% of the population but consume about one third of the National Health Service's drug expenditure. Clinical studies show that the adverse drug reactions become more common with increasing age. Thus in one study in the age group 41–50 years, 11.8% of patients experienced adverse reactions to drugs but in the 80+ years group the incidence increased to 25%. There are several reasons for this:

(a) They take more drugs. In one survey in general practice, 87% of patients over 75 were on regular drug therapy with 34% taking three to four different drugs daily. The most commonly prescribed drugs were diuretics (34% of patients), analgesics (27%), tranquillisers and anti-depressants (24%), hypnotics (22%) and digitalis (20%).

(b) Pharmacokinetics change with increasing age (see Fig. 6.1) and this may lead to higher plasma levels of drugs and thus an increased liability to side effects (see below).

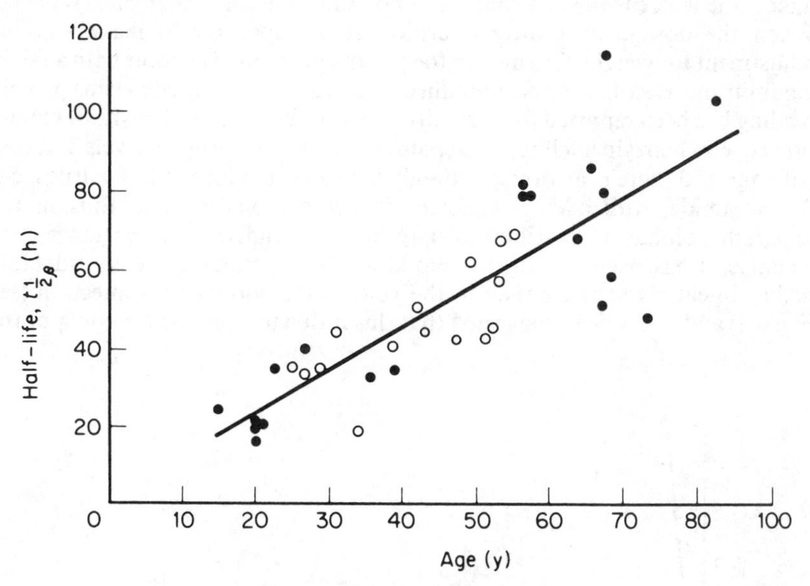

Fig. 6.1 Relationship between diazepam half-life and age in 33 normal individuals. Solid circles refer to non-smokers and open circles to smokers (From U. Klotz *et al.*, *J. Clin. Invest.*, **55**, 347 (1975).)

(c) Homeostatic mechanisms become less effective with advancing age, therefore drugs which interfere with homeostasis will produce increased effects.

(d) Some systems, particularly the central nervous system, become more sensitive to the action of certain drugs.

(e) Increasing age produces changes in the immune response and this may lead to an increased liability to allergic reactions.

Pharmacokinetics

1. Drug absorption in the elderly There is evidence of impaired absorption in old people but this is mainly concerned with complex transport systems which are necessary for the absorption of many nutrients. Thus iron, xylose, galactose, calcium and thiamine absorption are reduced in old people. Most drugs are absorbed by simple diffusion down the concentration gradient and this would not be expected to be impaired by age. Intestinal blood flow is reduced by up to 50% in the elderly and gastric motility is increased, probably due to the tendency towards reduced acid secretion in the old. Although these factors might be expected to alter drug absorption, such evidence as exists suggests that age does not affect drug absorption provided gastrointestinal function is normal.

2. Drug distribution Ageing is associated with loss of weight and lean body mass and an increased ratio of fat to muscle and body water. This enlarges the volume of distribution of fat-soluble drugs such as diazepam (Fig. 6.4) and lignocaine whereas the distribution of polar drugs such as digoxin is reduced. When the dosage of a drug is critical it is important to make suitable adjustment for weight. Changes in the plasma proteins also occur with a fall in albumin and a rise in gamma globulin concentrations. Reduced plasma protein binding has been reported for some drugs, e.g. tolbutamide, phenytoin, but not others, e.g. benzylpenicillin, diazepam. α_1-acid glycoprotein levels increase with age and there is a correspondingly increased binding of basic drugs, e.g. disopyramide, with ageing. Changes in protein binding and thus in the apparent volume of distribution may be of considerable importance. For instance, it has been shown that blood levels of pethidine are considerably higher in elderly subjects than in the young after intravenous injection (see Fig. 6.2) and it has been suggested that this is due to decreased binding of the

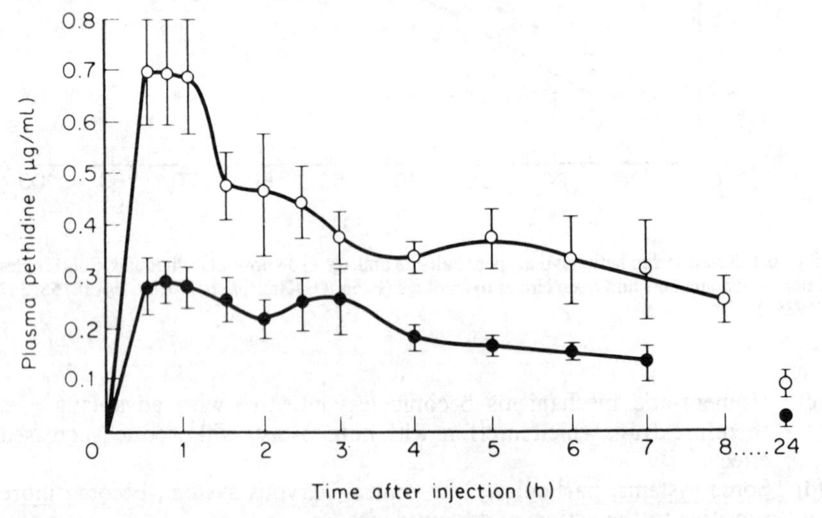

Fig. 6.2 Plasma pethidine concentrations following an intramuscular injection of 1.5 mg/kg to young, ● (16–40 years), and old, ○ (over 70 years), subjects (From K. Chan *et al.*, *Brit. J. Clin. Pharm.*, **2**, 297 (1975).)

pethidine to plasma protein (Fig. 6.3) and at other sites thus reducing the apparent volume of distribution. Similarly the fall in plasma protein which occurs with age causes an increase in the proportion of free and active drug in those drugs which are protein bound. With warfarin which is highly protein bound, there will be an excess of free drug in the plasma of elderly patients after a standard adult dose, and therefore an increased risk of bleeding. In the same way phenytoin clearance is greater in the elderly and this is associated with decreased plasma protein binding of the drug. The affinity of plasma protein for phenytoin does not alter with age and this decreased binding capacity reflects the decreased amount of albumin in the plasma of old people.

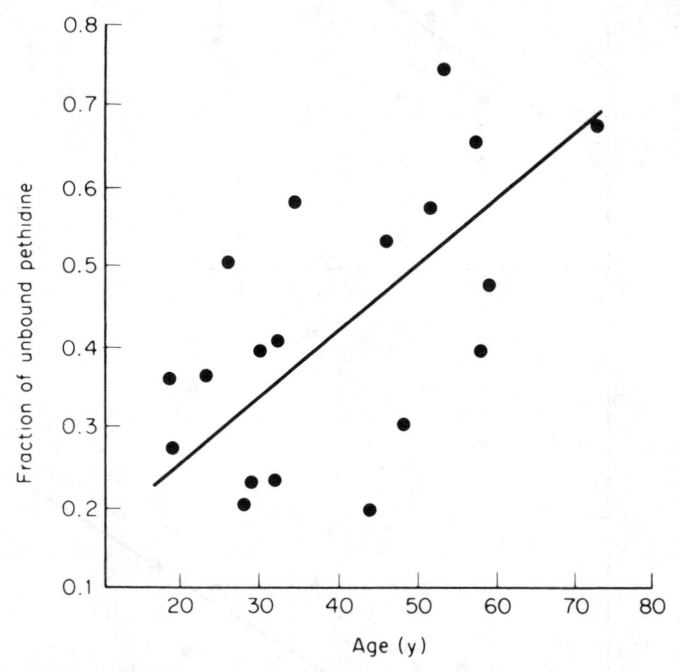

Fig. 6.3 Relationship of plasma binding of pethidine and age (From L. E. Mather *et al.*, *Clin. Pharm. Ther.*, **17**, 21 (1975).)

3. Metabolism Many drugs are metabolised in the liver to water-soluble compounds and then excreted via the kidneys. There is a general decrease in protein synthesis in the elderly so it would not be surprising if enzyme activity decreased concurrently. Indirect evidence suggests that there is a decrease in the rate of enzymic degradation of some, but not all, drugs with advancing age. Most of the studies depend on demonstrating a prolonged plasma half-life which could be secondary to an increased apparent volume of distribution (Fig. 6.4). Ideally changes in clearance with age should be documented to confirm that ageing reduces drug metabolism. Phase I oxidative drug metabolism has been shown to be significantly decreased in old age for some but not all drugs:

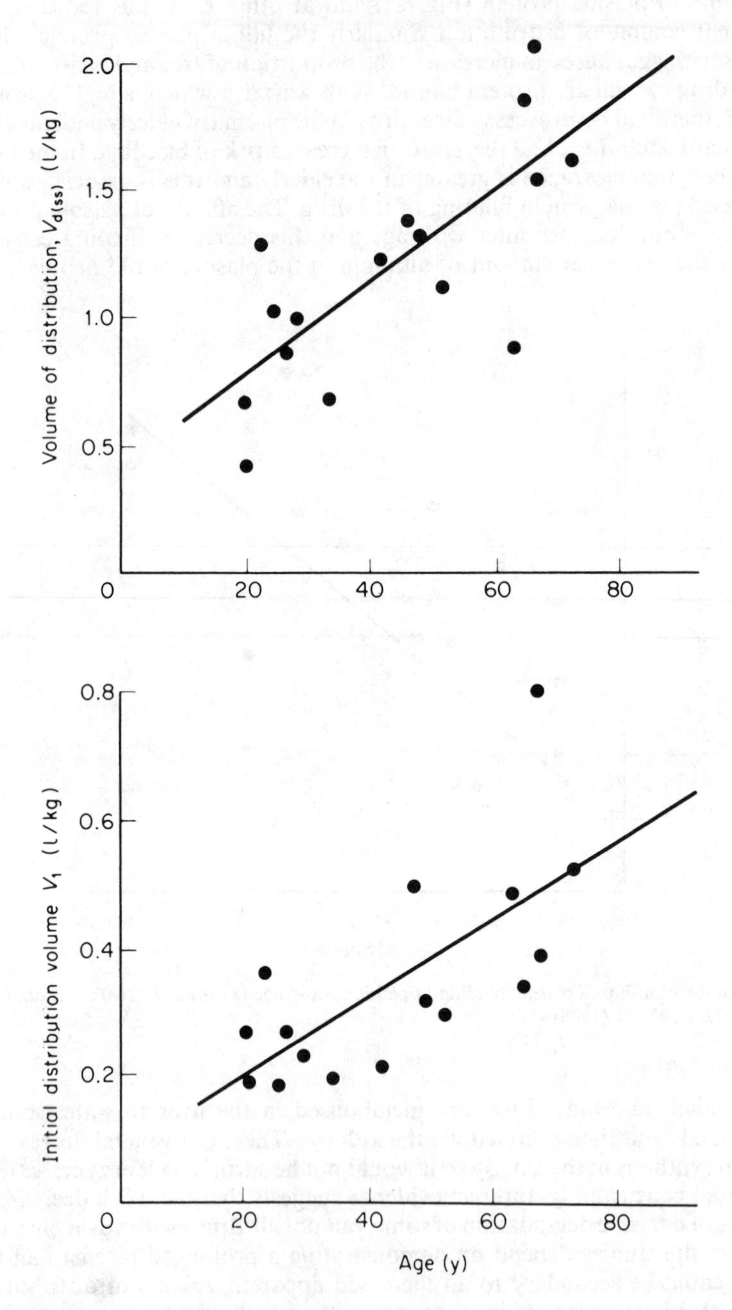

Fig. 6.4 Correlation of volumes of distribution of diazepam with age in normal volunteers (From U. Klotz *et al.*, *J. Clin. Invest.*, **55**, 347 (1975).)

Oxidation reduced with age	*Unchanged oxidation with age*
Alprazolam	Digitoxin
Clobazam	Ethanol
Chlordiazepoxide	Lignocaine
Chlormethiazole	Metoprolol
Diazepam and desmethyldiazepam	Prazosin
Midazolam	Warfarin
Propranolol	
Nortriptyline	
Theophylline	

In some cases the evidence is equivocal thus in the case of amylobarbitone, estimation of its main metabolite 3-hydroxy-amylobarbitone showed a reduced excretion in the elderly group (Fig. 6.5) which suggested a reduced rate of metabolism. Phase II conjugation processes are much less affected by ageing. Thus the acetylation of isoniazid and the glucuronidation of oxazepam, lorazepam and temazepam do not alter with age although there is some evidence that there is reduced formation of the glucuronides of indomethacin and ketoprofen in the elderly. One possible partial explanation of the

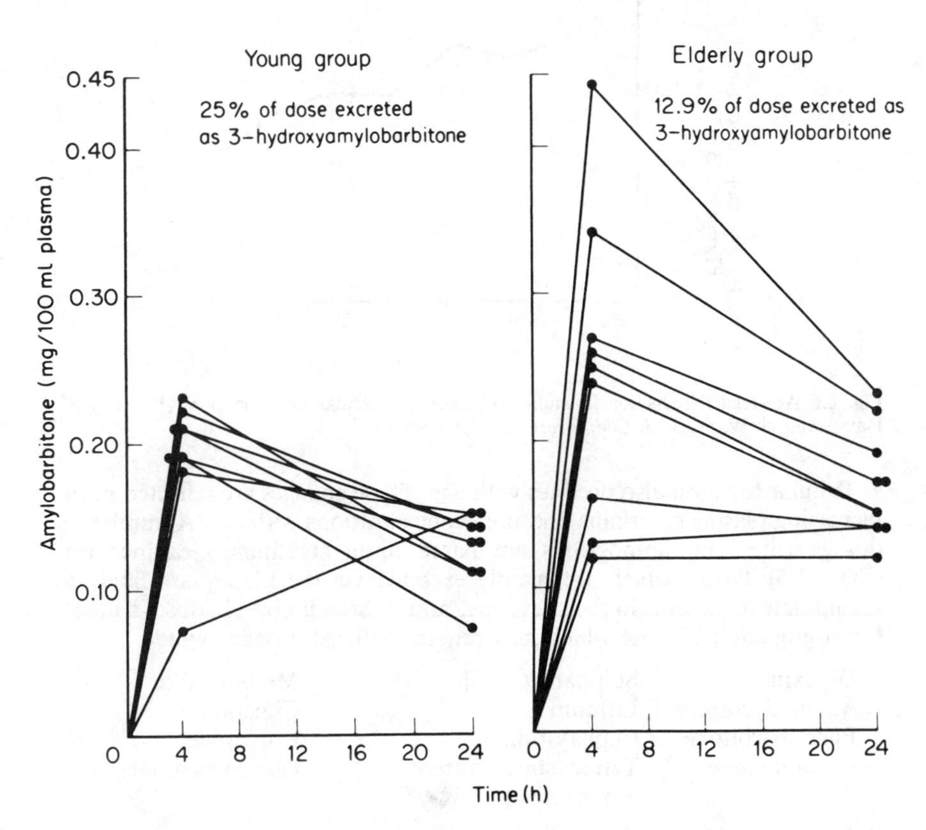

Fig. 6.5 Amylobarbitone plasma levels after a single 200 mg oral dose in a group of young (age 20–40) and old (over 65) subjects. (From R. E. Irvine *et al.*, *Brit. J. Clin. Pharm.*, **1**, 41 (1974).)

decreased ability of the aged to metabolise single doses of test drugs may be that the old smoke and drink alcohol less than the young, thus reducing the stimulus to hepatic enzyme induction. Furthermore, the elderly may be less able to respond to inducing stimuli than the young. Poor nutrition in the elderly may be another factor partly responsible for the decline in microsomal function with age.

4. Renal excretion Probably the most important cause of drug accumulation in the elderly is declining renal function. In patients over 80 the glomerular filtration rate has dropped to 60–70 ml/min (Fig. 6.6) although they may have other renal disorders associated with advancing years such as prostatic hypertrophy. The glomerular filtration rate falls at a rate of approximately 1 ml/min/1.73 m^2 each year after the age of 20. This is summarised by the relationship:

$$\text{GFR} = 153.2 - 0.96 \times \text{age}$$
$$= \text{inulin clearance (ml/min/1.73 m}^2\text{)}$$

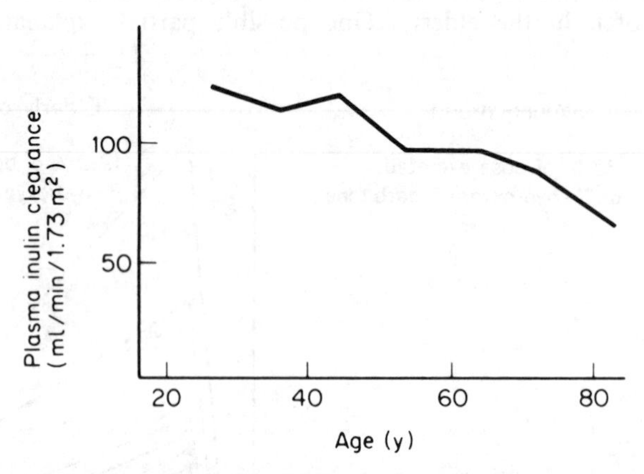

Fig. 6.6 Age-related reduction in inulin clearance (glomerular filtration rate) (From D. F. Davies and N. W. Stock, *J. Clin. Invest.*, **29**, 496 (1950).)

Tubular function also declines with age. These changes are reflected in the increasing plasma creatinine and urea concentrations with age. A number of dosage rules and nomograms are based upon creatinine clearance (see Chapter 5). Drugs which are mainly excreted via the kidney are likely to accumulate in patients in their seventies and eighties if given in doses suitable for young adults. Those which may require reduced dosage include:

Digoxin	Sulphamethazole	Methotrexate
Aminoglycosides	Lithium	Cimetidine
Phenobarbitone	Cephaloridine	Frusemide
Procainamide	Tetracyclines (except doxycycline)	Chlorpropamide

Polar drug metabolites are excreted by the kidneys and thus accumulate in the elderly. Many are inactive, but some, e.g. the hydroxylated metabolites of tricyclic antidepressants, have activity and accumulation of such metabolites can produce adverse effects.

Pharmacodynamic changes

Evidence that the elderly are intrinsically more sensitive to drugs than the young is scanty. It has been demonstrated that although the absorption, distribution and elimination of nitrazepam is unchanged by age, the sensitivity of the elderly as measured by psychometric tests is greater and the effects last longer than in the young. It is common clinical experience that nitrazepam given to the elderly in hypnotic doses used for the young may produce prolonged daytime confusion. Presumably this increased sensitivity reflects changes in the ageing brain. Similarly other drugs may expose physiological defects which are a normal concomitant of ageing. Thus the frequency and magnitude of postural hypotension increases with ageing. This presumably contributes to the increased incidence of postural hypotension resulting from the administration of drugs such as phenothiazines, β-blockers, adrenergic neurone blockers, tricyclic antidepressants and diuretics.

Several studies have shown that the increase in heart rate produced by isoprenaline is diminished in older patients and this and other evidence suggests that the sensitivity of the β-receptor response mechanism falls with age. Although there seems to be no change in the number of β-adrenoceptors on the leucocyte membrane these receptors have a reduced affinity for agonists with increasing age. If this were also true of cardiac muscle membrane receptors the declining response of the heart with ageing would be explained. Nevertheless, although the elderly may be less sensitive to drugs such as β-blockers at the cellular level, this effect may be balanced by the higher plasma drug levels resulting from decreased first-pass metabolism of some of these drugs. Similarly, studies on isolated myocardium suggest that aged heart muscle has decreased digoxin binding sites which could be one factor in the well-known sensitivity of the elderly to this drug. In the case of warfarin the aged liver shows a greater inhibition of clotting factor synthesis than in the young, and old people thus require lower warfarin doses for effective anticoagulation.

Compliance in the elderly

There is evidence that young adult patients fails to take their medicines as instructed even in diseases such as tuberculosis where there should be considerable motivation towards compliance. In the elderly there is evidence of non-compliance in about 60% of patients. This may be due to a failure of memory or to not understanding how the drug should be taken. In addition, patients may have previously prescribed drugs in the medicine cupboard which they take from time to time. It is therefore essential that the drug regime should be kept simple and should be carefully explained. There is scope for improved methods of packaging so that over- or under-dosage is prevented. Multiple drug regimes must be avoided if possible. Not only will such regimes confuse the patient but they will increase the risk of interactions (see p. 190), and they are usually unnecessary.

THE EFFECT OF DRUGS ON SOME SYSTEMS IN THE ELDERLY

Central nervous system

Cerebral function is easily disturbed in old people and results in disorientation and confusion. Drugs are one of the factors which may contribute to this state; sedatives and hypnotics can easily precipitate a loss of awareness and clouding of consciousness. Over-vigorous attempts to lower the blood pressure may produce cerebral ischaemia and confusion.

1. Night sedation Some degree of night sedation may be needed as sleeplessness and confusion are common. The common causes of insomnia should be remembered and treated if possible. They include:

(a) pain, which may be due to such causes as arthritis
(b) constipation—the discomfort of a loaded rectum
(c) urinary frequency
(d) depression
(e) anxiety
(f) left ventricular failure
(g) dementia

Benzodiazepines are widely prescribed in elderly patients but are not free of side effects. Most have a long half-life (see p. 210) and some degree of hangover with morning drowsiness is quite common. Abrupt withdrawal may precipitate an anxiety state. Many benzodiazepines have long half-lives and may have active metabolites. *Temazepam* (10–20 mg) or *triazolam* (125 mg) are short acting but may not be helpful if early wakening is a problem.

Chloral 0.5–1.0 g is also useful: it seldom produces delirium, has little habituation potential and does not disturb sleep patterns.

Chlormethiazole has a short half life (about 4 h) and is relatively safe. Its main disadvantage is that it produces a burning sensation in the nose soon after ingestion. The usual dose is 250–500 mg.

2. Tranquillisers Restlessness and agitated depression are common in old people and may be associated with some degree of dementia. These states can be ameliorated by phenothiazines, for example, thioridazine 10–25 mg or perphenazine 4–8 mg. Phenothiazine side effects must be remembered (see p. 247). Of particular importance are:

(a) The development of Parkinsonian symptoms and particularly slowness and rigidity, may be a problem and may require lowering the dose, stopping the drug, or occasionally concurrent use of anti-Parkinsonian drugs. The elderly are more prone to Parkinsonian syndromes but they are less likely to have dystonias than young patients. Tardive dyskinesia is commoner in the elderly and thioridazine, which has the lowest incidence of extrapyramidal effects of the phenothiazines perhaps because it is only a weak dopaminergic blocker, may be especially useful in these patients.
(b) Postural hypotension may complicate the use of phenothiazines.
(c) Hypothermia.

3. Antidepressants Although depression is common in old age and may indeed need treating, it should be remembered that the tricyclic antidepressants can cause constipation, urinary retention and glaucoma (all due to their parasympathetic blocking action), and also drowsiness, confusion and postural hypotension. More dangerously they can produce cardiac arrhythmias and may occasionally be responsible for unforeseen sudden death of elderly patients. The possibility that the depression results from a drug used in the treatment of another disease should be remembered. Examples are methyldopa, phenobarbitone, digoxin, propranolol and tranquillisers. Tricyclic antidepressants can produce worthwhile remissions of depression but should be started at very low dosage, e.g. amitriptyline 25 mg nocte, and only cautiously increased in dose. Alternatively mianserin or trazodone can be used. They are safer than the tricyclics but more expensive and certainly no more effective.

4. Anti-Parkinsonian drugs. The anticholinergic group of anti-Parkinsonian drugs (e.g. benzhexol, orphenadrine) quite often cause side effects in the elderly. Urinary retention due to prostatic enlargement and bladder neck fibrosis can be dangerous. Glaucoma may be precipitated or aggravated and confusion may occur with quite small doses. Levodopa can be effective but it is particularly important to start with a small dose. Levodopa 100 mg + carbidopa 10 mg (Sinemet) is a suitable initial dose and can be increased. In patients with dementia the use of anticholinergics, levodopa or amantidine may produce adverse cerebral stimulation, leading to complete decompensation of cerebral functioning with excitement and inability to cope.

Cardiovascular system

1. Hypertension There is considerable debate as to whether hypotensive drugs have a place in the treatment of patients over 70 or even over 60, and a clear answer awaits the results of further trials. As a rule, elderly patients do not tolerate hypotensive agents well. Postural hypotension can be dangerous with attacks of faintness and collapse which could result in fractured bones. Many of the centrally acting drugs such as methyldopa or clonidine produce excessive sedation and depression. Patients with poor peripheral circulation may find that β-blockers exacerbate their cold extremities and claudication, by reducing cardiac output and peripheral blood flow. In the present state of knowledge, it is preferable to confine the use of hypotensive drugs to those with severe and life-threatening hypertension.

Drugs are an important cause of *postural hypotension* in the aged. They include phenothiazines, tricyclic antidepressants, diuretics, vasodilators, levodopa and benzodiazepines.

2. Digitalis overdose is commoner in the elderly, presumably because of the reduced apparent volume of distribution and decreased renal elimination of digoxin (see p. 374). Confusion, toxic psychosis, depression and an acute abdominal syndrome resembling mesenteric artery obstruction are all more commonly seen in the old than in the young as features of intoxication. Hypokalaemia, due both to decreased intake (potassium-containing foods are expensive and sometimes outside the budget of the pensioner) and faulty homeostatic mechanisms resulting in increased renal loss, is commoner in the old and is a contributory factor in some patients. Digoxin is sometimes prescribed when there is no indication for it, e.g. for an irregular pulse which is due to multiple ectopic beats rather than atrial fibrillation. At other times the indications for initiation of treatment are correct but the situation is never reviewed and the drug stopped. In one series of geriatric patients on digoxin the drug was withdrawn in 78% without detriment.

3. Diuretics can be dangerous in the old since they may cause postural hypotension, produce hypovolaemia and intravascular thrombosis, precipitate hypokalaemia and potentiate digitalis. Too vigorous a diuresis may result in urinary retention in an old man with an enlarged prostate and necessiate bladder catheterisation with all of its attendant risks. In either sex, brisk diuresis associated with mental impairment or reduced mobility can result in incontinence. Loop diuretics should therefore be reserved for urgent indications and a thiazide or a thiazide + triamterene or spironolactone used. Moduretic (thiazide + amiloride) is popular but can cause both hyperkalaemia and hyponatraemia so care is required. Thiazide-induced gout is an important side effect to be remembered, particularly in those with a personal or family history of the condition.

Oral hypoglycaemic agents

Diabetes is common in the elderly and many patients are treated with oral hypoglycaemic drugs. It is probably better for elderly patients to be managed with diet if at all possible and to undertreat those who require drugs, so that symptoms of hyperglycaemia are relieved without any danger of hypoglycaemia. Tolbutamide, which has a short half-life (5 h) is preferable to the longer acting drugs such as chlorpropamide (half-life 36 h) which may cause prolonged hypoglycaemia, resulting in neurological sequelae.

Antibiotics

Antibiotics do not usually cause undue problems in old age as long as the decline in renal function is remembered when an aminoglycoside or tetracycline is used. Whether hypersensitivity rashes are more common, especially with ampicillin, is not known, but they can be troublesome and this drug is the commonest cause of drug rashes in the elderly.

Use of drugs in the elderly

There is little doubt that the commonest cause of iatrogenic disease in the elderly is the improper prescription of drugs. Common-sense rules for prescribing have been suggested (and apply not only for the elderly):

1. Know the pharmacological action of the drug employed.
2. Use the lowest effective dose.
3. Use the fewest drugs a patient needs.

4. Drugs should not be used to treat symptoms without first discovering the cause of the symptoms, i.e. first diagnosis, then treatment.
5. Drugs should not be withheld because of old age: but it should be remembered that there is no cure for old age either.
6. A drug should not be continued if it is no longer necessary.
7. Do not use a drug if the symptoms it causes are worse than those it is meant to relieve.
8. It is rarely sensible to treat the side effects of one drug by prescribing another drug.

In the elderly it is often important to pay attention to matters such as the formulation of the drug to be used: many old people tolerate elixirs and liquid medicines better than small tablets or capsules. Supervision of drug taking may be necessary since an old person with a serious physical or mental disability cannot be expected to comply with any but the simplest drug regimen. Containers require especially clear labelling and should be easy to open, since child-proof containers are often impossible for the grandparents to open as well.

Chapter 7
INTRODUCTION OF NEW DRUGS, CLINICAL TRIALS AND ADVERSE REACTION SURVEILLANCE

INTRODUCTION OF NEW DRUGS

In the aftermath of the thalidomide disaster the Minister of Health of the UK established in 1963 a Committee on Safety of Drugs since it was clear that some control over the introduction and marketing of drugs was necessary. These efforts at regulation culminated in the Medicines Act 1968 which provides for the licensing of all medicinal products (for both human and veterinary use) and controls their retail sale, supply and advertising. The Act is administered by:

(a) The Licensing Authority (the Ministers of Health and Agriculture)
(b) The Medicines Commission: an advisory body to the Ministers who also act as independent arbiters distinct from the Committee on Safety of Medicines.
(c) The Committee on safety of Medicines (CSM) which has succeeded the Committee on Safety of Drugs. This is an independent group of clinicians, clinical pharmacologists, toxicologists, pharmacologists, pathologists and others who advise the Licensing Authority. They judge whether a drug is safe, efficacious and of adequate quality for its intended use taking into account data from preclinical laboratory experiments, human volunteer studies and clinical trials in patients. On this basis advice is given as to whether marketing approval would be appropriate (if it is refused manufacturers may appeal to the Medicines Commission for their independent opinion to be given to the Licensing Authority).

The discovery of new drugs does not originate, however, with government but with major research-based pharmaceutical companies which exist to discover, develop, manufacture and market drugs. The place of academic units in the discovery of new drugs is small, since the cost involved is now beyond even the most lavishly funded university department. The development of a new drug now takes some 10 years and costs in excess of £50 millions. The success rate of new candidate drugs is low. The largest British-owned drug company, Imperial Chemical Industries, annually synthesises some 8000 different molecules for study of their pharmacological properties, of which 5–10 go on to preclinical evaluation, which eliminates at least half. The remainder undergo early trial in man and perhaps 1 in 20 substances reaching this stage will be suitable to undergo further clinical study. A company which produces a new product every couple of years is considered to be exceptionally successful.

The development of a new drug falls into four main phases (Fig. 7.1):

(a) discovery and synthesis;
(b) pharmacological and pre-clinical testing;
(c) clinical safety and efficacy testing;
(d) marketing

The original method for discovering drugs was by random screening of compounds which is a rather inefficient use of time and money. Increasing understanding of basic pharmacology has made the possibility of being able to design molecules to possess specific pharmacological effects more nearly a reality. When a compound with clearly recognisable pharmacological effect is isolated, it is usual to synthesise and examine a range of analogues, sometimes several dozen, to attain the optimal balance between activity and toxicity. Such a candidate molecule will then pass into the pre-clinical testing programme proper. Amongst many other tests the following will be studied:

(a) The dose of drug which, if given acutely by various routes, will kill 50% of a group of animals (LD_{50}).
(b) The efficacy of the drug and the dose–response relationship of its activity.
(c) The chronic toxicity over 3–6 months in at least two species, one of which is not a rodent.

Such tests in animals are of very little predictive value for man since the commonly used animals rarely handle the drugs in the same way as man. Laboratory models of many well-known drug effects in man, e.g. chloramphenicol-induced bone marrow aplasia, methyldopa-associated haemolytic anaemia, do not exist. More recently there has been a move towards shorter animal toxicity studies but with greater emphasis on detailed metabolic and pharmacokinetic studies of the new drug in several species in order that the most appropriate animal model may be chosen for the chronic studies. At high dose levels some changes are nearly always seen in animal studies. The problem is to estimate the relevance of these changes and at present there is no obvious way of doing this.

Reproduction studies are also carried out to assess the effect of the compound on the fertility of both male and female animals (rats being usually employed) and on their offspring. Males are dosed for 11 weeks (to ensure that drug is given during all stages of spermatogenesis) and at least three dose levels are used. The animals are then mated with undosed females and some of the females are killed and examined, some at the end of the first two thirds of pregnancy and some just prior to term. The number of live, dead and absorbed fetuses are determined and they are examined for abnormalities. Others are allowed to litter, the babies allowed to wean and then killed and examined for abnormalities. Similar studies are performed after mating dosed females with undosed males. Teratology studies are carried out usually with rats and rabbits and the animals dosed during the period of fetal organogenesis. Once again the real relevance to man of such expensive and time-consuming studies

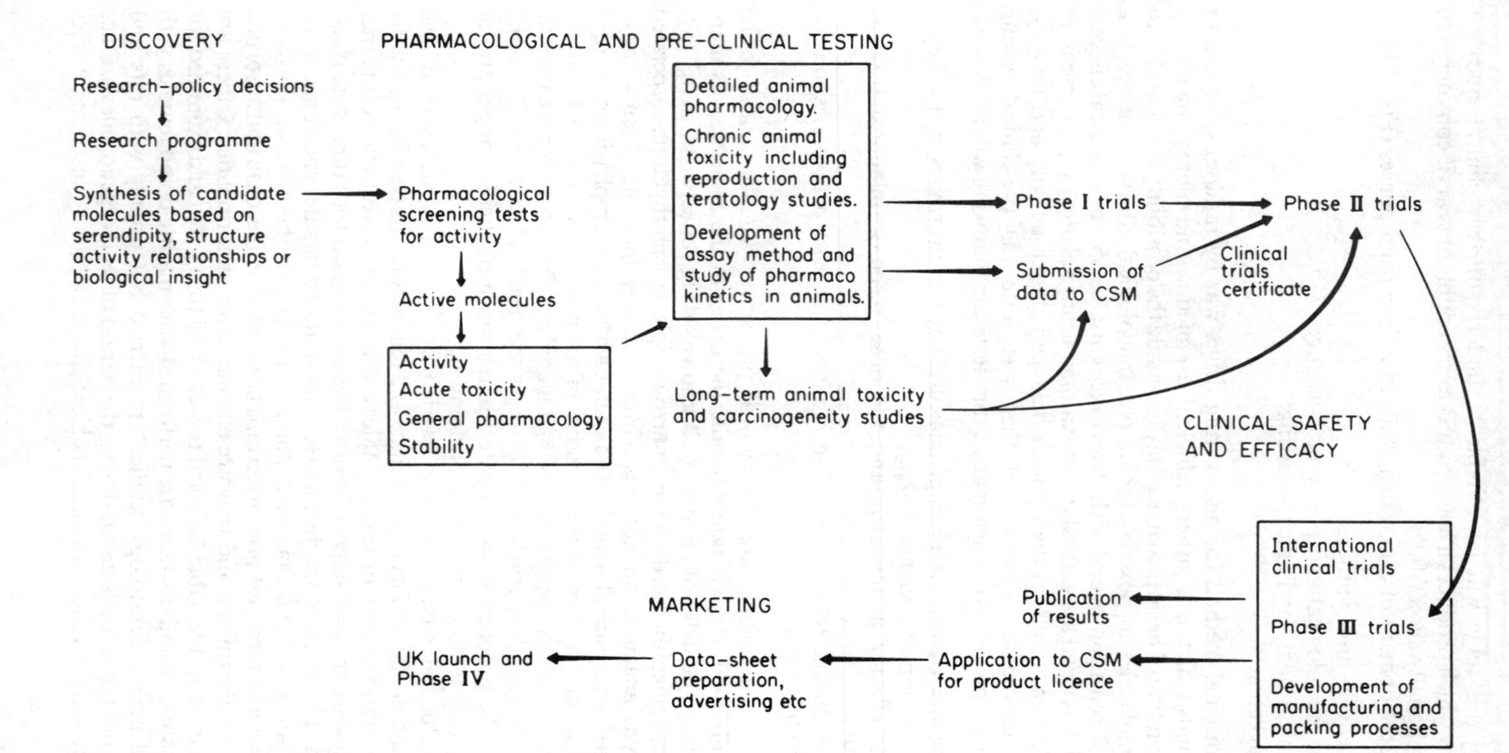

Fig. 7.1 Stages in the development of a new drug.

has never been completely established, although they are required by all drug regulation authorities. A present trend is towards fairly early testing of drugs in man under carefully controlled conditions. This frequently gives more useful information for the clinician, particularly about pharmacology and pharmacokinetics.

These studies in which the drug is first given to man are usually called *Phase I trials*. Volunteers, either normals or patients, depending upon the nature of drug, are used. Usually a dose of around one-thirtieth to one-twentieth of the minimum dose which produces an effect in animals is chosen as the starting dose. Depending upon the slope of the dose–response curve in animals the dose is then increased in subsequent volunteers until an effect is detected. The subjects are monitored carefully both clinically and by the laboratory and the nature, severity and duration of any side effects are carefully recorded. The effects of chronic dosing (say for 14 days) is subsequently studied once the safety of single doses is established.

These investigations are usually limited to special centres and the aim is to determine the pharmacology and pharmacokinetics, to note side effects and to take preliminary steps in delineating its place in therapy. There is at the time of writing considerable controversy over volunteer studies following the very occasional severe adverse reaction. However, despite apparent risks such tests are in reality remarkably safe. Recently the experience of 12 years of such tests carried out with normal prison volunteers, largely in the Michigan State prison service, was published. Over the years 1964–76, 29 162 participants took part in 805 studies involving 614 534 subject days. During this time 64 significant medical events occurred, of which 58 were definite adverse drug reactions. There was complete recovery in all but one case and no deaths occurred. Thus a significant medical problem occurred once every 26.3 years of individual subject participation. It is important however that:

(a) Studies are carried out by those who are experienced in this type of work.
(b) A full range of equipment is available for resuscitation should an emergency occur.
(c) Volunteers should be carefully screened before the experiment to exclude ill health and intercurrent drug taking.
(d) Volunteers are indemnified against any disability which may result from the experiment.
(e) It should be remembered that no experiment of this type is entirely without risk.

At the same time as Phase I trials are carried out, various chronic animal toxicity studies are being completed. If everything is satisfactory, an application for a *clinical trial certificate* is made in order that studies may be conducted in patients.

This application requires very comprehensive data on the chemistry, pharmacology, biological action and toxicity of the drug from both animal experiments and volunteer studies in man. In the past this has led to considerable delays in granting the certificate with subsequent financial loss to the company involved. In 1981 the Clinical Trials Exemption Scheme was introduced (See Medicines Act Leaflet No. 62.)

Under this scheme pharmaceutical companies may obtain exemption from the need to obtain a Clinical Trials Certificate before proceeding to a trial. The company is required to submit a summary of scientific evidence about the drug together with a statement as to ethical committee approval to the licensing authority and must undertake to inform the CSM of any problems arising in the trial. The licensing authority has 35 days to consider the submission and if exemption is not refused during this period the clinical trial may proceed.

Phase II studies are then undertaken in which aspects of the clinical pharmacology of the drug are studied by a small number of independent investigators. Often these studies are in patients and therefore the protocol will require approval by the pharmaceutical company, the hospital ethical committee and the CSM. These studies continue to define the therapeutic profile and dosage schedule of the drug for the next stage of Phase III trials.

Phase III is the phase of formal clinical trials in which the efficacy of the new drug is compared with either placebo or a reference drug of established efficacy. It is usual for possible drug interactions between the new compound and commonly prescribed drugs to be investigated at this time. During this stage the aim is to identify those patient groups who respond more and less well, to increase patient exposure in terms of numbers and duration of therapy and to identify less common adverse reactions. During this phase the results of very long-term animal studies usually become available. Life span studies in mice (21 months) and rats (24 months) are undertaken to determine any increase in susceptibility to tumours. Thus even at this late stage of drug development the project may have to be abandoned if such studies prove unfavourable. Also during this period the manufacturers will be setting up plant for large-scale manufacture and undertaking further pharmaceutical studies on drug formulation, bioavailability and stability. The medical advisers to the company will, in association with their pharmacological, pharmaceutical and legal colleagues be gathering together the large amount of data necessary to make formal application to the Licencing Authority via the CSM for a *product licence*. The size of the submission documents may extend to several hundredweights of paper. It is not therefore surprising that not less than six months and more often a year elapses before final permission is gained for the drug to be marketed. Marketing approval may be general or granted subject to certain limitations which may include restriction to hospital practice only, restriction in indications for use or a requirement to monitor some particular action or organ function in a specified number of patients. All prescribing doctors are provided with a factual *data sheet* giving information on each new medicine and the contents of this must be agreed with the CSM. It must provide all the information necessary to make a proper decision as to whether the drug is indicated (i.e. it is not an advertisement) and must also detail all known hazards of the drug. Doctors are also reminded (by means of an inverted triangle symbol) that this is a recently introduced drug and that any suspected adverse reaction should be reported to the CSM.

The stage of open release on prescription is sometimes called *Phase IV*. Although the previous phases of study may have been complex and searching it would be unlikely that more than a few thousand patients would have taken the drug prior to general release. During Phase IV an estimate of patient acceptibility may be made and the probable place of the drug in treatment can be assessed. The surveillance of adverse reactions mainly belongs to this phase.

CLINICAL TRIALS

Assessment of treatment by clinical impressions is no longer adequate and all procedures, whether medical or surgical, must be assessed by properly designed clinical trials. The first stage in any experiment is to *define objectives*. In the case of a clinical trial of a drug these may be of various levels of complexity: is it desired to show that the drug is effective, more effective than a standard drug, improves the patient's symptoms, enhances their prognosis, has fewer side effects than the usual therapy? These questions must be decided before the experimental protocol is drawn up. In general, it is better to have only a few precisely defined objectives of general interest and clinical relevance.

The *selection of patients* for clinical trial must be dictated by strict criteria. Firstly the informed consent of the patient must be obtained, preferably in writing. The patient must know the length of the trial and the extent of any investigations or inconveniences required. The diagnosis of the disease to be treated must be secure and carefully defined. *Exclusion criteria* must also be decided so that during a trial patients who require other treatment will be excluded from the final analysis. The *end-point of a study* must also be defined: this may be some change in the patient's condition or else a specified duration of treatment. The permissible *dose levels* of the drug during the trial must also be decided. It is necessary in any trial to establish detailed rules for the treatment of patients, since even when this treatment schedule is well defined there may be medical reasons for allowing specified departures from the intended regime. Once established, the criteria for entrance to and exclusion from the trial, the treatment policy, the criteria and times of assessment must be observed, otherwise there is a danger that arbitrary factors may influence the outcome.

Even with careful selection and monitoring the *default rate* of a trial (particularly a long-term trial) may approach 10–20%. To obtain good adherence to the trial the full understanding of the patient is essential and it is often useful to have a run-in period of 6–8 weeks on placebo. This period allows assessment of the patient's commitment to the project and exclusion of non-attenders, those who decline repeated examinations or investigations and patients who do not take their tablets regularly. Compliance may be monitored by tablet counting at each visit or more rarely by inclusion of a marker substances (e.g. riboflavin, isoniazid) in the tablets which can easily be detected in the urine.

In planning a trial a choice of a *fixed or variable dosage schedule* must be made. A fixed dosage is easier to administer but only answers the rather limited questions of the efficacy of that particular dose. Furthermore, in many cases giving a standard dose of a drug may produce different results in different patients since, due to variability in drug disposition, the steady-state drug levels may be extremely variable and the diseased state may likewise respond variably. The situation can become even more complex if the drug metabolites themselves have pharmacological activity, since these will be formed in various amounts in different patients. In trials involving more than one clinician further difficulties arise with a flexible dosage scheme, since some doctors may be less tolerant than others of their patients' side effects and alter dosages appropriately.

It is useful to distinguish between designs in which patients have only one of the alternative treatments so that *comparisons are made between subjects* and those in which more than one treatment is given to each patient and *comparisons are made within subjects*. The former design is usual in acute diseases for which the available treatment period is short, but may also be used in chronic disease when treatment is required over a long time to achieve an effect or when assessment of results follows a long time after application of the treatment. Within-subject comparison is more useful for chronic illness in which treatments may be serially applied.

It is standard practice to make *simultaneous comparisons* of treatments, for if treatments are applied at different times any apparent difference may be due not to treatment but to some other confounding factor. Thus the use of *retrospective controls* or of several groups of patients studied in different centres requires very stringent tests to ensure that like is being compared with like.

It is well known that 30–50% of patients, depending upon circumstances, will give positive responses of various sorts to *placebos*. It is not possible to identify and exclude placebo reactors from a trial and therefore if possible this part of the total variability must be minimised by using the patient as his own control.The design usually employed is the *crossover*. The patients are *randomised* into two groups, one to receive *placebo* or *reference drug*, the other receives these treatments in reverse order. Ideally randomisation is by allocation from random-number tables or by sealed randomly assorted envelopes. The use of randomisation by day of admission or surname may be biased by external events or in the latter case by the relationship of name to national or religious origins. The use of a *placebo* may produce ethical difficulties if the disease under study is severe but placebos are justified if there is real doubt about the benefits of a drug.

A problem which arises if patients cross over from one active treatment to another is the need for patients to be free of the first drug before embarking upon the second treatment so as to avoid *'carry-over' effects*. Some drug effects, e.g. monoamine oxidase inhibitors, take weeks to wear off so that a cross-over design is inappropriate unless a lengthy interval occurs between treatments. Other highly lipid soluble drugs like chlorpromazine are slowly released from deep body compartments for several weeks, which is why it takes a month or more before patients relapse after withdrawal of major tranquillisers. One approach to this problem is to withdraw the drug until relapse occurs and then to institute the alternative therapy. There are obvious ethical difficulties with this design and it is arguable whether this method can be justified.

If at all possible the trial is conducted so that the patients are unaware of what medication they are receiving, a so-called *blind design*. Ideally the physician administering the drug is also unaware of the nature of the treatment—a *double blind* trial. This is important when the criteria for assessment of improvement are subjective or require interpretation by the observer, e.g. improvement of anxiety, or when the attitude of the doctor or his expectation of drug effects contributes to the efficacy of the drug, e.g. improvement in exercise tolerance. Thus in the evaluation of meprobamate it has been shown that clinicians with an optimistic and enthusiastic approach to its use were able to demonstrate its superiority over placebo whilst those with a neutral attitude could not. Such effects are insidious since the observer is not usually aware of his influence or of the inevitability of bias unless the treatment is double blind. With orally administered drugs the double blind condition is maintained by using identical tablets for different treatment groups, the key to the code being held by a third person unconcerned with the trial but accessible in case the code needs to be broken. It is sometimes difficult to maintain the double blind condition either from the patient (e.g. a new antihistamine may produce sedation) or the doctor (e.g. a β-blocker will, if it is effective, produce bradycardia). Taste may be camouflaged by addition of a strong masking flavour, but even so an aftertaste may remain which will identify the drug to the subject. In a double blind study of placebo, a new anti-inflammatory drug and aspirin in rheumatoid patients, experienced observers were able to guess the period of aspirin therapy in 80% of the patients. Therefore sometimes patient assessments should be made by a 'blind' observer not concerned with the giving of treatment or the detection of side-effects.

Removal of bias in the data collected is sometimes difficult. For example, even in relatively objective assessment methods such as blood-pressure measurement, the observer can show digit preference or observer bias and a number of instruments have been devised to prevent this. In the random-zero sphygmomanometer the zero point of the mercury column randomly varies to compensate for observer bias, but not digit preference, whereas in the London School of Hygiene sphygmomanometer the mercury columns are hidden from the observer in a box, thus eliminating observer and digit bias.

Because suitable patients are not available at one centre a further complication may be added by making a *multicentre trial of treatment*. This is, however, a rather unsatisfactory method, since if many doctors participate each will contribute only a few patients and, because of variation between doctors in the interpretation of the trial protocol, the sample of patients studied will be more heterogeneous than expected, the measurements less precise and the power of the trial diluted. Some check should therefore be inserted into the protocol to ensure as uniform a between-centre variation as possible and a clinical co-ordinator should monitor the performance of each centre.

It is possible to calculate the number of patients required to establish a given difference between treatment at a *specified level of statistical confidence* and such estimates may be used to determine the size and duration of a trial. Statistics cannot completely answer the question as to when a randomised controlled trial should be stopped, however, and such trials may occasionally be inefficient if one treatment is greatly superior to the other, since this might be shown more quickly if assessments were able to be made during the trial. Clearly it is neither ethically nor economically reasonable to continue with a trial once the result has clearly favoured one alternative. A design of trial which permits timely and efficient termination of a comparison is the *sequential design*. In this design patients are paired so that the alternative treatments are represented in each pair. For each pair a judgement based upon agreed criteria is made as to the superiority of one of the treatments. This judgement is termed a preference. Pairs for which no preference for any one treatment can be made do not enter the analysis. The results of each preference are plotted on a chart such as that shown in Fig. 7.2. The shape of boundaries in the chart is drawn up using statistical criteria. When the line of preference crosses the upper or lower boundaries of the chart the trial may be terminated since at this point a clear difference at a previously decided level of statistical significance has been demonstrated. Pairing of successive entrants to a trial automatically removes variation due to gradual trends in response occurring throughout the trial, e.g. changes in natural history of the disease, altered standards of assessment of response. The use of sequential trials may rapidly obtain an answer to a problem, but on the other hand it must be recognised that if there is actually no difference, or only a small difference, between treatments the sequential trial requires more patients than non-sequential trials to establish this.

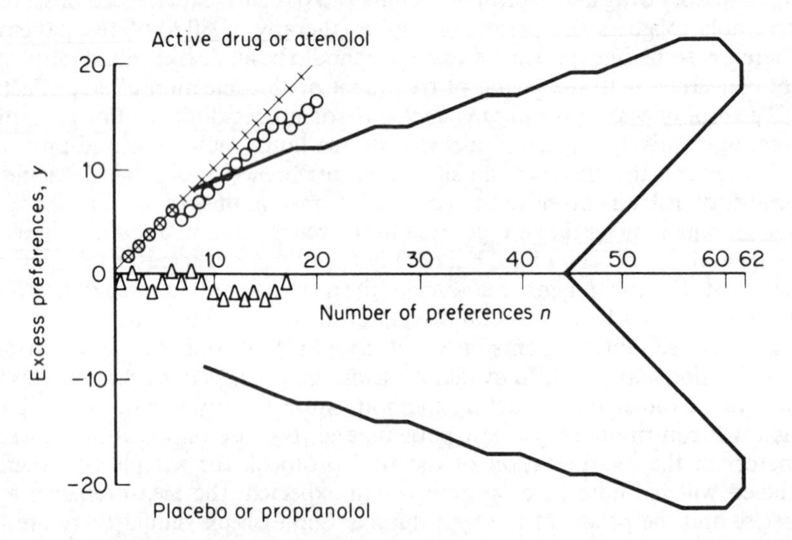

Fig. 7.2 Sequential analysis of a trial of the effects of atenolol (x) and propranolol (O) versus placebo in hyperthyroid patients using objective assessment of effects including heart rate. Both drugs are significantly better than placebo ($p = 0.05$) but a comparison of atenolol and propranolol (△) fails to distinguish between them in efficacy (From D. G. McDevitt and J. K. Nelson, *Brit. J. Clin. Pharm.*, **6**, 233 (1978).)

Sequential trials are not always suitable and an ethical dilemma which has not been satisfactorily solved is whether a trial should be stopped by breaking the double blind if the organisers suspect that a proportion of patients are responding well (or badly) to a new drug. To halt the trial before its planned conclusion would destroy its scientific validity but not to do so would prejudice the prognosis of some of the participants. A partial solution has been tried by the Anturane Reinfarction Trial Research Group who investigated the effects of sulphinpyrazone in preventing cardiac mortality following myocardial infarction (see p. 607). Based upon an average monitoring period of only 8 months they found a reduction of 48.5% in mortality in patients treated with drug as opposed to placebo. Although having no idea of long-term effects the organisers' solution to the problems was to inform all the patients of the results of the trial without breaking the double blind and to continue only with those patients giving informed consent on this basis. Patients were also offered the alternatives of sulphinpyrazone treatment or no treatment at all.

The design of clinical trials has now become extremely complex and the advice of a *statistician* is advisable before a trial protocol is set up to ensure that the trial is properly conducted and will yield analysable and meaningful results at its conclusion.

Ethics committees

In recent years there has been increasing concern over the ethical implications of some types of medical research and this includes the testing and trials of new drugs. This has led various institutions including medical schools, hospitals, pharmaceutical companies and some colleges to set up ethics committees.

The objective of these committees is to protect subjects of research and to preserve their rights and at the same time to facilitate research in the interests of society.

Membership In the UK there is no statutory structure for ethics committees. It is generally agreed that they should represent a wide range of expertise and sensible opinion but obviously cannot include experts in every branch of medical science. It is perhaps desirable that they should contain at least one layman and a representative of the nursing profession can be helpful. They should not be too large and about ten members would seem appropriate.

Applications for Ethics Committee Approval In general an application should state:

(1) Description and purpose of investigation.
(2) Number and type of patients/subjects/ likely to be involved and whether these include women likely to become pregnant.
(3) Duration and location of project.
(4) Procedures involved, hazards and degree of discomfort.
(5) Experience of investigator.
(6) Statement as to informed consent, whether oral or in writing and in the presence of a disinterested third party.
(7) Whether X-rays or radioactive substances will be used.
(8) Whether a Clinical Trial Certificate, a Product Licence or an Exemption has been issued for the drug.
(9) Whether the subject's GP will be informed.
(10) With a novel drug given in association with the pharmaceutical industry, whether indemnification against 'no fault liability' has been obtained.

Procedure The Ethics Committee should meet regularly. Most applications are approved without argument, a few will require further discussion and very rarely a project is rejected.

It is desirable that there should be some follow up of projects and if some ethical problem arises it should be referred back to the Ethics Committee.

It is difficult to decide to what degree an Ethics Committee should consider not only the ethical aspects of an application but also its scientific content. It could be argued that it is unethical to carry out a poorly designed study which will not give meaningful results. Most Ethics Committees take a mid-way stance on this problem and would only comment on the scientific validity of a project if it were obviously very bad.

Sanctions Ethics Committees are not statutory and there is no binding reason for an investigator to seek their consent before embarking on an experiment. However, if there were some accident, he would find himself in a very difficult position. In addition, many scientific journals now require a note as to whether consent has been obtained from an Ethics Committee before accepting a communication.

For further information the reader is referred to the Guidelines on the Practice of Ethics Committees in Medical Research published by the Royal College of Physicians of London.

COMPLIANCE

In most clinical trials it is usual, but not invariable, to ensure that patients do in fact take the drugs prescribed. Extrapolation from clinical trials to general clinical practice is thus only justified if the same degree of compliance with prescribing instructions exists. It is now apparent that this expectation is frequently unfulfilled. Even in hospital the administration of drugs may not be completely in accordance with the wishes of the prescriber. An early study (1962) showed that the average nurse made 1 error for every 6 drugs given. With improved methods of drug prescription and recording and altered nursing procedures the error rate is now nearer 1 in 50. Fortunately most errors are those of wrong time rather than of wrong drug or wrong patient. Nevertheless, it is important that high standards of care and good communication be established between nurses, pharmacists and prescribers. Outside hospital patients may fail to comply with instructions either because they do not understand their drug regime or, because despite full comprehension of the doctor's intentions, they fail to carry out instructions. Thus in a study of children given a 10 day course of penicillin for streptococcal infections it was found that over half had not been given the drug by their parents after 3 days, at 6 days this had risen to 71 % and by 9 days only 18 % were taking penicillin. This study revealed the unreliability of the interview for determining compliance since 83 % of the parents in this study claimed that all the drug had been given. It is believed that between 25 and 50 % of all outpatients drugs are not taken. This may be more pronounced in cases where treatment is prophylactic or suppressant and where the consequences of stopping the drug may be delayed. An element of complacency or boredom with treatment may thus be important, e.g. in tuberculosis treatment it was found that whilst at the end of one year 18% were non-compliant by the end of four years 61% had ceased to take treatment. Side effects may increase drug rejection but there is much evidence that drugs with neither side-effects nor subjectively obvious therapeutic action are also rejected.

There is no typical drug defaulter and a non-compliant patient is not readily identified and may not even be a consistent defaulter, i.e. the non-compliance may not be a constant feature of behaviour and under different circumstances he may be a model patient. No consistent personality type, social class, income group, sex, age, education level, occupation has been shown to be useful in predicting which patients will default from therapy. Even doctors may be drug defaulters! The magnitude of non-compliance problems, particularly in outpatients, makes its consideration mandatory for all conditions in which therapeutic failure has occurred. Although much is now known about the complex factors associated with failure of compliance (over 200 determinants of compliance have been described), the manoeuvres necessary to improve the situation are not worked out. Some factors which have been considered are as follows:

(a) *Patient education*: Over half of patients who leave hospital have been found to have a poor or erroneous understanding of their disease and its treatment. The value of educating patients to improve compliance has been studied, with variable results. There is general agreement that giving the patient further information and taking the time to ensure that this is properly understood is humane and helpful to the patient, but a consistent relationship between this knowledge and good compliance has not been demonstrated.

(b) *Reducing the number of pills to be taken*: Compliance has been shown to fall, as might be expected, with increasing number of pills. Results of trials in which this number has been reduced have given conflicting results, although a priori it might be imagined that using larger doses of drug less frequently or a combination tablet might help. Combination tablets containing a fixed ratio of drugs suffer from a number of disadvantages in that they restrict flexibility in individualising the dosage of the various components, it is easier to overlook possible contraindications of specific components, and if side effects occur it is difficult to know which component is responsible. On the other hand, the oral contraceptive pill is an impressive testimony for combination drugs and in many cases flexible dosing is unnecessary.

(c) *Reducing dose frequency*: Again common sense indicates that this should help compliance, and indeed a few studies suggest this is so by implication, although no formal study has considered this point. There is some evidence that compliance is virtually all or none, so that if an important effect is to be achieved measures must be potent enough to move individuals from virtually nil to full compliance.

(d) *Use of alternative drugs* for a condition may be of benefit, perhaps if side effects are a bar to full compliance. No strong evidence exists to show that this is true, however.

(e) *Use of parenteral and depot preparations* is probably helpful, although the poor compliance of many diabetics on self-injected insulin shows that the route of administration in unimportant. The use of long-acting phenothiazines has been helpful in the management of schizophrenics in the community. Injectable penicillin for rheumatic fever prophylaxis has been more successful than oral preparations in achieving favourable clinical outcomes.

(f) *Clear labelling of containers* with reminder devices does not obviously improve compliance. Possibly allowing patients to administer their own drugs in hospital may improve comprehension but there are no follow-up studies to show that such patients have good compliance on leaving hospital.

Although much of the above regarding improvement of compliance is negative, it is our belief that simple drug regimes with clear instruction given carefully and rehearsed by the patient may improve compliance in practice until further advances in drug delivery systems make compliance more effectively controlled.

ADVERSE REACTIONS TO DRUGS

Adverse reactions may be defined as the unintended effects of drugs used in the prevention, diagnosis or treatment of disease. They comprise a heterogenous collection of symptoms and signs. The classification proposed by Rawlins and Thompson (1977) has proved most useful. They divided them into Type A in which the adverse reactions are part of the drug's normal pharmacological effect and are therefore predictable; they are dose-related with a low mortality. Type B are novel reactions, are not predictable from the drug's known action, are not dose-related and may have a considerable mortality.

Examples	Type A	Type B
Beta-blockers	Bradycardia	Oculocutaneous syndrome
	Bronchospasm	(with practolol)
Thiazides	Gout	Thrombocytopenia
Chlorpromazine	Sedation	Hepatotoxicity

Type A reactions are usually due to incorrect dosage (too much or for too long) or to disordered pharmacokinetics, usually a failure of elimination. Type B reactions are unrelated to the drug's pharmacological action and in many instances the underlying mechanism is poorly understood. Sometimes this appears to be on an immunological basis. Another feature is that they occur infrequently (1 : 1000–1 : 10 000 treated subjects being typical).

Adverse reactions due to interactions between two or more drugs given together are considered in Chapter 8.

There are between 30 000 and 40 000 medicinal products available directly or on prescription to the public in the UK. A random survey found that around 80% of adults took some kind of medication during a two-week period. Therefore the degree of exposure to drug substances in the population is substantial and the incidence of adverse reactions must be viewed in this context. Several reports have suggested that the incidence of adverse reaction is extremely high, e.g. in the US it has been claimed that one-seventh of all hospital days is devoted to the care of drug toxicity. Another claim is that 1 in 10 of hospital inpatients in the US suffers an adverse drug reaction which increases their stay by one week and leads to the death of 6 % of those affected. It has been claimed that 140 000 Americans die annually from drug therapy (i.e. it is the fourth most common cause of death). Such figures are probably in gross error, being much too high as they are based upon extrapolation from highly selected data. More carefully collected data (from the BCDSP—see below) suggests that around 1 in 1000 medical inpatients die, at least in part, as a consequence of drug therapy. However, most of these patients are already suffering from severe illness and the incidence of preventable deaths is about 1 in 10 000 (the drugs involved were mainly potassium chloride or intravenous fluids). Further information is required to assess accurately the risks of non-fatal events due to drugs and to place these in the context of the benefits of drug therapy.

ADVERSE REACTION MONITORING

Once a new drug has been generally released, continued surveillance is required. It is obvious that the preliminary testing of medicines as described above, although excluding many ill effects of drugs, is a leaking sieve and that the use of drugs on a large scale could still carry risks due to initially undetected toxicity. To minimise this danger and to discover these actions before too much damage occurs, a variety of early detection methods have been introduced.

1. Discovery from close observations at the initial trials

Although early trials are important in assessing the efficacy of new drugs, they are not so useful in picking up side effects because there are usually only a limited number of subjects taking the drug in such a trial. Most untoward effects are relatively rare. Thus if some unforeseen side effect occurs in early trials, it will probably only occur once or twice and may therefore be overlooked or attributed to some other cause.

Formal clinical trials have had as their main objective the assessment of therapeutic benefits, and perhaps organisers are less alert to adverse reactions than they should be. The deficiencies of the trial as a detector of adverse reactions is demonstrated by the failure to demonstrate the serious toxicity of practolol before it was generally released, although a number of trials were undertaken during which some participants would have suffered adverse reactions. Clinical trials can potentially assess the incidence of adverse reactions and relate this to therapeutic benefit, although, particularly in early trials, the patients are carefully selected and undergo procedures which are not necessarily representative of normal clinical practice. However, some important adverse effects have been demonstrated in formal trials, e.g. the Coronary Drug Project showed that clofibrate was associated with arrhythmias (1 in 80), thrombophlebitis (1 in 300) and gall-bladder disease (1 in 400). Clinical trial protocols should require the recording of events without any judgement as to causation. Thus a patient who breaks a leg whilst on treatment may have been ataxic as a side effect or it might be merely a coincidence, but if the event is recorded it will eventually become apparent whether this is relevant.

2. Voluntary National Reporting

When a drug has been released for general use it is still necessary to continue surveillance. Untoward effects which have been missed in the early clinical trials become apparent when the drug is used on a wide scale.

In the UK, a Register of Adverse Reactions was started in 1964. Doctors and dentists were asked to report any adverse effects which they considered due to drugs. The CSM operates a system of spontaneous reporting by doctors on pre-paid postcards ('*yellow cards*').

Such an exercise consists of three stages:

(a) collection of data;
(b) analysis of data;
(c) feedback to the doctors of information.

Although this method of surveillance has proved useful, there are certain inherent difficulties. Under-reporting is a major problem: probably on average not more than 10% of adverse reactions are reported. This may be due partially to confusion about what events to report, in deciding whether a drug is responsible for an effect, or sometimes which of several drugs being taken by the patient is responsible. Furthermore there is often difficulty in correlating a particular disorder with the taking of a drug—particularly if there is some delay between cause and effect. A further problem is that if the drug is responsible for an increase in the incidence of some disease which is already common, e.g. gall-bladder disease, carcinoma of the bronchus, the changes in incidence must be very large before this can be detected, since cases due to drug therapy become obscured by cases due to other causes.

It must, however, be admitted that doctors are rather inefficient at detecting adverse reactions to drugs. For example, it took some 15 years for the relatively obvious interaction between barbiturates and oral anticoagulants to be described. In one study it was shown that even when the physicians within a hospital were counselled and requested to report all possible adverse reactions and when they knew that their performance was being monitored, the detection rate was only 7% of the total reactions detected by specialists. Furthermore, those reactions reported were in general the obvious or previously described and well-known reactions. Studies by the Oxford record linkage group have found that retrospective examination of the clinical records of patients taking practolol reveals that during treatment with this drug general practice consultations about eye problems increased 3.5 times and for skin problems the consultation rate doubled. All of these effects took place before the dangers of practolol were appreciated. Thus the information was there but its significance was not appreciated. Again, when the effects of practolol on eye, ear, skin and peritoneum were publicised the CSM was inundated by reports of similar cases: the so-called band-wagon effect. There have been some successes with the scheme, however. For example, the release of ibufenac, an anti-inflammatory analgesic, was rapidly followed by about 40 spontaneous reports of liver damage to the CSM, and the drug was subsequently removed from the market.

Although potentially the population under study by this system comprises all the patients using a drug, in fact under-reporting yields a population which is not uniformly sampled and thus data which are unrepresentative and difficult to work with statistically. This accounts for the lack of incidence of adverse-reaction figures for most drugs. The advantage of such systems is that they are relatively inexpensive and easy to manage and in theory at least ensure permanent monitoring of all drugs, all consumers and all types of adverse reaction.

The reports from drug regulatory bodies of 22 countries are in addition collated by the WHO Unit of Drug Evaluation and Monitoring in Geneva. This unit is an impartial international advisory agency and does not have any powers of drug regulation, nor does it serve as such to member states. The possibility of rapid access to reports from other countries should be of great value in detecting the rarer type of adverse reaction, although the same comments as apply to the national systems apply to this register.

There is also the fascinating question as to different prescribing habits and even differences in the pattern of untoward drug effects in different countries. This has hardly been studied at all but with increasing co-operation it may well become important.

3. Monitoring from national statistics

A great deal of information is available from death certificates, hospital discharge diagnoses and similar records. It may be possible from these data to pick out a change in disease trends and relate this to drug therapy. Perhaps the best-known example of this is the increased death rate in young asthmatics noted in the mid-1960s, which was ultimately traced to the over-use of bronchodilator inhalers containing drugs which were non-specific β-agonists. Although relatively inexpensive the difficulty of this method is obvious. Quite a number of patients must suffer before the change is sufficient to be noticed, particularly in diseases with an appreciable mortality. Data interpretation may also be particularly difficult when hospital discharges are used as a source of information, since sometimes diagnosis can only be provisional and may change as the patient's disease progresses.

4. Record linkage

Record linkage, although a very long-term project, may well produce some important results. The basic idea is that patient's medical records from both GP and hospital sources from cradle to grave should be kept and analysed. This method could be particularly useful when looking for really long-term ill-effects from drugs or from other factors, for instance, the increased incidence of leukaemia in those receiving radiation *in utero* or the occurrence of uterine adenocarcinoma in adolescents whose mothers had received stilboestrol during pregnancy.

Analysis of data is becoming more sophisticated with the use of computers to store information, but one must know what information is worth storing, and must ask the correct questions. Two main types of inquiry can be made:

(a) Follow-up of individuals who have received selected drugs to determine the adverse reactions attributable to the drug. This approach is of most value when a drug is already suspected of producing some particular effect and is not particularly suited to the discovery of unexpected adverse effects. A defect is the absence of a control group. It has been convincingly demonstrated that untreated subjects or those receiving placebo often experience symptoms commonly listed as side effects of drugs. Therefore the results of such studies can be biased by the preconceived ideas of the investigator or the effects on the patient of his enhanced interest.

(b) Follow-up of patients with specific diseases rather than those treated with specific drugs is sometimes easier to carry out since most clinicians categorise their patients under disease rather than treatment. Thus it is easier to review the frequency of adverse reactions to, say, phenytoin, by selecting all the records of epileptics from the records. One of the largest disease-oriented systems is that of the US Perinatal Study which received data on drug exposure and fetal outcome from over 50 000 consecutive pregnancies. From this has come evidence linking malformations and maternal exposure to phenytoin.

5. Case-control studies

One of the great difficulties in monitoring drugs for adverse effects is that if they occur relatively rarely (say, 1 in 1000 patients), very many patients have to be monitored before a particular side effect becomes apparent.

An alternative approach to the problem is to study a group of patients who have developed a particular symptom or syndrome and to compare the frequency of exposure to possible aetiologic agents with a control group. Although this method is comparatively easy to carry out, artefacts may occur as a result of faulty selection of patients or controls. In spite of these difficulties, this approach has had some success, such as the linking of stilboestrol with vaginal adenocarcinoma and of lincomycin with pseudomembranous colitis.

In its most simple form it is really an extension of the idea of the alert doctor (see below) but with the considerable amount of data now available in such studies as the Boston Drug Surveillance Program, it should be possible to use this method on a wider scale and in a more sophisticated manner.

6. Monitored release

There are a number of proposals at present being debated for various schemes of monitored release of new drugs, the principal feature of which is that the pharmaceutical company marketing a new drug should be responsible for obtaining accurate reports on all patients treated up to an agreed number. This is therefore an extension of the market research and limited toxicity monitoring carried out by some companies. Drugs undergoing monitored release would be given a provisional product licence by the CSM and any doctor would be free to prescribe them provided he co-operated in the monitoring scheme. This would involve registration of the patient with the CSM together with appropriate clinical information being placed on record. Suspected adverse reactions would be recorded in the usual way but after a suitable period the doctor would be asked to return a form recording any consultations requested by the patient. This would allow estimation of the incidence of adverse events, and long-term monitoring could be carried out with the help of the Office of Population Censuses and Surveys which holds records of death certificates, etc. The quota of patients to be studied would be variable—say 5000–10 000 for a commonly used drug—and once this had been completed a full product licence could be issued. Presently proposed schemes differ as to who would be responsible for follow-up and arrangements for confidentiality and data handling. Such a method ought to be particularly useful with drugs which are used only by certain specialised doctors, for example, anaesthetists. Successful studies are being carried out particularly by the Drug Surveillance Research Unit at the University of Southampton using prescription event monitoring. Prescriptions for certain drugs are being followed up and the prescribing doctor is asked to fill in a simple questionnaire recording *any* medical event which occurs in the patient. A serious weakness of the monitored release method is the lack of a suitable control group, since it would be difficult to interpret the incidence of a particular adverse reaction without knowing the incidence, determined by the same method, of this reaction in patients not treated with the new drug.

7. Patient questionnaires

These are being explored as a method both of intensive surveillance and of involving the consumer in the problem, so they are partially an educative exercise. Self-administered questionnaires have been used for outpatients attending hypertension and diabetic clinics and have detected previously unsuspected adverse effects, e.g. headache and weakness in the legs as effects of phenformin. They have also been used to show negative effects, e.g. that propranolol is not associated with any of the eye symptoms associated with the adverse effects of practolol.

8. Intensive monitoring

In the last few years a number of intensive monitoring programmes, usually hospital-based, have been started. The Aberdeen–Dundee Monitoring system abstracts data from some 70 000 hospital admissions each year, storing these on a computer file prior to analysis. An even more comprehensive system is the Boston Collaborative Drug Surveillance Program (BCDSP) which involves selected hospitals in several countries, including Scotland. In the BCDSP all patients admitted to specially designated general wards are included in the analysis. Specially trained personnel obtain the following information from hospital patients and records:

1. background information, i.e. age, weight, height, etc.;
2. patient's medical history,
3. patient's drug exposure;
4. side effects of drugs;
5. outcome of treatment and changes in various laboratory tests during hospital admission.

A unique feature of comprehensive drug-monitoring systems lies in their potential to follow up and investigate adverse reactions suggested by less sophisticated detection systems or by isolated case reports in medical journals. Furthermore, the frequency of side effects can be determined more cheaply than by a specially mounted trial to investigate a simple adverse effect, e.g. the risk of developing a rash with ampicillin was found to be around 7% by clinical trial and by the BCDSP which can determine these facts almost automatically from the data on file. Also new adverse reactions or drug interactions may be detected by multiple correlation analysis of the data. Thus, when an unexpected relationship arises, such as the 20% incidence of gastro-intestinal bleeding in patients treated with ethacrynic acid as compared to 4.3% of patients treated with other diuretics, there is little chance of bias arising from awareness of the hypothesis during data collection since the data are collected before the hypothesis is proposed. It is also possible to isolate factors predisposing patients to a particular complication; in the case of ethacrynic acid these were female sex, a high blood urea, previous heparin administration and intravenous administration of the drug. An important aspect of this type of approach is that negative associations may also be detected. Thus no significant association between aspirin and renal disease was found; indeed long-term aspirin consumption is associated with a decreased incidence of myocardial infarction, an association which may be of therapeutic importance.

In terms of *new* but uncommon adverse reactions, however, the numbers of patients undergoing intensive monitoring taking a particular drug are too small for the effect to be detected. Such monitoring therefore can provide information only about relatively common, early reactions to drugs used under hospital conditions. Patients are not in hospital long enough for detection of delayed effects which are just the reactions least likely to be spotted even by an astute clinician. There are plans to extend intensive drug monitoring to cover general practice, psychiatric, paediatric and obstetric patients. It should be recognised, however, that intensive monitoring is not a foolproof and comprehensive method of drug screening.

9. Feedback

There is no use in collecting vast amounts of data on adverse reactions unless it is analysed and important information reported back to the prescribing doctor. This has not proved easy for the CSM and there have been a number of instances in which leaks to the media have preceded the information reaching the doctor. In addition to articles in the medical press the CSM circulates to all doctors a 'Current Problems' information sheet which deals with important and recently discovered adverse reactions. If an acute problem arises doctors will usually receive notification from the CSM and often the pharmaceutical company involved.

Summary

It would appear from all this that there is as yet no perfect method of detecting ill effects from drugs. The methods used are largely complementary. Initial trials picking out the frequently occurring reactions, national reporting systems filtering out the rarer side effects, intensive monitoring finding a few adverse effects, but also giving an idea of their frequency in relationship to the amount of drug prescribed and record linkage looking for long-term effects. The feedback to doctors of information about adverse drug reactions and the general public is a difficult balancing act. Unfortunately, before it becomes clear that a drug is causing a certain ill effect, there is a period of suspicion when the case is not proven. Too rigid and early action under these circumstances will cause alarm which may or may not be justified and could lead to the withdrawal or reduced use of potentially valuable drug. Against this it is obvious that the earlier ill-effects can be detected and prevented, the better. The requirement of over-elaborate safety regulations before a new drug is released by protocols so strict that neither aspirin nor digitalis could possibly have been passed is also self-defeating and could lead to therapeutic stagnation. A situation approaching this may have occurred in the USA, where strict regulations have led to considerable delay in introducing such useful drugs as β-blockers and salbutamol.

Arguably some patients will receive inferior or unnecessarily dangerous drugs when better drugs are available elsewhere. The development of drugs under such a system also becomes extremely costly, and this hinders the provision of drugs for rare diseases or for tropical diseases limited to the poorer parts of the world. Companies are unwilling to hazard their reputations or risk litigation by supplying drugs which have not undergone the full multi-million pound testing programme if the eventual sales are unlikely to allow them to cover even the costs of the tests.

Unfortunately, many patients and the media seem to believe that any serious reaction to a drug necessarily implies negligence by the prescriber or inadequate testing by the manufacturer. The use of powerful drugs always carries an inherent risk. For most drugs the information required to determine accurate benefit-to-risk ratios is not available. There is no accepted definition of a 'significant risk' for drug therapy and clearly the apparent incidence of adverse reactions depends upon whether this term relates to a reaction which importantly influences the patient's clinical state or to a minor or transient effect. Most monitoring systems accept the opinion of a single observer, often with no particular expertise in the field, as to the relation of an untoward clinical event to drug therapy. As in other clinical judgements a degree of subjectivity enters into this assessment, since generally adverse drug reactions present no unique clinical or laboratory findings to delineate them from concurrent illness. In a study of 60 selected cases by three clinical pharmacologists, agreement was reached in only 50% of cases and nearly all of these were thought to be unrelated to drugs. In the other cases there was disagreement about the nature of the agent causing the adverse reaction, and complete agreement between the clinical pharmacologist assessors and the responsible physicians occurred in less than half the cases. Statements about adverse drug reactions should therefore be regarded with reservation unless the degree of certainty can be clearly stated. Ideally, adverse reactions should be fully accepted as drug-related only when the criteria for proof conform to the same rules as those required for beneficial effects.

In the prevention of drug-related illness there is one further agent which is worth remembering and that is the *alert doctor*. This means that when something odd occurs, not necessarily related to drugs, the doctor spends time discussing every possibility with the patient. It is salutary to remember that so far the majority of initial reports of the most serious adverse effects have come from the observations of individual doctors.

Proprietary and non-proprietary (generic) titles

When a new drug is released it has a *proprietary* name supplied by the pharmacological company introducing it and a *non-proprietary (generic)* title supplied by the British Pharmacopoeia.

Until the patent on a drug runs out it is usually only available from the company which introduced it. After this other companies can manufacture and market it, sometimes under their own proprietary name and sometimes under the generic title. When this happens the hospital pharmacist will usually shop around for the 'best buy'. If a doctor in hospital prescribes a drug by its proprietary name, the same drug but produced by another company may be dispensed. This can save a considerable amount of money. If, however, a general practitioner prescribes a drug by its proprietary name, the pharmacist must dispense that particular drug even though it may be more expensive than the same drug produced by other companies.

It would seem obvious then that to cut costs all drugs should be prescribed under their generic titles or the pharmacist should be at liberty to dispense a generic alternative. There are however arguments against this view:

(a) The actual formulation of a drug may differ between companies, perhaps affecting bioavailability (see p. 65).
(b) If a doctor prescribes a particular company's drug, it is only right that it should be dispensed, especially if that company has spent millions of pounds researching its discovery and introduction.

At present there is considerable pressure to introduce generic prescribing into general practice but it is being resisted by the pharmaceutical industry and others.

Formularies and restricted lists

In times when there were very few active drugs, mixtures were often prescribed containing agents of varying efficacy and usually unpleasant taste. Many hospitals had formularies which were essentially recipe books containing the mixtures preferred by the staff of that particular hospital. With the therapeutic revolution which occurred after the Second World War, when the older types of medicine were replaced by single active agents prepared by the pharmaceutical industry, the need for such formularies disappeared.

More recently the National Formulary and now the British National Formulary (BNF) were published. The BNF contains information about all drug preparations currently available together with advice on prescribing and is extremely useful.

The escalating drug bill and the bewildering range of drugs available has led some hospitals to introduce their own formularies again. These are essentially a restricted list of drugs in the hospital pharmacy and may also include information about the drugs and their use. Doctors are discouraged but not prevented from prescribing medicines not included in their hospital formulary.

The objects of these formularies are:

(a) To reduce spending by stocking 'best buy' drugs.
(b) To simplify purchasing and storage of drugs.
(c) To increase prescribing doctors' awareness of drug actions and cost.

It can be argued that formularies which are essentially restrictive interfere with the doctor's right to prescribe the drug he feels appropriate for his patient and may also limit innovation. It is therefore imperative that there should be continuing dialogue between those preparing and updating the formulary and those prescribing the drugs.

Chapter 8
DRUG INTERACTIONS

Drug interactions are pharmacological responses which cannot be explained by the action of a single drug but are due to two or more drugs acting simultaneously. Interactions may be harmful to the patient by increasing efficacy or toxicity or alternatively by decreasing the therapeutic effect of a co-administered agent. Occasionally therapeutic benefit may be obtained by an interaction which allows reduction of dose by enhanced efficacy without increased toxicity.

It is usual for patients in hospital to receive a number of drugs. At the Johns Hopkins Hospital one study showed an average of 14 drugs were prescribed to medical patients (one received 36 different drugs during one admission). The BCDSP obtained an average figure of 9.1 drugs/patient/admission for hospital in-patients in the USA as compared with 4.6 drugs/patient/admission in Scotland.

Outpatients similarly receive several drugs; sometimes these are supplemented by proprietary over-the-counter medicines, by drugs supplied by friends and relatives or even by drugs prescribed by other doctors without reference to the patient's own doctor. It is estimated that for patients taking 2–5 drugs, the incidence of potential interactions is overall 19 %, which rises to over 80 % for those taking 6 or more drugs. Thus the greater number of drugs prescribed, the more likely things are to go wrong (Fig. 8.1). One American writer has described the 'carrier-bag' syndrome whereby patients are obliged to bring a bag to the pharmacy to carry away all the various medicines prescribed. In one prospective study of over 25 000 days of hospitalisation, 4.7 % of the patients studied were found to have potentially interacting drug combinations but in only 6.2 % of these at-risk patients was any clinical evidence of the putative interaction detected. In the BCDSP around 7 % of adverse drug reactions appear to be due to drug interactions. Thus adverse drug interactions occur approximately in 0.5–2 % of hospital inpatients.

Several large compendia of drug interactions have been published. Unfortunately, many of the described interactions are based on animal or in vitro experiments, the results of which cannot be transferred uncritically to the clinical situation. The same problems exist for the detection of drug interactions as have been delineated for adverse drug reactions (Chapter 7). In addition, it is possible to carry out laboratory studies to supplement clinical observation. The clinician ideally requires information on the frequency of occurrence and the consequences for the patient of a given interaction: as with adverse drug reactions, this information is unavailable. In essence, every time a doctor prescribes a drug or drug combination, he is performing an experiment on that particular patient. Every individual has a peculiar set of characteristics which will determine his response to therapy. Even when potentially interacting drugs are prescribed adverse effects are not invariable.

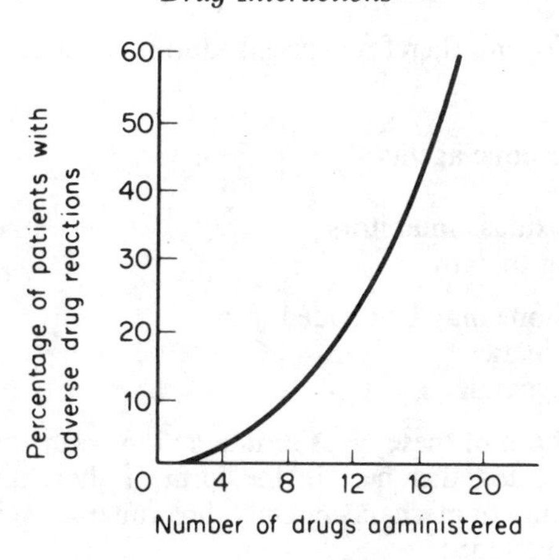

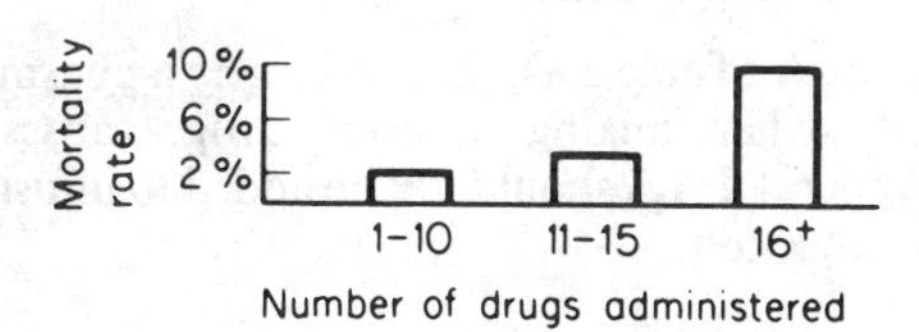

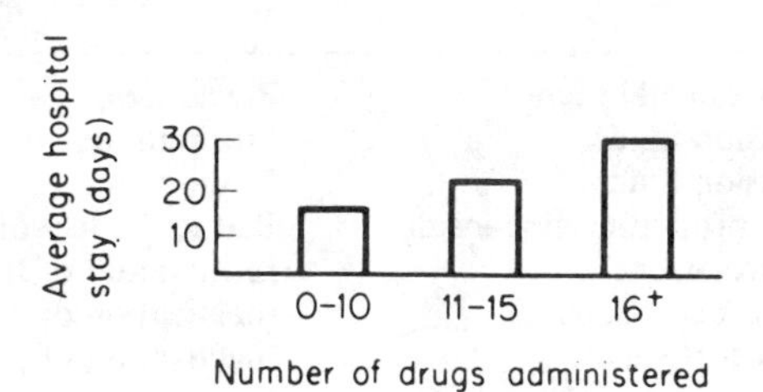

Fig. 8.1 Relationship of number of drugs administered to (a) adverse drug reactions; (b) mortality rate and (c) average duration of hospital stay (From J. W. Smith *et al.*, *Ann. Int. Med.*, **65**, 631 (1966).)

Thus, in a study of warfarin potentiation by chloral, only 25 % of patients receiving this combination showed a significant increase in anticoagulant effect. Similarly about the same proportion of patients receiving adrenergic neurone blockers (guanethidine, bethanidine) and a potentially interacting drug demonstrated any effect. The factors determining whether an individual patient will manifest a potential drug interaction are unknown.

It is impossible to remember even the simplified lists which comprise most of this chapter and it is assumed that prescribers will have access to suitable reference books to be able to check on a particular problem. Nevertheless there are certain drug groups where drug interactions are liable to cause dangerous results and therefore special caution is required with concurrent therapy:

anticoagulants
oral hypoglycaemic agents
digitalis
monoamine oxidase inhibitors
cytotoxic drug therapy

Drug interactions may be divided into

I. pharmacokinetic
II. pharmacodynamic.

Examples of both of these types of interaction occur throughout this text; they are grouped together here in the form of short illustrative tables to emphasise the unity of mechanism. Only those interactions of proven clinical importance are included.

1. Pharmacokinetic interactions

(a) *Outside the body* (Table 8.1): This is largely a pharmaceutical problem of incompatibility when mixing different drugs causes precipitation or inactivation. In general drugs should not be added to infusions and are better given by a bolus injection.

Table 8.1 Interactions outside the body

Mixture	*Result*
Thiopentone + suxamethonium	Precipitation
Diazepam + infusion fluids	Precipitation
Phenytoin + infusion fluids	Precipitation
Soluble insulin + protamine zinc insulin	Reduced effect of soluble insulin
Heparin + hydrocortisone	Inactivation of heparin
Kanamycin + hydrocortisone	Inactivation of kanamycin
Penicillin + hydrocortisone	Inactivation of penicillin

(b) *Interactions in the gut* (Table 8.2): See Chapter 2.

(c) *Drug displacement from binding sites* (Table 8.3) is often suggested as the underlying mechanism behind several interactions but in only a few cases has this been rigorously proven (Chapter 1) and the examples in Table 8.3 include some where the quantitative importance of displacement has not been established.

(d) *Interactions with drug metabolism*: Decreased effects of drugs may result from enzyme induction by a second agent (see p. 84). Clinically this is significant if the treatment of a patient requires accurate control or a threshold level of drug. Some clinically important interactions are shown in Table 8.4.

Inhibition of drug metabolism may produce toxicity or an exaggerated or prolonged response. The mechanisms may be competition for the same enzyme—e.g. the interaction of ethanol and trichloroethanol—or direct inhibition of the enzyme—e.g. the interaction of allopurinol with azathio-

Table 8.2 Interactions in the gut

Mixture	*Mechanism*	*Result*
Digoxin + metoclopramide	Altered gut motility	Reduced digoxin absorption
Digoxin + propantheline		Increased digoxin absorption
Prednisone + propantheline		Increased prednisone absorption
Tetracycline + sodium bicarbonate	Altered gut pH	Decreased tetracycline absorption
Tetracycline + Ca^{2+}, Mg^{2+}, Al^{3+}, Fe^{2+}	Chelation	Mutually reduced absorption
Para aminosalicylate + penicillin	Direct toxicity produces a malabsorption syndrome	Reduces absorption
Neomycin + penicillin		
Colchicine + penicillin		
Griseofulvin + phenobarbitone	? why absorption decreased	Low levels of griseofulvin

Table 8.3 Interactions due to drug displacement from binding sites

Bound drug	*Displacing drug*	*Result*
Bilirubin	Sulphonamides Vitamin K	Kernicterus
Tolbutamide	Salicylates Phenylbutazone	Hypoglycaemia
Methotrexate	Salicylates Sulphonamides	Agranulocytosis
Thiopentone	Sulphonamides	Prolonged anaesthesia
Warfarin	Salicylates Trichloroacetic acid Clofibrate	Haemorrhage

Table 8.4 Interactions due to enzyme induction

Primary drug	*Inducing agent*	*Effect of interaction*
Oral anticoagulants e.g. warfarin	Barbiturates Glutethimide Dichloralphenazone Rifampicin	Decreased anticoagulation
Tolbutamide	Phenytoin Alcohol Chlorpromazine	Decreased hypoglycaemia
Oral contraceptives	Rifampicin	Pregnancy
Prednisone and Dexamethasone	Barbiturates	Reduced steroid levels
Chlorpromazine	Barbiturates	Reduced phenothiazine levels
Doxycycline	Barbiturates	Reduced doxycycline levels
Quinidine	Phenytoin Barbiturates	Reduced quinidine levels

prine. Drugs which inhibit the metabolism of one drug do not necessarily inhibit the metabolism of another, e.g. allopurinol inhibits antipyrine metabolism but does not affect phenylbutazone or warfarin, drugs which are also oxidised by hepatic microsomes. In some cases it may be the balance of interactions in the individual patient which determines the interaction effect, thus diazepam has been shown to reduce phenytoin plasma levels, possibly by enzyme induction, but also to elevate them, possibly by competition for metabolism.

Inhibition of or competition for drug-metabolising enzymes may also occur, producing a prolonged or toxic response (Table 8.5). The time course of such interactions is often shorter than for enzyme induction, since it depends merely upon the attainment of a high enough concentration of the inhibiting drug at the metabolic site.

Table 8.5 Interactions due to enzyme inhibition

Primary drug	*Inhibiting drug*	*Effect of interaction*
Phenytoin	Isoniazid	Phenytoin intoxication
	Phenobarbitone	
	Phenylbutazone	
	Chloramphenicol	
	Disulphiram	
Oral anticoagulants	Allopurinol	Haemorrhage
e.g. warfarin	Nortriptyline	
	Quinidine	
Azathioprine	Allopurinol	Bone-marrow suppression
Tolbutamide	Phenylbutazone	Hypoglycaemia
Chlorpropamide	Chloramphenicol	Hypoglycaemia
	Dicoumarol	
Pethidine	MAOI	Prolonged sedation
Barbiturates	MAOI	Prolonged sedation

Table 8.6 Competitive interactions for renal tubular transport

Primary drug	*Competing drug*	*Effect of interaction*
Penicillin	Probenecid	Increased penicillin blood level
Methotrexate	Salicylates	Bone-marrow suppression
	Sulphonamides	
Salicylate	Probenecid	Salicylate toxicity
Indomethacin	Probenecid	Indomethacin toxicity
P.A.S.	Probenecid	P.A.S. toxicity
Lithium	Thiazide diuretics	Lithium toxicity
Chlorpropamide	Phenylbutazone	Hypoglycaemia
Digoxin	Spironolactone	Increased plasma digoxin levels

(e) *Interactions during renal excretion*: Many acidic drugs share a common transport mechanism in the proximal tubules and can therefore mutually reduce excretion by a competitive process (Table 8.6). Changes in urinary pH also alter drug excretion and administration of systemic alkalinising or acidifying agents or carbonic anhydrase inhibitors may change blood levels of these drugs (Table 8.7).

Such effects have, however, been of clinical significance extremely rarely, although they can be of value in the management of drug overdose (Chapter 22).

Table 8.7 Some drugs whose excretion is affected by alteration in urinary pH

Excretion enhanced by acidification	*Excretion enhanced by alkalinisation*
Fenfluramine	Salicylate
Amphetamine	Phenobarbitone
Pseudoephedrine	Barbitone
Quinidine	
Procainamide	
Mexiletine	
Pethidine	

2. Pharmacodynamic interactions may arise by:

(a) *Interaction at drug receptors*, e.g. the use of naloxone to reverse opiate intoxication, or less directly the reversal of muscular relaxation by tubocurarine by the indirect local increase of acetylcholine via cholinesterase inhibition with neostigmine. It is unusual for drugs without any intrinsic action on the receptor to be involved in this type of interaction. Possibly the increased anticoagulant effect of warfarin during d-thyroxine or clofibrate therapy is an example. These drugs are devoid of effect on clotting factors or their synthesis but may increase the affinity between warfarin and its receptor site in the liver.

(b) *Effects on drug transport mechanisms* may prevent drugs reaching their site of action upon receptors or else prolong their effect due to slow removal from the vicinity of receptors (Table 8.8).

(c) *Synergism of effects* of drugs acting at the same site or influencing the same physiological system is common and some examples are shown in Table 8.9.

Table 8.8 Some drug interactions secondary to inhibition of uptake or transport of drugs at their site of action

Primary drug	*Inhibiting drug*	*Effect of interaction*
Guanethidine Bethanidine Debrisoquine Clonidine	Tricyclic antidepressants Phenothiazines, especially Chlorpromazine	Reduction of hypotensive effect
Fenfluramine	Tricyclic antidepressants	Depression or prolonged sedation
Phenylephrine Adrenaline Noradrenaline	Tricyclic antidepressants Guanethidine	Potentiation of pressor effect of catecholamines

(d) *Alterations in fluid and electrolyte balance* induced by drugs may modify the responses of tissues to drugs. Some examples are shown in Table 8.10.

Table 8.9 Synergistic drug effects

Primary drug	*Interacts with*	*Resulting in*
Alcohol	Other CNS depressant drugs e.g. barbiturates antihistamines narcotics	CNS depression
Tubocurarine	Aminoglycosides e.g. streptomycin kanamycin Quinidine Procaine	Prolonged paralysis
Oral hypoglycaemia drugs	Salicylates Propranolol Monoamine oxidase inhibitors	Prolonged or excessive hypoglycaemia
Digitalis	Propranolol Guanethidine	Bradycardia due to unopposed vagal effects of glycoside

Table 8.10 Interactions secondary to drug-induced alteration of fluid and electrolyte balance

Primary drug	*Interacting drug effect*	*Result of interaction*
Digitalis	Diuretic-induced hypokalaemia	Digitalis toxicity
Lignocaine Quinidine Phenytoin	Diuretic-induced hypokalaemia	Antagonism of antiarrhythmic effects
Digitalis	Suxamethonium releasing potassium via depolarisation	Digitalis toxicity
Diuretics	Phenylbutazone induced salt and water retention	Antagonism of diuretic effects
Tubocurarine	Diuretic-induced hypokalaemia	Prolonged paralysis
Lithium	Thiazide-induced reduction in renal clearance	Raised plasma lithium levels

Interference of drugs with chemical diagnostic tests

A brief note is necessary concerning this 'interaction' since several drugs can interfere with chemical estimations performed on body fluids. Such interference may be due to biological interactions, e.g. alteration of binding protein, or technical, resulting from some interaction with the method used to carry out the test. Clinical chemists should always be told of the drug history of a patient before being asked to undertake lengthy, complicated and costly investigations, the results of which might be totally invalidated by the patient's treatment.

Table 8.11 Examples of biological interference with laboratory tests

Test	*Drug*	*Mechanism*	*Effect of drug*
Serum copper	Oestrogens (including the pill)	Increased binding protein	Increase
Serum cortisol	Oestrogens (including the pill)	Increased binding protein	Increase
Serum iron	Oestrogens (including the pill)	Increased binding protein	Increase
Serum thyroxine	Oestrogens (including the pill)	Increased binding protein	Increase
Serum thyroxine	Phenytoin Salicylates	Competition with thyroxine for binding to carrier protein	Decrease
Serum thyroxine	Androgen	Reduced binding protein	Decrease
Urinary 5-hydroxy-indoleacetic acid	MAOI	Reduced katabolism	Increase
Urinary ketones	Sodium valproate	Drug excreted as ketones	Positive
Urinary vanillyl-mandelic acid	MAOI	Reduced katabolism	Increase
Blood grouping and compatibility testing	Methyldopa Mefanamic acid Penicillin (> 20 000 units daily)	Antibody formation Antibody formation Antibody formation	Makes cross matching of blood difficult

Table 8.12 Examples to technical interference with laboratory tests

Test	*Method*	*Drug*	*Spurious effect*
Catecholamines	Fluorimetry	Tetracyclines	Raised
		Methyldopa	Raised
Cortisol	Sulphuric acid fluorescence	Fenfluramine	Raised
		Spironolactone	Raised
Digoxin	Radio-immunoassay	Spironolactone	Reduced
Folic acid	Microbiological	Antibiotics	Test invalidated
Ketones in urine	Ferric chloride	Salicylates Chlorpromazine	Positive
Protein-bound iodine	All methods	X-ray contrast media	Raised
		Clioquinol	Raised
Reducing substances in urine	Benedict's test or Clinitest	Nalidixic acid Salicylates	Positive
Vanillylmandelic acid in urine	Fluorescence	Methyldopa	Raised
Vitamin B_{12}	Microbiological	Antibiotics	Invalidated
Blood grouping and compatibility testing	Agglutination	High molecular weight dextrans; Methyldopa; Mefanamic acid	Rouleaux formation invalidates test

B. Systematic Considerations

Chapter 9
THE NERVOUS SYSTEM

PSYCHOTROPIC DRUGS

This is a mixed group of drugs affecting the mind which often possess overlapping pharmacological properties so that at a low dose for example a drug may be employed as a sedative and at a higher dose as a hypnotic. They may be broadly classified as:

(a) hypnotics;
(b) anti-anxiety agents (anxiolytics, sedatives, minor tranquillisers);
(c) anti-psychotic drugs (neuroleptics, major tranquillisers);
(d) anti-depressants;
(e) mood stabilisers;
(f) psychotomimetics.

HYPNOTIC DRUGS

Insomnia is common: in one survey 45 % of women and 15 % of men over the age of 45 in two Scottish cities regularly took prescribed hypnotics. There is no clear division between the occasional bouts of insomnia suffered by the average person at times of mental or physical stress and chronic pathological sleeplessness. It is important to exclude causes of insomnia which require treatment in their own right:

(a) pain, e.g. arthritis, peptic ulcer;
(b) dyspnoea, e.g. left ventricular failure, bronchospasm;
(c) cough;
(d) frequency of micturition;
(e) full bladder and/or loaded rectum in the elderly;
(f) excitatory drugs, e.g. caffeine, amphetamine derivatives;
(g) depression, in which disturbed, restless sleep, particularly with early morning awakening occurs;
(h) anxiety states when there may be difficulty in getting off to sleep.

There is a tendency for total sleep time to be reduced in the elderly and this is accompanied by more frequent awakening and decreased dreaming. Although about a third of our life span is spent in sleep the function of this state is not clearly understood. It is possible to distinguish two opposing states of sleep:

(a) *Non-rapid eye movement* (*NREM*) *or orthodox sleep* is associated with slow waves on the EEG. No eye movements apart from slow oscillations during the lighter stages of sleep occur. Cardiorespiratory activity is slow and steady and during the deeper phases growth hormone is secreted. During

NREM sleep mitosis of somatic cells is maximal and it has been postulated that body-repair processes occur at this time.

(b) *Rapid eye movement (REM) sleep* is associated with bursts of rapid eye movements and an EEG pattern characteristic of wakefulness. Cerebral blood flow is greater than when awake and heart rate, respiration and blood pressure become increased and variable. Erection of the penis occurs during REM sleep. If awoken the sleeper reports dreaming. Animal experiments show that cerebral synthetic processes are maximal during REM sleep.

Drugs may produce states which superficially resemble sleep but which lack the characteristic normal mixture of these two sleep states. Thus, for example, barbiturates suppress REM sleep and when discontinued there is an excess of REM sleep ('rebound') which is associated with restlessness, dreaming and insomnia. Consequently further drug may be required to suppress the symptoms of its withdrawal. The long-term use of hypnotics should be avoided because of their relative ineffectiveness and the risk of dependence. There may be a place for such drugs in the management of acute insomnia such as may occur during a period of stress or anxiety. Chronic insomnia is probably best approached by a combination of psychotherapy with as little recourse to drugs as is possible. Presently, the drugs of first choice are the benzodiazepines which have several advantages over other groups of drugs used as hypnotics. These drugs are a heterogeneous collection, the main ones comprising:

(a) chloral derivatives;
(b) piperidinediones, e.g. glutethimide;
(c) barbiturates;
(d) alcohols, e.g. ethanol, ethchlorvynol;
(e) phenothiazines, e.g. promethazine;
(f) quinazolines, e.g. methaqualone;
(g) chlormethiazole;
(h) benzodiazepines.

The main members of these classes will now be separately examined.

Chloral derivatives

These are halogenated alcohols. In aqueous media chloral is converted to chloral hydrate. This is a hypnotic but is mainly metabolised in the body to trichloroethanol, which is less polar and possibly more active than its precursor. Because of the rapid conversion of chloral hydrate to trichloroethanol *in vivo* it is difficult to compare the actions of the two substances—the actions of administered chloral derivatives appear to be due to trichloroethanol.

These are central depressants, but like other hypnotics, delirium and excitement can be produced, particularly in the elderly or if pain is present.

In therapeutic doses chloral derivatives are safe hypnotics and produce little change in respiration and circulation; however, in overdose dangerous respiratory and myocardial depression and hypotension develop. During recovery from overdose jaundice and proteinuria may occur.

Pharmacokinetics Chloral hydrate is well absorbed from the intestine but is rapidly reduced by the action of alcohol dehydrogenase in the liver, blood and other tissues to form trichloroethanol. Chloral hydrate is not normally detected in the blood or urine after oral administration. Some trichloroethanol is converted to trichloroacetic acid, the rest being conjugated with glucuronide to form urochloralic acid. The $t_{1/2}$ of trichloroethanol is 8 h, which is short enough to prevent much accumulation, but that of trichloroacetate is about 4 days, so that this metabolite accumulates substantially on chronic dosing. It is not clear that trichloroacetate accumulation is harmful (although it displaces warfarin from protein binding) however it is not desirable that any foreign compound should accumulate in patients. Excretion of metabolites is mainly renal but some urochloralic acid appears in the bile.

Clinical use Chloral hydrate is an effective, reasonably safe hypnotic, inducing sleep in 30–60 min. It has an unpleasant taste and should be given well diluted to minimise gastric irritation. For adults the usual hypnotic dose is 1–2 g. It is also useful in children although its bitter taste may pose problems: the usual dose is 15–30 mg/kg body weight.

Chloral can also be given as chloral hydrate capsules (250 and 500 mg) or as tablets of *dichloralphenazone* (*Welldorm*—650 mg dichloralphenazone) or elixir of either.

Adverse reactions

1. Large doses produce respiratory and cardiovascular depression. Death usually results from 10 g, i.e. ten times the therapeutic dose. Repeated use leads to tolerance and dependence. Occasionally patients become disorientated, confused, paranoid or somnambulistic. As with most hypnotics a period of hangover is experienced the next day.
2. Chloral is a gastric irritant and produces nausea and vomiting. Chloral hydrate is an unpleasant-tasting liquid and tablets of dichloralphenazone are less nauseating.
3. Rashes are not uncommon, and include erythematous, scarlatiniform, urticarial and scaling eruptions. The appearance of the rash may be delayed and usually begins on the face and limbs and then spreads to the trunk.
4. The drug is contraindicated in severe renal, hepatic, myocardial and respiratory disease.
5. **Drug interactions.** There is mutual potentiation of central nervous depression when given with other hypno-sedatives. This effect is seen with alcohol (the original 'Mickey Finn'). In this case an added effect is competition for the rate-limiting enzyme step, alcohol dehydrogenase, between ethanol and trichloroethanol which mutually reduces their metabolism.

   Chloral is one of several drugs which potentiate the effects of warfarin by displacing it from plasma-protein binding sites.

   Enzyme induction is not clinically significant with chloral hydrate. However, the phenazone moiety of dichloralphenazone induces hepatic enzymes and can for example, accelerate the rate of metabolism of warfarin.

Piperidinediones

Glutethimide

This non-barbiturate hypnotic was introduced in order to avoid the disadvantages of the barbiturates. Unfortunately glutethimide has turned out to be at least as hazardous as these drugs.

Glutethimide is a powerful sedative and hypnotic, but produces cardiovascular and respiratory depression even more readily than the barbiturates. In addition the drug is antitussive, antiemetic and anticholinergic, commonly producing a dry mouth.

Pharmacokinetics Glutethimide is highly lipid soluble and there may be considerable delay in absorption, although once dissolved the drug readily passes through lipid membranes. Glutethimide is completely metabolised. It is closely related to thalidomide but thalidomide is mainly hydrolysed whereas glutethimide is hydroxylated, the principal metabolite is itself a central depressant with a longer $t_{1/2}$ than glutethimide. The plasma $t_{1/2}$ of glutethimide has been variously reported as 5–20 h, but in overdose plasma levels correlate only poorly with the duration of coma, probably because of the central depressant effects of the hydroxylated metabolites.

Clinical uses Glutethimide has been used as a hypnotic in doses of 0.5 g. When given in doses of 0.125–0.25 g 6 hourly it has an anxiolytic action, but fatigue and sleepiness usually occur as well. This drug is obsolete.

Adverse reactions

1. Prolonged hangover, dry mouth and constipation are common side effects.
2. Dependence is similar to that due to barbiturates. On withdrawal there may be anxiety, restlessness, nausea, tachycardia, tonic muscle spasms and fits.
3. In overdose, there is respiratory depression and characteristically severe hypotension. A lethal dose for an adult is about 10 g. Mydriasis is a prominent feature (as opposed to the small pupils of chloral overdose). Dry mouth, paralytic ileus and urinary retention resulting from its anticholinergic properties may develop. Convulsions, sudden apnoea and cerebral oedema may occur during intoxication. Several studies have found glutethimide to have the highest mortality of all drug-induced comas, death being over ten times more frequent than in comparable barbiturate overdoses.
4. Glutethimide is a powerful inducing agent.

Barbiturates

These are valuable drugs in current use as anaesthetics, anticonvulsants and occasionally, hepatic enzyme inducers. As hypnotics, however, their use is rapidly diminishing due to drug toxicity, proneness to dependence, frequency of death from overdose and interactions with many other drugs. It should also be pointed out that like most other drugs prescribed as hypnotics, e.g.

glutethimide, chloral hydrate, meprobamate, the evidence that barbiturates are effective hypnotics is poor. Most of these drugs become ineffective when taken repeatedly over a two-week period. They are not analgesic and may even increase restlessness and other responses to pain due to a stimulant action on the thalamus.

Pharmacokinetics Common to all barbiturates:

1. Absorbed from gastric, small intestinal and rectal mucosae.
2. Metabolism by liver microsomal oxidising systems although phenobarbitone and barbitone have low enough pKa values, protein binding and lipid solubility to undergo significant renal elimination. Metabolites are inactive hydroxy and aldehyde derivatives and there is evidence in the case of amylobarbitone for a substantial genetic control over the rate and extent of this process.
3. Powerful enzyme inducers including autoinduction with chronic use.

The properties of these drugs are summarised in Table 9.1.

Table 9.1 Properties of barbiturates

Drug	$t_{1/2}$ (*h*)	*Other features*
Heptobarbitone (Medomin)	6–12	Eliminated by metabolism Renal excretion insignificant
Amylobarbitone (Amytal)	18–36	Eliminated by metabolism Renal excretion insignificant
Quinalbarbitone (+ amylobarbitone = Tuinal)	18–36	Eliminated by metabolism Renal excretion insignificant
Pentobarbitone (Nembutal)	24–48	Moderate lipid solubility 35% protein bound Eliminated by metabolism Renal excretion insignificant
Butobarbitone (Soneryl)	36–48	Eliminated by metabolism Renal excretion insignificant
Phenobarbitone	50–100	Low lipid solubility 20% protein bound 30% excreted in urine unchanged
Barbitone	Similar to phenobarbitone	Low lipid solubility 5% protein bound 65% excreted in urine unchanged

Clinical Uses Apart from their uses in anaesthesia and epilepsy, their use as hypnotics, anxiolytics and sedatives is not advised and they have been supplanted by the benzodiazepines which are safer for these purposes.

Adverse effects

1. Therapeutic doses of the barbiturates as hypnotics usually produce satisfactory sleep for the first one or two weeks; thereafter, because of nervous-system habituation, sleep is not so readily induced. Nevertheless, attempts to stop the drug result in anxiety, insomnia and

excessive dreaming. Barbiturates suppress that portion of sleep during which dreaming and rapid eye movements occur (REM or paradoxical sleep). When withdrawn, a period of excessive REM sleep occurs for some days which is associated with poor sleep (see Fig. 9.1) and the patient may request a further prescription of hypnotic, thus reinforcing the pattern of hypnotic-taking behaviour.

2. After barbiturate-induced sleep a prolonged hangover occurs with loss of mental activity during the first half of the following day.
3. Dangerous respiratory depression occurs with about 10 times a hypnotic dose. Patients with incipient or overt respiratory failure may die if given therapeutic doses of these drugs.
4. Drug dependence rapidly develops. Barbiturates are taken by addicts either orally or by injection, usually of ground-up tablets (commonly pentobarbitone, quinalbarbitone, amylobarbitone or Tuinal, a proprietary mixture of the last two drugs). Barbiturates are highly irritant to the tissues and extravasation causes sloughing ulcers.
5. Paradoxical excitement may occur in the young with barbiturates.
6. In the elderly barbiturates may cause depression, confusion, ataxia and a tendency to fall. A strong correlation has been observed between fracture of the femur and nocturnal falls associated with barbiturate hypnotics.
7. Barbiturate overdosage still accounts for a significant proportion of hospital admissions. Barbiturates are particularly lethal when taken with alcohol.

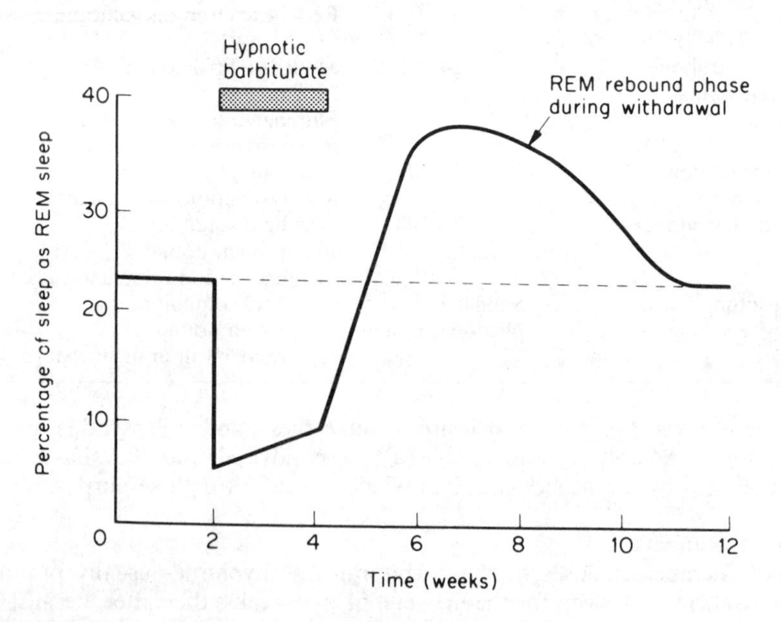

Fig. 9.1 Rebound of REM sleep following suppression by a course of a hypnotic dose of a barbiturate for two weeks.

8. Barbiturates are specifically contraindicated in myxoedema, chronic liver and renal failure, acute porphyria and senile dementia.
9. **Interactions** with other drugs are frequent—usually because of their powerful enzyme-inducing properties (see p. 84). Of particular note are the interactions with oral anticoagulants (diminished activity), vitamin D (osteomalacia) and the contraceptive pill (pregnancy).
10. Rashes.

Alcohols

Ethyl alcohol (see p. 848) Patients accustomed to taking alcohol in the evenings may find it difficult to sleep if the drug is suddenly withdrawn, as may happen on admission to hospital. A small dose of alcohol may help them to sleep. However, alcohol is a powerful drug of dependence, and even when used for therapeutic purposes patients can become dependent. Alcohol produces REM sleep suppression in much the same fashion as barbiturates. REM rebound may be responsible in part for continued ethanol consumption.

Phenothiazines

Promethazine (Phenergan) This phenothiazine derivative is an H_1 histamine receptor-blocking drug. As with many drugs of this type, it has antipruritic, hyoscine-like and sedative properties. In paediatric practice drugs such as promethazine or trimeprazine are widely used as sedatives and hypnotics—particularly if the child is suffering from an itching allergic condition such as urticaria and some forms of eczema.

As a hypnotic, the efficacy of promethazine shows great inter-individual variation which can lead to dangers. In patients who have failed to respond to the usual dose of promethazine, a further increase in the dose can lead to vertigo, excitement, delirium and respiratory depression. Because of this variability in response and production of excitement, the drug cannot be recommended as a hypnotic. However, as a premedicant before operations or medical investigations it can be useful: not only is sedation produced, but the hyoscine-like actions result in drying of salivary and bronchial secretions and suppression of vomiting.

Chlormethiazole (Heminevrin)

This is an acidic, water-soluble thiazole derivative. It has hypnotic and anticonvulsant properties. Because of its structural similarities to part of the vitamin B_1 molecule, it has been suggested that it acts by competing with this vitamin in neuronal energy-generating metabolic processes. No convincing evidence has been produced to support this hypothesis.

Pharmacokinetics Absorption following oral administration is rapid, peak plasma levels being attained at 60 min. The $t_{1/2}$ is 50 min. Sedation and sleep usually occur 30–60 min after taking the drug orally. When given orally, chlormethiazole undergoes extensive first-pass metabolism (85 %) which may be dose-dependent and results in low bioavailability by this route. In cirrhosis the oral bioavailability is increased about tenfold, although its elimination is only slightly retarded. This results from decreased first-pass metabolism by the damaged liver. Chlormethiazole should therefore be given in reduced oral dosage in patients with cirrhosis of the liver. (see Figs 5.11 and 5.12).

Clinical uses

1. This drug has gained acceptance as a sedative in the elderly. It appears to be effective but probably has no demonstrable advantage over the benzodiazepines. It is given in the form of syrup, tablets or capsules in a dose of 250–500 mg of the edisylate.
2. Acute withdrawal from alcohol, barbiturates and the narcotic analgesics can be treated with chlormethiazole but after one week some physicians change to a neuroleptic drug. Initial oral therapy may be 2 g of chlormethiazole edisylate 6 hourly on the first day, 1.5 g 6 hourly on the second day, 1.0 g 6 hourly on the third day and 500 mg 6 hourly for a further 3 days. If intravenous therapy is used, 40–80 ml (of a solution of chlormethiazole edisylate 8 mg/ml) may be given initially over 2–3 min and subsequent drug given more slowly. Severely affected patients may require 500–1000 ml over 6–12 h.

   The drug potentiates the respiratory and cardiovascular depressant effects of alcohol, barbiturates and neuroleptics and thus should be given particularly cautiously in patients who have taken these drugs.
3. Even though this drug is anticonvulsant, it has a short plasma half-life and is a powerful sedative. It is therefore unsuitable for the day-to-day prevention of fits. However, intravenous infusion (200–1500 ml of a 0.8 % solution) is effective in the treatment of status epilepticus.

Adverse effects

1. Before sedation is produced a tingling sensation is experienced in the nose. This may be accompanied by sneezing, conjunctival irritation and (with large doses) bronchorrhoea.
2. The acidic preparations of the drug can produce gastric irritation.
3. When large doses are being used in the treatment of delirium tremens, a fall in blood pressure may be produced, particularly after rapid intravenous administration.
4. Intravenous solutions of 0.8 % concentration usually produce no local toxicity, but 2 % solution can lead to thrombophlebitis and intravascular haemolysis.
5. Dependence is a problem which limits its use in alcoholics.

Benzodiazepines

The main actions of benzodiazepines are:

(a) anxiolytic;
(b) anticonvulsant;
(c) muscle relaxant.

(a) Although such hypnosedatives as meprobamate and the barbiturates are powerful anxiolytic agents, they are effective only in doses which produce drowsiness and impairment of mental and physical performance. The benzodiazepines exert a more specific effect on the limbic system, and can therefore reduce anxiety in doses which do not produce somnolence. Nevertheless, larger doses are sedative and one of their main uses is as hypnotics.

(b) Benzodiazepines raise the threshold for electrically induced fits and those due to leptazol or local anaesthetics in experimental animals. In clinical practice diazepam, clonazepam, lorazepam and nitrazepam are effective in several forms of epilepsy (see p. 275).

(c) Decreased voluntary muscle tone occurs in normal individuals and in patients with spasticity. In therapeutic doses, neuromuscular transmission is not affected but there is inhibition of polysynaptic reflexes within the spinal cord. This muscle relaxation is due to facilitation of inhibitory GABA receptors in the cord.

Although this action may be beneficial in spasticity and muscle spasm due to pain, post-anaesthetic respiratory depression can be prolonged in patients given curare and a benzodiazepine.

Benzodiazepine receptors This group of drugs appears to act on specific receptors which enhance the effects of inhibitory neurotransmitters – in particular γ-aminobenzoic acid – in the brain and spinal cord. The consequences of this in the motor system are an anticonvulsant action and reduction in muscle tone. In the limbic system such inhibition could result in alleviation in anxiety.

Specific antagonists of this receptor have been found. These cause feelings of emotional tension and can provoke panic. Their use is presently experimental.

Pharmacokinetics Some relevant data for commonly used drugs appear in Table 9.2. Pharmacodynamically the benzodiazepines are virtually identical: the differences between them arise due to their differing pharmacokinetics. Relationships between clinical effects and plasma concentrations of the benzodiazepines are relatively imprecise and weak although in general terms the higher the plasma level the greater the effect. At present there seems to be no benefit to be expected from routine measurement of plasma benzodiazepine levels in patients since no clearly therapeutic range has been established.

Benzodiazepines are well absorbed orally. Clorazepate is hydrolysed in the stomach to an active metabolite, desmethyldiazepam (nordiazepam), the rate of hydrolysis depending upon acidity. The rate but not the extent of total absorption of clorazepate as nordiazepam is reduced by antacids. The absorption of chlordiazepoxide has also been found to be slowed by antacid, although the total amount finally absorbed is unaffected, so that attainment of a steady-state level is unimpaired when the drug is given chronically.

The absorption of most benzodiazepines from intramuscular injections is less rapid and produces lower peak plasma levels when compared to oral administration. The unreliability of the intramuscular route is important when sedation of unco-operative patients is required, e.g. alcohol withdrawal or acute anxiety. However, lorazepam is reliably and rapidly absorbed following intramuscular injection.

Table 9.2 Pharmacokinetic properties of some benzodiazepines

Drug	*Therapeutic dose*	*Active metabolites*	$t_{1/2}$ *of parent compound (h)*	*Special features*
Longer acting				
Diazepam (Valium)	2–10 mg IV 2.5–20 mg	Desmethyldiazepam ($t_{1/2}$ = 36–200 h) Oxazepam	20–50	General 'all purpose' benzodiazepine but also useful i.v. in status epilepticus i.m. injection poorly absorbed
Chlordiazepoxide (Librium)	10–25 mg	Desmethylchlordiazepoxide Desmethyldiazepam Oxazepam	3–30	i.m. injection poorly absorbed (precipitates at injection site)
Chlorazepate (Tranxene)	15 mg	Desmethyldiazepam Oxazepam	30–60	Parent drug completely metabolised to desmethyldiazepam (i.e. is a pro-drug)
Clobazam (Frisium)	10–20 mg	N-desmethylclobazam	24	Claimed to produce no psychomotor impairment. Less hypnotic and muscle relaxant effects than diazepam
Nitrazepam (Mogadon)	5–10 mg	None	24	Hypnotic use but also anticonvulsant
Flurazepam (Dalmane)	15–30 mg	Desalkylflurazepam ($t_{1/2}$ = 40–250 h) Hydroxyethylflurazepam	2	Hypnotic – acts mainly as pro-drug
Alprazolam (Xanax)	250–500 μg		6–25	Triazolobenzodiazepine with anxiolytic and possibly antidepressant activity (not recommended for specific treatment of depression)
Clonazepam (Rivotril)	Oral 1–8 mg IV 1 mg	None	30	Used as an anticonvulsant

Table 9.2 *(Continued)*

Drug	*Therapeutic dose*	*Active metabolites*	*$t_{1/2}$ of parent compound (h)*	*Special features*
Shorter acting with no long-lived active metabolites				
Oxazepam (Serenid)	15–60 mg	None	5–20	
Lorazepam (Ativan)	1–2.5 mg	None	10–20	Useful i.v. in status epilepticus Well absorbed by i.m. injection – thus useful in delirium tremens
Temazepam (Euhypnos, Normison)	10–30 mg	None	5–20	Used only as hypnotic
Ultra short acting				
Lormetazepam (Loramet, Noctamid)	0.5–1 mg	None	10 (longer in elderly)	Hypnotic – particularly in elderly
Triazolam (Halcion)	125–250 μg	Hydroxytriazolam ($t_{1/2}$ = 7 h)	2–4	Used only as hypnotic Psychotic reactions have been reported
Midazolam (Hypnovel)	IV 2.5–7.5 mg	Hydroxymidazolam ($t_{1/2}$ = 1–1.5 h)	2	Used i.v. for profound psychosedation, e.g. for endoscopy

High blood levels are rapidly produced by the intravenous route. 10–20 mg diazepam intravenously results in a plasma concentration of 1 μg/ml in 4 min. During the next 30–60 min there is a rapid α-phase decline to about 0.25 μg/ml and then elimination slows (β-phase). Sometimes at 6 h there is a rise in blood concentration and reappearance of sedation. This phenomenon is possibly due to reabsorption of the drug excreted in the bile (enterohepatic recirculation).

The benzodiazepines are highly protein bound in the plasma, e.g. at therapeutic concentrations chlordiazepoxide is 87–88 % and diazepam is 95 % bound.

With the exception of chlorazepate the major site of metabolism of benzodiazepines is the liver. There is an interrelated pattern of benzodiazepine metabolites, many of which are pharmacologically active and are used therapeutically (Fig. 9.2). The central position of desmethyldiazepam can be appreciated from this scheme. This substance has a very long $t_{1/2}$ of 96 h and at steady state its levels may exceed those of its parent substance. This accumulation may therefore explain the frequently observed hangover effects of continued administration of diazepam for example (see Fig. 9.3). Temazepam which does not form this metabolite and is largely excreted unchanged as glucuronide has a shorter $t_{1/2}$ and appears to produce less

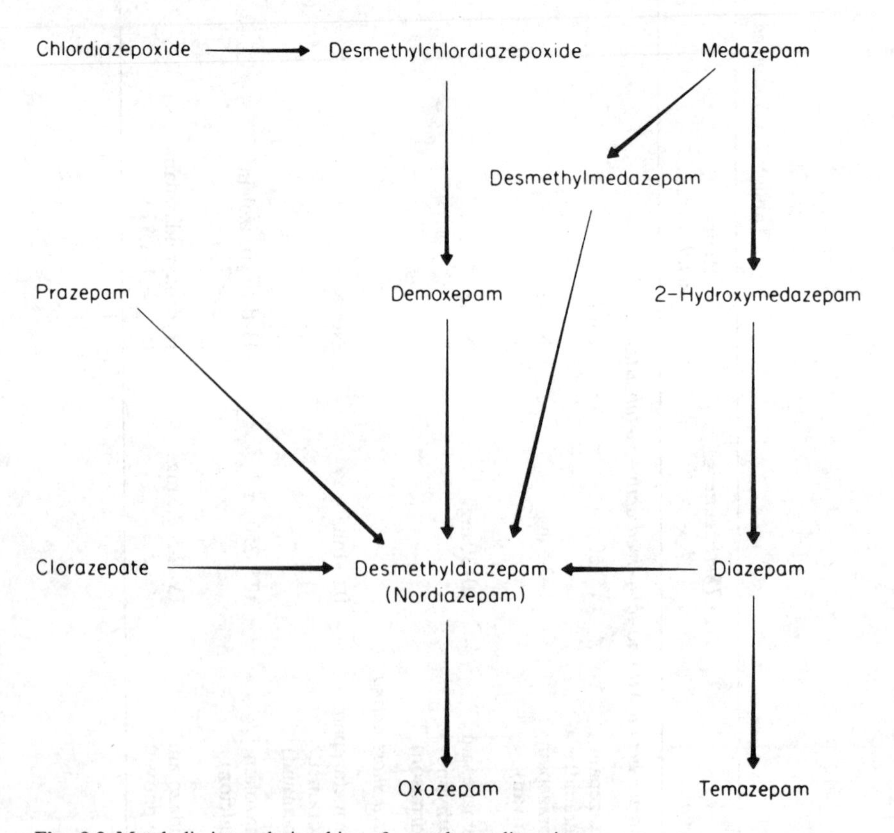

Fig. 9.2 Metabolic interrelationships of some benzodiazepines.

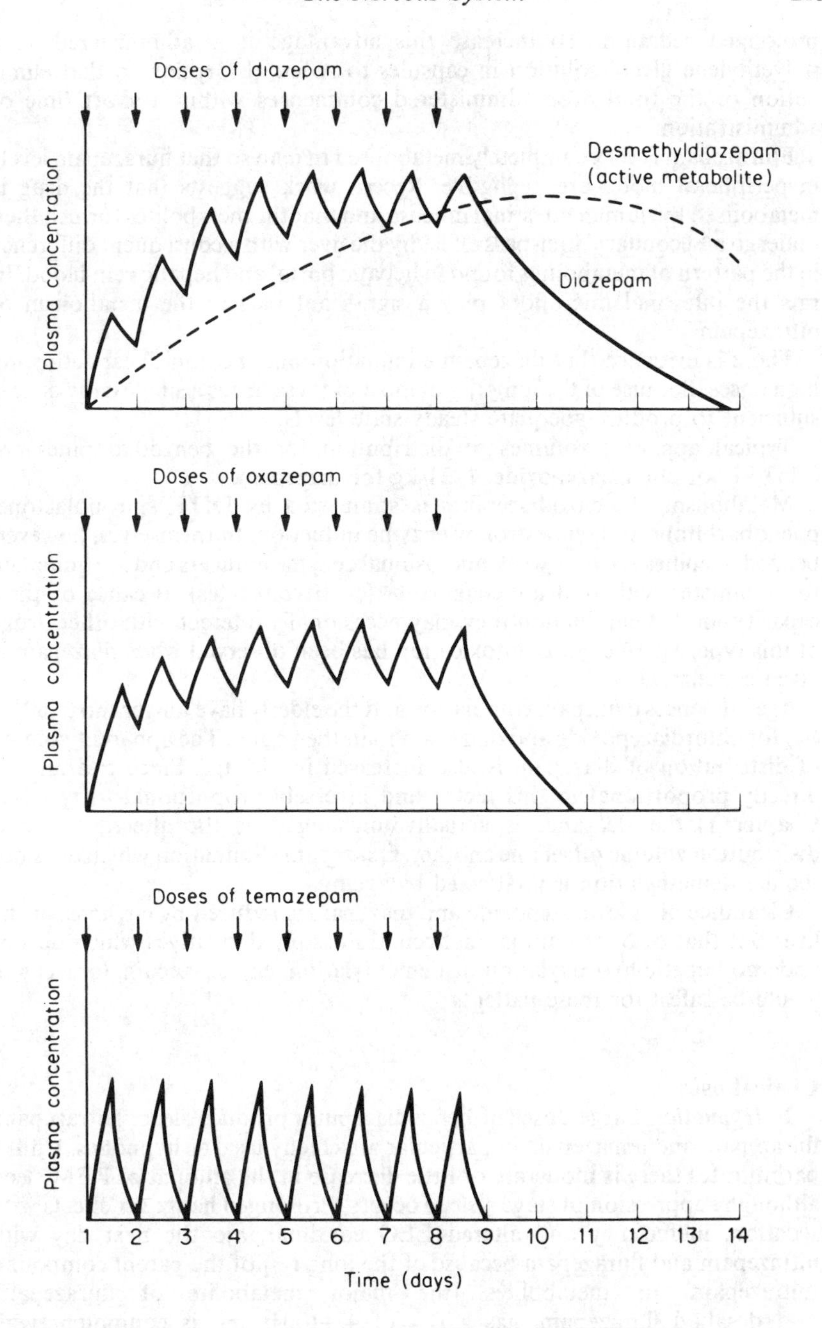

Fig. 9.3 Schematic diagram of plasma concentrations following daily dosage of three benzodiazepines. Note (a) the accumulation of both diazepam and its active metabolite; (b) the absence of accumulation and active metabolites for oxazepam and temazepam.

prolonged sedation. To increase this advantage it is administered as a polyethylene glycol solution in capsules to speed absorption so that elimination of the total dose administered commences within a short time of administration.

Flurazepam is very completely metabolised in man so that flurazepam levels in peripheral blood are negligible. Recent work suggests that the drug is metabolised by human intestinal mucosa and that the metabolites formed then undergo a 'secondary' first-pass effect by the liver with a consequent difference in the pattern of metabolites found in hepatic portal and hepatic vein blood. In rats the intestinal microflora play a significant part in the metabolism of nitrazepam.

There is evidence that diazepam elimination may be non-linear following high doses. Because of the long $t_{1/2}$ of most of these drugs a single daily dose is sufficient to produce adequate steady-state levels.

Typical apparent volumes of distribution for the benzodiazepines are 0.35 l/kg for chlordiazepoxide, 1–2 l/kg for diazepam.

Metabolism of benzodiazepines is stimulated by DDT, spironolactone, phenobarbitone and lynoestrol by enzyme induction. In themselves, however, benzodiazepines are only weak microsomal enzyme inducers and are quite safe to administer with oral anticoagulants (cf. barbiturates). Because of their capacity-limited elimination they may occasionally interact with other drugs of this type, e.g. phenytoin intoxication has been observed when diazepam is given concurrently.

Age influences diazepam elimination and the elderly have longer (up to 60%) $t_{1/2}$ for chlordiazepoxide and diazepam than the young. The apparent volume of distribution of diazepam is also increased in old age. Since clearance is directly proportional to this factor and inversely proportional to $t_{1/2}$ (see Chapter 1) the clearance is actually unchanged as the altered $t_{1/2}$ and distribution volume offset one another. Oxazepam elimination which does not require demethylation is unaffected by ageing.

Clearance of chlordiazepoxide and diazepam is reduced by cirrhosis of the liver but that of oxazepam is unaffected. Possibly derivatives which do not undergo hepatic hydroxylation or demethylation, e.g. oxazepam, lorazepam, would be safest for these patients.

Clinical uses

1. *Hypnotics* Large doses of benzodiazepines produce sleep. Nitrazepam, flurazepam and temazepam in particular are chiefly used as hypnotics. Unlike barbiturates there is moderate or little decrease in the amount of REM sleep although suppression of stage 4 sleep occurs. Prolonged hangover effects with sedation, inefficiency and altered EEG continue into the next day with nitrazepam and flurazepam because of the long $t_{1/2}$ of the parent compound (nitrazepam) or metabolites (the major metabolite of flurazepam, N-1-desalkyl flurazepam, has a $t_{1/2}$ of 47–100 h and is equipotent with flurazepam). This effect is less prominent with temazepam, which has a shorter $t_{1/2}$ and is probably the most suitable of this group as a hypnotic. There is no intrinsic reason why other benzodiazepines such as diazepam cannot be employed as hypnotics although their long $t_{1/2}$ is likely to cause hangover

effects. Careful evaluation of flurazepam and pentobarbitone under sleep laboratory conditions has shown that only the former is effective in producing sleep on chronic administration. Pentobarbitone only induces and maintains sleep on short-term administration but with regular use its effectiveness wanes. Although these are efficient hypnotics which do not induce tolerance, on withdrawal sleep usually becomes worse for up to six months, which may perpetuate the hypnotic habit.

Benzodiazepines cause less respiratory depression and nocturnal confusion in the elderly and also less drug dependence compared with the barbiturates, glutethimide, methaqualone and meprobamate. Death by drug overdose is not readily achieved using benzodiazepines on their own. When administered with alcohol or the barbiturates, there is a greatly increased chance of fatal respiratory and circulatory depression.

2. Diazepam, chlordiazepoxide, oxazepam, lorazepam, medazepam and other benzodiazepines are used as *anxiolytic agents* in acute and chronic anxiety states. In severe anxiety, including panic attacks, doses are given which produce sedation, but in less severe anxiety, anxiolytic effects may be achieved with much less sedation than equieffective doses of barbiturates or meprobamate and are perhaps less likely to produce drug dependence. Nevertheless, the prolonged use of large doses of the benzodiazepines produce psychological dependence and should not be used in the management of chronic anxiety.

3. The usefulness of the benzodiazepines in the treatment of *epilepsy* has not yet been adequately assessed. However, clonazepam and diazepam are effective in status epilepticus. Clonazepam is of proven value in petit mal and in akinetic attacks, and nitrazepam may be useful in salaam seizures (see also p. 275).

4. Diazepam is employed as a *premedicant* in surgery and for procedures such as endoscopy, ECT and cardioversion as a powerful psychosedative. In order to induce a state of sedation, relaxation and anterograde amnesia, intravenous diazepam is given slowly until dysarthria and ptosis occur. The dose producing this varies greatly (between 5 and 60 mg) and the state of maximum amnesia lasts for about 10 min. The particular advantage of this drug over the intravenous barbiturates is that the patient is rousable and can co-operate, yet his recall of the procedure is suppressed. Cardiovascular and respiratory depression is not usually clinically significant. Patients with obstructive respiratory disease should probably never be sedated, but those with impending liver failure tolerate benzodiazepines better than barbiturates.

Disadvantages of diazepam in this context include a relatively long induction period (60–90 s) without instantaneous control of the level of consciousness. Compared with the barbiturates, diazepam requires a prolonged recovery period. The patient should not drive or handle other dangerous machines for 24 h. Recovery is usually quicker after midazolam.

5. Diazepam reduces *spasticity* in the management of upper motor neurone paresis. A disadvantage of this treatment is that reduction of muscle tone can result in greater difficulty in weight-bearing by paretic legs.

6. *Muscle spasm* due to pain (as in vertebral disc prolapse) may be reduced by diazepam.

7. *Tetanus*. A continuous infusion of 3–10 mg/kg/per 24 h of diazepam or intermittent i.v. doses of 0.1–0.3 mg/kg can be used to control spasms.

Adverse effects These mainly involve the nervous system, but other forms of toxicity may be encountered.

1. *Central nervous system*

(a) Sedation: feelings of fatigue, sleepiness, mental slowing are usually dose dependent.

(b) Other consequences of CNS depression: ataxia, dysarthria, motor incoordination, diplopia, blurred vision, weakness, vertigo, increased proneness to motor vehicle and other accidents, confusion, apathy.

(c) States resembling Korsakoff's psychosis and alcoholic intoxication are sometimes produced. Occasionally these drugs precipitate outbreaks of rage and violence, presumably due to the release of anxiety-repressed hostility. Some patients taking triazolam (Halcion) have developed severe anxiety, depersonalisation, feelings of unreality, paranoia, hyperacusis and restlessness.

(d) Less common and more unpredictable effects are:

(i) Stimulation instead of sedation, similar to paradoxical excitement in children given barbiturates.

(ii) Antisocial behaviour, probably a consequence of alcohol-like intoxication.

(iii) Hypnogogic hallucinations during the induction of sleep. Nitrazepam has frequently been described as causing nightmares. These often involve stressful incidents in the patient's past.

(iv) Diazepam administration has occasionally been associated with the appearance of depression and suicide.

(v) Patients with organic brain disease may respond adversely to large doses of diazepam and develop tremulousness, crying episodes, impaired concentration, nocturnal confusion and agitation.

(vi) Diazepam inhibits stage 4 (slow wave) sleep and thus suppresses attacks of night terrors (which arise during this phase of sleep). The attacks may be displaced to the waking hours.

2. *Allergic reactions* are uncommon. Chlordiazepoxide has produced urticaria, angioedema and maculopapular eruptions. Light sensitivity dermatitis, fixed drug eruptions, non-thrombocytopenic purpura and swelling of the tongue have been described with benzodiazepine treatment. Acute anaphylaxis has also been reported.

3. *Other toxic effects* There is no convincing evidence that these drugs are toxic to haemopoietic tissues, liver or foetus. However, there is one report of a child born with absent first digits and a dislocated head of radius when the mother took diazepam in the first trimester of pregnancy.

4. *Intravenous diazepam*

(a) Cardiovascular and respiratory depression are uncommon. Patients particularly prone to develop hypotension or apnoea are those with serious underlying disease such as respiratory failure in chronic lung disease and those who have been previously given other central depressant drugs.

(b) Local pain is commonly experienced on repeated intravenous injections of diazepam. Phlebitis occurs after 3.7–7.0% of injections. The incidence of this complication is reduced by flushing the vein with 150–250 ml of isotonic saline.

'*Diazemuls*' is an emulsion of diazepam in intralipid. Following intravenous injection it is less irritating to the vein and to the perivenous tissues if leaking occurs. Diazepam emulsion injection is available in 10 mg vials.

Midazolam (Hypnovel) is a benzodiazepine which forms water-soluble salts. It is injected intravenously as a sedative prior to procedures such as endoscopy and dental treatment. Peak sedation is accompanied by anterograde amnesia. The elimination $t_{1/2}$ is 2 h and its active metabolite α-hydroxymidazolam has a $t_{1/2}$ of 1–1½ h. It is less irritant to veins than diazepam injection, but thrombophlebitis can occur. Rapid injection may result in hypotension, apnoea and respiratory obstruction. Repeated injections increase the half-life and may ultimately produce coma. The adult sedating dose is usually between 2.5 and 7.5 mg (0.07 mg/kg body weight).

Drug interactions

(a) *Acute potentiation* of the effects of alcohol, barbiturates and other hypnotics. The intravenous solution of diazepam contains propylene glycol and this contributes to the central depressant and hypotensive properties of the preparation.

(b) *Chronic effects* Although benzodiazepines are highly protein bound, in practice interactions are not observed due to displacement of other protein-bound drugs such as sulphonamides, minor analgesics and oral anticoagulants.

Benzodiazepines are weak inducers of hepatic metabolising enzymes, but do not produce a clinically significant effect. Some interactions occur whose mechanism is not completely understood. Some examples follow:

(i) An increase in plasma phenytoin levels in patients given a benzodiazepine. Phenytoin toxicity can result.
(ii) In one patient stabilised on a coumarin anticoagulant, benzodiazepine administration was followed by the appearance of ecchymoses.
(iii) One patient with Parkinsonism treated with levodopa experienced worsening of the tremor when given a benzodiazepine.

Drug dependence Early impressions that the benzodiazepines are not drugs of dependence have not been confirmed. Although these drugs less readily produce dependence than the barbiturates or alcohol, physical and psychological withdrawal states can occur. Dependence usually follows taking large doses for prolonged periods, but withdrawal states have also arisen after limited drug exposure. The full withdrawal picture appears after an interval of 3–8 days and consists of a cluster of features unusual in anxiety states, although frank anxiety and panic attacks commonly develop as well. Perceptual distortions (such as feelings of being surrounded by cotton wool), visual and auditory hallucinations, paranoid ideas, feelings of unreality, depersonalisation, paraesthesiae, headaches and other pains, blurring of vision, dyspepsia and flu-like symptoms are all characteristic. Depression and agoraphobia are also common. The syndrome may persist for many weeks.

ANXIOLYTIC DRUGS (MINOR TRANQUILLISERS)

This group of drugs allays feelings of tension and anxiety without producing undue sedation. In practice, all anxiolytics produce feelings of fatigue and sleepiness, and are hypnotics if given in sufficiently high doses. Conversely, in small doses all hypnotics are anxiolytics. Thus hypnotics and anxiolytics could be grouped together as *hypnosedatives*. Nevertheless, the benzodiazepines are unusual in that anxiolytic doses of these drugs produce much less sedation and ataxia than equieffective doses of drugs such as the barbiturates and meprobamate.

The drugs used in the treatment of anxiety include the following:

benzodiazepines (see p. 210);
meprobamate—no longer recommended for this purpose;
β-blockers (see p. 425);
antidepressants (see p. 221);
barbiturates (see p. 206)—no longer recommended for this purpose.

Meprobamate (Equanil; Miltown)

Although meprobamate possesses anxiolytic properties, it is also sedative and, unlike the benzodiazepines, cannot relieve anxiety without significant hypnotic effects. Meprobamate relaxes skeletal muscle tone, and is also anticonvulsant. This drug is now rarely used.

Pharmacokinetics Intestinal absorption is fairly rapid and peak levels in the blood are reached 1–2 h after oral administration. The $t_{1/2}$ is 10 h. The most abundant metabolite is the hydroxylated derivative which is pharmacologically inactive. Meprobamate produces significant hepatic enzyme induction.

Adverse effects Meprobamate is sedative and in small doses produces lack of concentration, feelings of tiredness and heaviness. The effects of other central depressants, including alcohol, are potentiated. Drug dependence is readily produced. Abrupt withdrawal results in insomnia, anxiety and convulsions. Allergic rashes and asthma occur in about 2% of patients. Bone-marrow depression is a recognised complication but is rare. Like the barbiturates, meprobamate can produce an exacerbation of acute intermittent porphyria.

The use of drugs in the treatment of anxiety

Although anxiolytic drugs are prescribed more frequently than any other group of therapeutic agents, the treatment of anxiety states remains unsatisfactory. Furthermore, these drugs are frequently misused in that they are prescribed inappropriately in such situations as interpersonal problems.

Much more successful is the treatment of panic attacks, phobic anxiety and physiological fear (such as of a surgical or investigatory procedure). Here powerful psychosedation can be successfully produced by intravenous diazepam. The dose required to abolish anxiety and produce anterograde amnesia varies widely, but in an adult this is usually 5–20 mg given over 5 min.

Long-term drug treatment is inappropriate and positively harmful in chronic anxiety. The benzodiazepines, however, may be useful intermittently when used in combination with other forms of supportive help in facing a temporary exacerbation. Anxiety states with predominantly peripheral manifestations such as tremor, tachycardia and angina may be greatly helped by using β-adrenoceptor blocking drugs.

The majority of patients with anxiety have some degree of depression as well, and many depressed patients have features of agitation and anxiety. In some of these, tricyclic antidepressant drugs may be of considerable value. Some physicians find the anxiolytic antidepressants (see p. 228) useful in these situations. Such drugs include:

dothiepin (Prothiaden);
doxepin (Sinequan);
iprindole (Prondol).

In general these drugs have tricyclic-type antidepressant activity with anxiolytic effects similar to those of the benzodiazepines. Although their anticholinergic properties are less marked than those of imipramine and amitriptyline, they are probably less effective antidepressants.

Phobic anxiety may respond to antidepressant drugs – in particular the monoamine oxidase inhibitors.

ANTIDEPRESSANT DRUGS AND THE TREATMENT OF DEPRESSION

The cause of depression remains unknown. The so-called amine hypothesis suggests that affective disorders result from disturbances in the availability of amines. Some of the evidence cited in favour of the theory is pharmacological:

1. Reserpine depletes brain amines and produces depression in some people.
2. Many drugs which are effective in the treatment of affective disorders change the synaptic concentrations of 5-hydroxytryptamine (5-HT), noradrenaline or dopamine.
3. 5-HT blocking drugs such as methysergide may produce depression.
4. Administration of the 5-HT precursor L-tryptophan may improve response to treatment in depression. Giving L-dopa in Parkinson's disease may alleviate depression.
5. Measurement of biogenic amine metabolites in depressed patients is difficult. It has been found that brain 5-HT levels are lower in depressed suicides than in controls dying from other causes but no change has been found in noradrenaline. Cerebrospinal fluid levels of the various metabolites of amines have been extensively investigated: generally 5-hydroxyindole acetic acid (5-HIAA) from 5-HT metabolism is found to be low in depression but equivocal data have been obtained for catecholamine metabolites.

The main treatments for depression have all been discovered by chance. There is no really adequate animal model for depression and whilst studies in normal individuals (particularly those of gloomy disposition) may be helpful, there is no efficient screening test for antidepressant drugs. Reserpine antagonism is often cited as a useful test in animals, but mianserin which is clearly effective in man does not produce antagonism in this model. Electroconvulsive therapy (ECT) has been shown to be one of the most effective treatments for severe depression: its mode of action on the brain is unknown. Drug treatments to be discussed below include:

tricyclics
miscellaneous structures including tetracyclics
monoamine oxidase inhibitors
L-tryptophan
thioxanthenes
lithium

As such this does not constitute a logical classification of these drugs: there is even dispute concerning the exact definition of a tricyclic antidepressant. In general, however, all the above list of drugs may affect brain amines in one way or another. MAOIs do not discriminate between 5-HT and noradrenaline but when the tricyclic and more recently introduced antidepressants are consid-

Table 9.3 Selective actions of antidepressants on amines

Drug	*Type of amine*	*Effect on cerebral amines*
Imipramine	3°	Equally powerful inhibition of NA and 5-HT uptake.
Desipramine	2°	Powerful inhibition of NA uptake. Little or no effect on 5-HT.
Trimipramine	3°	Powerful inhibition of 5-HT uptake. Some action on NA and DA uptake. (Desmethyl metabolite blocks NA uptake).
Clomipramine	3°	Powerful inhibition of 5-HT uptake.
Amitriptyline	3°	Powerful inhibition of 5-HT uptake. Some action on NA uptake.
Nortriptyline	2°	Powerful inhibition of NA uptake. Some action on 5-HT uptake.
Butriptyline	3°	Weak inhibition of NA and 5-HT uptake.
Mianserin	3°	No effect on uptake. Blockade of central α_2-receptors, enhancing NA release.
Nomifensine	1°	Powerful inhibition of DA and NA uptake. Some action on 5-HT uptake.
Maprotiline	2°	Powerful inhibition of NA uptake. Some action on 5-HT uptake.
Viloxazine	2°	Equally powerful inhibition of NA and 5-HT uptake.
Trazodone	3°	Low concentrations block 5-HT actions, high concentrations block 5-HT uptake.
Iprindole	3°	Blocks reuptake of NA in brain, but not peripherally.

NA = noradrenaline; 5-HT = 5-hydroxytryptamine; DA = dopamine.

ered it is seen that some may discriminate between amines at central synapses (Table 9.3). In general the tertiary amines appear preferentially to inhibit 5-HT re-uptake whilst the secondary amines inhibit noradrenaline re-uptake more readily.

It is alleged that the effects of inhibiting 5-HT uptake and thus raising the local synaptic concentration of transmitter 5-HT is to elevate mood and produce an increased sense of well-being whereas the effect of inhibiting noradrenaline re-uptake is to increase the general drive and motor activity of patients. Possibly drugs which preferentially affect noradrenaline uptake are associated with increased cardiovascular adverse effects.

Tricyclic antidepressants

Imipramine was fortuitously discovered to be an antidepressant although, as an analogue of chlorpromazine, it was initially tested as an antipsychotic agent. Tricyclic antidepressants were originally considered to be compounds containing two benzene rings fused to a central seven-membered ring. With the introduction of some other compounds such as iprindole this concept has been broadened. Tricyclic antidepressants are effective in terminating attacks of depression in about 70% of patients and appear to act by raising local concentrations of amine transmitters in the brain by inhibiting uptake into the cytoplasmic stores within the presynaptic neurone. The differences produced in inhibitory effect on 5-HT and noradrenaline uptake mechanisms by the presence of a secondary or tertiary amine in the side chain are shown in Table 9.3.

Improvement in depression with tricyclic drugs, as with MAOI, may take several weeks. Since depression is a recurrent disorder and trials indicate some prolonged benefit it is necessary to continue treatment with these drugs for at least six months following remission of depression to prevent relapse. In the majority of therapeutic trials, electroconvulsive therapy is found to be more effective than imipramine. The remainder demonstrated no difference in effectiveness between the two modes of treatment. ECT acts more rapidly and this may be of crucial importance in the suicidal patient. The disadvantages of ECT include temporary memory loss, transient confusion and (possibly) permanent intellectual changes. Thus, initially, many psychiatrists prefer tricyclic therapy for depressed patients. Also the recurrence rate of depression after ECT is about 20–45% after six months, whilst on amitriptyline or imipramine this is 15–17%. Thus even with patients given ECT, tricyclics may be helpful additional treatment. Comparisons of placebo and tricyclic therapy show that during the period of observation, 30–50% of depressed patients improve on a placebo, whilst 70% respond to tricyclic drugs.

Similar studies have shown that ECT is more effective than treatment with the monoamine oxidase inhibitor drugs, phenelzine and isocarboxazid. However, a minority of patients respond well and rapidly to a tranylcypromine–trifluoperazine combination.

In general there is no clear-cut difference in effectiveness between the two main types of antidepressant. However, the tricyclics are probably more effective than the MAOIs and are certainly safer. There appear to be some patients who respond optimally to monoamine oxidase inhibitors. This may be genetically determined, but some forms of the disease, particularly hysteria with secondary depression, may be helped by these drugs. Non-psychotic mixed anxiety-depression does not usually respond well to drugs. Doxepin and dothiepin are tricyclics with both anti-anxiety and antidepressant properties and are superior to placebo treatment in this condition, but equally effective to the benzodiazepines. Schizo-affective disorders do not usually improve with drug therapy, but rapidly improve during ECT. The choice of treatment for specific varieties of depressive illness and its integration with the equally important psychotherapy and social counselling are beyond the scope of this account.

Pharmacokinetics Tricyclic antidepressants, being lipid soluble, are readily absorbed from the gastrointestinal tract but are subject to considerable first-pass hepatic metabolism. Tricyclics themselves may delay their own absorption and that of other drugs, due to their anticholinergic effect in decreasing gastric emptying rate and intestinal peristalsis.

Protein binding of these drugs is high (e.g. imipramine 85%, clomipramine 90%) and thus they can interact with other highly protein-bound drugs. It is possible that differences in protein binding which determine the free and active drug may be one factor in the poor correlation between plasma levels of total drug and clinical response. The techniques for free drug estimation are, as yet, not clinically available. Their affinity for tissue and plasma proteins and their large apparent volume of distribution makes them poorly dialysable in cases of overdose.

Tricyclics are extensively metabolised before excretion. When administered orally there is considerable first-pass hepatic metabolism. The percentage of nortriptyline metabolised first-pass is estimated at 34–48% while that of imipramine is 53%. Protriptyline probably has the lowest first-pass effect of these drugs (10–25% of the oral dose) which may be related to its long $t_{1/2}$. As a general rule initial demethylation of the side chain occurs, thus imipramine is partly metabolised to desipramine and a proportion of amitriptyline is similarly converted into nortriptyline. These monomethyl derivatives are pharmacologically active. Ring hydroxylation, which abolishes activity, also occurs prior to conjugation and excretion. The extent of hydroxylation is governed by previous exposure to drugs (particularly stimulation of hydroxylation by inducing agents) and by genetic factors.

As with a large number of psychoactive drugs, the tertiary amine structure is associated with high lipid solubility and a large apparent volume of distribution, e.g. for imipramine it varies from 28–61 l/kg body weight and for nortriptyline from 25–55 l/kg body weight. These drugs are therefore present at very low concentrations in plasma after distribution. Studies in twins revealed a five-fold variation in $t_{1/2}$ for nortriptyline (18–93 h) and a two-fold variation in $V_{d\beta}$. No correlation exists between these variables in unrelated subjects, but there is good agreement within monozygotic twins, suggesting that inter-individual variability in these parameters is largely genetically determined. The plasma protein binding of nortriptyline varies to give a two-fold range of unbound drug and this may also be under genetic control and so contribute to the two-fold difference in $V_{d\beta}$. For imipramine it has been shown that apparent volume of distribution/fraction of free drug in plasma is a constant which demonstrates the dependence of apparent volume of distribution upon plasma–protein binding.

Given this degree of variability in pharmacokinetic disposition it is not surprising that there is a wide scatter (5–30 fold) in plasma steady-state levels between individuals on the same dose. Thus patients receiving imipramine 3.5 mg/kg/day have steady-state plasma concentrations of 95–1020 ng/ml and nortriptyline given in a dose of 100 mg at night produces steady-state levels varying between 120 and 681 ng/ml. Apart from variations in drug disposition another important factor appears to be the rate of hydroxylation, since there is a significant correlation between the elimination rate constant of nortriptyline (which because of the ease of measurement has been most widely studied) and the corresponding metabolic clearance to 10-hydroxy-nortriptyline. It is also correlated with the ability to hydroxylate other drugs such as phenylbutazone, and twin and family studies show this to be under polygenic control. Hepatic enzyme induction (see p. 82) is also important and lower plasma steady-state levels of tricyclic antidepressants are present in patients who smoke (nicotine and polycyclic hydrocarbons are inducing agents), drink alcohol or take barbiturates.

There is a good correlation between tricyclic blood levels and inhibition of noradrenaline re-uptake ($uptake_1$), blocking of tyramine pressor responses and degree of disturbance of ocular accommodation. Unfortunately the relationship between steady-state levels and antidepressant activity is not so well understood and different workers have produced conflicting evidence.

Only 70 % of depressed patients respond adequately to tricyclic antidepressants. One explanation may be the wide variation in individual plasma levels of these drugs which are attained by a given dose. Therefore the widely accepted notion that a fixed-dose scheme, e.g. 150 mg amitriptyline daily, constitutes a therapeutic trial is unlikely to be valid since this may be too small a dose for some patients and too large for others. It has not yet been established that the response of patients can be improved by monitoring plasma antidepressant concentrations. Most is known about nortriptyline since it is the most easily assayed of this group of drugs. Several, but not all, studies have suggested that nortriptyline levels below 50 ng/ml and above 200 ng/ml are ineffective. Thus for some patients it is possible that response could be improved by reducing rather than increasing the dose. Possibly the upper concentration limit may reflect the increasing importance of some toxic effect, e.g. inhibition of amine transmitter release produced by high concentrations of drug at central synapses.

As nortriptyline obeys linear kinetics it follows that it is possible to predict the steady state attained by multiple doses from the administration of a single oral dose and therefore to find the dose for optimal antidepressant effect. Thus, despite great variation in plasma $t_{1/2}$ and volume of distribution, equation (1.68) may be employed to individualise drug regimes (see Fig. 9.4):

$$\bar{C} = \text{average steady-state concentration} = \frac{1.44 \times \text{dose} \times t_{1/2}}{\text{dose interval} \times V_d}, \qquad (1.68)$$

$t_{1/2}$ and V_d being determined following a single dose.

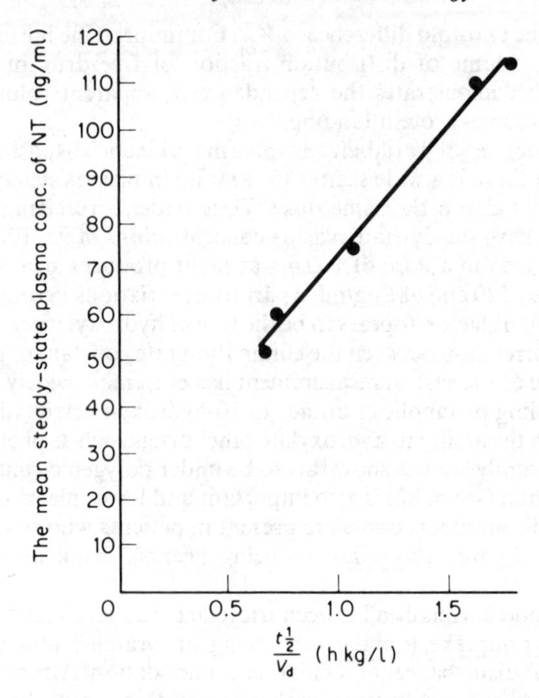

Fig. 9.4 Correlation between the steady-state plasma concentration of nortriptyline and the ratio between plasma $t_{1/2}$ and apparent volume of distribution of a single dose of nortriptyline in the same 5 individuals. Since plasma clearance $= \frac{0.693\ V_d}{t_{1/2}}$ the relationship of C to $1/_{\text{Clearance}}$ (eq. (1.69)) is demonstrated (From B. Alexanderson and F. Sjoqvist, *Ann. N. Y. Acad. Sci.* **179**, 739 (1971).)

For amitriptyline, which is more widely used in the UK, the relationship between plasma concentration and response is also not well defined. Several studies have suggested a linear relationship between these variables compared with the curvilinear relationship for nortriptyline. Others have suggested that there exists a therapeutic range of total plasma tricyclic concentration (amitriptyline plus its metabolite nortriptyline) which attains steady-state conditions after a few weeks chronic administration, 160–240 ng/ml being optimal. Most recently a multi-centre collaborative study organised by the WHO has failed to demonstrate any relationship whatsoever between plasma amitriptyline concentration and clinical effect. Presently therefore the measurement of tricyclic antidepressant levels in patients remains a research exercise whose usefulness has yet to be demonstrated.

Clinical use In the absence of individual pharmacokinetic data, these drugs are initially given in small doses (e.g. 25 mg for imipramine and amitriptyline) each evening and increased at weekly intervals until a therapeutic response has been produced. In order to establish that the patient is unresponsive to this type of antidepressant, the drug is usually given for about 6 weeks.

There is some evidence that systemic clearance of tricyclics is slower in the elderly who usually have longer half-lives for these drugs than the young. This may explain why the aged are particularly vulnerable to the anticholinergic side effects (especially constipation and hesitancy of micturition). In these patients only small doses should be used.

Combination of a tricyclic with a phenothiazine or other antipsychotic drug is probably only justified in some cases of psychotic depression. Such combinations, if used for mild depression, expose patients to an unnecessary risk of additive anticholinergic effects and tardive dyskinesia. If sedation is appropriate, either a sedative tricyclic (amitriptyline, doxepin) or an adjunctive benzodiazepine can be used. A number of drugs (methylphenidate, MAOIs, thyroxine) have been reported to increase the speed or efficacy of action of tricyclics: such combinations are experimental and may be dangerous and should only be used by experts. If a patient improves with a tricyclic compound it should be continued for at least six months before cautious reduction of the dose over several weeks is attempted. If depressive symptoms do not recur, the patient and family should be warned about the possibility of relapse and the patient observed periodically. If symptoms recur treatment should be continued: some patients appear to require maintenance therapy, often for years. In such cases regular attempts should be made to discontinue therapy so that the patient does not continue to take an unnecessary drug. A patient who does not improve on tricyclic drugs should be considered for therapy with either one of the newer tetracyclic compounds or nomifensine or an MAOI, lithium or ECT.

Imipramine in low dosage is sometimes used in the management of nocturnal enuresis.

Adverse effects may be classified as follows:

(a) *Autonomic* (*anticholinergic*) Dry mouth, constipation, tachycardia, paralysis of accommodation, aggravation of narrow-angle glaucoma, postural hypotension, vomiting, retention of urine, paralytic ileus (rare).

(b) *Central nervous system* Fine tremor, sedation, isomnia, decreased REM sleep, twitching, convulsions (*tricyclics are epileptogenic*), dysarthria, paraesthesia, ataxia. Uncommonly: confusion, mania, schizophrenic excitement. Anticholinergic and sedating actions are more pronounced with tertiary amine drugs than with secondary amines.

Abrupt termination of the drug can produce mild withdrawal reactions for 1–2 days. These include nausea, vomiting and malaise.

(c) *Cardiovascular system* In therapeutic doses these drugs may cause flattening of T waves, prolongation of the QT interval and ST depression. In large doses tachycardia, atrial fibrillation, ventricular flutter and atrioventricular or intraventricular block may result. Sudden death is commoner in patients taking tricyclics.

(d) *Allergic reactions* Skin reactions, intrahepatic cholestasis, agranulocytosis (very rare).

Drug interactions

1. Monoamine oxidase inhibitors may produce potentiation of both drugs. MAOIs should be stopped for a minimum of 14 days before beginning tricyclics.

2. Alcohol potentiates tricyclics—especially sedation.
3. Anticholinergic drugs—effect increased.
4. Anticonvulsants increase CNS depression, but their dose may need to be increased because tricyclics may provoke fits.
5. Anti-Parkinsonian drugs potentiate anticholinergics at toxic levels. May produce syndrome of hyperpyrexia, agitation and convulsions.
6. Antihypertensives
   (a) Clonidine—loss of hypotensive activity and possible hypertensive rebound.
   (b) Adrenergic neurone blockers, e.g. guanethidine—block of drug uptake into neurone and consequent loss of hypotensive effect.
7. Sympathomimetic amines (amphetamines, noradrenaline, adrenaline and phenylpropanolamine in 'cold cures'): effects of amines increased with hypertensive reaction.

Iprindole (Prondol)

This, whilst similar in structure to tricyclics, has an indole nucleus and a cyclo-octane ring. Like true tricyclics it inhibits cerebral noradrenaline $uptake_1$ but in contrast it does not show this effect in the peripheral nervous system. It also has only one-tenth of the anticholinergic effect of imipramine and so produces a lower incidence of atropine-like side effects. Antihistamine activity is also weak and there is little sedation or interference with REM sleep.

Few pharmacokinetic data are available and the compound appears to be extensively metabolised prior to elimination in the urine.

Trials indicate antidepressant efficacy near or equivalent to that of imipramine and amitriptyline. It is given in doses of 30 mg 8 hourly increasing if necessary to 60 mg 8 hourly. It is relatively well tolerated but some patients have developed urticaria, eosinophilia and cholestatic jaundice. Other adverse effects seen with tricyclics may be less common.

Anxiolytic tricyclic antidepressants

1. Doxepin (Sinequan)

Doxepin is a tricyclic dibenzoxapine antidepressant which also possesses considerable anxiolytic activity. Although it appears to be a less powerful antidepressant than imipramine or amitriptyline, it may be helpful in the treatment of patients suffering from mild depression with an overlay of anxiety.

Pharmacokinetics and clinical use Good absorption follows oral administration. The usual dose range is 50–150 mg given as a single evening dose. Steady-state levels of 9–45 ng/ml of doxepin and its main metabolite, desmethyldoxepin occur in patients taking 50 mg o.m. whilst after 150 mg nightly steady-state values of 47–131 ng/ml have been found. The peak plasma levels usually occur around 4 h after a dose and the $t_{1/2}$ varies from 8 to 20 h whilst that for the main metabolite, desmethyldoxepin, in 33–81 h. There is extensive first-pass hepatic metabolism which ranges from 55 to 87 % of the oral dose in different patients. In depression there appears to be a correlation between clinical response and concentration of doxepin plus desmethyldoxepin: most responders have levels above 110 ng/ml. The relief of anxiety does not correlate with plasma drug levels, however.

Adverse effects These are similar to the older tricyclic antidepressants: atropine-like effects, drowsiness, tachycardia and postural hypotension.

The antihypertensive action of guanethidine is reversed.

2. Dothiepin (Prothiaden)

This is a thio-analogue of amitriptyline which has comparable antidepressant activity to this drug with associated anxiolytic properties. Due to the latter effects a beneficial effect occurs within a few days of beginning treatment, whilst the antidepressant effect becomes apparent after about 10 days. The $t_{1/2}$ is 46–56 h. The side effects are similar in nature to those encountered with other tricyclics, but their incidence and severity is reportedly less. The therapeutic dose range is 75–200 mg daily.

Miscellaneous structures

Viloxazine (Vivalan)

This bicyclic antidepressant was serendipitously developed from a series of β-blockers. It is, however, free from β-blocking activity. As an antidepressant it appears to be similar in effectiveness to imipramine.

Pharmacokinetics Viloxazine is rapidly and completely absorbed from the gut and gives peak plasma concentrations at 1–4 h of 0.8 μg/ml/mg oral dose/kg. Thus after a dose of 80 mg a blood level of about 0.8 μg/ml is usually attained in an 80 kg patient. The average optimum daily dose is 200 mg, but as the $t_{1/2}$ is only 2–5 h, this is given in divided doses. No therapeutic plasma-level range has been established. Viloxazine is not highly protein bound. It is extensively metabolised by hydroxylation, the metabolites appearing in the urine as glucuronides. 98 % of the ingested drug is excreted in the urine mainly as metabolites. 2 % is excreted via the bile.

Adverse effects Viloxazine has much less anticholinergic and adrenergic activity than the tricyclics. However, there is a greater tendency to postural hypotension after an initial increase in blood pressure. The commonest toxic effect during therapy is nausea. Sedation is not produced and alcohol can probably be taken by patients on this drug. Larger therapeutic doses may produce headache and vomiting. Epileptic seizures have also been reported during therapy. In overdose, atrioventricular block has occurred but at present it is not possible to assess its safety in overdose compared to tricyclics.

Maprotiline (Ludiomil)

Although related to tricyclics the presence of a bridge across the central ring

Table 9.4 Some commonly used tricyclic antidepressants

Approved name	*Proprietary names*	$t_{1/2}$ *(hours)*	*Administration*	*Remarks*	*Special uses apart from depression*
Imipramine	Tofranil	4–18	Oral: slowly increase dose from 25 to 150–300 mg daily	Insomnia; moderately sedative	1. Phobic anxiety: prevents panic attacks. 2. Nocturnal enuresis.
Amitriptyline	Tryptizol	8–20 (N.B. nortriptyline is a metabolite)	Oral, but for more rapid effect i.v. preparation available. Slowly increase dose from 25 to 75–150 mg daily.	Sedating Powerfully anticholinergic.	
Desipramine	Pertofran	12–25	Same dosage as imipramine but response not more rapid.	Little sedation; less anticholinergic than imipramine.	
Nortriptyline	Aventyl	18–93	Same dosage as amitriptyline. Response not more rapid than imipramine.	Relatively non-sedative	
Protriptyline	Concordin	54–198	Oral 15–60 mg daily. May have marginally faster onset of action than imipramine.	Least sedative of the tricyclics; may be stimulant.	Depression with apathy or retarded features.

Table 9.4 (*Continued*)

Approved name	*Proprietary names*	$t_{1/2}$ *(hours)*	*Administration*	*Remarks*	*Special uses apart from depression*
Clomipramine	Anafranil	16–20 ?non-linear kinetics	Oral 10 up to 75 mg daily	Sedating.	
Butriptyline	Evadyne	65–135 (mainly metabolites)	Oral 25 up to 150 mg daily.	Moderately sedative; ?fewer anticholinergic effects. Marked first-pass effect	Anxiolytic

structure converts it into a three-dimensional tetracyclic structure. It shares many of the pharmacological and biochemical properties of the tricyclics.

Pharmacokinetics It is well absorbed from the gut. The $t_{1/2}$ is slightly longer than other secondary amine antidepressants at 27–58 h. The volume of distribution is 19–29 l/kg body weight. There is no obvious relationship between plasma concentration and antidepressant effect, but fits are most likely to occur on higher dose regimes (about 225 mg daily).

Maprotiline is extensively metabolised and probably undergoes hepatic first-pass metabolism: about 60% is excreted as metabolites in urine, the remainder in the bile. Inter-individual variation occurs in whole-body clearance and protein binding.

Clinical use The dosage range is usually 25–150 mg daily, preferably given as a single evening dose. In the elderly lower doses should be given initially. It appears to be as effective as imipramine as an antidepressant.

Adverse effects Side effects are anticholinergic (dry mouth, headaches, constipation, dizziness, palpitations) and in common with the tricyclics the effects of adrenergic neurone blocking anti-hypertensives are antagonised, epilepsy aggravated, postural hypotension produced and in overdose cardiac tachyarrhythmias can be induced. The drug should not be given concurrently with the monoamine oxidase inhibitors. The actions of directly acting sympathomimetic drugs are enhanced. Maprotiline is contraindicted in patients with ischaemic heart disease.

Mianserin (Bolvidon; Norval)

This piperazino-azepine is a truly tetracyclic compound. It has no effect on the uptake of biogenic amines by neurones, no sympathomimetic activity and no significant anticholinergic effects. Thus, whereas conventional tricyclic antidepressants inhibit uptake and reduce noradrenaline and 5-HT turnover in the brain (Table 9.3), mianserin increases noradrenaline turnover without affecting that of 5-HT or dopamine. One possible mechanism of action is that mianserin blocks the presynaptic α-adrenergic receptors modulating synaptic noradrenaline release, resulting in increased noradrenaline release. Mianserin is also a potent antagonist of 5-HT receptors in peripheral tissues and probably at central synapses of 5-HT neurones with noradrenergic neurones. These 5-HT neurones inhibit noradrenaline release and their blockade increases noradrenaline availability and turnover. Like many (but not all) antidepressants, mianserin is also a potent histamine H_1 receptor antagonist. Whether this action is involved in either the therapeutic or undesirable effects of these drugs is unclear but H_1-receptor block correlates well with their sedative action. Mianserin therefore acts in a different way to the tricyclic antidepressants and it can no longer be assumed that a compound must inhibit amine re-uptake mechanisms before it can be considered to be a potential antidepressant. Interestingly, mianserin causes a dose-dependent increase in the proportion of slow (<6 Hz) waves in the EEG (as do the tricyclic antidepressants).

Pharmacokinetics Mianserin is absorbed from the gut and gives peak plasma levels at 2–3 h, but much individual variation in plasma concentrations. There appears to be a relationship between plasma levels and therapeutic outcome. As with the tricyclics a poor response to treatment is associated with both low and high plasma mianserin levels. The effective plasma level is not yet clearly defined. Plasma mianserin levels also relate directly to the proportion of EEG activity below 6 Hz and inversely with 9–13 Hz and α-waves. The plasma $t_{1/2}$ is about 10 h at age 20–25 years but in the elderly (over 70 years), it increases variably to approximately 15–45 h. Thus on average steady-state concentrations in the elderly will be double those in younger patients and doses used for the young could cause excessive and protracted sedation in the old. Only small amounts cross the placental barrier due to a high proportion bound to plasma protein.

Clinical uses The usual total daily dose is 30–60 mg, which can be given at night and corresponds to 75–150 mg amitriptyline, being apparently equally effective. The lack of serious cardiovascular toxicity and interaction with adrenergic neurone blocking agents makes it particularly suitable for patients at risk of suicide and for those being treated with guanethidine or related drugs. It has also been given to patients with ischaemic heart disease without untoward effects.

Adverse effects Unwanted effects apart from drowsiness and sedation are uncommon. At usual doses there is little anticholinergic activity but large doses may decrease salivation although there is no constipation, tachycardia, dizziness, tremor or faintness. Epilepsy is probably exacerbated. An important feature is the apparent lack of cardiotoxicity in overdose (c.f. tricyclics which are very toxic in this situation). There is no interference with the uptake and effects of adrenergic neurone blocking drugs. It may cause considerable postural hypotension especially in the elderly.

Rarely agranulocytosis or aplastic anaemia develops in patients taking mianserin. Another uncommon adverse reaction is a polyarthropathy which may be accompanied by a rash or abnormal liver function tests.

Nomifensine (Merital)

This is unrelated to any of the foregoing, being a tetrahydroisoquinoline derivative. It causes both a release of dopamine and inhibits re-uptake of both dopamine and noradrenaline. There seems to be no effect on 5-HT re-uptake. The hydroxylated metabolite of nomifensine may have a direct agonist effect at dopaminergic synapses. It may therefore be regarded as showing both activating properties similar to amphetamines and antidepressant effects like tricyclics. Because of its possible dopamine agonist effects it has been tried in Parkinsonism with some remission of symptoms, but it has no useful effect in hyperprolactinaemia or acromegaly, unlike the dopamine agonist bromocriptine (see p. 610).

Pharmacokinetics Following oral administration of nomifensine peak levels are reached in 1–1½ h. However, the drug is extensively and rapidly metabolised. The plasma $t_{1/2}$ of unchanged nomifensine is 0.8–1.9 h and that of the conjugate only marginally longer. Less than 5% unchanged nomifensine is excreted in the urine.

In renal failure higher blood levels are reached and there is an increased incidence of toxicity. In anuric patients the $t_{1/2}$ extends up to 46 h and the drug should not be used in patients with a GFR of less than 25 ml/min.

Clinical uses The activating effect of nomifensine may be particularly useful in the treatment of patients with predominant features of retardation and apathy. On the other hand it should not be given to agitated depressive since it may make their agitation worse. It should be given together in these cases with a tranquilliser. Patients with schizoaffective disorders may also worsen if given nomifensine and require additional treatment with a neuroleptic. Nomifensine is usually given in doses of 25 mg 8 hourly (a single daily dosage is unlikely to be effective because of the short $t_{1/2}$) which is increased to 50 mg 8 hourly or more if necessary.

No objective evidence of more rapid responses than occur with tricyclics has been presented.

Adverse effects Nomifensine has no pronounced anticholinergic activity, but patients do experience dry mouth, palpitations, constipation and blurred vision. There is probably no effect on fit threshold. In 1986 the drug was withdrawn because of serious hypersensitivity reactions, in particular haemolytic anaemia, vasculitis and liver necrosis.

Trazodone (Molipaxin)

This compound has a unique structure – it is a triazolopyridine. It has some inhibitory action on uptake$_1$ of 5-HT as well as directly blocking 5-HT receptors. In addition it has a similar, but weaker, action to mianserin in promoting noradrenaline release by blockade of α_2-adrenergic receptors.

Pharmacokinetics Gastrointestinal absorption is more complete when the drug is taken with food. The elimination $t_{1/2}$ is 4 h.

Clinical uses Trazodone is an effective antidepressant and is also anxiolytic. The relative freedom from anticholinergic and cardiotoxic effects makes this a suitable drug for the elderly and in patients with cardiac disease. The oral daily dose is 50–600 mg in single or divided doses. For acute anxiety 50 mg may be injected intravenously.

Adverse effects Trazodone is sedating but has much less pronounced anticholinergic and cardiotoxic properties than the tricyclic antidepressants. Epilepsy may be aggravated.

Monoamine oxidase inhibitors (MAOI)

During the early 1950s when analogues of isoniazid were undergoing trial for the treatment of tuberculosis it was noted that one agent, iproniazid, was euphoriant. It was soon found that it inhibited MAO and that an 'amphetamine-like' action in rabbits occurred if reserpine was given after chronic iproniazid administration. A number of other MAOIs have appeared (Table 9.5) but their use has declined in recent years because of their dangerous reactions with certain foods and a wide range of drugs. They are mainly reserved for depressed patients who have not responded to other drugs, particularly tricyclic antidepressants. The MAOIs inhibit several oxidising enzymes including brain mitochondrial monoamine oxidase. In this way neuronal concentrations of amines, such as noradrenaline, dopamine and 5-HT, increase in the brain and thus elevate mood.

Release of noradrenaline from large intraneuronal stores in sympathetic nerve fibres leads to serious hypertensive reactions if indirectly acting sympathomimetic agents enter the circulation.

α-agonists acting on the vasomotor centre in the brain stem produce a reflex lowering of the blood pressure. MAOIs, by raising brain concentration of noradrenaline in this area, also lower the blood pressure and have been used as hypotensive drugs.

Pharmacokinetics The MAOIs are generally lipophilic and are well absorbed from the gut. They freely penetrate cell membranes and the blood–brain barrier. The hydrazine MAOIs produce irreversible inhibition of monoamine oxidase whilst the inhibition produced by the non-hydrazines is reversible. Thus with many of the MAOIs, even after cessation of treatment when the drug can no longer be detected in the body, the effects of treatment may persist and dangerous toxicity arise.

Multiple forms of monoamine oxidase exist in the body and the various MAOI drugs differ in their ability to inhibit the two principal forms of the enzyme.

The hydrazine MAOIs are partly metabolised by acetylation and acetylator status of the patients affects the proneness to toxicity: slow acetylators more frequently experience toxicity. Differences in therapeutic responsiveness can be detected between acetylator phenotypes. Blood-level studies relating to clinical effect are not available. However, in one trial depressed patients treated with phenelzine demonstrating an 80% inhibition of platelet monoamine oxidase were more likely to benefit than those with less enzyme inhibition. The relationship between peripheral and central inhibition of MAO is unclear.

It has been suggested that the response to MAOIs may be genetically determined and that the result could be predicted in a patient if the response of a first-degree relative to the same drug were known. This possible pharmacogenetic variation presumably reflects biochemical factors, but more evidence is required before it can be accepted.

The improvement of patients on MAOI, if it occurs, varies considerably and may be slow, some patients requiring treatment for 6–8 weeks before showing effect. The generally accepted order of clinical efficacy does not correspond to their efficacy in MAO inhibition. Some of the variations and contradictions in clinical trials of MAOIs may related to inter-patient pharmacokinetic differences.

Table 9.5 Monoamine oxidase inhibitors in general use

Approved name	*Proprietary name*	*Administration*	*Special features*
(A) Hydrazines			
Iproniazid	Marsilid	25 mg 12 or 8 hourly	Not now generally used because of hepatotoxicity. Peripheral neuropathy.
Phenelzine	Nardil	15 mg 8 hourly	? Most effective. Lowest incidence of reported hypertensive crises.
Isocarboxazid	Marplan	Initially 50 mg daily reducing to maintenance of 10–20 mg daily	
(B) Non-Hydrazines			
Tranylcypromine	Parnate	10 mg 8 hourly	? Acts more rapidly than hydrazine MAOIs. Implicated particularly in interaction with foodstuffs.
	in Parstelin (10 mg tranylcypromine 1 mg trifluoperazine)	1 tablet twice or three times daily	For depression with anxiety

Adverse effects These can be grouped as follows:

(a) *Mild effects*
autonomic phenomena are common
dry mouth (atropine-like effect)
orthostatic hypotension
hesitancy of micturition (atropine-like effect)
water retention
weight gain
dizziness
headache

(b) *More severe*
serious nervous system toxicity is uncommon
agitation, anxiety
hypomania
acute schizophrenic-like illness
acute confusion
dizziness
tremor
weakness
dysarthria
clonus, hyperreflexia
peripheral neuropathy (iproniazid)
oedema
hepatocellular necrosis resembling infectious hepatitis and occasionally producing liver failure

(c) *Serious overdose*
There is often a latent interval of about 6 h followed by agitation, fever and tachypnoea. The reflexes become brisk and there may be involuntary movements of the face. Serious poisoning leads to progressive dilatation of the pupils and coma. Treatment may include care of the unconscious patient (including control of fluid balance); acidification of the urine; chlorpromazine and β-blockers and possibly dialysis.

(d) *Drug interaction*

(i) hypertensive and hyperthermic reactions sufficient to cause fatal subarachnoid haemorrhage, particularly with tranylcypromine. Such serious reactions are precipitated by amines, including indirectly acting sympathomimetic agents (such as tyramine (in cheese), dopamine (in broad bean pods and formed from levodopa), amines formed from any fermentation process (as in yoghurt, beer, wine), phenylephrine (including that administered as nose drops and in cold cures), ephedrine, amphetamine (all can give hypertensive reactions); other amines: pethidine (excitement, hyperthermia), levodopa (hypertension); reserpine: (hypertension); tricyclic, tetracyclic and bicyclic antidepressants (excitement, hyperpyrexia).

(ii) failure to metabolise drugs which are normally oxidised: narcotic analgesics, barbiturates, alcohol (perhaps reactions with alcoholic drinks occur mainly because of their tyramine content). These drugs will have an exaggerated and prolonged effect.

(iii) enhanced effects of oral hypoglycaemic agents, anaesthetics, suxamethonium, caffeine, anticholinergics (including benzhexol and similar antiparkinsonian drugs).

The dangers of these reactions are such that it is advisable for patients to carry a printed card giving details of these and to receive adequate instruction from the doctor before being given an MAOI.

L-tryptophan (Optimax)

This essential amino acid is hydroxylated to 5-hydroxytryptophan (5-HTP) and then decarboxylated to 5-hydroxytryptamine (5-HT) which is a neurotransmitter probably contributing to the control of mood. 5-HT itself does not pass the blood–brain barrier, but provided there are adequate coenzyme (ascorbic acid and pyridoxal phosphate) levels in the brain, exogenous 5-HTP and tryptophan can be taken up and metabolised to 5-HT. This synthesis does not necessarily increase the level of 5-HT acting as neurotransmitter, however. There is some evidence for lowered plasma tryptophan levels in depressed patients but although this is not completely established there is controlled trial evidence that administration of tryptophan with monoamine oxidase inhibitors or imipramine will improve the response of patients to these drugs. Tryptophan alone (usually with pyridoxine) has been given to depressed patients in doses of 3–4 times the normal dietary intake (i.e. doses of 5–9 g daily). Tryptophan potentiates the effectiveness of the MAOI and tricyclic antidepressants. Its lack of side effects and safety in overdose are important features of its pharmacology.

Thioxanthenes

The thioxanthenes are triple-ring heterocyclic compounds which differ from phenothiazines in that the nitrogen of position 10 in the phenothiazine nucleus is replaced by a carbon atom. The side chains are similar to those of some of the neuroleptic phenothiazines but are attached to C_{10} by a double bond. The general pharmacology of the thioxanthenes is similar to that of the phenothiazines. Thus these drugs reduce spontaneous motor activity, are potent antiemetics, antagonise amphetamine-induced stereotypic behaviour in animals (an experimental model for testing antipsychotic drugs) and can induce catalepsy. However, thioxanthenes are less sedative and appear to have antidepressant activity.

Chlorprothixene (Taractan) is structurally analogous to chlorpromazine. It was the first of this group to be shown to have antipsychotic properties. Controlled trials in schizophrenics reveal it to be significantly more effective than placebo but probably (in the doses used) less effective than chlorpromazine, thioridazine or fluphenazine. In the dose range used in the treatment of schizophrenia (50–1000 mg/day) the sedative anticholinergic and cardiovascular side effects resemble those of chlorpromazine.

Clopenthixol has similar antipsychotic activity and side effects to perphenazine (equivalent doses are approximately 130 mg clopenthixol daily and 50 mg perphenazine daily). The incidence of drowsiness, motor restlessness and extrapyramidal signs are virtually the same. Despite clinical effectiveness the incidence of laboratory abnormalities has been found to be higher than expected and it has therefore not been marketed in the USA.

Flupenthixol is an antipsychotic drug which is available in oral and intramuscular long-acting forms. The depot preparation is given in single doses of 40–120 mg i.m. every two weeks. Extrapyramidal side effects occur.

The uses of the thioxanthenes. Although these drugs are primarily used to treat schizophrenia and other psychotic states, including organic psychosis, they have been used as antidepressants. For the treatment of depression the thioxanthenes are more effective than placebo but probably less successful than the tricyclics. The thioxanthenes have anxiolytic properties and may be of value in agitated depressive states.

Lithium

Lithium has proven efficacy in the treatment of mania and as a prophylactic agent in recurrent affective disorders, i.e. recurrent depressions (unipolar affective disorder) and manic depression (bipolar affective disorder). There is some evidence that it is useful in treating hyperactive children and possibly alcoholism. Other experimental applications include management of inappropriate ADH secretion and hyperthyroidism.

The mechanism of action of lithium is not understood and the biochemical changes produced are complex. Increased 5-HT synthesis and accelerated turnover of noradrenaline have also been demonstrated after acute lithium treatment, but chronic dosage decreases 5-HT and dopamine turnover. These findings cannot be accommodated by the amine theory of depression. Attention has recently focussed upon mechanisms which involve resetting of the post-synaptic amine receptors by lithium.

Pharmacokinetics Lithium is usually administered as the carbonate and is readily absorbed after oral administration so that injectable preparations are unnecessary. Peak plasma levels occur 3–5 h after dosing, the $t_{1/2}$ varies with age, being 18–20 h in young adults and up to 36 h in the elderly. Sustained release preparations are available, but in view of the long $t_{1/2}$ are not kinetically justified. The evidence that they produce more even plasma levels is not established, they are not always well absorbed in the upper gut and may thus produce lower intestinal upset. The long $t_{1/2}$ also means that it takes several days for the body to reach lithium balance and the first samples for plasma-level monitoring should be taken after about a week. Lithium elimination is almost entirely renal. Like sodium, lithium does not bind to plasma protein and readily passes into the glomerular filtrate; 70–80% is reabsorbed in the proximal tubules but, unlike sodium, there is no distal tubular reabsorption and its elimination is unaltered by diuretics acting on the distal tubule. Because the proximal reabsorption of sodium and lithium is competitive, sodium deficiency and sodium diuresis can increase lithium retention and toxicity. An important implication of the renal handling of lithium is that neither loop diuretics, thiazides nor spironolactone can enhance lithium loss in a toxic patient and they may even enhance toxicity. Osmotic diuretics or dialysis will, however, reduce elevated plasma lithium levels. As renal clearance of lithium varies from one patient to another it is necessary for lithium dosage to be determined individually and this is best achieved by monitoring plasma lithium levels, which are best taken 10–12 h after the last dose. During initiation of treatment levels are determined once or twice weekly, but after stabilisation this is usually required only every three months or so. The therapeutic range is 0.8–1.2 mmol/l. A successfully treated patient has no symptoms to remind him of the need for treatment and therefore measurement of lithium levels is a useful check on compliance.

Clinical use 300 mg of lithium carbonate is equivalent to 8 mmol and it is usual to begin treatment with 600–900 mg daily, but this may need reduction in patients with known renal impairment. This initial dose is increased slowly, depending upon the plasma level, doses of 1500–2400 mg/day being common. Response usually occurs after 2–4 weeks but full benefit may not be evident before 6–12 months. The commonest cause of failure of treatment is non-compliance. The duration of therapy is undecided, but may be lifelong in recurrent affective disorder, where relapse is almost certain within a few months of discontinuation of prophylaxis. Patients with schizoid symptoms or a short manic–depressive cycle do not respond well to lithium and may require treatment with additional drugs.

Adverse effects Lithium is a toxic drug and its adverse effects may be divided into

(a) *Dose dependent*
Plasma level
1.5–3 mmol/l—ataxia, weakness, drowsiness, thirst, diarrhoea.
3–5 mmol/l—confusion, spasticity, convulsions, dehydration, coma, death.

(b) *Dose independent*
1. Hypothyroidism (10% patients on chronic therapy). Initiation of lithium therapy should be preceded by assessment of thyroid function. Inhibition of adenyl cyclase may result in decreased synthesis of thyroid hormone and a goitre due to increased TSH release. Chronic lithium therapy has also been reported to produce thyrotoxicosis.
2. Nephrogenic diabetes insipidus—possibly due to interference by lithium with stimulation of adenyl cyclase by ADH. Polyuria and polydipsia thus can occur with chronic lithium therapy. There may also be an increase in aldosterone secretion.

3. Cardiac effects may occur when lithium plasma levels are within the therapeutic range. The commonest are reversible T-wave changes (attributed to replacement of intracellular potassium by lithium which is only slowly extruded from the cell). Arrhythmias have also been recorded but if there is psychiatric need, cardiac disease is not a contraindiction to lithium.
4. Loss of bone calcium and density—possibly due to interference with parathormone effects mediated by cyclic AMP.
5. Weight gain—possibly due to insulin release by lithium.

Although lithium is teratogenic in the rat no increase in fetal abnormalities has been convincingly demonstrated in man. It should not be used in the first trimester of pregnancy and only with caution in the later months.

Drug interactions with lithium are rare:

1. Extrapyramidal complications and tardive dyskinesia associated with haloperidol and phenothiazines may be commoner when they are used in conjunction with lithium. Tricyclics and MAOIs may be used safely with lithium.
2. Thiazides may precipitate lithium toxicity by reducing lithium clearance.
3. Non-steroidal anti-inflammatory agents can also reduce lithium clearance and produce toxicity, probably because they cause sodium retention.

ANTIPSYCHOTIC DRUGS (NEUROLEPTICS), MAJOR TRANQUILLISERS

These are agents which are effective in excited or agitated psychotic states such as acute episodes of schizophrenia, hypomania and delirium. They have revolutionised the management of schizophrenia and are sometimes called 'tranquillisers'. This is a misnomer since it implies that they merely act as sedatives in the manner of say, benzodiazepines. Rather they exert unique antipsychotic properties and form the only generally recognised drug therapy for schizophrenia with demonstrated efficacy and relative safety.

Recently a correlation has been demonstrated between the therapeutic potencies of a wide range of antipsychotic drugs and their ability to block dopaminergic receptors *in vitro*. Dopamine receptors are classifed as types D_1 and D_2: D_1 receptors activate adenyl cyclase, whilst stimulation of D_2 receptors has no effect on adenyl cyclase. The antipsychotic activity of the neuroleptics is due to blockade of D_2 receptors. A theory that D_1 receptors are involved has not been substantiated. Sulpiride, a selective D_2 blocker, has antipsychotic activity. Dopamine blockade produces a number of effects in the CNS including extrapyramidal disorders in man and analogous catalepsy in animals. These effects are not reversible by levodopa since the dopamine formed from this exogenous source is insufficient to overcome the powerful, albeit competitive, blockade by these agents. After prolonged use tardive dyskinesias may develop (see p. 255) and may be due to a compensatory oversensitivity to dopamine (analogous to denervation supersensitivity) which becomes more apparent when the drug is withdrawn. Their anti-emetic properties also result from dopaminergic blockade in the chemoreceptor trigger zone (note that apomorphine, a powerful emetic, is a dopaminergic agonist). Serum prolactin levels are also elevated by their action on the inhibitory tubero-infundibular pathway (see p. 610).

Many of these agents also block other types of receptor. This, and differences in drug distribution, may explain why some specific dopaminergic blocking drugs such as metoclopramide produce virtually no antipsychotic effects but may give rise to extrapyramidal symptoms. Attempts to relate the development of extrapyramidal reactions in patients to the efficacy of antipsychotic drugs have not been very rewarding. Extrapyramidal effects may be inversely proportional to their affinity for central muscarinic cholinergic receptors and a drug such as thioridazine may possess enough anticholinergic effect to compensate for its interference with dopamine binding and the consequent perturbation of the extrapyramidal balance between dopamine and acetylcholine.

The crucial importance of dopaminergic blockade in the action of antipsychotic drugs is revealed by comparison of the clinical effects of the two optical isomers of flupenthixol. This thioxanthine exists as a cis (α) form which has dopamine blocking activity and a trans (β) isomer which does not block dopamine receptors. In most other respects, in particular cholinergic, noradrenergic and opiate receptor-blocking potencies, these isomers are identical. In a clinical trial in schizophrenia, however, only patients on cis-flupenthixol improved and those on the trans isomer did no better than those on placebo. In this trial it was found that positive symptoms (e.g. hallucinations, delusions, incongruity of affect) showed rapid improvement whereas negative features such as flattening of affect and uncommunicativeness did not improve.

Although it is clear that dopaminergic blockade is involved in their antipsychotic effect, their site of action is unclear since there are relatively few known dopaminergic pathways in the brain. The mesolimbic area and projections from the midbrain nuclei to forebrain cortex are currently suggested as possible loci. In animal studies antipsychotic activity is closely related to actions on dopamine levels in the mesolimbic system and extrapyramidal effects to those in the corpus striatum.

The time course of dopaminergic blockade does not clearly relate to improvement of schizophrenic symptoms. This is shown by the fact that the increase of prolactin levels due to dopaminergic blockade occurs within a few hours of the first dose of drug whilst the time course of the therapeutic response is much slower and often takes several weeks. Thus whilst dopaminergic blockade appears to be essential for antipsychotic efficacy, it may be necessary for some slower adaptive process to occur, and it is this change which is related to symptom improvement.

Presently there is no evidence that dopaminergic systems are overactive in the schizophrenic brain, although this hypothesis is technically difficult to substantiate. However, it is possible that the abnormality may occur not presynaptically but postsynaptically and that in schizophrenia certain key dopaminergic synapses show receptor supersensitivity. There is also some post-mortem evidence suggesting that in some areas of some schizophrenics'

Table 9.6 Antipsychotic drugs

Chemical group	*Examples*
1. Phenothiazines—Aliphatic side chains	Chlorpromazine Promazine
—Piperidine side chains	Thioridazine
—Piperazine side chain	Trifluoperazine Prochlorperazine Perphenazine Fluphenazine
2. Butyrophenones	Haloperidol Benperidol Droperidol Trifluperidol
3. Thioxanthenes	Chlorprothixine Thiothixine Flupenthixol
4. Diphenylbutylpiperidines	Pimozide Fluspirilene
5. Dihydroindoles	Molindone
6. Dibenzodiazepines	Loxapine Clozapine
7. Orthopramides	Sulpiride

brains there are increased numbers of dopamine receptors as compared to normal.

Controversy still rages around the specificity of these drugs, but many agree that in some respects they have a more specific effect in combating schizophrenic (and particularly paranoid) symptoms than in other psychotic illness. If they are specifically antischizophrenic agents, their mode of action may give insight into the pathology underlying such states.

Antipsychotic drugs comprise several different chemical groups (see Table 9.6).

Phenothiazines

The antipsychotic phenothiazines have central antihallucinatory and calming activity. Although tiredness and sedation are produced, the most characteristic central action is diminution of emotional responsiveness and indifference to environmental changes. This is called the *ataractic* state. Other central effects include inhibition of the chemoreceptor trigger zone of the medullary vomiting centre and inhibition of hypothalamic function (including loss of temperature control, increased prolactin release leading to galactorrhoea, amenorrhoea and delayed menstruation and weight gain). Many have powerful extrapyramidal effects and in addition to blocking dopamine receptors also block muscarinic cholinergic receptors (with atropine-like effects), histamine (H_1) receptors and α-adrenergic receptors. This latter action plays a part in the production of postural hypotension which is also due to central impairment of cardiovascular reflexes (see Table 9.7).

Phenothiazines have tricyclic structures in which two benzene rings are linked by sulphur and nitrogen atoms. Three classes of phenothiazines are formed according to the substitution in the side chain attached to the nitrogen: aliphatic chains, piperidine or piperazine groups.

The *aliphatic* chains contain dimethylaminopropyl groups. Drugs of this class (e.g. chlorpromazine) are sedating and have considerable α-adrenoceptor blocking activity. They show relatively greater peripheral effects (dry mouth, hypotension, tachycardia) than other members of the group.

The *piperazines* on a weight-for-weight basis are more powerfully antipsychotic and produce less sedation. Some members of this group (e.g. trifluoperazine) may have stimulant properties. Extrapyramidal side effects are produced more readily than with the aliphatic type of drug. These compounds also possess useful antiemetic properties.

The *piperidines* (e.g. thioridazine) are also more potent than the aliphatic type but sedation is usually prominent. Extrapyramidal side effects are less common than in the other two groups. They have powerful α-adrenergic blocking (and hence hypotensive) and anticholinergic actions.

Pharmacokinetics In contrast to the antidepressants, these compounds have been little studied pharmacokinetically because of the multiplicity of metabolites. Their large apparent volumes of distribution (e.g. for chlorpromazine $V_d = 22$ l/kg) result in low plasma levels which present technical difficulties in estimation.

Most is known about chlorpromazine. When given orally it is incompletely absorbed with a bioavailability of about 30%. This is further decreased by the presence of food or by simultaneous administration of anticholinergic drugs and some antacids. Animal studies suggest considerable degradation of chlorpromazine in the gut before entering the portal circulation (a prehepatic first-pass effect). Peak plasma levels are reached in 2–3 h but the $t_{1/2}$ varies between 2 and 24 h in different individuals. The plasma steady-state levels are reached in around one week and have been reported as ranging from 10 to 1200 ng/ml in psychotic patients. Changes of dose more often than every five days are therefore inadvisable, and daily dosing is adequate in most patients. A single night-time dose will increase compliance and the sedative effects of the drug are maximal when they are most needed. Plasma levels only poorly correlate with dosage, generally a specific level may be attained with a lower dose in young patients or those beginning treatment as compared with the elderly or those undergoing prolonged treatment, suggesting that age and enzyme induction may influence its disposition. After intramuscular injection absorption is irregular, possibly due to local precipitation of drug and its effects upon the vascular system in muscle.

Chlorpromazine is an unstable molecule which rapidly forms an inactive sulphoxide on exposure to light. It has 168 potential metabolites, 70 of which have been identified in man. The general routes of metabolism are:

(a) Demethylation producing nor_1- and nor_2-chlorpromazine, which are sedative and enter the brain.

Table 9.7 Commonly used phenothiazines

Approved name	*Proprietary name*	*Antipsychotic dose (mg) per day*	*Extrapyramidal effects*	*Anti-emetic effects*	*Sedative effects*	*Hypotensive effects*	*Remarks*
Chlorpromazine	Largactil Chloractyl	100–2000	+ +	+ +	+ +	+ +	Phenothiazine for general purposes
Promazine	Sparine	100–1500	+ +	+ +	+ +	+ +	
Thioridazine	Melleril	100–800	+	+	+ + +	+ + +	Used in elderly. Greatest tendency to produce retinopathy and cardiac toxicity
Trifluoperazine	Stelazine	3–30	+ + +	+ + +	+	+	Antiemetic
Prochlorperazine	Stemetil	50–150	+ + +	+ + +	+	+	Commonly used as anti-emetic
Fluphenazine	Modecate Moditen	2–20	+ + +	+ + +	+ +	+	Used in depot preparations
Methotrimeprazine	Nozinan	25–100	+	+ + +	+ + +	+ + +	Not used as antipsychotic but has powerful analgesic action

(+ + + = high; + + = moderate; + = low)

(b) Oxidation producing sulphoxides and N-oxides, which are pharmacologically inactive.
(c) Hydroxylation producing 3-hydroxy- and 7-hydroxychlorpromazine. Although 7-hydroxychlorpromazine has been implicated in the production of skin pigmentation, it appears to be an important antipsychotic metabolite and is probably more active than the parent substance.
(d) Conjugation with glucuronic acid and sulphate.

Metabolism is primarily by hepatic microsomes although the brain, kidneys, lungs and gut also play a part.

Chlorpromazine is 90–95% bound, mainly to albumin and is concentrated in some tissues, e.g. brain concentration is 4–5 times that of plasma.

Following a single dose, a clear relationship has been established between the peak plasma level and effects such as sedation, pulse, pupil size, salivary secretion and orthostatic hypotension, although the threshold for response varies from patient to patient. With chronic administration a tolerance develops to the sedative effects. The plasma chlorpromazine level may fall while the antipsychotic effect becomes manifest. Possibly this results from increased metabolism due to self-induction or else the known anticholinergic effect of chlorpromazine results in delay in absorption and increased gut metabolism. The relationship between plasma levels and therapeutic effect is not well established, but levels of 35–350 ng/ml have been associated with clinical improvement and severe toxicity is seen above 600 ng/ml. Quantitation of metabolites may be necessary for the pattern of therapeutic response to emerge but the patients who respond usually have higher ratios of 7-hydroxychlorpromazine + chlorpromazine to chlorpromazine sulphoxide than unresponsive patients.

Thioridazine has been partially investigated but presents most of the same problems as chlorpromazine. The $t_{1/2}$ varies from 10 to 36 h with a tendency to prolongation in the elderly. A diurnal variation in metabolism (some metabolites are active) has been described, elimination being slowed during sleep.

Clinical uses:

1. The effectiveness of these drugs in schizophrenia has been demonstrated in a number of double blind clinical trials. Not only are acute episodes terminated, but general deterioration in chronic schizophrenia is prevented and the need for hospitalisation is greatly reduced. Minimal effective doses should be used. Signs of tardive dyskinesia are indications to stop piperazine or propylamino-phenothiazines and if continued medication is needed to control psychotic behaviour, thioridazine or clozapine should be used.
2. Hypomania and other excited psychotic illnesses usually respond well to these drugs although they may induce depression. However, in the agitated state due to alcohol withdrawal, phenothiazines may precipitate fits. They may be effective in elderly agitated patients and in violent individuals.

3. Severe anxiety and panic may occasionally respond inadequately to anxiolytic agents and require additional treatment with phenothiazines.
4. Painful terminal illness. Perhaps their main benefit in these circumstances is to reduce the emotional response to pain. In addition phenothiazines potentiate some of the central effects of the narcotic analgesics.
5. α-adrenoceptor blockade may be of value in the treatment of shock, and in hypertensive reactions complicating monoamine oxidase inhibitor and tricyclic antidepressant therapy.
6. The anti-emetic properties of the phenothiazines are valuable in vomiting complicating metabolic disturbances, terminal illness, narcotic administration, radiation, and antitumour drug therapy.
7. Prochlorperazine is used to suppress vestibular function in Ménière's disease.
8. Even though the neuroleptic drugs can cause dyskinesias, they may also be used to treat them, e.g. they can suppress chorea in Huntington's chorea.
9. Hiccough which is otherwise intractable may be terminated by chlorpromazine.
10. Control of some of the manifestations of withdrawal from addictive drugs.
11. Some of the phenothiazines with powerful antihistamine activity, e.g. promethazine, trimeprazine, are useful anti-pruritic agents but suffer from the tendency to produce sedation and sometimes other phenothiazine side effects. These antihistamines are not antipsychotic agents.

Adverse effects

1. The commonest are dose-dependent extensions of pharmacological effects:
   (a) Anticholinergic: dry mouth, nasal stuffiness, constipation, urinary retention, blurred vision.
   (b) Postural hypotension due to peripheral α-adrenergic blockade, which is rarely severe. Gradual build-up of dose aids the development of tolerance.
   (c) Sedation (which may be desirable in agitated patients), drowsiness and confusion. Tolerance usually develops after several weeks on a maintenance dose but can be overcome by an increased dose. Depression may develop, particularly following treatment of hypomania.
2. Abnormal involuntary movements including tremor, seizures, Parkinsonism, dystonia, dyskinesia, uncontrollable restlessness (akasthisia) and tardive dyskinesia (see p. 255). All but the last of these are reversible. Acute dystonias can appear within a week of beginning the drug but the other reactions can be delayed for months. There seems to be no relationship between dose and their appearance. Their pathogenesis probably results from blockade of dopamine receptors, although tardive dyskinesias may involve actual structural damage.
3. Jaundice occurs in 2–4% of patients taking chlorpromazine, usually during the second to fourth weeks of treatment. It is due to intrahepatic

cholestasis and is a hypersensitivity phenomenon associated with eosinophilia. Substitution of another phenothiazine may not reactivate the jaundice.

4. Ocular disorders observed during chronic administration include corneal and lens opacities and pigmentary retinopathy. This may be associated with cutaneous light sensitivity. Recent studies implicate the hydroxylated metabolites of chlorpromazine as the culprit in the ocular disorders.
5. Another type of hypersensitivity reaction involves the skin. 5% of patients develop urticarial, maculopapular or petechial rashes. These disappear on withdrawal of the drug and may not recur if the drug is reinstated. Contact dermatitis and light sensitivity are common complications. Abnormal melanin pigmentation may develop in the skin.
6. Chlorpromazine consistently raises serum cholesterol levels. Glucose tolerance tests may also be impaired.
7. Blood dyscrasias are uncommon but may be lethal, particularly leucopenia and thrombocytopenia. These usually develop in early days or weeks of treatment. The estimated incidence of agranulocytosis is approximately 1 in 10 000 patients receiving chlorpromazine.
8. Sudden cardiac arrhythmia and arrest occurs with phenothiazines in the absence of gross structural damage although mitochondrial abnormalities have been noted in heart muscle. T-wave abnormalities and increased frequency of ventricular premature beats are noted on the ECG.
9. The malignant syndrome is another rare and potentially fatal complication of neuroleptics. Its clinical features are rigidity, hyperpyrexia, stupor or coma, and autonomic disorders.
10. Fits can be precipitated—particularly in alcoholics. Pre-existing epilepsy may be aggravated.

The BCDSP (q.v.) indicates that adverse reactions are commonest in patients receiving high doses and tend to occur soon after starting treatment. The commonest serious reactions noted were fits, coma, severe hypotension, leucopenia, thrombocytopenia, and cardiac arrest.

Drug interactions

1. Chlorpromazine potentiates the effects of alcohol both by an additive sedative effect and via inhibition of alcohol dehydrogenase. Other centrally depressant drugs, e.g. barbiturates, are potentiated. Respiratory depression due to narcotics is enhanced.
2. Anticholinergic effects affect the absorption of paracetamol, levodopa, digoxin and lithium.
3. Hypotensive drugs are potentiated.
4. Chlorpromazine inhibits the metabolism of tricyclic antidepressants, increasing their plasma levels.
5. The hypotensive actions of guanethidine and other adrenergic neurone blockers are antagonised.
6. Chlorpromazine is a moderately effective enzyme inducer.

Butyrophenones (see Table 9.8)

Haloperidol The first member of the butyrophenone group to be used clinically. It is an effective alternative antipsychotic drug to the phenothiazines.

The main actions of haloperidol are similar to those of the piperazine phenothiazines. Thus it is less sedative than chlorpromazine but more powerfully anti-emetic and more prone to produce extrapyramidal effects. Although haloperidol is an α-blocker, it has weaker autonomic actions than the phenothiazines.

Pharmacokinetics The drug is well absorbed after oral administration, the bioavailability being approximately 60% by this route. The $t_{1/2}$ for elimination is 12–38 h and so steady-state levels are reached within a week on a steady maintenance dosage. There is a linear relationship between dose and plateau plasma levels (cf. chlorpromazine). Haloperidol is oxidised in the liver via oxidative dealkylation and does not apparently form pharmacologically active metabolites. Metabolism may show a diurnal rhythm, being slowed in sleep. There is no relationship between age and plasma levels attained by a given dose. The relationship between plasma level and therapeutic effect is not established: 3–10 ng/ml has been suggested as the therapeutic range.

Adverse effects

1. CNS: sedation, which is potentiated by other central depressants. Extrapyramidal syndromes; depression—particularly in patients treated with this drug for hypomania.
2. Hypotension—less severe than with chlorpromazine.
3. Leucopenia, agranulocytosis and jaundice have been reported but appear to be uncommon.

Pimozide (Orap) This is a long-acting antipsychotic, $t_{1/2} = 18$ h. In the maintenance treatment of schizophrenia pimozide is given as a single daily dose (2–10 mg). Sedation is not a prominent feature of its activity and at antipsychotic doses extrapyramidal effects are negligible and autonomic effects virtually absent. Pimozide is usually unsuccessful in the acute management of psychomotor agitation, aggression and manic excitement. It is of most value in apathetic and withdrawn patients.

Adverse effects include depression, extrapyramidal effects (in large doses), aggravation of epilepsy.

Fluspirilene is a long-acting injectable neuroleptic (see below). The preparation for injection is in a microcrystalline form of low solubility. This results in slow absorption from the injection site. In doses of 1.25–10 mg per injection, powerful antipsychotic activity persists for 6–15 days. The drug is usually started at a dose of 2 mg i.m. weekly, increasing the dose by 2 mg each week until acute symptoms are controlled or toxicity arises. Extrapyramidal signs are not usually troublesome and only occur 12–48 h after each injection unless high doses are used. Fatigue and postural hypotension may also occur.

Table 9.8 Some clinically useful butyrophenones

Approved name	*Proprietary name*	*Dose*	*Special uses apart from in psychosis*
Haloperidol	Haldol Serenace	Oral: 0.5–5 mg, 12 or 8 hourly. i.m.: Up to 30 mg 6 hourly may be needed to control acute excitement. Usually given with antiparkinsonian drug, e.g. procyclidine (Kemadrin).	Anaesthetic pre-medication. Alcohol withdrawal syndromes. Gilles de la Tourette syndrome.
Benperidol	Anquil	Oral 0.25–1.5 mg daily in divided doses.	Deviant and anti-social sexual behaviour.
Droperidol	Droleptan	Oral 5–20 mg i.m. 5–10 mg i.v. 5–15 mg	With narcotic analgesic for neuroleptanalgesia. Anaesthetic premedication. Anti-emetic.
Trifluoperidol	Triperidol	0.5–2.5 mg daily oral	Acute behavioural disorders. Mania.

Controlled trials indicate that fluspirilene is as effective as long-acting phenothiazines and as oral trifluoperazine in controlling acute schizophrenia.

Dihydroindoles

These are antipsychotic drugs with an indole structure. The group includes oxypertine (Integrin) and molindone (Muban). Oxypertine is given orally in a daily dose of 80–120 mg (divided).

The dihydroindole neuroleptics are sedating. They show little extrapyramidal toxicity and very little α-receptor blockade.

Dibenzodiazepines

Clozapine is a non-phenothiazine dibenzodiazepine with a piperazine side chain. Preliminary experience with this substance suggests high antipsychotic efficacy and few extrapyramidal side effects, but its place in therapy is not yet established.

Orthopramides

This group of drugs include sulpiride (Dolmatil). The general properties are similar to those of the dibenzodiazepines. Sulpiride blocks D_2, but not D_1, dopamine receptors in the brain. It has little or no action on 5-HT, adrenergic α_1 and α_2, cholinergic and γ-aminobutyric acid receptors. The drug also inhibits D_4 receptors—this results in an increase in glutamate release and dopamine transmission. Sulpiride can cause motor and mental arousal and relieve depression in schizophrenia.

Parkinsonism is probably less commonly produced than with the older neuroleptics. Acute dystonic reactions and tardive dyskinesias are not usually produced.

The starting oral dose is 200–400 mg twice daily.

Effects of major tranquillisers on schizophrenia

Spontaneous recovery (social remission) of schizophrenia is about 20%, whilst drug therapy leads to a social recovery rate of 50–60% for patients who have been ill for less than 3 years. It is principally the florid symptoms of the disease which respond. These are thought insertion, thought broadcasting, thought block, delusions, feelings of passivity and auditory hallucinations.

Modern drug treatment has not increased the number of symptom-free patients but has shifted patients with overt psychotic symptoms into the group with residual symptoms. Although maintenance therapy has been shown to be more effective than placebo the relapse rate during treatment may be as high as 25% during one year. Studies have shown that it is reasonable for long-term therapy of such patients to be managed by their family physician: such patients do no worse than those attending a psychiatric outpatient department. At times because of severe psychotic episodes, imminent risk of suicide or injury or social problems at home, it becomes necessary to admit such patients and to intensify their medical treatment. Very infrequently are locked wards or physical restraint necessary since drug therapy proves so effective. Prolonged and intensive analytical psychotherapy aimed at changing the patient's personality has not been shown to be an effective primary mode of treatment for severe schizophrenia. Active supportive psychotherapy is humane and may allow schizophrenics and their families to cope with a relapsing and socially crippling disability. There is no convincing evidence that ECT is of value in the management of schizophrenia.

Discontinuation of treatment results in relapse of 75–95% of patients within 1 year and 25% relapse within 1 week. Maintenance therapy with depot phenothiazines may therefore need to be considered as extending over many years. The long-term effects of such treatment are, of course, unknown at the present time. All drugs should be used in smallest effective doses. In some schizophrenic patients lithium is more effective than a neuroleptic.

Tetrabenazine has a similar action to reserpine and so has antipsychotic effects but can produce depression. It does not cause tardive dyskinesias.

Depot neuroleptics

Fatty acid esters of phenothiazines are increasingly used for maintenance therapy. Single injections may last for 2–4 weeks. The ester link is broken by tissue esterases to liberate free drug which is then absorbed from the injection site. The rate of hydrolysis is further reduced by using the ester in an oily solution. Acute dystonic reactions may follow initial doses suggesting that early release of drug may be considerable.

Drugs of this type are:

fluphenazine decanoate (Modecate)
fluphenazine enanthate (Moditen enanthate)
flupenthixol decanoate (Depixol)
perphenazine enanthate
fluspirilene (Redeptin)
pipothiazine undecylenate and palmitate (Piportil)

The commonest cause of relapse in chronic schizophrenia is failure to take neuroleptic therapy. The long-acting neuroleptics have proved successful in reducing hospitalisation by preventing such relapses. These agents can also used in manic and acutely disturbed psychotic patients but are unsuitable for the initiation of therapy.

In addition to improved compliance, depot neuroleptics improve the bioavailability of these drugs since neuroleptics are subject to erratic oral absorption and a significant gut and hepatic first-pass metabolism. Depot preparations bypass gut and hepatic metabolism and a relatively higher concentration of unaltered drug is available to the CNS.

Fluphenazine decanoate is efficacious and safe in the majority of patients and is injected intramuscularly every 2–3 weeks. In acute illness the drug is injected daily, initially in small doses. In the elderly initial injections of 0.1 ml (2.5 mg) are given because of the risk of Parkinsonism. Doses may be built up to 100–500 mg, but the general rule is as soon as possible to give the minimum dose as infrequently as possible. The average dose is 25 mg every 3 weeks.

When a patient is being given a long-acting preparation after a short-acting neuroleptic, it may be helpful to have a one week 'drug holiday' to reduce the chance of toxicity. There is a considerable variation in the response of patients to depot neuroleptics and the drug regimen must be individually tailored and periodically reviewed, partly because of the occurrence of side effects with time and partly because dosage reduction will be required when the patient improves.

Adverse effects of depot neuroleptics There is no evidence that toxic effects are more frequent with injection as compared to oral neuroleptics.

Extrapyramidal effects—akinesia, acute dystonic reactions, oculogyric crises, akathisia and tardive dyskinesia—are the most troublesome, and about 30% of patients experience them, depending upon the dosage regime employed. Anticholinergic drugs may be helpful and benzodiazepines can relieve akathisia, but levodopa is ineffective since these side effects result from blockade of dopaminergic receptors. Anti-Parkinsonian drugs may only be needed during the first few days following an injection when neuroleptic plasma levels are highest, and it may be possible to discontinue them during the remainder of the dosage interval. Parkinsonian symptoms remain a problem throughout treatment and do not decrease with the duration of therapy, so that patients must be frequently reviewed.

Other important adverse effects include: lens and corneal opacities; skin reactions (mild) and epilepsy (large doses of phenothiazines can induce fits even in normal subjects). The so-called 'malignant syndrome' consists of hypertonia, dyskinesias, pallor, hyperthermia and pulmonary congestion.

Drug interactions occur with other centrally acting depressant drugs, e.g. alcohol, to cause increased sedation.

Choice of depot neuroleptic There is little evidence upon which choice may be made. A double-blind comparison of flupenthixol and fluphenazine showed that the former is more effective in schizophrenic patients with lowered mood or history of depression, whilst fluphenazine is more appropriate in elated or acutely disturbed patients.

Fluspirilene is probably less useful than the alternatives since weekly injections are nearly always required.

MOTOR DISORDERS AND THEIR TREATMENT

SPASTICITY

This is the increase in muscle tone which accompanies decrease in voluntary muscle power due to damage to the corticomotoneurone pathways in the brain or spinal cord. Drugs which have been used to reduce spasticity include diazepam, baclofen, dantrolene, thymoxamine, orciprenaline and phenothiazines.

Diazepam acts on spinal-cord neurones, by facilitating GABA effects. Although spasticity and flexor spasms may be diminished, sedating doses are needed to produce this.

Baclofen (Lioresal) also reduces spasticity and flexor spasms by stimulating presynaptic GABA receptors. In adequate doses (5–20 mg t.d.s.) less sedation is produced than equieffective doses of diazepam (15–50 mg daily) but there may also be vertigo, nausea and hypotension. Fits may occur with larger doses.

Dantrolene (Dantrium) acts directly on striated muscle and inhibits excitation–contraction coupling. Although it appears to be effective in reducing spasticity in the clinical situation, it is probably less useful than baclofen, in that muscle power is reduced as spasticity is relieved. The drug is initially given in small doses—25 mg daily—and then slowly increased to 50–100 mg 6 hourly. Toxic effects include drowsiness, vertigo, malaise, weakness and fatigue.

Other therapy has not yet been adequately assessed: thymoxamine, an α-adrenergic antagonist, inhibits spinal monosynaptic reflexes, possibly by blocking spinal noradrenaline receptors; orciprenaline diminishes tetanic fusion by increasing the rate of muscular relaxation; phenothiazines, particularly dimethothiazine, depress fusimotor activity, perhaps by inhibiting spinal noradrenergic bulbospinal pathways.

CHOREA

In Huntington's chorea there are changes in GABA metabolism in the basal ganglia, including a net decrease in the concentration of the transmitter. No drug is available which can increase GABA levels or actions in the brain. In both Huntington's and Sydenham's chorea there is an intact nigrostriatal dopaminergic system, and thus there is a relative imbalance characterised by excessive dopaminergic stimulation of a depleted cell population in the striatum (see Fig. 9.5). Although neuroleptics and tetrabenazine are equally effective, the neuroleptics are best avoided in these conditions as they can themselves induce permanent dyskinesias. *Tetrabenazine* is given in doses of 25 mg b.d. increasing to 50 mg t.d.s. or q.d.s. If this drug produces depression, then pimozide 2 mg daily or thiopropazate 5 mg t.d.s. may be substituted. Drowsiness may be countered by giving amphetamine without exacerbating the abnormal movements, although when given alone amphetamine, like anticholinergic agents, and levodopa, can provoke chorea in the predisposed.

DYSKINESIAS

Neuroleptic drugs can produce any type of dyskinesia which may occur spontaneously. These are:

drug-induced Parkinsonism;
acute dystonic reactions;
akathisia;
chronic tardive dyskinesias.

Drug-induced Parkinsonism is due to a reduction in dopamine effects in the striatum (see p. 256). Phenothiazines and butyrophenones vary in their propensity to produce Parkinsonism. Those with high anticholinergic activity are less likely to produce this reaction. Uncommonly metoclopramide and domperidone can produce Parkinsonism.

Acute dystonic reactions can be induced by a number of antipsychotic drugs. About 2–10% of patients treated with phenothiazines (especially of the piperazine type), butyrophenones and the thioxanthines develop dystonia. The antiemetic metoclopramide also causes dystonic reactions. The condition may be due to an increase in transmitter turnover. It usually occurs in younger patients, and rapidly develops, usually within 48 h of the start of treatment. There is abrupt onset of retrocollis, torticollis, facial grimacing, dysarthria, laboured breathing and involuntary movements. Accompanying these may be scoliolis, lordosis, opisthotonus and dystonic gait. The signs can be abolished by intravenous injection of 2 mg benztropine or 10 mg diazepam.

Akathisia is a state of motor restlessness and can be provoked by all the neuroleptic drugs and by levodopa. There may be inability to keep the limbs still or a compulsion to walk or run and an inability to remain seated. Akathisia may begin within days, weeks or months of starting treatment. The pharmacological basis of akathisia is unknown, but is presumably an extrapyramidal disturbance as it may occur with idiopathic Parkinsonism. When drugs have provoked akathisia, it may resolve before or after cessation of drug therapy. Anticholinergic drugs such as benztropine may help.

Chronic tardive dyskinesias consist of oro-facial chewing and sucking movements, often accompanied by distal limb chorea and dystonia of the trunk. About 15% of patients treated with neuroleptics for over 2 years develop this complication. If treatment is continued, the syndrome persists, but stopping the neuroleptics results in slow improvement in only 40% of patients and sometimes dyskinesia worsens. Tardive dyskinesia is thought to result from the development of 'denervation hypersensitivity' in the dopaminergic post-synaptic receptors of the nigrostriatal pathway following chronic receptor blockade by neuroleptics. It is therefore due to a relative preponderance of dopaminergic effects, so explaining its exacerbation by drug discontinuation which removes the receptor blockade and allows more dopamine to stimulate the sensitised receptor. Administration of haloperidol, pimozide or thiopropazate (all dopamine antagonists) initially improves tardive dyskinesia, but the use of these drugs may produce an escalating dosage situation where more and more drug is required to suppress the dyskinesia. Anticholinergic drugs worsen and may precipitate tardive dyskinesia in patients on chronic neuroleptic treatment (cf. Parkinson's) and enhancement of cholinergic effects with physostigmine or deanol (2-dimethylaminoethanol), a putative acetylcholine precursor, is beneficial. Neither tetrabenazine nor reserpine causes tardive dyskinesias (presumably because they do not prevent dopamine receptor stimulation) and tetrabenazine is sometimes effective in this complication. A recent experimental approach which has achieved limited success is the oral administration of choline, which probably increases brain acetylcholine levels, thereby redressing the dopaminergic preponderance in the brain.

PARKINSONISM AND ANTIPARKINSONIAN DRUGS

The principal features of Parkinsonism are tremor, rigidity and akinesia. The major types are idiopathic Parkinson's disease, toxic (phenothiazines, butyrophenones, manganese and carbon monoxide poisoning) and post-encephalitic.

The Parkinsonian syndrome arises because of an abnormality in the nigrostriatal projection and its connections. The nigrostriatal projection consists of very fine nerve fibres travelling from the zona compacta of the substantia nigra to the corpus striatum. This pathway is dopaminergic and inhibitory (see Fig. 9.5). Parkinsonism arises because of deficient transmission at D_2 receptors. Other fibres terminating in the corpus striatum include excitatory cholinergic nerves.

The apparently antagonistic effect of dopamine and acetylcholine within the striatum have suggested that Parkinsonism may result from an imbalance between these two systems of neurotransmitters (see Fig. 9.6). Thus improvement of symptoms might occur if effects of these transmitters could be modified. Damage to the dopaminergic fibres facilitates oscillatory bursts of activity in the thalamus which in turn excites cells in the motor cortex. Thus

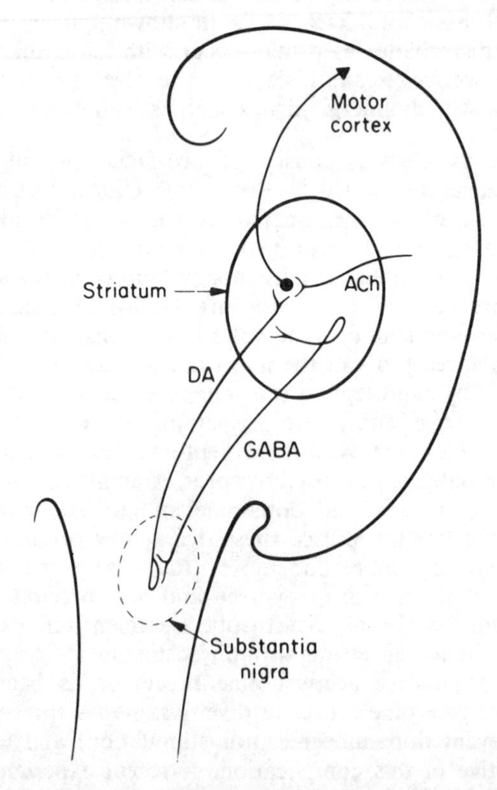

Fig. 9.5 Representation of relationships between cholinergic (ACh), dopaminergic (DA) and GABA-producing neurones in the basal ganglia.

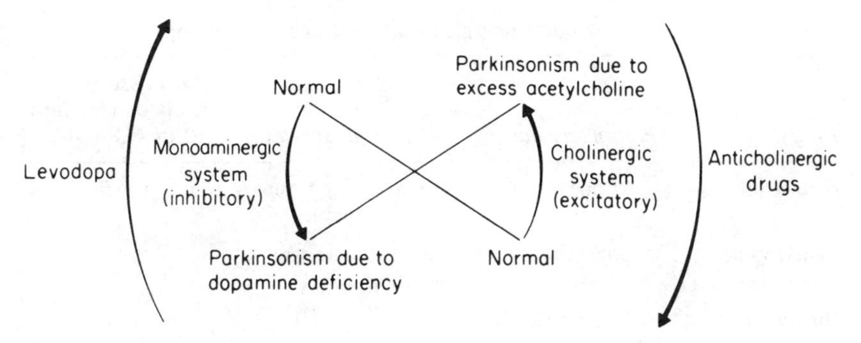

Fig. 9.6 Antagonistic actions of the monoaminergic and cholinergic systems in the production of Parkinsonian symptoms.

loss of inhibitory dopaminergic fibres (or alternatively increased activity in cholinergic excitatory fibres) can lead to tremor. An excessive output of nerve impulses from the corpus striatum will increase the drive to gamma-fusimotor neurones and may explain Parkinsonian regidity.

The treatment of the syndrome should ideally start with removal of the cause, but in most patients with chronic progressive Parkinsonism, the cause cannot be found. Exposure to toxic agents has been considered. One possibility is 1-methyl-4-phenyl-1,2,5,6-tetrahydropyridine (MPTP) which might gain access to the brain following accidental exposure. Drugs producing Parkinsonism, such as neuroleptics, methyldopa, metoclopramide, procaine, reserpine and tetrabenazine may be withdrawn, and this usually leads to cessation of the disability. Symptomatic control by drug therapy is usually required.

Drug treatment in general decreases the excessive striatal activity either by decreasing cholinergic excitatory activity or by increasing dopaminergic inhibitory activity.

A. Anticholinergic Drugs

Cholinergic activity in the striatum can be blocked by atropine. Synthetic anticholinergic drugs have a similar action and those used for Parkinsonism are said to produce more powerful central effects with less peripheral atropine-like effects. In addition these drugs may block dopamine uptake into the corpus striatum.

Anticholinergic drugs reduce rigidity but generally do not improve tremor or akinesia. Table 9.9 lists some of the drugs of this type in common use. They are usually given in divided doses, which are increased every 2–5 days until optimum benefit is achieved or until toxic effects occur. Peripheral toxicity includes dry mouth, blurred vision, possible precipitation of glaucoma, urinary retention and constipation. Central effects such as confusion and excitement occur most commonly in the elderly. These are contraindicated in some forms of glaucoma and in the presence of obstructive prostatic hypertrophy.

Table 9.9 Anticholinergic drugs used in Parkinsonism

Drug	*Proprietary name*	*Special features*	*Daily dose (mg)* (usually divided into 3 or 4 doses)
Benzhexol	Artane	Long acting preparation available	1–15
Benztropine	Cogentin	Single daily dose; sedating	0.5–6
Biperiden	Akineton		2–12
Orphenadrine	Disipal	Antihistamine; some central stimulation	150–400
Procyclidine	Kemadrin		7.5–60

B. Drugs affecting the dopaminergic system

Dopaminergic activity can be enhanced by:

1. administration of levodopa alone;
2. administration of levodopa with peripheral decarboxylase inhibition;
3. release of endogenous dopamine;
4. stimulation of the dopamine receptor;
5. inhibition of monoamine oxidase type B.

1. Levodopa

The nigro-striatal deficiency of dopamine cannot be corrected by giving dopamine itself, because this does not penetrate the blood–brain barrier. Levodopa can enter the brain and then undergo decarboxylation to form dopamine.

Pharmacokinetics Levodopa is absorbed from the proximal small intestine and is subject to breakdown both by decarboxylases in the intestinal wall and by the gut flora. Oral absorption is therefore somewhat variable. Malabsorption of levodopa occurs in some Parkinsonian patients due to delayed gastric emptying which allows increased gastric destruction and can lead to therapeutic failure. Absorption is improved by antacids, metoclopramide or co-administration of decarboxylase inhibitors. The plasma $t_{1/2}$ following intravenous infusion is short (30–60 min) and is only moderately prolonged (by about 30%) by decarboxylase blockade. Following oral administration of 15 mg/kg of levodopa, peak levels of about 2 μg/ml are reached at 1 h. Therapeutic levels are thought to lie in the range 0.5–1 μg/ml. There is, however, a poor correlation between plasma levels at any moment and improvement in disability. Nevertheless dyskinetic reactions to the drug correspond to high levodopa blood levels.

Overall 75–80% of patients obtain some benefit from levodopa and in 20% the response is dramatic, although maximum benefit may not be obtained for up to two years. The reasons for failure to respond are obscure; in some cases unacceptable toxic effects of the drug are responsible.

Clinical use The initial daily dose is 500 mg, increasing by 250 mg every second or third day until toxic effects appear. This dose is maintained until tolerance develops (usually about one week) and then increments are resumed. The average maximum dose is 2–3 g/day but some patients require (and can tolerate) 8 g/day. The drug is given in three or more divided doses. Maximum improvement may take 6 months to be attained.

Adverse effects These include:

nausea and vomiting;
postural hypotension;
involuntary movements (dystonic reactions);
psychological disturbances.

In addition there may occur

cardiac arrhythmias;
sweating;
darkening of urine;
vaginal discharge.

Metabolic changes produced by levodopa include stimulation of growth-hormone release, suppression of prolactin release, increased blood cholesterol and diminished glucose tolerance.

Nausea may be helped by metoclopramide, by giving levodopa with meals and by administration of smaller doses more frequently than 6 hourly.

Postural hypotension does not usually persist after the first few weeks, but excessive hypotension may result if antihypertensive treatment is given concurrently. For such hypotensive reactions elastic stockings may be helpful. Cerebral and myocardial infarction occurring during treatment has been attributed to this fall in blood pressure.

The involuntary movements include:
akathisia (abnormal restlessness and inability to keep still); chorea
jerking of the limbs (myoclonus)
facial grimacing and chewing movements
spasmodic torticollis and dystonic spasms

Involuntary movements may become worse as treatment is continued and may necessitate a reduction in dose. There is evidence to suggest that the dopamine receptors responsible for involuntary movements differ from those in the striatum which are implicated in Parkinson's disease. Some partially selective antagonists of these 'dyskinetic receptors' have been found but none are yet suitable for clinical use. Further research is in progress to produce such selective antagonists which would allow dopamine to be used in larger doses in suitable patients. In some patients useful antidepressant actions occur or there is an increase in libido.

Psychological disturbances which can be produced by levodopa are:

vivid and disturbing dreams;
agitation (may be improved with benzodiazepines);
paranoia;
elation;
confusion;
hallucinations;
depression (may be helped with tricyclic antidepressants);
dementia (uncertain if treatment plays causal role).

Drug interactions

Pyridoxine (which enhances peripheral dopa decarboxylase activity, so reducing circulating levodopa levels) interferes with the action of levodopa.

Phenothiazines and butyrophenones (dopamine antagonists)

Monoamine oxidase inhibitors—given concurrently may produce a hypertensive reaction. (The hypotensive actions of other drugs are potentiated by levodopa.)

Contraindications to levodopa include cardiac arrhythmias, recent myocardial infarction, hypomania and schizophrenia.

In patients who cannot tolerate long-term therapy, the overall mortality ratio is about 2.4 : 1, whilst in patients who can remain on long-term therapy, life expectation is normal. Treatment failures in the first 3 months are due to toxic confusional states, nausea, response failure and choreiform movements. Despite this effect on life expectancy, levodopa has not fulfilled initial hopes that the natural progression of Parkinson's disease could be prevented and in

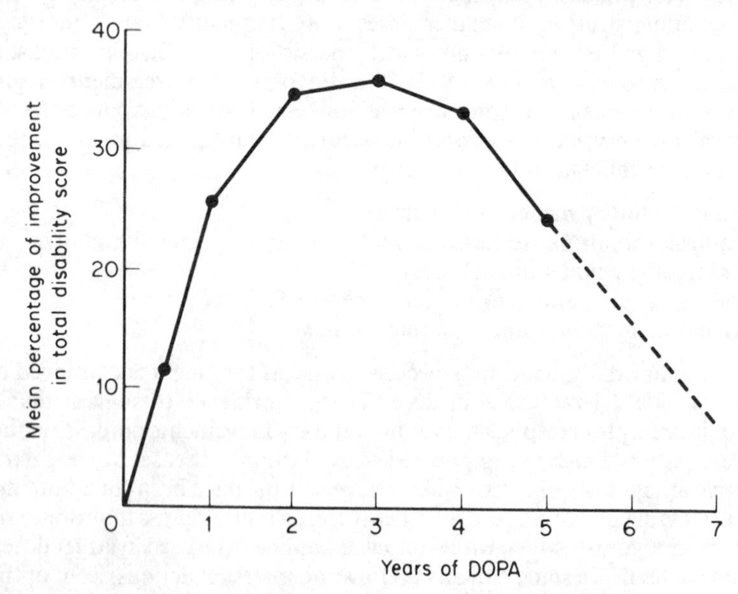

Fig. 9.7 Average outcome of chronic levodopa therapy (From C. D. Marsden and J. D. Parkes, *Lancet*, 1, 345 (1977).)

the long term many patients on chronic levodopa therapy lose the initial benefits of the drug (Fig. 9.7). In general, at 5 years about one-third of patients have lost all of the initial benefit, one-third have a reduced response and the remaining third are maintained at an improved functional level. In the deteriorated third, either the disabilities of the Parkinson's disease reassert themselves or increasingly severe fluctuations in clinical response occur ('on–off' phenomena). In the latter the beneficial effects of each dose last for increasingly short periods and disability due to Parkinson's disease (the 'off' period) reappears. This episodic Parkinsonism is often modified so that one feature, e.g. akinesia, predominates. The patient eventually suffers violent swings from good to bad control and requires levodopa more and more frequently to maintain mobility. This end-of-dose deterioration occurs in some form in up to 40% of patients on levodopa for 5 years, and several theories have been proposed to explain the phenomenon:

(a) Competition between levodopa and amino acids in protein foodstuffs may explain the alleged precipitation of an attack by a meal, thus a low protein diet has been suggested.
(b) Minor dopamine metabolites may compete for dopaminergic receptors.
(c) 'Off' periods coincide with low plasma levodopa levels although the use of sustained-release preparations of levodopa has proved disappointing. Continuous infusion of levodopa reduces on–off swings, whereas meals lower peak plasma levodopa concentrations. Feeding high protein meals or phenylalanine, leucine and isoleucine reduces the beneficial effects of levodopa infusions without altering plasma levels.
(d) Changes in dopaminergic receptor sensitivity or dopamine synthesis may occur as manifestations of progressive damage to the basal ganglia.

Other late complications are dementia, psychotic episodes, nightmares, depression, and painful cramps of the hands and feet.

2. Levodopa with peripheral decarboxylase inhibitors

Peripheral decarboxylase inhibitors reduce the extracerebral conversion of levodopa into dopamine. The combination of decarboxylase inhibitors with levodopa has several advantages:

(a) 4–5 fold reduction in levodopa dosage;
(b) clinical benefit appears early (in 1–2 weeks);
(c) incidence of vomiting is reduced from 80% to 15%;
(d) incidence of cardiac arrhythmias is reduced or prevented;
(e) pyridoxine intake does not affect treatment.

The neurological and psychiatric adverse effects are not made less frequent by this combined therapy and the 'on-off' phenomenon may begin earlier in the treatment.

The available inhibitors of L-aromatic acid decarboxylase are:

1. methyldopa hydrazine (Carbidopa);
2. N-DL-seryl-N (2,3,4,-trihydroxybenzyl)-hydrazine (Benserazide).

Without these inhibitors, 95% of levodopa is metabolised outside the brain.

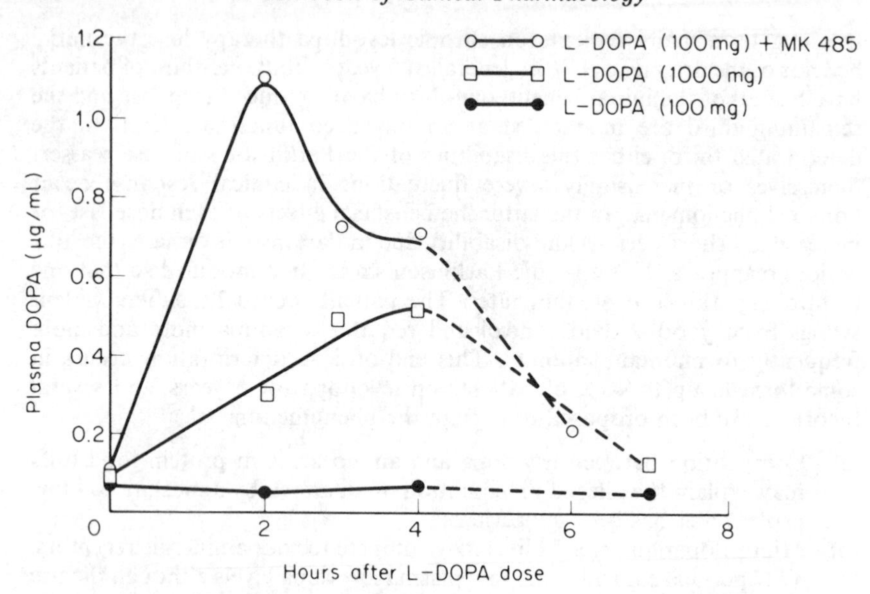

Fig. 9.8 Increased plasma DOPA concentrations following combination with a peripheral dopa decarboxylase inhibitor in one patient (From D. L. Dunner *et al.*, *Clin. Pharm. Ther.*, **12**, 213 (1971).)

In their presence, levodopa levels rise (see Fig. 9.8) and the excretion of dopamine and its metabolites falls. The two inhibitors have similar properties, are equally effective in reducing the incidence of vomiting and allow the same reduction in levodopa dosage.

Administration Levodopa (250 mg) with Carbidopa (25 mg) tablets (Sinemet 275) are given in divided doses, starting at ½–1 tablet and increasing to 8 tablets daily. Levodopa (100 mg) with Benserazide (25 mg) (Madopar 125) is also given in divided doses, up to 8 capsules daily. For greater convenience in adjustment of dose other sizes of tablets are available: Sinemet-110 (carbidopa 10 mg plus levodopa 100 mg); Madopar 62.5 (benserazide 12.5 mg plus levodopa 50 mg); Madopar 250 (benserazide 50 mg plus levodopa 200 mg).

3. Release of endogenous dopamine

This is increased by amphetamine and by amantadine.

Amantadine (Symmetrel) has similar actions to levodopa in Parkinsonism in that it reduces tremor, rigidity and akinesia, but the magnitude of the benefit is usually less and only 60 % of patients obtain some benefit. The effect appears rapidly, but the optimal results (which may appear after several days) may not last beyond two months in 30–40 % of patients.

The $t_{1/2}$ varies from 10 to 30 h and so steady-state levels are reached after 4–7 days treatment. The improvement in extrapyramidal signs is related to amantadine plasma levels more closely than is the case for levodopa.

Presumably failure of response to amantadine results from abnormalities of the basal ganglia. Serious toxicity is not common but the following may occur: nightmares, insomnia, dizziness, hallucinations, convulsions, peripheral oedema, livido reticularis (possibly a physiological response of the skin to depleted catecholamine stores in peripheral nerves).

Amantadine is given as a 100 mg capsule daily for one week and then 200 mg thereafter. Its use is largely confined to those patients in whom levodopa is contraindicated and in early Parkinsonism before levodopa is used.

4. Stimulation of dopamine receptors

This can be achieved by agonists other than dopamine; it is an action of:

piribedil;
apomorphine and norpropylapomorphine;
bromocriptine;
lergotrile.

Because of their dopamine-like effects, these drugs not only benefit Parkinson's disease but can also produce nausea, neurological and psychiatric complications, stimulation of growth-hormone release and inhibition of prolactin release. Piribedil and apomorphine have unacceptable toxic effects in man. Bromocriptine (see p. 610) shows great individual variation in its effects. It is usually as effective as levodopa and has similar toxic effects. In a minority it is helpful in reducing on-off swings. This may be related to its longer half life (6–8 h). Bromocriptine improves rigidity, tremor and akinesia, but lergotrile may have a preferential action on tremor.

5. Inhibition of monoamine oxidase type B

Two forms of monoamine oxidase are known: type A has 5-hydroxytryptamine and tyramine as substrates, whilst type B is active against benzylamine and tyramine. Whereas drugs such as pargyline inhibit mainly type A, the B enzyme is inhibited by phenylisopropylmethylpropionylamine (Selegiline). Enzyme A appears to destroy neurotransmitters such as adrenaline, noradrenaline and 5-hydroxytryptamine, but the physiological function of the B form is not understood. Both types of enzyme can destroy dopamine. Thus inhibition of the B enzyme could raise brain dopamine levels without affecting other major transmitter amines. This has been utilised in the treatment of Parkinsonism. Selegiline (Eldepryl) is used with levodopa and a decarboxylase inhibitor. As it selectively inhibits MAO-B, it does not produce a hypertensive reaction with cheese or other sources of amines. Given in doses of 5–10 mg daily with levodopa it may improve patients who are suffering dyskinesias or on-off phenomena. Selegiline is metabolised first to an active metabolite (which inhibits MAO-B) and then to amphetamine and methamphetamine. Toxicity includes involuntary movements, agitation, confusion and insomnia.

The use of drugs in Parkinsonism

Over two thirds of patients with Parkinson's disease improve with levodopa, the reduction in disability being 40–50%. By comparison, amantadine is one sixth and anticholinergics one third as effective (measured as average reduction in disability). However these two agents may be used in the early stages of the disease. In particular anticholinergics may alleviate troublesome muscle pain which is experienced by many patients (especially at night) before frank rigidity develops.

The majority of patients with Parkinson's disease are best treated with levodopa combined with a decarboxylase inhibitor. If low doses of levodopa are sufficient to control the syndrome, there is no advantage in adding the decarboxylase inhibitor. Despite theoretical disadvantages persistent nausea can be treated with 10 mg metoclopramide 8 hourly. Swings in response may be reduced by adding a longer-acting drug such as bromocriptine or norpropylapomorphine.

Unacceptable and uncontrollable toxic effects from levodopa are an indication for a trial of anticholinergic drugs. Also, mildly affected patients may do well on the anticholinergic drugs or amantadine. There is no objective evidence that the combinations of anticholinergics with levodopa or with amantadine are advantageous.

Levodopa treatment may fail because of:

1. non-compliance;
2. unacceptable toxicity;
3. failure of absorption;
4. severe, advanced Parkinson's disease, particularly due to underlying neurological conditions such as cerebral atherosclerosis and progressive supranuclear palsy.
5. incorrect diagnosis and patient has striatonigral degeneration, olivoportocerebellar atrophy, Shy–Drager syndrome or progressive subranuclear palsy.
6. pyridoxine (possibly in a tonic or 'health' preparation).
7. a neuroleptic or metoclopramide is being taken.

Parkinsonism due to neuroleptics cannot be treated with levodopa, as this antagonises all main actions of the neuroleptic and can aggravate the psychotic state for which the drug is being used. Anticholinergic drugs are usually used, but there is no objective evidence that they are effective.

EPILEPSY AND ANTI-EPILEPTIC DRUGS

The term 'epilepsy' covers a range of paroxysmal disorders of brain function which may be caused by many neurological and metabolic conditions. Precise diagnosis of the clinical type of epilepsy is important from several points of view, in particular as an indication of the type of drug treatment likely to be helpful. Table 9.10 illustrates some of these.

Despite the remarkable efficacy of the anticonvulsant drugs their mode of action is not understood. These agents are not all sedative, but selectively block repetitive discharges at concentrations below those which block normal impulse conduction. Some of the anticonvulsants act on the GABA receptor complex. GABA acts as the inhibitory transmitter by opening the chloride channel. The benzodiazepines increase the effectiveness of GABA thus enhancing neuronal inhibition. The barbiturates and phenytoin act by

Table 9.10 Drug treatment of various forms of epilepsy

Type of epilepsy	*Drugs most likely to be successful*
Petit mal absences with a 3 Hz spike and wave pattern in the EEG	Ethosuximide, Trimethadione, Clonazepam, Valproate
Hypsarrhythmia with salaam attacks—a form of myoclonic epilepsy in early childhood with generally poor prognosis	Nitrazepam, Corticotrophin
Myoclonic and akinetic attacks with a 2 Hz spike and wave pattern on the EEG	Nitrazepam, Clonazepam, Valproate
Grand mal	Phenytoin, Phenobarbitone, Primidone, Valproate, Carbamazepine
Partial seizures (focal fits) including psychomotor and psychosensory epilepsy	Phenytoin, Phenobarbitone, Primidone, Valproate, Carbamazepine

N.B. Treatment is begun using one drug, and if tolerated, this is increased in dosage to its maximum efficacy (guided by blood levels) before adding or substituting another drug.

blocking the picrotoxin receptor. This latter receptor reduces the action of GABA.

Phenytoin appears to prevent the propagation of epileptic discharges rather than suppressing the excitability of the primary focus, whereas phenobarbitone decreases general neuronal excitability. This may explain why phenytoin is effective in controlling grand mal but is less so in preventing minor seizures originating from a focal discharge.

There is good evidence that the seizure threshold is altered by the levels of cerebral monoamines, especially 5-hydroxytryptamine (5-HT), noradrenaline and dopamine. Elevation of 5-HT levels by several anticonvulsants, including valproate and clonazepam, has been demonstrated. Increasing cerebral 5-HT concentrations experimentally by administering the 5-HT precursor, 5-hydroxytryptophan, potentiates the action of anticonvulsants: this observation cannot yet be exploited clinically.

Although many effects on the function of central transmitters have been observed with anticonvulsants, the most convincing evidence that such mechanisms are of direct relevance to anticonvulsant activity is that benzodiazepines appear to potentiate the central actions of the inhibitory transmitter GABA. Sodium valproate inhibits enzymes catabolising the inhibitory transmitter GABA and prevents its uptake by nerves, thus elevating brain GABA levels in animals. Conversely, substances decreasing GABA levels (such as isoniazid) are epileptogenic. At dose levels likely to be achieved in clinical practice, however, this mechanism would not appear to be important.

These observations, although they hint at some underlying common pathway involving derangement of transmitter function, cannot yet be incorporated into a unifying theory of action of anti-epileptic action.

General principles of treatment of epilepsy with drugs

Before any treatment is prescribed, the answers should be known to the following questions:

1. Are the fits truly epileptic and not due to some other disorder (e.g. syncope, cardiac arrhythmia)?
2. Is the epilepsy caused by a condition which requires treatment in its own right?
3. Are there remediable or reversible factors which aggravate the epilepsy or precipitate individual attacks?
4. Is there a significant risk of fits if the patient is left untreated?

The ideal anticonvulsant is that which will completely suppress all clinical and electroencephalographic evidence of the patient's epilepsy while producing no immediate or delayed side effects.

In the UK at least 24 anticonvulsant preparations are available (some are duplicates and others contain more than one drug). The ideal drug does not exist and the choice of a drug must depend on the balance between efficacy and toxicity.

Control should initially be attempted using a *single drug*, which should be chosen from knowledge of the type of epilepsy. The dose is increased until either the seizures cease or the blood drug concentration is in the toxic range and/or signs of toxicity appear. It should be stressed that some patients have epilepsy which is controlled at drug blood levels below the usual therapeutic range and others do not manifest toxicity above the therapeutic range. Thus estimation of drug plasma concentration is to be regarded as a guide but not an absolute arbiter. The availability of plasma level monitoring of anti-epileptic drugs has allowed the more efficient use of individual drugs. In a recent study of phenytoin monotherapy for grand mal and focal epilepsy only 10% of new patients required the addition of a second drug although it was estimated that 54% might have done so if levels had not been measured. Similar results have been obtained with carbamazepine. Seizure control is better correlated with the attainment of an optimal plasma level for one drug rather than with the number of drugs consumed, and many patients would probably be better off being treated with one drug rather than with the more usual polypharmacy. If a drug proves to be ineffective it should not be suddenly withdrawn since this may provoke status epilepticus. Another drug should be introduced in increasing dosage whilst the first is gradually withdrawn.

Few studies have investigated the advantages of combined drug therapy although this is sometimes necessary. In most, but not all, cases the effects are additive. Combinations of three or more drugs probably do more harm than good by increasing the chances of adverse drug reaction without improving seizure control. It has been suggested, largely on the basis of anecdote, that ethosuximide and troxidone can precipitate major seizures when given to patients with petit mal. This has induced some physicians to use these drugs with prophylactic phenytoin or phenobarbitone. The efficacy of this procedure has never been proven and we believe that drug administration of any type should be kept to the minimum; we would not therefore advocate this practice.

INDIVIDUAL ANTIEPILEPTIC DRUGS

Ethosuximide (Zarontin)

This is one of a group of succinimide drugs and is presently the treatment of choice for petit mal absences. It is more effective and less toxic than the oxazolidines such as trimethadione.

Pharmacokinetics It is well absorbed following oral administration. Plasma $t_{1/2}$ is 70 h in adults but only 30 h in children. Thus ethosuximide need be given only once daily and steady-state values are attained within 7 days.

Blood-level estimations are not usually required, but effective concentrations lie in the range 40–120 μg/ml. The average dose which will attain this is 20 mg/kg/day. In practice 500 mg is given as the initial dose and this is increased by 250 mg every week until the attacks are prevented. Extensive hepatic metabolism produces two major metabolites which are inactive. No significant plasma–protein binding occurs and the CSF drug concentration is similar to that in plasma.

Clinical use Ethosuximide is continued into adolescence and then gradually withdrawn over several months. If a drug for grand mal is being given concurrently, this is continued for a further 3 years. The daily dose usually lies between 0.5 and 2 g.

Adverse effects Apart from dizziness, nausea and epigastric discomfort, side effects are rare and there are few doubts about its safety. Ethosuximide and trimethadione have been suspected of making grand mal worse, but this has not been confirmed in a controlled trial. However, grand mal and petit mal may coexist in the same child, and a drug such as phenytoin may be added to the ethosuximide treatment.

Trimethadione or Troxidone (Tridione) was an alternative drug for the treatment of petit mal and is only rarely used only for patients who cannot tolerate ethosuximide. The dose is 0.6–1.2 g/day.

The main metabolite is dimethadione which is also pharmacologically active. The demethylation reaction (trimethadione to dimethadione) is fast, and at peak levels the plasma ratio of dimethadione/trimethadione is about 20. The plasma $t_{1/2}$ of active substances is 16 h and pharmacological activity rests largely with dimethadione. Above levels of 700 μg/ml (expressed as dimethadione) toxic effects are frequent. Even with chronic administration of submaximal doses, sedation and blurring of vision in bright light (hemeralopia) are frequent. Other toxic effects are:

scotomata (indication for stopping the drug);
rashes—acneiform and morbilliform;
blood dyscrasias, neutropenia (common), agranulocytosis (rare);
pancytopenia (rarest);
nephrotic syndrome;
hepatitis.

Phenytoin; DPH; Diphenylhydantoin (Epanutin)

This is one of the drugs of choice in the treatment of grand mal and partial (focal) seizures, including psychomotor attacks.

Pharmacokinetics Intestinal absorption is variable and a single case of isolated phenytoin malabsorption has been described. There is wide variation in the handling of phenytoin, and in a group of patients taking the same dose there is a 50-fold variation in steady-state plasma levels (see Fig. 1.26). The following factors contribute to the variation of plasma levels:

(a) Age: phenytoin clearance increases with age and this is correlated with the lower protein binding and plasma albumin levels found in the elderly. Young children may metabolise the drug faster than adults, possibly because they have less steroidal hormones to compete for metabolism.
(b) Body weight: reflects the volume of distribution (0.6 l/kg).
(c) Sex: makes a small contribution, steady-state levels being lower in females.

Although these each play a part in the inter-individual variation, their contribution is small. Of greater importance is phenytoin metabolism which is under polygenic control and varies widely between patients.

Phenytoin is extensively metabolised by the liver, mainly to 5-parahydroxyphenyl-5-phenylhydantoin and less than 5% is excreted unchanged. The enzyme responsible for elimination becomes saturated at concentrations within the therapeutic range and phenytoin exhibits dose-dependent kinetics which, because of the low therapeutic index of phenytoin makes clinical use of the drug difficult. Because the metabolic handling of the drug reaches a maximum rate, increasing the dose beyond this limit results in a steep increase in plasma concentration (see Fig. 9.9). The clinical implications of such behaviour are:

(a) Dosage increments should be 50 mg or less once the plasma level is within the therapeutic range.
(b) Fluctuations above and below the therapeutic range occur relatively easily due to changes in the amount of drug absorbed or by forgetting to take a tablet. This behaviour also magnifies bioavailability differences and clinical intoxication has resulted from alteration of the excipient in phenytoin capsules from calcium sulphate to lactose (see Fig. 2.6).
(c) Drug interactions are common since administration of a second drug such as sulthiame which inhibits phenytoin metabolism, or carbamazepine which enhances it, result in clinically important interactions.

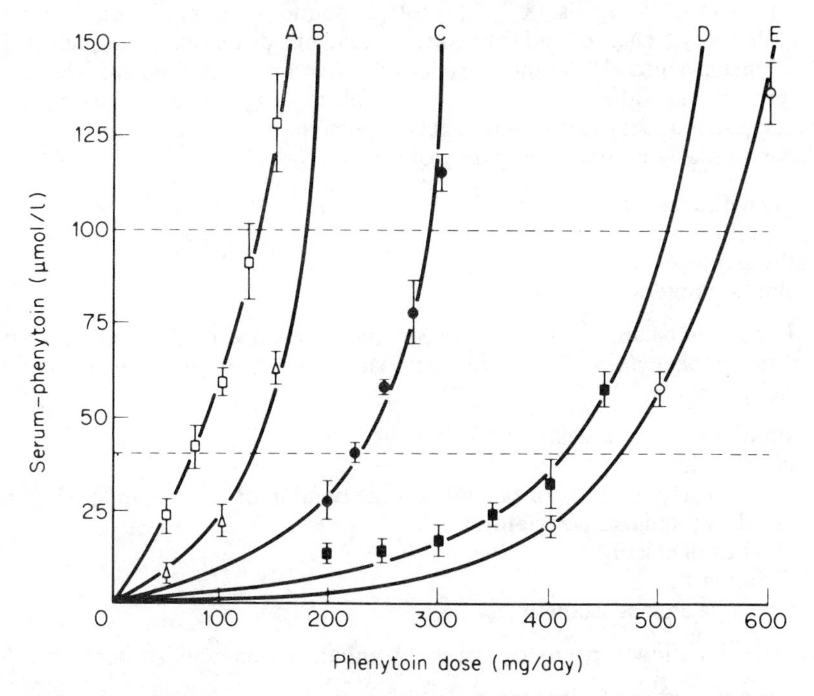

Fig. 9.9 Relationship between daily dose of phenytoin and resulting steady-state serum level in five patients on several different doses of drug. The curves were fitted by computer assuming Michaelis–Menten kinetics (From A. Richens and A. Dunlop, *Lancet*, **2**, 247 (1975).)

(d) Changes in enzyme activity, as might occur in infections, might produce a critical change in enzyme activity.

The saturation kinetics of phenytoin make it invalid to calculate a $t_{1/2}$, since the rate of elimination depends upon the plasma level and enzyme saturation (Fig. 1.17). After a single dose of phenytoin the $t_{1/2}$ is around 10–17 h, but in patients on continuous phenytoin therapy the $t_{1/2}$ of an isotopically labelled tracer dose of phenytoin may be as long as 140 h. Practically, this means that the time to reach a plateau plasma concentration is longer than is predicted from the $t_{1/2}$ of a single dose of the drug. Hence a loading dose of 800–1000 mg can safely be given. Furthermore, the usual dosage suggested of, say, 100 mg 8 hourly is unnecessary and its replacement by 300 mg as a single daily dosage is of proven efficacy.

Absorption from the gut is slow (peak levels at 2 h) but is even slower and more erratic with a lower peak after intramuscular injection. Phenytoin is extremely insoluble and crystallises out in intramuscular injection sites. For the rapid attainment of therapeutic plasma levels intravenous injection is needed. Because of its poor solubility the parenteral preparation has a pH of 10 and precipitation of the free acid occurs if the injection is added to intravenous infusion fluids. The high pH is irritant to veins and tissues. Phenytoin should not be given at rates of greater than 50 mg/min because at higher rates of administration cardiovascular collapse, respiratory arrest and seizures may occur.

At therapeutic levels 90% is protein bound to albumin and to two α-globulins which also bind thyroxine. In uraemia, displacement of phenytoin from plasma protein binding results in lower drug requirements. Sodium valproate, like other fatty acids, can displace drugs from plasma–protein binding sites and it increases the effects of phenytoin by this mechanism. Other drugs similarly potentiating phenytoin include:

phenylbutazone;
salicylic acid;
diazoxide;
sulphonamides.

Other important interactions occur via alterations in the hepatic metabolism of phenytoin. Drugs which impair metabolism and can precipitate toxicity include:

sulthiame (after a delay of 10–20 days);
pheneturide;
isoniazid (about 10% of patients on the combination develop toxicity: all are slow isoniazid acetylators);
chloramphenicol;
dicoumarol;
benzodiazepines (sometimes).

Drugs which lower phenytoin levels by enhancing metabolism are:

benzodiazepines (sometimes);
ethanol;
carbamazepine.

Phenytoin elimination is impaired in liver disease. Chronic renal disease may result in unusually low levels—possibly because of hypoalbuminaemia, displacement of protein-bound phenytoin by accumulated endogenous metabolities or hydroxyphenylhydantoin or by changes in the drug-binding characteristics of plasma protein or by induction of phenytoin metabolism (see Fig. 5.7).

Clinical use For adults the usual dose is 300 mg/day given as a single dose. Blood levels (ideally) are then measured after 2 weeks. According to response and level, adjustments should be 50 mg at a time and no more frequently than every 4–6 weeks. Salivary phenytoin levels may become available soon for routine drug monitoring. With grand mal the majority of patients are best controlled with phenytoin alone. Multiple drug therapy is rarely required. Phenytoin illustrates very well the usefulness of drug blood levels, but it should be stressed that not all patients require a plasma phenytoin level within the therapeutic range of 10–20 μg/ml for optimum control of their seizures, some will require less. Therefore the correct dose of the drug is that which suppresses their fits, not necessarily one which produces the recommended blood level.

Adverse effects These may be classified as follows:

1. *Nervous system* (see Fig. 9.10): High levels produce a cerebellar syndrome (ataxia, nystagmus, intention tremor, dysarthria), involuntary movements and sedation. Seizures may paradoxically increase with phenytoin intoxication. High levels may also result in psychological disturbances.

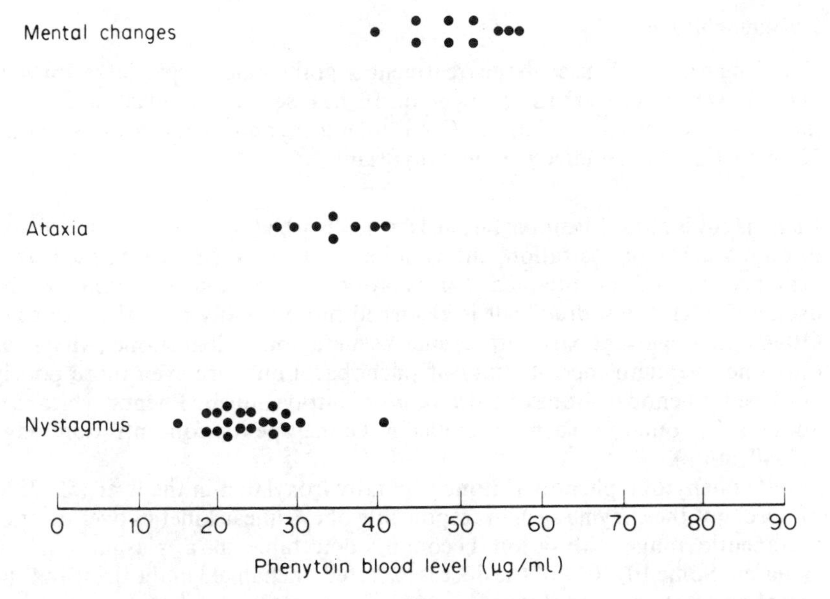

Fig. 9.10 The onset of nystagmus, ataxia and mental changes in relation to phenytoin blood levels (From H. Kutt *et al.*, *Arch. Neurol.*, **11**, 642 (1964). Copyright 1964. American Medical Association.)

2. *Allergic:* Rashes, hypersensitivity hepatitis, drug fever.
3. *Collagen changes:* Coarse facial features, gum hypertrophy.
4. *Haematological:* Megaloblastic anaemia which responds to folate; rarely aplastic anaemia; lymphadenopathy (which rarely progresses to lymphomatous change).
5. *Effects on fetus* (difficult to distinguish from effects of epilepsy): Increased perinatal mortality, possibly raised frequency of cleft palate, hare lip, microcephaly and congenital heart disease.
6. *Endocrine:* Inhibition of ADH release, aggravation of diabetes mellitus, acne has been traditionally thought to be aggravated by phenytoin but this has not been confirmed in a formal controlled investigation.

N.B. phenytoin displaces thyroxine and to a lesser extent triiodothyronine from thyroid hormone-binding globulin, so increasing peripheral clearance of thyroid hormone. This may interfere with interpretation of *in vitro* tests of thyroid function without producing clinical hypothyroidism.

Drug interactions:

(a) Other drugs affecting phenytoin metabolism (see above).
(b) Phenytoin induces liver enzymes and increases rate of metabolism of oral contraceptives, oral anticoagulants, dexamethasone, nortriptyline, pethidine.

Also active vitamin D is more rapidly destroyed resulting in a reduced effect and consequent anticonvulsant-induced osteomalacia (see p. 278).

Phenobarbitone

This drug was widely used in the treatment of grand mal and partial seizures. It may, however, exacerbate petit mal. It has several disadvantages over phenytoin, especially sedation, CNS tolerance and withdrawal seizures. Nevertheless it is an effective anticonvulsant.

Pharmacokinetics Phenobarbitone is well absorbed (80–90%) after oral and intramuscular administration, but by either route up to 6 h may elapse before peak plasma levels are attained. This is probably due to the insolubility of the drug although the sodium salt is absorbed more rapidly than the free acid. Other anticonvulsant barbiturates such as methylphenylbarbitone (which has only one twentieth the solubility of phenobarbitone) are even more poorly absorbed. Phenobarbitone can also be given intravenously. Phenobarbitone is about 50% bound to plasma proteins in the therapeutic concentration range (15–40 μg/ml).

Like phenytoin, phenobarbitone is parahydroxylated in the liver (55–75% of dose) but the enzyme system responsible obeys linear kinetics over most of therapeutic range, saturation becoming detectable at a plasma level of 70 μg/ml. Some 10–40% of the dose is excreted unchanged in the urine but the actual amount excreted depends upon urinary pH and volume.

Plasma $t_{1/2}$ is 100 h for adults and 40 h for children. The drug need therefore be given only once daily.

Clinical use The usual dose of phenobarbitone is 60–180 mg daily. Alterations are not normally made more frequently than every 3 weeks. Barbiturates should never be withdrawn suddenly, but the dose slowly reduced over the course of months. The relationship between plasma phenobarbitone levels and its effects on the nervous system are less well correlated than is the case with phenytoin. Tolerance may occur to the effects of phenobarbitone and one patient may be sedated by a level of 20 μg/ml whilst another functions normally at a chronically maintained level of 50 μg/ml. There is no clear toxic threshold for the drug and phenobarbitone estimations are clinically less helpful than those for phenytoin. The usually quoted therapeutic range of plasma phenobarbitone concentrations is 10–25 μg/ml but this is generally recognised to be only a guideline.

Adverse effects Phenobarbitone is frequently sedating in therapeutic doses. Increasing doses produce a cerebellar syndrome, the initial sign being nystagmus on lateral gaze. Children are often able to tolerate higher plasma levels than adults without any evident toxic effects. Other possible CNS effects include mental retardation, apathy, depression, hyperkinesia (especially in children) and severe convulsions on rapid drug withdrawal.

Other effects:

Allergy: rashes, anaphylaxis;
Haematological: folate deficiency, anaemia, aplastic anaemia (rare);
Congenital abnormalities.

Drug interactions Hepatic enzyme induction: the following are more rapidly metabolised:

oral anticoagulants	vitamin D (anticonvulsant osteomalacia)
dexamethasone	doxycycline
oral contraceptives	phenylbutazone
nortriptyline	digitoxin
diazepam	metyrapone
	DDT

Other drug interactions: impaired gastrointestinal absorption of griseofulvin and coumarins.

Phenobarbitone metabolism is inhibited by:

sulthiame	isoniazid
pheneturide	chloramphenicol

Primidone (Mysoline)

This is as effective as phenobarbitone in the treatment of grand mal and partial epilepsy (including psychomotor attacks) but is not now used as a first line drug because of sedation and ataxia.

Pharmacokinetics Primidone is metabolised to two main products—phenobarbitone and phenylethylmalonamide (PEMA). All three compounds are anticonvulsant. After a therapeutic dose of primidone, the plasma concentration of phenobarbitone is 2–6 times that of unchanged primidone.

The conversion of primidone into phenobarbitone probably obeys Michaelis–Menten kinetics and is therefore saturable whilst the kinetics of the conversion to PEMA are apparently first order. Thus the ratio of these three compounds varies with the dose of primidone. The $t_{1/2}$ of primidone is 3–12 h and of PEMA is 29–36 h, but the drug need only be given once daily because the main active metabolite (phenobarbitone) has $t_{1/2}$ of 100 h.

The presence of three active substances in the blood renders blood-level monitoring too complex for routine use.

Clinical use The initial dose is usually 125–250 mg given in the evening to avoid day-time sedation. This is increased until control is gained or adverse effects occur.

Adverse effects These are common, particularly at the start of treatment and since phenobarbitone levels in the plasma are not detected until at least 24 h the early CNS toxicity is probably due to primidone itself rather than its metabolites.

Nervous system:
- sedation
- cerebellar syndrome
- severe convulsions on rapid drug withdrawal
- intellectual deterioration
- hyperactivity in children.

Haematological changes: folic acid deficiency, aplastic anaemia (rare).

Drug interactions occur because of enzyme induction by primidone and by the inhibition of primidone and phenobarbitone metabolism by sulthiame, carbamazepine and isoniazid.

Carbamazepine (Tegretol)

This is structurally related to the tricyclic antidepressants although it has a similar spatial molecular configuration to phenytoin.

In addition to its effectiveness in grand mal and temporal lobe epilepsy, carbamazepine may also benefit trigeminal neuralgia. Petit mal is not helped. Carbamazepine is now one of the drugs of choice for tonic-clonic epilepsy.

Pharmacokinetics The drug is slowly but well absorbed following oral administration. The plasma levels fluctuate widely during absorption and a direct effect of the drug on gastric motility has been suggested. The plasma $t_{1/2}$ after a single dose is 25 to 60 h but on chronic dosing this falls to 10 h, possibly due to enzyme induction. This is shorter than the $t_{1/2}$s of phenytoin and phenobarbitone and thus carbamazepine should be taken 12 hourly in order to avoid large swings in blood levels. The approximate therapeutic range is 4–10 μg/ml plasma. There is no constant relationship between dose and blood levels. Interpretation of plasma levels is complicated by the formation of carbamazepine-10, 11-epoxide which has antiepileptic properties, but a shorter $t_{1/2}$ than carbamazepine (2 h). Marked interindividual variation exists in the ratio of carbamazepine to epoxide and probably it will be necessary to estimate the blood levels of both substances to control therapy adequately, although it is not established that the epoxide enters the brain in adequate concentration to exert a therapeutic effect.

At therapeutic concentrations carbamazepine is 75% bound to plasma protein and it is feasible to use salivary carbamazepine concentrations to monitor the unbound drug in the plasma as an alternative to blood analysis.

Clinical use 100–200 mg twice daily followed by a slow increase in dose until seizures are controlled. Often 1200 mg daily is required.

Adverse effects are common, but they are not usually severe. Sedation, ataxia and giddiness occur early and nystagmus, diplopia and slurred speech are found in 50% of patients with plasma levels over 8.5 μg/ml. Initial leucopenia is common but this is usually transient. Carbamazepine may cause hyponatraemia and water intoxication due to an antidiuretic action which has been capitalised upon for the treatment of diabetes insipidus. Water retention may adversely affect epilepsy and could explain some cases of therapeutic failure.

Carbamazepine is an effective enzyme inducer: phenytoin levels are reduced by concurrent carbamazepine treatment and the actions of warfarin and oral contraceptives are impaired.

Benzodiazepines (see p. 210)

The benezodiazepines, *diazepam*, *lorazepam* and *clonazepam* have anticonvulsant properties in addition to their anxiolytic and other actions. Unfortunately on prolonged usage tolerance to their antiepileptic properties tends to develop. Clonazepam (Rivotril) was introduced specifically as an anticonvulsant: its chief uses are as maintenance therapy and in status epilepticus in which diazepam or clonazepam given intravenously is the treatment of choice. Lorazepam has recently been introduced for status epilepticus. Clonazepam has a wide spectrum of activity, having a place in the management of the minor motor seizures of childhood, particularly petit mal and infantile spasms. It is also useful in psychomotor and myoclonic epilepsy but it is unlikely to replace phenytoin in the management of grand mal or focal motor seizures except in patients with resistant epilepsy. Despite this wide activity spectrum clonazepam is not effective in all cases of any one kind of disorder: selection of suitable patients may be made on the basis of the normalisation of the EEG in response to intravenous clonazepam. Sometimes seizure suppression by clonazepam declines with continuous treatment and this may be overcome in some patients by temporary discontinuation followed by reinstitution of treatment. Clonazepam may be given in conjunction with other drugs such as phenytoin.

Pharmacokinetics Clonazepam is well absorbed orally and the $t_{1/2}$ is about 30 h. Neither therapeutic nor adverse effects appear to be closely related to plasma levels, control of most types of epilepsy occurs within the range 30–60 ng/ml. Clonazepam is extensively metabolised to mainly 7-aminoclonazepam and 7-acetaminoclonazepam which then undergo hydroxylation and/or conjugation with sulphate and glucuronide. All these metabolites lack anticonvulsant activity.

Clinical uses Clonazepam is given in divided doses of 4–8 mg/day in adults. The intravenous dose is 0.5–2 mg.

Lorazepam (Ativan) is only used intravenously in status epilepticus in a dose of 4 mg. It may be slightly safer than either diazepam (Valium) or clonazepam since it possibly produces less hypotension or respiratory depression. Its place in therapy has however, to be established.

Nitrazepam (Mogadon) has a specialised use in the treatment of salaam attacks and other unusual forms of epilepsy in childhood.

Adverse effects are frequent and about 50 % of patients experience lethargy, somnolence and dizziness with clonazepam. This is minimised by starting with a low dose then gradually increasing it. In many cases sedation disappears on chronic treatment. More serious effects are muscular incoordination, ataxia, dysphoria, hypotonia and muscle relaxation, increased salivary secretion and hyperactivity with aggressive behaviour.

Sodium valproate (Epilim)

This is sodium dipropylacetate and is of great interest in that it is effective against several forms of epilepsy: grand mal, petit mal, psychomotor epilepsy (but not other forms of partial epilepsy), and myoclonic epilepsy.

Pharmacokinetics It is well absorbed when given orally (95–100 % bioavailability). Like fatty acids and phenytoin it is highly bound (approximately 90 %) to plasma protein, showing a two-fold inter-individual variation in the amount of free drug. Like phenytoin, there is a reduction in binding in uraemia and the unbound drug shows good correlation with serum creatinine and urea but, unlike phenytoin, not with plasma protein levels. The plasma $t_{1/2}$ is 7–10 h. Little progress has been made in identification of metabolites. Possibly the presence of active metabolites explains the relatively slow onset and long time course of action. Because of low lipophilicity the brain–plasma ratio is low (0.3) and a large dose (800–1400 mg/day) is necessary. There appears to be substantial interindividual variation in the handling of the drug and plasma level estimation may be helpful. A therapeutic range of 40–80 μg/ml has been suggested. Sodium valproate can be used on its own or in combination with other drugs.

Clinical use Dosage starts at 600 mg daily in divided (8 hourly) doses and is increased every 3 days by 200 mg/day, until control is achieved. This is generally in the range 1000–1600 mg/day but may be up to 2600 mg/day. The onset of effect is slow and may take several days. This could be due to the accumulation of an unidentified metabolite or to the elevation of a neurotransmitter in the brain. Other drugs may be used in conjunction with valproate which may reduce their clearance and elevate their plasma levels.

Adverse effects most commonly involve the alimentary system. Toxic effects include:

nausea, vomiting, diarrhoea, abdominal pain (may be reduced by enteric-coated tablets);
enhancement of sedatives (including alcohol);
temporary hair loss;
false positive ketone test in urine which may cause confusion in the management of diabetes has been reported;
teratogenic effects have been reported: therefore its use should where possible be avoided in pregnancy;
rarely hepatic necrosis has developed in children taking high doses;
acute pancreatitis is another rare complication.

Drug interactions

potentiation of MAOIs;
potentiation of phenytoin (protein binding displacement);
potentiation of phenobarbitone and primidone (probably inhibition of metabolism).

Enzyme induction is less likely with valproate because of its simple chemical structure.

Chlormethiazole (Heminevrin) (see also p. 209)

Chlormethiazole is a powerful anticonvulsant which can be given intravenously in the treatment of status epilepticus. When given orally it has a short half-life (1 h) and is therefore not convenient to use in the day-to-day treatment of epilepsy.

Sulthiame (Ospolot)

Sulthiame, a carbonic anhydrase inhibitor, does not have convincing anti-epileptic activity of its own. Its efficacy with phenytoin is probably due to the ability of sulthiame to inhibit phenytoin metabolism. Toxic effects include sedation and paraesthesiae.

Status epilepticus

Status epilepticus of the grand mal type is a medical emergency with a mortality of at least 20% and with neurological and psychiatric sequelae in many of the survivors. The management should:

1. *Terminate the fits as soon as possible.* The longer the fit continues the more difficult it is to stop. Intravenous benzodiazepines are the most effective treatment. Clonazepam is probably the best choice since it is more effective than diazepam in abolishing experimentally induced fits in animals and photo-induced seizures in man. This experimental evidence is supported by trials which show that clonazepam may work when diazepam has failed. 1–2 mg of clonazepam or 10 mg diazepam are given intravenously over 2 min. Apnoea is

uncommon after benzodiazepine administration unless the patient has previously been given a barbiturate or other respiratory depressant. The airway must be maintained and if necessary artificial respiration given. If fitting does not cease within 5 min a further dose should be given. A rapid fall in benzodiazepine levels occurs 30–60 min after intravenous administration. Thus repeated doses may be required. Clonazepam has a longer duration of action than diazepam, which is another advantage. If clonazepam fails chlormethiazole may be tried: a 0.8 % solution is infused at a rate of 500 mg in 6–8 h. Hypotension and respiratory depression are the main complications likely to occur with this drug. Single intravenous injections of chlormethiazole (1 mg), lorazepam (5 mg), phenytoin (400 mg at a rate of 50 mg/min), or an intramuscular injection of paraldehyde (10 ml as two separate 5 ml i.m. injections) are also effective.

If these drugs are not effective, short-acting barbiturates such as 150–750 mg thiopentone sodium intravenously may be necessary, but facilities for artificial ventilation should be available. Failure to control the fits may necessitate curarisation and ventilation. Further drug therapy is then controlled by EEG monitoring since it is thought that paralysis is not sufficient by itself to prevent cerebral damage.

2. *Determine the cause of the fits.* A common cause of status epilepticus is failure to take maintenance anticonvulsants. Blood levels of drugs should be measured in a sample taken before the start of emergency treatment.

3. *Recommence normal drug therapy as soon as possible.* If the patient is not already on anticonvulsants a loading dose of phenytoin (15 mg/kg) either via a nasogastric tube or by slow intravenous infusion with ECG monitoring at a rate not faster than 50 mg/min. Repeated drug levels are measured until the therapeutic range has been reached. High levels may themselves lower the convulsion threshold as a manifestation of toxicity.

A note on anticonvulsant osteomalacia

An important consequence of anticonvulsant therapy is induction of hepatic mixed-function oxidases (see p. 82). These enzymes increase catabolism of both dietary and endogenously produced vitamin D into biologically inactive substances. This reduces serum 25-hydroxycholecalciferol and decreases production of the active, 1, 25-dihydroxycholecalciferol which is synthesised by the kidneys. Sub-clinical or symptomatic rickets or osteomalacia then develop due to deficient active vitamin D. The increased demand for vitamin D is around 500–1500 units/day and the deficit is increased by the poor diet and lack of sunlight which is the lot of many institutionalised epileptics. The associated hypocalcaemia may increase the tendency to fits. At present, however, the place of prophylactic vitamin D with its attendant dangers is not established, but good dietary habits should be encouraged in epileptics.

DRUGS USED IN THE TREATMENT OF MIGRAINE

Although the cause of this common condition affecting about 5 % of the population is not understood, it is clear that disturbance of cerebral blood flow is involved. The early aura phase is associated with vasoconstriction which is mainly intracranial and presumably causes localised cerebral ischaemia and consequent dysfunction. This much is known from angiographic and isotopic blood-flow studies. Shortly after this phase the extracranial vessels dilate and pulsate, changes which are associated with local tenderness and the classical headache, which is characteristically unilateral, being in the territory of one or other carotid artery.

The initial stimulus to vasoconstriction is unknown. Noradrenaline has been suggested as a mediator of this effect but noradrenaline-secreting tumours (phaeochromocytoma) are not notably associated with migraine and depletion of noradrenaline stores with reserpine does not influence migraine. One hypothesis is that migraine patients inherit an inherently unstable cerebral vasculature prone to excessive contraction and dilatation when stimulated by factors which in normal subjects produce only minor effects. Thus ingestion of vasoactive amines in food by a migraine sufferer may bring about such inappropriate circulatory responses of the intra- and extracranial vessels. Serotonin (or 5-hydroxytryptamine, 5-HT) is a potent vasoconstrictor of the extracranial vessels in man and although migraine is not a feature of the carcinoid syndrome (where 5-HT levels may be very high) it has been postulated that serotonin released from platelets in migraine causes vasoconstriction. This summates with the effects of kinins and histamine (produced as a response to ischaemia) to increase the pain sensitivity of the affected arteries. Enhanced platelet aggregation has been demonstrated in migraine and this could enhance the effects of vasoconstriction in producing the aura. Absorption and metabolism of 5-HT by blood vessels reduces circulating 5-HT concentration and removes this counterbalance to circulating vasodilator substances such as kinins, prostaglandin E_1 and histamine. These then act upon the unstable vasculature to produce inappropriate vasodilatation and pain. The initial stimulus to platelet 5-HT release is unknown: fatty acids and immune complexes are current suggestions. Several other precipitating factors have been clinically recognised although in some cases, e.g. precipitation by chocolate, they are not easily demonstrated scientifically. They include:

- physical trauma, e.g. 'heading' a football;
- local pain from sinuses, cervical spondylosis, etc.;
- sleep (too much or too little);
- foods, e.g. those containing vasoactive amines such as tyramine in cheese, or phenylethylamine;
- allergy, e.g. to wheat, eggs, fish;
- stress or alternatively relaxation after stress;
- travel;
- hormonal changes, e.g. menstrual cycle;
- fasting and hypoglycaemia.

Some of the most effective prophylactic drugs against migraine inhibit 5-HT re-uptake by platelets, thus maintaining plasma 5-HT levels and so preventing loss of tone in the vessels. In addition they may have antihistamine and anti-5-HT activity which blocks the permeability-increasing actions of these transmitters.

These largely unproven hypotheses involving many postulated mediators have prompted the use of numerous drugs in this condition, many of them having powerful pharmacological effects. Clinical trials in migraine are bedevilled by the fact that migraine is paroxysmal and no stimulus exists which will reproducibly initiate an attack. Spontaneous migraine is notoriously subject to variations in frequency which might give an erroneous impression of efficacy. Similarly migraine symptoms are of variable severity even within the same patient. Therefore the benefits or otherwise of many of the treatments advocated depend upon rather dubious evidence. They may be divided as follows.

A. DRUGS USED IN TREATING THE ACUTE ATTACK

1. Analgesics Narcotic analgesics are never indicated for migraine since the need for repeated administration might encourage dependence and the gastrointestinal effects would be disadvantageous. Aspirin 900 mg or paracetamol 1 g are useful in treatment of the headache, and may be rational if prostaglandins are indeed involved in the mechanism of headache production. There is evidence these are effective in about three-quarters of patients. During a migraine attack gastric stasis occurs and this reduces drug absorption. It is therefore suggested that a soluble aspirin preparation be employed and this may be usefully coupled with metoclopramide which acts both as an anti-emetic (useful if nausea is a prominent symptom) and enhances gastric emptying (Fig. 9.11). It is combined with aspirin in Migravess (metoclopramide 5 mg + aspirin 325 mg) and paracetamol in Paramax (metoclopramide 5 mg + paracetamol 500 mg).

2. Anti-emetics have a useful role in their own right if gastrointestinal symptoms are troublesome. Although no controlled studies comparing their efficacy have been performed it is reasonable to avoid anti-emetics with sedative properties, e.g. antihistamines, phenothiazines, and on this account metoclopramide (p. 560) or domperidone would appear to be the best choice, since its lack of sedative effect allows patients to resume their usual activities very soon after treatment with oral aspirin and i.m. metoclopramide.

3. Ergotamine

This is an alkaloid derived from ergot. It has partial α-adrenergic agonist (vasoconstrictor) actions with α-blocking effects at supratherapeutic doses. Structurally the lysergic acid moiety of the molecule resembles both 5-HT and noradrenaline and it may block 5-HT uptake by platelets and blood vessels thus allowing 5-HT to activate vasoconstrictor receptors. It is believed to act by vasoconstriction in migraine but if given during the migraine aura it can aggravate sensory and motor defects.

Pharmacokinetics Ergotamine probably shows marked inter-individual variations in absorption when administered orally. Several preparations are available:

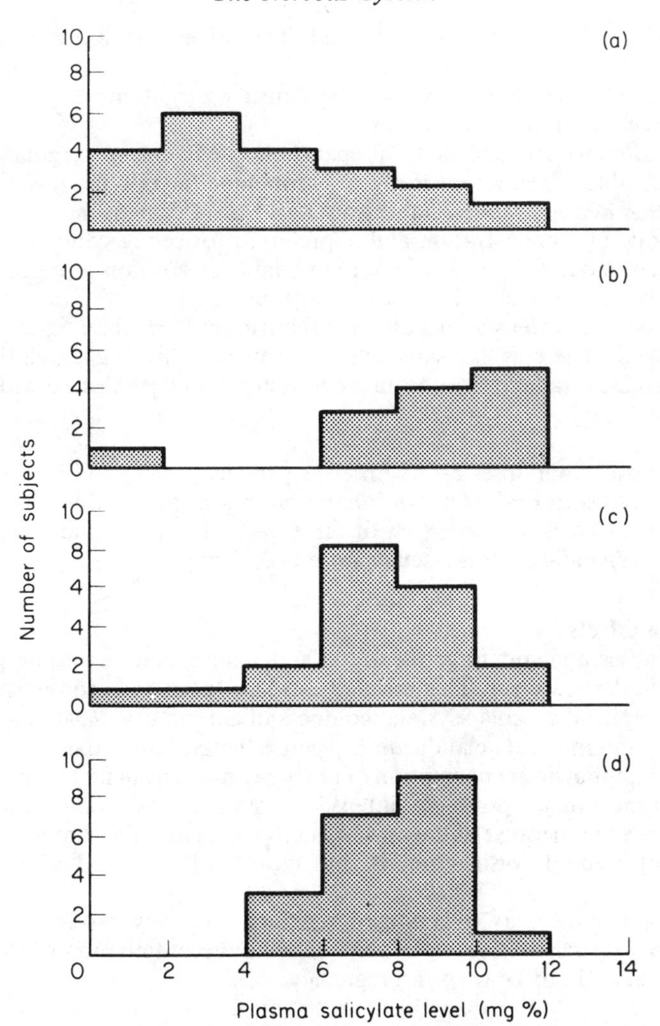

Fig. 9.11 Comparison of the distribution of plasma salicylate levels 30 min after ingestion of 900 mg effervescent aspirin: (a) migraine patients during attack – aspirin alone; (b) migraine patients between attacks – aspirin alone; (c) migraine patients during attack – metoclopramide before aspirin; (d) non-migrainous volunteers – aspirin alone (Modified from G. N. Volans, *Brit. J. Clin. Pharm.*, **2**, 57 (1975).)

(a) *Oral*, e.g. Cafergot, Migril, which contain other substances such as caffeine (in trivial amounts from the point of view of effects on the CNS but which might improve ergotamine absorption according to some studies), atropine or cyclizine. The oral dose of ergotamine is 1 mg.

(b) *Sublingual* (Lingraine containing 2 mg ergotamine alone). Although these tablets have a relatively rapid dissolution time less than 20 % of the drug is absorbed in 5 min and it is probable that much of the benefit is obtained from the drug that is swallowed. The tablets are bitter and may be unpalatable to some patients.

(c) *Rectal*: Cafergot suppositories contain 2 mg ergotamine and some other largely irrelevant substances.

(d) *Inhalation*: an inhaled preparation (Medihaler—ergotamine) is available. It delivers 0.36 mg of ergotamine tartrate per dose.

(e) *Parenteral*: intramuscular injection of 0.25–0.5 mg is the most effective mode of administration and is preferred for severe conditions such as migrainous neuralgia, where the variable absorption of ergotamine by other routes would be disadvantageous.

It undergoes extensive hepatic metabolism and less than 5% is excreted unchanged. There is no satisfactory assay for this drug and the $t_{1/2}$ is undetermined: radioactivity from labelled ergotamine is cleared with a $t_{1/2}$ of 34 h.

Clinical use High doses can themselves produce nausea and headache. It is advisable to start oral, rectal or inhalation treatment at a dose of 1 mg only (e.g. half a Cafergot suppository or three puffs of an ergotamine Medihaler). The corresponding intramuscular dose is 0.25 mg.

Adverse effects

1. Nausea and vomiting, due to too high a dose, may be misinterpreted as due to undertreatment. This mistake can have disastrous consequences.
2. Peripheral vascular system: coldness of extremities, Raynaud's phenomenon, intermittent claudication, paraesthesiae and digital gangrene. Ergotism, following consumption of rye bread made from flour contaminated with ergot fungus produces intense vasospasm and was known as St Anthony's fire (because of the burning limb pains) in earlier times. Treatment of ergot-induced vasospasm is by means of a vasodilator such as nitroprusside.
3. Ergotamine may, when used regularly, actually produce headaches which may persist for several days following discontinuation of the drug.
4. It should not be used in pregnancy.

4. Cyproheptadine (Periactin) is a powerful antihistamine and anti-5-HT agent with mild anticholinergic properties. It also has a tranquillising effect. There is some evidence that it is of benefit in migraine and vascular headache but the mechanism of action is obscure. It can be used both symptomatically, when the benefit often occurs within an hour, or prophylactically. It is given in an initial dose of 4 mg which is repeated, if necessary, after half an hour. This dose should not be exceeded within a 6 hour period. The maintenance dose is 4 mg 6 hourly. The chief adverse effects are drowsiness, anticholinergic effects (dry mouth, blurred vision, etc.), increased appetite and rarely allergic rashes and CNS stimulation.

5. Anxiety. Some patients feel agitated during an attack, and find that an anxiolytic allows them to relax and sleep off the headache. Diazepam 5–10 mg or clorazepate 15 mg are effective.

B. DRUGS USED FOR MIGRAINE PROPHYLAXIS

Prophylactic therapy is not used unless more than two attacks occur each month.

1. Pizotifen (Sanomigran) is probably first choice in migraine prophylaxis. It is related to the tricyclic antidepressants. It has some antidepressant action and potentiates catecholamine effects although its main effect is as a 5-HT and histamine-blocking drug. It also has anticholinergic properties which result in atropine-like side effects. It may also cause weight gain, dizziness and muscle pain.

The dose is 1.5 mg at night or 0.5 mg 8 hourly, adjusted according to response within the range 0.5–6 mg daily.

2. Methysergide (Deseril) This has powerful anti-5-HT activity and also some anti-inflammatory and vasoconstrictor effects.

Clinical uses

Many do not use this drug because of its toxic effects.

1. It has no effect on the acute attack of migraine and is used solely prophylactically, in a dose of 1–2 mg two or three times daily with meals. Initially 1 mg is given at night and the dose is slowly increased up to 2 mg six hourly. Its use is indicated only in patients who, despite other attempts at control, experience such severe migraine as to interfere with their work or social activities. Because of the toxicity of methysergide it is wise to use the smallest dose that suppresses about 75% of the headaches rather than to increase the dose to a high level in an attempt to suppress all headaches. It will give relief in up to 80% of patients but its side effects are so troublesome that half of these will discontinue its use.

2. In the carcinoid syndrome high oral doses of 12–20 mg/day are required to suppress diarrhoea.

Adverse effects

1. Gastrointestinal disturbances: nausea, vomiting, diarrhoea and abdominal pain are most common. They usually appear within a day or so of beginning treatment but their appearance may be delayed by several weeks.
2. Neurological disturbances: mild euphoria, dissociation, experiences of unreality, hyperaesthesia.
3. Weight gain and oedema.
4. Vasoconstriction of large or small arteries which is usually reversible on discontinuing the drug. May produce angina, intermittent claudication, abdominal angina, etc.
5. Non-specific fibrotic changes in peritoneum and thorax. Retroperitoneal fibrosis was the first and commonest syndrome to be described. These changes are not dose-related and fortunately regress when the drug is withdrawn.

3. Clonidine (Dixarit) is also used in hypertension (see p. 442). It causes blood vessels to become less capable of responding to, or sustaining, the vasoconstrictor and vasodilator effects of catecholamines, which may be the mechanism involved in migraine prophylaxis. The dosage used is lower than that employed in hypertension, being 50 μg twice daily increasing to 75 μg twice daily if there is no remission after two weeks. Adverse effects include drowsiness, depression, dry mouth and thirst. At these low doses no interference with control of hypertension should occur.

4. Propranolol and other **β-adrenergic blockers** (timolol, atenolol, pindolol, acebutolol) have been shown to have prophylactic efficacy as compared to placebo. Their action is uncertain but they may act by paradoxically dilating constricted cerebral vessels and by preventing dilatation of extracranial vessels. It has been suggested that a subgroup of patients with mitral valve prolapse, tissue dysplasia (vertebro-thoracic deformities, phakomata, facio-corporal asymmetry) and poor response to ergotamine constitute a sub-group of patients who achieve complete and reproducible remission on propranolol. Propranolol is given in a maintenance dose of 80–160 mg/day in divided doses. β-blockers will potentiate the peripheral vasoconstriction due to ergotamine and should not be given concurrently with this drug.

5. Other drugs which may have prophylactic value in migraine are anti-depressants and anticonvulsants. Dihydroergotamine has been used to prevent migraine. Continuous therapy with lithium carbonate is effective in preventing cluster headache.

DRUGS USED IN MYASTHENIA GRAVIS

This syndrome of increased fatiguability and weakness of striated muscle probably results from an immune process which reduces the number of available acetylcholine receptors at the neuromuscular junction. Myasthenics possess antibodies which interact with post-synaptic cholinergic receptors and which can be passively transmitted to produce a myasthenic syndrome either by transfer of a purified immunoglobulin fraction from their serum to another individual or across the placenta to produce a myasthenic neonate. Indeed, plasmapheresis, which reduces the amount of antibody present, has experimentally produced striking clinical improvement. The antibodies vary from patient to patient and are often directed against sites on the muscle not involved in neurotransmitter binding. However, when bound at these sites, complement is also bound and the final result is an increased rate of receptor clearance from the muscle surface. Reduction of the number of available receptors results in low-amplitude end-plate potentials which in some fibres may be below threshold and so fail to trigger muscle-action potentials, thus reducing the power of the whole muscle.

An immunological cross-reactivity may exist between antigens in the thymus and the cholinergic receptor but the stimulus to the production of antibody is unknown. A fall in antibody titre occurs after thymectomy but only slowly, and this operation may work by reducing the number of circulating T lymphocytes capable of assisting B lymphocytes to produce antibody. A fall in antibody titre also occurs after treatment with corticosteroids and immunosuppressive drugs.

Anticholinesterase drugs

The defect in neuromuscular transmission following the action of antibody may be redressed by cholinesterase inhibitors which inhibit acetylcholine breakdown and increase the concentration of transmitter available to stimulate the receptors.

Neostigmine and pyridostigmine are the basis of treatment. Physostigmine was initially used but produces CNS toxicity because it crosses the blood–brain barrier. **Neostigmine** is initially given in doses of 15 mg 8 hourly but usually requires more frequent administration (up to 2 hourly) because of a short duration of action (2–6 h) and tolerance. It is rapidly inactivated in the gut so that the corresponding parenteral dose (1–2 mg) is much smaller. Cholinesterase inhibitors enhance both muscarinic and nicotinic cholinergic effects. The former results in increased bronchial secretions, abdominal colic, diarrhoea, miosis, nausea, salivation and lachrymation. Some of these effects may be blocked by giving atropine or propantheline. These toxic effects are valuable indicators of overdosage when assessing the optimum treatment regime.

Pyridostigmine is another non-selective anticholinesterase. It has a more prolonged action than neostigmine and it is rarely necessary to give it more frequently than 4-hourly. 60 mg pyridostigmine is equivalent to 15 mg neostigmine and it is initially given in a dose of 60 mg 8 hourly, although individual requirements vary and some patients need up to 2000 mg in a day. It has been shown that despite differing oral maintenance doses in patients the final plasma concentration is maintained within a relatively narrow range: for optimal response the peak plasma levels fall between about 45 and 85 ng/ml despite an 11-fold difference in oral dosage. This suggests that the different dosage requirements in myasthenic patients is partly related to differences in absorption, metabolism and excretion as well as to the variable nature of the disease. Pyridostigmine contains a quarternary nitrogen and is charged at all pH values rendering it poorly absorbed across all membranes. Its absorption does not obey first-order kinetics and a significant hepatic first-pass effect further complicates its pharmacokinetics. The $t_{1/2}$ is about 1–2 h. Because of its slow rate of absorption patients who tend to be weak on waking may benefit from a dose of the quicker acting (within 30 min) neostigmine being given with the first dose of pyridostigmine.

Although marked improvement may follow treatment most patients must accept some residual disability. Increasing anticholinesterase drug dosage above the maximum response level may result in increased weakness rather than the anticipated improvement possibly by the drug itself acting as a competitive inhibitor of acetylcholine at the cholinergic neuromuscular receptors. If this becomes severe it is known as a *cholinergic crisis* (see below).

Ambenonium (Mytelase) and distigmine (Ubretid) are similar drugs with parasympathomimetic toxicity. These effects may be abolished by atropine or propantheline.

Alternative drugs

The immunosuppressant **azathioprine** (2.5 mg/kg) has been successfully used either on its own or combined with steroids. **Ephedrine** which acts by increasing the presynaptic release of acetylcholine, has had limited success. More recently spectacular remissions of symptoms have been obtained using oral administration of **prednisolone**. Increased weakness may occur at the beginning of treatment which must therefore be instituted in hospital. This effect has been minimised by the use of alternate day therapy with 25 mg prednisone with a gradual increase of dose to 100 mg alternate days. With such high doses the usual side effects of corticosteroids (see p. 639) are to be expected. Therefore the dose is reduced by 5 mg each month for as long as improvement is maintained.

The indications for thymectomy which is probably most beneficial to the young adult female myasthenic are outside the scope of this book.

Plasmapheresis provides short-term relief by removing the motor end-plate antibody.

Myasthenic and cholinergic crisis

Severe weakness leading to paralysis may result from either a deficiency (myasthenic crisis) or an excess (cholinergic crisis) of acetylcholine at the neuromuscular junction. Clinically the distinction may be difficult and an injection of the very short-acting anticholinesterase **edrophonium (tensilon)**, 10 mg i.v., may aid diagnosis. This transiently improves a myasthenic crisis and aggravates a cholinergic crisis. Because of its short duration of action any deterioration of a cholinergic crisis is unlikely to have serious consequences, although facilities for artificial ventilation must be available. It is important that the strength of essential (respiratory or bulbar) muscles be monitored during the test rather than that of non-essential (limb or ocular) muscles, since a cholinergic and myasthenic crisis may coexist in the same patient and it is the response of the important muscle groups which determines the patient's prognosis.

Myasthenic crises may develop as a spontaneous deterioration in the natural history of the disease, or as a result of infection or surgery. Drugs should not be forgotten as a cause and include:

1. *Aminoglycosides*, e.g. neomycin, streptomycin, which impair conduction in the terminal motor nerve fibres.
2. *Other antibiotics*: polymyxin, colistin and bacitracin.
3. *Curare* sensitivity may be increased 100-fold and myasthenics are also sensitive to other drugs with neuromuscular blocking activity like *ether*, *gallamine* and *pancuronium*. There is reduced sensitivity to suxamethonium.
4. *Quinine* and *quinidine* which reduce the excitability of the muscle membrane. There is enough quinine in tonic water to cause decompensation.

5. Respiratory depressants such as *barbiturates*.
6. *Antiarrhythmic* drugs reduce the excitability of muscle membrane and *lignocaine*, *procainamide* and *propranolol* may increase weakness.

Treatment of: (a) *Myasthenic crisis* is with neostigmine (0.5 mg i.m.) repeating this every 20 min with frequent edrophonium tests.
(b) *Cholinergic crisis*: Treatment of myasthenia with anticholinesterases can be usefully monitored by observation of the pupil (a diameter of 2 mm or less in normal lighting would suggest overdose). Overdosage produces a cholinergic crisis and further drug should be withheld. Atropine may be given to block excessive muscarinic activity.
A cholinesterase reactivator such as *pralidoxime* (1–2 g i.v. over 2–4 min) is also useful.

The myasthenic syndrome of Eaton and Lambert

This rare myasthenic syndrome occurs in patients with (usually) bronchial carcinoma and resembles the syndrome occurring after botulism or with aminoglycoside overdose. Unlike myasthenia gravis where repetitive stimulation of a motor nerve causes responses of decreasing amplitude, in this syndrome the converse occurs and successive stimuli facilitate acetylcholine release. The defect is believed to lie in an abnormality of acetylcholine release, although the quanta of acetylcholine stored in the vesicles at the nerve endings are of the normal size. The clinical response to edrophonium is often less than in myasthenia gravis and anticholinesterases are not very effective treatment. In these cases *guanidine* given in oral divided doses (20–30 mg/kg/day) is used. The onset of effect is slow and the drug dosage should be increased until benefit or toxicity (restlessness, agitation, diarrhoea, anorexia) occur. Many of the side-effects can be corrected by the administration of atropine.

Chapter 10
ANALGESIC AND ANTIRHEUMATIC DRUGS

ANALGESICS AND THE RELIEF OF PAIN

Pain is a common symptom and is important as it may indicate that something is wrong and may give a clue as to the nature of disease. In addition, pain is unpleasant for the patient and its relief is one of the most important duties of a doctor. Although analgesic drugs and pain have been studied for many years, a number of questions remain unanswered.

Mechanism of pain

Peripheral sensation may be transmitted to the spinal cord via large-diameter myelinated nerves (A delta fibres) or by the non-or thinly myelinated nerves (C fibres). A delta fibres are rapidly conducting, and innervate mechanoreceptors that may be activated by minimal stimulation (i.e. touch). They relay in the deeper layers of the dorsal horn and cross over to ascend in the spino-thalamic tract. The free endings of the slowly conducting C fibres are only activated by more intense stimulation which may be mechanical, thermal or chemical. They relay in the more superficial part of the dorsal horn, i.e. lamina I and lamina II (substantia gelatinosa), and also ascend in the crossed spino-thalamic tract and will ultimately subserve the appreciation of pain. The transmitter used by neurones concerned with these impulses in the dorsal horn is not known but a neuropeptide, substance P is the most likely candidate.

The transmission of pain impulses, at this level can be modified in two ways (Fig. 10.1):

1. Stimulation of A delta fibres in the same segment as that receiving painful stimuli decreases the appreciation of pain. This is the basis for the use of counter-irritants and of vibro-massage machines to relieve pain. A similar effect can be achieved by applying opioids or metenkephalin locally to the appropriate segment of the spinal cord.

   It is postulated that stimulation of A delta fibres causes local release of enkephalin which combines with the opioid receptors on the terminal neurones of fibres subserving pain preventing the release of substance P and thus inhibiting transmission.
2. Transmission of impulses subserving pain can also be inhibited in the dorsal horn by fibres projected from above.

   Electrical stimulation or the injection of opioids into the peri-aqueductal grey matter (PAG) or the nucleus raphé magnus (NRM) leads to the relief of pain. The PAG projects on to the dorsal horn via the NRM (see Fig. 10.1) and it seems probable that activation of this system

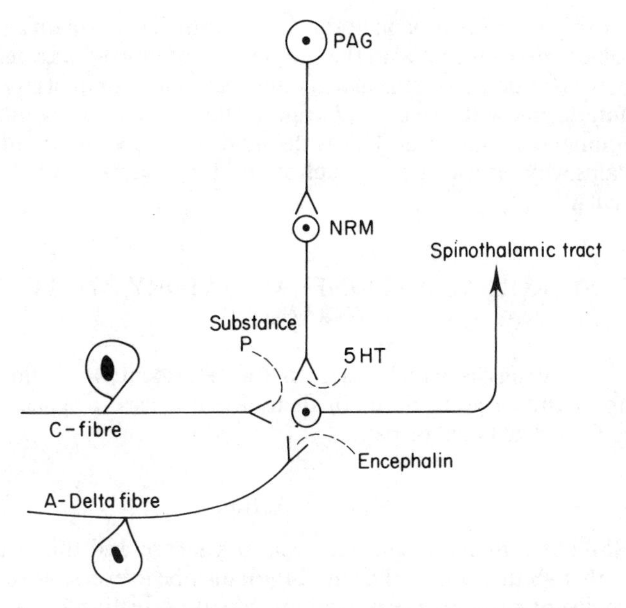

Fig. 10.1 Proposed pain pathways of the dorsal horn. PAG = Periaqueductal grey matter; NRM = Nucleus raphe magnus; 5-HT = 5 hydroxytryptamine.

also inhibits transmission of impulses subserving pain. The mode of inhibition at the dorsal horn is not clear but at present 5-hydroxytryptamine and noradrenaline seem likely to be involved.

Whether sensory data are felt as pain depends on their interpretation by the brain. Sensory impulses may ascend in the spinal cord via the oligosynaptic ascending system which terminates in the postcentral gyrus and is concerned with the localisation of pain, or the multisynaptic ascending system which joins the limbic system and is concerned with the emotional concomitants of pain. These systems interact with each other, with other aspects of cerebral activity such as memory and reflect back to modulate dorsal horn mechanisms (see above). They may also stimulate motor activity.

The importance of these ideas in terms of clinical pharmacology is that inhibiting and facilitating mechanisms are to some degree controlled by the higher centres and thus emotional and other factors have a considerable effect on the appreciation of pain. It should be remembered that several areas in the brain are concerned with the appreciation of pain and that the sensation of pain itself has several components. What the patient feels is the result of the interaction between the stimulus and the response of the nervous system.

Theoretically pain can be relieved:

1. By removing the peripheral stimulus. This may be done pharmacologically and is perhaps largely responsible for the analgesic action of the NSAI group of drugs.
2. By blocking transmission in peripheral nerves as with local anaesthetics.

3. By modifying transmission at the dorsal horn. This explains some of the actions of opioids and also the mechanism of vibro-massage, electrical transcutaneous nerve stimulation and perhaps acupuncture.
4. By interfering with the central appreciation of pain or by inhibiting its emotional concomitants. This is the mode of action of opioids and also explains why the use of drugs such as antidepressants may help in certain patients.

NON-STEROIDAL ANTI-INFLAMMATORY ANALGESICS (NSAIAs)

This group of drugs is widely used in the treatment of rheumatoid and osteoarthritis and of gout. Some of them are also used as general purpose analgesics for other types of pain.

Mode of Action

All the NSAIAs inhibit the enzyme cyclo-oxygenase and this is their most important therapeutic action. The inhibition may be irreversible (e.g. aspirin, indomethacin) or reversible (e.g. propionic acid derivatives).

Cyclo-oxygenase plays a major role in the synthesis of prostaglandins, prostacyclin and thromboxanes (see Fig. 18.2). Some of these substances play an important part in the erythema, oedema, pain and fever associated with inflammation either by direct action or by sensitising the appropriate tissue to other substances released by tissue damage such as bradykinin. By inhibiting prostaglandin synthesis both inflammation and pain are reduced. In addition to the above, some NSAIAs may suppress inflammation by other actions:

(a) inhibition of phosphodiesterase: this reduces the production of superoxides which damage tissues;
(b) inhibition of leucocyte migration;
(c) removal of toxic hydroxyl residues.

The NSAIAs share several other properties:

1. *antipyretic* (see under 'Aspirin' below);
2. *inhibition of platelet aggregation* (see p. 605);
3. *prolongation of labour and relief of dysmenorrhoea* probably because by inhibiting prostaglandin synthesis, NSAIAs remove the stimulus to uterine contraction;
4. many of the group (phenylbutazone, azapropazone and aspirin) *potentiate the effect of anticoagulants.*

NSAIAs and Renal Function

(See also analgesic nephropathy p. 307).

It seems probable that prostaglandins, particularly prostacyclin and prostaglandin E_2, play a rôle in the autoregulation of renal blood flow and glomerular filtration rate.

If cyclo-oxygenase inhibitors are given to normal subjects, there is no measurable alteration in renal function except salt and water retention. However, in the following circumstances they can cause marked changes:

1. Seriously reduced renal function due to kidney disease.
2. Compromised renal perfusion due to volume depletion, sodium deficiency, cardiac failure, nephrotic syndrome, or cirrhosis.
3. Active inflammation, e.g. sepsis, systemic lupus erythematosus.

It appears that under these circumstances prostaglandins are responsible for vasodilation and maintenance of renal perfusion and inhibition of their synthesis by NSAIAs causes:

(a) Fall in GFR and renal perfusion;
(b) Fall in renin production;
(c) Rise in blood pressure;

Clinically this may cause acute renal failure but this must be a rare occurrence bearing in mind the widespread use of NSAIAs even in those with impaired renal function.

Practically all NSAIAs cause salt and water retention. This is partly due to reduced renal perfusion but in addition prostaglandins may inhibit chloride and sodium reabsorption in the ascending limb of the loop of Henle and their inhibition by NSAIAs thus reduces salt excretion. As a consequence the response to diuretics is reduced in those taking NSAIAs, some hypotensive drugs including β-blockers become less effective and heart failure may be made worse.

Finally, NSAIAs can rarely cause an interstitial nephritis usually presenting as the nephrotic syndrome which is reversible on withdrawing the drug.

NSAIAs and gastrointestinal bleeding All NSAIAs cause indigestion and sometimes gastrointestinal bleeding because they depend on the inhibition of prostaglandin synthesis to produce their effects. Prostaglandins inhibit gastric secretion and promote vasodilation so that preventing their production causes gastric ischaemia and hyperacidity – circumstances which can promote ulceration.

The newer NSAIAs are less liable to cause bleeding than aspirin but it is not clear whether there are differences within the group. Paracetamol does not cause bleeding as it has only a weak peripheral action. NSAIAs may cause a haematemesis or, with prolonged use, oozing leading to iron-deficiency anaemia (see also p. 297). Bleeding is more likely in patients over 60.

NSAIAs and bronchospasm Bronchospasm is precipitated in a small number of asthmatics taking NSAIAs and the food additive, tartrazine. This is believed to be due to the inhibition of synthesis of prostaglandins of the E series which normally act as bronchodilators. The safest minor analgesic for asthmatics is paracetamol, although even this can very rarely cause an attack. Aspirin can also exacerbate giant urticaria.

The use of NSAIAs is considered on page 313.

Classification of NSAIAs

There is no entirely satisfactory method of classification; the following is based on chemical structure:

1. Salicylates and related substances
2. Indoleacetic acids
3. Propionic acids
4. Anthranilic acids
5. Phenylacetic acids
6. Oxicams
7. Pyrazolones

Salicylates

Aspirin

Salicylic acid is usually administered as sodium salicylate or acetylsalicylate (aspirin). It is one of the oldest drugs in use, having been known to the Greeks and Romans. In all pharmacological tests, including analgesia and inhibition of prostaglandin synthesis, the acetylsalicylate ion is more effective than the salicylate ion. Unfortunately the hepatic conversion of acetylsalicylate into salicylate is rapid and acetylsalicylate has a $t_{1/2}$ of only 20–30 min and it is subject to considerable first-pass metabolism in the liver (see Fig. 10.2). Indeed, if this rapid conversion did not occur, aspirin would be an even more effective agent. One way to increase acetylsalicylate plasma levels is to give aspirin in solution as the calcium or sodium salt which increases the rate at which plasma acetylsalicylate levels rise and the maximum level attained (see Fig. 2.11) It is convenient to consider aspirin (acetylsalicylate) and the other salicylates under one heading.

Actions of salicylates Salicylates have three main therapeutic actions though two of them may be identical and will be considered together.

Analgesic/anti-inflammatory Salicylates are mild analgesics and particularly effective in the rheumatic diseases, including rheumatoid arthritis and acute rheumatic fever where they appear to have a specific effect on the disease process. It is also useful in a wide range of minor pains and discomforts.

There is now little doubt that salicylates produce their major analgesic effect by peripheral mechanisms at the site of pain production. Whether they have some additional central analgesic action is unclear. Their peripheral action has been largely elucidated and depends essentially on reducing the production of certain prostaglandins by inhibiting cyclo-oxygenase (see p. 605). There is evidence that in man the turnover of prostaglandin is reduced by about 80% by a therapeutic dose of aspirin.

Antipyretic Salicylates have a marked antipyretic action and will reduce the temperature if it is raised. This is usually accompanied by profuse sweating and is believed to be due to inhibition of the synthesis and subsequent release of prostaglandin E in the pre-optic nucleus of the hypothalamus, which is the site of the temperature-regulating area. Prostaglandin E_1 has a powerful

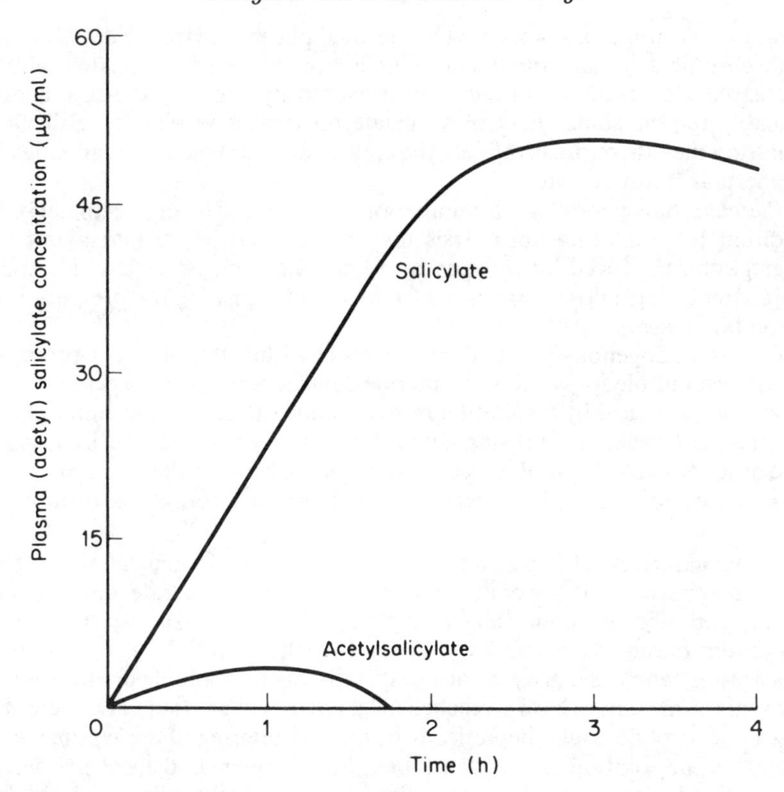

Fig. 10.2 Plasma levels of salicylate and acetylsalicylate following 650 mg aspirin given orally, demonstrating rapid conversion of acetylsalicylate to salicylate.

pyrogenic action and is thought to be released in the brain by circulating pyrogens. The level of this prostaglandin rises in the cerebrospinal fluid during fever, and this rise is blocked by aspirin.

Other actions of salicylates

Central actions Salicylates increase respiratory rate and volume by two mechanisms: by a direct action on the respiratory centre and by uncoupling oxidative phosphorylation causing increased oxygen utilisation and production of carbon dioxide. Even in full therapeutic doses the increased respiratory rate can be appreciated at the bedside and it becomes very obvious after aspirin over-dosage. As a secondary effect it leads to a respiratory alkalosis which is part of the acid–base disturbance produced by aspirin (see p. 876).

Stomach (see under adverse effects p. 297).

Kidney (see also p. 290) Aspirin causes shedding of the tubular epithelial cells into the urine; this usually lasts only a few days even with continued administration of aspirin. Whether prolonged salicylate dosage can cause permanent renal damage in man is still argued. An apparent reduction in creatinine clearance accompanied by elevated plasma creatinine levels occurs with chronic salicylate treatment. This is not, however, associated with a decreased glomerular filtration rate measured by other methods and presumably reflects some effect of salicylate on creatinine kinetics. Salicylate ingestion may therefore invalidate the creatinine clearance test as an index of glomerular filtration rate.

Platelets Salicylates have a number of actions on platelets (see p. 605). In addition to promoting fibrinolysis they reduce platelet stickiness and the aggregation produced by collagen or adrenaline. This effect lasts for some days after a single dose and has led to the use of aspirin in the prevention of thrombosis (see p. 607).

Uterus Endogenous prostaglandin release within the uterus is probably partly responsible for causing the uterine contractions which expel the fetus. Abortion produced by instillation of hypertonic saline into the amniotic sac may be due to release of prostaglandins from damaged decidual cells. Aspirin and other NSAIAs by inhibiting cyclo-oxygenase prolong the duration of this process and in animals have been shown to prolong normal parturition.

Pharmacokinetics The gastrointestinal absorption of salicylates is rapid, with an apparent half-life of absorption of 5–15 min. The rate and extent of absorption depend upon many factors. With ordinary aspirin tablets maximum plasma salicylate levels are not reached until about 1½–2 h after absorption, whereas if given as one of its salts, such as soluble or effervescent aspirin, the maximum level is reached in less than half an hour. This increased rate of absorption could theoretically be due to buffering of the aspirin which increases the solution rate of the tablet, but the increased local pH delays absorption by increasing drug ionisation, so in practice it is doubtful whether this makes much difference although there may be less gastric irritation. The higher absorption rate observed with effervescent preparations may be explained as an effect on gastric motility mediated through a slight alkalinisation of gastric contents. It has never been demonstrated that a faster rate of achievement of a given plasma salicylate level is of any clinical benefit. The presence of food in the stomach may more than double the half-life of aspirin absorption. Alteration of gastric emptying by drugs may also alter aspirin absorption (see Fig. 9.11). Aspirin suppositories produce slow and relatively unreliable absorption. As mentioned above, acetylsalicylic acid is subject to considerable first-pass hepatic metabolism (50–60 %) to salicylate and once in the blood further hydrolysis occurs due to plasma and red-cell esterases which contribute about 20 % of total aspirin hydrolysis.

Salicylates are widely, but unevenly, distributed throughout the body, highest levels occurring in liver and kidney. The concentration in synovial fluid is about 50 % of the plasma concentration. The apparent volume of distribution is about 0.17 l/kg, indicating mainly distribution into extracellular water, but the V_d is dose dependent and is larger at higher doses. The uneven distribution is partly determined by pH-dependent passive diffusion and partly by other factors, including an active transport system across the choroid plexus. Salicylates are considerably bound (80–85 %) to plasma protein, mainly to albumin which is acetylated by aspirin. Protein binding of salicylates is dose dependent, since for plasma concentrations of

100–200 μg/ml the free fraction is 15–20 %, whilst at over 400 μg/ml the free fraction is 40–50 %. This phenomenon is even more marked and may produce clinical toxicity in hypoalbuminaemia. Salicylates may also affect the protein binding of other drugs (see interactions).

Salicylate is metabolised largely in the liver by four main parallel pathways, two of which are saturable, and it is also excreted unchanged in the urine by a first-order process. This is summarised by the scheme shown in Fig. 10.3. The formation of salicylurate is interesting since it is one of the few drug metabolism mechanisms which occur in mitochondria and is an easily saturable process. Because of the saturable nature of some of these pathways the percentages of products formed is variable and those in the scheme above are only approximations. For dosages lower than 4 mg/kg the plasma disappearance of salicylate follows first-order kinetics with an apparent $t_{1/2}$ of 2–4 h but for higher doses the elimination is overall non-linear and the $t_{1/2}$ may be 15–30 h. Clinically this means that for example doubling the daily dose from 2 to 4 g given in four divided doses raises the plateau level of salicylate in the body from 1.3 to 5.3 g, a fourfold increase. It will also require a longer time to reach steady state using a larger daily dose, since the effective $t_{1/2}$ is prolonged (see Fig. 10.4). Salicylate elimination is influenced by urinary pH, the loss being greater if the urine is alkaline (see p. 876). When used in rheumatoid arthritis, levels of about 200–250 μg/ml are required. This is close to the level at which clinical signs of salicylism appear (300 μg/ml). The level for adequate analgesia has not been established.

Clinical uses The dose of aspirin varies, depending upon the type of pain being treated. For the multitude of minor pains which afflict humanity the usual dose for an adult is 600 mg (2 tablets) and this may be repeated four to six hourly if required.

In acute rheumatic fever, adults require 5–8 g daily and the plasma salicylate level should be kept between 250 and 300 μg/ml. This high dosage which may produce side effects is necessary to suppress the rheumatic process.

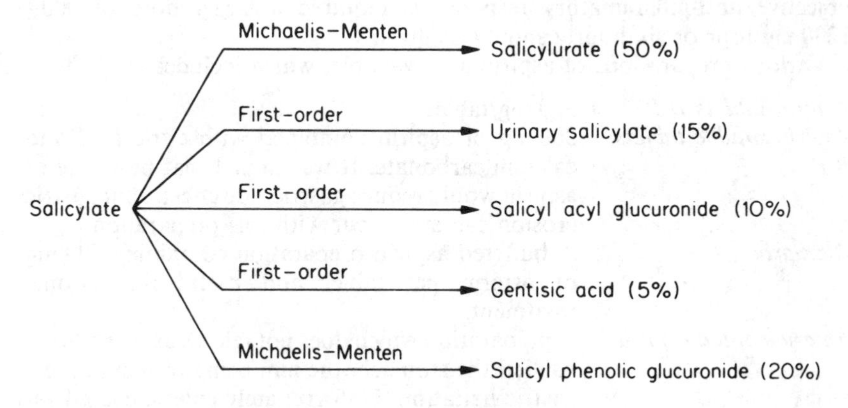

Fig. 10.3 The four main pathways of salicylate metabolism.

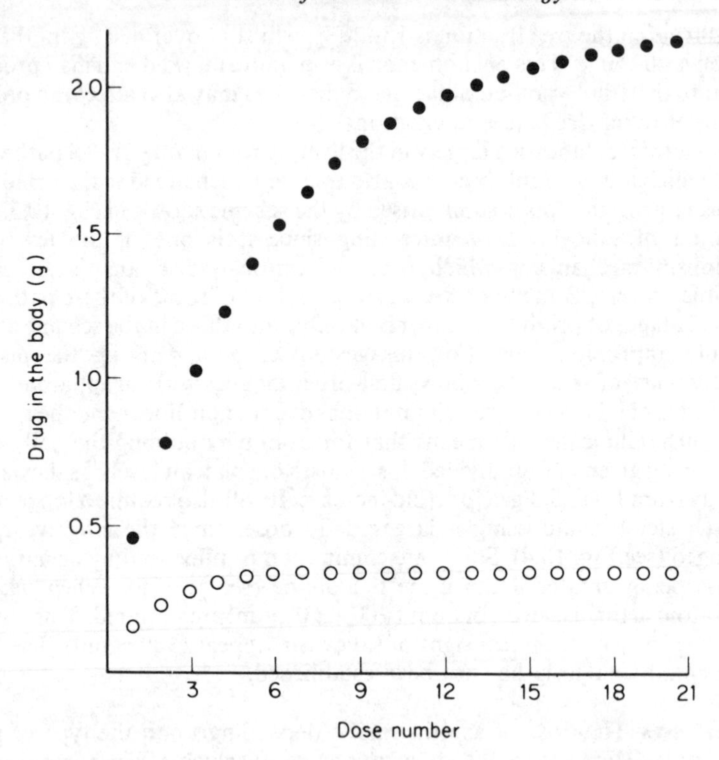

Fig. 10.4 Simulation of accumulation of salicylic acid in the body as a function of the dose number when 0.5 g (open circles) or 1.0 g (closed circles) is given orally every 8 hours. The drug is assumed to have a rapid absorption rate ($t_{1/2}$ 10 minutes) and the ordinate shows amounts in the body immediately before the next dose (From G. Levy and T. Tsuchiya. Reprinted with permission from the *New Eng. J. Med.*, **287**, 430 (1972).)

In rheumatoid arthritis, 600 mg four hourly will relieve symptoms but if an objective anti-inflammatory response is required a larger dose of 900–1200 mg four or six hourly should be given.

Various preparations of aspirin are available, which include:

Aspirin tablets B.P.	300 mg/tablet
Aspirin soluble tablets B.P.	300 mg of aspirin combined with citric acid and calcium carbonate. It was hoped that buffering of aspirin would reduce gastric side effects, but gastric erosion can still occur with this preparation.
Aloxiprin	A buffered aspirin preparation containing 500 mg of aspirin per tablet and useful for chronic treatment.
Enteric-coated aspirin	A preparation which does not release aspirin until it has left the stomach, the aim being to reduce local gastric irritation. Unfortunately enteric-coated aspirin has variable bioavailability.

Choline magnesium trisalicylate — A salicylate compound claimed to have the analgesic and anti-inflammatory effects of salicylate without the gastric side effects and without causing platelet deaggregation. 500 mg of salicylate/tablet: dose 2–3 tablets twice daily.

Adverse effects:

1. *Salicylism*: High therapeutic or excessive doses of salicylates will cause tinnitus, deafness, nausea, vomiting and occasionally abdominal pain and flushing.
2. *Dyspepsia and blood loss from the stomach* (see also p. 532) is rather more common with aspirin than with other NSAIAs, particularly if high doses are used and treatment is prolonged, but it rarely causes serious trouble if it is taken for short periods in analgesic doses for minor pain.

   Dyspepsia occurs in about 2–6% of patients taking aspirin. Examination of the faeces will show traces of blood but the loss is usually less than 15 ml/day although about 10% of individuals lose more.

   Bleeding is increased if aspirin is taken with alcohol and reduced if taken with alkali; however, it can occur even in the achlorhydric patient. With prolonged treatment blood loss may be sufficient to cause an iron deficiency anaemia.

   Acute severe gastric bleeding is much less common occurring in about 15 per 100 000 regular users. Aspirin can also rarely cause chronic ulcers (10 per 100 000 users).

   Aspirin should not therefore be given to patients with active peptic ulceration; it should not be given at the same time as anticoagulants and preferably should be taken with or after meals. Buffered aspirin reduces the risk of bleeding but it can still occur.
3. *Wheezing*, sometimes accompanied by urticaria and rhinorrhoea, occurs in some aspirin-sensitive asthmatics (possibly as many as 2% of asthmatics). This is associated with the presence of nasal polyps and similar reactions to other NSAIAs (see p. 291) and tartrazine (a yellow food dye).
4. Salicylates may provoke *gout* due to their effects on uric acid excretion (see below).
5. *Toxic effects on the liver* have been reported in a number of patients being treated for rheumatoid arthritis, rheumatic fever and systemic lupus erythematosus. It is dose-dependent and usually requires a plasma concentration of more than 250 μg/ml. The main changes are elevation of the serum enzymes. Histological change is minimal and liver-function tests revert to normal on stopping the drug. The cause is not known, but there is no evidence of immunological abnormalities.
6. It has been suggested that *Reye's syndrome*, a rare encephalopathy complicating viral infection in children may be precipitated by aspirin.

Drug interactions

The salicylates potentiate gastric irritation by some other drugs such as alcohol and phenylbutazone.

They may potentiate the effects of oral hypoglycaemic agents and oral anticoagulants by their effects on the protein binding of these drugs.

Corticosteroids appear to induce their metabolism and it is often difficult to attain therapeutic levels with usual salicylate doses in patients concurrently receiving steroids.

Benorylate (Benoral)

This is the acetylsalicylic ester of paracetamol and therefore has analgesic, antipyretic and anti-inflammatory properties. It may be regarded as a prodrug of both acetylsalicylate and paracetamol. It is administered orally, absorbed from the gut intact and hydrolysed by hepatic and plasma esterases to its constituents. Benorylate itself has a plasma $t_{1/2}$ of about 1 h. The purpose of this formulation is to reduce gastric irritation which appears to be partly achieved, although benorylate may cause nausea, indigestion and heartburn, gastric bleeding is rare. Benorylate is available as tablets or suspension and can be used in osteoarthritis, musculo-skeletal pain and rheumatoid arthritis. The usual adult dose is 1.5 g (as tablets) three times daily, or 4 g (as suspension) twice daily, but larger doses may be needed to achieve anti-inflammatory salicylate concentrations in rheumatoid arthritis when the dose is best judged by monitoring salicylate plasma levels.

Diflunisal (Dolobid)

This is 5-(2, 4-difluorophenyl)-salicylic acid, i.e. a close relative of aspirin which has anti-inflammatory, antipyretic and analgesic properties probably mediated by prostaglandin synthetase inhibition. It may be slightly more effective as an analgesic than aspirin. It is well absorbed from the gut, peak blood levels being achieved in 2–4 h. It is excreted in the urine as unchanged or conjugated drug. The plasma $t_{1/2}$ is 8 h after 250 mg but it appears to obey dose-dependent non-linear kinetics since it is 11 h after 500 mg.

The usual dose is 250 mg twice daily and may be increased to a maximum of 750 mg daily.

Although gastric side effects appear less common than with aspirin, diflunisal should be avoided in peptic ulceration. Tinnitus has occasionally been reported. Some interaction does occur with anticoagulants with increased risk of bleeding, but is probably unlikely with oral hypoglycaemic agents. In general, diflunisal may be better tolerated than aspirin but its place in treating osteoarthritis and rheumatoid arthritis as well as more general and non-specific causes of pain has yet to be determined.

Indoleacetic acids

Indomethacin
Tolmetin
Sulindac

Indomethacin (Indocid)

Indomethacin is an indoleacetic acid derivative with anti-inflammatory, antipyretic and analgesic effects, unrelated to but somewhat similar in action to phenylbutazone, although less toxic.

Pharmacokinetics It is readily absorbed by mouth or from suppositories, and by the latter method it produces about 75 % of the levels expected from oral administration of the same dose. Indomethacin is about 90 % bound to plasma proteins and the plasma-protein binding is not saturable within the therapeutic dose range. Indomethacin undergoes extensive hepatic metabolism and both parent compound and metabolites take part in an enterohepatic circulation. The $t_{1/2}$ is 7–10 h but is prolonged in biliary obstruction since the bile is a major excretory route which may allow continued administration in renal failure. In normal circumstances indomethacin and its metabolites are excreted in the urine. It has been claimed that there is a clear relationship between plasma level and clinical effect with adverse effects predominantly over 10 μg/ml.

Clinical uses Indomethacin has a considerable anti-inflammatory action, probably as a result of inhibition of prostaglandin synthesis. It has only weak analgesic action. It is used in treating rheumatoid arthritis and associated disorders, ankylosing spondylitis and gout. It is of little use in relieving pains which are not associated with inflammation.

Side effects are rather common so it is best to start treatment with a single dose of 25 mg daily and increase this gradually up to 25 mg three times daily. Further increase in dosage is unlikely to increase effectiveness. In acute gout the initial dose is 50 mg orally repeated after 4 hours and then 6 hourly for a few days.

It can also be given as a suppository (100 mg) at night to relieve morning stiffness in rheumatoid arthritis and a slow release preparation containing 75 mg of indomethacin per capsule is available.

Adverse effects Indomethacin produces some side effects in at least 25 % of patients taking the drug. The most common are headaches and occasionally other central nervous symptoms such as light-headedness, confusion or hallucination. Gastric bleeding can occur (see p. 532). Activation or masking of infections in a fashion similar to corticosteroids has also been reported. Indomethacin may be dangerous in patients with impaired renal function and/or cardiac failure. Deterioration of renal function with hyperkalaemia and salt and water retention may occur. This is probably due to changes in renal haemodynamics which are the result of decreased prostaglandin synthesis.

Interactions Indomethacin should not if possible be combined with anticoagulants. It may also reverse the effect of some blood pressure lowering drugs.

Indomethacin in neonates Prostaglandins appear to prevent closure of the ductus arteriosus and indomethacin has been used to facilitate closure in infants with symptomatic patent ductus. Success in closure appears related to the plasma level of indomethacin which may vary considerably.

Tolmetin (Tolectin)

This is a pyrrole acetic acid derivative with analgesic, anti-inflammatory and some antipyretic activity. It inhibits prostaglandin synthetase being more active in this respect than aspirin or naproxen but less effective than diclofenac or mefenamic acid. It is a competitive but reversible inhibitor of this enzyme as compared to aspirin and indomethacin which are irreversible inhibitors.

Pharmacokinetics It is almost completely absorbed after oral administration and plasma levels peak at 20–60 minutes. It is eliminated largely by metabolism to inactive metabolites which are excreted in the urine. It is very highly protein bound (> 99 %) and has a low apparent volume of distribution.

Clinical uses are as for other non-steroidal anti-inflammatory drugs. Most adults respond to a total daily dose of 600–1800 mg in divided doses 3–4 times a day.

Adverse effects It causes less gastrointestinal bleeding than aspirin. Headache, tinnitus, vertigo, peptic ulcer, sodium retention and skin rashes (i.e. all the adverse effects of other members of the group) have been reported.

Sulindac (Clinoril)

This is an indene unrelated to salicylate, phenacetin, pyrazolone or aryl-alkanoic acids. It is well absorbed when given orally and is approximately half as potent as indomethacin on a weight basis, but the safety ratio (in animal tests) between the dose causing intestinal perforation or haemorrhage and the anti-inflammatory dose is several times higher than for indomethacin. Sulindac, which is itself inactive, undergoes irreversible conversion to inactive sulphone and a reversible conversion to an active sulphide after ingestion. The sulphide is approximately as active as indomethacin and has a $t_{1/2}$ of 18 h as compared to a $t_{1/2}$ of 1.5–3 h for the parent compound. Sulindac is therefore a prodrug which reduces local exposure of the intestinal mucosa to active compound, thereby reducing irritation. Enterohepatic recycling of sulindac followed by conversion back to sulphide contributes to the maintenance of high-plasma levels of active compound. Sulindac should, however, be avoided in the presence of active peptic ulceration.

Sulindac is used in rheumatic conditions of all types including gout. The dosage is 100–200 mg twice daily. It is protein bound and should be used cautiously with oral anticoagulants and hypoglycaemic drugs. Generally well tolerated, the main adverse effects are gastrointestinal disturbance, hypersensitivity rashes and central nervous system effects such as sweating and vertigo.

Propionic acids (see Table 10.1)

This large group of drugs is probably the most generally useful, particularly in the treatment of rheumatoid arthritis with a relatively low incidence of side effects.

Table 10.1 Propionic acid derivatives currently available in the UK

Approved name	*Proprietary name*	$t_{1/2}$ *(h)*	*Protein binding (%)*	*Metabolism*	*Dose*	*Side effects and special features*
Fenbufen	Lederfen	15	98	++	600 mg nocte	Indigestion, avoid in peptic ulceration.
		(metabolite)			300 mg mane	Produces a therapeutically active metabolite. Rashes rather frequent.
Fenoprofen	Fenopron	2.5–3	99	+	300–600 mg	Indigestion, avoid in peptic ulceration.
					8 hourly or 6 hourly	Rashes. Avoid in renal failure.
Flurbiprofen	Froben	2.5–6.0	99	++	50–100 mg,	Indigestion, avoid in peptic ulceration.
					8 hourly	Rashes. Relatively active.
Ibuprofen	Brufen	1.9	99	++	400–800 mg	Indigestion, avoid in peptic ulceration.
	Elbufac				6 hourly	Rashes. Low incidence of side effects but not so active as some of the group.
Ketoprofen	Orudis	1.6–1.9	95	+	50 mg two–four	Indigestion, avoid in peptic ulceration.
					times daily.	Rashes.
Naproxen	Naprosyn	12–15	99	++	500 mg	Indigestion, avoid in peptic ulceration.
	Synflex				12 hourly	Rashes. Relatively active. Twice daily dosage.

Key: ++ Largely hepatic; + partially hepatic.

Anthranilic acids

Mefenamic acid
Flufenamic acid

Mefenamic acid (Ponstan)

This is another non-steroidal anti-inflammatory drug. It is absorbed rather slowly from the intestine, reaching peak concentration in 2–3 h. It is 98.5% bound to plasma proteins. Metabolites are produced without analgesic properties. It is used as a mild analgesic and the usual dose is 500 mg three times daily. It is also used by some for dysmenorrhoea and in children.

Adverse effects Diarrhoea may occur. Other side effects are rare but include dizziness, rashes, depression of the white blood count and autoimmune haemolytic anaemia in which antibody is directed against normal red cells (for this reason it can interfere with blood cross-matching). There are a number of reports of non-oliguric renal failure in patients taking mefenamic acid. This usually occurs in older patients especially if they are dehydrated, and usually improves when the drug is stopped. Overdosage with mefenamic acid is particularly liable to cause fits: this symptom relates poorly to the plasma level of the drug. Like some other drugs affecting prostaglandin synthesis it has been found to prolong the abortion time in patients undergoing induction by hypertonic saline.

Flufenamic acid (Arlef)

This is another member of the group which is perhaps slightly more rapidly absorbed than mefenamic acid. The $t_{1/2}$ is 3 h and the usual dose is 400–600 mg daily in divided doses.

Phenylacetic acids

This group is similar to the propionic acids and is represented in the UK by diclofenac (Voltarol). This has a $t_{1/2}$ of 1–2 hours and undergoes extensive metabolism. It is 95–98% protein bound.

The usual dose is 75–150 mg/day in divided doses. It may also be given by deep intramuscular injection (75 mg once or twice daily). A suppository form is also available.

Like other NSAIAs it may cause dyspepsia and aggravates peptic ulcers.

Oxicams

Piroxicam (Feldene) Actions, use and side effects are the same as the other NSAIAs. It is largely metabolised and has a long half-life (35–60 h) so a once-daily dose of 20 mg is sufficient. For the treatment of acute pain (i.e. gout or soft tissue injuries) 40 mg daily should be given for the first two or three days.

Pyrazolone compounds

Phenylbutazone
Oxyphenbutazone

The earliest members of this group were antipyrine (now used in experimental work as a marker for enzyme induction) and aminopyrine (still used in Europe but not much in the UK because it can cause blood dyscrasia).

Phenylbutazone (Butazolidine); Oxyphenbutazone (Tanderil)

Pharmacokinetics Phenylbutazone is almost completely absorbed when given orally. Phenylbutazone has a small apparent volume of distribution (approximately 120 ml/kg) and is about 98 % bound to plasma proteins when it is given in low doses. With high doses the binding sites become saturated and the fraction of bound drug decreases. This means that a relatively small increase in dosage (say from 200 mg to 600 mg daily will cause a considerable increase in the amount of free drug in the plasma and in the incidence of side effects. The steady-state plasma concentration in subjects receiving repeated administrations of the drug do not show a linear relationship (see Fig. 10.5) above doses of 100 mg/day. This is because at higher doses the proportion of

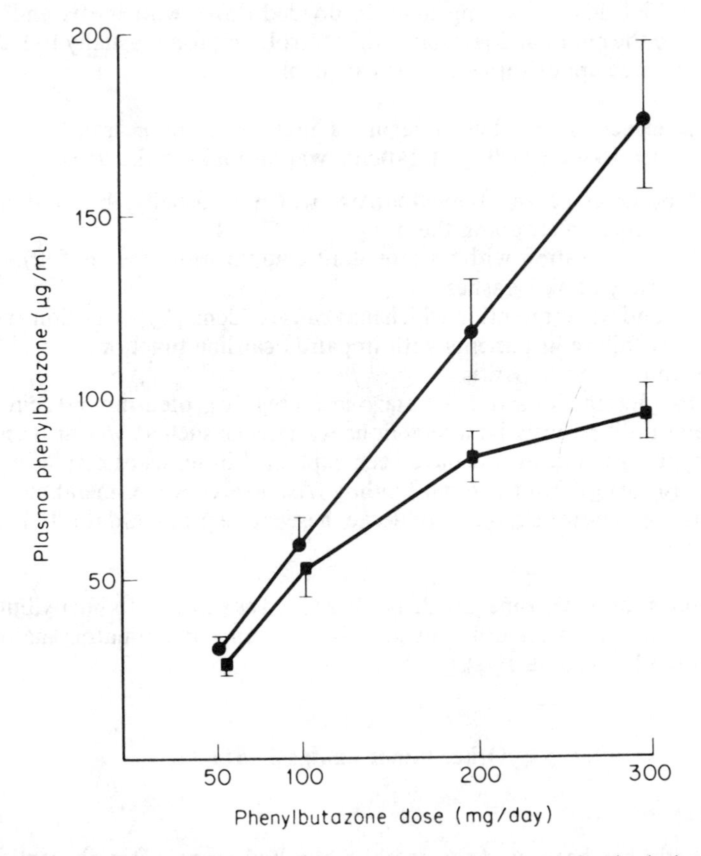

Fig. 10.5 Predicted phenylbutazone plasma concentration on the assumption that it obeys linear kinetics (●) and observed plasma levels (■) after dosing to steady state with different doses of drug in seven patients (From M. L'E. Orme *et al.*, *Brit. J. Clin. Pharm.*, **3**, 185 (1976).)

phenylbutazone free in plasma is greater and the apparent volume of distribution larger so that the plasma level falls relative to the increase in dose. Doses of 800 mg and 1600 mg daily for 3 weeks give the same steady-state level, although the plasma $t_{1/2}$ is similar at both dose levels. The metabolic clearance is therefore also increased.

Phenylbutazone is extensively metabolised in the liver, the most important reactions being glucuronide formation and hydroxylation to oxyphenbutazone which has similar properties to phenylbutazone. The $t_{1/2}$ is 56–86 h and it takes about 3 weeks to reach steady state.

No consistent relationship has been demonstrated between the plasma level of phenylbutazone and its clinical or toxic effects.

Clinical uses Although phenylbutazone is a powerful anti-inflammatory agent, it is a rather weak analgesic. It also has some uricosuric action. Serious side effects (see below) are frequent and in the UK its use is restricted to hospitals where it still has some place in the treatment of ankylosing spondylitis.

The initial dose is 400 mg daily in divided doses with meals and this is reduced to the minimal dose which will control symptoms, usually 100–200 mg daily. 250 mg suppositories are also available.

Adverse effects Phenylbutazone has a number of unpleasant side effects which affect about 10–20% of patients who are taking the drug.

1. Depression of the bone marrow which is usually, but not always, reversible on stopping the drug.
2. Peptic ulceration with its attendant complications (see p. 532).
3. A variety of skin rashes.
4. Salt and water retention which may cause oedema, hypertension and even heart failure in patients with impaired cardiac function.
5. Jaundice and hepatitis.
6. Drug interactions: phenylbutazone is a highly protein-bound acidic drug and until recently its interactions with drugs such as warfarin and oral hypoglycaemic agents have been explained in terms of displacement of these drugs from protein-binding. A more complex metabolic explanation is now believed to underlie these interactions and this is discussed on p. 596.

Azapropazone/feprazone are distantly related chemically to phenylbutazone but have a somewhat different spectrum of anti-inflammatory activity in animal models (Table 10.2).

Other minor analgesic drugs

Phenacetin

Phenacetin has been used for nearly a hundred years. After absorption it is largely metabolised to paracetamol and some minor metabolites. The plasma $t_{1/2}$ is 35–105 min.

Table 10.2

Approved Name	*Proprietary name*	$t_{1/2}$ (*h*)	*Protein binding*	*Dose*	*Side effects and special features*
Azapropazone	Rheumox	20	98 %	300 mg 6–8 hourly	Gastrointestinal disturbances Rashes May potentiate warfarin Salt and water retention, uricosuric and is effective in acute gout.
Feprazone	Methrazone	–	–	200 mg 8 hourly	As above

It is an effective analgesic and antipyretic. In the 1950s it became apparent that the prolonged use of analgesic/anti-inflammatory drugs in high doses was associated with renal damage of a fairly characteristic type which was named 'analgesic nephropathy' (see below). Phenacetin may also produce haemolytic anaemia in G6PD deficiency and methaemoglobinaemia. Because of these problems it has now been withdrawn in the UK.

Paracetamol

This is derived from phenacetin and has analgesic and antipyretic properties but is not anti-inflammatory and has no effect on platelets or blood-clotting mechanisms. Its site of analgesic action is incompletely understood. It is a weak inhibitor of some peripheral cyclo-oxygenases and is as potent as aspirin in inhibition of the brain cyclo-oxygenase. It has therefore been suggested that a central site of action is involved. It is anti-pyretic, presumably due to its effects on brain prostaglandins.

Pharmacokinetics Absorption of paracetamol following oral administration is rapid and has been comprehensively investigated. The absorption rate and relative bioavailability are increased by concomitant administration of metoclopramide and there is a significant relationship between gastric emptying and absorption. Diurnal variations in the absorption rate, with reduced absorption at night, have been demonstrated. A high carbohydrate meal reduces absorption, whereas exercise increases absorption rate. Paracetamol is rapidly metabolised in the liver and has a plasma $t_{1/2}$ of 75–180 min. The major metabolites are sulphate and glucuronide, which are excreted in the urine in proportion of about 25% and 75% of the dose accompanied by 1–4% unchanged drug. When paracetamol is taken in overdose the capacity of these conjugating mechanisms is exceeded and a reactive metabolite is formed which produces hepatocellular damage (see p. 868). Under these circumstances the plasma $t_{1/2}$ is prolonged, liver damage being likely if it exceeds 4 h and coma being almost invariable if it is greater than 12 h. Paracetamol is 25–50% bound to plasma proteins and is evenly distributed throughout the body.

Clinical uses Paracetamol is a mild analgesic with antipyretic effects but little, if any, anti-inflammatory properties. It has no irritant effect on the gastric mucosa. It may therefore be employed in place of aspirin although it is by no means without its own specific problems and it should not be regarded as a universal aspirin substitute. It is useful in paediatrics since, unlike aspirin, it can be formulated into a stable suspension which is pleasing to children. The usual adult dose is 0.5–1 g (1–2 tablets) repeated at 4–6 hourly intervals to maintain analgesia.

Adverse effects Drug rashes, methaemoglobinaemia and blood dyscrasias have been occasionally reported but the evidence for nephrotoxicity is slim (see below). The most important toxic effect is liver damage which occurs after overdose and is considered on p. 868. Rarely it can cause chronic active hepatitis.

Analgesic nephropathy

Non-narcotic analgesics have been used for many years: phenacetin was introduced in 1887, paracetamol in 1893 and aspirin in 1899. It was not, however, until 1953 that post-mortem studies revealed an increased incidence of chronic renal disease with papillary necrosis, interstitial fibrosis and tubular atrophy. These changes correlated with a high consumption of non-narcotic analgesic drugs. At that time, in certain countries, particularly on the European mainland, the habit had emerged of taking mixtures, usually containing phenacetin, caffeine and other analgesics, for a variety of minor ailments and as an aid to dealing with the stresses of life. Abuse of these drugs, which could be obtained easily over the counter, escalated until huge quantities were being consumed by some individuals. Since then this relationship between analgesic abuse and renal disease has been confirmed throughout the world. Its incidence varies widely from country to country, being particularly high in Scandinavia, South Africa and Australia, where it is the second most common cause of end-stage renal disease and responsible for about one-fifth of all renal transplants. In the UK it is relatively uncommon, being responsible for only 1–2% of transplants. The reasons for these differences in geographical distribution are unknown. It has been suggested that it may be due to genetic differences in drug response. In South Africa and Australia dehydration may be a factor since this increases renal damage in animals.

Although there has been a considerable amount of work to identify the causative agent and elucidate the pathogenesis, the problem is not completely solved. The main difficulties are:

(a) Several analgesics are often taken together as a mixture, making it difficult to identify the culprit.
(b) The usual problem of relating the results of animal experiments to man.

Phenacetin was originally thought to be the causative agent, but more recently it has been realised that other minor analgesics can be nephrotoxic and may also be implicated. The drugs most frequently involved are:

1. *Phenacetin*: About 80% of administered phenacetin is metabolised to paracetamol but a number of other metabolites are formed by deacetylation and hydroxylation which could be toxic to the kidney. A manufacturing contaminant, acetic-4-chloranilide, has also been implicated but the evidence is slight. In man it has been calculated that about 1.0 g of phenacetin daily for three years is required before nephropathy develops, but many subjects can take much more without adverse effects.

2. *Paracetamol*: This is the main metabolite of phenacetin. In animals large doses (up to 7.0 g/kg/day) only produce minor tubular changes. In dehydrated dogs, however, a concentration gradient develops between the medulla and papilla, similar to that found for sodium. It is tempting to believe that the high paracetamol concentration achieved in the renal papilla also occurs in man and is responsible for papillary necrosis, but the epidemiological evidence implicating paracetamol in producing nephropathy in man is weak.

3. *Aspirin*: Prolonged administration of large doses of aspirin (500 mg/kg/day) to animals causes papillary necrosis and renal fibrosis, although, unlike paracetamol, there is no medullary/papillary aspirin concentration

gradient. The mechanism which produces these changes is unknown but aspirin inhibits prostaglandin synthesis and prostaglandins act as vasodilators in the kidney. Possibly this interferes with the blood supply to the loops of Henle. Aspirin uncouples oxidative phosphorylation which also promotes renal damage. In man, aspirin in doses of .6 g daily produces a shower of renal tubular epithelial cells in the urine. These cells are shed largely by the proximal tubule, however, and their relevance to the development of papillary necrosis is doubtful.

Although acute renal failure can occur with aspirin overdosage, this situation is complicated by the general toxic effects of aspirin and dehydration. The hypothesis that aspirin taken alone is an important cause of chronic renal damage in man is not established.

4. *Analgesic mixtures*: There is accumulating evidence that analgesic mixtures are more likely to produce renal damage than single agents. This is not surprising in view of the many ways outlined above in which these drugs can affect the kidney and a combination of direct cytotoxicity and altered blood flow could produce analgesic nephropathy.

Renal changes in man The early and essential lesion in analgesic nephropathy is papillary necrosis associated with medullary fibrosis and tubular atrophy. The cortex is relatively spared. Initially the kidneys are not decreased in size but as the disease progresses, shrinkage occurs. Inflammatory changes are absent unless infection is superimposed. About one-third of patients with analgesic nephropathy show evidence of renal infection. In these patients infection may contribute to progressive deterioration in renal function. It is not, however, the initial cause of the disease and progressive renal damage from analgesics can certainly occur in its absence.

Clinical course Analgesic nephropathy occurs most commonly in middle-aged women who have had heavy consumption of analgesics over several years. This is more likely to be due to some form of dependence on the drugs than to ordinary medical reasons such as treatment of chronic arthritis. Many patients are unwilling to admit to taking analgesics and the history may therefore be difficult to elicit.

The disease presents with progressive renal failure, hypertension is a common feature and the course may be punctuated by recurrent episodes of infection. Sometimes the onset is sudden with acute papillary necrosis causing colic and haematuria. Anaemia is common, not only due to renal failure but also from chronic gastric blood loss caused by aspirin. There is moderate proteinuria together with casts and red and white cells. As the disease advances the glomerular filtration rate progressively falls and the ability to concentrate and acidify the urine is lost relatively early. Pyelography may show detachment of the papillae or outline of spaces formed by the disappearance of the pyramids. Occasionally the papillae are calcified.

Treatment Analgesics must be stopped. This prevents further deterioration of renal function and sometimes function may improve. Treatment is otherwise symptomatic.

Prevention Phenacetin has been banned in the UK. This step is unlikely to abolish analgesic nephropathy entirely as other analgesics are probably implicated. Although newer anti-inflammatory drugs have not been shown to cause nephropathy, their mode of action on prostaglandin synthesis suggests that this is a possibility. It would be wise to keep an open mind until more information is available.

The occasional taking of minor analgesics is very unlikely to cause renal damage. Although results are conflicting, retrospective studies of patients in the UK treated with minor analgesics over long periods for rheumatoid arthritis and allied conditions suggests that these patients do not have a high incidence of renal failure. The reason for this must be that analgesic mixtures are not commonly used for this purpose and, although quite large doses are given, they are not as high as in patients who abuse these drugs. It seems reasonable, therefore, to continue to treat such patients with single minor analgesics but to avoid mixtures, and to remember the possibility of nephropathy. Particular care should be taken with patients who already have renal disease and those liable to develop papillary necrosis such as diabetics.

DRUGS WHICH SUPPRESS THE RHEUMATOID PROCESS

The following drugs are not analgesics but they appear to suppress the inflammatory process in rheumatoid arthritis. Except for the steroid hormones their action is not dramatic but they have a part to play in the management of some patients with rheumatoid arthritis. They are not effective unless there is evidence of active disease. Their mode or modes of action are not fully understood.

Gold salts (Chrysotherapy)

Gold was originally introduced as an agent which was thought to be effective against the tubercle bacillus but although having little, if any, therapeutic action in tuberculosis, it was found to be antirheumatic and is now used mainly in the treatment of rheumatoid arthritis.

Gold has a number of actions which could be responsible for its effects in rheumatoid arthritis. It inhibits prostaglandin synthesis and lysosomal enzymes and it binds to immunoglobulin and complement. It is not known which, if any, of these actions is important therapeutically.

Pharmacokinetics Gold compounds are poorly and irregularly absorbed from the intestine and must therefore be given by intramuscular injection. It becomes bound to plasma proteins and the plasma half-life increases with repeated administration and may vary from one day to several weeks. Its distribution in the body is complex but it appears to be concentrated in inflamed areas. It is mainly excreted in the urine and a small amount is lost in the faeces. Total clearance from the body takes a very long time and after a course of gold treatment, gold is excreted in the urine for up to one year.

Clinical uses Gold is used in courses of weekly deep intramuscular injections but the optimal dose is still not settled. Sodium aurothiomalate is given:

Week 1 1.0 mg
2 5.0 mg
3 10.0 mg
4 50.0 mg injections weekly until a total of 1.0 g has been given.

Thereafter 50.0 mg should be given monthly to a total of 3.0 g. Further maintenance treatment can be given. A therapeutic response will not be seen for 4–8 weeks after starting treatment.

Gold therapy should not be undertaken lightly because of its toxicity. It is recommended for seropositive cases of rheumatoid arthritis with persistent disease of moderate severity following adequate trial of non-steroidal anti-inflammatory drugs. About 75% of patients will improve with reduction in joint swelling, disappearance of rheumatoid nodes and a fall in ESR.

Adverse effects from gold can be troublesome and sometimes dangerous. Some adverse effect occurs in up to 50% of patients: in half of these effects are severe. They are associated with HLA antigen DR3.

(a) *Skin rashes* are an indication for stopping treatment as exfoliation can occur. Photosensitive eruptions, urticaria and erythematous reactions have been reported. They may be preceded by itching.
(b) *Renal damage*, which takes the form of a nephrotic syndrome. Gold should not be used in patients with renal disease. Urine should be tested before each gold injection and if more than a trace of protein is present, gold must not be given. The urine is then tested one week later and treatment not resumed until the urine is protein free. It is best to restart at a lower dose.
(c) *Blood dyscrasias* may occur suddenly and in spite of routine blood counts. They should be treated with steroids, antibiotics and transfusion if necessary, and dimercaprol (see p. 867).
(d) *Stomatitis*.
(e) Rarely patients complain of an *exacerbation of symptoms* after each injection.

Oral gold A gold preparation (Auranofin) is now available for oral use. It is poorly absorbed from the gastrointestinal tract producing lower plasma levels than after injection. The $t_{1/2}$ is 10–30 days.

Clinical use The dose is 3.0 mg twice daily and it is perhaps a little less effective than parenteral gold.

Adverse effects Diarrhoea is the commonest, other adverse effects are similar to those for parenteral gold but less common.

Penicillamine

Penicillamine is the name given to an amino acid β, β-dimethylcysteine found in penicillin hydrolysates. The drug has been used in a wide variety of conditions including Wilson's disease, cystinuria, lead poisoning, chronic active hepatitis, morphoea, and scleroderma. More recently, however, it has found a place in the management of rheumatoid arthritis..

There are several actions of penicillamine including metal chelation, but in rheumatoid arthritis and other autoimmune states it appears to dissociate certain macroglobulins. It may also inhibit release of lysosomal enzymes in connective tissue. Controlled clinical trials have demonstrated the benefit of the drug on severe uncontrolled rheumatoid arthritis and it is probably of equal potency to gold therapy.

Pharmacokinetics The drug is well absorbed from the gut in the fasting state. Iron interferes with absorption. Initially there is rapid excretion of a number of metabolites of penicillamine, but some of the active substance is tightly bound to plasma proteins and tissues and is slowly excreted over several months.

Clinical uses The drug is given orally between meals and is now given in amounts lower than hitherto. The initial dose is 250 mg daily, and the first increment of 250 mg daily is made only after 8 weeks. Further increments are made even more slowly and the maximum dose is usually 750 mg daily. Even smaller maintenance doses are at present under trial. Improvement starts after a few weeks and reaches a maximum in about six months. Results are similar to those obtained with gold.

Initially weekly blood and urine tests are carried out, and then monthly during maintenance treatment. The tests should include platelets and white counts and urine protein and blood screening.

Adverse effects These are common with penicillamine and can be dangerous. They are associated with the poor sulphoxidation phenotype (see p. 110).

(a) *Bone marrow hypoplasia:* Thrombocytopenia is common. If it occurs, treatment must be stopped and recovery usually occurs within two weeks. Penicillamine may then be started at a lower dose. If further thrombocytopenia occurs, the drug must be abandoned. Leucopenia is less common and is an indication for stopping the drug. Full blood count with platelets is necessary every two weeks for the first three months of treatment and then at monthly intervals.

(b) *Proteinuria*: Mild proteinuria is common and occurs in 30% of patients. If it occurs the drug should be stopped until the urine clears and then treatment resumed at a lower dose. Heavy proteinuria is an indication to give up the drug.

(c) Other side effects include *mammary hyperplasia*, *haemolytic anaemia*, *mucous membrane ulceration*, *systemic lupus erythematosus*, *myasthenic syndrome* and *loss of taste* which usually appears early and may disappear with continued treatment.

The toxicity of penicillamine is such that it can only be used confidently by clinicians with experience of the drug who are willing to follow up patients meticulously. Some patients derive no benefit from the drug, others respond for several months and then relapse. These may respond again if the dosage is further increased, but not necessarily so. This late-acquired resistance to penicillamine does not occur in Wilson's disease when the drug is administered chronically and so its cause does not therefore result from any change in penicillamine kinetics.

Chloroquine (see p. 757)

This antimalarial 4-aminoquinoline has been found to have beneficial effect in rheumatoid arthritis comparable with gold. It is also used in systemic lupus erythematosus. The mode of action is uncertain. It is not analgesic or anti-inflammatory. Various mechanisms have been proposed and perhaps the most relevant is that chloroquine may stabilise lysosomal membranes which may therefore limit tissue damage by katabolic enzymes.

Clinical uses Like gold, chloroquine accumulates in the body slowly and whilst plasma concentrations are very variable and often low, progressive tissue binding occurs and it is this tissue binding with nucleoprotein and melanin which probably produces many of the toxic effects. Remission of symptoms in rheumatoid arthritis occurs after 2–3 months treatment with 75–300 mg chloroquine daily. Many toxic effects are known (see p. 757) but the most serious side effect of chloroquine is due to deposition of the drug in the uveal tract which leads to macular degeneration. This does not usually occur until treatment with 250 mg or more has been continued for over one year. An early symptom is the appearance of coloured haloes when the patient looks at a light. Patients having chloroquine should therefore either stop treatment after a year or have regular ophthalmic examinations.

Sulphasalazine (see p. 535)

This drug, whose major rôle is in the management of ulcerative colitis, was originally introduced for arthritis. Recent re-evaluations suggest that it is as effective as penicillamine in reducing disease activity used as a 'second-line' agent when NSAIAs have failed. In these cases it is not apparently acting as a NSAIA. In the doses required (0.5 g/day initially increasing to 2 g daily) it produces frequent side effects although it may still be less hazardous than gold or penicillamine. Further work is required to define its place in rheumatoid arthritis treatment.

Azathioprine

This immunosuppressive drug may be used in patients with resistant rheumatoid arthritis and in SLE and polymyositis.

Clinical use The usual starting adult dose is 100 mg daily. Allopurinol delays the breakdown of the drug and necessitates a reduction in the dose.

Side effects Bone marrow depression is the most common side effect and monthly blood counts are required. It rarely causes hepatitis and rashes. (See also p. 817).

Corticosteroids (see p. 634)

Steroids produce a rapid improvement in the symptoms of rheumatoid arthritis by virtue of their anti-inflammatory action. They do not, however, alter the course of the disease.

With prolonged use their side effects become troublesome (see p. 639). They may be given into the joint to try to minimise systemic side effects and this produces short-term relief of symptoms.

The use of drugs in rheumatoid arthritis

The treatment of rheumatoid arthritis by medication consists of deploying the available drugs to the best advantage, so a flexible approach is necessary.

The non-steroidal anti-inflammatory (NSAIA) drugs play a major part in controlling symptoms but do not alter the underlying disease process. There are certain general principles which apply to their use in rheumatoid and osteoarthritis:

1. There is considerable inter-person variation in the response to these drugs and if the symptoms have not improved after two weeks treatment it should be changed to another drug in the group.
2. There is little point in raising the dose as this does not usually increase efficacy but may increase toxicity – the exception is aspirin which is analgesic in low doses and becomes in addition anti-inflammatory in higher doses.
3. There is no advantage in giving more than one of these agents at a time.
4. In rheumatoid arthritis, stiffness and pain is often worse on rising. This can be relieved by using a long-acting drug or by giving a suppository last thing at night. Alternatively, a rapidly absorbed drug such as soluble aspirin or ibuprofen can be given first thing in the morning.
5. All NSAIAs have a gastric-irritant effect in some patients and should be given directly after meals. They should be avoided in patients with peptic ulceration or serious dyspepsia. If, however, they cannot be withheld, they may be combined with cimetidine or ranitidine. The less-powerful drugs such as low-dose ibuprofen may be preferred. Suppositories of indomethacin or naproxen can be used but even these can occasionally cause gastric bleeding.
6. NSAIAs can cause fluid retention and reverse the action of hypotensive drugs. They also cause some slight deterioration in renal function. This is usually of no importance but can be serious in patients with renal failure (see p. 290).
7. NSAIAs displace warfarin from its protein-binding sites and may precipitate bleeding, so careful control is necessary if they are used together and this should be regarded as a calculated risk. They can also increase the effects of oral hypoglycaemic agents.
8. A history of bronchospasm caused by an NSAIA should preclude the use of any drug in the group.
9. There is no consensus of opinion as to the best buy. Treatment may be started with a standard drug (i.e. aspirin or indomethacin) or with one of the cheaper more recent introductions which usually have a lower incidence of side effects.

When the disease is resistant and progressive in spite of these measures, the suppressive group of drugs may be added to the therapeutic regime, although side effects can be troublesome.

The place of steroid hormones in treatment has changed over the years. There is no doubt that they suppress the inflammatory process and produce rapid and dramatic relief. However, prolonged use may require escalation of the dose, and as the dose increases side effects become more and more prominent. They are now only used when other measures have failed and in the elderly where a rapid therapeutic response is required to prevent the patient becoming permanently bed-ridden. No patient should, however, be allowed to become permanently disabled without at least a trial of steroids being considered.

NARCOTIC ANALGESICS (OPIOIDS)

OPIOID RECEPTORS

Stereospecific receptors with a high affinity for opioid analgesics are present in neuronal membranes obtained from brain. They are found in high concentrations in the periaqueductal grey matter, the limbic system, the pulvina of the thalamus, the hypothalamus, medulla oblongata and the substantia gelatinosa of the spinal cord. In addition to opioids, narcotic antagonists (particularly naloxone) and certain analgesic peptides specifically bind to these receptors.

These peptides which are widely distributed throughout the nervous system are concerned with important neurological mechanisms. They can be divided into three groups:

1. The encephalins, leu-encephalin and met-encephalin, which contain five amino acids and differ in only one of them.
2. Dynorphins which are extended forms of the above and are more potent in binding to opioid receptors and more powerful analgesics.
3. Endorphins. These peptides are derived from larger precursors (pro-opiomelanocortin, pro-encephalin and pro-dynorphin) and may act as neurotransmitters or as longer-acting neurohórmones.

It would appear that there are several networks in the brain using opioid receptors with peptide neurotransmitters. The population of nerve cells within these networks is not cytochemically homogenous and at least three types of opioid receptors have been recognised.

μ receptors— Interact with morphine and similar opiates, and possibly met-enkephalin, and are blocked by naloxone. Cause miosis, bradycardia and central analgesia. Dependence, euphoria and respiratory depression are also produced.

κ receptors— Interact with morphine and possibly dynorphins.
Not blocked by naloxone.
Cause pupillary constriction, sedation and spinal analgesia.

σ receptors— Interact with pentazocine and possibly phencyclidine and leu-encephalin. Not blocked by naloxone. Cause dysphoria, hallucinations, respiratory and vasomotor stimulation.

The exact rôles played in man by these different networks has not been clarified nor has the relationship between the various peptide agonists and the differing populations of receptors.

Blocking opioid receptors with naloxone has little effect on normal individuals but in patients suffering from chronic pain it produces hyperalgesia. This suggests that a pre-existing stimulus is required to activate the pain-inhibiting function of the opioid system.

Electrical stimulation of areas of the brain rich in encephalins and opioid receptors (such as the periaqueductal and periventricular grey matter), elicits analgesia which is abolished by naloxone. Thus such electrically induced analgesia is probably due to liberation of endogenous opioid peptides. Of particular interest is the observation that physical and emotional stress can produce analgesia which is reversed by naloxone. The evolutionary significance of these systems might be a mechanism whereby an adaptation could be made to adverse environments and allow the individual to continue functioning (and perhaps escape to a more friendly environment) activated by increased secretion of encephalins within the brain.

In clinical medicine otherwise intractable pain can be ameliorated by electrical stimulation of the periventricular or periaqueductal grey matter using implanted electrodes. Also pain relief by acupuncture may be mediated by encephalin release, because it is antagonised by naloxone. β-endorphin has been successfully used as an analgesic when administered to patients suffering from the pain of terminal cancer. In animals endorphins produce dependence and tolerance in the same way as opioids.

Narcotic analgesics are believed to exert their effects by entering the brain and binding to opioid receptors. The resulting pattern of pharmacological activity will depend on their affinity for the various receptors and whether they are simple or partial agonists. Important evidence to support this was the discovery that the receptor affinities of all narcotic analgesics which have been tested parallel their analgesic potency.

In addition to their involvement in brain function the opioid peptides may well play a neuro-endocrinological rôle. Administration in man suppresses the pituitary-gonadal and pituitary-adrenal axis and stimulates the release of prolactin, TSH and growth hormone.

In addition, high concentrations of opioid peptides are found in the sympathetic ganglia and in the adrenal medulla. Their function has not been elucidated but they may play an inhibitory rôle in the sympathetic system.

Following repeated administration of an exogenous narcotic, the sensitivity of the receptors may decrease and thus necessitate increases in dose to produce a constant effect. On sudden withdrawal of the drug, endogenous opioids are not sufficient to stimulate the insensitive receptors and this may be the physiological basis for the initiation of the withdrawal state. Autonomic disturbances occur because of a failure of the normal inhibition that the endogenous opioid system exerts on the hypothalamus.

Because the distribution of opioid receptors in the brain is not only in the main pain pathways but also in the limbic system (which is involved in emotional responses) the possibility that encephalins are disturbed in psychiatric disease is being investigated. Increased levels of β-endorphin have been found in the CSF of schizophrenics and in manic patients. Also in animals catatonia has been produced following intraventricular injection of β-endorphin. In the light of these observations, naloxone has been used in schizophrenics. Although conflicting reports have been made of the efficacy of such treatment, the weight of evidence at present suggests that with adequate doses naloxone can be of some benefit in this disease. In hypomanic patients naloxone reduces the level of euphoria.

There are preliminary reports that the portions of the β-lipotrophin molecule which lack analgesic activity appear to be antipsychotic and improve schizophrenia.

Opium

This is derived from the dried milky juice exuded by incised seed capsules of the poppy *Papaver somniferum* which is grown largely in Turkey, India and S. E. Asia. As long ago as the third century BC its medicinal properties were recognised. Homer refers to it in the Odyssey as 'nepenthes', a drug given to Odysseus and his followers 'to banish grief or trouble of the mind'. Sydenham introduced laudanum (tincture of opium) into English medicine in the 17th century and wrote that 'few would be willing to practice medicine without opium'. Osler referred to it as 'God's own medicine'. Opium is a complex mixture of alkaloids, the principal components being morphine (9–17%), codeine (0.5–4%), noscapine (2–9%), papaverine (0.5–%1) and thebaine (0.1–0.8%). Morphine is by far the most powerful and so the actions of opium are those of morphine.

Morphine

Actions of morphine within the CNS

Analgesia Morphine relieves nearly all types of pain, but is most effective when the pain is prolonged rather than occurring in short-lived spasms.

There are two aspects to the suffering caused by pain: firstly there is the appreciation of the painful stimulus itself, then there is the reactive anguish which follows this appreciation. The mental reaction to pain is very variable and is considerably influenced by the circumstances in which the pain is felt. Fear, depression and preoccupation with the pain will all tend to exacerbate its apparent severity whereas elation or an intense interest in something else can reduce and sometimes completely abolish the awareness of pain. This is one reason why it is notoriously difficult to relate the results obtained from testing an analgesic on normal volunteers using experimentally produced pain to its effectiveness in the clinical context.

Morphine appears to relieve both aspects of the suffering from pain and this is the main reason why it is so useful in medical practice. In terms of experimental pain, morphine has some effect in raising the threshold, although this is not as marked as might be expected. In addition, morphine increases pain tolerance so that the sensation is not unpleasant and no longer produces suffering. This is very important in clinical medicine when a patient suffers severe pain as associated with serious illness or trauma and thus with anxiety. The relief of this aspect of suffering is a crucial part of the usefulness of the narcotic drugs. Euphoria may also occur in patients with clinical pain (and in addicts) but is less marked in normal subjects. Dependence upon morphine and tolerance to its effects is of great importance and is considered on p. 838.

Other suppressant central effects Morphine will produce drowsiness and, with larger doses, sleep. Unlike barbiturates there is no incoordination and little confusion. Overdose leads to coma. Morphine depresses the sensitivity of the respiratory centre to carbon dioxide but not to hypoxia, thus causing a progressively decreased respiratory rate. This effect is dose-related, but certain categories of patient are more susceptible to this action and include those with decreased respiratory reserve from asthma, bronchitis, emphysema and hypoxia. Bronchoconstriction occurs, usually only to a minor degree, which is mediated by histamine release. This is only marked in asthmatics, in whom morphine is best avoided because of its depressant effect on the respiratory centre. Morphine also depresses the cough centre and for this reason has been used in small doses to treat a troublesome cough. Cough suppression does not involve the endorphin receptor and this property of opiates is not stereo-specific, so that d-isomers, e.g. dextromethorphan, are effective antitussives.

Central stimulating actions Morphine causes vomiting in 10–15% of patients by stimulation of the chemoreceptor trigger zone. For this reason it may be combined with a phenothiazine (see p. 562) such as prochlorperazine 12.5 mg by injection. This action is not mediated by the endorphin receptor but appears to involve dopaminergic receptors.

Fits may be provoked by morphine.

Morphine causes pupillary constriction by stimulating the Edinger–Westphal nucleus in the midbrain. This action is not of pharmacological importance but provides a useful diagnostic sign in narcotic overdosage.

Morphine releases ADH but inhibits ACTH, FSH and LH release.

Actions of morphine outside the CNS

Cardiovascular system Morphine dilates capacitance and resistance vessels by both neurally and locally mediated mechanisms. The former results from withdrawal of efferent sympathetic vasoconstrictor discharge causing attenuation of the tonic α-adrenergic stimulation of the peripheral circulation. Morphine also causes peripheral histamine release and thus vasodilation. In some patients it may also cause bradycardia due to stimulation of the vagal centre in the medulla. If this effect becomes dangerous (as may occur in the period immediately following a cardiac infarct), it can be reversed by giving atropine.

Gastrointestinal and urinary tracts Morphine increases the muscle tone throughout the gastro-intestinal tract, which is combined with decreased peristalsis. This is believed to result from an action on the ganglion plexus in the gut wall. The result is constipation with a hard dry stool and for this reason morphine is used in the symptomatic relief of diarrhoea. The increase in muscle tone also involves the sphincter of Oddi. In therapeutic doses morphine causes a variable rise in intrabiliary pressure which may last for 2–3 h. Increased blood lipase and amylase levels may occur.

In man its effect on the smooth muscle of the ureters is variable, but there may be some increase in tone. There is also some evidence that labour may be prolonged by morphine but its effect on uterine contraction is inconsistent.

Pharmacokinetics Like other organic bases opiates are well absorbed from peripheral sites by diffusion and morphine can be given orally or by subcutaneous, intramuscular or intravenous injection. After intramuscular injection the peak therapeutic effect is achieved in about 1 h and it lasts for 3–4 h (Fig. 10.6). The duration of this action depends on the dose of morphine and upon the severity of the pain. 4 hourly dosage may be required to control severe pain whereas 6 or 8 hourly dosage may suffice in lesser cases.

Morphine is metabolised largely by combination with glucuronic acid but also by N-dealkylation and oxidation, about 10% being excreted in the urine as morphine and 60–70% as the glucuronide. It has long been considered that this takes place mainly in the liver and gut wall and in an investigation of patients with cancer having long-term oral treatment its bioavailability was found to be between 16 and 64%. In addition, for an individual, the dose/plasma relationship for morphine and its main metabolite is linear over a wide range of oral dosage and independent of the duration of treatment. There is also a strong clinical impression that patients with liver disease are particularly sensitive to the actions of morphine. This is unlikely to be the whole story—it is now recognised that those with renal failure are also sensitive to the drug and that morphine clearance is closely related to both plasma creatinine and creatinine clearance. The part played by the kidney in morphine metabolism is not known but it is possible that the tubules are capable of glucuronidation. Morphine is a base and a sufficient amount of the undissociated molecule exists at pH 7.4 to penetrate cells so that it disappears rapidly from the circulation. Thus blood levels are low whilst the drug becomes

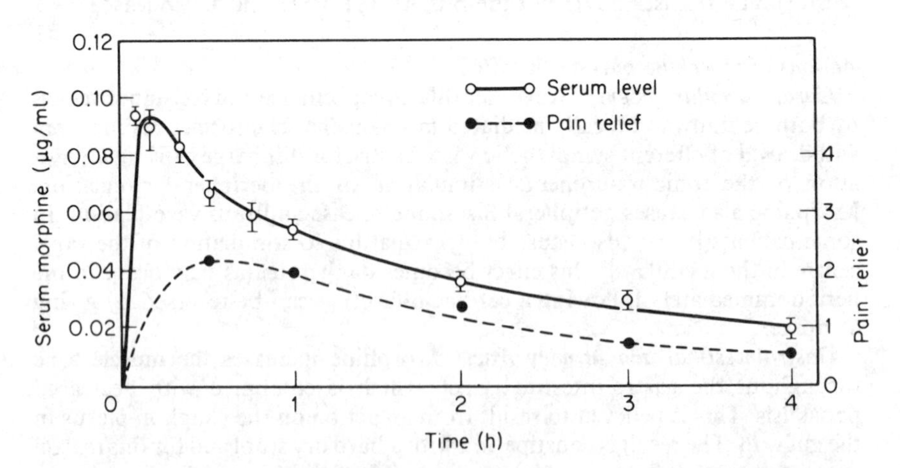

Fig. 10.6 Relationship of serum morphine concentration (after 10 mg/70 kg morphine sulphate intramuscularly) and analgesia in surgical patients. Note that analgesic effect lags behind serum concentration. Analgesia assessed on subjective score of: 0, none; 1, slight; 2, moderate; 3, lots; 4, complete. (From B. A. Berkowitz *et al.*, *Clin. Pharm. Ther.*, **17**, 629 (1975).)

concentrated in the tissues, especially liver, kidney, lung, muscle and spleen. The plasma level of morphine depends upon its redistribution back into the blood from this peripheral compartment, as well as an enterohepatic circulation. It is possible to construct multiphasic plasma concentration–time curves which require the postulation of several pharmacokinetic compartments. The distribution $t_{1/2}$ is about 2 min and the apparent volume of distribution is 3–4 times body weight indicating considerable tissue uptake. This is succeeded by other phases of variable $t_{1/2}$ and the elimination $t_{1/2}$ ranges from 18 to 60 h.

The birth of opiate-dependent babies born to addicted mothers demonstrates the ability of the drug to cross the placenta. The plasma protein binding of morphine is unusual in that it appears to be largely to globulin (rather than albumin) which has the characteristics of an immunoglobulin. Unlike diamorphine only small amounts of morphine cross the blood–brain barrier and its potent central effects reflect extraordinary receptor sensitivity.

Repeated doses lead to tolerance of morphine. This is largely due to the central nervous system becoming less sensitive to the action of the drug (see p. 315).

Clinical uses

1. *Pain* The most important use of morphine is for pain relief. For acute pain following injury, myocardial infarction or in the immediate postoperative period, the average adult will require 10 mg subcutaneously or intramuscularly repeated at 4–6 hourly intervals. A large patient suffering severe pain may need 15–20 mg.

Morphine may be given intravenously if rapid relief is required and the usual dose is 5.0 mg. Alternatively, it can be given continuously by an infusion pump. This method is very effective and relatively small doses are required to procure good analgesia.

Morphine is effective orally although rather larger doses may be needed owing to the first-pass effect. Oral morphine produces a smoother and more prolonged analgesic action and it is particularly useful in terminal malignant disease (see p. 323). It is usually given as an elixir of morphine, the dose and frequency of administration depending on the severity of the pain. Morphine is also available as a sustained release preparation (MST Continus, 10, 30, 60 and 100 mg tablets) and twice daily dosage may be adequate.

2. *Premedication for anaesthesia* (see p. 353).

3. *Left ventricular failure* (see p. 385). Morphine is very effective in the relief of acute left ventricular failure. How this is achieved is still not known, but it seems probable that it is due to several actions including depression of the stretch reflexes from the lungs, lowering of the peripheral resistance and dilatation of the capacity vessels of the circulation, thus causing venous pooling (see p. 381). The dose is usually 10 mg by injection.

4. *Diarrhoea* The constipating action of morphine and other opiates makes them useful for treating diarrhoea. Morphine, usually in the form of tincture of opium, was widely used in the past but at present codeine phosphate 30 mg three times daily is preferred.

5. *Cough* Opiates suppress the cough reflex and many older cough

mixtures contained morphine. Codeine appears to be as effective and is preferable on other grounds.

Adverse effects

1. *Dependence* The most important ill effect of morphine is the rapid development of drug dependence. This is particularly liable to occur if the drug is used for the pleasurable feeling it produces rather than in a therapeutic context. Morphine produces both psychological and physical dependence. The subject is further considered on p. 838.

2. *Nausea and vomiting* occur in about 15% of subjects and are less likely to occur if the patient rests. It can be controlled by a phenothiazine anti-emetic (prochlorperazine 12.5 mg by injection or chlorpromazine 25–50 mg orally). *Constipation* occurs in 100% of patients and often requires the use of a laxative. Sedation is dose related and occurs in about 30% of patients on an average dose. *Nightmares* occurs in about 1% of patients and can be helped by haloperidol 2–4 mg at night.

3. *Respiratory depression* is not usually a problem when morphine is used to control pain in terminal cancer. It is dangerous in overdose and in patients who are unduly sensitive to the drug (see below).

4. *Acute retention* Patients with prostatic hypertrophy may suffer acute retention of urine as morphine increases the tone in the sphincter of the bladder neck.

5. *Allergic phenomena* These are rare but rashes and even acute anaphylaxis have been described.

Certain types of patient appear particularly sensitive to the pharmacological actions of morphine. These include the *very young*, the *elderly*, those with *chronic lung disease and patients with myxoedema*. In *chronic liver disease* it might be expected that morphine would be metabolised more slowly with resulting accumulation and signs of overdosage. However, if used carefully, practical experience suggests that it is not absolutely contraindicated. Similarly, its actions are prolonged in chronic renal failure. *Morphine should not be used during an attack of asthma.* Although sometimes successful it may cause a fatal respiratory arrest.

Interactions Morphine will augment the action of other central depressants (i.e. phenothiazines, tricyclic antidepressants and various hypnotics) and should not be combined with MAO inhibitors.

OTHER NARCOTIC ANALGESICS

During the last hundred years it has been realised that opium was not without disadvantages, particularly the development of dependence and other side effects. A great deal of work has gone into synthesising morphine analogues in the hope of producing a drug with the therapeutic actions of morphine but without its disadvantages. However, the analgesic action of narcotics appear to be closely related pharmacologically to their side effects and it is only recently that there has been some success in producing useful drugs which are more or less free from these problems. It is possible that with better understanding of the central action of narcotics and in particular the three-dimensional aspects of their structure–action relationship, new and better drugs will become available. However, it should be recalled that the history of developments in this field has not been encouraging in that morphine was introduced as a non-addictive alternative to opium and this in turn was superseded by heroin which was believed to be non-addicting. Newer drugs such as dextropropoxyphene and pentazocine which were originally thought to lack abuse potential are now known to possess such features.

Diamorphine (Heroin)

Diamorphine is diacetylmorphine. Its actions are similar to those of morphine although it is about 2.5 times more potent as an analgesic when given by injection. There is a clinical impression that side effects including vomiting are less common with heroin than with morphine and that it has a greater euphoric effect and is thus to be preferred in the management of terminal disease. This is not supported by evidence (see Fig. 10.7) and the drugs are very similar. Diamorphine is also said by some to have greater addictive potential than morphine and it is banned from use in the USA. Again this is unsupported by evidence.

Pharmacokinetics After *injection* diamorphine is hydrolysed (deacetylated) to form 6-acetylmorphine and morphine. Both diamorphine and 6-ac-

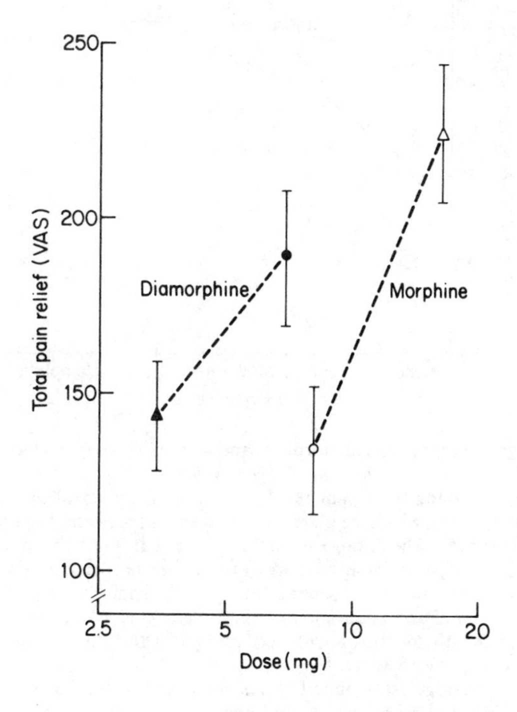

Fig. 10.7 (a)

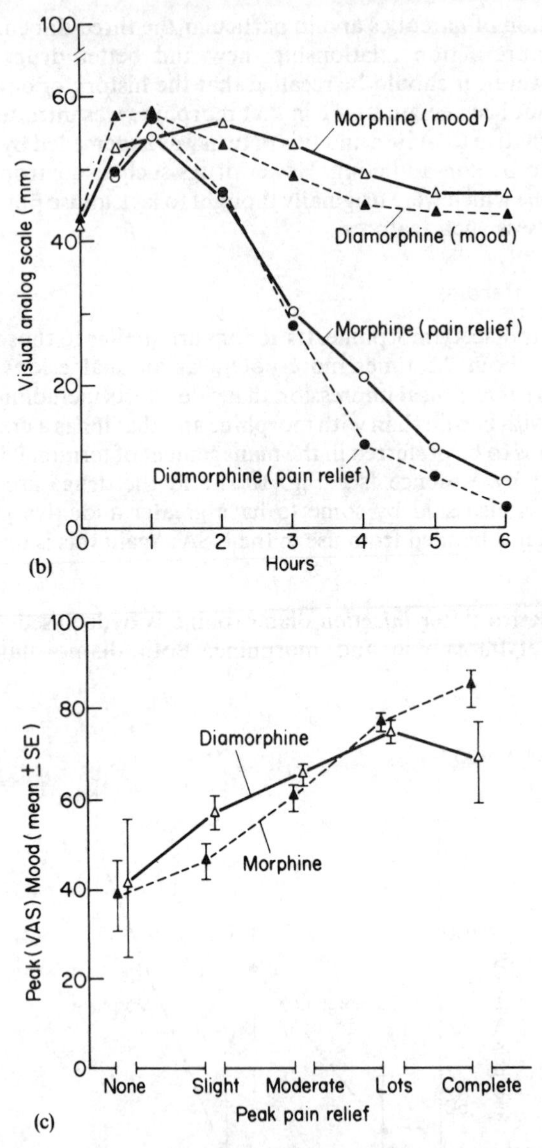

Fig. 10.7 Comparison of the actions of morphine and diamorphine (reproduced with permission from Kaiko R. F., *et al.* (1981). *New Eng. J. Med.* **305,** 1501.)
(a) Dose response curves for total pain relief as measured by visual analogue scale (VAS) consisting of a 100 mm line on which the patient marked a point between 'no relief' on the left and 'complete relief' on the right. The distance from the extreme left was the VAS score for that dose. 50 patients received the upper diamorphine dose (●) and lower morphine dose (○); another 50 received the lower diamorphine dose (▲) and the upper morphine dose (△).
(b) Time action curves for diamorphine and morphine. Pain relief VAS as for (a); Mood VAS was 'worst I could feel' on the left and 'best I could feel' on right. The distance from the extreme left to the patient's mark was the VAS score.
(c) Mean peak visual analogue scale mood scores associated with peak pain relief scores after diamorphine (solid line) and morphine (dashed line).

etylmorphine are metabolised very rapidly, the half-life of diamorphine after intravenous injection being about 3 minutes. This occurs in the liver and other organs including the brain. Morphine thus formed is, however, more slowly metabolised. Diamorphine and 6-acetylmorphine (which is pharmacologically active) enter the brain more rapidly and in greater amounts than morphine and thus account for the more rapid clinical effect of diamorphine, although the persistent effects are due to morphine formed in the CNS and elsewhere. 50–70% of the injected dose can be recovered from the urine, mostly in the form of conjugated morphine. After *oral administration* morphine only appears in the blood, presumably due to the considerable first-pass effect transforming both diamorphine and 6-acetylmorphine. Further the amount of circulating morphine after oral diamorphine is about 20% less than that obtained by an equivalent dose of oral morphine, suggesting that giving oral diamorphine is really an inefficient way of giving morphine.

Clinical uses Diamorphine is used for the same purposes as morphine. It can be given intravenously when it is effective within a few minutes, the dose being 2.5–5.0 mg. Given subcutaneously or intramuscularly, it is effective in about 15–20 minutes and the dose is usually 4–8 mg. It is more soluble than morphine and this may be an advantage if large doses are being given by injection.

It is also used orally, particularly in the management of terminal disease. It is effective within 30 minutes and is usually given as an elixir containing 5 mg diamorphine in 5 ml. The analgesic action lasts about 4 hours but depends on the severity of the pain and the dose. It can usefully be combined with prochlorperazine to control vomiting.

Adverse effects are as for morphine.

Analgesics in terminal disease

The relief of pain in terminal disease, usually cancer, requires careful use of analgesic drugs and there are certain rules to remember.

1. Use a large enough dose to relieve the pain completely.
2. Drug dependence is not a problem in this type of patient.
3. It is much easier and requires a smaller dose of the drug to keep the patient free from pain than to relieve pain and its attendant anxiety when it has fully developed. Therefore in chronic pain and terminal illness *regular administration is necessary*. In this context the relatively short duration of action of morphine and diamorphine must be remembered and the drug will probably have to be given at least four times daily. Strict adherence to 4 or 6 hourly injection regimes when the patient is requesting 3 hourly relief is inhumane and poor medicine.
4. If possible it is best to use oral medication. In addition to convenience this produces a smoother control of pain without peaks and troughs of analgesia.
5. Although tolerance to the analgesic action of the drug may develop it is not usually essential to escalate the dose to keep the patient comfortable.

A variety of analgesic drugs may be used depending on the severity of the pain and the preference of the patient and the physician. For mild pain paracetamol 1.0 g, aspirin 600 mg or tabs codeine co two tablets are usually satisfactory. Doses should be adjusted so that the patient is kept pain-free.

Rarely, *Buprenorphine*, 0.2–0.4 mg dissolved under the tongue is useful for more severe pain and it has the advantage of a rather longer action than most powerful analgesics. For short-term analgesia to cover dressings etc., *dextromoramide*, 5.0 mg orally or by injection is effective for 2–3 hours. *Diconal* (dipipanone + cyclizine) can be used orally but the cyclizine may make it rather sedative.

For severe pain *morphine* or *diamorphine* are the drugs of choice. They are given as elixirs or in aqueous solution. The dose will depend on the severity of the pain but it is usual to start with 5–10 mg of morphine or 4–8 mg of diamorphine and increase as required. The addition of cocaine to the elixir is of no benefit but chlorpromazine or prochlorperazine reduce vomiting and may increase analgesia. *Methotrimeprazine*, 25 mg three times daily can be used for the same purpose. Morphine is also available as *slow release tablets* (MST Continus) which last about 10 hours and are a useful substitute.

If night pain is a problem an *oxycodone* (30 mg) suppository gives relief for about 8 h. Doses should be adjusted so that the patient is kept pain-free. Rarely because of vomiting or the severity of the pain, morphine requires to be given by injection. Narcotic drugs are constipating and most patients require regular danthron or a similar aperient and sometimes suppositories. About 25% of patients with terminal cancer have some degree of endogenous depression. A trial of an antidepressant is worthwhile if this is suspected, but patients on opioids should be started on a low dose (i.e. imipramine 25 mg) which is increased as required.

Bone Pain There is some evidence that the pain caused by secondary deposits in bone is due to the release of prostaglandins. Various prostaglandin synthetase inhibitors have been used including aspirin up to 4.0 g daily or flurbiprofen 50 mg t.d.s. but results appear to be variable.

Intrathecal and epidural opioids

Injection of opioids intrathecally in animals produces local analgesia, presumably due to a direct effect on μ opiate receptors in the substantia gelatinosa of the spinal cord. This observation has now been extended to man. Opioid agonists can be injected intrathecally but this leads to a high incidence of side effects. Epidural injection is more satisfactory when presumably a small amount of opioid leaks into the CSF. It is probable that an epidural injection produces a combination of local and systemic effects due to some escape of the opioid into the circulation. Analgesia is more localised and lasts longer than with systemic administration alone and can be reversed by a local injection of naloxone. Analgesia occurs within 2–3 minutes of injection.

Side effects with epidural injection of opiates are:

Systemic— Respiratory depression
Nausea and vomiting
Somnolence and itching
Segmental— Urinary retention

The drugs used are:

Pethidine 25–100 mg

Fentanyl 100–200 mg
Morphine has a high incidence of systemic reactions.

Clinical use Epidural opioids have been used in a variety of acute and chronic pains and particularly in childbirth.

Pethidine

The actions of pethidine are in many ways similar to those of morphine. Although pethidine is often considered to be a weaker analgesic than morphine this is largely a matter of dosage, and if enough of the drug is given, effects equianalgesic with morphine can be obtained, 10 mg morphine intramuscularly being equivalent to 75 mg pethidine intramuscularly.

Pethidine in equianalgesic doses causes about the same degree of respiratory depression and smooth muscle spasm as morphine. It does not constrict the pupil or suppress cough but may cause vomiting. It produces little euphoria but may cause dependence.

Pharmacokinetics Pethidine can be given parenterally or by mouth. Although well absorbed from the gut there is a considerable first-pass hepatic metabolism (50 %) so that about double the parenteral dose is required to produce the same effect. Like many opioids the plasma concentration–time curve after oral dosing often shows a double peak, which may be interpreted as being due to either enterohepatic recycling or an effect of the drug on its own absorption mediated via its ability to delay gastric emptying and reduce gut motility. It is known that pethidine is also recycled back into the stomach from the circulation. Hepatic metabolism is the main elimination route, since less than 50 % is excreted unchanged in the urine. The major metabolites are the N-demethylated product, norpethidine and the hydrolysis product, pethidinic acid and its conjugates. Norpethidine, which only appears in the blood after multiple doses, is about half as active as an analgesic as pethidine but has twice its convulsant activity.

The $t_{1/2,\beta}$ of pethidine is 3–4 h and the initial $t_{1/2,\alpha}$ is about 10 min, indicating rapid extensive tissue distribution. The elimination $t_{1/2}$ is approximately doubled by cirrhosis and acute viral hepatitis. Higher plasma pethidine concentrations also occur in elderly patients and probably reflect decreased systemic clearance. Approximately 30 % of pethidine is free in plasma in younger patients but in the elderly this is increased to about 60 %. Taking these two factors together, the free pethidine concentration in patients over the age of 70 may be some four times higher than in younger patients. Therefore the initial parenteral dose used in the aged should not exceed 25 mg.

Pethidine is commonly used for obstetric analgesia as it is short acting. It can cross the placenta, and the placental blood may contain a higher concentration of pethidine than maternal blood. Pethidine or its metabolites may be responsible for respiratory depression of the neonate and this is exacerbated by the prolonged elimination $t_{1/2}$ in neonates of about 22 h (seven times longer than in healthy adults).

A correlation has been established between the plasma pethidine concentration and its pharmacological effects:

0.1–0.2 μg/ml	lethargy, dry mouth, tranquillisation;
0.2–0.4 μg/ml	mild analgesia, euphoria;
0.4 μg/ml	moderate analgesia;
0.5 μg/ml	marked respiratory depression;
0.6 μg/ml	potent analgesia.

Clinical uses Pethidine can be used in treating moderately severe pain, the usual dose being 25–100 mg parenterally or 50–150 mg orally. It is quite widely used in obstetrics as it does not appear to reduce the activity of the pregnant uterus during childbirth.

Drug interactions
(a) Monoamine oxidase inhibitors: a syndrome characterised by rigidity, hyperpyrexia, excitement, hypotension and coma has occurred when these drugs are given together. Its mechanism is unknown.
(b) Pethidine may, like other opiates, delay gastric emptying and intestinal transit time, thus interfering with the absorption of co-administered drugs.

Methadone

Methadone differs structurally from morphine but has very similar actions. Its analgesic action is about the same and it also causes respiratory depression and increases the tone of intestinal smooth muscle, but it produces rather less euphoria and drowsiness. It is a drug of dependence and can suppress the symptoms of morphine withdrawal.

Pharmacokinetics Although methadone is often given parenterally it is well absorbed after oral administration, and requires approximately double the parenteral dose to produce the same effect. After oral dosage, the peak blood level is achieved in about 4 h. It is 40% protein bound to albumin and the plasma $t_{1/2}$ is about 25 h. The metabolism of methadone seems rather variable, particularly with repeated doses, so that with prolonged administration accumulation can occur. This persistence of methadone in plasma is consistent with the slow onset and long duration of the abstinence syndrome occurring in subjects withdrawn from methadone.

Methadone is extensively metabolised, mainly in the liver, and the metabolites are excreted in the urine and sweat.

Clinical uses Methadone can be used for the relief of pain in a similar way to morphine. The dose is 5–10 mg by injection and its effect lasts from 4 to 6 h. There may be some local tissue reaction at the site of injection. If given orally the dose is 5–15 mg, and the onset of analgesia is delayed by about 45 min.

Methadone is also used to replace morphine and diamorphine when these drugs are being withdrawn in the treatment of drug dependence (see p. 842).

Phenazocine (Narphen)

This is an orally active analgesic which is approximately three times more potent than morphine and is useful for the rapid relief of severe pain. It is particularly useful in terminal care since it can be given orally or sublingually in doses of 5 mg (up to 20 mg is sometimes needed) to produce rapid analgesia lasting for 5–6 h. It can also be given by injection in doses of 1–2 mg and may be used in premedication, for postoperative pain and in obstetrics. It produces minimal sedation and tolerance is slow to develop.

Codeine

This is the methyl ether of morphine but (unlike diacetylmorphine) has only about one tenth of the analgesic potency of morphine. Although it is converted to morphine in the body before acting it produces little euphoria and is of low addiction potential. As a result it has been used for many years as an alternative to aspirin for treating less severe pain and as a cough suppressant.

Pharmacokinetics It can be given orally or by intramuscular injection. The oral : parental analgesic potency ratio is 1 : 1.5. Codeine itself has a plasma $t_{1/2}$ of 2.4 h but free morphine also exists in the plasma and it has been suggested that codeine acts as a slow-release prodrug (q.v.) producing low but sustained levels of morphine. The resulting morphine levels in the brain may be adequate to produce analgesia but inadequate to induce abuse.

Clinical uses

1. Analgesia as Codeine phosphate tablets B.P. (15, 30 and 60 mg) in doses of 15–60 mg up to 4 hourly. Many over-the-counter preparations containing codeine in combination are also available.
2. Cough suppression as Codeine linctus B.P.C. containing 15 mg codeine phosphate in a dose of 5 ml.
3. Diarrhoea is controlled using codeine phosphate tablets.

Adverse effects Constipation and nausea are the most commonly encountered problems.
Other opiates commonly used in practice appear in Table 10.3.

Dextropropoxyphene (Co-proxamol)

Dextropropoxyphene is similar structurally to methadone but it is a weaker analgesic. Although it is not at present classed by the WHO as a narcotic it has several properties in common with that group of drugs. It is well absorbed after oral administration and is partially metabolised and partially excreted in the urine. Its elimination half-life is 12–24 hours and the half-life of its active metabolite norpropoxyphene is 24–48 hours.

Dextropropoxyphene may be used alone as a mild analgesic in doses of 65 mg three or four times daily, but in the UK it is commonly combined with paracetamol as Co-proxamol (and other similar preparations), which contains 32.5 mg of dextropropoxyphene and 325 mg of paracetamol per tablet. Distalgesic is effective in the control of pain of moderate severity, the usual dose being one or two tablets. Although the combination is very widely used there is no clear evidence that it is superior to other mild analgesics given alone. Further, the disparity in half-lives of the two components may be a

Table 10.3 Other opioids in common use

Approved name	*Proprietary name*	*Dosage*	*Analgesic efficacy*	*Dependence liability*	*Special features*
Dextromoramide	Palfium	5–20 mg orally or by injection.	Equivalent to morphine.	Equivalent to morphine	Duration of action 2–3 h. Useful oral drug for severe pain of short duration.
Dihydrocodeine	DF118	30–60 mg orally or by injection.	Equivalent to codeine.	May occur particularly with high doses.	Mild to moderate pain. No good for dental pain. Constipating.
Dipipanone	Diconal (10 mg with cyclizine 30 mg)	10–25 mg intramuscularly. Diconal given orally.	25 mg equivalent to 10 mg morphine.	Equivalent to morphine.	Useful powerful analgesic which can be given orally.
Ethoheptazine	Combined with aspirin and meprobamate in Equagesic.	Not used alone.	Equivalent to codeine.	None.	For mild to moderate pain.

Table 10.3 (continued)

Approved name	*Proprietary name*	*Dosage*	*Analgesic efficacy*	*Dependence liability*	*Special features*
Levorphanol	Dromoran	1.5–3 mg orally. 2–4 mg by injection.	3–4 times that of morphine.	Equivalent to morphine.	Only clinically available member of the morphinan series. No advantages over morphine.
Papaveretum	Omnopon	10–20 mg orally or by injection.	Half as effective as morphine by weight.	Equivalent to morphine.	Contains total opium alkaloids standardised to equivalent of 50 % anhydrous morphine. Claimed to produce fewer side effects but evidence unconvincing.
Oxycodone	Proladone	30 mg as suppository at night	30 mg suppository = 20 mg morphine orally	Similar to morphine	Useful in producing night-long analgesia.

disadvantage when single doses are used but is less important with long-term administration.

Co-proxamol is not free from risk since overdose can be fatal particularly if alcohol is taken in addition (see p. 874).

Dextropropoxyphene in high doses produces euphoria and abuse and dependence may occur, although injection of the drug is limited by deleterious effects on soft tissue and veins at the site of injection. Dependent subjects may take larger doses of sometimes 1.0 g or more daily and symptoms may follow withdrawal.

Even Co-proxamol in therapeutic doses may cause drowsiness and light-headedness and therefore care must be taken with ambulant patients undertaking tasks such as driving which require concentration.

Analgesic mixtures

There are a large number of analgesic mixtures which usually contain aspirin or paracetamol combined with a mild opioid. There is some debate as to whether such mixtures are better than single drugs but they are widely used and often appear effective. Among those available are:

Aspirin & Codeine tablets Dispersible (Co-codaprin)	—Aspirin 400 mg codeine 8 mg
Codeine & Paracetamol tablets	—Codeine 8 mg paracetamol 500 mg
Dihydrocodeine & Paracetamol tablets (Co-dydramol)	—Dihydrocodeine 10 mg paracetamol 500 mg
Aspirin, Paracetamol & Codeine tablets	—Aspirin 250 mg paracetamol 250 mg codeine 6.8 mg
Equagesic tablets	—Ethoheptazine 75 mg meprobamate 150 mg aspirin 250 mg

OPIATE ANTAGONISTS

Minor alterations in the chemical structure of narcotic analgesics can produce substances which displace the narcotic drugs from their receptor sites and thus reverse their actions. Some of these substances are themselves weak agonists and can produce some of the actions of the narcotic drugs.

Naloxone (Narcan) (see p. 868)

Naloxone has no agonist action and therefore completely reverses the action of narcotics. In addition it is effective against pentazocine and dextropropoxyphene. It can be given intravenously or intramuscularly, the dose being 0.8–2.0 mg for the treatment of narcotic poisoning. Its effect is very rapid and if a satisfactory response has not been obtained in 3 min the dose may be repeated to a maximum of 10 mg. If the patient does not respond, the diagnosis of opioid overdose should be reconsidered. The action of some opioids (methadone, dihydrocodeine, dextropropoxyphene) may outlast those of naloxone which has a $t_{1/2}$ of an hour although its peak effect may only last 10 minutes and an infusion of up to 5 mg/hour may be needed. It can also be used to reverse the effects of morphine post-operatively, or in the management of the apnoeic infant after birth when the mother has received an opioid during labour. Naloxone can precipitate acute withdrawal symptoms in opiate-dependent patients.

Partial agonists

There are several drugs available which act as partial agonists at opioid receptors. Nalorphine is one of these but is now little used clinically.

The newer introductions are effective analgesics but seem only to have weak addictive properties. They are becoming increasingly used for the control of moderately severe or severe pain. Those which will be considered are listed below but there will no doubt be further introductions.

- Pentazocine
- Buprenorphine
- Nalbuphine
- Butorphanol
- Meptazinol

Pentazocine (Fortral)

Pentazocine is about half as effective as morphine as an analgesic. It produces some respiratory depression and sedation but less than morphine. It raises the systemic and pulmonary arterial blood pressure with a resulting increase in heart work. Therefore it is not a good drug to use when the heart is under stress (for example, immediately following a myocardial infarct).

It can be used to treat moderate to severe pain in doses of 30–60 mg by injection or 25–100 mg orally.

Pharmacokinetics Pentazocine can be given by injection but orally only 20% is available. After oral administration the peak blood level occurs in about 2 h. Pentazocine is extensively metabolised by oxidation in the liver and only a small percentage is excreted as glucuronide. The $t_{1/2}$ is about 2 h. Analgesic effect correlates with plasma levels and high plasma levels are associated with more side effects. There is a threefold inter-subject variation in urinary elimination of unchanged drug, and this is related to the state of enzyme induction of the individual: smokers metabolise 40% more pentazocine than non-smokers.

Adverse effects 7–10% of patients receiving pentazocine in usual therapeutic doses experience some form of central nervous system disturbance. Bizarre effects such as hallucinations, euphoria and feelings of depersonalisation have been reported. Dysphoria and nausea also occur but vomiting is less frequent than after administration of morphine. Although dependence is unusual it has been reported and withdrawal symptoms, generally milder than those of morphine, are known. If given to abusers of opiates with physical dependence pentazocine, because of its antagonist properties, may provoke a withdrawal syndrome.

The injection is irritant and changes of intramuscular site are necessary to prevent damage to subcutaneous tissues and skin.

Buprenorphine (Temgesic)

This has a more complex structure than morphine, being related to thebaine. A related drug is *diprenorphine* which is used in veterinary practice to produce a catatonic state for capture of wild animals or for surgery which can be reversed by naloxone. This drug has been used for suicide in man. Buprenorphine has powerful agonist activity but almost equivalent antagonist effects so that it has self-limiting opiate actions including a low liability to dependence.

Pharmacokinetics Like other opiates it is subject to a considerable hepatic first-pass metabolism if administered orally. It is metabolised by dealkylation and glucuronidation before excretion predominantly in the bile. The duration of pain relief may be a little longer than morphine (6–8 h after 0.4 mg given by intramuscular injection). Buprenorphine crosses the placental barrier and is not recommended in pregnancy until more is known of its effects.

Clinical uses The recommended dosage is 0.3–0.6 mg by slow intravenous or intramuscular injection repeated every 8 h for post-operative pain. It can also be given sublingually in doses of 0.2–0.4 mg and given this way is useful in controlling chronic pain of various types. When changing from buprenorphine to a pure opioid agonist such as morphine, large doses of morphine may be required initially to displace the buprenorphine on the opioid receptors.

Respiratory depression is rare except in patients with pre-existing carbon dioxide retention.

Adverse effects Because it has antagonist properties it can precipitate mild withdrawal symptoms in narcotic addicts.

Buprenorphine has few cardiovascular effects but sometimes causes drowsiness which may be potentiated by other central depressant drugs. Respiratory depression is less than with morphine but may occur if given in overdose. The effects of buprenorphine are not reversed by nalorphine but naloxone is effective in larger doses than usual (i.e. 4.0 mg). Doxapram (q.v.) is also useful to stimulate respiration in doses of 50–100 mg followed by 1.0 g by infusion over 6–8 h.

Euphoria has occasionally been observed and addicts find the subjective effects morphine-like. Chronic administration of buprenorphine blocks the subjective and pupillary responses to morphine and withdrawal of the drug causes mild abstinence syndrome. Physical dependence liability is low.

Meptazinol (Meptid)

This drug is related structurally to the opioids. However, it differs in that:

(a) It has only a weak affinity for opioid receptors.
(b) Binding sites are largely in the spinal cord and cortex.
(c) Its actions are only weakly inhibited by naloxone.

(d) It has less respiratory-depressing effect than morphine or pethidine. The dose ratio for respiratory depression compared with pethidine is 1 : 1.8.

It appears to be a rather unusual mixed agonist/antagonist at μ opioid receptors with possible action at other receptor sites.

Pharmacokinetics The $t_{1/2}$ of meptazinol is 2 h (only $3\frac{1}{2}$ h in the fetus), the drug being 95 % metabolised by the liver. Only 27 % is bound to the plasma protein. It is absorbed after oral dosage with a bioavailability of 9 % (due to the first-pass effect) and the peak blood level is reached after $1\frac{1}{2}$ h.

Clinical use It is a potent analgesic, 100 mg by injection being equivalent to 100 mg of pethidine or 10 mg of morphine. It is effective for about 3 h. It has proved useful in the control of post-operative pain and in obstetrics where its short half life in the fetus and relatively minor effect on respiration should prove useful. The usual dose is 75–150 mg by injection. Dependence potential is very low. It is also effective orally in doses of 200 mg 3–6 hourly.

Adverse effects Similar to opioids: nausea, vomiting and drowsiness.

Butorphanol (Stadol)

This is a partial agonist similar to buprenorphine but has a more rapid onset of effect and shorter duration of action (3–4 hours). It is more sedative than pentazocine.

Clinical use Similar to buprenorphine but more rapid effect. The dose is 1–4 mg and 2 mg = 10 mg of morphine.

Nalbuphine (Nubain)

This is a partial agonist. It is approximately equipotent with morphine but with a low dependence potential. The usual dose is 10–20 mg by injection.

Nefopam (Acupan)

This is a member of a new class of analgesics and is chemically unrelated to any other known analgesic, being a cyclised analogue of orphenadrine. Beyond its analgesic effects it shares no pharmacological properties with the non-steroidal anti-inflammatory agents. It is not a central nervous system or respiratory depressant like the opioids; indeed, enhancement of some reflexes occurs. The mechanism by which it produces analgesia is obscure, but it has some actions on peripheral tissues similar to the opioids.

Pharmacokinetics It is rapidly absorbed (15–30min) following oral administration, and may also be given by i.m. or i.v. injection (60 mg orally ≡ 20 mg parenterally). The plasma $t_{1/2}$ is 4–8 h. It is extensively metabolised by the liver to inactive compounds excreted in the urine. There is probably a significant first-pass hepatic metabolism.

Clinical uses It is not indicated for minor aches and pains but is effective in moderate to severe pain. 20 mg nefopam has a similar time—effect curve to 12 mg morphine when given intramuscularly. There is little increase in analgesia above this dose. Clinical studies have shown that nefopam can relieve post-operative pain, the pain of terminal malignancy and pain associated with musculo-skeletal disorders, but its place in clinical practice has not yet been established. At present there is not enough experience to recommend its use in myocardial infarction.

Adverse effects Neither tolerance nor drug dependence has been demonstrated. Sedation is not a problem with nefopam although the mild relaxation effect that it produces when relieving pain may result in sleepiness. Constipation and gastrointestinal irritation are also absent. The side effects which do occur are similar to those of other strong analgesics and include nausea (less frequent than with opioids), sweating, nervousness, dry mouth and insomnia. Since nefopam is not an opioid, treatment of overdosage with naloxone will be ineffective and management should therefore be supportive only with administration of diazepam if excitation occurs.

HYPERURICAEMIA AND GOUT

Uric acid is the end product in the metabolism of the purines adenine and guanine. About two thirds is excreted in the urine. The remainder is excreted into the gut and is broken down by the intestinal bacteria. The blood level of uric acid reflects the total amount in the body, and in a normal population is dependent on age and sex.

Hyperuricaemia may arise for three reasons:

(a) As a result of a genetically determined defect of metabolism as occurs in primary gout, causing overproduction of uric acid.
(b) As a result of increased breakdown of nuclear material which is seen in leukaemia and similar disorders, particularly when treated by cytotoxic drugs.
(c) When excretion is decreased, as occurs in renal failure or when tubular excretion of uric acid is diminished by diuretic or by small doses of salicylates.

Hyperuricaemia is associated with a number of pathological states:

(a) Gout—monosodium urate crystals are precipitated in the synovial fluid of the joint and elsewhere.
(b) Uric acid nephropathy—damage to the kidney occurs as a result of urate crystals in the renal parenchyma.
(c) Uric acid renal stones.

To prevent these complications it may be necessary to lower the plasma uric acid levels.

Production of uric acid

The final stages in the production of uric acid are shown in Fig. 10.8. Two of these stages are dependent on the enzyme xanthine oxidase.

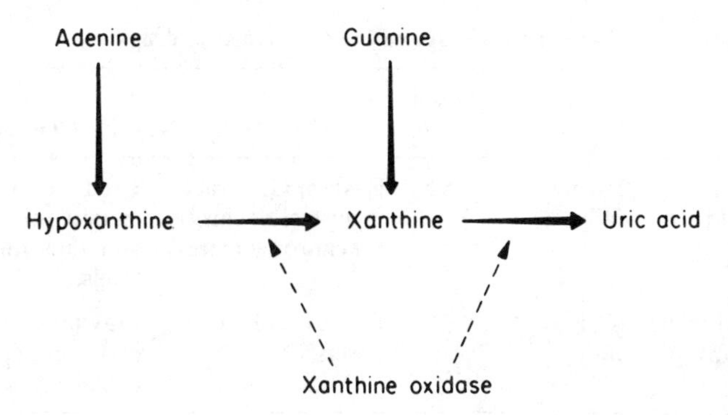

Fig. 10.8 The final stages in the production of uric acid.

In lower animals uricase converts uric acid into allantoin which is rapidly eliminated by the kidneys, but man has suffered an apparently disadvantageous evolutionary mutation and uricase has been lost so that the less soluble uric acid must be excreted.

Renal excretion of uric acid

Uric acid is filtered by the glomerulus but 98% is actively reabsorbed in the proximal tubule. It is also excreted into the distal tubule via an active transport system. It is more soluble in an alkaline urine and one factor in the development of uric acid stones is an impairment of the ability to excrete alkaline urine.

It is thus possible to lower the plasma uric acid concentration by increasing renal excretion of uric acid or by inhibiting its synthesis.

TREATMENT OF GOUT

1. Uricosuric agents

These drugs (see Table 10.4) inhibit the active transport of organic acids by the renal tubules. Their main effect on the handling of uric acid by the kidney is to prevent the reabsorption of filtered uric acid by the proximal tubule, thus greatly increasing excretion (see Fig. 10.9).

These drugs are largely excreted in the urine via the renal tubule.

After a week the initial dose may be increased stepwise until a satisfactory plasma level of uric acid is obtained. An acute attack of gout may be precipitated if treatment is started with a large dose. It is a good idea to give concurrent treatment with an anti-inflammatory drug, e.g. indomethacin (25 mg 8 hourly) or with colchicine (0.5 mg 8 hourly) for three months until this risk is past. In order to lessen the risk of renal stones which may develop following the increased excretion of uric acid, for the first month the patient should be given enough water to have a urine output of 2 l/day and sodium

Table 10.4 Commonly used uricosuric drugs

Drug	*Initial dose*	*Plasma half-life*	*Adverse effects*	*Other uses*
Probenecid (Benemid)	250 mg daily	8 h	Rashes, G.I. tract upsets, nephrotic syndrome (rare).	Used to block excretion of penicillin and thus raise blood levels.
Sulphinpyrazone (Anturan)	100 mg daily	3 h	Rashes, G.I. tract upsets.	May prevent myocardial infarction (see p. 606).

bicarbonate to keep the urinary pH above 7.0. Salicylates are uricosuric but the high doses required make them unacceptable for this purpose. Low doses of salicylates actually raise plasma urate and may antagonise the action of probenecid and sulphinpyrazone.

Other uricosuric drugs Phenylbutazone, indomethacin and large doses of salicylates will increase the excretion of uric acid but are rarely used for this purpose.

2. Prevention of urate synthesis

Allopurinol (Zyloric)

Allopurinol is a xanthine oxidase inhibitor and provides an excellent example of the logical use of a drug to correct metabolic abnormality. It decreases the production of uric acid so that the end products of purine metabolism are now three substances (hypoxanthine, xanthine and uric acid), each with its own solubility. Precipitation into joints or elsewhere is therefore much less likely and uric acid is actually mobilised from deposits which slowly disappear.

Pharmacokinetics Allopurinol is rapidly and well absorbed from the intestine. Its plasma half-life is about 3 h. It is largely converted to oxypurinol which is itself a weak xanthine oxidase inhibitor (Fig. 10.10).

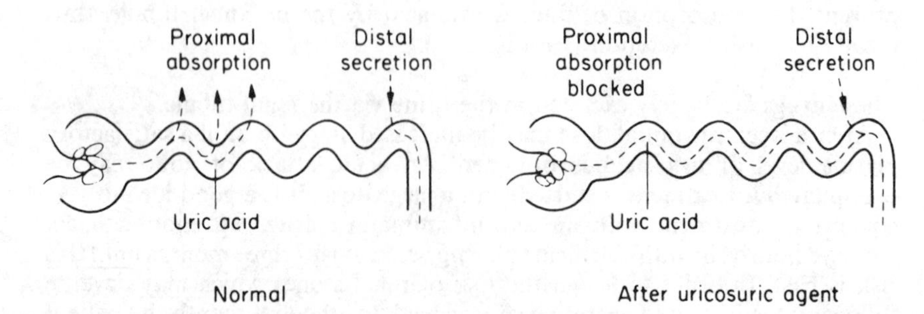

Fig. 10.9 Effect of uricosuric drugs on uric acid elimination by the renal tubule.

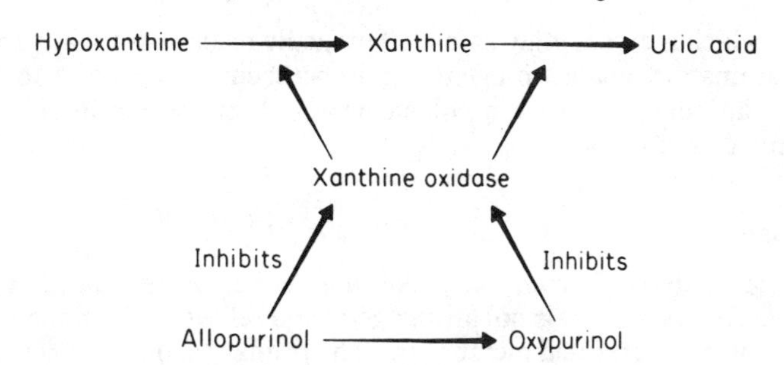

Fig. 10.10 Inhibitory actions of allopurinol.

Clinical uses Allopurinol is used as a long-term medication to treat hyperuricaemia and its complications. If possible the plasma uric acid concentration should be kept below 0.42 mmol/l. The initial dose is 200 mg daily and may be increased to 600 mg daily.

Allopurinol is of no use for the treatment of acute gout and its use may provoke acute gout during the first few weeks of treatment. Concurrent indomethacin or colchicine is therefore indicated for the first month of treatment. In early uncomplicated gout there is probably little to choose between allopurinol and uricosuric drugs, but allopurinol alone or in combination with uricosurics is particularly indicated in:

(a) gout uncontrolled by uricosurics;
(b) severe tophaceous gout;
(c) urate renal stones;
(d) gout with renal failure;
(e) acute urate nephropathy;
(f) gout with high levels of urinary urate;
(g) intolerance to uricosuric drugs;
(h) treatment of leukaemias and lymphomas with cytotoxic drugs.

Adverse effects are infrequent. The theoretical risk of forming xanthine stones has not proved to be a practical problem although crystals of xanthine, hypoxanthine and oxypurinol (which appear to be harmless) are found in the muscles of allopurinol-treated patients.

Skin rashes and more serious hypersensitivity reactions can occur and appear to be dose related: they are particularly liable to occur if allopurinol is given to a patient with renal failure and are presumably due to accumulation of metabolites. Rarely it may also cause myelosuppression.

Allopurinol decreases the rate of breakdown of 6-mercaptopurine and azathioprine. If these drugs are combined the dose of 6-mercaptopurine should be reduced (see p. 794). It may also interfere with the inactivation of oral anticoagulants.

Acute gout

The acute attack is due to the precipitation of monosodium urate crystals in the joint. These are irritant and there is a resultant acute inflammatory response which is exceedingly painful. This acute reaction is usually treated by anti-inflammatory analgesic agents (indomethacin 50 mg t.d.s.) for a short time. An alternative is to use colchicine which is specific in relieving the symptoms of acute gout.

Colchicine

Colchicine is derived from the seeds and corm of the meadow saffron (*Colchicum autumnale*). It is not an analgesic and relieves only the pain of gout. It has no effect on uric acid metabolism. The primary action of colchicine is to bind to the microtubular protein of cells, causing polymerisation and interfering with their function. The most important results of this are:

(a) The arrest of cell division at the metaphase. Although this phenomenon is not used therapeutically it is a useful tool in research.
(b) In acute gout sodium monourate crystals precipitate in the joint. Leucocytes migrate into the area and engulf the crystals. This leads in turn to increased production of lactic acid, a fall in pH and further precipitation of urate. Colchicine inhibits the migration of leucocytes and thus breaks the cycle and reduces inflammation and pain.

Pharmacokinetics Colchicine is rapidly absorbed from the gastrointestinal tract. The $t_{1/2}$ is 30 min. It is partly metabolised and a major portion is excreted via the bile and undergoes enterohepatic circulation, which may account for its toxic effects on the gastrointestinal tract.

Clinical uses Colchicine is given in doses of 0.5 mg orally every 2 h until the pain is relieved. Unfortunately it causes diarrhoea and vomiting and this may be severe enough to stop the treatment. No more than 6.0 mg should be given during the first 72 h. Colchicine can also be used prophylactically in doses of 0.5 mg three times daily.

It should be used with care in old or feeble patients and in those with renal, cardiac or gastrointestinal disease.

Adverse effects The most important side effects are nausea, vomiting and diarrhoea, probably due to a direct effect on the intestinal mucosa. There is considerable variation in individual sensitivity to these effects and a few patients cannot tolerate colchicine.

Precipitation of gout by drugs

1. Diuretics: Thiazides (via their action the distal tubule which inhibits urate secretion), ethacrynic acid, frusemide and bumetanide. But not triamterine, amiloride or spironolactone.
2. Pyrazinamide
3. Clofibrate
4. Aspirin (low doses)
5. Chemotherapy for leukaemia and lymphomas.

Chapter 11
GENERAL AND LOCAL ANAESTHETICS; MUSCLE RELAXANTS

GENERAL ANAESTHETICS

These may be considered in two groups:

A. Inhalational anaesthetics
B. Intravenous anaesthetics.

A. INHALATIONAL ANAESTHETICS

These include halogenated hydrocarbons:

enflurane
isoflurane
halothane
trichlorethylene
ethyl chloride } almost obsolete as general
chloroform } anaesthetics in the UK

and non-halogenated agents:

nitrous oxide
ether
cyclopropane.

Halothane

Halothane is 2-bromo-2-chloro-1,1,1-trifluoroethane. It is a potent inhalational anaesthetic which at room temperature is a colourless liquid. The boiling point is 50° and saturated vapour pressure at 20° is 243 mm Hg.

It is decomposed by light, and is stored in amber-coloured bottles, stabilised by 0.01 % thymol. It does not react with soda lime and is non-inflammable and non-explosive.

Pharmacokinetics Partition coefficients are:

blood–gas	2.5
fat–blood	60.0
brain–blood	2.6

It is soluble in blood at 37° 1.16 % w/v.

The minimal alveolar concentration for anaesthesia is 0.75 vols %. The vapour is non-irritant and not unpleasant to smell. For induction of anaesthesia 2–4 % vapour is administered and for maintenance 1–2 % is used.

Halothane is metabolised in the liver and in some species is a hepatic enzyme inducing agent. The metabolites produced include bromide and chloride ions, trifluoracetylethanolamide, chlorobromodifluoroethylene and trifluoroacetic acid which are found in the urine. Metabolites are slowly cleared from the body over the course of three weeks.

Clinical uses In low concentrations on its own it is a poor analgesic, but with nitrous oxide and oxygen it is very useful for many purposes. Whilst apparently simple to use, its therapeutic index is relatively low and overdosage is easily produced. Warning signs are bradycardia, hypotension and tachypnoea. Unfortunately, unlike ether which initially produces respiratory depression in toxic doses (this can be easily treated), halothane may induce cardiovascular collapse, which is a more difficult situation to retrieve.

Particular aspects of the use of halothane relate to the following:

1. Moderate muscular relaxation is produced: it is rarely sufficient for major abdominal surgery. The effect of d-tubocurarine is potentiated at the motor end plate and at ganglia and hypotension can result. Gallamine is less likely to produce the latter effect with halothane.
2. Heat loss is accelerated and may aid hypothermic techniques.
3. It is particularly indicated:
   (a) when quiet spontaneous respiration is required;
   (b) when muscle relaxants are contraindicated;
   (c) when hypotension would be useful to reduce bleeding at the site of operation;
   (d) in bronchitic and asthmatic patients;
   (e) for external version in obstetrics.

Adverse effects

1. *Cardiovascular*

(a) Increased myocardial excitability, ventricular extrasystoles, ventricular tachycardia and ventricular fibrillation may occur. Predisposing factors include carbon dioxide retention, adrenaline administration, atropine and sensory stimulation during light anaesthesia. Ventricular extrasystoles can be controlled by intravenous β-adrenoceptor blockers.

(b) Bradycardia mediated by the vagus and hypotension. This may be treated with a slow intravenous injection of atropine. Deaths have occurred from myocardial failure.

(c) The blood pressure usually falls during halothane anaesthesia. This is probably due to ganglion blockade, central vasomotor depression and myocardial depression.

2. *Respiratory depression* commonly occurs resulting in decreased alveolar ventilation. Respiratory centre depression usually precedes myocardial depression and is dose dependent. Although the depth of respiration is decreased there is tachypnoea.

Halothane produces bronchodilatation and is suitable for bronchitic and asthmatic patients.

3. *Central nervous system*. Despite generalised CNS depression, the drug is not a good analgesic and also may lead to convulsions.

Psychological changes may persist for over a week after administration.

4. *Liver*. Halothane can produce massive hepatic necrosis or subclinical hepatitis following anaesthesia. However, the incidence of massive necrosis due to halothane is very low. Patients most at risk are middle aged, obese or have previously (within 28 days) had halothane anaesthesia. The basic lesion appears to be a hypersensitivity type of hepatitis which is independent of halothane dose.

5. *Uterus*. Uterine atony or postpartum haemorrhage may result from halothane.

Enflurane

Enflurane is 2-chloro-1,1,2-trifluoroethyl, difluoromethyl ether; it is a volatile liquid with a pleasant ethereal smell when vapourised (boiling point 56.5°C).

Pharmacokinetics The partition coefficients are:

blood–gas	1.8
fat–blood	36
brain–blood	1.4

A suitably calibrated vapouriser is used to provide accurate concentrations. For induction an initial inspired concentration of 1 % is gradually increased to 4.5 % in oxygen or a nitrous oxide–oxygen mixture. For maintenance 1–3 % concentration is used.

As it is poorly soluble, only a small fraction, approximately 2.5 %, is metabolised. However, free fluoride ion is released by this process and during prolonged anaesthesia this may lead to nephrotoxicity in susceptible patients.

Clinical uses Enflurane is a potent anaesthetic which has the potential advantage of producing direct muscle relaxation and reversible potentiation of muscle relaxants. It is increasingly used in anaesthetic practice, particularly if multiple anaesthetics are necessary (as liver dysfunction is very rare) or rapid recovery is important.

Adverse effects

1. *Cardiovascular* it produces depression of myocardial contractility to a relatively greater extent than halothane. However it does not sensitise the myocardium to catecholamines, unlike halothane.

2. *Respiratory depression* is common, but is only a problem if, during deep anaesthesia, spontaneous ventilation is allowed.

3. *CNS*. High concentrations may produce spike and wave activity in the EEG, particularly in children. In the presence of hypocapnia this may lead to grand mal fits.

4. *Uterine tone* may be reduced and promote post-partum haemorrhage.

Isoflurane

Isoflurane is 1-chloro-2,2,2-trifluoroethyl, difluoromethyl ether; it is a volatile liquid (boiling point 48.5°C).

Partition coefficients are:		
	blood–gas	1.4
	fat–blood	45
	brain–blood	2.6

This is the less-soluble isomer of enflurane. Less than 1% undergoes metabolism so fluoride accumulation is not seen. It produces respiratory depression but less myocardial depression than enflurane or halothane and EEG abnormalities have not been seen. Hypotension occurs due to peripheral vasodilatation. Thus isoflurane appears to have the advantages of enflurane as an anaesthetic but probably with less toxicity.

Nitrous oxide

This is a colourless gas which is 1½ times heavier than air. It is neither flammable nor explosive but supports combustion. Nitrous oxide is stable and unaffected by soda-lime. This anaesthetic gas is not irritating to the mucous membranes. Although it is a powerful analgesic it is a weak anaesthetic.

Pharmacokinetics The solubility in plasma is 45 volumes %—i.e. it is 15 times more soluble than oxygen. The partition coefficients are:

0.47	between blood and gas (cf. 0.013 between blood and nitrogen)
1.0	between brain and blood
3.0	between fat and blood

Anaesthesia is induced rapidly due to the low partition coefficient between blood and nitrous oxide. Unconsciousness is not usually attained unless the concentration of inhaled gas is above 70%, however less than 30% inhaled oxygen may result in a PaO_2 below 80 mm Hg. (10.5 k Pa).

Nitrous oxide is eliminated unchanged from the body, mostly via the lungs. Despite its high solubility in fat, following anaesthetic administration, most is eliminated within minutes.

Clinical uses

1. General anaesthesia after premedication, thiopentone induction and with a volatile or intravenous supplement. There is poor muscular relaxation, and muscle relaxants may be required.

2. A 25% concentration of nitrous oxide in oxygen is a good analgesic, perhaps as effective as morphine in relieving post-operative pain.

Pre-mixed nitrous oxide and oxygen in equal volumes (Entonox) can be administered on a demand system and has been used as an analgesic in labour, myocardial infarction, postoperative physiotherapy, changing of surgical dressings and removal of drainage tubes.

Adverse effects

1. Nitrous oxide on its own, like nitrogen, produces progressive hypoxia and can result in death or permanent neurological sequelae.

With adequate (20 % or more) oxygen, nitrous oxide does not depress the respiration but nitrous oxide potentiates respiratory depression due to barbiturates and narcotic analgesics.

2. Nitrous oxide in the alveolar gas will equilibrate with the pulmonary capillary blood whilst nitrogen will leave the circulation and pass into the alveoli. Because of the big difference in their blood–gas partition coefficients, much more nitrogen will leave the circulation compared with the nitrous oxide entering. Thus pressure will increase in the gut, lungs, middle ear and sinuses, and ear complications and pneumothorax may occur.

After cessation of administration of nitrous oxide, the rapid outflow into the alveoli can result in diffusion hypoxia, i.e. the gas diffuses out very quickly, and can account for up to 10 % of the expired volume; this displaces alveolar air so that the patient is left a hypoxic mixture to breathe.

3. Prolonged administration (as in tetanus treatment) has resulted in megaloblastic anaemia, due to interference with the action of vitamin B_{12}, and agranulocytosis.

Other inhalation anaesthetics
These are reviewed in Table 11.1.

Occupational hazards of inhalational anaesthetics
Apart from the obvious risks to patients, the effects of prolonged exposure to these agents on anaesthetists and other theatre personnel has to be considered. Among postulated hazards are abortion, low birthweight infants, congenital disorders and cancer in adults. Although much of the evidence is controversial it is becoming clear that such exposure may be hazardous and that all possible precautions to ensure efficient removal of anaesthetic gases from the environment must be taken. A recent survey of anaesthetists in the West Midlands found that one in ten of their children had a congenital anomaly, the birthweights of children were below normal (more so when the mother was an anaesthetist) and there was an excess of infertility and cancer both in the adults and their children.

B. INTRAVENOUS ANAESTHETICS

1. Sodium thiopentone (Intraval; Pentothal)

Thiopentone is ethyl (1-methyl butyl) thiobarbiturate. The sodium salt dissolves in water and a 5 % solution has a pH of 10.8. 1.6 % sodium carbonate is added to the powder in order to prevent the formation of the free acid on exposure to atmospheric carbon dioxide. It is therefore an extremely irritant solution.

Pharmacokinetics A dose of 4 mg/kg intravenously produces loss of consciousness within 10 s and general anaesthesia for about 5 min. The plasma $t_{1/2\beta}$ of the drug is 6 h but the rapid course of action is explained by its high lipid solubility coupled with the rich cerebral blood flow which ensures rapid penetration into the brain. The short-lived anaesthesia results from the rapid

Table 11.1 Properties of some inhalational anaesthetics

	Boiling point (°C)	Flammability	Reaction with soda lime	Partition coefficients Blood–gas	Fat–blood	Oil–water	Metabolism	Elimination	Potency
Cyclopropane	−32.9	Very explosive	Does not decompose	0.46	20.0	34.4	Very little metabolised	Most excreted in 10 min. Complete desaturation much longer	Very potent: can be used with more than 20% O_2. Rapid induction by 7–23 vols % vapour for general anaesthesia
Ether	35	Very explosive and inflammable	Stable	12.0	33	3.2	10–15% metabolised	Most excreted unchanged via the lungs	3–20 vols % vapour for general anaesthesia
Chloroform	61	Non-flammable but forms phosgene when heated	Decomposed by alkalis, but can be used with soda lime	8.4	68.5	100	Small amount metabolised to methylene chloride	Most excreted unchanged via lungs. Complete desaturation takes many hours	Potent anaesthetic. 4% vapour for induction. 2% for maintenance of general anaesthesia.

Table 11.1 (continued)

	Boiling point (°C)	*Flammability*	*Reaction with soda lime*	*Partition coefficients*			*Metabolism*	*Elimination*	*Potency*
				Blood–gas	*Fat–blood*	*Oil–water*			
Trichlorethylene	87	Not explosive but will burn in oxygen	Decomposes to dichloracetylene	9.0	106.7	400	Small amount metabolised to trichloroacetic acid	Most drug excreted unchanged via lungs	A relatively weak anaesthetic agent. Not used to produce deep anaesthesia. Slow but smooth induction 0.2–2.0 vols % vapour for general anaesthesia.
Ethyl chloride	12.5	Burns in air or oxygen to give HCl fumes.	Hydrolysed	2.0	40				Anaesthetic concentration 3–4.5 vols % vapour. Narrow safety margin.
Cyclopropane	Non-irritating. Can cause laryngospasm. Powerful respiratory depressant. CO_2 retention.		BP well maintained. Vascular resistance increased. Cardiac output raised. Bradycardia and ventricular ectopics. Adrenaline contraindicated	Nil			Good	Inhibited only in deep anaesthesia	Cyclopropane shock emergence delirium

Table 11.1 Properties of some inhalational anaesthetics (continued)

	Respiratory system	*CVS*	*Organ damage*	*Muscle relaxation*	*Uterine contraction*	*Analgesia*	*Recovery from anaesthesia*
Ether	Moderate irritation. Initial increase in respiratory volume then progressive fall with deep anaesthesia.	Initial tachycardia, then normal rate. Fall in BP. Fall in peripheral resistance. Arrhythmias rare	Temporary depression of liver function and of biliary secretion.	Good	Relaxed	Some early analgesia	Nausea and vomiting common
Chloroform	Depression of respiratory centre. Prolonged breathing of 2% vapour may give respiratory arrest. Non-irritant.	Progressive fall in BP. Ventricular arrhythmias common. Sudden cardiac arrest. Light anaesthesia accompanied by vasoconstriction. Adrenaline contraindicated	Toxic hepatitis may develop 1–3 days after anaesthetic: esp. repeated administration.		Complete relaxation during deep anaesthesia	Good analgesia in sub-anaesthetic doses	50% patients have post-operative nausea and vomiting
Trichlorethylene	Moderately irritating. Tachypnoea and shallow breathing. Fall in PO_2, rise in PCO_2.	BP well maintained. Bradycardia and ventricular ectopics. Adrenaline contraindicated	Nil	Poor	0.5 w/v. Good analgesia for obstetrics		Slow recovery. Post-operative nausea and vomiting

Table 11.1 (continued)

	Respiratory system	*CVS*	*Organ damage*	*Muscle relaxation*	*Uterine contraction*	*Analgesia*	*Recovery from anaesthesia*
Ethyl chloride	Slightly irritating. Respiratory centre depressed after initial stimulation.	Initial bradycardia followed by tachycardia. Adrenaline increases myocardial irritability, but ventricular fibrillation is rare		Poor. Muscles may go into spasm.			Nausea and vomiting common

fall (α phase) of the blood concentration, which occurs due to distribution of drug into the tissues when the drug is transferred rapidly out of the brain to maintain equilibrium (see Fig. 11.1). The main early transfer is into the muscle. In the hypovolaemia and vasoconstriction occurring in shock this transfer is reduced and sustained high concentrations develop in the brain and heart, producing prolonged and sometimes fatal depression of these organs. These facts were unknown during the early use of the drug when the mortality from thiopentone use in trauma, for example after the Pearl Harbour attack, was as high as 1 in 80. Relatively little enters fat initially because of its poor blood supply, but 30 min after injection the thiopentone concentration continues to rise in this tissue. Such absorption by fat is responsible for the termination of anaesthesia from 0.5–2 h following injection if sufficiently large doses of thiopentone have been given to attain equilibrium between an anaesthetic concentration in the brain and a similar concentration in the blood. Following administration of even larger doses, sustained blood levels result in prolonged anaesthesia due to saturation of tissue stores and slow metabolism. The latter occurs at only 10–15 % per hour. The depth of anaesthesia depends not only on the plasma concentration but on the duration of exposure of the brain to the drug.

Thiopentone is 75 % bound to plasma proteins, thus only about 25 % of the total plasma drug concentration is in equilibrium with the extravascular fluids. Hypocapnia, and the associated rise in pH, increases the proportion of

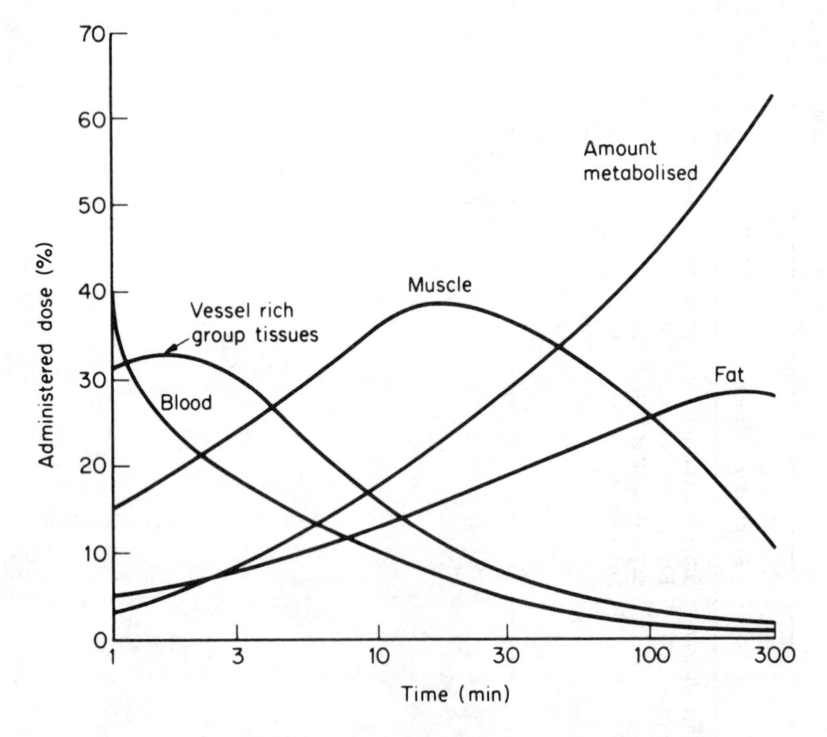

Fig. 11.1 Tissue distribution of thiopentone following intravenous injection.

unbound drug and thus prolongs the anaesthetic action. Sulphonamides, aspirin, phenylbutazone and naproxen may also have the same effect. Thiopentone binding is also reduced in uraemia and hepatic failure and this may explain in part the sensitivity of such patients to the drug.

Metabolism is almost complete, mainly side-chain oxidation, and occurs in the liver, muscles and kidneys. The metabolites are excreted via the kidneys. Reduced doses are used in the presence of impaired liver or renal function.

General effects

Central nervous system Depression of many central functions leads to sedation, hypnosis, surgical anaesthesia and respiratory depression. Subanaesthetic doses are not analgesic and produce hyperalgesia. Thiopentone is anticonvulsant.

Cardiovascular system The force of cardiac contraction is reduced and cardiac output is reduced. Cardiac arrest can occur in patients with preexisting heart disease. There is dilatation of peripheral capacitance with a fall in blood pressure and reduction in renal blood flow.

Respiratory system In addition to centrally mediated respiratory depression, there is an increased tendency to laryngeal spasm. Bronchospasm may also occur.

Pregnant uterus Thiopentone has no effect on uterine tone.

Clinical uses for thiopentone include: induction for general anaesthesia; general anaesthesia for short operations, reduction of fractures and examinations; status epilepticus or fits following local anaesthetic; as an aid to psychiatric investigation and electroconvulsive therapy.

Adverse effects Allergy can manifest as urticaria or anaphylactic shock. Necrosis of tissue and peripheral nerve injury can occur due to accidental extravascular administration and arterial spasm if accidentally injected into an artery. Post-operative restlessness and nausea are common.

Contraindications include children under 4 years, shock, anaemia, uraemia, myocardial ischaemia, dyspnoea due to pulmonary or cardiac disease, obstructive airways disease, acute intestinal obstruction, porphyria, alcoholics taking disulfiram.

2. Methohexitone (Brietal)

Methohexitone is sodium 1-methyl-5-allyl-5-(1-methyl-2-pentynyl) oxybarbiturate. The pH of a 2% solution is 11.1. By weight it is more than 2½ times as potent as thiopentone. Recovery of consciousness is more rapid than with thiopentone and is explained by the same mechanism, i.e. redistribution of the drug from the CNS into muscle. Its hepatic clearance is much greater than that of thiopentone and the $t_{1/2}$ is only 70–125 min.

Methohexitone is less irritating to the tissues compared with thiopentone and can be injected intramuscularly, but both drugs are equally hazardous when injected intra-arterially.

It is not anticonvulsant and can possibly produce fits during anaesthesia.

Type I allergic reactions may occur. Methohexitone (in a dose of about

1 mg/kg) can be used to induce anaesthesia. Other uses of this barbiturate include: dental and other short operations; electroconvulsive therapy; pre-anaesthetic sedation can be produced by intramuscular or rectal administration of methohexitone.

3. Ketamine

Ketamine is 2-O-chlorophenyl-2-methylaminocyclohexanone hydrochloride. It is soluble in water and supplied as 1, 5 and 10% solutions.

Pharmacokinetics Ketamine is rapidly absorbed after oral and intramuscular administration although it is commonly given intravenously. The plasma $t_{1/2}$ is 2.5–4 h. It is 5–10 times more lipid soluble than thiopentone and rapidly passes the blood–brain barrier. An intravenous dose of 2 mg/kg produces anaesthesia within 30 s which lasts for 5–10 min, whilst 10 mg/kg given intramuscularly is effective in 3–4 min. Although anaesthesia wears off within 10–20 min, complete recovery is more protracted. Unconsciousness is probably terminated by redistribution of the drug from the brain to other tissues as with thiopentone.

The role of metabolism in the elimination of ketamine is particularly important since some of the metabolites have pharmacological activity which may be responsible for post-anaesthetic hallucinations. The main metabolites are alcohols produced by N-demethylation or hydroxylation of the cyclohexanone ring. Other drugs can interfere with ketamine metabolism, e.g. diazepam and barbiturates inhibit demethylation and prolong the $t_{1/2}$ although, because the duration of anaesthesia is determined by redistribution, this does not influence anaesthetic effect. Halothane slows the uptake and redistribution of ketamine as a result of its depressant effect on the cardiovascular system.

Clinical uses Ketamine is used as a parenteral anaesthetic. The state produced is different from conventional anaesthesia—there is profound sedation and analgesia but there may be dreaming and muscle tone is increased. However, visceral pain may be experienced. It has been used successfully in short operations, induction prior to other anaesthetics, unpleasant therapeutic and diagnostic precedures in children, operations in shocked patients, open-heart surgery, operative delivery in obstetrics. Ketamine may also be given as an intravenous infusion (3 μg/kg/min) to produce continuous sedation and analgesia in patients on ventilators in the intensive care unit.

It has been used for management of mass casualties or for anaesthesia of trapped patients to carry out amputations, etc.

Because of its ease of administration and safety, in countries where there are few skilled anaesthetists its use is widespread.

Adverse effects *Central nervous system:* vivid, unpleasant, brightly coloured dreams of a hallucinatory character occur in some 15% of patients during recovery and are often accompanied by delirium. Dreams are not uncommon after anaesthetics but those after ketamine are peculiar and resemble the effects of a hallucinogen. They are minimised by sedative premedication, by using ketamine only for induction and by ensuring a peaceful and undisturbed recovery.

Intracranial pressure is increased by ketamine and its safety in patients with raised intracranial tension has been questioned.

Cardiovascular system: the blood pressure is raised by 25–30 mm Hg and the pulse by 10–15 beats/min, which may be dangerous in hypertensive patients or in those with heart failure or a history of cerebrovascular accident. Ketamine has antiarrhythmic properties.

Respiratory system: respiration is mildly stimulated and salivation is increased, producing a risk of fluid aspiration into the lungs. Pharyngeal and laryngeal reflexes are unimpaired.

4. **Benzodiazepines** (see p. 210)

Diazepam has been used for induction and to supplement nitrous oxide anaesthesia. Despite the possession of a good amnesic effect and producing less cardio-respiratory depression than the ultra-short-acting barbiturates, it is not popular for induction. It is slow to act, can cause pain during injection and ensuing thrombophlebitis, unpredictable cardiovascular depression may occur and full recovery is prolonged. Despite these drawbacks, it is used as a psychosedative for minor procedures such as dentistry, endoscopy and cardioversion.

The incidence of thrombophlebitis with i.v. diazepam has been substantially reduced by using a preparation made up in soya bean oil (Diazemuls).

Midazolam (Hypnovel) (see p. 219) is a newer benzodiazepine with a short plasma half-life (approximately 2.5 hours) and no active metabolites (unlike diazepam). It rarely produces thrombophlebitis and onset of hypnosis is more rapid than with diazepam. Recovery times after single doses of diazepam and midazolam are similar but midazolam seems to produce a greater degree of amnesia which may be useful after procedures such as endoscopy or bone marrow trephine. It should not be given in repeated doses as accumulation has been reported.

5. Etomidate (Hypnomidate)

This is an induction agent which allows rapid recovery without hangover and causes less hypotension than similar agents. Used alone it produces severe injection pain and involuntary muscle movements. These can be reduced by using large veins for injection and premedication (e.g. with opioids like pethidine or fentanyl). The usual induction dose is 300 μg/kg by slow injection.

Although useful for induction this drug should not be used by repeated bolus injection or infusion to produce prolonged anaesthesia. Like other imidazoles (e.g. ketoconazole) it inhibits certain cytochrome P_{450}-dependent enzymes concerned with adrenal steroidogenesis. Thus etomidate is associated with increased mortality related to low plasma cortisol concentrations when used to provide chronic sedation, e.g. for patients on ventilators. The effect of etomidate on other cytochrome P_{450} enzymes such as those for drug metabolism has not been reported.

6. Ethyl alcohol (see p. 848)

Alcohol is occasionally used as an intravenous anaesthetic. It has been employed in obstetrics and is a powerful inhibitor of uterine contractions. In patients dependent on alcohol, operations under general anaesthesia can precipitate the abstinence syndrome. This is prevented by i.v. alcohol before the operation.

Solutions of 5–10% w/v are infused: the amount required varies widely but a typical dose is 500 ml of an 8% solution given over 2–3 h. Induction of anaesthesia may take 15–20 min.

Toxicity includes emergence delirium, hangover (nausea, headache), local thrombophlebitis.

NEUROLEPTANALGESIA

Neuroleptanalgesia is a state which consists of depression of activity, lack of initiative and reduced response to external stimuli. Symptoms of psychomotor agitation disappear and the patient is in a state of analgesia and sedation although able to understand and answer simple questions and obey commands. This state can be useful in complex diagnostic procedures although nitrous oxide may be added to induce unconsciousness. Neuroleptanalgesia is commonly produced by a combination of droperidol and fentanyl or phenoperidine.

1. Droperidol (Droleptan)

This is a butyrophenone (see p. 249) which may therefore produce extrapyramidal effects. It is also a potent α-adrenergic blocker and has quinidine-like properties which may explain the cardiovascular stability of patients undergoing surgery under its influence. It has a rapid distributive (α-) phase with a $t_{1/2,\alpha}$ of minutes. It is given orally or more usually by intramuscular or intravenous injection, these two latter routes being almost equivalent in speed of onset of action due to the rapid absorption of droperidol. The rapid distribution results in rapid onset of action. The plasma elimination $t_{1/2\beta}$ is 2–3 h but droperidol has a depressant effect on behaviour for up to 48 h when given in usual doses (10 mg). This is probably related to its accumulation and retention in the brain and in animals its neuroleptic activity is well correlated with the brain level of unchanged drug. About 10% of the drug is excreted unchanged, the rest undergoes hepatic metabolism to inactive products.

2. Fentanyl (Sublimaze)

This is the narcotic analgesic commonly employed with droperidol to produce analgesia. It is exceptionally potent having approximately 100 times the analgesic activity of morphine. It is also used to depress the respiration in patients requiring prolonged assisted ventilation.

It rapidly distributes into the tissues following injection accounting for its rapid action. The $t_{1/2}$ is 2–4 h. Fentanyl is rapidly and extensively metabolised but the short duration of action (the peak effect lasts only 20–30 min is probably due to redistribution of drug from brain to tissues (cf. thiopentone). Particular care should therefore be taken after relatively large or multiple injections when accumulation of the drug would probably occur because of saturation of tissue stores.

As with other opioids, respiratory depression may occur which can be reversed by naloxone. Bradycardia can be antagonised by atropine and muscular rigidity (an opioid effect) can be relieved by muscle relaxants.

3. Phenoperidine (Operidine)

Phenoperidine is an alternative to fentanyl in neuroleptanalgesia or to depress respiratory drive in patients on ventilators. It is an opiate and the same remarks apply as for fentanyl.

4. Alfentanil (Rapifen)

This is a new opioid with a short half-life of 1.5–2 hours. Onset and duration of action and recovery time are shorter than with fentanyl. However, like fentanyl, it also causes respiratory depression.

SEDATION IN THE INTENSIVE CARE UNIT

These remarks apply to patients who require prolonged mechanical ventilation.

Such patients usually require sedation not only on humanitarian grounds, but also to reduce the responses to stress, e.g. hypertension, tachycardia, which may be dangerous in patients with cardiac or neurological disease. Ideally sedation would be achieved with no depression of respiration and allow rapid reversal. Benzodiazepines, e.g. diazepam, lorazepam (but not midazolam—see above), are widely used but prolonged recovery may be a problem. The development of benzodiazepine antagonists in the future may usefully circumvent this.

Narcotic analgesics are particularly useful when the patient has pain, e.g. after major surgery or trauma. Intravenous infusions of pethidine or morphine produce excellent analgesia with less respiratory depression than after intermittent doses. Recovery may be prolonged however, especially if metabolism is impaired. Short-acting opioids, e.g. phenoperidine, fentanyl, alfentanil, are effective analgesics when infused (or given as frequent boluses) and recovery is usually rapid.

Two agents which were previously popular in this setting, etomidate and 'Althesin' (alphoxolone and alphadolone) have recently been withdrawn. The former because of serious depression of the adrenal cortex and the latter due to anaphylactoid reactions to the solvent.

PREMEDICATION FOR ANAESTHESIA

Premedication was originally introduced to facilitate the induction of anaesthesia with agents such as chloroform and ether which are irritant and have long induction times. Modern induction methods are simple and not unpleasant and the chief aim of pre-medication is now to allay anxiety in the patient awaiting surgery. Inadequate premedication may lead to the administration of larger doses of anaesthetic than would otherwise have been required, often resulting in delayed recovery from anaesthesia. Anaesthetic premedication usually comprises two drugs, a sedative and an antiparasympathetic drug:

1. Sedatives Apart from allowing the patient to feel less tense about the impending operation, these drugs may provide a degree of amnesia for pre- and post-operative events and reduce the incidence of unpleasant dreams during emergence from anaesthesia.
(a) *Opioids* are probably the most commonly used premedicants. Their main drawbacks are:

(i) respiratory depression;
(ii) failure to provide pre- or post-operative amnesia although they enhance this property of hyoscine or diazepam;
(iii) increased post-operative nausea and vomiting.

Many opioids have been used, Omnopon (papaveretum injection B.P.C.) is often employed by anaesthetists. This contains about half its weight as morphine, the rest being other opium alkaloids. It is usually given as 20 mg intramuscular injection and in this dose causes the same frequency of post-operative vomiting and nausea as 10 mg morphine. Pethidine is also employed although it is less sedative in the usual 100 mg dose than 10 mg morphine. It is powerful suppressant of bronchial reflexes and its quinidine-like action on the heart diminishes the risk of arrhythmia.

(b) *Butyrophenones* Droperidol, often in conjunction with fentanyl (doses 2.5 mg and 0.05 mg respectively) is sometimes used. This mixture is especially useful for intravenous use where quick sedation is required.

(c) *Phenothiazines* produce useful sedation and are antiemetic but are antianalgesic and therefore need to be given in conjunction with analgesics. Other unwanted effects are hypotension and extrapyramidal tremors. Promethazine is commonly used in doses of 25–50 mg intramuscularly; it has an atropine-like effect which may render the use of that drug unnecessary, although pethidine is added for analgesia. Trimeprazine (Vallergan) is a useful pre-medicant phenothiazine in children. It can be given orally or intramuscularly $1\frac{1}{2}$–2 h before anaesthesia. The dose is 3 mg/kg.

(d) *Benzodiazepines* provide good relief from pre-operative anxiety, do not depress respiration or cause nausea, and diazepam can be given orally or intravenously. Given intravenously, diazepam has an intense but short-lived amnesic action. Benzodiazepines have no analgesic properties and therefore an opioid is often given with them, although the respiratory depressant effects of such drugs are potentiated by benzodiazepines. The anticonvulsant activity of benzodiazepines may also be of benefit and these drugs are safe and reliable premedicants.

2. Antiparasympathetic drugs These are used to dry secretions and to prevent over-activity of the parasympathetic nervous system and in particular of the vagus. Although nitrous oxide and halothane, unlike ether, do not produce copious secretion from the respiratory tract, succinylcholine is associated with parasympathetic overactivity.

(a) *Atropine* is the traditional agent. It is a mild cerebral stimulant and produces a dry mouth and tachycardia. These effects occur maximally at around 1 h after intramuscular injection of 0.6 mg. Many anaesthetists would give the drug during induction to achieve high blood levels at the appropriate time and to spare the patient the unpleasant experience of a dry mouth and a thirst during the pre-operative phase when tranquillity is desired. At least 2 mg of atropine are required to produce complete parasympathetic blockade so that complete protection against parasympathetic effects cannot be guaranteed when usual doses are employed. Atropine should not be used where marked tachycardia is present due to disease, e.g. hyperthyroidism, fever. The possibility of precipitating acute closed-angle glaucoma should also be remembered.

(b) *Hyoscine* differs from atropine in having a lesser effect on heart rate. It is also a cerebral depressant and may cause confusion in the elderly, so that atropine is the better drug for this age group. Hyoscine is antiemetic.

LOCAL ANAESTHETICS

The three main groups of local anaesthetics are:

Amides:	lignocaine prilocaine mepivacaine bupivacaine etidocaine cinchocaine
Benzoic acid esters:	cocaine piperocaine
p-aminobenzoic acid esters:	procaine amethocaine benzocaine

Lignocaine (Xylocaine; Lidocaine) (see p. 405)

Lignocaine is N-diethylaminoacetyl 2,6-xylidine hydrochloride. It is currently the most widely used local anaesthetic in the UK. Lignocaine is chemically stable and like most local anaesthetics, it is a weak base with a pK_a of 7.86. The un-ionised form is lipid soluble and spreads through tissues penetrating cell membranes. This necessary conversion to the un-ionised form explains why local anaesthetics are less active (or inactive) if injected into an inflamed area (local tissue acidosis) or in acidotic patients. Local anaesthetics act on the plasma membranes of excitable cells. The resting transmembrane potential is unaffected but the rapid inflow of sodium ions, which is the ionic basis of the initial rapid upstroke of the action potential, is prevented. Local anaesthetics produce this effect by displacement of membrane bound calcium from sites on membrane phospholipids, leading to expansion of the membrane lipids resulting in distortion and constriction of the sodium channels. Pressure reverses both expansion of the membrane and local anaesthesia.

Unlike the majority of other local anaesthetics, lignocaine is not a vasodilator. It diffuses more readily in the tissue compared with other similar drugs. Like other local anaesthetics the small, unmyelinated fibres are depressed first and the larger myelinated fibres last. The order of loss of function is therefore: pain, temperature, touch, proprioception and skeletal muscle tone.

Pharmacokinetics Although the local anaesthetics are lipid-soluble bases which can enter hydrophobic components of neuronal cell membranes, the soluble form prepared for injection must be an ionisable molecule. Lignocaine is thus manufactured as a hydrochloride. The thicker the nerve fibre, the higher the concentration of local anaesthetic required to block the transmission of action potentials. The onset of action is rapid. It is absorbed into the circulation from sites of injection and is metabolised by the liver microsomal amidases. The local action is prolonged by the simultaneous administration of a vasoconstrictor. The local anaesthetic action of 1 % lignocaine lasts about 1 h but with adrenaline this is increased to $1\frac{1}{2}$–2 h.

Toxic concentrations can be reached in the blood following tissue infiltration of lignocaine although lower levels are produced with vasoconstriction. A rough guide for maximum local administration is 7 mg/kg with adrenaline and 3 mg/kg without adrenaline. Naturally toxicity can readily result from accidental intravenous administration of lignocaine.

Local anaesthesia of mucous membranes can be attained by topical application. Absorption may be very rapid (from the larynx, bronchi and urethra) and levels in plasma may be reached similar to those after intravenous injection.

Adverse effects Toxicity is not great but cardiovascular and central nervous complications can occur. Systemic allergy is uncommon.

Central nervous system signs are essentially stimulation followed by depression. These are restlessness, anxious behaviour, drowsiness, amnesia, vertigo, tremor, convulsions, respiratory failure. Treatment should include artificial ventilation and i.v. administration of thiopentone, diazepam or suxamethonium to control convulsions.

Cardiovascular system Hypotension, pallor, sweating, bradycardia, low output cardiac failure, cardiac arrest. Cardiac massage may be necessary. For acute hypotension, raise the legs, give oxygen and administer intravenous fluids.

Respiratory depression may have a delayed onset.

Systemic allergy bronchospasm, urticaria, angio-oedema. Contact dermatitis is not uncommon in medical staff handling lignocaine and in patients following local administration to the skin. Reactions to vasoconstrictor drugs include pallor, anxiety, tachycardia, tachypnoea and hypertension. Methaemoglobinaemia due to lignocaine is rare.

Clinical use For subcutaneous or submucous infiltration 0.25–0.5 % lignocaine solutions are used containing adrenaline 1/200 000. For topical mucosal analgesia a 4% solution, 1 and 2% jelly and 5% ointment are available. Solutions of 2% with 1/80 000 adrenaline are used for nerve block. A 4% solution dropped into the conjunctival sac produces good analgesia without cycloplegia, mydriasis or vasoconstriction. A 1 or 2% solution of plain lignocaine is used for procedures such as lumbar puncture or bone marrow trephine: it is used to anaesthetise the skin and deeper pain-sensitive membranes such as the periosteum.

In addition to its uses as a local anaesthetic, lignocaine is used in the treatment and prevention of ventricular arrhythmias (see p. 405).

Prilocaine

Prilocaine is similar in structure and actions to lignocaine, but is less likely than lignocaine to produce toxic effects.

Pharmacokinetics Prilocaine is metabolised by amidase in the liver, kidney and lungs. The rapid production of oxidation products, particularly o-toluidine and nitrosotoluidine, may give rise to methaemoglobinaemia. This is of no clinical importance unless there is severe anaemia or circulatory failure.

Clinical uses Prilocaine is most useful when a high concentration or large total amount of local anaesthetic is needed, e.g. for injection into vascular areas such as the perineum or face. For topical analgesia a 4% solution is used. In extradural analgesia the onset is slower but the duration and intensity of action are greater.

Adrenaline has a smaller effect in prolonging the duration of analgesia with prilocaine than with lignocaine.

Excessive doses can lead to CNS and CVS toxicity. This is dependent on the plasma concentration of the drug. An approximate guide to maximal dosage is 10 mg/kg.

In dental procedures prilocaine is often used with the peptide vasoconstrictor felypressin.

Cocaine

Cocaine is the major local anaesthetic alkaloid in the leaves of the coca plant (*Erythroxylon spp.*) which grows in South America. It is too toxic to be injected and therefore is used only topically. It inhibits noradrenaline uptake by peripheral nerves but the action of cocaine on the brain is not fully understood. The central effects of cocaine are believed to result from depression of cerebral inhibitory pathways rather than a true stimulation.

Pharmacokinetics Cocaine is readily absorbed from all mucous membrane surfaces. Concentrated solutions may be absorbed more slowly than dilute ones due to its powerful vasoconstrictor action. In the body it is metabolised by esterases in various organs, particularly the liver, and some is hydrolysed by plasma esterases. About 10% is excreted unchanged via the kidneys.

Acute intoxication Restlessness, anxiety, confusion, tachycardia, angina, cardiovascular collapse, convulsions, coma, death.

Central nervous system Initial stimulation gives rise to excitement and raised blood pressure, followed by vomiting. This may be followed by fits and CNS depression. Small doses produce central respiratory stimulation; larger doses depress respiration.

Clinical use A 4% solution is a powerful surface anaesthetic in the eye. Vasoconstriction and mydriasis occur but the pupil still responds to light and accommodation is not affected. The cornea may become clouded and corneal ulceration can develop. Although a small reduction in intraocular tension usually occurs, an acute attack of glaucoma is occasionally precipitated. The maximum analgesic activity lasts 20–30 min. Cocaine solution (4%) and paste (25%) can be used together in nasal operations. A reasonable dose for surface analgesia is 3 mg/kg with a maximum total of 200 mg. Because of its inhibitory effects on amine uptake, cocaine potentiates adrenaline so that addition of a vasoconstrictor is unnecessary and may be dangerous.

Adverse effects Drug dependence is readily produced (see p. 843).

Procaine (Novocain)

Procaine is p-aminobenzoyl-diethylaminoethanol. It is presented in a solution as the hydrochloride. Only highly concentrated solutions (20% and above) produce surface anaesthesia since it is not absorbed through mucous membranes. It is therefore useless as a surface anaesthetic. For infiltration 0.25–1% solutions are used. The toxicity is about one-quarter that of cocaine. It has a relatively short action because of hydrolysis by serum cholinesterase but this may be prolonged by up to 45–90 min when adrenaline is added. Like amethocaine it inhibits the antibacterial action of sulphonamides.

Benzocaine

This is a surface anaesthetic which is comparatively non-irritant and has a low toxicity.

Compound Benzocaine lozenges BPC (containing 100 mg benzocaine) are used to prevent nausea and vomiting during the taking of dental impressions and for the passage of bronchoscopes and oesophagoscopes in the conscious patient. They can also be used to alleviate the pain of local oral lesions such as aphthous ulcers, acute pharyngitis, lacerations and carcinoma of the mouth. As an insufflation it has also been used for painful throat conditions.

It is an ester which on hydrolysis produces p-aminobenzoic acid so that it should not be used in patients being treated with sulphonamides.

Other local anaesthetics: See Table 11.2.

MUSCLE RELAXANTS

The drugs which are called muscle relaxants are reversible muscle paralysers. They are usually grouped as:

1. Non-depolarising agents (competitive blockers), such as tubocurarine,

pancuronium, gallamine, benzquinonium and alcuronium, which bind to the motor end plate cholinergic receptor and prevent depolarisation by acetylcholine.

2. Depolarising agents, such as suxamethonium and decamethonium halides, which prevent the motor end plate responding to acetylcholine by maintaining it in a constant state of depolarisation. In practice, drugs of this second group can also exert a curare-like action after an initial phase of depolarisation.

All of the muscle relaxants are highly charged molecules and do not pass through plasma membranes into cells. They are therefore administered intravenously and are distributed by blood flow and diffusion throughout the body. Changes in muscle blood flow or cardiac output can thus alter the speed of onset of neuromuscular blockade.

1. Non-depolarising agents

Tubocurarine

Curare, an arrow poison used by South American Indians, is derived from the plant *Chondrodendron tomentosum.* The active alkaloid, tubocurarine, is an isoquinoline derivative which has neither analgesic nor anaesthetic properties but can release histamine and is a weak ganglion blocker.

Pharmacokinetics Curare is not absorbed when taken orally; hence the Indians could use it to paralyse game animals. Tubocurarine is absorbed following administration intramuscularly, subcutaneously, intraperitoneally, sublingually or rectally, but in practice it is given intravenously. The $t_{1/2}$ is about 100 min.

The duration of paralysis is influenced not only by drug elimination but also by the rate of drug dissociation from the cholinergic receptor at the end plate. The $t_{1/2}$ for dissociation from the receptor appears to be about 12 s in man. Some tubocurarine is metabolised in the muscles but 30% is excreted unchanged in the urine. Renal excretion is by glomerular filtration and no secretion or reabsorption takes place via the tubular epithelium because of the high degree of ionisation of the drug. However, there must be an alternative pathway for the elimination of d-tubocurarine since little or no prolongation of blockade occurs in patients with renal failure. Biliary excretion occurs in dogs but has not yet been demonstrated in man.

Plasma-protein binding appears to be to globulins rather than albumin. Patients with liver disease may require larger doses of tubocurarine because of raised levels of plasma globulins and also (possibly) due to increased amounts of end-plate acetylcholine due to deficient esterase synthesis.

After intravenous administration, the effect comes on rapidly, reaches a maximum at 3 min and persists for 20–30 min, although following repeated administration a more prolonged effect results. The action is prolonged in acidotic patients, and shortened in alkalosis. Volatile anaesthetics, such as ether and halothane, intensify and prolong the action of tubocurarine.

There is only poor penetration of the placental barrier and usual doses do not affect the fetus. The blood–brain barrier is not crossed.

Table 11.2 Properties of some local anaesthetics

Local anaesthetic	*Potency*	*Toxicity*	*Uses*
Amethocaine (*Tetracaine*)	10–20 times that of procaine. 0.5% for surface analgesia 0.025–0.05% for infiltration	Cardiac asystole. Ventricular fibrillation. Maximum dose 300 mg NB: rapid absorption through mucous membranes can produce systemic toxicity.	Infiltration. Surface anaesthesia in mouth and skin. Corneal analgesia. Not for bronchoscopy or cystoscopy.
Bupivacaine (*Marcain*)	4 times more potent than lignocaine. 0.25–0.5% solution for infiltration	Safer than lignocaine for extradural block. Maximum dose 25–30 ml of 0.5% solution	Very long action (5–16 h). Infiltration. Extradural block. Epidural block.
Etidocaine (*Duranest*)	0.25–5% solutions	Safer than lignocaine and bupivacaine. Motor block readily produced in extradural analgesia	Long-acting, rapid onset. Extradural, topical and infiltration.

Clinical uses 6–30 mg intravenously is the usual dose range. Initial effects are ptosis and extraocular muscle paresis followed by weakness of the muscles of the face, jaw and neck. Small doses of the drug may produce weakness of the limbs without impairment of respiration; however, clinically useful amounts of the drug produce apnoea and inhibition of laryngeal movements and cough.

The drug is used for muscular relaxation during operations under general anaesthesia, tracheal intubation, facilitation of assisted ventilation and prevention of coughing and laryngospasm during anaesthesia.

At the end of the procedure, the patient should be given intermittent positive-pressure ventilation until breathing starts spontaneously or the effect of tubocurarine is reversed by an injection of the anticholinesterase neostigmine (1–2.5 mg) which increases the amount of acetylcholine at the end plate. This should be preceded by atropine (0.6 mg) to prevent the parasympathetic effects of the acetylcholine by blocking the muscarinic cholinergic receptors. Excess neostigmine may cause neuromuscular block by depolarisation which may be confusing unless the possibility is considered. This is usually the reason for a patient relapsing after neostigmine administration despite an initial recovery from paralysis.

Adverse effects Slight hypotension (rarely hypertension) due to autonomic ganglion blockade; occasionally bradycardia; histamine release can cause flushing of the face and upper chest and very rarely bronchospasm and circulatory collapse; persistent diplopia for several days; prolongation of neuromuscular blockade may occur in the presence of respiratory acidosis, myasthenic syndromes, concurrent administration of β-receptor blockers, aminoglycosides, frusemide and some tetracyclines.

Pancuronium (Pavulon)

Pancuronium is a bisquaternary amino-steroid. It is a non-depolarising muscle relaxant with rapid onset of action, a peak effect at 2–3 min and duration of action of 20–30 min. Weight for weight, it has about 5 times the potency of d-tubocurarine.

Pharmacokinetics The $t_{1/2}$ is approximately the same as d-tubocurarine (100 min). It is partly metabolised by hepatic microsomes, 30% undergoes renal excretion and 25% is eliminated in the bile (33% of this as the hydroxylated metabolites). The monohydroxy metabolite has some muscle-relaxant properties but the dihydroxy metabolite is inert. Since a large fraction of pancuronium is eliminated by the kidneys, patients with reduced renal function show reduced elimination and prolonged neuromuscular blockade.

In plasma only about 13% of pancuronium is free, much being bound to gamma globulin and albumin. The apparent volume of distribution for both pancuronium and tubocurarine varies with the levels of these proteins and influences the duration of neuromuscular blockade. Pancuronium like tubocurarine does not pass the blood–brain or placental barriers.

The action of pancuronium is antagonised by hyperkalaemia. Muscular paralysis is prolonged and enhanced by coadministration of volatile anaesthetics, but not affected by changes in body-fluid pH.

Adverse reactions Histamine release, noradrenaline release, minimal CVS activity, occasionally a small rise in blood pressure.

Gallamine triethiodide (Flaxedil)

This is 1,2,3-tri-(β-diethylaminoethoxy)-benzene-triethyl iodide. It has a muscle-paralysing effect similar to that produced by tubocurarine, but with a shorter action of 15–20 min.

Pharmacokinetics Gallamine crosses the placental barrier. Excretion is as unchanged drug via the kidney and in renal failure a compensatory increase in biliary excretion does not occur. In renal failure prolongation of neuromuscular blockade occurs.

Clinical use 20 mg of gallamine triethiodide are equivalent to 3 mg of tubocurarine chloride when given intravenously. Gallamine can be administered intramuscularly with hyaluronidase. It may be used in operations on patients with heart block. The drug is contraindicated in renal failure, tachycardia and for obstetric anaesthesia.

Adverse reactions Tachycardia due to vagal blockade and β-receptor stimulation. Occasional mild hypotension due to minimal sympathetic blockade is seen but often a slight rise in blood pressure occurs which may result in increased bleeding during anaesthesia. Less histamine is released than by tubocurarine. Muscle paralysis is potentiated by hypocapnia.

Some other non-depolarising neuromuscular blockers are shown in Table 11.3.

2. Depolarising agents

Suxamethonium (Scoline)

Suxamethonium is the dicholine ester of succinic acid and thus structurally resembles acetylcholine. Solutions of suxamethonium halides (chloride, bromide and iodide) are available for injection. These are unstable in warm environments and must be stored at 4°. They also lose activity if mixed with thiopentone since the solutions of these drugs are incompatible.

Pharmacokinetics The action of suxamethonium is terminated by metabolism by plasma enzymes: serum pseudocholinesterase first converts it into succinyl monocholine. This is also a depolarising muscle blocker but has only 1/20th of the potency of the parent compound. Succinyl monocholine is further hydrolysed to choline and succinic acid by both acetylcholinesterase and serum pseudocholinesterase. This second reaction occurs much more slowly than the first hydrolysis. The plasma $t_{1/2}$ of succinylcholine is 2–4 min. In the absence of any enzyme activity, non-enzymic hydrolysis continues at a rate of 5% per hour.

In about 1 in 2800 of the population a genetically determined abnormal plasma pseudocholinesterase is present which has poor catalytic activity (see

Table 11.3 Other non-depolarising muscle relaxants

Drug	*Potency compared with tubocurarine*	*Duration of action*	*Special features*
Alcuronium (Alloferin)	2.0	Rapid onset 15–20 min	Widely used. No histamine release. Can cause hypotension Little effect on heart rate. Care in renal impairment.
Fazadinium (Fazadon)	0.25	40 min	Very rapid onset of action. Tachycardia. Reduce dose in severe renal disease.
Atracurium besylate (Tracrium)	0.5	15–40 min	Non-enzymic degradation (unstable at pH 7.4 and 37°) so safe in renal or hepatic impairment. Does not accumulate on repeated dosing. Action prolonged by hypothermia.
Vecuronium bromide (Norcuron)	2.0–2.5	20–30 min	Predominantly biliary excretion. Does not accumulate on repeated dosing.

Chapter 4). Slow hydrolysis of suxamethonium in these patients produces prolonged apnoea, sometimes lasting several hours.

Acquired deficiency of cholinesterase may be due to malnutrition, dehydration, electrolyte disturbances, anaemia, liver disease (parenchymatous and obstructive), carcinomatosis, radiation, poisoning (e.g. organophosphorus). Even very low blood cholinesterase levels acquired due to these diseases only prolong suxamethonium apnoea by several minutes.

Clinical uses Because of the muscarinic actions of suxamethonium, atropine is usually given before its use. Administration is usually intravenous but it may be given intramuscularly with hyaluronidase. A weak solution, 1% or less, is given in order to minimise fasciculations. A single adult dose of 50 mg produces paralysis for 2–4 min. Apnoea lasting more than 15 min is considered abnormal. Children are given 1–2 mg/kg, but neonates up to 6 weeks may be resistant and require a non-depolarising blocker.

Suxamethonium is used for abdominal closure, orthopaedic manipulation, tracheal intubation, bronchoscopy, electroconvulsive therapy.

Adverse reactions Prolonged apnoea (see above, and Chapter 4), muscular fasciculations are often produced several seconds after injection of suxamethonium. This may be the cause of muscular pains after anaesthesia. Occasionally hypertonicity develops for 3–5 min and is then replaced by hypotonicity. Rarely this hypertonicity may develop into malignant hyperpyrexia (see below and Chapter 4).

Positive and negative chronotropic effects can be produced on the heart in an analogous manner to the actions at the myoneural junction. Low doses may produce bradycardia, whilst repeated doses produce tachycardia. In hyperkalaemic patients the drug may precipitate ventricular fibrillation. Furthermore, suxamethonium itself promotes potassium release from striated muscle.

Muscarinic actions of suxamethonium cause increases in salivary and gastric secretions, and the drug is contraindicated in severe glaucoma because it produces a rise in intraocular pressure.

Suxamethonium has produced anaphylactic reactions. It is contraindicated in severe liver disease, and in patients with extensive burns.

Neostigmine (which reverses the effects of curare) inhibits cholinesterase and may prolong the action of suxamethonium by increasing depolarisation.

Malignant hyperthermia (see p. 113)

This is a rare but potentially lethal complication of anaesthesia: it has occurred with many anaesthetics, including halothane and suxamethonium. It produces a rapid increase in body temperature accompanied by tachycardia and generalised muscle spasm. Severe acidosis and hyperkalaemia lead to serious arrhythmias.

Treatment includes the following:

1. Cool the patient with ice.
2. Administer intravenous sodium bicarbonate to correct acidosis and treat serious arrhythmias promptly.
3. Give 50% glucose and insulin to correct hyperkalaemia.
4. Administer dantroline sodium intravenously: this inhibits excitation–contraction coupling in striped muscle thus relieving muscle spasm. Intravenous boluses of 1 mg/kg are given as required at 5–10 minute intervals to a maximum of 10 mg/kg. Susceptible individuals may be given dantrolene orally as a protective measure.

Chapter 12
CARDIOVASCULAR DRUGS

HEART FAILURE

Heart failure occurs when the heart can no longer fulfil its function as a pump to deliver adequate amounts of oxygenated blood to the tissues.

An understanding of the various modes of treatment which may be used to treat heart failure requires some knowledge of the factors which normally determine the performance of the heart. These are: preload, afterload, myocardial contractility and heart rate.

1. Preload This describes the filling pressures of the left ventricle which determine the extent of stretch of myocardial fibres at the end of diastole.

The Frank–Starling relationship shows that stroke volume increases with end-diastolic pressure (see Fig. 12.1). The major influences on preload are blood volume (which increases in heart failure due to sodium and water retention (Fig. 12.2.)) and systemic venous tone. In heart failure, the ventricular function curve is depressed, so a lower output results from any filling pressure. The effect of various agents which may alter this relationship is also shown in Fig. 12.1 and will be discussed later.

2. Afterload describes the tension which develops in the ventricular wall in order to eject the stroke volume. It is principally determined by the systemic peripheral resistance, and the lower this is, the less the impedance to ventricular emptying. In patients with heart failure, reduction in afterload may improve cardiac output (and thus perfusion of essential organ systems).

3. Myocardial contractility This describes the intrinsic capacity of the heart muscle fibres to contract. It is often described as the inotropic state, and positive inotropes can improve cardiac performance by increasing contractility (Fig. 12.1).

4. Heart rate Increased heart rate will usually improve output and reduce preload. However, when there is coronary artery disease, coronary blood flow is determined by:

(i) the pressure difference between diastolic aortic pressure and the left ventricular end diastolic pressure, and
(ii) the time spent in diastole during which flow can occur. Tachycardia reduces this time.

Three particularly important features of heart failure occur as follows:

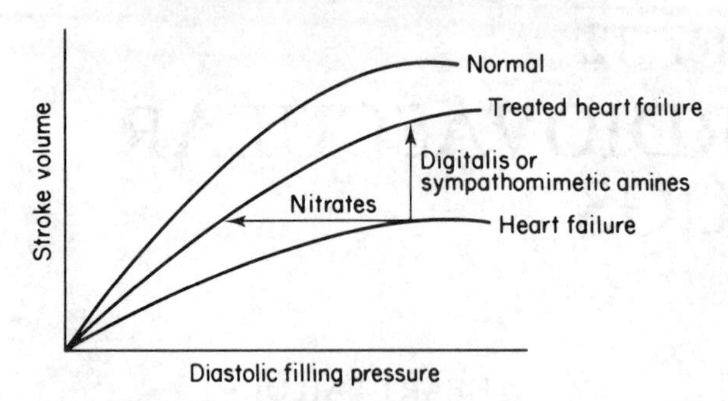

Fig. 12.1 Relationship between stroke volume and diastolic filling pressure. These measures are directly related to cardiac output and venous pressure respectively.

1. Reduced cardiac output activates baroreflexes leading to *increased sympathetic tone*, producing tachycardia, and peripheral vasoconstriction. Cardiac catecholamine stores become depleted with time, and the failing heart becomes reliant upon circulating catecholamines from the adrenals. There is also evidence to show a reduction in β-adrenergic receptors in the failing heart. These facts explain how mild cardiac failure may worsen if β-blockers are administered, as these drugs block compensatory reflex tachycardia.

2. Reduced cardiac output leads eventually to *decreased renal perfusion*, which activates *renin release*, with the production of *angiotensin II* (which increases peripheral resistance) and *aldosterone*. Aldosterone induces sodium and water retention but this is not the sole cause of the expanded blood volume in heart failure, as some patients have normal aldosterone levels. Loss of the retained fluid into tissues, exacerbated by raised pulmonary and peripheral venous pressure, leads to pulmonary and peripheral oedema respectively.

Fig. 12.2 shows the complex way in which the compensatory responses to heart failure interact.

3. Recently, a hormone called *atrial natriuretic factor* has been characterised which is released from the atrium in response to atrial distension, and leads to increased sodium (and water) excretion and to vasodilation. The role of this factor in heart failure and its possible involvement in therapy have yet to be determined.

Management of congestive cardiac failure

Left ventricular failure (LVF) is most commonly due to hypertension, coronary heart disease or valvular disease. When uncontrolled it commonly progresses to congestive cardiac failure (CCF) when right ventricular failure (RVF) occurs secondary to LVF. The other common cause of RVF is chronic lung disease (cor pulmonale).

Detection and treatment, if possible, of the underlying cause is essential for specific treatment, e.g. pacemaker insertion for complete heart block, control of thyrotoxicosis, surgery for ventricular aneurysm, but in many cases little can be done to treat the underlying disease, and management is aimed at relieving symptoms and optimising cardiac performance.

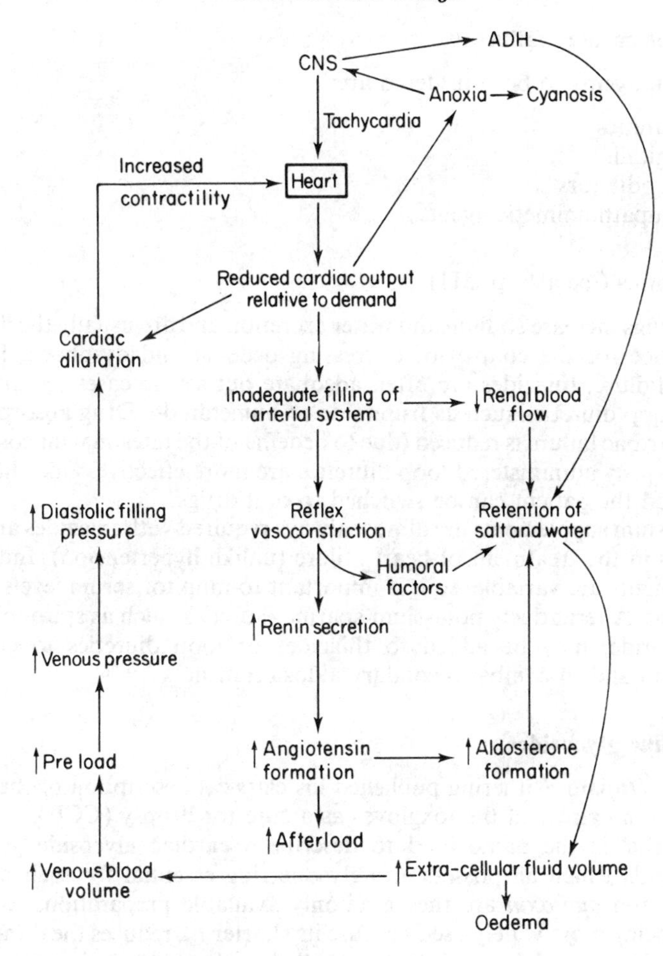

Fig. 12.2 Compensatory responses to heart failure.

General measures

These include:

1. Bed rest: improves renal blood flow.
2. Reduction in sodium intake to less than 2 g/day: this reduces pulmonary and peripheral oedema.
3. Anticoagulants: bed rest and low cardiac output predispose to deep venous thrombosis and anticoagulation reduces this risk.
4. Withdrawal of drugs which aggravate cardiac failure, e.g. β-blockers, verapamil, non-steroidal anti-inflammatory drugs.
5. Oxygen, if hypoxia is evident.

Drugs for cardiac failure

The main agents to be considered are:

1. Diuretics
2. Digitalis
3. Vasodilators
4. Sympathomimetic agents.

1. Diuretics (see also p. 511)

These drugs increase sodium and water excretion and are usually the drugs of first choice for the control of distressing oedema and dyspnoea. In mild cardiac failure, thiazides are often adequate but severe cases require more potent loop diuretics such as frusemide or bumetanide. Drug absorption in severe cardiac failure is reduced (due to oedema of the intestinal mucosa), and intravenously administered loop diuretics are more effective. Once failure is controlled the patient can be switched to oral drugs.

Potassium supplements are almost always required with thiazides and loop diuretics in the treatment of heart failure (unlike hypertension). Individual requirements are variable, so it is important to monitor serum levels during treatment. Alternatively potassium-sparing diuretics, such as spironolactone or amiloride, may be added to thiazides or loop diuretics to conserve potassium and to combat secondary aldosteronism.

2. Cardiac glycosides

In 1785, William Withering published his classical description of the use of digitalis (an extract of the foxglove) as a cure for dropsy (CCF).

'Digitalis' is the name used to describe a cardiac glycoside group of compounds which all possess an aglycone ring essential for their activity. *Digoxin* and *digitoxin* are the commonly available preparations, with the former being more widely used because its shorter $t_{1/2}$ reduces the duration of any toxicity and makes it easier to use. *Both drugs have identical cardiac effects.*

Until recently, digitalis was considered to be the mainstay of treatment in CCF, but its use has been re-evaluated because in many cases it has been difficult to demonstrate sustained benefit. Thus it is important to review all patients on maintenance treatment, as many are being unnecessarily exposed to the dangers of digitalis toxicity. The only undisputed indication for chronic digitalis therapy in heart failure is control of ventricular rate in rapid atrial fibrillation.

Mechanisms and effects of digitalis

1. Digitalis inhibits the membrane-bound enzyme Na^+, K^+, Mg^{2+}-ATPase which is responsible for the active expulsion of sodium from myocardial cells (the 'sodium pump'). This results in accumulation of intracellular sodium ions which displace bound calcium ions. The rise in free intracellular calcium is thought to account for the *positive inotropic activity*, i.e. increased myocardial contractility, with return of the Starling curve towards normal (see Fig. 12.1) and reduction in cardiac size.

2. Reduction of the membrane potential towards zero (due to increased intracellular sodium) may account for the *arrhythmogenic potential* of cardiac glycosides since this displaces the membrane potential towards the threshold potential for spontaneous discharge, and increases the slope of diastolic depolarisation. The ECG may reflect these effects with shortening of the QT interval and sagging of the ST segment (see Fig. 12.3).

3. *Slowing of the ventricular rate* results from 4 main mechanisms.

(a) *Delayed conduction through the atrioventricular node* (in particular) and the bundle of His. This is particularly important in *atrial fibrillation* where the atria discharge at very high rates (350/min) and the ventricles follow irregularly with some degree of block, for example at 120/min. Delaying A-V conduction increases the degree of block, reduces the ventricular rate and thus improves cardiac output. Progress may be assessed from the pulse rate: successful control is judged to be gained at rates of 70–80/min. In toxic doses, complete heart block may occur.
(b) *Improved cardiac haemodynamics* due to the positive inotropic effect reduces sympathetic tone, and thus the compensatory tachycardia.
(c) Small doses of digitalis *sensitise the sino-atrial node to vagal impulses.*
(d) Larger (often toxic) doses directly *depress the S-A node* and can cause sinus arrest.

4. Direct vasoconstriction of peripheral arterial and venous smooth muscle increases peripheral resistance and accounts for the failure of cardiac output to rise when digitalis is given to normal subjects. However, in heart failure, peripheral vasoconstrictor tone is already high and improvement in haemodynamics due to digitalis allows reduced sympathetic nervous activity and overall vasodilatation to occur.

5. Diuresis due to inhibition of renal tubular $Na^+ K^+$-ATPase. However, this is a minor effect, the major reason for diuresis is improved cardiac output.

Pharmacokinetics The properties of digoxin (from *Digitalis lanata*, the white foxglove) and digitoxin, (from *Digitalis purpurea*) are summarised in Table 12.1.

Absorption is mainly from the small intestine, and is variable in the case of the relatively water-soluble digoxin. Absorption from tablet preparations of digoxin is greatly influenced by their pharmaceutical characteristics, and in the past, differences between preparations have led to marked variation in bioavailability (Fig. 12.4) and even to cases of digoxin toxicity. Modern manufacturing processes ensure that the currently available preparations disperse rapidly and uniformly. In 1969 in the UK an apparently trivial change in the Burroughs Wellcome brand of digoxin 'Lanoxin' reduced the bioavailability from these tablets. The bioavailability was not restored to the previous levels of 65–70 % until 1972. That this had an important effect on the steady-state plasma digoxin levels of patients can be seen from Fig. 12.4. Whilst no major toxicity was detected in the UK, a similar variation in bioavailability due to altered manufacture appears to have been responsible for an outbreak of digoxin intoxication in Israel. The chief factor in determining bioavailability from tablets appears to be drug-particle size. Attempts to improve the consistency of absorption by using tablets with very

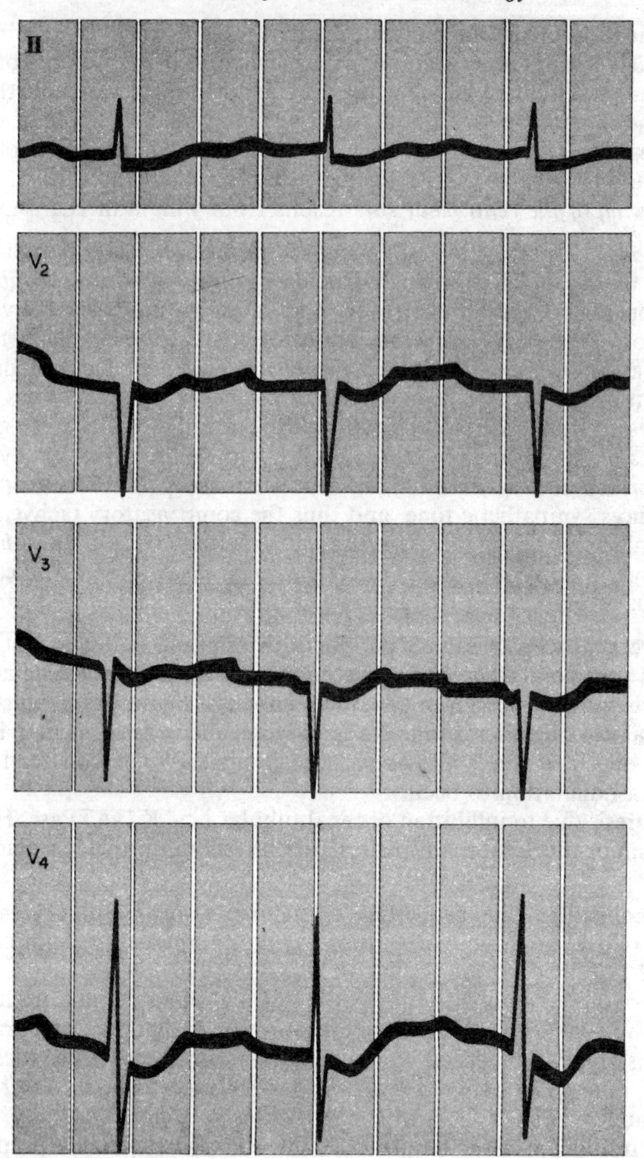

Fig. 12.3 Digitalis effect and probable toxicity. Note (a) the sagging ST segment not only in leads with dominant R waves (II, V_4) but also in those with dominant negative ventricular deflections; (b) prolonged P–R interval (first-degree heart block).

high dissolution rates or gelatin capsules filled with digoxin solution are based upon the assumption that the problem lies solely in the properties of the drug dosage form. The results of such studies suggest that the limiting and variable factor with the present generation of digoxin tablets is the individual patient's

Table 12.1 Comparison of the pharmacokinetic properties of the two most commonly used cardiac glycosides

	Digoxin	*Digitoxin*
Absorption from gut	Variable 20–80% (bioavailability may be a therapeutic problem)	100%
Hepatic metabolism	Minimal	90% (thus sensitive to induction of mixed function oxidase by other drugs)
Renal excretion	80% (a relatively water-soluble drug)	Minimal (therefore safer than digoxin in renal failure)
Protein binding	25%	95%
Lipid solubility	Relatively low (therefore obese patients should not be dosed on the basis of their body weight)	High (hence dosage in obese patients is based on body weight since the volume of distribution is increased by obesity)
$t_{1/2}$	$1\frac{1}{2}$ days	6 days
Time to peak effect (hours)	$1\frac{1}{2}$	4–12
Therapeutic levels (ng/ml)	1–2	20–35

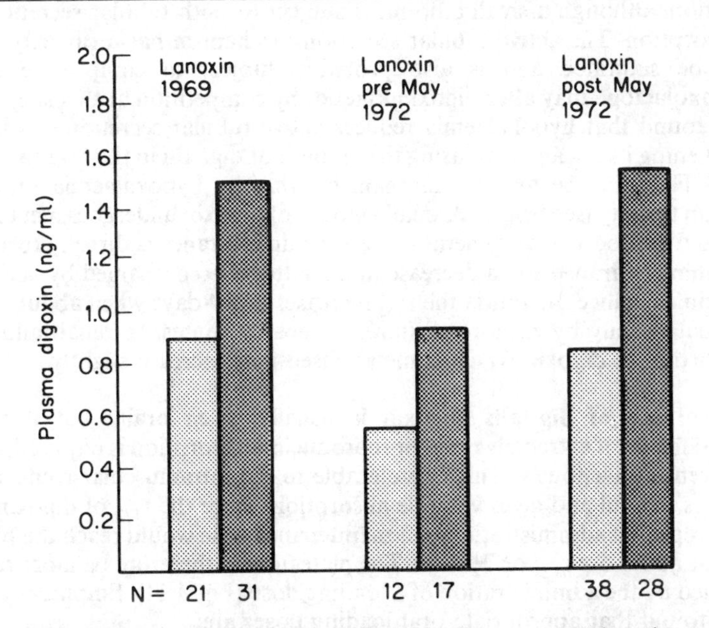

Fig. 12.4 Mean plasma digoxin levels in patients using Lanoxin (light columns 0.25–0.375 mg/day, dark columns 0.5 mg/day). N = number of patients in each group. (From T. R. D. Shaw, *Postgrad. Med. J.*, **50**, 92 (1974).)

absorptive capacity and not the properties of the formulation. Even using digoxin elixir the inter-individual variation in absorption is wide, being 57 to 96% of the administered dose in one study. Thus, using tablets which dissolve even more rapidly than those in current use may not further improve the consistency or reproducibility of absorption.

Digoxin absorption probably occurs over a relatively small area of intestine ('window effect'), and may be enhanced by drugs which reduce intestinal motility, e.g. propantheline (an anticholinergic drug). Conversely, absorption is reduced by drugs which increase motility, e.g. metaclopramide (see Fig. 12.5). However, with the rapidly dissolving digoxin preparations currently available, these interactions are no longer of importance clinically. Non-absorbed drugs which can bind digoxin such as cholestyramine, kaolin, pectin, and some antacids, can significantly reduce digoxin bioavailability.

Digoxin pharmacokinetics appear to require at least a two-compartment model and the drug is widely distributed throughout most of the tissues excepting fat. Digoxin can enter the CNS, thus accounting for the CNS toxic symptoms. Some recent evidence has suggested that the cardiac arrhythmias of digitalis toxicity may also be mediated through neural mechanisms. Binding to plasma proteins is relatively unimportant and hypoalbuminaemia or the displacement of digoxin from binding by other drugs or cholesterol which occur *in vitro* are not clinically important. The apparent volume of distribution varies from about 4 to 12 l/kg and is reduced in renal failure, myxoedema and the elderly, which partly accounts for the difficulties in the use of the drug in these cases.

80% of digoxin is excreted unchanged in the urine, mainly by glomerular filtration, although a small amount is subject to both tubular secretion and reabsorption. The active tubular secretion mechanism has a capacity which may be saturated and is also probably subject to competitive effects (spironolactone may alter digoxin kinetics by competition at this site). It has been found that hypokalaemia reduces active tubular secretion of digoxin, lengthening its $t_{1/2}$ and increasing the amount of digoxin in the body at steady state. This may be another mechanism whereby hypokalaemia promotes digoxin toxicity (see below). A small amount of digoxin undergoes metabolism to inactive products. In general terms digoxin clearance is directly related to creatinine clearance and a decrease in the latter is accompanied by decreased digoxin clearance. In anuria the $t_{1/2}$ increases to 4.4 days when about 14% is eliminated daily by extra-renal (mainly hepatic) routes. In renal failure the proportion of digoxin which is metabolised may increase slightly.

Clinical use of digitalis Digoxin is usually given orally but if this is impossible, or if extremely rapid or reproducible absorption is required, it may be given intravenously. This is preferable to the intramuscular route, as the latter is painful and gives variable absorption. Since the $t_{1/2}$ of digoxin is $1\frac{1}{2}$ days, repeated administration of a maintenance dose would reach the plateau level at about $5 \times t_{1/2}$ or $7\frac{1}{2}$ days. The plateau may therefore be more rapidly attained by the administration of a loading dose (Fig. 1.11). Empirically it has been found that appropriate oral loading doses are:

for a patient in sinus rhythm 12 μg/kg, which carries a 5% risk of toxicity;
for a patient in atrial fibrillation, 20 μg/kg which carries a 9% risk of toxicity.

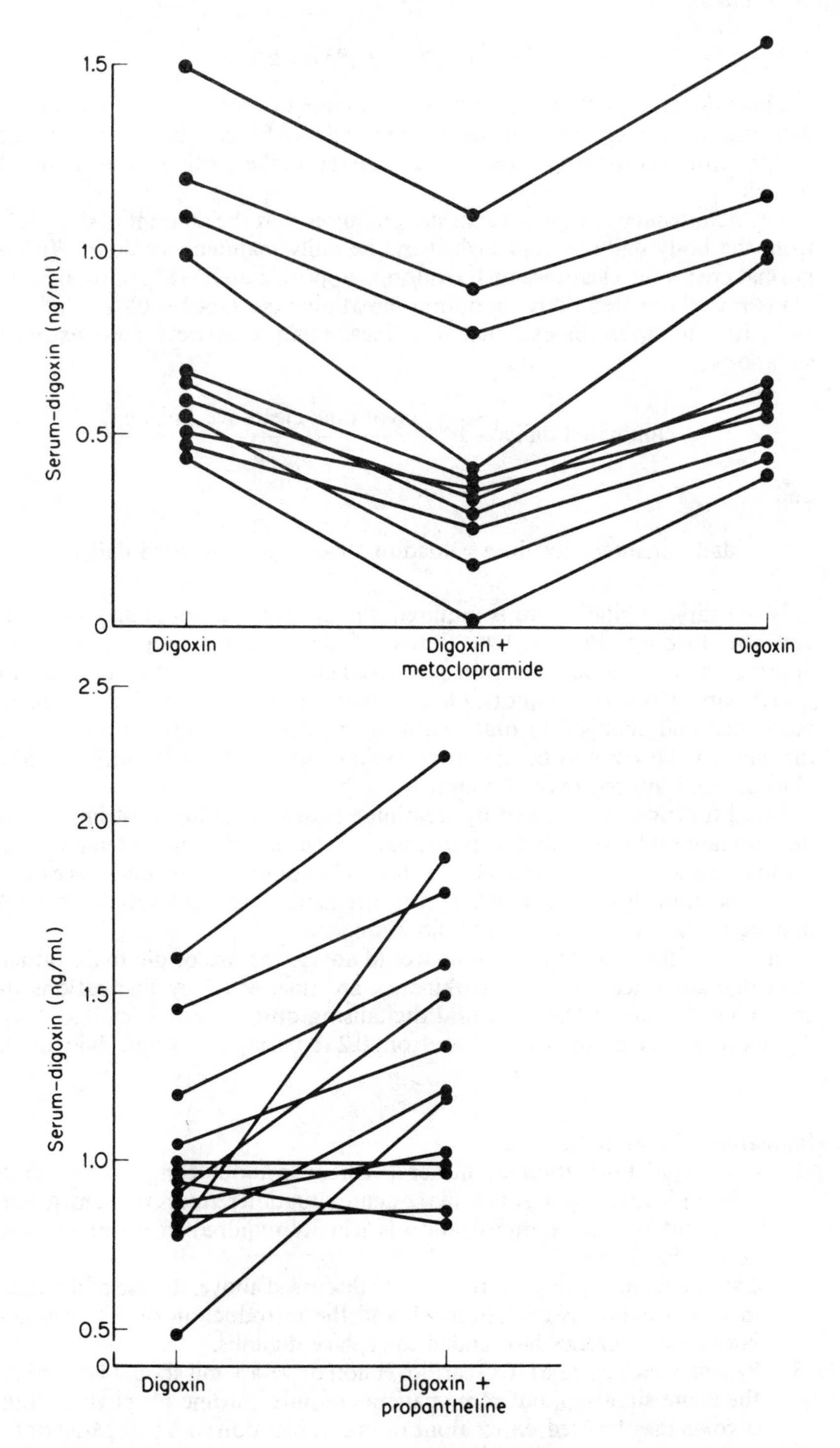

Fig. 12.5 Serum digoxin concentrations during treatment with (a) digoxin and metoclopramide; (b) digoxin and propantheline (From V. Manninen *et al.*, *Lancet*, **1**, 398 (1973).)

These doses are administered in 3 or 4 divided doses at 5 hourly intervals with examination before each dose for toxic effects. In renal failure the volume of distribution is apparently reduced and therefore the loading dose is reduced by half.

The maintenance of the plateau state requires that the amount of drug lost from the body daily be replenished by the daily maintenance dose. With a normal creatinine clearance of 100 ml/min, approximately 34% of total body digoxin is eliminated daily. In anuria (creatinine clearance = 0) this falls to 14%. Relying upon the existence of a linear relation between these extreme situations,

$$\%\text{ eliminated daily} \simeq 14 + \frac{\text{creatinine clearance (ml/min)}}{5}$$

and

$$\text{daily maintenance dose} = \text{loading dose} \times \%\text{ eliminated daily.}$$

When rapid digitalisation is required, the intravenous route may be used, and the loading dose is two thirds of that recommended orally, i.e. approximately 13 μg/kg for a patient in atrial fibrillation. It is probably best to give the first 0.5 mg in 2 aliquots, 2 hours apart. After this, the patient should be reassessed and changed to oral treatment if possible. Intravenous doses of digoxin may be given as boluses over 5 min or diluted (in 0.9% saline or 5% glucose), and infused over 30 minutes.

Renal function (as assessed by creatinine clearance) is the most important determinant of digoxin dosage, particularly in the elderly, and in renal failure the loading dose should be reduced by half. The subsequent maintenance dose should be individually assessed, and measurement of plasma levels (see below) may be particularly useful in this situation.

In renal failure, some physicians would advise the use of digitoxin rather than digoxin since its pharmacokinetics are unaffected by fluctuations in creatinine clearance. The total oral digitalising dose ranges from 1 to 2 mg digitoxin and the maintenance dose from 0.2 to 0.5 mg as a single daily dose.

Indications for digitalis

1. Fast atrial fibrillation or flutter (with or without congestive cardiac failure). Rapid digitalisation in the acute situation reduces the ventricular rate, and chronic administration is usually required to maintain it at acceptable levels.
2. Cardiac failure with sinus rhythm. As discussed above, the use of digitalis in this situation is controversial, and the introduction of new vasodilators and diuretics has tended to replace digitalis.
3. Re-entry tachycardias. DC cardioversion or verapamil should be used in the acute situation, but some patients require chronic prophylaxis and digoxin may be used, either alone or in combination with verapamil or β-blockers. Digoxin should be *avoided* in the Wolff–Parkinson–White syndrome (see p. 419).

Contraindications

1. 2nd or 3rd degree heart block or sinus bradycardia.
2. Hypertrophic obstructive cardiomyopathy. Digoxin increases the efficiency of contraction and may worsen outflow tract obstruction.
3. Wolff–Parkinson–White syndrome: see p. 419.
4. DC cardioversion: digitalised patients are at risk of developing serious ventricular arrhythmias, possibly because leakage of potassium coupled with catecholamine release enhances digitalis toxicity. If possible, digoxin should be withheld for 24 hours and digitoxin for 72 hours prior to cardioversion, and the smallest possible shock required to produce reversion to sinus rhythm employed. In an emergency however, digitalisation is no bar to electrical cardioversion.

Adverse effects Digitalis has a very low therapeutic index and at least 60% of the toxic dose is required to produce a therapeutic effect. Because of this narrow safety margin it has been argued that if it were to be introduced as a new drug today it would be regarded as too dangerous for clinical use. Several studies of the prevalence of intoxication have yielded figures of 15–20% for hospital in-patients on digoxin. This contrasts with the figure of 5% obtained in a prospective study of digitoxin intoxication, indicating that the latter may be the safer drug, notwithstanding its longer half-life which renders accumulation likely.

The clinical features of digitalis intoxication are detailed in Table 12.2. As digoxin preparations have become more pure the incidence of gastro-intestinal symptoms as the harbinger of toxicity, as they were in Withering's time, has decreased. Today the initial indication of intoxication may be a fatal cardiac arrhythmia. In a study of an accidental intoxication of 179 patients with three times the prescribed dose of digitoxin which occurred in the Netherlands, the following symptom incidence was recorded:

Table 12.2 Clinical manifestations of digitalis intoxication

A. *Gastrointestinal*	Common—anorexia, vomiting, diarrhoea, abdominal pain. Unusual—haemorrhagic bowel necrosis.
B. *Cardiovascular*	Any type of arrhythmia Any type of conduction defect Cardiac arrest Increasing cardiac failure.
C. *Neurological*	Common—headache, drowsiness, fatigue, blurred vision, altered colour vision, confusion visual aberrations Unusual—neuralgia, paraesthesiae, coma, optic neuritis producing scotomata or blindness, paresis of ocular muscles.
D. *Others*	Unusual—Skin rashes due to allergy, gynaecomastia.

95%	Fatigue and lethargy
82%	Muscular weakness with difficulty in walking or raising arms
80%	Anorexia and/or nausea
95%	Hazy vision with difficulty in reading and/or alteration in the colour of objects
100%	Abnormalities of red–green hue discrimination although these changes were too subtle to be detected by the standard Ishihara chart used for clinical testing of colour vision. Many patients also complained of visual aberrations, e.g. glittering vision, photophobia, seeing moving spots. As Na^+ K^+-ATPase activity is important for colour vision: these visual anomalies are thus a direct measure of the pharmacodynamic action of digitalis.
65%	CNS disturbances—7% developed frank psychosis
65%	Abdominal pain

With these numerous features it is hardly surprising that the clinical diagnosis of digitalis intoxication is often missed and the symptoms attributed to intercurrent illness or worsening of the cardiac condition. In these circumstances estimation of the digoxin or digitoxin plasma level may be helpful. The digitalis effect on the ECG (sagging depression of the ST segment often with prolongation of the PR interval) does not of itself indicate intoxication. When such changes are seen in leads with predominantly negative QRS complexes this may suggest overdosage and the situation requires urgent review (see Fig. 12.3). The common arrhythmias associated with intoxication and their frequency from one series of cases are:

(a) *Premature ventricular ectopic beats* (33%). These frequently follow a normal sinus beat: bigeminal rhythm. N.B. this is not pathognomonic of digitalis intoxication and can occur in any form of heart disease.
(b) *Atrial tachycardia* which may be associated with varying degrees of heart block (10%).
(c) *Nodal tachycardia* (29%).
(d) *Sinus bradycardia, sinoatrial block, or sinus arrest* (2%).
(e) *A–V block* of any degree, the Wenkebach type being the most commonly detected by the bedside. Second- and third-degree heart block constitute 18% of digitalis-related arrhythmias, although first-degree block is electrocardiographically commoner.
(f) *Ventricular tachycardia* (8%).

There is a great individual variation in digitalis tolerance: some patients may require and take a maintenance dose four or five times that which produces toxicity in another patient. Numerous factors predispose to toxicity and are shown in Table 12.3.

Treatment of digitalis toxicity involves the following:

(a) Discontinuation of the drug may be sufficient, particularly if the signs of toxicity are confined to the gastrointestinal tract. If there are serious cardiac manifestations active treatment may be needed.
(b) Antidotes
   (i) potassium chloride given at the rate of 0.5 mmol/minute intravenously under constant electrocardiographic monitoring. This is

Table 12.3 Predisposing factors to digitalis intoxication

1. Electrolyte disturbances Hypokalaemia Hypercalcaemia Hypernatraemia Hypomagnesaemia Alkalosis	3. Disease states Hypothyroidism Hypoxia Renal failure (digoxin) Myocarditis Recent cardiac surgery Severe heart disease Severe pulmonary disease
2. Drugs Potassium-depleting diuretics Carbenoxolone Corticosteroids Reserpine Quinidine Catecholamines Amiodarone Nifedipine, verapamil	4. Old age (decreased muscle mass reduces ATPase binding sites, thus reducing apparent volume of distribution, and decreased renal function reduces digoxin elimination) 5. D.C. Cardioversion

safer than oral potassium since the drip may be stopped at the first sign of potassium excess. It is contraindicated in the presence of conduction disturbances.

(ii) EDTA as disodium edetate which chelates calcium may be used in the presence of block.

(iii) Antiarrhythmic agents in particular phenytoin, propranolol and lignocaine are useful in controlling arrhythmias. Propranolol should not be used in the presence of AV block since this may be exacerbated. DC countershock is used only as a desperate last resort if ventricular fibrillation or tachycardia unresponsive to other measures has occurred. Occasionally intracardiac pacing is required for heart block.

(iv) Severe cases of digoxin poisoning have been successfully treated with the Fab fragments of sheep digoxin-specific antibodies. This treatment is expensive and available at only a few centres in the United Kingdom.

Monitoring digoxin plasma levels A moderate correlation exists between the dose of digitalis administered and the resulting plasma level, and the toxic effects of digitalis are dose-related. Digoxin (and digitoxin) plasma levels may thus be of use clinically, and have become available in many hospitals. In practice (unless toxicity is suspected), a blood sample should not be taken less than 7 hours after an oral dose (4 hours after an i.v. dose) and the normally accepted therapeutic range for digoxin is 1–2 ng/ml, although toxicity may occur at levels over 1.5 ng/ml.

As potassium competes with digitalis for myocardial binding sites, drug levels must be interpreted in the light of the current plasma potassium. Hypokalaemia may lower the level of digitalis at which toxicity arises.

A recent study found that patients with digoxin-induced gastrointestinal symptoms had high serum drug levels whereas those with arrhythmias had therapeutic concentrations. In the latter cases however the Ca^{2+}/K^{+} ratio was higher (0.38) than in the former (0.31). Thus mild hypercalcaemia may contribute to digitalis toxicity as may also hypomagnesaemia.

Measurement of erythrocyte $Na^{+}K^{+}$ ATPase inhibition during treatment indicates the pharmacodynamic effect of digoxin and the therapeutic response of patients with atrial fibrillation correlates better with this measurement than with plasma digoxin concentrations (see Fig. 12.6). Nevertheless the correlation is by no means perfect and further work will be necessary to find a method of predicting tissue response from plasma digoxin levels.

At present, therefore, estimation of plasma digoxin levels is most useful in the diagnosis of therapeutic overdosage and in checking patient compliance rather than in controlling therapy.

Drug interaction with digitalis

1. Interaction involving absorption (see above, p. 372).
2. Drugs causing hypokalaemia (e.g. diuretics, carbenoxolone) may exacerbate toxicity.
3. Quinidine (?displacement from tissue binding sites), verapamil, β-blockers, amiodarone and nifedipine may all potentiate the action of digitalis on the myocardium.
4. Barbiturates, phenylbutazone and phenytoin may reduce maintenance plasma digitoxin levels (possibly due to hepatic enzyme induction).

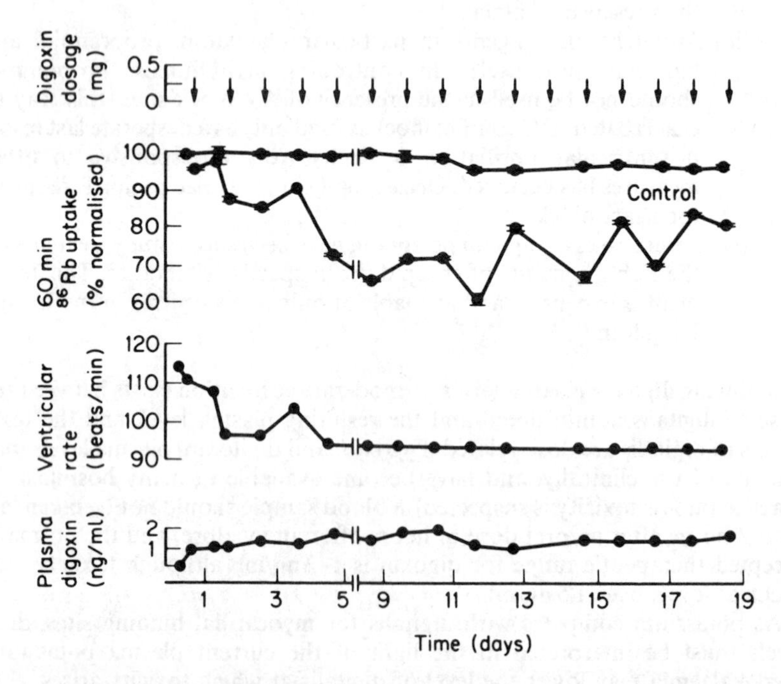

Fig. 12.6 Response of atrial fibrillation to digoxin showing relationship to plasma digoxin concentration and to a measure of ATPase inhibition (^{86}Rb uptake) (From J. K. Aronson *et al.*, *Brit. J. Clin. Pharm.*, **4**, 213 (1977).)

3. Vasodilators in the treatment of heart failure

Effective inotropic therapy with digitalis may produce a greater stroke volume for any given ventricular end-diastolic pressure (preload) and thus shifts the Starling curve towards normality (see Fig. 12.1). Diuretics relieve symptoms of congestion by reducing preload but with no effect on ventricular function. Vasodilators represent a third modality of treatment in which preload, afterload or both are reduced with consequent improvement in cardiac function.

Venodilators act primarily by increasing venous capacitance, thus venous return diminishes and preload is reduced. Reduction of pulmonary capillary pressure relieves pulmonary oedema and improves tissue oxygenation which in turn also improves myocardial function. Left ventricular dilatation is also relieved and this is important for several reasons: firstly, increase in ventricular volume leads to a rise in wall tension and myocardial oxygen consumption, reduction in the radius of the ventricular cavity thus improves oxygenation by reducing oxygen consumption. Secondly, with severe ventricular dilatation functional mitral and tricuspid regurgitation occur due to widening of the atrioventricular valve rings. By reducing ventricular dilatation regurgitation may be abolished.

Arterial vasodilators primarily reduce afterload i.e. they decrease the resistance to ventricular ejection. In the presence of heart failure, reflex vasoconstriction occurs which is largely mediated by the sympathetic nervous system. The diseased ventricle is therefore subjected to a greater than normal resistance to outflow which results in a vicious circle of increasing failure followed by increasing vasoconstriction. Left ventricular dilatation also contributes to the problem by increasing myocardial oxygen consumption and reducing contractility. Thus afterload becomes an important determinant of cardiac output and if it is reduced, the improved stroke volume and ventricular emptying which result lead to reduced end-diastolic pressure and volume (Fig. 12.7). Note that when the left ventricle is normal, a reduction in arterial impedance does not lead to much increase in stroke volume, but instead results in a reflex tachycardia to compensate for the fall in arterial pressure.

Clinical use of vasodilators Vasodilators are being increasingly used in the treatment of both acute and chronic congestive cardiac failure in patients who fail to respond adequately to diuretics. Many specialists would now turn to vasodilators before using digoxin.

The choice of vasodilator is determined by the clinical features. Thus if the main problem is pulmonary congestion, (with dyspnoea and raised pulmonary wedge pressure) a venodilator is the appropriate choice. If the problem is reduced cardiac output (with fatigue, syncope, etc.) or mitral regurgitation, then an arterial vasodilator is most effective. Arterial dilators are less useful if there is a fixed obstruction to arterial flow, e.g. aortic stenosis, hypertrophic cardiomyopathy. When both low cardiac output and pulmonary congestion are present, a mixed (or 'balanced') arterial and venous dilator is most useful.

The vasodilators available may be classified according to their primary site of action (see Table 12.4).

There are several potential problems associated with the use of vasodilators:

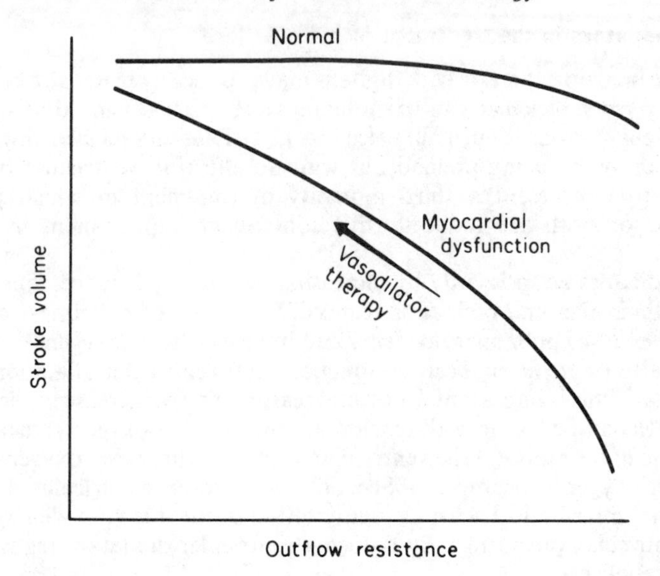

Fig. 12.7 Relationship of left-ventricular stroke volume to systolic outflow resistance in normal and diseased hearts. With myocardial dysfunction blood pressure is no longer directly determined by outflow resistance because stroke volume and resistance are inversely related.

1. An excessive fall in filling pressure with venodilators may produce a dangerous fall in cardiac output, particularly in patients who had normal or only slightly elevated wedge pressures when treatment was commenced. Alternatively, arterial dilators may lead to excessive systemic arterial hypotension, and may precipitate angina as coronary perfusion falls. Thus, particularly in acute heart failure, vasodilator therapy is not

Table 12.4 A classification of commonly used vasodilators according to their site of action

Arterial vasodilators	*Venodilators*	*Mixed arterial/venous vasodilators*
1. *Smooth muscle relaxants*	*Nitrates*	1. *α-blockers*
Minoxidil	Glyceryl trinitrate	Phentolamine
Hydralazine	Isosorbide	Phenoxybenzamine
	Isosorbide mononitrate	Prazosin
2. *β_2-agonists*		2. *Converting enzyme inhibitors*
Salbutamol		Captopril
Pirbuterol		Enalapril
Terbutaline		
		3. *Sodium nitroprusside*
		4. *Calcium antagonists*
		Nifedipine

without risk and careful intensive observation is essential. In this situation most clinicians would recommend the use of a Swan–Ganz catheter to measure pulmonary wedge pressures (and cardiac output in some cases), and an intra-arterial catheter for continuous systemic pressure recording.

2. The development of tolerance to vasodilators can occur with long term use. It may be drug-specific (i.e. not seen when the patient is changed to another vasodilator) e.g. with hydralazine or nitrates. It may be non-specific and due to such factors as reflex sympathetic stimulation leading to tachycardia and vasoconstriction, and activation of the renin-angiotensin-aldosterone system also producing vasoconstriction and salt and water retention. These effects counteract the action of vasodilators. Another problem altering the apparent efficacy of these drugs with chronic use is progression of the underlying disease.

Arterial Vasodilators The smooth muscle relaxants hydralazine, and minoxidil (see p. 443) are potent vasodilators, but tolerance may develop over time limiting their long-term use. Reflex tachycardia is a problem in hypertensive patients (requiring combined treatment with a β-blocker), but is less common in heart failure. Exacerbation of fluid retention usually requires additional diuretic treatment. They may be usefully combined with nitrates so that preload as well as afterload are reduced. The β_2-receptor stimulants also have some direct positive inotropic action due to stimulation of β_1-receptors (see following section).

Venodilators The nitrates (see p. 389) have an additional coronary vasodilator effect which make them particularly useful in acute LVF associated with myocardial infarction where there is pulmonary congestion. In this situation, intravenous administration allows careful titration against systemic blood pressure (which may fall) and heart rate. In chronic heart failure they may be used alone or combined with arterial dilators such as hydralazine.

Mixed arterial/venous dilators The α-receptor blockers, phentolamine and phenoxybenzamine block both postsynaptic (α_1) and presynaptic (α_2) receptors (see p. 447), thus they have the disadvantage of causing reflex tachycardia and postural hypotension. Prazosin, however, blocks only α_1-receptors (see p. 446) minimising these adverse effects. However, its use in chronic treatment of heart failure is often restricted by the development of tachyphylaxis (decreasing clinical effect from the same dose over time).

Angiotensin converting enzyme inhibitors (captopril and the more recently developed enalapril, see p. 452) have become increasingly popular in the treatment of refractory cardiac failure—particularly as tachyphylaxis is rarely seen. All other groups of vasodilators tend to increase stimulation of the already activated renin–angiotensin–aldosterone system, but these drugs reduce both afterload (peripheral resistance) by reducing renin production, and preload by reducing aldosterone production which in turn decreases sodium and water retention. However, no correlation between pre-treatment levels of plasma renin activity and the degree of acute haemodynamic effect resulting from treatment has been found. It is notable that reflex tachycardia is rarely seen. The incidence of first dose hypotension is much reduced by starting with a very low dose and ensuring that the patient is not salt depleted by diuretics.

Sodium nitroprusside (see p. 448) has a direct action on the smooth muscle of arteries and veins. It is given intravenously and its action commences within a few minutes of commencing an infusion, disappearing just as quickly when the infusion is stopped. There is almost invariably some fall in blood pressure and increase in heart rate associated with its use, but by using an infusion pump to control rate of delivery flexible control of blood pressure can be achieved. It has been successfully used in cardiogenic shock with severe peripheral hypoperfusion.

Nifedipine (see p. 395) is a calcium antagonist which relaxes the smooth muscle of coronary and systemic arteries, and peripheral veins, but unlike verapamil has no effect on cardiac conduction. It has been effective in heart failure, particularly in the presence of angina or hypertension (for which it is also commonly used).

Sympathomimetic agents

These are used in heart failure for their cardiac inotropic and peripheral vascular effects. The responses of the cardiovascular system to sympathomimetics are mediated by both α- and β-receptors:

1. α-receptor stimulation leads to vasoconstriction.
2. β_1-receptors are located in the heart and stimulation leads to increased heart rate, contractility and conduction through the atria and A–V node. There is also increased automaticity of the A–V node and the His-Purkinje system.
3. β_2-receptor stimulation dilates both peripheral and coronary arteries and arterioles.

Before these agents are employed to treat severe hypotension from any cause, hypovolaemia must be corrected, preferably using colloid solutions such as plasma or albumin. This requires careful monitoring, particularly when the cause is severe heart failure (cardiogenic shock) where volume overload could be fatal.

These agents should be given by a central line, if possible, to avoid peripheral vasoconstriction (α effect) though this does not apply to salbutamol or isoprenaline. Adrenaline and noradrenaline may cause tissue necrosis if they extravasate (if this occurs it should be promptly treated with α-blocking agents).

The differing properties of the sympathomimetic agents available are shown in Table 12.5.

Adrenaline This agent has predominantly α and β_1 effects and is the drug of choice in cardiac arrest with asystole (see p. 419) and in acute anaphylaxis. It is not used as an inotrope in cardiac failure because excessive β_1 stimulation markedly increases heart rate with high risk of tachyarrhythmias, together with a marked increase in myocardial oxygen demands.

Table 12.5 Cardiovascular actions of sympathomimetic agents

Drug	*Vascular receptors* α	β_2	*Cardiac receptors* β_1
Adrenaline	++	+	+++
Noradrenaline	++++	0	++
Isoprenaline	0	++++	++++
Dopamine*	++	±	++
Dobutamine	+	+	++
Salbutamol	0	++++	+

* Also stimulates dopaminergic receptors (see below)

Noradrenaline (Levophed) This is the neurotransmitter of the sympathetic nervous system and its major effect is on α-receptors although at low doses its β_1 effects predominate. At higher doses α-mediated vasoconstriction becomes evident with increased blood pressure and secondary reflex bradycardia (mediated by the vagus nerve). Thus despite increase in cardiac contractility, there is usually a decrease in cardiac output due to the α effects, and noradrenaline is rarely used in severe cardiac failure having been supplanted by newer agents.

Isoprenaline (Isuprel, Saventrine) This is a pure β-receptor stimulant and is effective in increasing heart rate and cardiac output in bradycardia or A–V block. However, it increases myocardial oxygen demands (which can precipitate angina) and may cause serious ventricular arrhythmias, and these effects limit its use. It is usually given by i.v. infusion at a rate of 0.2–6 μg/min (see also p. 470).

Dopamine (Inotropin) This is the metabolic precursor of noradrenaline. It activates both α- and β-receptors and also has vasodilator effects on the renal and mesenteric beds mediated via dopaminergic receptors which may also mediate coronary vasodilatation. The cardiac stimulant effect of dopamine is mediated directly via dopaminergic receptors and indirectly by release of noradrenaline from sympathetic nerve endings in the heart.

The cardiovascular response to dopamine depends on the dose infused:

(a) Low dose dopamine (2–5 μg/kg/min): stimulates renal dopamine receptors producing increased renal perfusion and urine output. Dopamine at this dose is often combined with frusemide (2–4 mg/min, max 1.5 g/24 h) in acute renal failure to stimulate glomerular filtration and produce a diuresis. Cardiac output is slightly increased and peripheral resistance is slightly decreased, so mean blood pressure is hardly altered.

(b) High dose dopamine (5–20 μg/kg/min): increasing inotropic activity occurs and the renal effect is lost. Blood pressure and cardiac output rise and tachycardia may be severe enough to cause angina or precipitate arrhythmias.

(c) At doses > 20 μg/kg/min, α-receptor stimulation increases peripheral resistance reducing both renal and skin blood flow, which can lead to gangrene of the extremities.

The $t_{1/2}$ of dopamine is about 2 min, and so it can only be given by intravenous infusion. It is rapidly metabolised by monoamine oxidase and dopamine β-hydroxylase.

In severe congestive cardiac failure dopamine is most beneficial at low doses and the addition of a vasodilator improves cardiac output to a greater degree than an increased dose of dopamine.

Contraindications: dopamine should not be used in the presence of ventricular arrhythmias, during the use of cyclopropane or halogenated hydrocarbon (e.g. halothane) anaesthetics or in the presence of phaeochromocytoma. Patients on monoamine oxidase inhibitors should receive one tenth of the usual dose.

Dobutamine (Dobutrex) This is a modification of isoprenaline which is predominantly a β_1-receptor stimulant. Unlike dopamine it does not stimulate the heart indirectly by releasing noradrenaline from nerve endings, which may explain why it is less prone to cause arrhythmias than dopamine.

It exerts a more prominent inotropic than chronotropic action as compared to isoprenaline, but the reason for this difference in response is unknown. Although it causes some peripheral vasodilation it does not dilate the renal vasculature. Thus in the clinical situation of severe cardiac failure associated with hypotension, oliguria and severe peripheral vasoconstriction (cardiogenic shock), the *combination* of dobutamine with low-dose dopamine (2–5 μg/kg/min) (for its renal effect) has been found to be very effective. Dobutamine also has a very short $t_{1/2}$ (2 min) and is mainly eliminated by hepatic metabolism to glucuronides and 3-O-methyldobutamine. The usual dose range is 5–10 μg/kg/min, but doses up to 40 μg/kg/min may be used if necessary.

Dobutamine reduces left ventricular filling pressure and raises cardiac output which is useful in acute left ventricular failure associated with myocardial infarction. However, particularly at higher doses (> 20 μg/kg/min), tachycardia intervenes and may extend the area of ischaemia. Ventricular tachyarrhythmias contraindicate the use of dobutamine.

Salbutamol (Ventolin) (see p. 471) This agent predominantly stimulates β_2-receptors and its beneficial effect in severe cardiac failure is mainly due to the resulting arteriolar vasodilation. By reducing afterload it improves cardiac output and may reduce ventricular filling pressures. Unlike dopamine and dobutamine it has the advantage of not increasing myocardial oxygen requirements, provided the dose is kept at a level which does not cause more than a small increase in heart rate: generally in the range of 0.15–0.4 μg/kg/min as an i.v. infusion.

Recent developments in the treatment of severe heart failure

Intra-aortic balloon counterpulsation is an invasive technique developed for use in cardiogenic shock to reduce cardiac work and improve coronary perfusion. It is most successful when used temporarily to support the circulation prior to, or after, definitive cardiac surgery.

Amrinone is a new inotropic drug which can raise cardiac output and lower ventricular filling pressures. Its mode of action is unknown, but possibly it acts at the level of excitation–contraction coupling to improve calcium release. It has the advantage of being effective orally, but its use may be limited by serious side effects (nausea and thrombocytopenia).

Pirbuterol is another recent introduction for the treatment of acute and chronic heart failure. It can be given both i.v. and orally. It has seven-fold higher specificity for β_2-receptors than salbutamol. Its principal actions are vasodilation of both systemic and pulmonary vascular beds, and a lesser positive inotropic effect. When given in acute heart failure it increases cardiac output while heart rate, blood pressure and myocardial oxygen consumption are relatively unchanged. It may also be effective in chronic airflow obstruction with pulmonary hypertension.

Its use in chronic heart failure has yielded conflicting results, and tachyphylaxis has been seen in some studies. Dysrrythmias are rare with pirbuterol.

Summary of the management of acute left ventricular failure

1. Sit the patient up.

2. Oxygen The hypoxia of cardiac failure is largely due to ventilation–perfusion imbalance with perfusion of under-ventilated alveoli. Oxygen therapy is therefore beneficial. The highest available oxygen concentration may be employed provided no contraindications to such therapy are present, e.g. chronic obstructive airways disease with raised pCO_2.

3. Frusemide 20–40 mg i.v. is usually adequate. The earliest haemodynamic changes may reflect venous dilatation rather than diuresis and it is effective in anuric patients with acute left-ventricular failure. However, diuresis is also important and both mechanisms reduce pulmonary oedema.

4. Opioids Diamorphine (3.5–5 mg i.v.) or morphine (8 mg i.v.) relieve the severe dyspnoea by several mechanisms:

(a) relief of anxiety.

(b) peripheral venous dilatation: this reduces venous return and thus relieves pulmonary oedema (this effect is equivalent to venesection). Morphine has no direct action on vascular smooth muscle, but the mechanism of vasodilatation may involve reduction in α-adrenergic tone.

(c) reduced sensitivity of the respiratory centre to reflex stimulation from the stiff congested lungs.

However, the danger of fatal depression of the respiratory centre must be remembered, particularly in patients with chronic obstructive airways disease. The sensitivity of the respiratory centre to opiates may also vary with time in the same patient, so a previously safe dose of opioid is no guarantee of safety in the future. Thus many prefer to reserve opioids until the effect of other less hazardous drugs has been assessed. Severe respiratory depression may be reversed with naloxone, and opioid-induced vomiting avoided by giving an antiemetic, e.g. prochlorperazine 12.5 mg i.v.

5. Salbutamol Given intravenously this may relieve both cardiac failure (see above) and the severe bronchospasm which often accompanies severe LVF. Aminophylline may also be effective in this situation but is more hazardous to use.

6. Digitalis This is particularly indicated in the presence of atrial tachyarrhythmias (see above).

7. Intermittent positive pressure ventilation may be required to treat intractable left ventricular failure.

CIRCULATORY SHOCK

Shock states are associated with alteration in the functioning of both the heart and the peripheral vasculature and result in life-threatening impairment of perfusion of vital organs such as the brain, kidneys and liver. The main types of shock are:

1. *hypovolaemic*: in which the repletion of volume with blood, plasma, dextran or crystalloid is the main therapeutic approach;
2. *endotoxic*: where administration of appropriate antibiotics, steroids and fluid therapy is employed;
3. *cardiogenic*: which requires augmentation of myocardial contractility, although in many patients the pump is irreversibly damaged and no therapy can be expected to improve the prognosis.

In all forms of shock secondary changes occur in the peripheral vessels resulting in redistribution of blood flow and inadequate perfusion of vital organs. In endotoxic shock this may be associated with inappropriate perfusion of non-essential tissue beds, e.g. the skin.

Initially shock results in increased tone of both pre- and postcapillary sphincters, thus maintaining blood pressure, but as the tissues become anoxic the arteriolar sphincters relax earlier than the venous sphincters and consequently pooling occurs in the capillary beds. Anoxic changes in cells induce release of a number of substances which further depress the functioning of the cardiovascular system. Drugs used in shock have been largely directed towards modifying autonomic responses. Some of these agents have been discussed earlier and include:

(a) *α-adrenoceptor blockers* such as phenoxybenzamine and chlorpromazine.

(b) *Pressor agents*, e.g. noradrenaline, have been used, but most authorities now believe that the use of vasoconstrictors is deleterious since although the arterial blood pressure is increased this is achieved by an increased peripheral resistance at the expense of further tissue anoxia.

(c) *Inotropic agents*, e.g. dopamine, isoprenaline, salbutamol, may be helpful (see above).

(d) *Vasodilators* may produce increased cardiac output by reducing afterload.

(e) *Corticosteroids* have been given in shock for many years on the basis that a prolonged high corticosteroid secretion rate such as occurs in shock could theoretically result in functional exhaustion of the adrenal cortex. It has been found that only glucocorticoids are possibly beneficial in shock: mineralocorticoids are ineffective or aggravate the state. Furthermore, they should be given in large amounts, i.e. in excess of that required to treat adrenal insufficiency. Doses of 4–8 mg/kg dexamethasone or 20–30 mg/kg methyl-prednisolone appear to be optimal. Benefit is only likely if steroids are given early, say within 4–6 h of the onset of shock.

The mechanism of action of corticosteroids is complex and ill-understood. Vasodilatation, α-adrenergic blockade and a positive inotropic effect have all been postulated, but no convincing evidence exists for any of these hypotheses. A potentiating effect on certain cardiovascular actions of catecholamines has also been suggested but careful experiments have failed to demonstrate this. Some of the improvement of tissue perfusion may result from their prevention of platelet aggregation and of lysosomal enzyme mediated capillary damage and vasoconstriction. These membrane-stabilising effects of steroids probably also prevent tissue damage and release of vasodepressor substances which promote deterioration in shock.

(f) *Insulin, glucose and potassium* have been used in some patients with severe congestive cardiac failure unresponsive to digitalis and diuretics. Glucose (1 litre of 50% glucose/day) and insulin (100 units soluble insulin) supply additional substrate to the myocardium and reduce the high levels of free fatty acids found in ischaemic myocardium. Potassium (200 mmol potassium chloride/day) reverses the efflux of potassium ions which occurs in ischaemia. This combination is possibly also capable of enhancing the activity of the sodium pump. The results of this therapy have been variable but any benefit usually occurs within 24 h of its institution.

The treatment of shock is at present difficult and mortality is in the region of 70–90%. Many of the drugs employed are ineffective and only a few agents, such as inotropes and corticosteroids, appear to be modestly useful. A new approach is urgently required.

ANTI-ANGINAL DRUGS

Angina pectoris is the most frequent symptom of ischaemic heart disease and results from a temporary relative imbalance of oxygen demand and supply in the myocardium. The characteristic central chest pain which radiates into the neck, arms and epigastrium is believed to be due to metabolites produced by ischaemic working muscle. The major determinants of myocardial oxygen consumption are:

1. Left-ventricular systolic wall tension which is related to the systolic intraventricular pressure and left-ventricular size by the Laplace law

$$T = \frac{PR}{D},$$

where T is the tangentially directed wall tension, P is the intraventricular pressure, R is the radius of the chamber and D the wall thickness. A large heart is therefore a demanding heart and reduction of heart size may benefit patients with angina.
2. Time spent in systole which is determined by the heart rate and ejection time.
3. The inotropic state of the myocardium which determines the rate of rise of ventricular pressure and is increased by sympathetic stimulation.

Normally coronary flow can increase five-fold to meet demand but in angina this capacity is limited. The onset of pain is preceded by myocardial dysfunction due to hypoxia which results in reduced left-ventricular contractility, dilatation of the ventricle and a rise in end-diastolic pressure. In cases where angina appears to be unrelated to effort a paroxysmal tachycardia may be the underlying cause. Angina may also result from reduced oxygen content of the coronary blood in anaemia, anoxia or smoking (where high levels of carboxyhaemoglobin may be responsible). Rarely it is due to increased demand due to fever, thyrotoxicosis or other high-output states such as arteriovenous fistula or Paget's disease of bone. In such circumstances treatment is obviously removal of the cause.

Three principal types of angina may be recognised clinically:

1. *Chronic stable angina* The majority of patients fall into this group. Cardiac pain is brought on by exertion and relieved by rest, and in any given patient pain appears at a fairly constant level of exercise. Pain may also be precipitated by cold environments, emotional stress and following meals.

The ECG may be normal at rest but typically on exercise testing (e.g. on a treadmill or bicycle ergometer) S-T segment depression develops in at least two bipolar leads. Coronary arteriography will usually confirm the presence of one or more fixed stenoses of the major coronary arteries.

2. *Unstable angina* This diagnosis applies to patients who often have a past history of chronic stable angina, but whose symptoms change and anginal attacks either increase in frequency, occur at rest or last a long time and are not relieved by rest or sublingual glyceryl trinitrate. They show ST or T wave changes in the ECG but there is no evidence of infarction either in the ECG or in serial enzyme estimations. Management includes immediate hospital admission, bed rest and treatment with nitrates (see below) in the first instance.

3. *Prinzmetal (variant) angina* Coronary artery spasm. Pain occurs at rest and has been shown to be due to coronary artery spasm (either in the presence or absence of 'fixed' coronary atherosclerotic lesions). It is becoming increasingly evident that spasm may account for severe myocardial ischaemia which can progress to infarction and even death. During attacks there is often

ST segment elevation on the ECG which returns to normal when the episode resolves.

The drugs employed in angina are discussed below.

A. Nitrates

Used for over a century, inorganic nitrate is pharmacologically inactive but organic nitrates and inorganic and organic nitrites are all effective as directly acting smooth-muscle relaxants. This direct action on arteries and veins is not blocked by the usual pharmacological receptor-blocking drugs. Two general hypotheses concerning the mode of nitrate action are current:

(a) nitrates act at specific receptors possibly involving—SH groups on the membranes of smooth muscle.
(b) nitrates enter smooth muscle cells where they form nitrite ions which induce relaxation.

They have several pharmacodynamic actions all of which contribute to the overall clinical effect:

(a) *Venodilation* This reduces venous return by producing peripheral pooling of blood and thus reduces left ventricular end diastolic pressure and volume. The resulting reduction in ventricular wall tension reduces cardiac workload and thus oxygen demand. In addition, coronary blood flow improves due to the decreased left ventricular end diastolic pressure which presents reduced obstruction to forward flow in the coronaries.
(b) *Increased blood flow to ischaemic areas* Total coronary blood flow is little altered and appreciable dilation occurs in normal rather than diseased vessels. However, there is evidence of increased perfusion of ischaemic areas of myocardium from collateral vessels.
(c) *Mild reduction in arterial tone* This also contributes to myocardial oxygen demand.

After nitrate treatment cardiac output usually falls, although patients with a severely compromised left ventricle may suffer little reduction in output as a result of the balancing improvement in myocardial function. In the erect position particularly, blood pressure falls as a result of reduced cardiac output and arterial dilatation. Since the baroceptor reflexes are unimpaired, a reflex tachycardia occurs but this is usually insufficient to compensate completely. Note that nitrates can relieve the pain of oesophageal spasm, biliary colic and renal colic in some cases and this can cause diagnostic confusion.

Glyceryl trinitrate (Nitroglycerin)

This remains the most widely used drug in the treatment of angina.

Pharmacokinetics Glyceryl trinitrate (GTN) is absorbed from the oral mucosa and through the skin but it has almost 100% first-pass hepatic metabolism which makes it ineffective if swallowed. Even when taken by the sublingual or dermal routes, it is very rapidly metabolised by hepatic glutathione-organic nitrate reductase to nitrate metabolites and inorganic nitrate which have much lower biological potency. The $t_{1/2}$ of GTN is 1–2 min.

There is little evidence that repeated use of nitrates produces tolerance to circulatory effects (as may occur in animals). Whether withdrawal of sustained nitrate effects can lead to vasoconstriction, as has been postulated to explain the high frequency of myocardial infarction among explosive workers, has yet to be determined.

Adverse effects (These apply to *all* nitrate preparations) Flushing, headaches, palpitations, dizziness and syncope may occur. In practice a dose of glyceryl trinitrate which relieves pain without major side effects can be secured by the patient swallowing the remainder of the sublingual tablet as soon as pain is relieved. Tolerance to the headache sometimes occurs but does not imply loss of therapeutic effect, although cross-tolerance may occur for this side effect with other nitrates. The mechanism of the headache is probably stretching of meningeal structures due to cerebral and meningeal vasodilatation.

Methaemoglobinaemia can occur with excessive dosage. Marked anaemia and raised intraocular or intracranial pressure contraindicate the use of nitrates.

Note that the effectiveness of GTN in some patients is decreased by a very marked reflex tachycardia and this may be reduced if the patient is also given a β-blocker.

The following preparations are available:

1. *Sublingual preparations*

(a) *Sublingual GTN tablets.* This is the usual method of administration. The patient is instructed to take one tablet (0.3 mg or 0.5 mg) as often as necessary symptomatically, or preferably, prophylactically (e.g. prior to undertaking angina-provoking exercise). They should be warned that use may cause headache or hypotension so that taking them sitting down may be advisable. Since glyceryl trinitrate is an explosive oily liquid that easily evaporates from the tablets, patients must be told to store tablets in a dark bottle out of sunlight or heat. Other tablets or cotton wool should not be put into the bottle since they may take up some of the glyceryl trinitrate. Tablets should be discarded when there is no longer a burning feeling when the tablet is put under the tongue. The tablets may be used for up to 8 weeks after opening the bottle and should be labelled with the date of expiration.

(b) *Sublingual GTN spray (Nitrolingual)* This contains 0.4 mg GTN per spray. Its advantages over tablets are that it has a more rapid onset of action, 30 s as compared to 1–2 min for the tablets, and it is chemically stable for at least 3 years. Only a few patients benefit from these effects however and its higher cost precludes general use.

2. *Sustained release GTN*

(a) *Suscard* This is a buccal slow release GTN preparation which is placed between the gum and upper lip above the incisor teeth. Its onset of action is longer than sublingual tablets and more variable. It presents problems during speaking and eating and absorption is variable. It may be effective for 3–5 h.

(b) *Sustained release GTN for oral absorption (Nitrocontin Continus,*

Sustac) Tablets of 2.4 mg, 6.4 mg and 10 mg are available but even in a dosage of 12.8 mg t.d.s. (the maximum recommended) the pronounced first-pass effect means that plasma levels are generally not high enough for continuous therapeutic effect.

3. *Preparations for transcutaneous absorption*

(a) *2% GTN in lanolin ointment* (*Percutol*) This is used for angina prophylaxis with each application lasting around 4–8 h. The usual dose is 1.25–5 cm of cream (approx. 8–32 mg of GTN) which is applied to the chest wall under wax paper and occluded by a dressing (the cream is not rubbed in). Patients vary in their response and it is best to allow individual patients to find the optimum dose which protects against pain but leaves them relatively free from side effects. Its disadvantages are that it is expensive, inconvenient, can cause skin irritation and absorption is variable.

GTN ointment may be useful as an aid to venepuncture since a small amount (approx. 2.5 mg) applied over the skin of the back of the hand or forearm leads to local venous dilatation without systemic side effects. This can be particularly useful in children and patients requiring frequent venepunctures, e.g. those undergoing cancer chemotherapy.

(b) *GTN patch* (*Transiderm-Nitro*) This is a slow-release GTN reservoir (25 mg) in a plastic patch (see p. 60) which is applied daily (which aids compliance) and is less messy than the ointment. Approximately 5 mg of drug is absorbed from the reservoir per 24 h. Skin irritation can be minimised by varying the site of application each day. It is too expensive to recommend for routine use but is useful for patients with variant angina (coronary artery spasm) who often experience unpredictable episodes of pain and it has been shown to prevent ST segment elevation as well as relieve symptoms.

4. *Intravenous GTN* (*Nitrocine, Tridil*) At rates of 0.6–12.0 mg/h it may be effective in acute left ventricular failure and unstable angina. The comments below on i.v. isosorbide dinitrate (q.v.) also apply.

Isosorbide dinitrate

Pharmacokinetics Isosorbide dinitrate (ISDN) is subject to a large and variable (20–70%) first-pass metabolism to mononitrates which also have vasodilator activity. The $t_{1/2}$s of the dinitrate itself and of the 2- and 5-mononitrate metabolites are 0.5, 1.5 and 4.5 hours respectively. Because of slow but variable absorption and because of the long half-life of the 5-mononitrate metabolite, it can produce a sustained effect, unlike GTN.

Adverse effects See GTN above.

The preparations available include:

1. *Oral ISDN* (*Cedocard, Isordil, Sorbitrate, Vascardin*) This is widely used for angina prophylaxis. The tablets are usually swallowed but may be chewed for a more rapid (but shorter lasting) effect. A dose of 10–60 mg is given every 4–6 hours, though up to 2-hourly administration may be necessary in some cases. The onset of action is 20–30 min after ingestion (but 2 min if the tablet is chewed).

2. *Slow-release ISDN* (e.g. Isoket Retard; Sorbid S.A.). These preparations give more sustained blood levels thus reducing both frequency of adminis-

tration and side effects. Twice daily administration is adequate and the dose range is 40–160 mg daily.
3. *Intravenous ISDN* (*Cedocard, Isoket*) This is used to treat unstable angina, severe post-infarction pain and severe cardiac failure. The dose is 1–10 mg/h (normally 4–7 mg/h) and is titrated against response in terms both of pain relief and haemodynamic measurements, particularly heart rate and blood pressure. Hypotension is the chief adverse effect. The infusion may be given in 0.9% saline or 5% dextrose or preferably via a syringe pump, using glass or polythene syringes or containers and polythene tubing as there is a loss of drug activity if polyvinyl chloride containers or tubing are used. The infusion should not be stopped suddenly as severe rebound pain may occur. The above comments (apart from dose) also apply to GTN infusions.

Isosorbide 5-mononitrate (Elantan, Ismo 20) This is an active metabolite of isosorbide dinitrate which does not undergo first-pass metabolism. It is well absorbed with a $t_{1/2}$ of 4–6 hours. It is excreted by the kidney both as unchanged drug and the inactive glucuronide. Inter-patient variation in plasma levels is much less than with GTN or ISDN and it appears to be just as effective. The dose is 20–40 mg t.d.s.

Pentaerythritol tetranitrate (Cardiacap, Mycardol, Peritrate) This is similar to ISDN although the efficacy in angina is less well documented. It is given orally and slow-release preparations are available.

Amyl nitrite This is now obsolete in the treatment of angina due to its expense, inconvenience and unpleasant smell. It is given by inhalation of a volatile liquid from crushable glass ampoules. Its main use now is in the management of cyanide poisoning (see p. 871).

B. β-adrenergic blocking drugs

Sympathetic stimulation increases cardiac rate and work and myocardial oxygen consumption. Increased cardiac sympathetic activity is associated with some of the conditions which precipitate angina, e.g. exercise, emotion, cold and thus β-adrenergic blockade might be anticipated to reduce attack frequency. β-blockers reduce the heart rate (Fig. 12.8), systolic intraventricular pressure and the inotropic state of the myocardium, all factors which will reduce myocardial oxygen demand. The reduced heart rate also allows a longer diastolic period for filling of the coronary circulation. These beneficial effects are slightly antagonised by a longer ejection period and cardiac dilatation but overall there is a reduced oxygen demand for any given work load after β-blockade (see Table 12.6).

Theoretically, β-blockers might also reduce coronary blood flow by direct interference with the adrenergic control of coronary resistance vessels. These vessels have both α-adrenergic receptors mediating constriction and β_2-adrenergic receptors, producing relaxation of the coronary vessels. These mechanisms appear to be of little importance, however, in the overall regulation of coronary vascular resistance, which is mainly determined by vasodilator metabolites from the myocardium in many patients. However, in

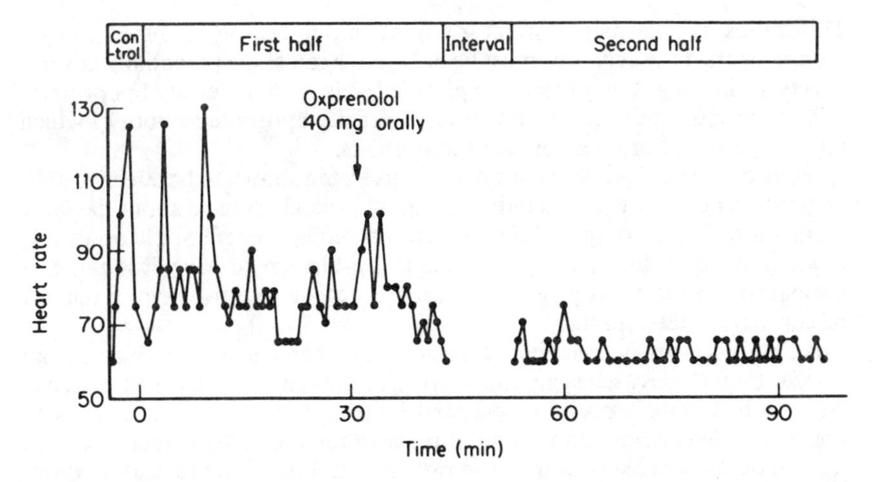

Fig. 12.8 Effect of 40 mg oxprenolol on heart rate in a patient with angina watching a televised live football match (From S. H. Taylor and M. K. Meeran in *New Perspectives in Beta Blockade*, Ciba, 1973.)

Table 12.6 Effect of nitrates and β-blockers on factors influencing myocardial oxygen consumption. Effect of each factor is shown in the main body of the table, effect on oxygen consumption appears in brackets

Factor	*Nitrate*	*β-blockers*
1. Left-ventricular systolic tension		
(i) Systolic intraventricular pressure	↓(−)	↓(−)
(ii) Ventricular size	↓(−)	↑(+)
2. Heart rate	↑(+)	↓(−)
3. Ejection time	↓(−)	↑(+)
4. Inotropic state of myocardium	↑(+)	↓(−)

patients with coronary artery spasm (variant angina), β-blockade is *contraindicated* because it may allow unopposed α-adrenergic coronary vasoconstriction to occur and thus actually promote spasm. As the contribution of coronary artery spasm to angina is recognised in increasing numbers of patients, other agents (principally nitrates and calcium antagonists) have become more widely used. A patient who is already taking β-blockers however, should not stop them suddenly for fear of provoking a withdrawal reaction (see below).

In addition to these haemodynamic effects, β-blockers might also beneficially influence myocardial glucose metabolism. They can reduce myocardial fatty-acid uptake with a consequent relative rise in carbohydrate utilisation.

This raises the cardiac respiratory quotient, indicating reduced oxygen requirements. However, this must be balanced against the potentially adverse effects in the long term of lowered plasma levels of high density lipoproteins and raised levels of triglycerides and low density lipoproteins both of which may increase the progression of atherogenesis.

Many different β-blockers (see p. 430) have been shown to be effective anti-anginal agents. Most studies indicate that all β-blockers have about the same therapeutic efficacy despite differing pharmacological profiles. Theoretically, it would be appropriate for an anti-anginal β-blocker to have little intrinsic sympathomimetic activity and to be relatively cardioselective (avoids the risk of coronary artery spasm).

All β-blockers may precipitate cardiac failure if an adequate cardiac output is reliant upon increased sympathetic tone. Although this risk is undoubted in patients following a major myocardial infarct, it is small in patients with uncomplicated angina. Prevention of myocardial anoxia by reducing cardiac oxygen demand is likely to improve rather than impair myocardial performance. Patients considered to be at risk by this complication may be cautiously treated with β-blockers after adequate therapy with diuretics and digitalis if this is considered essential to control angina.

Stopping β-blockers β-blockers should not be rapidly withdrawn from patients with angina since in some cases this provokes a rebound increase in the frequency and severity of the pain and has occasionally provoked myocardial infarction. Withdrawal is sometimes associated with sweating, tremor and palpitations. This does not appear to be due to increased catecholamine release, and recent work suggests that an increased plasma triiodothyronine concentration may be responsible.

The *dosage of β-blocker* varies with the drug and from patient to patient: the maximum tolerated dose is considered to be the optimum and with most drugs this is determined by initial administration of a small dose, e.g. 10 mg propranolol 6 hourly followed by a gradual increase determined by the pulse rate and the patient's symptoms. The dose of β-blocker is increased until the resting heart rate has fallen to 50–55 beats/min. Although β-blockade is not reliably estimated from the resting pulse rate, in most patients this is an adequate measurement. When failure of β-blocker treatment is suspected however, it is sensible to conduct a supervised exercise test, since this offers a physiological stress which will establish whether optimum β-blockade has been established. Failure of treatment may be assumed if on a maximal exercise test the heart rate is within the range 100–125 beats/min, yet the patient remains disabled by angina. Although β-blockers may not completely relieve pain, they may allow more pain-free exercise and such attacks of angina as occur may be treated with glyceryl trinitrate.

C. Calcium-ion antagonists

This heterogenous group of compounds competitively inhibit the slow passage of calcium ions through the cell membranes of the myocardium and vascular smooth muscle. This effect occurs principally in phase 2 (the plateau phase, see p. 401) of the action potential and reduces contractility in these tissues. Free calcium ion is also made available to contractile protein by release from stores in the sarcoplasmic reticulum, but these stores are minimally developed in myocardial and vascular smooth muscle, which may explain the susceptibility of these tissues to calcium antagonists. These drugs have no effect on striated muscle.

Calcium antagonists have the following main effects:

1. Relaxation of venous smooth muscle leads to peripheral venous pooling and reduction of preload.
2. Peripheral arteriolar dilatation also reduces afterload.
3. Reduction of myocardial contractility (negative inotropic effect) occurs to some extent but this is usually a minor effect and is offset by 1. and 2.
4. Relaxation of coronary vascular smooth muscle increases coronary blood flow and also has a protective effect against coronary vasospasm.
5. Effect on heart rate and cardiac conduction:
   (a) Nifedipine has no effect on cardiac conduction and its administration results in a mild increase in resting heart rate as a reflex response to peripheral vasodilatation.
   (b) Verapamil, diltiazem, lidoflazine, prenylamine and perhexiline are able to depress the cardiac conducting system. Reduction of sinus node automaticity usually produces a mild resting bradycardia. Prolongation of conduction through the atrioventricular node accounts for the anti-arrhythmic effects of these drugs, particularly verapamil and diltiazem.

Note that in contrast to β-blockers, calcium antagonists may be given safely to patients with asthma, chronic bronchitis and peripheral arterial disease.

Nifedipine (Adalat)

Pharmacokinetics Nifedipine is rapidly and almost completely absorbed orally but an even speedier onset of action (within 5 min) can be achieved by biting a 10 mg capsule and retaining the contents in the mouth for absorption through the buccal mucosa. The plasma $t_{1/2}$ is 4–5 hours, although clinically its duration of action is 8–12 hours. It is metabolised by the liver to inactive metabolites which are excreted by the kidney. The rate of nifedipine oxidation may be polymorphically inherited (see p. 109).

Clinical use Nifedipine is a very potent coronary arterial vasodilator and has no obvious effects on intracardiac conduction (unlike verapamil). It is particularly useful for coronary artery spasm (variant angina). The usual dose is 10–20 mg t.d.s., although it is wise to start with 5 mg t.d.s. in the elderly. There is also a sustained release preparation which aids compliance (the dose being 20 mg b.d.). It is light-sensitive and there is no satisfactory intravenous preparation. It may usually be safely combined with β-blockers, nitrates, digoxin, diuretics and other antihypertensive agents.

Adverse effects Peripheral vasodilation may cause flushing, headache and postural hypotension, usually about 30 min after ingestion (as plasma levels increase rapidly). Occasional patients experience an attack of angina at this time, which has been attributed to lowered systolic blood pressure inducing a particularly marked reflex tachycardia. This may be managed either by adding a β-blocker (to prevent the tachycardia) or by changing to another calcium antagonist such as verapamil which has a sinus node depressant effect. Peripheral oedema and facial swelling may occur, and this may not respond to diuretics since it reflects selective dilatation of the pre-capillary resistance vessels with consequent elevation of capillary filtration pressure. Occasionally severe hypotension and even cardiac failure occur when nifedipine is combined with a β-blocker but this is rare. Muscle tremor, muscle weakness, glucose intolerance and hypersensitivity reactions have also been reported occasionally. In some patients nifedipine has a diuretic action.

Verapamil (see p. 416)

Diltiazem (Tildiem)

These two agents share very similar properties in that they both inhibit cardiac conducting tissue resulting in a mild resting bradycardia as well as having vasodilator activity. Diltiazem appears to be less negatively inotropic than verapamil.

The usual oral dose of diltiazem is 60 mg 8 hourly and if necessary the divided dose can be increased to 360 mg/day. Like verapamil there is marked pre-systemic elimination and the bioavailability is thus variable, the mean being around 40% which accounts for inter-individual dose differences. Diltiazem may increase the plasma levels of β-blockers having low bioavailability due to high first-pass effects like propranolol. The $t_{1/2}$ is 4–7 hours: it is extensively metabolised but only one minor metabolite has antiarrhythmic activity.

Bradycardia and heart block occur infrequently, often in patients with pre-existing sino-atrial disease. Ankle oedema has also been noted (q.v. nifedipine).

Lidoflazine (Clinium)

The exact mode of action of this drug is unclear but it can block slow calcium channels in vascular smooth muscle and the myocardium. It has no major effect on intracardiac conduction although the Q-T interval is prolonged. During chronic administration, resting heart rate and blood pressure fall slightly. Lidoflazine undergoes hepatic metabolism with a long $t_{1/2}$ of 1–2 days. A major disadvantage of this drug is the delay of 4–6 weeks before the onset of clinical effect and its full benefit is not seen for 2–3 months.

Adverse effects Dizziness, tinnitus, headache and gastrointestinal disturbance are the commonest problems but tend to remit with time. Prolongation of the QT interval predisposes to ventricular tachycardia particularly in patients taking potassium depleting drugs, digoxin, β-blockers or other anti-arrhythmic drugs.

Perhexilene (Pexid)

This calcium antagonist also has a weak quinidine-like and natriuretic properties. It undergoes hepatic metabolism with excretion of metabolites via the kidney and in bile, and has a long $t_{1/2}$ of 2–5 days. Its use is limited by side effects. These include headache, unsteadiness (severe enough to affect driving skills), nausea and vomiting and rashes. More serious neurological adverse effects include raised intracranial pressure, peripheral neuropathy and myopathy. These are reversible on stopping the drug. Poor metabolisers of debrisoquine (p. 109) have increased susceptibility to these effects. Weight loss is common and may be severe so patients must be weighed before and at regular intervals during treatment. Liver dysfunction and hypoglycaemia may also occur.

Prenylamine (Synadrin)

This calcium antagonist also inhibits uptake and release of catecholamines from sympathetic nerve endings. Its use is declining. Side effects include dizziness, mild sedation and diarrhoea. It may provoke serious ventricular arrhythmias and should be avoided in patients on potassium-depleting drugs or with pre-existing conduction defects.

General management of angina

In addition to drug therapy it should be remembered that angina may be greatly helped by a number of general measures which include:

(a) Avoidance of heavy meals, exposure to cold or wind.
(b) Stopping smoking: apart from being an important risk factor for the development of coronary artery disease, the pharmacological effects of smoking may increase cardiac output, cause coronary constriction, provoke increased catecholamine secretion and so induce angina in the susceptible ('tobacco angina'). In addition, recent data have shown that smoking interferes with the efficacy of both selective and non-selective β-blockers and nifedipine in angina.
(c) Reduce body weight if overweight.
(d) Stress may play a part in the precipitation of anginal attacks. β-blockers have a useful sympatholytic action in this situation, although in unstable angina conventional sedatives may also be indicated.

In *chronic stable angina* medical treatment with a combination of nitrates, β-blockers or calcium antagonists is usually successful. Younger patients, particularly if serious coronary artery disease is present (i.e. triple vessel disease or left anterior descending artery stenosis) and patients whose symptoms remain severe with maximal medical therapy are considered for coronary artery by-pass grafting or transluminal coronary angioplasty.

Unstable angina is best managed by admitting the patient to hospital for strict bed rest (with sedation if necessary) and treatment with nitrates. If the pain does not resolve calcium antagonists or β-blockers may be added. There is no indication for emergency open heart surgery and patients should be investigated when their symptoms have resolved, by exercise testing possibly followed by coronary angiography.

Patients with *variant angina* should *not* be given β-blockers which allow unopposed coronary vasoconstriction. Calcium antagonists and nitrates are the most effective treatment. Urgent open heart surgery is unnecessary and may be dangerous.

Management of acute myocardial infarction

Approximately 40% of deaths from this extremely common disease occur within an hour of the initial attack: the majority before medical attention has arrived. Therefore it is likely that the most significant reduction in mortality will result from:

(a) prevention of the underlying lesion—a difficult and controversial aim at the present time;
(b) wider availability of defibrillation facilities outside hospitals with instruction of the general public in their use: an expensive and possibly dangerous exercise although such schemes have been shown to be feasible in the USA.

At present we have chosen to concentrate upon the provision of specialised coronary care units in designated hospitals. This has, however, only reduced over-all mortality from the condition by around 5–10%. The chief principles of management are:

1. Relief of pain with an opioid. Apart from humanitarian virtues in reducing fear and distress, this will reduce catecholamine release which may decrease the tendency to ventricular arrhythmias. Their vasodilator effects will reduce afterload and could conceivably reduce infarct size and improve cardiac failure. Pethidine and pentazocine have adverse haemodynamic effects and diamorphine or morphine are the drugs of choice, although their depressant effects on the respiratory centre must be remembered.
2. Arrhythmias are treated as described below.
3. The use of drugs for the prophylaxis of arrhythmias in the absence of any rhythm abnormality is controversial. Lignocaine, quinidine, procainamide and phenytoin have all been subjected to careful trials. Treated patients have fewer arrhythmias but paradoxically no improvement in overall survival. In the absence of conclusive demonstration of benefit, the use of antiarrhythmic drugs for prophylaxis in the coronary care unit is unwarranted since it exposes patients to the added risks of drug toxicity. It is, however, important to keep the plasma potassium level above 4.5 mmol/l as this decreases the incidence of arrhythmias.

Although it was once believed that fatal ventricular fibrillation was always heralded by warning arrhythmias such as ventricular ectopic beats, it is now apparent that primary ventricular fibrillation may occur without warning in up to 50% of cases. Even when ventricular premature beats do occur, they are not necessarily followed by fibrillation. Recent studies have cast doubt upon the efficacy of lignocaine as an effective treatment for ventricular premature beats occurring early in diastole (i.e. near the preceding T wave). Possibly the pathogenesis of these early extrasystoles is beyond control by presently available drugs.

4. Oxygen is given routinely in most hospitals to patients with complicated myocardial infarction and in many units it is also given for the first few hours after infarction. There appears to be no evidence of benefit from the practice although there is none of harm either.

5. Low-dose heparin (q.v.) has recently been shown to reduce the incidence of significant deep-vein thromboses and consequent pulmonary emboli in patients after a myocardial infarction.

6. The use of streptokinase infused either systemically or directly into the coronary arteries in an attempt to lyse acute coronary artery thrombosis has shown some promising results. To be effective this treatment should be started as soon as possible after the onset of symptoms. Thrombolytic drugs are further discussed on p. 602.

7. Reduction of infarct size has been the goal of a number of investigators. Drugs which have been claimed to produce such effects include corticosteroids, β-blockers, intravenous nitroglycerine, frusemide and hyaluronidase. Catecholamines and digitalis on the other hand may extend the infarcted area.

β-Blockers for the survivors of acute myocardial infarction

In recent years many large multicentre trials have been carried out to assess the potential benefits of β-blockers in these patients. To understand the rationale for this treatment, the fate of patients surviving an acute myocardial infarction (MI) should first be examined. Mortality is highest within the first year of leaving hospital, and three groups of patients can be recognised:

1. High risk group (1/6 of patients). They have evidence of left ventricular dysfunction and frequent ventricular ectopics on 24 hour ECG recordings taken after the infarction. First year mortality is 20–40% in this group.
2. Low risk group (2/6 of patients). This is the first infarction and there was no history of cardiac symptoms preceding it. They have no heart failure or ventricular ectopy and the submaximal exercise test performed post-infarction is negative. First year mortality is 2%.
3. Intermediate risk group (3/6 of patients). They have some but not all of the features of the high risk group. First year mortality is 10%.

Evidence suggests that the largest single cause of first year mortality is sudden death, probably due to ventricular fibrillation. β-blockers reduce sympathetic nervous stimulation of the heart and may decrease the incidence of potentially fatal re-entry ventricular arrhythmias.

Two schedules of β-blocker administration have been examined:

(a) *Early* Arbitrarily defined as administration (usually intravenous) within 72 h of acute MI. Treatment is continued (orally) for a variable time after this.

(b) *Late* Administration commences after 72 h and continues for at least a year.

Results of early administration Acute intravenous administration of the cardioselective β-blockers metoprolol and atenolol has been shown to reduce the incidence of arrhythmias and probably to limit the eventual infarct size. Timolol and sotalol (non-selective β-blockers) also appear to show this effect. Surprisingly these agents actually reduce the incidence of heart failure rather than increase it as might be expected, probably due to the beneficial effect on infarct size. However, there have been other trials which have not shown benefit from early β-blockade and at present their use in this way is still regarded as controversial by many clinicians.

Results of late administration The evidence is now strong that administration of certain β-blockers for 12–18 months after an acute MI results in an overall 20–30% reduction in first year mortality. Some of the best results so far have been obtained with the non-selective β-blockers timolol (10 mg b.d.) and propranolol (80 mg b.d. or t.d.s.) and evidence suggests that the survival advantage comes from the lower incidence of sudden death in treated patients.

The question as to whether all survivors of an acute MI should be treated is controversial as the mortality of the low risk group is very low and as these drugs have side effects, many clinicians would not give β-blockers to this group of patients. Similarly, severe left ventricular dysfunction may contraindicate their use in the high risk group, thus it is the intermediate risk patients who are perhaps most likely to benefit. β-blockers are an obvious choice in patients who also have angina, hypertension or supraventricular arrhythmias (approximately one-third of survivors of acute MI). Many clinicians would start a β-blocker (provided there are no contraindications) at the first outpatient visit following discharge from hospital. At present there is no obvious benefit in continuing treatment for longer than 12–18 months unless, of course, there is another indication for β-blockade.

It is hoped that further clinical trials will identify more precisely those patients who would benefit from β-blockade, and the optimum time of starting and duration of therapy.

ANTIARRHYTHMIC DRUGS

Myocardial cells, like other cells, show a negative intracellular resting potential (65–75 mV for atrial fibres; 90–95 mV for ventricular fibres). When depolarised by a propagated action potential originating in the conducting system, a complex action potential ensues (Fig. 12.9) which is conventionally divided into four phases.

In the resting state the negative intracellular potential is maintained by concentration gradients of ions across the cell wall, potassium being the predominant intracellular ion and sodium and calcium being predominantly extracellular. The cells of the cardiac conducting system show spontaneous depolarisation and when this reaches the critical threshold potential an action potential is initiated which is then conducted to the myocardial cells.

The sino-atrial node (SA node) normally has the fastest rate of spontaneous depolarisation and thus acts as the 'pacemaker' of the heart. The wave of depolarisation then spreads across the atria to the atrioventricular node (AV

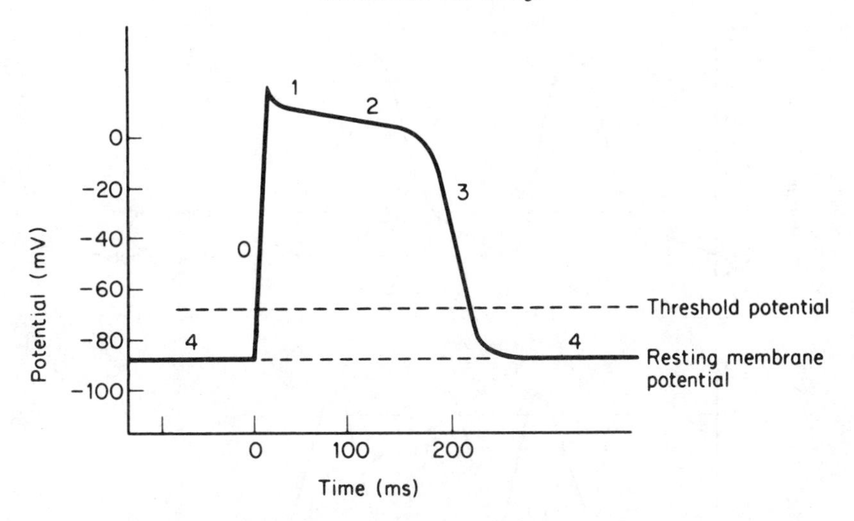

Fig. 12.9 Phases of the action potential in a myocardial cell. Phase 0, rapid influx of Na^+ ions into the cell. Phases 1 and 2, slower influx of Na^+ and Ca^{++} ions. Phase 3, passive efflux of K^+ ions to restore resting potential. Phase 4, restoration of resting ionic gradients across the cell membrane. In conducting cells (Fig. 12.10a) a slow net inward leak of Na^+ ions leads to spontaneous depolarisation.

node) through the atrioventricular septum in the bundle of His, and then via the right and left bundle branches and Purkinje fibres to the ventricular muscle.

Arrhythmias may develop from abnormalities of automaticity or conduction or a combination of the two. Abnormal automaticity may result if there is an increase in the rate of firing of a pre-existing pacemaker which then 'captures' and drives the heart at its own rate and this may also occur if an ectopic pacemaker develops. Ectopic pacemakers may be due to (Fig. 12.10):

(i) change in rate of diastolic depolarisation (phase 4);
(ii) change in maximum negative diastolic potential;
(iii) change in threshold

These changes may occur singly or in combination. They can be provoked by many stimuli including catecholamines (stress), injury, hypoxia, acidosis increased extracellular potassium or calcium. Many of these factors are present adjacent to a myocardial infarct.

The common arrhythmias

Certain stimuli are recognised to increase the chance of developing an arrhythmia (and should always be corrected if possible) e.g. hypoxia, acidosis, hyper- or hypokalaemia, hypercalcaemia, hypomagnesaemia, infection. The following is intended as a simple guide to the common arrhythmias:

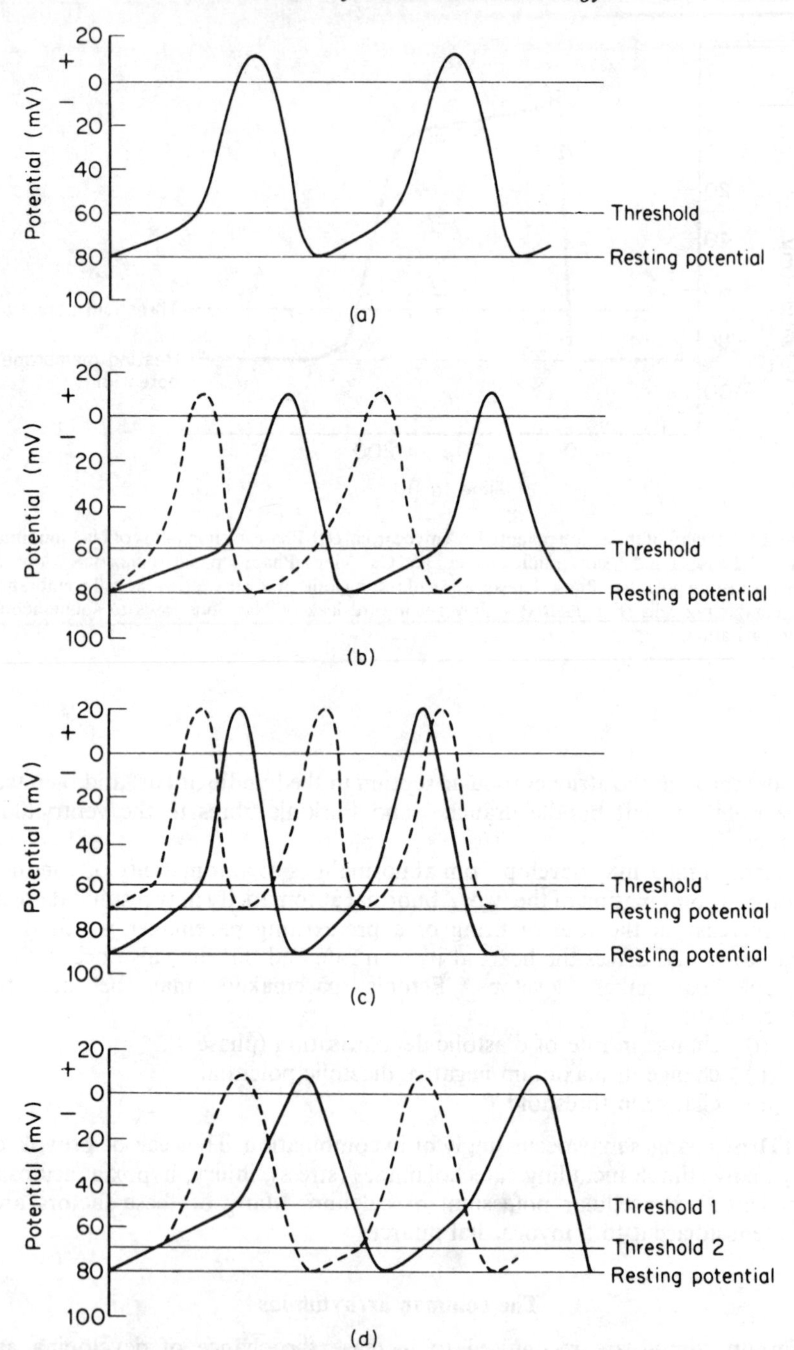

Fig. 12.10 (a) action potential of spontaneously discharging pacemaker cell; (b) effect of change in rate of diastolic depolarisation; (c) effect of change in resting potential; (d) effect of change in threshold potential.

A. Arising from the sinus node.

1. Sinus tachycardia: the rate is 90–150/min with normal P waves and PR interval. (Treatment is directed to the underlying cause e.g. pain, left ventricular failure).
2. Sinus bradycardia: the rate is less than 60/min with normal complexes. It is a common finding in athletes and patients taking β-blockers.

B. Atrial arrhythmias

1. Atrial fibrillation: the atrial rate is > 350/min with variable ventricular conduction, thus this arrhythmia is irregularly irregular.
2. Atrial flutter: the atrial rate is 250–350/min with a fixed ventricular conduction e.g. atrial rate 300/min with 3 : 1 block gives a ventricular rate of 100/min.

C. Nodal arrhythmias (i.e. arising at the A–V node)

1. Atrioventricular block:
   1st degree: prolongation of the PR interval.
   2nd degree: is of 2 types, *Mobitz Type I* in which the PR interval lengthens progressively until a P wave fails to be conducted to the ventricles (Wenckebach phenomenon) and *Mobitz Type II* in which there is a constant PR interval with variable failure to conduct to the ventricles.
   3rd degree: complete A–V dissociation with emergence of an idioventricular rhythm (usually < 50/min).
2. Nodal tachycardias: these are usually due to re-entry circuits and lead to rapid, narrow complex tachycardias at rates > 150/min (see Fig. 12.11). There are two groups:

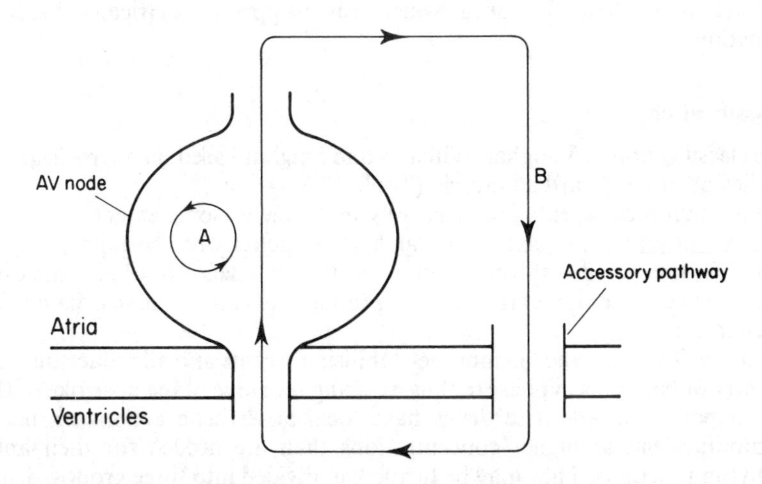

Fig. 12.11 Re-entry circuits involving A–V node. A, intranodal; B, extranodal.

(i) Intranodal. Fibre tracts in the AV node are arranged longitudinally and if differences in refractoriness develop between adjacent fibres then an atrial impulse may be conducted antegradely through one set of fibres and retrogradely through another leading to a re-entry ('circus') tachycardia.

(ii) Extranodal. An anatomically separate accessory pathway is present through which conduction is faster and the refractory period shorter than in the AV node. Ectopic atrial impulses may initiate a re-entry tachycardia. In sinus rhythm the ECG shows a shortened PR interval sometimes with a widened QRS complex with a slurred upstroke—the delta wave (Wolff–Parkinson–White (W.P.W.) syndrome) or a normal QRS complex (Lown–Ganong–Levine syndrome).

D. Ventricular arrhythmias

1. Ectopic beats: irregularly occurring abnormal QRS complexes originating from ectopic foci within the ventricles.
2. Ventricular tachycardia: the ECG shows rapid, regular, wide QRS complexes. Independent P waves (unrelated to QRS complexes) may be seen.
3. Ventricular fibrillation: the ECG shows a completely irregular rhythm with wide complexes, circulatory arrest results.

Antiarrhythmic drugs

The number and availability of these agents over the past 20 years has substantially increased but none provides the ideal combination of convenient administration, efficacy and minimal toxicity. There has also been greater awareness of the value of electrophysical testing of patients under controlled conditions to aid selection of the appropriate drug. The principle of this method is to find the drug which can suppress electrically induced arrhythmias.

Classifications

The classification of Vaughan Williams and Singh is based on microelectrode studies of isolated cardiac muscle (Table 12.7).

Note that most agents are negatively inotropic to some extent.

In recent years a 5th class of antiarrhythmic activity has been proposed in which chloride ion flux through anion selective channels is blocked. Alinidine (a derivative of clonidine) is a new drug thought to cause bradycardia by this mechanism.

Class I These are the 'membrane-stabilising' agents and all reduce the rate of entry of Na^+ ions in phase 0, thus reducing the slope of the upstroke of the action potential. All these drugs have local anaesthetic actions on nerve membranes but at higher concentrations than are needed for their anti-arrhythmic actions. They may be further subdivided into three groups: drugs in group 1A lengthen the duration of the action potential, those in 1B lead to

Table 12.7 Classification of antiarrhythmic drugs according to Vaughan Williams and Singh

Class I	*Class II*	*Class III*	*Class IV*
A. Quinidine Procainamide Disopyramide Ajmalin*	β-blockers Bretylium	Amiodarone Disopyramide Sotalol	Verapamil
B. Lignocaine Mexiletine Tocainide Phenytoin			
C. Lorcainide* Flecanide			

* Not widely available in the UK.

an overall shortening of the action potential and those in 1C do not alter action potential duration.

Class II Anti-sympathetic agents acting either by interfering with noradrenaline release from sympathetic nerve endings or by competitive blockade of the cardiac β-receptors.

Class III These drugs prolong the duration of the action potential (and thus the refractory period) but do not depress membrane responsiveness (i.e. they have little effect on phase 0 depolarisation).

Class IV These drugs inhibit the slow inward movement of calcium ions which is particularly important in the cells of the A–V node where this influx produces most of the depolarisation. Thus the A–V node is particularly susceptible to this type of agent.

This classification is useful for improving understanding of mechanisms of action but it does not have much direct clinical relevance. Table 12.8 based on the major sites of action of these agents, may be more useful.

Clinical pharmacology of selected antiarrhythmic agents

Class I agents

Lignocaine (Xylocard, Lidocaine)

Lignocaine is a class I agent which reduces the rate of rise of the action potential and also suppresses automaticity by decreasing the slope of phase 4 depolarisation. It has no effect on the S–A or A–V nodes.

Pharmacokinetics Lignocaine given orally is hydrolysed in the gastrointestinal mucosa and extensively metabolised on its first pass through the liver to monoethylglycylxylidide (MEGX) and glycylxylidide (GX) which possess less antiarrhythmic action than lignocaine. These metabolites are probably responsible for some of the CNS toxicity of this drug. As the oral

Table 12.8 Sites of action of antiarrhythmic agents

Site of action	*Drugs*	
Atria	Disopyramide Amiodarone Quinidine Procainamide Ajmalin	
A–V node and S–A node	Digoxin (see p. 368) β-blockers Verapamil	
Accessory pathways	Disopyramide Amiodarone Quinidine Procainamide Ajmalin	
Ventricles	Lignocaine Mexiletine Phenytoin Tocainide Lorcainide Flecainide	Disopyramide Amiodarone Quinidine Procainamide Ajmalin Bretylium

bioavailability is so poor (30%) the drug is given parenterally. The intramuscular route produces very variable drug levels, depending partly on the site used, e.g. injections into the deltoid muscle achieve higher levels than those into the buttock or thigh, and thus the intravenous route is preferred.

The half life is 2 hours in normal subjects with an apparent volume of distribution of 1.5 l/kg. 75% of the drug is metabolised by the liver but when hepatic blood flow falls, clearance decreases. Thus after an uncomplicated myocardial infarction the half life increases to 4–6 hours and in cardiac failure it rises to 10 hours (with a fall in volume of distribution to 0.5 l/kg) which may lead to accumulation if standard doses are used.

Clinical use The therapeutic range in plasma is 1.5–4.0 mg/l and this is most rapidly achieved (in the absence of cardiac failure) by giving a bolus of 50–100 mg i.v. over one minute followed by an infusion of 4 mg/minute for ½–1 h reducing to 2 mg/min for 2 h and to 1 mg/min thereafter for a period not usually exceeding 36–48 h. In patients with shock and poor peripheral circulation or severe hepatic dysfunction the initial infusion should not exceed 1 mg/min. As the difference between therapeutic and toxic plasma levels is small for lignocaine, it is particularly important to try to tailor the dose correctly to each patient.

If the patient shows no signs of lignocaine toxicity and break-through ventricular tachycardia or fibrillation occur, then a further 100 mg bolus may be given over 2 min and the infusion rate increased to 4 mg/min as appropriate to suppress the arrhythmia.

Lignocaine remains a drug of first choice for the treatment of ventricular tachycardia and fibrillation. In common with other class I agents it is most effective when the plasma potassium concentration is maintained at the upper end of the normal range, i.e. 4.3–5.0 mmol/l.

Adverse effects

1. CNS: drowsiness, twitching, paraesthesia, nausea and vomiting, focal followed by grand mal seizures.
2. CVS: bradycardia, cardiac depression (negative inotropic effect), asystole. Lignocaine is contraindicated in the presence of second- or third-degree heart block since it may increase block or abolish the idioventricular pacemaker which is maintaining cardiac rhythm.

Mexiletine (Mexitil)

This drug has very similar actions to lignocaine, the chief differences being that it is active orally and it is sometimes effective in arrhythmias resistant to lignocaine.

Pharmacokinetics Well absorbed orally (cf. lignocaine) but absorption delayed after myocardial infarction. $t_{1/2}$ 16–18 h in normal subjects but in patients with myocardial infarction this may increase to 25 h or more, possibly due to reduced hepatic metabolism (cf. lignocaine). Only 10 % is excreted in the urine so that renal failure is of minor importance in its clinical use. The effective plasma level is 0.6–2.5 μg/ml. Absorption is enhanced by metoclopramide and delayed by narcotic analgesics.

Clinical use Intravenous (as with lignocaine a reducing infusion rate is required after the initial bolus).

Bolus:	100–250 mg slowly over 5–10 min
Infusion:	250 mg in first hour 250 mg over next two hours Then 0.5–1 mg/min until oral therapy established.
Orally:	Initial loading dose is 400 mg (600 mg if absorption reduced in myocardial infarction) Followed after 2 h by the maintenance dose of 200 mg 6–8 hourly. A slow-release preparation for twice daily dosage is also available.

Adverse effects

Low therapeutic index like lignocaine
Gastro-intestinal tract: nausea, vomiting, hiccoughs, indigestion
CNS: drowsiness, confusion, ataxia, paraesthesia
CVS: hypotension, bradycardia.

Phenytoin (Epanutin) (see p. 268)

Although mainly used as an anticonvulsant, phenytoin has class I anti-arrhythmic activity. It has two particular uses:

(i) It shortens a prolonged QT interval, e.g. in complete heart block with ventricular ectopy.
(ii) It increases A–V nodal conduction but suppresses ventricular excitability making it valuable in digoxin overdoses.

It is also effective in ventricular arrhythmias although lignocaine is usually preferred.

Quinidine (Kinidin Durules, Kiditard, Quinicardine)

Quinidine is the dextro-rotary isomer of quinine. In addition to class I activity, quinidine has significant anticholinergic activity which blocks the vagal influence on the A–V node, thus facilitating A–V conduction. In atrial flutter or fibrillation such enhanced A–V conduction may result in dangerously increased ventricular rates. Pre-treatment with digoxin to increase the A–V block must thus be given prior to any attempt to convert these arrhythmias with quinidine. The major effect of quinidine on the ECG is prolongation of the QRS and QT intervals. (It should be stopped if QRS duration exceeds 0.14 s or widens by $>50\%$).

Pharmacokinetics Quinidine is well absorbed orally and has a half life of 5–7 h. Most of the drug is hydroxylated to less active metabolites in the liver. Only 10–15% is excreted unchanged in the urine. However, renal excretion may be usefully increased if the urine is acidified and this can be utilised in cases of overdose. Conversely, heart failure or administration of antacids or thiazides may lead to metabolic alkalosis and cause toxicity.

Intoxication may also occur in cardiac failure associated with a smaller volume of distribution for the drug, most likely due to decreased perfusion of the body tissues with a consequent increase in the amount of drug in the central (plasma) compartment. This reduced distribution volume rather than altered elimination kinetics is probably the usual cause of intoxication in cardiac failure.

Slow-release preparations are available but their bioavailability may be lower than that of the standard formulation. The drug is 80% bound to albumin. Therapeutic plasma levels are 4–6 mg/l.

Clinical use Quinidine is not commonly used now due to its unpleasant and potentially dangerous adverse effects. It is almost exclusively given orally as the sustained-release preparation (500 mg b.d.) and an initial test dose should be given to detect hypersensitivity (see below). The intravenous route is very dangerous and is thus avoided. Quinidine is mainly used for treatment of recurrent ventricular arrhythmias.

It is contraindicated in heart block, hyperkalaemia, digitalis intoxication, heart failure and hypotensive states.

Adverse effects

1. CVS effects are the most important since they can be fatal; they include atrioventricular and ventricular block, ventricular arrhythmias and depressed myocardial contractility. Quinidine syncope is due to ventricular tachycardia and can occur with plasma concentrations within or

below the therapeutic range. This may be due to depressed conductivity, allowing re-entry rhythms or a decreased membrane potential which enhances automaticity. Serious conduction disturbances are more likely when pre-existing conduction abnormalities are present.

2. Cinchonism—a syndrome of tinnitus, headache, nausea, visual disturbances including altered colour perception, diplopia and night blindness, vertigo and decreased auditory acuity—occurs with large doses.
3. Gastrointestinal disturbances (nausea, diarrhoea and vomiting) are the most common problems in clinical use.
4. Hypersensitivity producing a reversible thrombocytopenia is due to antibodies against a plasma protein–quinidine complex. Bone-marrow suppression also occurs as a direct effect on the marrow.

Drug Interactions

1. Concurrent administration with digoxin leads to a 2–3 fold increase in plasma digoxin levels (possibly due to decreased renal clearance or displacement from tissue binding sites) so the maintenance dose of digoxin *must* be reduced.
2. Potentiation of coumarin anticoagulants and drugs with hypotensive activity may also occur.
3. Phenobarbitone and phenytoin reduce plasma quinidine levels and efficacy. This interaction is due to enzyme induction and probably occurs with other enzyme inducing agents.

Procainamide (Procainamide Durules, Pronestyl)

This drug is similar to quinidine in its cardiac actions.

Pharmacokinetics 80% of an oral dose is rapidly absorbed and peak levels occur within 1 hour. The $t_{1/2}$ is 2–3.5 h which is too short to make oral dosing convenient. 90% is excreted in the urine, 60% as unchanged drug and the rest as N-acetylprocainamide (NAPA) which also has antiarrhythmic activity (acetylation is governed by acetylator status—see below). Like quinidine, increasing urinary pH retards excretion and may lead to toxicity.

The therapeutic range is 4–10 mg/l and ideally plasma levels should be monitored, particularly in renal failure and congestive cardiac failure where excretion is impaired.

Clinical use The need for very frequent dosing has led to the development of slow-release formulations of the drug. It is effective in a wide range of atrial and ventricular arrhythmias but is not generally a first line drug, possibly because of its wide spectrum of side effects. The oral loading dose is 1 g followed by 250–500 mg up to 3 hourly or 1.0–1.5 g of the sustained-release preparation every 8 hours. Intravenously, boluses of 100 mg are given over 5 min and repeated until the arrhythmia is controlled or 1 g has been given. This may be followed by a maintenance infusion of 1–3 mg/min.

Although resembling quinidine in its anti-arrhythmic actions, the two drugs are not always interchangeable since some patients tolerate one drug better than the other. Procainamide is potent and has a wide anti-arrhythmic spectrum. It is used for:

(a) Premature atrial beats, paroxysmal atrial tachycardia and atrial fibrillation of recent onset.
(b) It is only moderately effective in converting atrial flutter or fibrillation into sinus rhythm but has a place in maintaining sinus rhythm after electrical conversion.
(c) Ventricular premature beats or tachycardia after myocardial infarction will often respond to procainamide.

Adverse effects

1. CVS: hypotension, reduced cardiac output, increased ventricular ectopic beats. Dosage is excessive if QRS is prolonged by 30%.
2. GI: dose-related nausea, vomiting and diarrhoea usually occur with doses in excess of 4 g/day.
3. Drug-induced systemic lupus erythematosus syndrome: usually reversible. On chronic therapy 80% patients develop antinuclear antibodies and 5–15% will become symptomatic. Coombs' positive haemolytic anaemia and thrombocytopenia also occur. Symptoms disappear within a few days or weeks when the drug is discontinued but the antinuclear factor may persist for many months.

Tocainide (Tonocard)

This agent has similar actions to lignocaine (both are class IB drugs) and can be given both orally and i.v.

Pharmacokinetics Bioavailability is nearly 100% when given orally and the $t_{1/2}$ is 11–15 hours. About 60% is metabolised in the liver (mainly to inactive metabolites) and the rest excreted unchanged in the urine (thus if the GFR falls below 30 ml/min, a 25–50% reduction in dose is indicated). The therapeutic range in plasma is 6–12 mg/l.

Adverse effects

1. CVS: SA or AV blockade may occur. Negative inotropic effects are generally *not* seen at therapeutic levels.
2. GI tract: Anorexia, nausea, vomiting, constipation and abdominal pain.
3. CNS: Drowsiness, tremor, fits.
4. Other: Rashes and interstitial pulmonary fibrosis may rarely occur.

Clinical use The initial oral dose is 400 mg t.d.s. (or 600 mg b.d.) up to a maximum of 2.4 g daily. When required intravenously, 500–750 mg is infused over 15–30 minutes and the patient is started on oral maintenance treatment immediately.

Lorcainide

This new agent has quinidine-like activity on the conducting system and leads to widening of the QRS complex, followed by prolongation of the PR interval and suppression of the ventricular ectopics.

Pharmacokinetics The $t_{1/2}$ is 5–8 hours but is prolonged in heart failure. Oral administration of a single 200 mg tablet results in presystemic elimination of 60% of the dose; however, this first pass metabolism is saturable and after several days of chronic administration oral bioavailability rises to over 90%. The metabolites also have antiarrhythmic properties. Dose reduction is not generally required in renal failure.

Clinical use The intravenous dose is up to 200 mg (in 200 ml saline) given over 20 min with reduction in the rate of infusion once the desired antiarrhythmic effect is achieved. Orally, 200–400 mg/day in 2–4 divided doses is usually effective. Individual titration of drug effect to the ECG is the best way to optimise treatment, the aim being to find a therapeutic dose that does not widen the QRS complex by more than 25%.

Adverse effects

1. CNS: Sleep disturbance (especially nightmares) in 18%, dizziness.
2. GI tract: Nausea, vomiting.
3. CVS: Negative inotropic effects are rare at therapeutic doses, intracardiac conduction defects may occur.

Flecainide (Tambocor)

Flecainide acetate is another new antiarrhythmic agent with class IC activity, i.e. it has no effect on the duration of the action potential. It is the first agent in this class to be available in the UK. It has been used successfully in the treatment of re-entry nodal tachycardias (it prolongs retrograde refractoriness in accessory pathways) and in suppression of ventricular ectopic beats and ventricular bradycardia.

Pharmacokinetics and clinical use The $t_{1/2}$ is 14–20 hours and this makes it suitable for twice (or even once) daily administration. Therapeutic plasma levels are in the range 0.2–1.0 mg/l. Flecainide is almost completely absorbed orally and treatment should commence with daily doses of 200–400 mg reducing after 3–5 days to the lowest dose that maintains control of the arrhythmia. Intravenously, a bolus of 100–150 mg may be given over 10–30 min, followed by an infusion of 1.5 mg/kg/h for one hour reducing to 0.25 mg/kg/h thereafter. It may be diluted in 5% dextrose but not in normal saline as it precipitates in this diluent at concentrations above 30 g/l.

Adverse effects CVS: It is contraindicated in patients with cardiac failure (negative inotropic effect) and in those with pacemakers (as it increases endocardial pacing thresholds). It may induce arrhythmias in a small proportion of patients. Dizziness, blurred vision, nausea and vomiting may occur. Other drugs: digoxin levels may rise by 15%. It is compatible with β blockers and anticoagulants.

Disopyramide (Dirythmin, Rhythmodan)

This agent has similar electrophysiological properties to quinidine, although at therapeutic doses it has little effect on PR, QRS or QT durations. However, by slowing conduction in accessory pathways it can be used to treat re-entry tachycardias with wide QRS complexes. It should be avoided in supraventricular tachycardias with narrow QRS complexes (e.g. atrial flutter) as it has pronounced *anticholinergic* activity which can lead to a paradoxical increase in the ventricular rate. This is due to conduction of a greater proportion of atrial beats, and prior treatment with digoxin (to block the A–V node) will prevent this (cf. quinidine).

Disopyramide may be used to treat ventricular tachycardia resistant to lignocaine and DC cardioversion.

Pharmacokinetics The effective plasma level is 2–4 mg/l. The $t_{1/2}$ is 4–6 h in normal subjects, but is prolonged and the volume of distribution reduced in patients with myocardial infarction, which predisposes these patients to toxicity. Conversely, patients with myocardial infarction achieve lower plasma levels when given the drug orally as compared to normals.

Disopyramide is readily absorbed, peak levels occurring within 2 h. The main site of metabolism is the liver and excretion is via the kidneys, 60% as unchanged drug, the rest mainly as the N-mono-dealkylated metabolite, which is only slightly less active than the parent compound against atrial arrhythmias, although it is inactive against ventricular arrhythmias.

Approximately 25% of the drug is bound to plasma proteins, but this binding is saturable and depends upon both the plasma disopyramide and metabolite concentrations. This non-linear binding complicates the clinical use of the drug.

Clinical use Intravenously, a bolus of 100 mg should be given over 15 min, followed by an infusion of 10 mg/h. Continuous ECG monitoring with facilities for cardiopulmonary resuscitation should be available, due to the possibility of a severe negative inotropic effect (see below).

The oral dose is 100–200 mg 6 hourly. A slow-release formulation is available. The drug is well absorbed and 60% is excreted unchanged in the urine so the dose should be reduced in renal failure.

Adverse effects Peripheral anticholinergic effects may be seen at therapeutic doses and may lead to dry mouth, blurred vision, raised intra-ocular pressure (thus glaucoma is a contraindication), urinary hesitancy and constipation.

Negative inotropic activity may be pronounced and severe cardiac failure (either intercurrent or in the past) is a contraindication. QT prolongation and various intracardiac blocks may occur (the presence of the latter being a contraindication to the use of this drug).

Interactions

1. Hypokalaemia antagonises the action of the drug and every effort should be made to keep the plasma potassium at the upper range of normal (i.e. 4.5–5.0 mEq/l).
2. Disopyramide potentiates the action of coumarin anticoagulants. Unlike quinidine, it does not alter digoxin levels.

Ajmalin

This new agent with class IA activity (thus prolonging the action potential) has been successfully used in ventricular and nodal tachycardias and for the prophylaxis of re-entry tachycardias.

Pharmacokinetics The $t_{1/2}$ is 5 hours, 50% of a dose is metabolised in the liver and the rest excreted unchanged in the urine. The intravenous dose is 1 mg/kg over 10 min (which may be repeated after 30 min) followed by an infusion if necessary. Oral bioavailability is 80% and the recommended starting dose is 100 mg 4–5 times daily which may be reduced to a maintenance dose of 50 mg 3–4 times daily.

Adverse effects Intracardiac blocks, nausea, constipation and visual disturbances may occur. Intrahepatic cholestasis with pyrexia is a rare but recognised adverse effect.

Class II agents (drugs with antisympathetic activity)

β-adrenoceptor blockers (see also p. 425)

β-blockade reduces sino-atrial rate and increases A–V node refractory period and conduction time. At therapeutic doses β-blockers do not alter ventricular conduction and QRS duration is unchanged. These drugs are particularly useful in the treatment of supraventricular arrhythmias associated with increased levels of circulating catecholamines (e.g. post-myocardial infarction, in phaeochromocytoma and for arrhythmias induced during anaesthesia) or due to increased sensitivity to catecholamines (thyrotoxicosis).

β-blockers are contraindicated in digoxin toxicity as complete A–V block may result, but with therapeutic digoxin levels a useful additive effect may be achieved to slow the ventricular response in atrial fibrillation or flutter. They may also terminate re-entry tachycardias (e.g. WPW syndrome) although newer agents are usually preferred, e.g. verapamil.

Recently, important evidence has emerged that intravenous β-blockade, commenced as soon as possible (within 6 hours) after acute myocardial infarction (provided there are no contraindications), may reduce the incidence of arrhythmias and reduce infarct size, with a decrease (rather than an increase) in the incidence of heart failure. This benefit has been shown with both selective (atenolol, metoprolol) and non-selective (timolol, sotalol) agents. Oral β-blockers should be commenced at the same time and probably continued for at least one year as evidence suggests appreciable reductions in post-infarct mortality may be achieved (see p. 399). Not all studies however have shown this beneficial effect.

Pharmacokinetics (see p. 430) Agents available for intravenous use include:

Propranolol 0.5–1.0 mg over 1 minute, repeated every 2 min up to a maximum of 10 mg.

Atenolol 2.5 mg over 2.5 min, repeated at 5 minute intervals as needed to a maximum total dose of 10 mg.

It is advisable that there should be continuous ECG monitoring with facilities available for resuscitation when i.v. β-blockers are given. In particular, i.v. atropine sulphate should be to hand for use as needed.

Adverse effects (see p. 435).

Bretylium (Bretylate)

This class II agent is proposed to act by accumulating in sympathetic nerves and reducing noradrenaline release. It is most widely used in the USA where many antiarrhythmics used in Europe are not available. Initially it may cause hypertension (probably due to displacement of noradrenaline from post-ganglionic receptors) and this is usually followed by sustained hypotension which may be severe. It is used as a second-line drug to treat severe ventricular arrhythmias. It is not effective in supraventricular arrhythmias.

Pharmacokinetics It is poorly absorbed orally and thus is only available for parenteral use. It is eliminated unchanged in the urine with a $t_{1/2}$ of $7\frac{1}{2}$ h. A bolus of 500 mg i.v. is given over 10 min, but a problem with this drug is that the full antiarrhythmic effect may take several hours to develop. One advantage of this drug is that it is a positive inotrope.

Amiodarone (Cordarone X)

This relatively new antiarrhythmic agent is highly effective but its use is limited by a high incidence of side effects. It is a class III agent, prolonging the duration of the action potential but with no effect on the rapid upstroke (phase 0) of the action potential. It prolongs repolarisation by reducing the permeability of the cell membrane to outward potassium current. It also reduces the slope of diastolic depolarisation and at the sinus node this action accounts for reduction in resting heart rate. It also delays atrial and A–V nodal conduction but has no effect on ventricular conduction.

Pharmacokinetics Amiodarone and its main metabolite, desethyl amiodarone (which exceeds the concentration of the parent drug in plasma), are highly lipid soluble. This is reflected in the very high volume of distribution of approximately 5000 l. The drug is highly plasma protein bound (> 90%) and accumulates in all tissues, particularly the heart. It is only slowly eliminated through the liver with a $t_{1/2}$ of 28–45 days. Antiarrhythmic activity may continue for several months after the drug is stopped.

The drug is variably absorbed (20–80%) and measuring plasma levels (therapeutic range 0.5–1.5 mg/l) may be useful to determine the minimum effective dose.

Clinical use Amiodarone may be effective in a wide variety of arrhythmias including:

(a) Supraventricular: resistant atrial fibrillation or flutter, nodal tachycardias (e.g. in WPW syndrome).
(b) Ventricular: recurrent ventricular tachycardia or fibrillation.

Amiodarone administration does not preclude the use of DC cardioversion and may be used to maintain sinus rhythm if cardioversion is successful. Note that the ECG may show U waves or deformed T waves but this is not an indication to discontinue amiodarone.

The drug is contraindicated in the presence of sinus bradycardia and A–V block. Care should be taken in patients with heart failure but it is not contraindicated. Patients with thyroid disease should not receive this drug.

Intravenously, amiodarone should be given via a central line to avoid thrombophlebitis. Initially 5 mg/kg in 250 ml of 5% glucose is infused over 20 min–2 h (to avoid hypotension) and may be repeated as needed up to 15 mg/kg/24 h. In extreme emergencies it may be given as a slow injection of 150–300 mg in 10–20 ml over 1–2 min.

Oral treatment should be started as soon as response is established. For patients who have not received i.v. treatment 200 mg t.d.s. for 7 days (or until the desired effect is achieved) helps to establish adequate tissue levels quickly and this is then reduced to the lowest daily dose which maintains effect, usually 200–800 mg daily.

Adverse effects These are many and varied and are common with plasma amiodarone concentrations exceeding 2.5 mg/l. They lead to a reduction in dose or discontinuation in a substantial number of patients.

1. The eye: Corneal deposits occur eventually in almost all patients. Electron microscopy shows deposits (possibly of drug or metabolite) in tissue macrophages. These deposits form linear opacities radiating in a fan-like manner throughout the corneal epithelium from a point below the centre of the cornea (described as 'une image de la moustache du chat'). Occasionally patients report coloured haloes in their field of vision but no change in visual acuity occurs. The deposits are seen only on slit lamp examination and gradually regress if the drug is stopped. As the deposits are generally benign opinion varies as to the necessity of regular ophthalmic examination.

2. The skin: Photosensitivity rashes are seen in 10–30% of patients. They are a phototoxic response to wavelengths in both the long ultraviolet (UVA) and visible light parts of the spectrum so ordinary sunscreens (which only protect against UV below 320 nm) are ineffective. Topical compounds which reflect both UVA and visible light are needed, e.g. zinc oxide, and patients should be advised to wear suitable clothing when exposed to bright sunlight. A reduction in drug dosage may also help. Occasionally patients develop a blue–grey pigmentation of exposed areas—this is a separate phenomenon from phototoxicity.

3. Thyroid gland: Amiodarone contains 37% iodine by weight and may precipitate hyperthyroidism in susceptible subjects. Amiodarone alters the results of some classical thyroid function tests (PBI, ^{131}I) and specific methods must be used. Usually there is a rise in T4 and reverse T3 (rT3) with a normal or low T3 and a flat TSH response to TRH. Thyroid function (T3, T4 and TSH) should be assessed prior to amiodarone administration and at 6 monthly intervals thereafter.

4. The lung: Pulmonary infiltration may develop with high doses which reverse on stopping the drug (this may be accelerated with prednisolone).

5. The liver: Transient elevation of hepatic enzymes may occur but occasionally severe hepatitis develops.

6. Nervous system: Peripheral neuropathy may develop in the first month of treatment, and reverse on stopping the drug. Proximal muscle weakness, ataxia and tremor may occur. The tremor may be helped by a small dose of propranolol. Nightmares, insomnia and headache are also reported.

In general, gastrointestinal intolerance and negative inotropism are not major problems.

Interactions

1. Potentiation of coumarin anticoagulants.
2. Precipitation of digoxin toxicity (the dose should be reduced by 50% when amiodarone is added).
3. Precipitation of severe bradycardia with β-blockers or calcium antagonists.

Calcium ion antagonists

This group includes verapamil, diltiazem, nifedipine, perhexilene, prenylamine and lidoflazine. They differ in their tissue specificities, verapamil is an antiarrhythmic with class IV activity because of its effect on the cardiac conducting system. All agents of this group have variable antihypertensive and coronary vasodilator (antianginal) properties. (See p. 394 for a fuller discussion of their mechanisms of action.)

Verapamil (Cordilox)

In common with other calcium antagonists verapamil relaxes the smooth muscle of peripheral arterioles and veins and the coronary arteries and it also has intrinsic negative inotropic activity. As an antiarrhythmic agent its major effect is to slow intracardiac conduction, particularly through the A–V node. This reduces ventricular response in atrial fibrillation and flutter and abolishes most re-entry nodal tachycardias, e.g. in WPW syndrome. It is now the drug of choice for treatment and prophylaxis of paroxysmal supraventricular tachycardias. A mild resting bradycardia is seen in many patients, together with prolongation of the PR interval on the ECG. Verapamil has negligible activity in ventricular arrhythmias.

Pharmacokinetics Verapamil is a racemic mixture of (−) and (+) verapamil. The (−) racemate is much more potent than the (+). Although the drug is very well absorbed orally the bioavailability is only 10–20% due to presystemic elimination which is stereoselective with the (−) isomer being preferentially metabolised. This explains the observation that even when equivalent total verapamil levels are achieved, the effect on the PR interval is greater for the same plasma level after an i.v. dose compared to an oral dose—this is due to higher levels of the more active (−) isomer after an i.v. dose.

Verapamil is highly protein bound in plasma. It is metabolised in the liver, one of the metabolites (norverapamil) being active. The $t_{1/2}$ is 3–7 h but is significantly prolonged in the presence of liver disease.

Clinical use Intravenous verapamil should only be given to closely monitored patients. A bolus of 10 mg over 2 min may be given, followed if necessary by a further 5 mg after 5 min. Alternatively an infusion of 5–10 mg/h may be given to a maximum dose of 100 mg per 24 h.

The oral dose is 40–120 mg t.d.s., note that this is about 10 times the i.v. dose due to the large first-pass effect. It is probably wise not to withdraw it suddenly but rather to decrease gradually over about 4 days.

Intravenous verapamil must not be given to a patient who has received β-blockers as this may result in severe A–V block and asystole. There is, however, a place for the cautious addition of oral verapamil to β-blocker therapy (or vice versa) and this combination may be very successful in patients with angina or hypertension that is otherwise difficult to control. In this case, the dose of the second drug should be gradually increased at two-weekly intervals until the optimum effect is achieved or side effects supervene.

Oral verapamil may be given as an alternative to a β-blocker to patients in whom digoxin alone has failed to control the ventricular rate in atrial fibrillation. However verapamil can reduce digoxin excretion and the dose of digoxin should be reduced, probably by 50 %, if the two drugs are combined. Verapamil is contraindicated in the presence of *digoxin toxicity* as there may be a potentially fatal additive effect on the A–V node.

Adverse effects and contraindications

CVS: Verapamil is contraindicated in severe cardiac failure as the negative inotropic effect combined with vasodilation may lead to severe hypotension and low cardiac output. This effect is rare in mild failure where the reduction in afterload tends to improve output and offset the negative inotropism. Verapamil is also contraindicated in the presence of the sick sinus syndrome or an intracardiac conduction block.

Verapamil may precipitate hypotension, 1st or 2nd degree A–V block or other bradyarrhythmias and if these cause serious cardiovascular embarrassment the patient may be resuscitated with calcium gluconate, atropine and/or isoprenaline.

GI tract: One third of patients experience constipation, this can usually be managed successfully with advice about a high fibre diet and laxatives if necessary.

Others: Headache, dizziness and facial flushing may be seen and are symptoms common to all the calcium antagonists. Drug rashes, pain in the gums and a metallic taste in the mouth are rare side effects.

Atropine

This is a natural alkaloid which is a highly selective antagonist of acetylcholine at muscarinic receptors. Parasympathetic blockade produces widespread effects: reduced salivation and sweating, decreased secretions in the gut and respiratory tract, initial bradycardia with atrioventricular dissociation followed by tachycardia, urinary retention, constipation, reduced airways resistance, pupillary dilatation and ciliary paralysis.

Pharmacokinetics It is completely absorbed after oral administration but probably undergoes some first-pass hepatic metabolism since the ratio of unchanged drug to metabolites is higher after intravenous dosing compared to oral administration. The $t_{1/2}$ is 13–38 h and although it is an ester of tropic acid and tropine, hydrolysis of the ester bond does not appear to be an important metabolic route and the drug is mostly N-demethylated and glucuronidated. Between 33 and 50% appears in the urine unchanged.

Clinical uses

1. Bradycardia – see below.
2. Premedication – see Chapter 11.
3. Ophthalmology – topically to produce mydriasis (NB. it is contraindicated in glaucoma).
4. In gastroenterology – see Chapter 15.
5. In organophosphorus poisoning – see Chapter 22.

Treatment of specific arrhythmias

These cannot be treated in isolation and various precipitating factors should be sought and treated where possible. These may range from thyrotoxicosis, electrolyte imbalance, pulmonary embolism, anoxia, infection, ventricular aneurysm, or merely the pain from a distended bladder in a stuporose patient.

Treatment of specific arrhythmias

1. Atrial fibrillation/flutter

(a) When rapid and uncontrolled: DC cardioversion is often the treatment of choice, particularly when the patient is hypotensive and in shock. Anticoagulation prior to this procedure is advisable and should be continued long-term after cardioversion if fibrillation persists or further intermittent episodes of arrhythmia occur. Digoxin (orally or i.v.) may be used if the patient is not in shock. It slows the ventricular rate by increasing A–V block. As an alternative, or if digoxin is not fully effective, verapamil i.v. may be used. In about 50% of patients with flutter digoxin restores sinus rhythm.

If DC cardioversion is attempted in a patient who is already digitalised dangerous ventricular arrhythmias may result. To avoid this, at least 48 h should elapse after the last dose of digoxin, but if cardioversion is required as an emergency 200 mg of phenytoin i.v. may be protective.

(b) For long-term control: Digoxin is the drug of choice but in some patients (despite therapeutic drug levels) digoxin is not enough to control ventricular rate and verapamil or a β-blocker may be added.

2. Paroxysmal supraventricular tachycardia

These almost always comprise a re-entry circuit involving the A–V node, e.g. WPW syndrome.

Vagal stimulation (e.g. carotid sinus massage, Valsalva manoeuvre) may be effective. Verapamil, 10 mg intravenously, is the drug of choice (provided that the patient is not β-blocked). If it is contraindicated or ineffective, or the patient is shocked, DC cardioversion is indicated. Disopyramide may also terminate the arrhythmia. Digoxin is contraindicated because it may dangerously accelerate anterograde conduction and thus increase the ventricular rate. Note that attacks of ventricular flutter/fibrillation may occur in WPW syndrome and delta waves may not be obvious on the ECG. The rapidity of the ventricular response may warn the clinician that this is the case, and thus that digoxin is contraindicated.

Recurrence may be prevented by propranolol, verapamil, procainamide or quinidine. Overindulgence in caffeine or smoking should be avoided.

3. Ventricular arrhythmias

Ectopic beats These occur commonly after myocardial infarction but their ability to predict ventricular fibrillation is poor and so long as the patient is carefully observed (ideally in an intensive care unit) they should probably not be treated. The exceptions are three or more consecutive ectopics or those in which the R wave of the ectopic beat falls close to the T of the preceding complex ('R on T' phenomenon). If these occur more than 48 h after a myocardial infarction they are predictive of ventricular fibrillation and treatment is indicated.

Lignocaine remains the drug of choice though many other agents in class I or III may be effective. If long-term prophylaxis is required disopyramide or amiodarone may be used.

Ventricular tachycardia

If the rate is less than 170/min and the blood pressure well maintained, a bolus of 50–100 mg lignocaine may be used. If the tachycardia is refractory or poorly tolerated, DC cardioversion followed by a lignocaine infusion is the treatment of choice. If these measures fail, the choice lies between amiodarone or disopyramide.

Ventricular flutter and fibrillation/asystole

(a) DC countershock (200 J) is required immediately (if available).
(b) An airway must be established as soon as possible and ventilation with 100% oxygen commenced.
(c) If DC shock is not immediately effective external cardiac massage must be continued while reliable intravenous access is established.
(d) 8.4% sodium bicarbonate 50 ml is infused to counter acidosis.
(e) Lignocaine 100 mg stat is given and DC shock repeated. Repeat after 30 s if unsuccessful using 400 Joules.
(f) If lignocaine fails, disopyramide or amiodarone may be tried.
(g) If the amplitude of the fibrillation decreases it should be coarsened by giving calcium gluconate and adrenaline (see below) and defibrillation attempted again. Note that calcium salts should not be given into the same line as sodium bicarbonate as this combination results in precipitation in the line.
(h) If there is primary asystole then ventricular fibrillation should be provoked, e.g. with 10 ml of 10% calcium gluconate and 10 ml of 1 in 10 000 adrenaline. Fibrillation is then treated as above.

Bradyarrhythmias

Sinus bradycardia

1. Raising the foot of the bed may be successful.
2. Atropine 0.3–0.6 mg i.v. given rapidly. If there is no response, another 1 mg should be given (full atropinization requires 0.04 mg/kg i.v.). The maintenance dose is 0.6–1 mg i.v. every 4–6 h, but it should be remembered that this drug can precipitate ileus or glaucoma and exacerbate urinary obstruction in patients with prostatism. Some patients may become psychotic after atropine.

   Also in 60 % of people atropine causes an initial reduction in heart rate lasting a couple of minutes probably due to a central effect which is followed by the anticipated increase in heart rate.

   The main problems of atropine treatment are:

   (i) difficulty in accurate adjustment of the heart rate so that unwanted tachycardia may result which may require control by a β-blocker.
   (ii) encouragement of ventricular fibrillation due to disorganization of normal conduction pathways leading to re-entry phenomena.
3. Isoprenaline i.v. may also be successful and if chronic treatment is required an oral slow-release preparation may be used.
4. Digoxin, β-blockers and verapamil which exacerbate bradycardia should be discontinued or the dose reduced.
5. Pacemaker insertion is indicated if the bradycardia is unresponsive to atropine/isoprenaline and is causing significant hypotension.

(i) The sick sinus syndrome (tachycardia–bradycardia syndrome) Treatment is difficult. If the patient is symptomatic from bradycardia, atropine or isoprenaline may be used. Digoxin or other drugs may be used for the tachycardias. However, drugs useful for one rhythm state often aggravate the other and a pacemaker is often used to control bradycardia so that the tachycardias can be treated with drugs as necessary.

Atrioventricular conduction disturbances producing bradycardia

1. First-degree heart block by itself does not require treatment, but if associated with sinus bradycardia may be treated with atropine.
2. Second-degree heart block

   Mobitz type I (Wenckebach block) is relatively benign and often transient. If complete block occurs the escape pacemaker is situated relatively high up in the bundle so that the rate is 50–60/min with narrow QRS complexes. Atropine or a temporary pacemaker is all that is required. Mobitz type II block is more serious and may unpredictably progress to a complete block with a slow escape ventricular rate. The only reliable treatment is a pacemaker.
3. Third-degree heart block may be associated with cardiac failure (q.v.). Atropine or isoprenaline either i.v. or 2 hourly as 20 mg tablets or the slow release preparation (Saventrine) in doses of 30–150 mg 4 hourly. Drug treatment is disappointing, however, and the present trend is to employ a temporary or more likely permanent pacemaker.

HYPERTENSION

The level of arterial blood pressure has a continuous distribution in the population and it is impossible to define a precise division of the population into hypertensives and normals. Although there is no point at which normal and high blood pressure can be divided, actuarial tables show a steady increase in age-adjusted death rate with increasing systolic and diastolic pressures. One definition of hypertension might therefore be a level of blood pressure above which investigation and treatment do more good than harm. None of our present treatments of hypertension offer cure; they reduce blood pressure without alleviating its cause. Presently a cause of hypertension can be ascertained in approximately 10% of patients. It is salutary to recall that studies have shown that in the UK only about half of hypertensives are diagnosed, of these only half are treated and only half of this group have adequate reduction of blood pressure. Therefore only about one-eighth of all hypertensive patients are receiving satisfactory treatment: we can and should do better.

Because treatment is not curative, the decision to treat hypertension means lifelong treatment for the patient. This decision has pharmacological, toxicological and economic implications and treatment must be demonstrated to favourably influence prognosis in order to justify its imposition. When ganglion blockers were introduced in the 1950s, it was rapidly established that reduction of blood pressure in malignant hypertension was life-saving. Renal failure was prevented and cardiac failure and retinal lesions regressed. These facts were determined by trials involving less than 100 patients without controls or elaborate double-blind conditions, since the prognosis of untreated malignant hypertension was poor. The expected one-year survival rate of less than 5% was improved to over 50% by treatment. For patients not in the malignant phase with diastolic pressures in excess of 110 mm Hg, the benefits of treatment required more elaborate trials involving 100–1000 patients. It has been established that in this group control of hypertension will prevent the advent of cardiac or renal failure and stroke even before the development of symptoms or any complication. The benefits are however less certain for the prevention of coronary artery disease, which is important, since the mortality and morbidity of this complication make a major contribution to the risks of hypertension. Recent research has shown that haemorrhagic stroke is commoner among patients with untreated hypertension whereas cerebral infarction is commoner in patients with treated hypertension. This is consistent with the concept that haemorrhage (from Charcot Bouchard aneurysms) is prevented by control of hypertension but such treatment does not alter the progression of atheroma.

Views on the indications for treatment in mild hypertension are still evolving since they must be based on the results of large-scale (>35 000 person years of observation) whose results are still being analysed. Most experts would agree that treatment is advisable in patients under 65 years with a systolic pressure >160 mm Hg and/or a diastolic pressure >100 mm Hg. Most controversy arises when treatment at pressures below these levels is considered. If treatment of blood pressure at this level is found to be beneficial, the number of potential patients, most of whom will be asymptomatic, may be as many as 1 in 10 of the adult population. Thus unless those who can profit most from therapy and those who will come to no harm if left untreated are defined, the overall population benefit could be achieved at the expense of many previously asymptomatic individuals, who would experience drug-induced side effects and derive no benefit. The total cost of treatment including drugs might also be prohibitive.

Before initiating drug treatment the diagnosis must be as accurate as possible. Cushing's syndrome, phaeochromocytoma, some forms of hyperaldosteronism (Conn's syndrome), coarctation of the aorta, some types of renal artery stenosis and renal disease are best treated by surgery or a combination of surgery and drugs. Drug-induced hypertension should also be considered and the responsible agent withdrawn if possible. Drugs causing chronic hypertension include:

(a) Oral contraceptives raise blood pressure in all women possibly by increasing plasma renin substrate. This rise is more marked in those already having a raised blood pressure, renal disease or a history of pre-eclamptic toxaemia. The major effect is related to the oestrogen component of the pill but progestogens can cause salt and water retention, thus contributing to the pressure rise. If the pill is discontinued, the elevated blood pressure usually returns to normal within a few weeks but may take several months to resolve completely.
(b) Corticosteroids (see p. 639).
(c) Carbenoxolone and liquorice derivatives cause sodium retention and hypertension with a clinical picture resembling that of primary hyperaldosteronism.
(d) Other drugs producing salt and water retention, e.g. non-steroidal anti-inflammatory agents, occasionally produce hypertension.
(e) Alcohol.

Non-drug control of blood pressure

A number of drugs are available for control of hypertension and these will be considered individually below. Non-drug techniques used to control hypertension include:

(a) Weight reduction: a loss of 9.5 kg was associated with falls of 26 mm Hg systolic and 20 mm Hg diastolic pressure in a group of mild hypertensives. Obesity probably accelerates vascular disease because it leads to hypertension: the association with hyperlipidaemia in population studies is relatively minor.
(b) Sodium restriction to 50 mmoles daily or less. This modest restriction has hypotensive effect alone and permits diuretics and β-blockers to work more effectively.
(c) Yoga, so-called transcendental meditation and relaxation techniques probably act by altering sympathetic nervous system activity. The fall in blood pressure is modest, 10–15 mm Hg, and not all subjects respond, possibly due to differing motivation. The long-term efficacy of such therapy is unproven.

DRUG TREATMENT OF HYPERTENSION

Diuretics

Many diuretics have antihypertensive properties although their mode of action is incompletely understood. A correlation exists between their natriuretic and hypotensive effects but an extremely powerful diuretic such as frusemide is a less powerful antihypertensive agent than the weaker diuretic thiazides. During the early stages of treatment both plasma and extracellular fluid volumes decrease and the antihypertensive effect may be reversed by re-expanding the plasma volume with dextran. Diuretics, at least initially, cause renin release and hyperaldosteronism, probably related to the extent of volume depletion. With prolonged treatment, however, although the hypotensive action persists, the plasma volume slowly returns towards normal (Fig. 12.12) which suggests some other mode of action. Excessive salt intake or a low glomerular filtration rate also interferes with the antihypertensive effect. With chronic treatment the total peripheral resistance, which is initially raised at the onset of treatment, slowly falls, suggesting an action on peripheral blood vessels. This could be an autoregulatory change in response to the altered

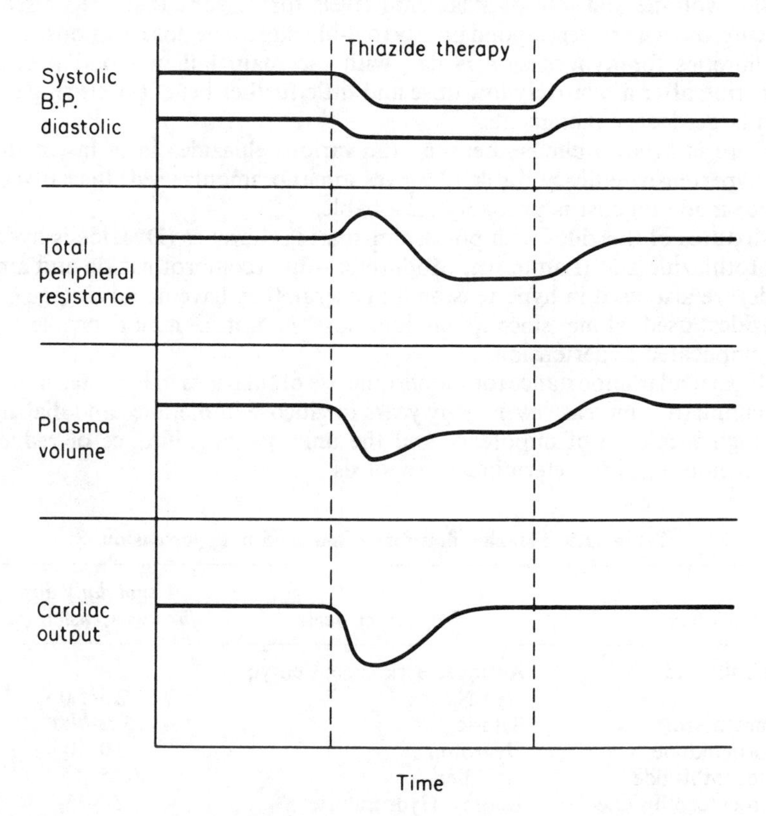

Fig. 12.12 Relationship between blood pressure, total peripheral resistance, plasma volume and cardiac output during thiazide therapy for hypertension.

blood volume and changes in tissue flow. The vasoconstrictor response to noradrenaline is also attenuated and some believe that depletion of sodium from arterial walls reduces their response to pressor stimuli, thereby reducing peripheral resistance. Alternatively there is some *in vitro* evidence for a direct vasodilator action of thiazides. The powerful vasodilator diazoxide (see p. 450) is a non-diuretic thiazide-like compound. Against the direct vasodilator theory is the fact that thiazides are ineffective in anephric patients.

Clinical uses Thiazide diuretics (see p. 495) are among the most widely used drugs for mild hypertension and may be given in conjunction with other agents, e.g. β-blockers and vasodilators. High-ceiling diuretics such as frusemide are less effective hypotensive agents than less powerful diuretics such as chlorthalidone or bendrofluazide. Thiazides used alone control about 40 % of patients with diastolic pressures less than 120 mm Hg and are seldom effective alone for pressures above this range. Because they elevate renin levels, some physicians would initiate therapy in the elderly, who often have low renin hypertension, with a diuretic but would prefer a β-adrenergic blocker for the young (and often high-renin) hypertensive. Diuretics may have higher efficacy in black patients whose hypertension is often associated with an expanded plasma volume and low plasma renin levels for reasons that are presently obscure and who often respond poorly to β-blockers. The dose–response curve of diuretics for hypotension is flat, with the main fall in blood pressure occurring after a relatively low dose and little further benefit occurring even with large dosage increments.

There is little to choose between the various thiazides in terms of their antihypertensive efficacy. Table 12.9 gives some commonly used alternatives. A choice made on cost is probably reasonable.

Mixtures of thiazides with potassium-sparing diuretics (Dyazide is hydrochlorothiazide and triamterine; Moduretic is hydrochlorothiazide and amiloride) are also used in hypertension. In general, they have no advantage over thiazides used alone since potassium loss is not a major problem in uncomplicated hypertension.

Of particular importance for the chronic use of thiazides in hypertension are the cumulative increase over many years in glucose intolerance and diabetes, the high incidence of impotence and the unknown significance of reduced HDL-cholesterol in determining prognosis.

Table 12.9 Thiazide diuretics often used in hypertension

Approved name	*Proprietary name*	*Usual daily dose for hypertension (mg)*
Bendrofluazide	Aprinox; Berkozide; Centyl; Neo-Naclex.	2.5–5.0
Chlorothiazide	Saluric	500–100
Chlorthalidone	Hygroton	50–100
Cyclopenthiazide	Navidrex	0.25–0.5
Hydrochlorothiazide	Esidrex; Hydrosaluric.	50–75
Polythiazide	Nephril	1–2

Piretanide (Arelix) This is a loop diuretic which is administered in a slow-release formulation and at a dose (6–12 mg/day) which produces only a mild diuresis. Given in this way its antihypertensive activity is similar to that of a thiazide. It has similar, if less severe, adverse reactions to other loop diuretics and its place in therapy is yet to be established.

Indapamide (Natrilix) is an indoline thiazide derivative which in large doses is a long-acting diuretic but which in smaller doses (2.5–5 mg daily) has rather greater antihypertensive properties than a thiazide without marked diuretic effect or potassium loss. This compound represents an effort to separate the diuretic effect from the vasodilator effect on blood vessels.

Spironolactone (Aldactone) has particular benefit in primary hyperaldosteronism where it rapidly corrects the biochemical abnormalities and restores a normal blood pressure. In essential hypertension, especially of the low-renin variety, spironolactone is as effective as thiazides.

Potassium depletion by diuretics in hypertension

Thiazide treatment of hypertension causes a dose-related fall in total body potassium and often in plasma potassium concentration. Magnesium loss may complicate this deficiency and hinder its correction. Ventricular extrasystoles are significantly increased by thiazide treatment and may be secondary to this hypokalaemia although the recent MRC mild hypertension trial found no significant association. The clinical significance of thiazide-induced ventricular extrasystoles is unclear. Insurance statistics and epidemiological data show that otherwise healthy individuals with ventricular extrasystoles have an increased risk of sudden death and are associated with coronary heart disease. Perhaps the sensible course is to minimise potassium loss by using small doses of diuretic and restricting sodium intake. Potassium chloride supplements are ineffective unless given in large (>60 mmoles/day) doses. Potassium-conserving diuretics are effective in correcting both potassium and magnesium deficiencies but can cause dangerous hyperkalaemia in patients with renal impairment. Concurrent β-blocker or converting enzyme inhibitor therapy may also moderate thiazide-induced hypokalaemia.

Adverse effects (see p. 498). Unlike many antihypertensives diuretics do not usually cause postural hypotension.

β-adrenoceptor blockers

Adrenergic receptors are classified into two groups, α and β, based on the effects of sympathomimetic amines on a variety of tissues. A further subdivision has been made into β_1-receptors, mainly in the heart, and β_2-receptors in the peripheral vessels, bronchi (and also, possibly, the heart). The distribution of some of these receptors is shown in Table 12.10.

β-adrenergic blocking drugs are competitive antagonists of synthetic agonists such as isoprenaline and of the natural neurotransmitter noradrenaline at β-adrenoceptors. Because they are competitive inhibitors their effects may be overcome by increasing the agonist concentration.

Table 12.10 Distribution of some adrenoceptors

Organ	*Receptor type*	*Effect of stimulation*
Heart	β_1	Increased heart rate
		Increased contractility
		Accelerated A–V conduction
	β_2	Coronary vasodilatation
	α	Coronary vasoconstriction
Blood vessels	α	Constriction (particularly skin and viscera)
	β_2	Dilatation (particularly striated and cardiac muscle)
Bronchi	β_2	Dilatation
Gastrointestinal tract	α and β	Reduced motility
Kidney	β_1	Renin release
Eye	α	Pupillary dilatation
	β_2	Pupillary constriction (weak)
Pancreas	(?β_1) β_2	Insulin release
Adipose tissue	β_1	Free fatty-acid release
Liver	α	Glycogenolysis
	β_2	Gluconeogenesis
Uterus	α	Contraction
	β_2	Relaxation
Mast cells	β_2	Inhibition of mediator release

Cardioselective β-blockers inhibit β_1-receptors but exert little influence on the bronchial and vascular β_2-receptors when employed in low doses. However, no tissue possesses exclusively one type of β-adrenoceptor, merely a preponderance of one type. Also, the absolute receptor number varies from time to time, e.g. they are increased by administration of β-blockers. In addition, the sensitivity of a patient may change so that when for example the bronchial calibre is highly dependent upon sympathetic tone as happens sometimes in asthmatics, even a cardioselective β_1-blocker may possess enough β_2-blocking potency to produce severe bronchospasm. Therefore even cardioselective β-blockers should not be given to asthmatics. Although cardioselectivity is not the only determinant of muscle blood flow, cardioselective agents may produce less peripheral circulatory disturbance than non-selective drugs. Since skeletal muscle fibres are largely supplied with β_2-receptors it is theoretically possible that selective agents could produce a lesser impairment of exercise performance.

There are also metabolic differences between selective and non-selective β-blockers. The metabolic response to insulin-induced hypoglycaemia depends upon hepatic glycogen breakdown (mediated via α-adrenoceptors) and gluconeogenesis (mediated by β_2-adrenoceptors). Thus a β_1-selective blocker is less likely to blunt the metabolic response of a diabetic who has received excess insulin. Adrenaline induces hypokalaemia via β_2-receptors linked to Na, K-ATPase and thus plays a part in short-term control of plasma potassium levels. In acute myocardial infarction plasma adrenaline rises to levels sufficient to produce significant hypokalaemia. It is also known that low plasma potassium levels are associated with life-threatening ventricular arrhythmias. The prevention of hypokalaemia could contribute to the cardioprotective effect of β-blockers in these circumstances and theoretically a non-selective blocker would be more suitable for this purpose. However, there is presently little evidence to support this contention.

Because β-selectivity is only relative, in practice cardioselectivity diminishes at high doses. Atenolol, metoprolol, acebutolol, betaxolol and practolol (available only for acute injection in arrhythmia treatment) possess cardioselectivity.

Some β-blockers may also weakly stimulate β-adrenoceptors whilst blocking the effect of injected catecholamines: this is the so-called *partial agonist* or *intrinsic sympathomimetic effect*. Theoretically drugs possessing intrinsic sympathomimetic activity might be less liable to induce cardiac failure, peripheral vasoconstriction, depressed A–V conduction or marked bradycardia. Excessive intrinsic activity is undesirable and such drugs, e.g. dichloroisoprenaline, para-oxprenolol, may actually cause tachycardia or hypertension and are therefore therapeutically useless. In man, partial agonist activity is difficult to demonstrate, but drugs with intrinsic activity reduce resting heart rate less than those without it. On exercise, increasing doses of β-blockers without partial agonist activity produce increased slowing of the heart rate, whereas drugs with intrinsic activity show a flattening of the dose–response curve at higher doses.

Drugs with partial agonist activity are probably slightly less effective in reducing the peripheral manifestations of thyrotoxicosis. There is some evidence that such drugs are less likely to cause cold hands and feet or to worsen Reynaud's phenomenon and partial agonism may be more important than β_1-selectivity in determining skin blood flow. There is no evidence that they cause less muscular fatigue than other β-blockers. Beta-blockers also decrease high density lipoproteins and increase low density lipoproteins which is possibly adverse for patients with coronary artery disease. Pindolol, which has the highest partial agonism of drugs currently commercially available, does not produce this detrimental lipid pattern.

These properties may be of relatively little practical importance in hypertension, although this opinion is disputed. In studies of β-blockers possessing intrinsic activity and/or selectivity, in doses producing similar reductions in exercise tachycardia the hypotensive effect is essentially similar and the possession of any particular combination of these properties does not influence the antihypertensive effect.

Some β-blockers, such as propranolol and oxprenolol (but not sotalol, timolol, and practolol), have local anaesthetic properties and a quinidine-like (Vaughan Williams Class I) effect (see p. 404) on the heart. These properties are included in the term '*membrane-stabilising activity*'. In the past there has been controversy as to the contribution of this property to the effects of β-blockers in arrhythmias and angina. Pharmacokinetic studies show that drug concentrations producing membrane stabilisation *in vitro* are not attained with usual clinical doses of β-blockers and are in excess of those producing β-blockade.

β-blockers produce numerous effects, which include:

(a) *Effects on carbohydrate metabolism* Hypoglycaemia releases adrenaline which stimulates glycogenolysis and gluconeogenesis (see above) and β-blockers (particularly the non-selective group) may inhibit this process. Further, the diabetic on β-blockers will be less able to recognise the autonomic responses associated with hypoglycaemia (tachycardia, tremor, pallor and sweating) which are mediated by catecholamines. These catecholamines may occasionally produce hypertension in such circumstances via unopposed α-adrenoceptor-mediated vasoconstriction. There is no evidence that chronic β-blockade increases the risk of developing diabetes nor that it leads to deterioration in diabetic control.

(b) *Lipolysis in adipose tissue* is reduced and therefore stress does not raise plasma free fatty acids. This could theoretically minimise the atherogenic effects of stress and probably contributes to the anti-arrhythmic effects of these drugs since free fatty acids are arrhythmogenic.

(c) *Platelet aggregation* is reduced and fibrinolysis enhanced by β-blockers, which may be beneficial in atherosclerosis and may protect against coronary artery occlusion by platelet thrombi.

(d) *Plasma potassium* is slightly increased by β-blockers and total body potassium gradually increases with chronic administration. These drugs can offset the hypokalaemic effects of diuretics and these two groups of drugs complement their actions when used in combination.

(e) *The central actions of β-adrenergic blockers* There is much evidence that in animals β-adrenergic receptors are widely distributed through the central nervous system. Studies with radioactively labelled β-adrenergic antagonists show that the main sites of these receptors are the cerebellum, the limbic forebrain, the hypothalamus and extrapyramidal areas. In general the effects of these drugs on the nervous system are inhibitory and depressant. In man, however, there is very little established information on the effects of these drugs. In normal subjects the EEG is unchanged, sleep patterns unaltered and although there is a strong clinical impression that at least some of these drugs have a central depressant action, the results of psychomotor tests are conflicting.

β-blockers are used for the treatment of:

(i) *Essential tremor*: most patients respond to small doses (40 mg, 8 hourly) of propranolol. The mechanism is unknown.
(ii) *Anxiety* symptoms mediated by the sympathetic nervous system are relieved by β-blockers. These include tachycardia, sweating and gastrointestinal tract disturbances. Present evidence suggests that this is predominantly a peripheral effect.

(f) *Long-term cardioprotection* Several studies with various β-blockers have demonstrated a reduced recurrence of myocardial infarction and/or sudden death in patients following infarction. There is presently little evidence that β-blockers can prevent a first myocardial infarction (primary prevention).

Mechanism of action of β-adrenergic blockers in hypertension Their mechanism of action in hypertension is undecided. Its existence is surprising since on pharmacological grounds blockade of vasodilation-mediating β-receptors might be anticipated to raise blood pressure. More than one of the following hypotheses may be correct:

(a) *Reduction in cardiac output* occurs when some β-blockers are given, but in acute experiments the blood pressure remains unchanged because the decreased output is offset by reflex vasconstriction. On continued administration the pressure falls because the peripheral resistance eventually decreases to pre-treatment levels. This reduction may be due to metabolic control mechanisms mediating the blood supply to the organs. Several β-blockers with intrinsic sympathomimetic activity, e.g. oxprenolol, pindolol, produce minimal effects on cardiac output but are hypotensive. Furthermore, high cardiac output hypertension is not particularly sensitive to β-blockers.

(b) There is often a delay in the attainment of the full antihypertensive effect and it has been suggested that attenuation of the cardiac response to pressor stimuli results in a *conditioning of the baroreceptors* to produce their inhibitory responses at a lower level and so the mean pressure gradually falls. This is analogous to the fall in pressure occurring when a hypertensive patient is put to bed which reduces the sensory input to the cardiovascular system and results in a resetting of the baroreceptors. It appears, however, that in man the baroreceptors are not responsible for the long-term control of blood pressure.

(c) A *central action of β-blockers* has been suggested. Clonidine (q.v.) is a centrally acting α-agonist and so β-blockade might result in unopposed α-adrenoreceptor stimulation of the same sites. Intracerebral injections of propranolol lower blood pressure in conscious animals. But similar injections of isoprenaline, a β-agonist, likewise result in hypotension and β-blockers injected into brain fail to antagonise rises in blood pressure provided by electrical stimulation of the medulla, although the associated tachycardia is blocked. Such experiments are artificial and only limited conclusions may be drawn from them. If propranolol were acting centrally a reduction in central efferent discharge might be expected and this has been demonstrated. The central action hypothesis does not explain the time lag between beginning treatment and the onset of effect, since no accumulation of drug appears to occur with time. Nor does it explain why drugs such as practolol, atenolol and metoprolol, which penetrate into the CNS very little, are effective hypotensive agents.

(d) *Renin release* is decreased by blockade of β_1-adrenoceptors. This could block an abnormal or inappropriate renin release producing hypertension via either a direct vascular effect of angiotensin or secondarily by aldosterone-mediated sodium retention. Renin secretion consequent to fixed obstruction of the renal artery or to parenchymal renal disease might be expected not to respond to β-blockers. However, a fall in renin activity may occur in renal hypertension after propranolol. This could explain how β-blockers lower blood pressure in the small group of younger hypertensives with high renin levels in whom these drugs are most effective. However, in the larger group of patients with low or normal renin levels β-blockers are also effective. No correlation of hypotensive effect with basal renin activity or lowering of renin levels has been found. The effects on renin release occur almost immediately and so this cannot explain the often delayed effects of β-blockade on hypertension. Furthermore, the dose required to lower renin maximally is often several times lower than the therapeutic dose and no suppression of renin occurs with pindolol, which sometimes increases renin levels. Thus in many cases inhibition of the renin–angiotensin system is probably not the main mechanism.

(e) *A vascular site of action* has been proposed. This supposes that elevated catecholamine levels associated with hypertension overstimulate vascular adenyl cyclase and result in subnormal sensitivity of the relaxation apparatus of the blood vessels. Chronic β-blockade thus allows the intracellular cyclic-AMP levels to fall and the relaxation mechanism slowly regains sensitivity to other mediators of relaxation such as histamine and prostaglandin PGE_2, which balance the unopposed α-vasoconstrictor tone. Because β-blockade only restores the normal relaxation ability of the vascular smooth muscle, excessive dosage does not produce hypotension.

Pharmacokinetics (see Table 12.11) An important determinant of their pharmacokinetics is their lipid solubility. Propranolol, timolol, oxprenolol

Table 12.11 Properties of some β-adrenergic blocking drugs

	Propranolol	*Practolol*	*Oxprenolol*	*Pindolol*	*Sotalol*
Cardioselectivity	0	+	0	0	0
Intrinsic sympathomimetic activity	0	++	++	+++	0
Membrane-stabilising effect	++	0	+	+	0
β-blockade potency compared to propranolol	1	0.3	1	10	0.3
$t_{1/2\beta}$ *(hours)*	2–4	8–12	1–2	3–4	12–16
First-pass hepatic metabolism (%)	60–70	0	40	15	15
% dose excreted unchanged in urine	<5	85	<5	40	75
CNS penetration	+	0	+	++	0
Effect on renin release	↓	0	↓	↑ or 0	↓
Recommended daily dosage (mg)					
(i) *Hypertension*	120–1000	Not recommended	160–480	15–45	160–600
(ii) *Angina*	120–480	Not recommended	120–480	2.5–15	160–480
Proprietary name	Inderal	Eraldin	Trasicor	Visken	Sotacor Beta-Cardone

Table 12.11(*Contd*)

	Betax-olol	*Tim-olol*	*Acebut-olol*	*Metopr-prolol*	*Aten-olol*	*Nad-olol*
Cardioselectivity	+	0	±	+	+	0
Intrinsic sympathomimetic activity	0	0	+	0	0	0
Membrane-stabilising effect	+	0	+	0	0	0
β-blockade potency compared to propranolol	4	6	0.3	1	1	1
$t_{1/2\beta}$ *(hours)*	12–22	4–6	6–8	3–4	6–9	16–24
First-pass hepatic metabolism (%)	10	Present	Present	50	50	0
% *dose excreted unchanged in urine*	10	20	40	3	10	100
CNS penetration	?	±	±	0	0	?
Effect on renin release	↓	↓	↓	↓	↓	↓
Recommended daily dosage (mg)						
(i) *Hypertension*	20–40	15–60	400–1200	100–400	50–200	80–240
(ii) *Angina*	Not yet approved	15–45	400–1200	100–300	50–200	40–240
Proprietary name	Kerlone	Bloca-dren; Betim	Sectral	Betaloc; Lopresor	Teno-rmin	Corgard

and metoprolol are the most lipid soluble and the least lipophilic are atenolol and sotolol. Acebutolol and pindolol have intermediate solubilities. The more lipophilic a drug the more extensive and rapid is absorption from the gut but also the higher is its first-pass metabolism in the gut wall and liver so that these drugs have short half-lives (usually 2–4 hours). Inter-patient variability in metabolic rate and thus effect is also greater for this group which also have a greater potential for drug interactions. Lipophilic β-blockers also enter the brain and can produce CNS side effects such as nightmares and hallucinations. Water-soluble β-blockers tend to be excreted via the kidneys without metabolism, to have longer half-lives (e.g. sotolol 12–16 h; nadolol 16–24 h) and will accumulate in renal failure.

Some β-blockers exhibit non-linear pharmacokinetics following oral absorption since the availability of small doses is low, but as the dose is increased progressively more reaches the systemic circulation (see Fig. 3.5) due to saturation of tissue binding in the liver. Drugs exhibiting this phenomenon include propranolol, alprenolol and possibly metoprolol. Propranolol, metoprolol, acebutolol and nadolol all produce higher plasma concentrations after chronic dosing than in the short-term, i.e. they apparently reduce their own metabolic rate. This could be due to reduced hepatic blood flow and first-pass effect secondary to a decreased cardiac output. Some of the metabolites of β-blockers are pharmacologically active. Thus propranolol forms 4-hydroxypropranolol which has β-blocking properties and a shorter $t_{1/2}$ than the parent compound. The major metabolite of acebutolol, acetylacebutolol is also active and is present in concentrations several times larger than acebutolol itself following oral administration but in much lower concentrations after intravenous injection, this pattern being consistent with the high hepatic extraction ratio and first-pass effect. The $t_{1/2}$ of acetylacebutolol is at least twice that of acebutolol and its accumulation probably determines the β-blocking properties of the drug.

Lipophilic β-blockers are usually highly protein bound, e.g. propranolol is 85–96% bound largely to α_1-acid glycoprotein (which carries 75% at therapeutic plasma concentrations) and also albumin and lipoproteins. Hydrophilic β-blockers have low protein binding, e.g. atenolol is less than 5% bound. A raised ESR, whether associated with chronic inflammation such as rheumatoid arthritis or acute infections, may produce increased plasma concentrations of highly protein bound β-blockers, e.g. metoprolol, propranolol, but not of the hydrophilic drugs like atenolol. Although age in itself may have little effect on β-blocker kinetics, in the population of symptomatic elderly patients seen by doctors, higher plasma levels of some of these drugs, e.g. oxprenolol, propranolol, acebutolol, are produced using lower doses than in the young. This is probably because such patients have high ESRs. Receptor density in the elderly is however reduced thus decreasing tissue sensitivity and so dose reduction is not usually needed.

Generally, good correlation can be demonstrated between most effects of β-adrenoceptor antagonists and the logarithm of the plasma concentration. The effective propranolol level to reduce exercise tachycardia appears to be at least ten times less than that which reduces diastolic blood pressure, although the correlation between antihypertensive effect and plasma level is poor. The dose–response curve is relatively flat compared to similar curves for other properties of β-blockers. The antihypertensive effect also achieves a maximum which cannot be exceeded by further dosage increments. Theoretically sustained plasma concentrations of β-blocker would be best in angina.

In the case of hypertension the pharmacological effects appear to be longer lasting than the plasma levels. Thus successful control of hypertension has been reported with once daily administration of atenolol, pindolol and sotalol. Slow release preparations are also employed, e.g. Slow Trasicor (oxprenolol), to prolong effective $t_{1/2}$, reduce the frequency of drug administration and hopefully to improve patient compliance. Single daily dose administration may also help control side effects: e.g. a patient who experiences nightmares with pindolol may be satisfactorily treated with a single morning dose. Compounds with short half-lives and no active metabolites, e.g. metoprolol, may be preferred in unstable angina and threatened infarction when an unwanted negative inotropic effect may require rapid discontinuation of β-blockade.

Clinical use β-blockers are useful drugs for the treatment of essential and renal hypertension of all grades of severity. They offer control throughout 24 h and do not produce postural hypotension since they smooth out swings of pressure due to posture, stress and exercise. There is a marked circadian variation in blood pressure and heart rate in both hypertensive and normal subjects. The highest readings occur during the morning and the lowest during the middle of the night. These circadian variations appear to depend upon an underlying neurohumoral rhythm. β-adrenergic blockade does not entirely alter this rhythm and appears to be less effective during the night and early morning (Fig. 12.13). Some account may need to be taken of these spontaneous fluctuations in blood pressure when considering the rational design of antihypertensive drug regimes.

Sexual dysfunction with β-blockers is uncommon.

Propranolol has been shown to give similar control to that obtained with guanethidine, bethanidine and methyldopa and has been more extensively studied than other β-blocking drugs. There is some evidence that black patients respond less satisfactorily to β-blockers than white patients. Choice may be made on the basis of the following facts:

(a) Propranolol has been the most widely used drug and as yet no evidence of important long-term toxicity has emerged.

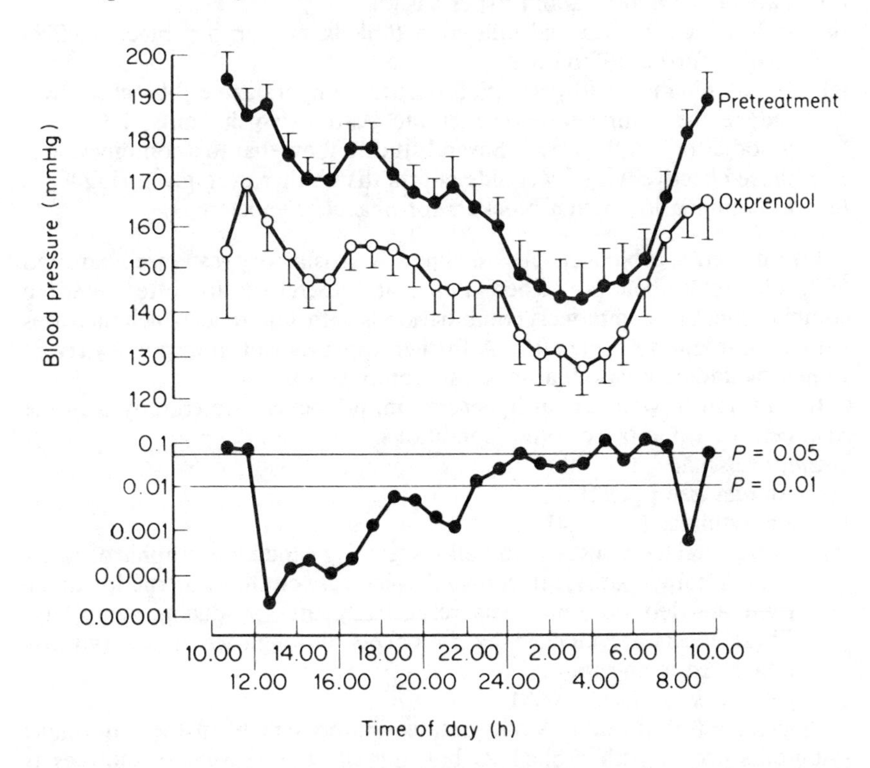

Fig. 12.13 Hourly mean systolic blood pressure obtained in 20 patients (by continuous monitoring via an indwelling arterial catheter) before treatment and after 6 weeks therapy with oxprenolol taken three times daily (mean dose 344 mg/day). The lower panel shows probability (P) for each hour of a significant difference between group means and control (From M. W. Millar-Craig *et al.*, *Clin. Sci.*, **55**, 3915 (1978).)

(b) There is a twenty-fold variation in plasma propranolol levels between different individuals given the same chronic dosage which presumably reflects differences in hepatic first-pass effect. Practically this means that a prolonged period of titration of dosage will be required for some patients. Some other drugs, e.g. atenolol, have a much smaller dose–response range and on this account may be more convenient to use.

(c) Side effects may limit the use of some β-blockers, e.g. a patient who experiences distressing nightmares when treated with say, pindolol, may be better treated by a drug which does not penetrate into the brain, e.g. atenolol.

With all β-blockers it is necessary to titrate the dosage according to individual requirements. It is useful to measure the pulse and blood pressure at rest supine, after standing up and following exercise. It should also be remembered that maximum antihypertensive effects may be exerted only after 2–4 weeks' therapy and that after this time hardly any additional anti-hypertensive effect can be anticipated.

β-adrenergic blockers would be particularly indicated in the following cases:

(a) Patients with angina and hypertension.
(b) Following a myocardial infarction β-blockers exert a protective effect against further infarction.
(c) In combination with vasodilators such as hydralazine β-blockade will reduce the compensatory reflex tachycardia which limits the use of vasodilators on their own. Several studies show that this combination is more effective with fewer side effects than either drug given singly.
(d) In combination with α-blockers for phaeochromocytoma.

Like diuretics, β-blockers elicit a clinically satisfactory response in around 60% of cases when prescribed alone, and therefore are often used in combination. The commonest combination is with a diuretic, which increases the response rate to some 80%. A further improvement in response may be gained by adding a vasodilator to this combination.

In addition to wide use in hypertension, β-blockers are employed in the treatment of a number of other conditions:

Cardiovascular

(a) Angina (see p. 392).
(b) Arrhythmias (see p. 413).
(c) Congenital heart disease: In Fallot's tetralogy and hypertrophic obstructive cardiomyopathy, catecholamines increase outflow obstruction in the right and left outflow tracts respectively thus producing symptoms. These effects are blocked by β-blockers although whether survival is influenced is uncertain.

Hyperthyroidism (see p. 668).

Psychiatry (see p. 221). Anxiety states—improvement in the autonomic symptoms occurs with β-blockers but any effect on psychic symptoms is secondary. A related use is the attenuation of the physiological effects of normal mental stress, e.g. public speaking, driving in heavy traffic.

Migraine There is evidence for a prophylactic effect (p. 284).

Essential tremor may be improved by β-blockers.

Chronic simple glaucoma β-blockers cause a fall in intraocular tension when administered locally or systemically. The mechanism is obscure and unexpected since β-agonists reduce the formation of aqueous humour and also reduce intraocular tension. Propranolol has local anaesthetic properties which make it unsuitable for topical use but timolol drops (Timoptol) are widely used. It is possible for drugs given in this way to be systemically absorbed and to produce adverse effects, e.g. bronchospasm.

Adverse effects

1. *Cardiovascular system* β-blockers will precipitate *heart failure* if used in patients requiring sympathetically mediated tachycardia to maintain an adequate output. In this they resemble other agents like reserpine which decrease the effectiveness of this compensatory mechanism. The most dramatic reduction in catecholamine effect occurs at the initiation of treatment and thus even small doses of β-blocker can be dangerous. Once treatment has been successfully initiated even a 25% dose increment represents only a small change in anti-sympathetic effect because of the shape of the dose–response curve and doses may be increased cautiously. Hypertensives with a history of cardiac failure should first receive treatment with diuretics and possibly digitalis before a β-blocker is used.

Bradycardia and *heart block* are increased by β-blockers.

Peripheral vascular disease and *Raynaud's phenomenon* are worsened or may be precipitated by these drugs. Approximately 5% of patients complain of cold hands or feet when given β-blockers; drugs with partial agonist properties may be less liable to cause this problem.

2. *Respiratory system*: *Bronchospasm* occurs in 2–5% of patients given non-selective β-blockers, the incidence being reduced if selective drugs are used. They should not be given to patients with a recent or past history of asthma since bronchospasm may occur even in those whose last attack of asthma was in childhood many years earlier.

Decreased respiratory centre sensitivity to carbon dioxide has been demonstrated experimentally following propranolol administration. This appears to result from β-blockade since it was not found with d-propranolol which has no β-blocking properties. This suggests an additional risk may operate in treating with propranolol patients with high pCO_2. Babies of mothers treated with propranolol during labour show respiratory depression.

3. *Central nervous system* effects occur particularly in those β-blockers known to penetrate the blood–brain barrier. The main problems are tiredness, nightmares, sleep disturbances and depression, but hallucinations have also been reported.

4. *Practolol* (which has now been withdrawn for long-term oral administration) was responsible for a particularly severe and specific syndrome which included a psoriasiform rash; xerophthalmia due to lachrymal gland fibrosis and which sometimes resulted in corneal destruction; secretory otitis media leading to deafness; fibrinous peritonitis causing ureteric and intestinal obstruction and a syndrome resembling systemic lupus erythematosus. These changes sometimes appeared or progressed following practolol withdrawal and were often associated with positive antinuclear factor and a wide range of

autoantibodies. This reaction was not predicted by animal tests and its incidence was too low to be detected in pre-marketing trials. Its appearance illustrates the need for vigilance by doctors as to the significance of even trivial symptoms with drug therapy. No similar syndrome has been reported with other β-blockers, although pustular psoriasis is occasionally precipitated by these drugs in individuals with psoriasis.

5. *Diabetics* on oral hypoglycaemic agents or insulin should be treated with caution because of the hypoglycaemia and insulin-potentiating action of β-blockers.

6. Minor side effects such as rashes, gastrointestinal disturbances (usually diarrhoea), muscle fatigue on exercise and cramps occasionally occur.

It is worth mentioning that as a group, β-blockers do not produce many of the disabling side effects associated with antihypertensive therapy in general. Thus postural hypotension, depression, drowsiness and impotence are unusual. There is no effect on plasma uric acid so that gout is not precipitated. In addition, tricyclic antidepressants and phenothiazines may be administered without interference with control of hypertension.

Drug interactions

1. Hepatic metabolism of more lipid-soluble β-blockers, e.g. propranolol, may be increased by enzyme-inducing drugs and reduced by inhibitors such as cimetidine.
2. Increased hepatic blood flow decreases the bioavailability of the highly metabolised β-blockers by reducing their first-pass metabolism. Food and hydralazine both act in this way.
3. β-blockers inhibit drug metabolism both directly and indirectly by decreasing hepatic blood flow secondary to decreased cardiac output. Propranolol and metoprolol reduce the clearance of lignocaine by both mechanisms and have produced lignocaine toxicity. Propranolol also inhibits the metabolism of chlorpromazine and warfarin.
4. Pharmacodynamic interactions: increased negative inotropic effects occur with verapamil (giving both intravenously can be fatal), lignocaine, tocainide and disopyramide.
   Postural hypotension with prazosin is potentiated.
   Rebound hypertension following clonidine withdrawal is potentiated and β-blockers may occasionally produce hypertension in patients taking sympathomimetic amines like phenylpropanolamine for nasal congestion.
   Exaggerated hypoglycaemia with insulin and oral hypoglycaemic drugs (see above).
5. The antihypertensive effect of β-blockers is antagonised by several NSAIDs. possibly due to salt and water retention although inhibition of prostaglandin synthesis may be involved. Sulindac, which has no effect on renal prostaglandin synthesis, has least effect on patients taking β-blockers.

Diuretic/beta-blocker combinations for hypertension

Most of the β-blockers marketed in the UK are available as combined preparations with a diuretic. These may be useful to improve compliance if the appropriate dosage ratio of diuretic and β-blocker is available. They are also cheaper for the patient but not for the NHS. Inflexibility in dose limits their use to those patients who require a small dose of β-blocker. They should never be used as first-line therapy nor should their dose be titrated up to obtain a large dose of β-blocker. Examples include Inderetic (propranolol 80 mg + bendrofluazide 2.5 mg), Co-Betaloc (metoprolol 100 mg + hydrochlorothiazide 12.5 mg), Tenoretic (atenolol 100 mg + chlorthalidone 25 mg).

Labetalol (Trandate)

Reduction of vasoconstrictor tone using α-blockers such as phentolamine has been used to treat hypertension but causes postural hypotension. Labetalol has mixed α- and β-competitive blocking properties, being approximately three times less active at α-receptors. This ratio of α- and β-blocking activities may be important for its pharmacological effects, which are those of vasodilatation (α-blockade) without tachycardia (β-blockade). The baroreceptor reflexes remain sufficiently active to avoid side effects associated with postural hypotension. Thus, unlike a pure β-blocker, labetalol reduces blood pressure primarily by reduction in peripheral resistance without changes in cardiac output at rest or on exercise. The heart rate at rest is usually unchanged, although exercise-induced tachycardia is attenuated. Labetalol has no intrinsic sympathomimetic activity and is a non-selective β-blocker. Although in normal subjects there are negligible effects on respiratory function it cannot be given to asthmatics without risk of producing bronchospasm. No important change in glucose metabolism occurs.

Pharmacokinetics Labetalol is almost completely absorbed from the gut but there is extensive first-pass hepatic metabolism so that it is only about 33% bioavailable, resulting in a wide variability of the effective oral dose between individuals. In chronic liver disease this first-pass effect is reduced and the availability may be doubled, resulting in increased pharmacological effects. The plasma $t_{1/2}$ is 3–4 h and it obeys linear kinetics. It is only 50% protein bound and thus has a relatively large apparent volume of distribution (approximately 10 l/kg). The major metabolites are inactive glucuronides. A linear relationship exists between plasma labetalol levels and the inhibition of exercise-induced tachycardia but the relationship of blood levels to the hypotensive effect is less clear.

Clinical use It is given orally in doses of 200–2400 mg daily divided 8 hourly. Unlike β-blockers its α-blocking action produces an immediate hypotensive effect. It is used in moderate and severe hypertension and additive effects have been demonstrated when it is combined with a diuretic or methyldopa. In low dosage for moderate hypertension its main action is as a β-blocker. In higher dosage there is more likelihood that α-blockade will produce postural effects.

Because of its immediate effect, unlike pure β-blockers, it may be used intravenously to achieve rapid control of hypertensive crises (see p. 459).

Labetalol is ideally suited for control of blood pressure in patients with phaeochromocytoma before and during surgery, because of its mixture of α- and β-blocking properties.

Its place in routine antihypertensive therapy is undecided; in some senses it has all the disadvantages of a fixed combination of drugs. Some authorities would prefer to alter independently the ratio of α- and β-blocking effects to suit individual patients.

Adverse effects Postural hypotension and those of β-blockade.

Adrenergic neurone-blocking agents

These drugs are taken up by adrenergic nerve terminals by the active transport process responsible for noradrenaline uptake. Once within the terminal they inhibit noradrenaline release by interference with the calcium ions coupling action potentials in the terminal membrane with neurotransmitter secretion. Guanethidine, but not the other members of the group, deplete noradrenaline from adrenergic terminals in blood vessels and the myocardium. Thus if this drug is given rapidly by intravenous injection the sudden catecholamine release may exacerbate hypertension: an effect particularly dangerous in patients with phaeochromocytoma who have large amounts of chromaffin tissue.

As with ganglion-blocking drugs (see below) the maximum hypotensive effects are achieved in the upright posture. Vasodilatation in response to exercise, digestion or heat, for example, causes further falls in blood pressure since compensatory venoconstriction mediated by the sympathetic neurones is absent. Reduced venous return such as during Valsalva's manoeuvre or defaecation may also cause undesirable hypotension due to the absence of compensatory reflexes. A pronounced diurnal swing in blood pressure is also seen in some patients reflecting diurnal variation in blood volume which is normally minimised by variations in sympathetic tone. Patients may complain of postural dizziness on rising in the morning which wears off later in the day. The blood pressure rises throughout the day so that control may be unsatisfactory in the evening despite low values in the morning. The failure of the cardiovascular system to respond to marked fluctuations in blood pressure is shown in Fig. 12.14, and postural hypotension is a marked feature of blood-pressure control with these agents.

Pharmacokinetics There are three main members of this group

(a) **Guanethidine (Ismelin)** The individual variation in dosage requirement for this drug is wide. Guanethidine is very slowly and incompletely absorbed from the gastrointestinal tract and undergoes a variable first-pass hepatic metabolism. Absorption varies from 3 to 45 % of the orally administered dose but is fairly constant for any one individual. Hepatic clearance of the drug is high but its $t_{1/2}$ is several days since the apparent volume of distribution is large. Hepatic metabolism terminates its action since the metabolites are inactive. The long $t_{1/2}$ means that accumulation to plateau level takes a long time and therefore changes in dose cannot be made more frequently than every 4–5 days, otherwise toxic levels may be reached. Adequate control therefore requires titration of dose over several weeks. The dose need only be given once daily.

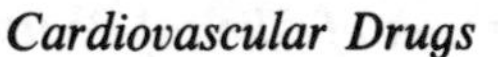

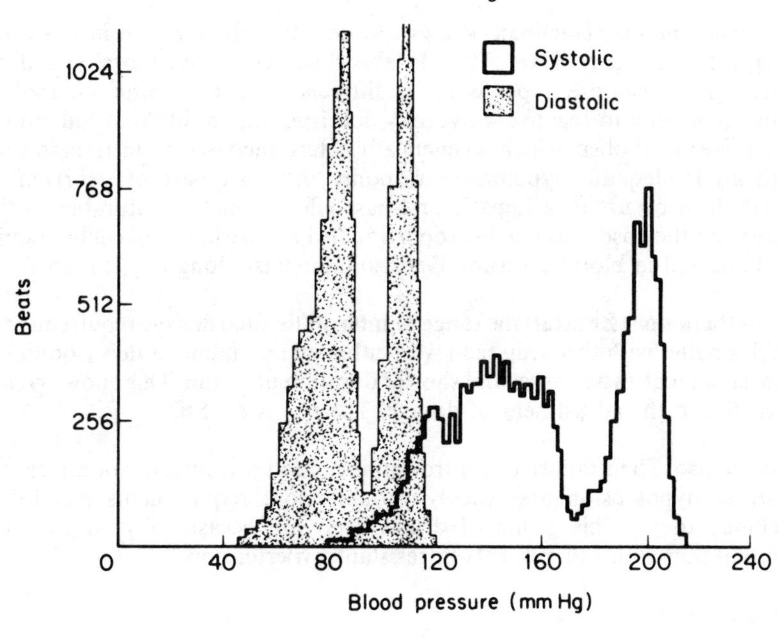

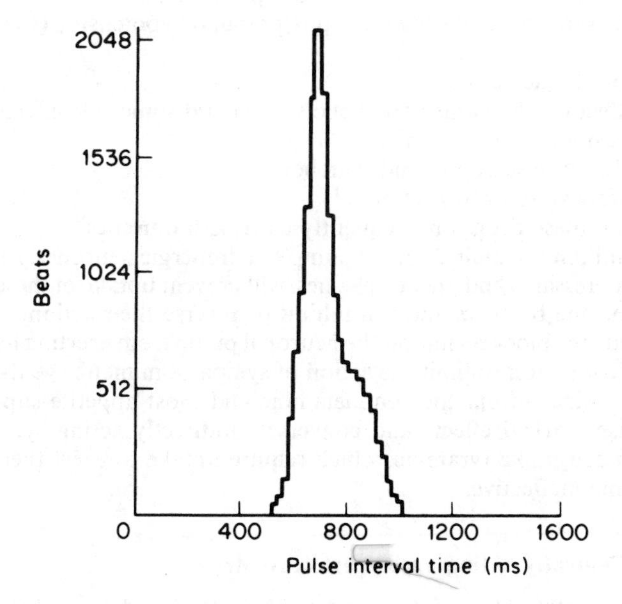

Fig. 12.14 Systolic and diastolic pressures and heart rate recorded over a 3-hour daytime period by continuous intra-arterial monitoring represented as incidence histograms. This shows the effect of bethanidine which produces a bimodal pattern for both systolic and diastolic pressures. Thus the systolic pressure fluctuates between a low of 80 mm Hg and rises as high as 220 mg Hg. With such fluctuations in pressure the heart should ideally be able to compensate by altering its rate during treatment with bethanidine; however, such compensation does not occur and the histogram of heart rate is unimodal with a narrow base. (From A. D. Goldberg and E. B. Raftery, *Lancet*, **2**, 1052 (1976).)

(b) **Debrisoquine (Declinax)** shows a wide (40-fold) variation in individual dosage requirement. Over 75% is absorbed when given orally and the variation in response depends upon differences in its hepatic metabolism, which is mainly to inactive 4-hydroxy debrisoquine in different individuals. Extensive metabolism which is genetically determined (see p. 109) is associated with an inadequate hypotensive response. At least part of debrisoquine metabolism occurs as a hepatic first-pass effect, which is saturable so that increasing the dose causes a disproportionate increase in plasma debrisoquine level and fall in blood pressure. Debrisoquine has a long $t_{1/2}$ (11–26 h).

(c) **Bethanidine (Esbatal)** the range of inter-individual dosage requirements is much smaller with this drug than with either guanethidine or debrisoquine. It also has a much faster onset and shorter duration of action. This allows greater flexibility in the adjustment of dosage. The $t_{1/2}$ is 8–15 h.

Clinical use Their failure to control supine blood pressure, the occurrence of postural hypotension and widely variable dose requirements has led to declining use of this group of drugs. They are occasionally employed in combination with other agents in resistant hypertension.

Adverse effects

1. The effects of adrenergic inhibition are often prominent:
   (a) postural, exertional and sometimes postprandial hypotension (Fig. 12.14);
   (b) inhibition of ejaculation.
2. There is no effect on the parasympathetic system and some side effects result from its unopposed action:
   (a) increased gastric secretion and diarrhoea;
   (b) nasal stuffiness and obstruction.
3. Fluid retention: these drugs are frequently used with diuretics.
4. Drugs which inhibit the amine uptake pump of adrenergic neurones, i.e. tricyclic antidepressants and phenothiazines, will prevent uptake of these adrenergic neurone blockers and can inhibit or reverse their action.
5. Adrenergic neurone blockers inhibit the neuronal pump from exerting its normal uptake function to limit the action of sympathomimetic agents. Thus noradrenaline, adrenaline, amphetamine and most appetite suppressants cause marked effects and conversely indirectly acting sympathomimetic drugs like tyramine, which require uptake to exert their activity, become ineffective.

Centrally acting antihypertensive drugs

The central nervous system plays an important rôle in the regulation of the peripheral circulation. Stimulation of certain α_2-adrenergic receptors in the brain stem pontomedullary area decreases sympathetic nervous outflow to the periphery which produces a fall in blood pressure. The hypotensive effects of methyldopa and clonidine are attributed to this central action. In addition this indirect central hypotensive effect mediated via α_2-adrenoceptors has been demonstrated for the following drugs when injected into the brain in animals:

(a) tricyclic antidepressants and cocaine—which inhibit noradrenaline re-uptake.
(b) monoamine oxidase inhibitors which inhibit noradrenaline catabolism.
(c) reserpine which liberates noradrenaline, although the hypotensive action of low-dose reserpine is predominantly a direct peripheral effect.

Methyldopa (Aldomet)

Methyldopa is taken up into the brain and converted into α-methyldopamine and then α-methylnoradrenaline in central adrenergic neurones. This latter metabolite is a potent α_2-adrenoceptor agonist and stimulates medullary α_2-receptors to lower blood pressure via a reduction in peripheral sympathetic tone. The hypotensive effect is slightly more pronounced in the erect than in the supine position. The cardiac output falls without change in peripheral resistance after chronic administration. This is unaccompanied by significant changes in renal blood flow or glomerular filtration rate.

Pharmacokinetics The major metabolite is the O-sulphate and its formation is dose-dependent, being much greater after an oral than an intravenous dose, suggesting first-pass metabolism as the drug crosses the gut wall and liver. Unchanged drug and metabolite are excreted by the kidneys and the drug has a plasma $t_{1/2}$ of 1.7 h, although there is evidence that its antihypertensive effect may be obtained by a single bedtime dose rather than by the more usual 6 to 8 hourly regime.

Clinical use One-half to two-thirds of hypertensives are controlled by methyldopa in doses which range from 0.75–4 g given usually (but perhaps not necessarily) in divided doses. There is some evidence that increasing the dose above 1.5 g daily contributes little further effect. Tolerance can occur to its action and at high doses side effects are prominent.

Adverse effects Although methyldopa produces minimal postural hypotension, it has numerous side effects. In one series 72% of patients noted adverse effects, in another 20% of patients found the drug unacceptable. Therefore the use of methyldopa is decreasing.

1. CNS effects are common (approximately 50% of patients) and often limit the use of the drug: drowsiness, dizziness (both postural due to hypotension and non-postural), nightmares, depression and rarely Parkinsonian features.
2. Interference with sexual function: decreased frequency of intercourse and failure of ejaculation.
3. Liver damage occurs due to hepatitis which in some cases progresses to chronic active hepatitis.
4. A positive Coombs test due to the production of IgG has been reported in 20% of patients on methyldopa for more than six months and 0.2% of these develop a symptomatic haemolytic anaemia whilst in others the

Coombs factor may interfere with cross-matching of blood. Reversible leucopenia and thrombocytopenia may also occur. Patients who suffer this reaction should stop the drug: the reaction is reversible.

5. Fluid retention is not infrequent and may precipitate heart failure. Thus thiazides are often useful adjunctive treatment.
6. Drug fever.
7. Hypertensive rebound has been reported following methyldopa withdrawal (cf. clonidine) but this is relatively mild.

Clonidine (Catapres)

Clonidine produces a fall in blood pressure and heart rate associated with a decreased cardiac output but unchanged peripheral resistance. The reduced cardiac output results from the combination of decreases in rate, stroke volume and venous return. Clonidine has little or no effect on renal blood flow or glomerular filtration rate. The cardiovascular effects of clonidine result from its central α-agonist properties. Vasoconstriction of peripheral blood vessels is counterbalanced by a reduction in central sympathetic outflow due to activation of α-receptors in the medulla. This centrally mediated, reduced sympathetic activity also produces bradycardia and reduced venous return. Prolonged clonidine treatment appears to reduce vascular reactivity by an action on the vessels and the direct effects of adrenaline, noradrenaline and angiotensin are much reduced.

Pharmacokinetics Hypotension (and sedation) are closely related to plasma clonidine concentration at low plasma levels but when the concentration rises the hypotensive response becomes disproportionately smaller. There is inter-individual variation in sensitivity to the effects of clonidine. The maximum effect develops at around 2 h following administration regardless of route of administration. The $t_{1/2}$ varies from 6 to 11 h.

Clinical use Clonidine is a potent agent and dosage is commenced at 0.05–0.1 mg 8 hourly. The dose is then increased until control of blood pressure is attained or side effects become limiting. Clonidine may be used with a diuretic, in which case the dose required is usually reduced or, like hydralazine, may be used in combination with a β-blocker.

Adverse effects Clonidine resembles the β-blockers in not producing postural hypotension. The incidence of other side effects is however moderately high and of the same degree as with methyldopa. About 10% of patients are unable to tolerate clonidine. The principal problems are:

1. Sedation and drowsiness: at least 50% of patients notice these effects but many gain tolerance as treatment proceeds, usually over the course of a few weeks. The antihypertensive and sedative actions appear to be linked: both depend upon α_2-adrenoceptor agonism. Depression may also occur with clonidine.
2. Dryness of the mouth persists for longer than sedation and results from excitation of presynaptic α_2-receptors which inhibit cholinergic transmission to the salivary glands.

3. Constipation, another anticholinergic side-effect, may be troublesome.
4. Sexual impotence is probably due to central reduction of sympathetic tone but other mechanisms may also be responsible.
5. An interesting but potentially dangerous effect may occur when clonidine therapy is abruptly withdrawn. There is rebound hypertension associated with anxiety, sweating, tachycardia and extrasystoles, and rarely a hypertensive crisis may be provoked. This reaction is relatively common and is disturbing since it makes clonidine an unsuitable drug for any patient whose ability to be compliant is in doubt. It has been suggested that this withdrawal syndrome can be prevented by gradual dose reduction over several days, but cases of severe rebound hypertension have been reported despite this precaution. Although perhaps commoner after chronic therapy, rebound phenomena have been reported after interruption of clonidine treatment of only 6–30 days duration.

   The mechanism of rebound hypertension is unclear: the effect resembles a phaeochromocytoma and is accompanied by large amounts of catecholamines in the plasma and urine (Fig. 12.15). It is treated either by an α-adrenergic blocking drug or by further clonidine. It has been suggested that clonidine produces increased catecholamine storage in nerve terminals by stimulating presynaptic α-receptors, which inhibit neurotransmitter release. When clonidine is withdrawn these stored catecholamines are released.
6. Concurrent administration of tricyclic antidepressants which have α-adrenoceptor antagonist properties may antagonise the action of clonidine.

These frequently occurring adverse effects have resulted in the infrequent use of clonidine.

Vasodilators

Hypertension is characterised by increased total peripheral resistance. It would seem logical to treat it with drugs acting on vascular smooth muscle to relax resistance vessels. Until recently the compensatory sympathetic outflow accompanying vasodilatation resulted in a restricted use for such drugs since this produced tachycardia and increased cardiac output (up to 75% increase). These reflex increases caused palpitations and angina which were unacceptable. Recently the use of β-blocking drugs to control these undesirable effects has resulted in a renaissance of the use of vasodilators in the treatment of hypertension.

(a) Hydralazine (Apresoline)

Hydralazine exerts a hypotensive action by reducing arterial resistance by up to 75% through a direct relaxation of arteriolar smooth muscle. Vascular resistance is decreased mainly in renal, cerebral, splanchnic and coronary circulatory beds, precapillary resistance vessels being more affected than the post capillary capacitance vessels. There is no direct effect on the heart or

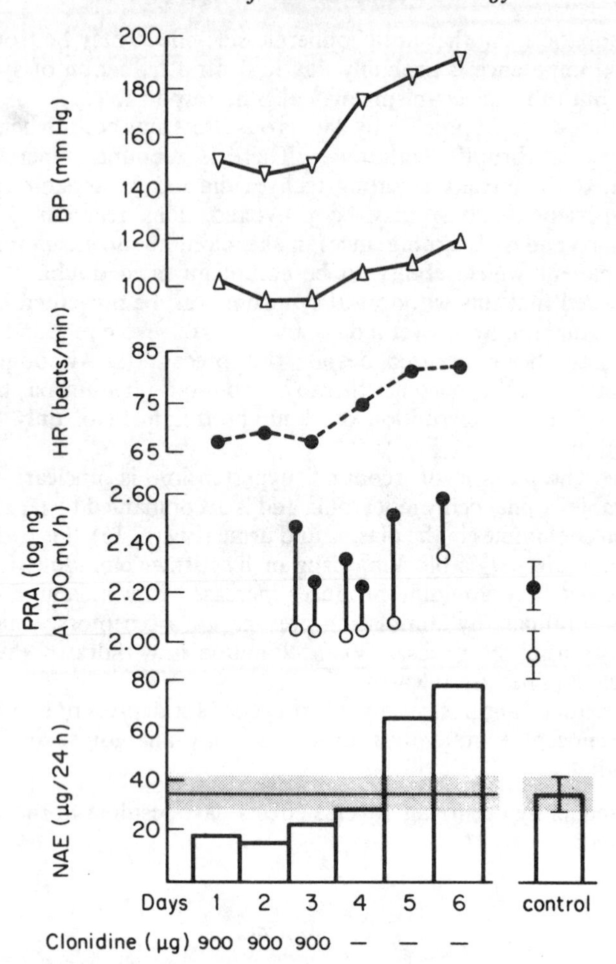

Fig. 12.15 Average daily blood pressure, heart rate (HR), plasma renin activity (PRA, ● upright, O recumbent) and urinary noradrenaline excretion (NAE) of seven patients during clonidine withdrawal. Hatched area indicates average ± s.d. of urinary noradrenaline excretion. (From G. G. Geyskes *et al.*, *Brit. J. Clin. Pharm.*, **7**, 55 (1979).)

circulatory reflexes, hydralazine is equally effective in upright and supine positions and severe postural hypotension is avoided. The effects of hydralazine alone are limited by reflex tachycardia (and accompanying palpitations) and the hypotensive effects are countered by homeostatic reflexes. It is therefore best combined with a β-blocker which limits tachycardia and increases cardiac output. Like other vasodilators, hydralazine causes salt and water retention accompanied by increased peripheral renin concentration. Weight gain and oedema can be limited by coadministration of a diuretic; increases in renin activity are effectively minimised by a β-blocker. This combination therapy has allowed wider and safer use of hydralazine.

Pharmacokinetics Hydralazine is rapidly and fairly completely absorbed after oral administration, peak levels being reached within 1 h of dosing. It distributes in about 50% of body water and 85% is protein-bound in plasma. Tissue binding also occurs, particularly in the walls of muscular arteries. This presumably explains why, despite a short plasma $t_{1/2}$ of 1.5–4 h, the half-offset time of the hypotensive effect is 30–140 h following discontinuation of treatment. It is therefore unlikely that a simple relationship exists between plasma hydralazine level and the circulatory effects of the drug.

Metabolism occurs by hepatic acetylation, the rate of which is dependent upon the genetically determined activity of N-acetyltransferase (see Chapter 4). The systemic availability of oral hydralazine is less than when it is given intravenously due to acetylation in the liver and gut wall (first-pass effect). The pharmacogenetic difference in acetylation is particularly prominent when the drug is given orally. Fast acetylators have lower steady-state plasma concentrations, less reduction in blood pressure and a reduced incidence of side effects. Acetylation is a saturable process and hydralazine exhibits dose-dependent kinetics on oral but not intravenous administration, which result from saturation of the acetylating system. Hydralazine differs from isoniazid (see p. 100) in that clear-cut differences between the $t_{1/2}$'$_{\beta}$ of the fast and slow acetylators are not discernible. Therefore the major pathway of hydralazine elimination does not show polymorphic characteristics.

Clinical use The most appropriate use is in patients whose blood pressure remains elevated despite adequate therapy with a β-blocker and thiazide (Fig. 12.16). It is usually given twice daily in doses less than 200 mg/day.

Rapid (within 15 min) reduction of severe hypertension may be achieved by i.v. administration of doses not exceeding 20 mg. The dose and frequency of administration of subsequent doses are variable; a slower reduction is achieved by i.m. administration.

Hydralazine is also used in the treatment of severe congestive cardiac failure (see p. 381).

Adverse effects

1. Related to direct or reflex-mediated haemodynamic actions: flushing, nasal congestion, headache, dizziness, palpitations, angina, oedema, weight gain. These effects are reduced by coadministration of a β-blocker and diuretic.
2. Lupus erythematosus syndrome. This is almost always reversible when hydralazine is stopped, although months may be required for complete disappearance of the reaction. The incidence is dose-dependent and higher in females and slow acetylators. Although it is usually recommended that maximum doses of 200 mg/day be given to slow and 300 mg/day to fast acetylators a recent study showed a 3 year incidence of lupus of 19.4% in women taking 200 mg/day suggesting that this dose could be too high.
3. Peripheral neuropathy. This is dose related and probably due to pyridoxine deficiency due to formation of a pyridoxine–hydralazine complex which inactivates the coenzyme. The neuropathy is corrected by pyridoxine supplements.

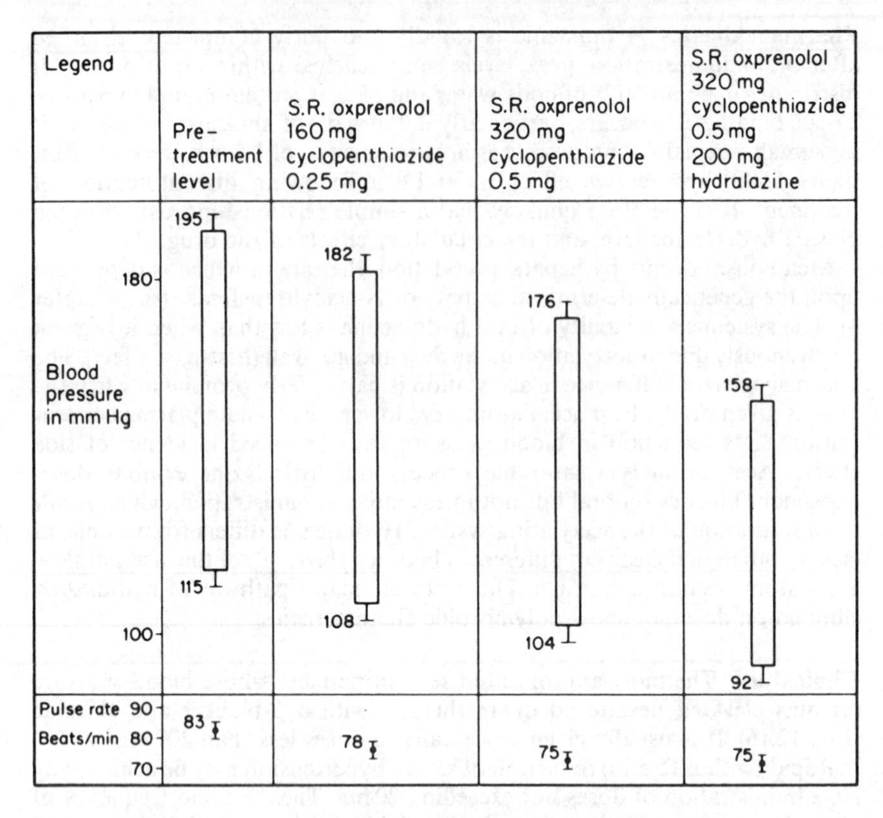

Fig. 12.16 Mean blood pressure levels and heart rate in stepwise trial in general practice of triple therapy in 397 previously untreated hypertensives (From W. A. Forrest, *Brit. J. Clin. Pract.*, **32**, 326 (1978).)

4. Blood dyscrasias: anaemia, agranulocytosis and leucopenia are rarely seen with the presently used low-dose therapy.

(b) Prazosin (Hypovase)

Prazosin is a phosphodiesterase inhibitor 20 times more powerful than theophylline, but the relationship of this to vasodilatation is obscure since the dose of prazosin used is very much smaller than one twentieth of the vasodilator dose of theophylline. The most important property appears to be that of post-junctional α_1-blockade. Unlike some α-blockers, e.g. phenoxybenzamine, it does not block the presynaptic α_2-receptors which are normally stimulated by the released neurotransmitter noradrenaline and which inhibit further transmitter release (see Fig. 12.17). Thus there is no interference with this negative-feedback pathway and relatively little tachycardia or increased cardiac output occurs during prazosin therapy as compared to phenoxybenzamine or hydralazine treatment. Unlike hydralazine, it does not raise renin levels.

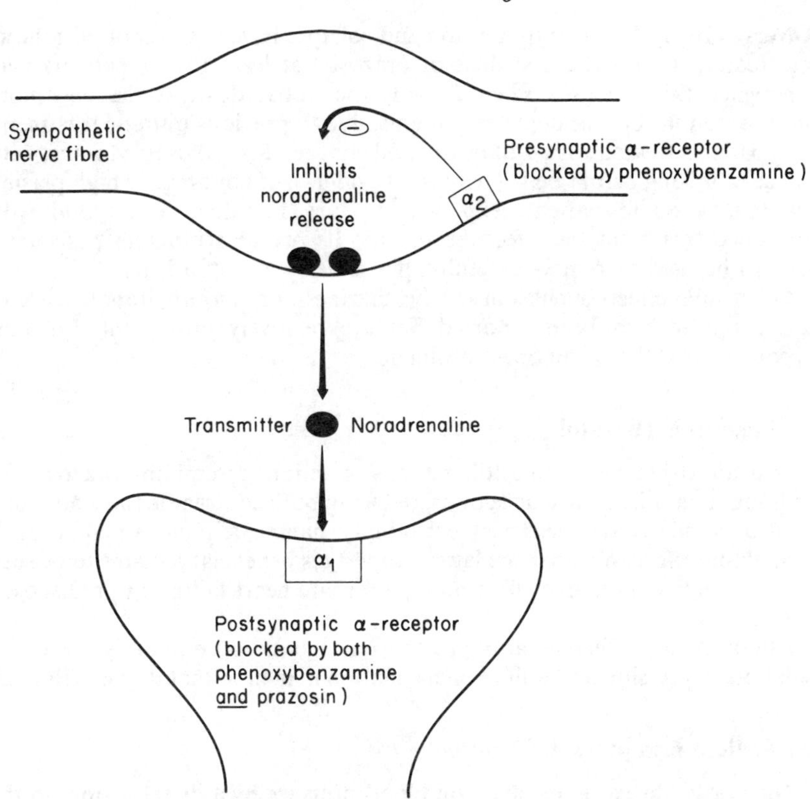

Fig. 12.17 Negative feedback control of noradrenaline release is modulated by presynaptic α_2–receptors, which are not blocked by prazosin (unlike postsynaptic α_1–receptors, which are blocked by this drug which is a pure postsynaptic α_1–blocker).

Pharmacokinetics Prazosin has a $t_{1/2}$ of 3 h, but provides satisfactory control of blood pressure in clinical practice when given twice daily. This may reflect a differing time course of tissue drug concentration from plasma and there is some evidence that the drug is concentrated in blood-vessel walls. There is a pronounced (40–50%) first-pass hepatic metabolism and some metabolites of prazosin are also hypotensive. Renal dysfunction does not affect its elimination.

Clinical use Treatment is begun with a low dose of 0.5 mg t.d.s. and increased slowly on the basis of patient tolerance and blood-pressure response. Most patients are maintained on doses of less than 20 mg/day. Prazosin may be used in conjunction with diuretics, methyldopa or other agents and is particularly effective when given with β-blockers. This latter combination may cause substantial reduction in blood pressure and should be initiated cautiously.

Prazosin reduces preload and afterload and augments cardiac performance in patients with congestive heart failure (see p. 381).

Adverse effects Severe hypotension and collapse have been reported following treatment with the first dose of prazosin: at least 1% of patients may experience this reaction when 2 mg is the initial dose. It may be more pronounced in sodium-depleted patients, due to previous diuretic treatment, or in patients treated with β-blockers, and it is therefore advisable to start with a dose of 0.5 mg before bed. There is no evidence of abnormally high plasma prazosin levels in patients experiencing this 'first-dose' effect and with continued treatment the effect disappears. Its prevalence makes prazosin a drug to be used extremely carefully, particularly in outpatients.

Other mild effects such as headache, dizziness, dry mouth, impotence, and pruritus have also been reported but are relatively infrequent. Postural hypotension is the commonest problem.

(c) Indoramin (Baratol)

This is an α_1-blocker with antihypertensive actions resembling prazosin. In addition it has direct cardiac actions, reducing both contractile force and rate. It also stabilises the electrical excitability having a lignocaine-like antiarrhythmic effect. Whether the latter property is beneficial remains to be seen but its negative inotropic effect may exacerbate heart failure in predisposed patients.

Although an effective antihypertensive agent, it commonly produces sedation, depression and failure of ejaculation in men so that its use is limited.

(d) Sodium nitroprusside (Nipride)

Nitroprusside exerts its effect on blood pressure by a direct action on the smooth muscle of arteries and veins. This action may involve binding of calcium to cellular or membrane storage sites which produces relaxation. Tachycardia is associated with the hypotensive effect. Cardiac output may be improved after myocardial infarction or in heart failure.

Pharmacokinetics The action of nitroprusside is immediate and evanescent so that to maintain constant hypotension it must be given by infusion. This also allows rapid reversal of its effects. Each nitroprusside ion liberates five cyanide ions by a non-enzymic reaction with haemoglobin. One of these is absorbed by reacting with the resultant methaemoglobin and the remainder are metabolised by rhodanase, a mitochondrial enzyme system in liver and kidney which is a sulphydryl transferase converting cyanide to thiocyanate. Vitamin B_{12} may be a rhodanase co-factor. Although the $t_{1/2}$ of nitroprusside is of the order of seconds, the thiocyanate formed has a $t_{1/2}$ of about a week and is excreted largely unchanged.

Clinical use Nitroprusside is used for the immediate reduction of blood pressure in hypertensive crises, to reduce afterload in the management of cardiogenic shock and in hypotensive anaesthesia.

It is administered intravenously, the initial dose being 0.5–1.5 μg/kg/min. As soon as a response is obtained the dose is adjusted to individual requirements, which are variable: usually within the range of 0.5–8 μg/kg/min. A maximum dose limit of 800 μg/min is recommended to avoid cyanide intoxication. The usual response to nitroprusside is an immediate fall in blood pressure by 30–40 %. Only rarely has tachyphylaxis been encountered. Because of its shortlived action, flexible control of blood pressure is easily achieved and can be varied using an infusion pump or microdrip regulator. It should only be used in intensive care facilities.

Degradation of nitroprusside occurs in the presence of light or acid yielding sodium ferrocyanide and cyanide. Fortunately this changes the colour of the resulting solution from the normal brownish-pink to blue or dark brown. The stock solution should be diluted only in 5 % dextrose: other diluents may produce toxic products. The infusion bottle should be covered with silver paper to prevent photodeactivation.

Adverse effects Side effects are usually due to a too rapid reduction in blood pressure and disappear with slowing of the infusion rate. Other effects are nausea, palpitation, dizziness, apprehension and muscle twitching, but generally its use is associated with a low incidence of toxicity. Prolonged or excessive dosage has resulted in deaths due to cyanide accumulation or in hypothyroidism from thiocyanate toxicity. Vitamin B_{12} levels fall with continued nitroprusside infusion and it is contraindicated in B_{12}-deficient patients.

(e) Minoxidil (Loniten)

This is the most effective of all known directly acting vasodilators. It is often effective in controlling blood pressure in patients who have not been satisfactorily managed on any other hypotensive regime. Minoxidil selectively relaxes arteriolar smooth muscle and reduces both systolic and diastolic pressures. Reflex increase occurs in heart rate which is largely prevented by β-blockers. It also produces marked fluid retention which not only antagonises the antihypertensive effect but can also precipitate cardiac failure. It must therefore always be given with a diuretic. Thiazides alone may be ineffective and frusemide administered twice daily is usually required. The mechanism of fluid retention is at least partly mediated by increased renin secretion.

Pharmacokinetics Gastrointestinal absorption is rapid and amounts to at least 95 % of the dose. Minoxidil does not bind to plasma protein or enter the CNS. The $t_{1/2}$ is about 1.5 h and it is eliminated by glucuronide formation followed by renal excretion. Plasma drug concentration is not correlated with effect and the hypotensive action declines at about 30 % per day so that once or twice daily dosing is adequate.

Clinical use Initially 5 mg daily in one or two doses is used and this is increased by 5–10 mg every 3 days to a maximum of 50 mg daily.

Adverse effects

1. Hair growth with elongation, thickening and enhanced pigmentation of fine body hair occurs in nearly all patients and is a serious drawback to use in women who may refuse to take it solely because of hirsutism. The mechanism is unknown: it is not a reflection of an endocrine abnor-

mality. There have been reports, as yet unsubstantiated, of its efficacy in alopecia and male-pattern baldness when applied topically.

2. 60–75% of patients have reversible flattening or inversion of the T waves in their electrocardiogram. These are asymptomatic and disappear on continued treatment.
3. Pericardial effusion has been reported, usually in patients with renal impairment and fluid overload.
4. Other effects: rash, gastrointestinal intolerance and breast tenderness.

(f) Diazoxide (Eudemine)

Diazoxide is an analogue of the thiazide diuretics but as a powerful vasodilator paradoxically has sodium-retaining properties rather than natriuretic ones. It is an arterial vasodilator via a direct action on arterial smooth muscle. It does not affect capacitance vessels and has no direct cardiac effects, nor does it impair cardiovascular reflexes. Thus when the blood pressure falls a sympathetically mediated tachycardia and increased cardiac output occurs. Diazoxide additionally causes catecholamine release by a direct action.

Pharmacokinetics The drug is mainly eliminated by glomerular filtration, although some undergoes hepatic metabolism. Its long $t_{1/2}$ of 20–30 h reflects the fact that 90% of the drug is protein bound and so protected from glomerular filtration. The $t_{1/2}$ is at least three times longer than its hypotensive action and when used at the usual dosage interval 4–12 h it accumulates extensively in the body. There is no correlation between the total plasma concentration of diazoxide and its hypotensive action since the latter depends upon the initial concentration of free drug in the resistance vessels. This being the case, the degree of blood pressure lowering is highly dependent upon the rate of injection and a slow infusion of diazoxide is less effective than a rapid injection of the same dose (Fig. 12.18). When the drug is injected rapidly, the plasma albumin drug binding capacity is temporarily exceeded, allowing a higher free-drug concentration to interact with the arterial smooth muscle and produce relaxation.

Clinical use Although maximum effects occur if a large dose is given rapidly, the response is unpredictable and dangerous hypotension can occur. In hypertensive crises (see p. 459) 50–150 mg are given slowly at first and larger doses given faster are used only if necessary. Alternatively it is given by constant infusion at rates of 15–30 mg/min when the desired effect is usually obtained within 30 minutes.

Oral diazoxide is only rarely used in severe and resistant hypertension because of its numerous adverse effects.

Adverse effects

1. Sodium retention may exacerbate cardiac failure and in patients with cardiac or renal impairment diazoxide should be administered with a powerful diuretic such as frusemide.
2. Hyperglycaemia is common and due mainly to direct inhibition of insulin release by pancreatic β-cells in the Islets of Langherhans.

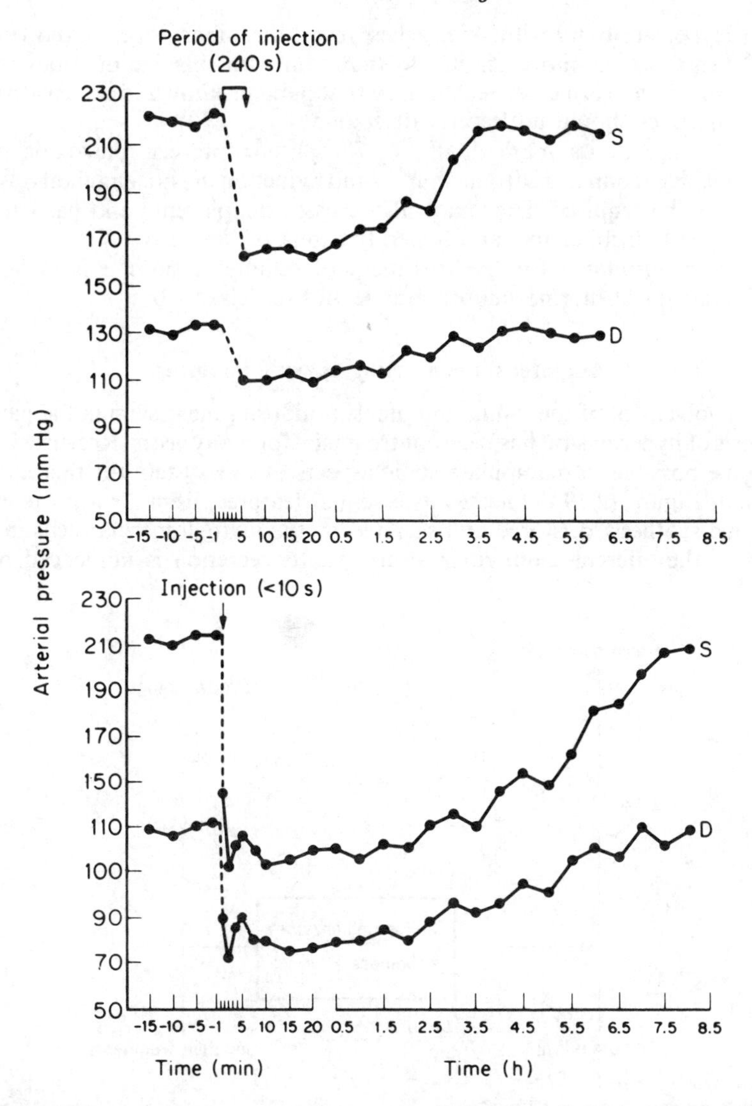

Fig. 12.18 Effect of injection rate on the hypotensive effect of diazoxide in a hypertensive subject (From E. M. Sellers and J. Koch-Weser, *Ann., N.Y. Acad. Sci.*, **226**, 319 (1973).)

Adrenaline release and a direct effect on the liver, mediated via increased intracellular cyclic AMP, result in increased glucose release. Blood sugar should be monitored in patients with impaired carbohydrate tolerance or renal failure since hyperosmolar, non-ketotic hyperglycaemic coma has been produced in a few instances by diazoxide. The hyperglycaemic action of the drug may be turned to good account in the management of hypoglycaemia due to an islet-cell tumour of the pancreas.

3. Hypersensitivity with skin rashes, fever, thrombocytopenia and leucopenia occurs and is similar to that seen with thiazide diuretics, with which there is a cross reaction, so that patients known to be sensitive to thiazides should not receive diazoxide.
4. Because of its marked affinity for plasma protein, diazoxide may displace coumarins from albumin and reduction in anticoagulant dosage may be required. Diazoxide also crosses the placenta and has caused hyperbilirubinaemia and hyperglycaemia of the fetus.
5. It is unsuitable for the treatment of eclampsia since it is powerful relaxant of uterine smooth muscle and so delays labour.

Angiotensin converting enzyme inhibitors

The involvement of the renin–angiotensin–aldosterone system in the pathogenesis of hypertension has been controversial for many years. Recently it has become possible to manipulate some aspects of this system for therapeutic benefit. Figure 12.19 delineates its essential features. Renin is a proteolytic enzyme synthesised, stored and secreted by the juxtoglomerular cells in the wall of the afferent glomerular arterioles. Its secretion is influenced by a

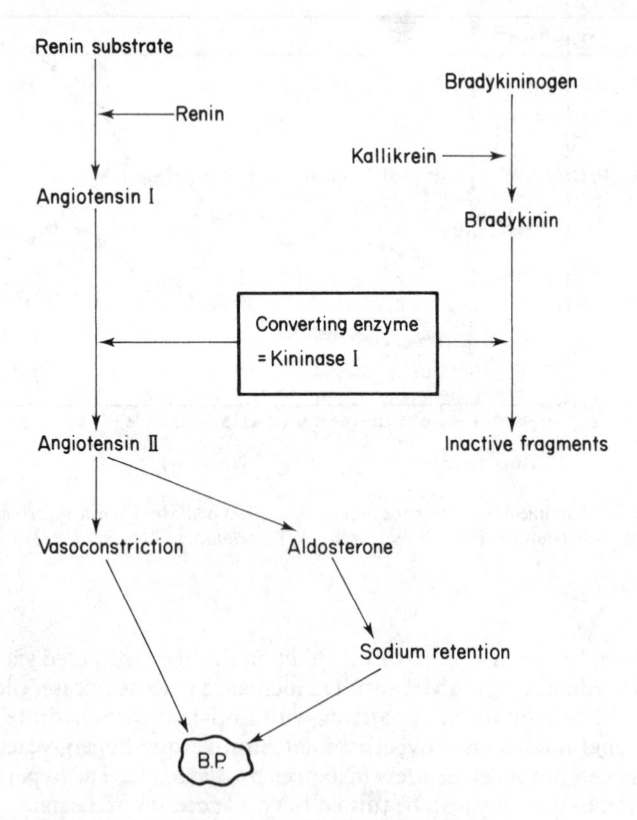

Fig. 12.19 Renin-angiotensin axis-role of converting enzyme.

number of factors including decreased blood pressure or volume and sodium depletion. Renin splits a circulating α_2-globulin substrate of hepatic origin to produce an inactive decapeptide angiotensin I. This is rapidly converted by a converting enzyme into angiotensin II which is by weight the most powerful vasoconstrictor known. Converting enzyme is a dipeptidyl carboxypeptidase identical with kininase II, an enzyme which degrades kinins such as bradykinin which has effects opposite to angiotensin II, namely vasodilatation and hypotension, natriuresis and diuresis. Converting enzyme is located mainly in the lungs but also occurs in plasma, blood vessels and the kidney. Angiotensin II, probably via its metabolite angiotensin III, releases aldosterone from the adrenal cortex which causes sodium retention with attendant volume expansion. Thus the renin–angiotensin axis affects both vasoconstrictor and volume components of blood pressure control.

In some hypertensives the role of these components is separated. Pure volume hypertension associated with low circulating renin levels occurs in primary hyperaldosteronism and in some cases of renal failure when the kidney is unable to excrete excess volume. Pure vasoconstriction hypertension with high renin levels occurs in some patients with severe renal parenchymal disease and in malignant hypertension. In such patients inhibition of the renin–angiotensin axis would be logical treatment.

Patients with essential hypertension may also be separated in terms of their renin–sodium profile into those with high renin (15%), low renin (30%) and normal renin activity (55%). It has been postulated that seemingly normal renin levels could be inappropriate in relation to the sodium retention suggesting that here also a treatment which could block angiotensin II might lower blood pressure.

Saralasin is an octopeptide analogue of angiotensin II which is a competitive inhibitor for the vascular receptors for angiotensin II and will lower the blood pressure in patients with high renin activity. As it requires infusion and has some partial agonism thus raising the blood pressure in patients with low renin activity, it remains a research tool.

Several *angiotensin converting enzyme* (ACE) inhibitors are now available. Captopril is a competitive inhibitor of the enzyme. It is an effective antihypertensive agent in renovascular disease and as monotherapy in essential hypertension it has comparable potency to thiazide diuretics or β-blockers. It is effectively combined with frusemide in treating more severe hypertension. Although its action is potentiated by concurrent administration of thiazides, the addition of β-blockers to captopril does not produce a further fall in blood pressure.

The extent of the fall in blood pressure after the initial dose in some but not all studies is proportional to the pretreatment renin and angiotensin II concentrations but after three or four doses many patients lose this effect and their blood pressure drifts back to pretreatment levels. On continued treatment over 3–4 weeks, there is a fall in blood pressure which has little relationship to pretreatment renin levels. This later fall may result from some other aspect of the pharmacology of the drug, e.g. prolonged survival of tissue kinins, resetting of baroceptors, but at present it must be admitted that only part of its effects is explicable in terms of ACE inhibition. Other questions remain such as why ACE inhibitors are effective in patients with normal renin levels and how they act in anephric patients. In some cases perhaps circulating renin may be unimportant and effective angiotensin II levels in the arterial wall may determine blood pressure.

Captopril

Pharmacokinetics Lack of suitable assays has limited knowledge of captopril kinetics. Following oral administration absorption is rapid with peak blood levels occurring at about one hour. Some 70% is absorbed but this is reduced to 30% by food so it should be taken before meals. Approximately 60% is recovered unchanged in the urine with the remainder accounted for by various inactive metabolites. Protein binding is approximately 30%. Protein binding decreases and half life (normally about 4 h) increases in patients with renal impairment so that dosage adjustment is required for renal failure.

Clinical use The initial oral dose is 2.5 mg 12 hourly which is increased to 50 mg 8 hourly after 2 weeks if a satisfactory reduction in blood pressure is not attained. A diuretic is often added and if this is not effective the dose is increased to 100 mg 8 hourly (maximum).

Captopril is also used in severe congestive heart failure (see p. 381).

Adverse effects

1. First dose effect: excessive hypotension with the danger of cerebral ischaemia may occur after the first dose particularly in diuretic pretreated (i.e. sodium and volume depleted) patients. The event cannot be predicted. Therefore any severely hypertensive patient who has received other antihypertensive drugs should have close medical supervision for at least three hours after the initial dose.
2. Renal effects: Proteinuria of greater than 1 g/day occurs in about 1% of patients with pre-existing renal disease and 0.5% in those without. It is recommended that the urine be tested for protein monthly. Only rarely is a true nephrotic syndrome produced. Usually proteinuria is reversible. Some patients with renal disease, particularly renal artery stenosis have developed acute renal failure following captopril, probably due to inadequate renal perfusion.
3. Neutropenia and agranulocytosis have occurred, mainly in patients with renal failure and on treatment with immunosuppressant drugs, usually for auto-immune collagen disorders. Such patients should not receive captopril unless there is no alternative and weekly white blood cell counts are recommended during the first 3 months of therapy in this patient group. All patients should be told to report the warning signs of agranulocytosis immediately.
4. Hyperkalaemia may occur secondary to reduced aldosterone production especially in patients with renal impairment. Potassium supplements or potassium conserving diuretics should be avoided with captopril.
5. A pruritic maculopapular rash, sometimes with fever, occurs in some 10% of patients. This may disappear if treatment is continued.

6. Gastrointestinal: Diminution or loss of taste (ageusia) occurs in some 5% of patients and is reversible and self-limiting in 2–3 months despite continued therapy.

Other ACE inhibitors

Many of the adverse effects of captopril are similar to those of other drugs containing –SH groups, e.g. penicillamine and heavy metal antagonists. Newer agents have been devised and one of these, enalapril (Innovace), is now available in the U.K. It is a prodrug forming the active acid form, enalaprilat, in the liver. Therapeutically it is similar to captopril. Adverse effects are perhaps a little less common but with the low doses of captopril now used there is little difference. A once daily dose of 10–20 mg enalapril is satisfactory in hypertension. Reduced dosage is required with renal impairment.

Calcium channel inhibitors (see also pp. 394, 416)

Contraction of vascular smooth muscle such as that of coronary and systemic arterioles depends upon the binding of calcium ion to a small binding protein called calmodulin. The Ca^{2+}–calmodulin complex activates muscle myosin kinase which in turn phosphorylates myosin and permits myosin to interact with actin producing contraction and vasoconstriction. In smooth muscle, unlike skeletal muscle, calcium ion stores are minimal and contraction thus depends upon transmembrane Ca^{2+} flux which can be blocked by calcium channel blocking drugs. Arterial smooth muscle, and in particular that of the coronaries, is more sensitive than venous smooth muscle so these drugs are predominantly arterial vasodilators. Although the aetiology of hypertension is obscure, calcium metabolism may in some way be linked to genesis. Thus a recent epidemiological study of over 9000 men showed a positive correlation between calcium concentrations and blood pressure. Calcium may be the final common link between several aetiological factors and vasoconstriction and calcium channel antagonists, by acting at this site, may interrupt this process. The reduction in blood pressure produced is *graded* and the higher the pretreatment pressure the greater the resulting decrease: there is little or no effect on the blood pressure of normotensives. This is in contrast to other vasodilators like nitroprusside or hydralazine and suggests that calcium channel blockers act on a functional abnormality of vascular smooth muscle.

Nifedipine (see p. 394) is given as a slow release 20 mg preparation (Adalat Retard) to overcome the short half-life of this drug. The dose is 20 mg twice daily which can be increased to 40 mg twice daily. Because of the graded action of the drug it can be used in all grades of hypertension from mild to severe without the fear of excessive hypotension. It has also been used in the treatment of hypertensive crisis although its place in this condition is not yet established. It cannot be advocated at present for the treatment of hypertension in pregnancy.

Unlike other vasodilators there is no significant change in heart rate after chronic administration: this has been attributed to resetting of the baroreflex arc to a normal level accompanied by increased baroreceptor sensitivity. This results in improved buffering of transient blood pressure surges.

Nifedipine may be used alone or in combination with a β-blocker where the action is additive rather than synergistic. Postural hypotension and heart failure have been recorded with such combinations although nifedipine, having no action on cardiac conduction is probably less dangerous than verapamil when used in this way. It should be noted that unlike β-blockers calcium channel antagonists are safe in asthmatics and may even improve this condition since they could block the calcium ion-dependent release of the mediators of bronchoconstriction from sensitised cells.

Verapamil (see p. 416) There is less experience with this drug in hypertension than nifedipine. It has been used as monotherapy in doses of 80–160 mg 8 hourly in mild to moderate hypertension. However, the need to avoid patients with sick-sinus syndrome, heart block or bradycardia and the theoretical danger of concurrent β-blocker therapy makes it less flexible than nifedipine in practice.

Ganglion-blocking agents

These block autonomic ganglia by competitive antagonism of the nicotinic cholinergic receptors. The effects on sympathetic ganglia include reduced transmission of excitatory impulses to the heart, blood vessels and adrenal medulla. Heart rate and peripheral resistance fall and blood pressure, which is only slightly decreased in the supine position, falls precipitately on standing up. This postural hypotension results from the gravitational pooling of blood in the veins in the absence of the compensatory reflex vasoconstriction which usually occurs. An additional consequence is decreased venous return which lowers cardiac output and may produce dizziness or fainting. Reduced flow to the coronaries, intestines and kidneys may also occur, resulting in further ischaemic damage. The non-selective effect on autonomic ganglia results in parasympathetic blockade and adverse effects which make these drugs unacceptable for general use.

Clinical use Although the first effective antihypertensive drugs, they are now rarely used for the emergency treatment of hypertensive encephalopathy or eclampsia (although more suitable drugs exist) and for hypotensive anaesthesia.

Trimetaphan (Arfonad) has a swift onset of action and a single dose lasts only a few minutes so that it is given either as an intravenous infusion at 3–4 mg/min or by intermittent injections of 10 mg. Trimetaphan also relaxes arteriolar smooth muscle, releases histamine and can reduce both cardiac output and stroke volume. It has found a place in the medical management of aortic dissection.

Reserpine

Derived from an Indian plant Rauwolfia, reserpine depletes stored catecholamines and 5-hydroxytryptamine in the brain and adrenergic nerves. This results from a specific inhibition of formation of storage complexes of catecholamines with ATP so that the free amine is destroyed by monoamine oxidase and other catabolic processes.

It is uncertain whether central or peripheral effects are more important in the treatment of hypertension. Consequences of the central effects are sedation and an increased parasympathetic outflow. The peripheral effect is to depress responses to adrenergic nerve activity so that bradycardia accompanies the hypotensive effect.

Pharmacokinetics Only 30% of an oral dose is absorbed. The $t_{1/2}$ is 2–4.5 h.

Clinical use An effective agent for mild to moderate hypertension either alone or in combination with thiazides, it has declined in use because of its unacceptable side effects. Doses of 0.25–0.5 mg daily are used. The onset of hypotensive effect is gradual and may not be apparent for 2–3 weeks, suggesting an indirect mode of action. Effects may persist for up to 6 weeks after the drug is stopped.

Adverse effects Unopposed parasympathetic effects produce nasal stuffiness, increased gastric acid production (it may exacerbate peptic ulcer) and diarrhoea. It causes minimal postural hypotension.

Heart failure is precipitated in patients reliant upon increased sympathetic tone to maintain an adequate cardiac output (cf. β-blockers). Central effects result in sedation and nightmares. Large doses produce an extrapyramidal syndrome. It is also epileptogenic. Severe depression culminating in suicide has resulted from chronic reserpine therapy.

The Boston Collaborative Drug Surveillance Program (see p. 185) has found the incidence of breast cancer is 3–4 times greater in hypertensive women treated with reserpine. Two other studies have supported these findings although other series have not detected this problem. The case must be regarded as being incompletely proven at present.

An approach to the management of hypertension

This section is titled thus because there is no unanimity amongst clinicians as to the best way to control blood pressure in essential hypertension. It is important first to establish the need for treatment by measuring the blood pressure on at least three occasions. This allows time for reduction of the patient's anxiety and tension about the procedure which can contribute to an elevated blood-pressure reading. Table 12.12 shows actuarial data for normal blood pressure limits in the UK population. Treatment is advisable in patients under the age of 65 years with systolic pressure $>$ 160 mg Hg and/or diastolic pressure $>$ 100 mg Hg and probably also of benefit in patients over this age limit.

It is irrational to treat hypertension aggressively without attempting to modify the patient's other risk factors. Thus patients must be advised to *stop smoking* and to *reduce weight* if obese. *Diabetes mellitus* must be sought and if present controlled by diet or drugs. Excessive *alcohol intake* must also be curbed since several population and clinical studies have demonstrated a relationship between alcohol intake and blood pressure, and alcohol itself

Table 12.12 Mean plus 2 standard deviations of systolic and diastolic blood pressures (mm Hg) for men and women of different age groups

	Men		*Women*	
Age (years)	*Systolic*	*Diastolic*	*Systolic*	*Diastolic*
15–19	132.5	86.1	128.5	84.9
20–29	136.8	88.8	131.2	86.5
30–39	139.5	90.9	136.4	89.3
40–49	144.3	93.2	145.9	92.7
50–59	150.3	94.7	152.8	94.8
60–69	153.8	95.2	155.8	95.1

has a pressor effect. *Exercise* may also be beneficial. The results of controlling salt intake, hypercholesterolaemia and hyperlipidaemia are presently controversial.

Drug treatment of hypertension should be as simple as possible. Once-daily dosing is preferable.

Assuming that no contraindications are present, we would begin treatment with a β-adrenergic blocker in patients below the age of 60 or a diuretic above that age. Over the age of 65–70, depending upon circumstances, we are not convinced that the benefits of treatment outweigh the dangers, unless the blood pressure is very high. Established stroke is not of itself an indication for therapy since treatment does not appear to improve prognosis in old age. The syndrome of progressive dementia punctuated by minor strokes which is often associated with mild hypertension is also best left untreated since with or without drugs the outlook is poor.

The object of treatment is to reduce the blood pressure to within the normal range of Table 12.12. If an inadequate response occurs to monotherapy with a diuretic or a β-blocker the alternative diuretic or β-blocker is added as appropriate. Patients who do not respond to this dual therapy (comprising less than 20 % in hospital practice) may be given a vasodilator in addition (so-called 'triple therapy') (see Figs 12.16 and 12.20). Our preference is for hydralazine but prazosin is equally effective providing it is introduced at low dosage.

The place of calcium entry blockers and converting enzyme inhibitors in the strategy of management of hypertension has not yet been completely established. One suggested scheme (see Fig. 12.20) employs monotherapy with β-blockers or converting enzyme inhibitors in younger patients who often have high renin levels and respond best to these agents. A diuretic and calcium antagonist are then sequentially added in poor responders. Older patients, who often have low renin levels, respond less well to β-blockers but particularly well to calcium entry blockers which are used initially. Failure to respond is countered by addition of a diuretic and possibly a third agent if this is ineffective.

Patients refractory to triple therapy probably constitute less than 1 % of the total population of hypertensive patients. Poor compliance and secondary, e.g. renal, causes of hypertension must be excluded. Minoxidil is usually effective in such patients and should always be given with a loop diuretic and usually a

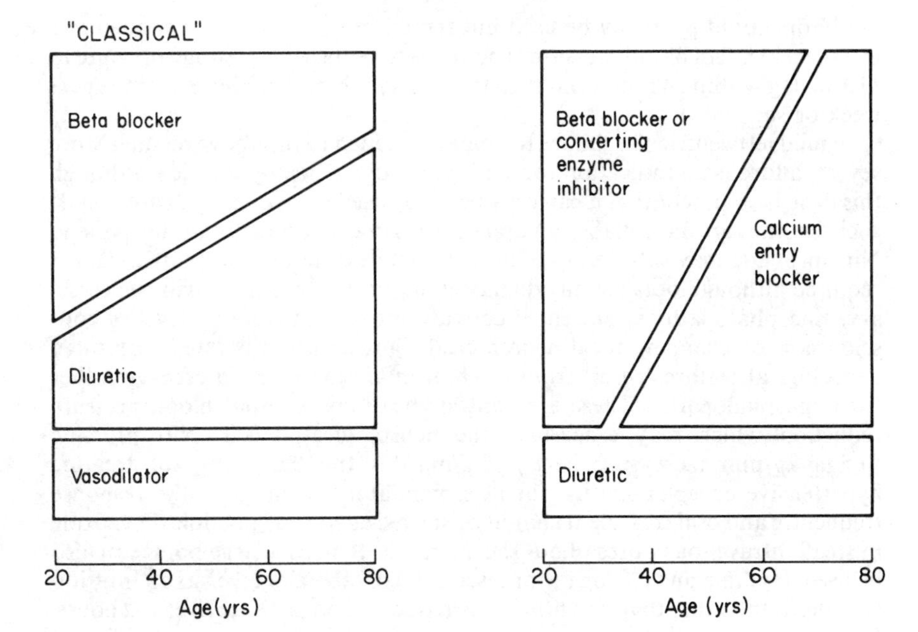

Fig. 12.20 Effect of age on strategies of antihypertensive therapy.

β-blocker as well. The combination of captopril and a diuretic is also an effective treatment for severe hypertension. Both of these regimes usually require hospital admission and if the blood pressure is only modestly elevated on standard triple therapy of diuretic, β-blocker and hydralazine a low dose of prazosin (0.5 mg 8 hourly increasing to a maximum of 5 mg 8 hourly) can be added in outpatients. Such 'quadruple therapy', although complicated, is well-tolerated and effective.

Malignant hypertension

Malignant hypertension is diagnosed on the basis of high blood pressure accompanied by papilloedema. Hypertension with grade III retinopathy (exudates and/or haemorrhages) is sometimes called accelerated hypertension. Both conditions are associated with arteriolar lesions in brain and kidneys and progression to death within one year in 90% of cases if untreated. Although a serious situation, over-zealous treatment producing rapid blood pressure reduction may be hazardous. Renal, cerebral or myocardial infarction or blindness may follow a precipitate fall in blood pressure. In most patients the blood pressure should be reduced over days rather than hours and the only indications for parenteral drugs are severe left ventricular failure or hypertensive encephalopathy. If these are absent the patient should be put to bed and oral treatment commenced with a β-blocker or labetalol. If these are contraindicated, nifedipine (20 mg), which unlike other drugs may not reduce cerebral perfusion, seems to be safe. Oral hydralazine, clonidine or methyldopa have also been used in this situation. Angiotensin converting enzyme inhibitors could probably be used but there is a possibility of a sudden and unexpected fall in blood pressure. The aim is to reduce the diastolic pressure to 110 mg Hg within 24 hours and then to normalise blood pressure over the next week or so.

In mild left ventricular failure frusemide is added to the above regime. More severe failure is an indication for sodium nitroprusside by infusion although this drug is so potent that it can only be safely used in an intensive care unit. If such facilities are unavailable, an oral drug regime may be safer for the patient. Nitroprusside may sufficiently reduce afterload so that no other treatment is required although occasionally diamorphine and/or frusemide will be necessary. Encephalopathy is present if convulsions or a fluctuating level of consciousness or changing focal neurological signs occur. It is rare. Very often neurological features result from cerebral infarction or haemorrhage rather than encephalopathy. These are contraindications to rapid blood pressure reduction which may exacerbate the neurological deficit. Nitroprusside (0.5 μg/kg/min increasing to 8 μg/kg/min) is the best drug for treating hypertensive encephalopathy but it is mandatory to monitor the response frequently and oral treatment should be started as soon as possible. Diazoxide in small intravenous doses of 50–150 mg rather than as a large bolus can also be used. Hydralazine (20 mg intramuscularly) or labetalol given as an infusion (1–3 mg/min) rather than as a bolus may reduce blood pressure over 1–2 hours. Intravenous clonidine or methyldopa can induce a precipitate fall in blood pressure and should be avoided.

Initial treatment of malignant hypertension is often easier than it becomes subsequently perhaps because at this stage many patients are mildly salt depleted. After treatment with powerful vasodilators they become relatively sodium overloaded and this renders control more difficult. Nevertheless, it is not always the case that patients presenting with malignant hypertension will require complex treatment regimens with large amounts of drugs once the emergency is past.

Acute aortic dissection

Dissection is encouraged by a wide pulse pressure and a rapid rate of rise of this pressure. This is worsened by vasodilators such as hydralazine. β-blockers and the ganglion blocker trimetaphan which decrease the rate and force of myocardial contraction are currently drugs of first choice in this condition.

Hypertension and pregnancy

When a hypertensive woman becomes pregnant it may be difficult to control the blood pressure and there is an increased incidence of pre-eclamptic toxaemia and of maternal and fetal morbidity in such patients. The presently favoured regime includes bed rest, hydralazine and/or methyldopa, although few controlled evaluations of various treatment regimes have been made. It has been suggested that the use of β-blockers might be associated with placental insufficiency and increased perinatal mortality. There is, however, no evidence to support this view and in fact a comparison between methyldopa and oxprenolol in controlling hypertension in pregnancy suggested that both were effective in lowering blood pressure and that oxprenolol offered an advantage over methyldopa in terms of fetal growth and well-being.

The hypertension of eclampsia is best treated by delivery of the fetus, if necessary by Caesarian section. Prompt reduction of blood pressure with intravenous hydralazine may prevent cerebral and retinal damage. Under these circumstances diazoxide has the additional effect of inhibiting labour (although this can be overcome by an oxytocin infusion) and so would be a less suitable drug. Frusemide given intravenously in large doses is usually given as well to reduce cerebral oedema and an anticonvulsant (diazepam or chlormethiazole) may be needed to prevent seizures.

Diuretics should not be used in pregnancy hypertension. They may further reduce plasma volume resulting in hypoperfusion of kidney and placenta. The only indication for diuretics is pulmonary oedema.

Hypotensive drugs in renal insufficiency

Although most patients with hypertension have normal or near-normal renal function, hypertension is a well-known complication of renal failure and the clinician may have to treat patients with severe hypertension and low glomerular filtration rates. Hypertension that co-exists with renal failure is often severe: before the introduction of effective drug therapy, 50 % of cases of malignant hypertension were due to renal disease.

Although good control of blood pressure is not easy in many patients with renal failure, it should be sought vigorously as uncontrolled hypertension accelerates the deterioration of renal function and good control may delay the need for dialysis.

There are, however, two problems:

(a) In the normal kidney, renal blood flow is maintained at a steady level over a wide range of perfusion pressure; this is brought about by changing the vascular resistance and may be effective down to a pressure of 60 mm Hg. Thus a fall in blood pressure, unless severe, does not reduce glomerular filtration. In the diseased kidney, however, presumably due to structural changes in the arterioles, renal blood flow and thus glomerular filtration may be much more dependent on perfusion pressure. If the blood pressure is lowered, therefore, in patients with severe impairment of renal function, it must be done slowly with frequent assessment of renal function, since renal function may initially deteriorate during treatment.

(b) A number of blood pressure lowering drugs are excreted via the kidneys, so that their use in renal failure will be followed by drug retention and subsequent evidence of overdose.

There is no real consensus as to how to treat hypertension in renal failure. A reasonable programme would seem to be:

Mild hypertension This may respond to a β-blocker with a thiazide diuretic. Propranolol is largely metabolised and so accumulation should not occur. If central effects prove troublesome with propranolol, and they may be a problem with higher doses, atenolol is satisfactory. There have been reports that β-blockers are particularly prone to increase the degree of renal failure, but we have not found that this is a problem. Thiazide diuretics are also useful, as they are unlikely to cause changes in plasma volume in renal failure.

Severe hypertension In this circumstances, prazosin or hydralazine will have to be added to the regime. Prazosin, starting with 0.5 mg three times daily (look out for postural hypotension), may be increased to a maximum of 20 mg daily. If this fails, hydralazine can either be substituted or added to the regime, the initial dose being 50 mg twice daily and increased to a maximum of 200 mg daily. Hydralazine should always be combined with a β-blocker to prevent tachycardia. Serious accumulation of these drugs should not occur.

Although thiazides are more effective hypotensive agents than loop diuretics in patients with moderate hypertension it has been found that in severe hypertension frusemide may be more effective than thiazides when it is used in reasonably large doses (80 mg/day with normal renal function; 250–1500 mg/day in renal failure). Potassium-retaining diuretics such as amiloride or spironolactone should be avoided in renal failure because of the danger of hyperkalaemia.

The blood pressure of patients on chronic dialysis can usually be controlled by slow removal of water and sodium during dialysis and by water and sodium restriction between dialyses. In some patients this provokes excessive renin secretion (due to decreased plasma volume) and a β-blocker with or without a vasodilator is additionally required.

VASODILATOR DRUGS IN PERIPHERAL VASCULAR DISEASE

Although many drugs are used in the treatment of peripheral vascular disease, their usefulness is difficult to assess because of spontaneous variation in the course of the condition and a significant placebo effect. Also, other therapy is often given at the same time. Thus a patient with intermittent claudication may be encouraged to stop smoking, diabetic control may be improved, a polyunsaturated fatty acid and low cholesterol diet recommended and an exercise programme started. All of these may benefit the condition. Another difficulty in assessing the therapeutic effectiveness of vasodilators is that the response in normal limbs may be different from that in ischaemic limbs. Indeed if normal vessels are more readily dilated, then blood can be 'stolen' from diseased parts of the limb to more healthy regions and the perfusion pressure which is already too low to adequately perfuse the limb may be still further reduced.

Three types of vasodilators are:

1. smooth-muscle relaxants;
2. α-blockers;
3. β-agonists.

1. Smooth muscle relaxants

Papaverine is a benzo-isoquinoline found in crude opium unrelated chemically or pharmacologically to the narcotic analgesics. It is a generalised smooth muscle relaxant and acts by inhibiting intracellular phosphodiesterase to increase cytoplasmic cAMP. The consequence of this is dilatation of arterioles and larger vessels with consequent fall in peripheral resistance.

Papaverine is little used in therapy although injections of papaverine are used in blood-vessel surgery and in the local treatment of acute vascular spasm, such as following accidental intra-arterial injection of thiopentone.

Nicotinic acid and nicotinylalcohol have identical pharmacological actions. They are vasodilators which in high doses can produce skin flushing, hypotension and syncope. The amounts of nicotinic acid required to treat hyperlipoproteinaemias are often sufficient to produce unpleasant sensations of heat and vasodilation in the skin of the face (see p. 577).

Tetranicotinoyl fructose (Bradilan) is broken down in the intestine to nicotinic acid and fructose. In doses of 500 mg q.d.s. the drug is effective in producing vasodilatation in the skin and muscles of arm and legs of patients with occlusive vascular disease. Controlled trials have indicated that there is symptomatic relief in over 50% of patients with Raynaud's disease.

Inositol hexanicotinate (Hexopal) has identical effects to nicotinic acid.

Oxpentifylline (Trental) is a xanthine derivative with mild α-adrenergic antagonism which causes vasodilatation and has a more prominent effect in reducing whole-blood viscosity which, for unknown reasons, is often raised in peripheral and cerebral vascular disease, myocardial infarction and diabetes mellitus. The reduced viscosity apparently results from increased erythrocyte flexibility and could improve blood flow through the microcirculation promoting better tissue nutrition. There is some uncontrolled evidence for the efficacy of the drug in peripheral vascular disease, but no convincing double-blind trials of adequate size or design have been reported.

Naftidrofuryl (Praxilene) has papaverine-like vasodilator activity and some ganglion-blocking effect. In animals it alters cellular metabolism and increases glucose uptake, possibly enhancing energy production despite impaired oxygen supply. Several uncontrolled investigations suggest benefit in some patients with cerebral vascular disease and in peripheral occlusive vascular disorders, but controlled trial evidence of efficacy is lacking. The usual oral dose is 100–200 mg 8 hourly. Toxicity is uncommon but occasionally the following have been reported: headache, nausea, epigastric pain, diarrhoea, neuropathy, insomnia and vertigo.

Nifedipine (see pp. 394, 455) acts as a peripheral arteriolar vasodilator by virtue of its calcium channel blocking effect. In several controlled double-blind trials it has been shown to improve Raynaud's phenomenon when given in doses of 10–20 mg 8 hourly.

2. α-blockers

Tolazoline (Priscol) This drug has been widely used in peripheral vascular disease. Its actions are complex and not fully understood.

(a) Vasodilation: This is due to both a direct action on the arteriole wall and to α-adrenergic blockade. In the usual therapeutic dose it appears that the direct action is the more important.
(b) Tachycardia, which is adrenergic in origin, is associated with a rise in cardiac output so that the effects on blood pressure are variable.
(c) Increased acid secretion by the stomach.

Tolazoline is well absorbed from the intestine and largely excreted unchanged by the kidney.

Clinical use Tolazoline in doses of 25 mg three times daily by mouth is used in vascular disease. In large-vessel atherosclerosis it is not usually effective. It may well produce vasodilatation, particularly of skin vessels, but because of the fixed obstruction in the major vessels, the blood supply to the limb cannot be increased and so muscle blood supply may actually suffer at the expense of the skin with subsequent failure to relieve intermittent claudication.

In Raynaud's disease, it is more effective and, used in association with other measures such as the use of gloves and keeping the body warm, helps to relieve vasospasm.

Adverse effects Tachycardia and cardiac arrhythmias are the most important. Occasionally the increase in cardiac work will precipitate angina in patients with coronary artery disease. Increased gastric acid secretion may exacerbate peptic ulceration.

Thymoxamine (Opilon) and **phenoxybenzamine (Dibenyline)** have not been shown to benefit peripheral vascular disease. After intravenous administration of thymoxamine, skin blood flow transiently increases in limbs affected by occlusive vascular disease and in Raynaud's phenomenon. Such an effect is not seen after an oral dose of 100 mg, perhaps because the intestinal absorption of thymoxamine is very poor.

3. β agonists

Isoxuprine (Duvadilan) Isoxuprine increased blood flow in the calf muscles of normal volunteers after an oral dose of 40 mg. However, there is no constant effect on blood flow in the muscles of subjects with vascular disease. Double-blind trials have indicated no beneficial effects on the clinical state of patients with peripheral vascular disease. Isoxuprine also inhibits uterine contractions via its β-agonist activity, although in high doses it also has a direct papaverine-like action on uterine smooth muscle. It is usually infused intravenously at a rate of 0.2 mg/min initially and the rate increased up to 0.5 mg/min until labour is inhibited. When labour has been arrested oral therapy may be given.

CEREBRAL VASODILATORS

Cerebral vessels differ from systemic vessels in their control mechanisms and reactivity. The tone of cerebral arteries is mainly controlled by the arterial pCO_2, a raised partial pressure causing dilatation, a low partial pressure causing constriction. Acutely ischaemic areas may show decreased reactivity so that raising pCO_2 causes vasodilatation, not in the ischaemic area but in the normal vessels, resulting in shunting of blood away from the affected area. Cerebral blood flow is normally subject to autoregulation and is unaffected by changes in mean arterial pressure within a range of 80–140 mm Hg. Therefore minor changes in systemic blood pressure do not alter cerebral blood flow in health. Autoregulation may be impaired by ischaemia so that blood flow through the vessels of an ischaemic area passively follows changes in blood pressure and a fall in systemic pressure may result in infarction. There is also evidence for neural regulation of cerebral blood vessels and parenchymal and pial arteries have an abundant nerve supply. The smooth muscle of these vessels has α- and β-adrenergic, cholinergic, serotoninergic and H_1 and H_2 histamine receptors but their function is at present unknown.

The use of cerebral vasodilators to improve dementia and other features of cerebral atherosclerosis is not fully established as an effective treatment. Studies which purport to show increased blood flow to the brain following drug treatment are irrelevant since the ischaemic areas responsible for symptoms may not share in this improved flow. Moreover, neurones in such areas may already have suffered irreversible changes and therefore it is unlikely that improvement could follow. The most effective method of evaluation at present is the properly controlled study of the functional improvement following drug therapy. The following drugs are sometimes employed:

1. **Hydergine (dihydroergocornine, dihydroergocristine and dihydroergokryptine mesylates)** is alleged to act by increasing the glycolytic rate in astrocytes which reduces their constricting effect on cerebral capillaries. Cerebral blood flow is only moderately increased although controlled trials showed moderate improvement in some measures of daily activity in geriatric patients.

2. **Cyclandelate** modestly increases cerebral blood flow and after administration of 400 mg 6-hourly for several weeks psychological testing showed improvement in elderly patients having diffuse cerebrovascular disease as compared with controls.

The clinical value of these drugs therefore cannot be regarded as proven, although in some cases a therapeutic trial may be justified, since there is so little which can be done for patients with diffuse atherosclerotic cerebrovascular disease.

Treatment after subarachnoid haemorrhage

Patients surviving the initial subarachnoid haemorrhage remain at risk during the next three weeks because of recurrent haemorrhage and cerebral arterial spasm. Many pharmacological agents have been implicated in the aetiology of cerebrovascular spasm including blood, serotonin, catecholamines and some prostaglandins. Recent clinical studies have shown protection against spasm and subsequent disablement or death from early administration of:

(a) propranolol and phentolamine but more likely the β-blocker is the important agent.
(b) propranolol 80 mg 8 hourly.
(c) a calcium entry blocking drug (nimodipine) given in high dose. Studies with other agents e.g. nifedipine are in progress.

Chapter 13
RESPIRATORY SYSTEM

DRUGS USED IN THE TREATMENT OF ASTHMA

Attacks of asthma are due to airways obstruction caused by constriction of the circular muscle in the bronchial wall, oedema of the mucosa lining the small bronchi and plugging of the bronchi with sticky mucus. The whole process is reversible but may ultimately be complicated by secondary changes in the lungs and bronchi which result in irreversible airways obstruction.

Two forms of asthma are recognised. In *allergic asthma* extrinsic allergens produce a Type I allergic reaction in atopic subjects, and a Type III late asthmatic reaction in non-atopic subjects. Type I reactions are associated with the presence of reaginic antibodies (IgE) on the surface of mast cells. When a specific antigen comes into contact with such sensitised cells, chemical mediators of the asthmatic reaction are released. These include histamine, 5-hydroxytryptamine, acetylcholine, prostaglandins, kinins and SRS–A (slow-reacting substance of anaphylaxis). The latter is a mixture of leukotrienes, the most powerful bronchoconstrictor of which is LTD_4 (see Fig. 18.2). Type III reactions are mediated by precipitating antibodies (IgG) which initiate an immune complex reaction usually involving complement activation. Patients with *non-allergic asthma* do not appear to be sensitive to any well-defined antigen although infection often precipitates an attack. As a group they respond poorly to bronchodilator drugs although corticosteroids may induce a remission.

Other factors of pharmacological relevance which must be taken into account are:

(a) Asthmatic subjects have diminished physiological and metabolic responsiveness to adrenergic stimulation. Bronchodilatation is related to the rise in intracellular cyclic 3′,5′-adenosine monophosphate (cyclic AMP) following β-adrenergic receptor stimulation. Lymphocytes from asthmatics show an attenuated rise in intracellular cyclic AMP when exposed to β-agonists like isoprenaline. Similarly asthmatics produce a smaller rise in plasma cyclic AMP than normals following isoprenaline inhalation. In addition to bronchodilatation, increased concentrations of cyclic AMP within mast cells have a stabilising effect, thereby reducing the release of mediators such as histamine and the production of leukotrienes.

(b) Reflex bronchoconstriction involving vagal pathways activated either peripherally by some irritant reflex originating in the airways or centrally seems to play a part in the production of the clinical phenomenon of the asthmatic attack. This may be the case even in the presence of an established allergen.

There are a number of ways in which the asthmatic process might be reversed (see Fig. 13.1):

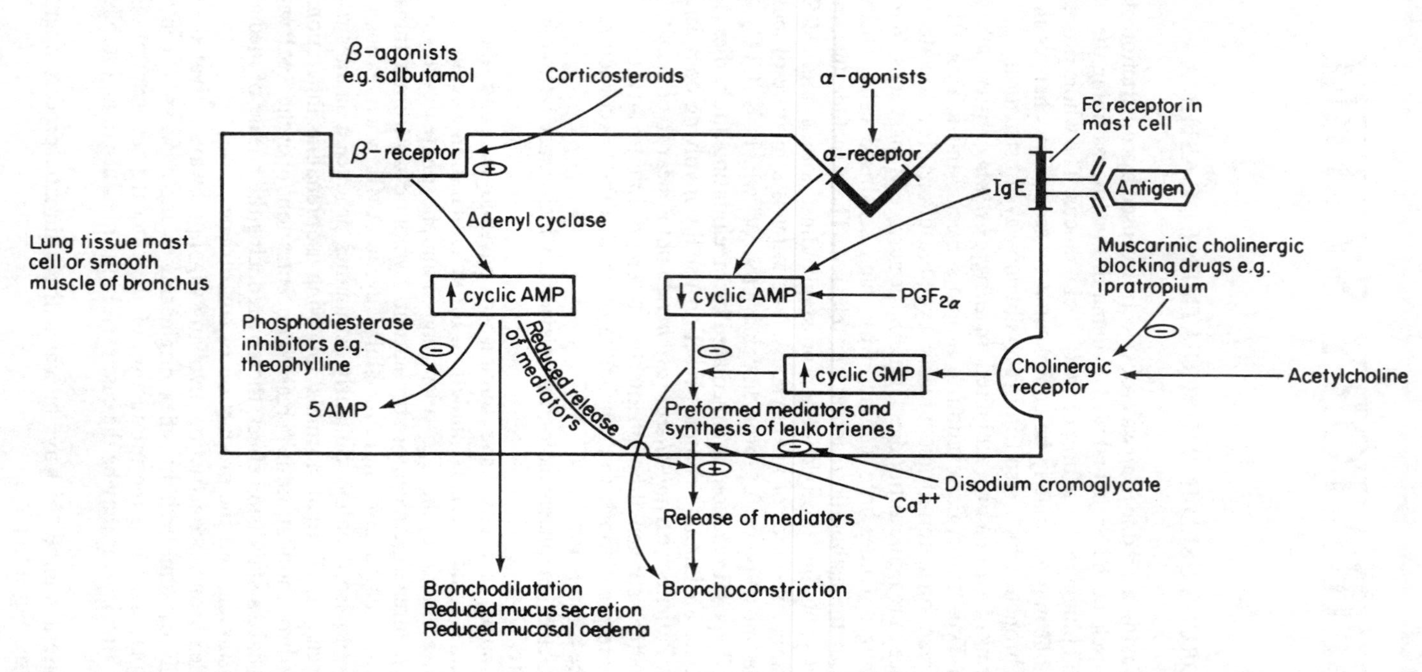

Fig. 13.1 Schematic representation of some of the pharmacological controls of bronchial tone and release of chemical mediators.

1. Increasing intracellular cyclic AMP concentration would relax the bronchiolar smooth muscle and also diminish the release of various chemical mediators from mast cells (see above).
   This can be achieved either by stimulation of β-receptors which increases intracellular cyclic AMP or by reducing its destruction by phosphodiesterase by inhibiting this enzyme with the xanthine group of drugs.
2. Corticosteroids have a complex action which includes
   (a) increasing intracellular cyclic AMP
   (b) decreasing capillary permeability and thus reducing bronchial oedema and congestion.
   (c) block of the high-capacity, low-affinity uptake mechanism for catecholamines (uptake$_2$) thereby increasing the efficacy of endogenous and exogenous catecholamines.
   (d) inhibition of phospholipase which decreases formation of both prostaglandins and leukotrienes which are important mediators in asthma.
3. Stabilising mast cells reduces the release of chemical mediators of the asthmatic reaction and is achieved by sodium cromoglycate. This prevents the calcium inflow which is required for mediator secretion. Attempts to block the action of chemical mediators (e.g. antihistamines) or to prevent the synthesis of prostaglandins (e.g. indomethacin) have been disappointing.
4. Anticholinergic drugs which block vagal reflexes can also prove beneficial.

β-adrenergic agonists

These drugs are all derivatives of phenylethylamine. The results of β-receptor stimulation include:

1. relaxation of bronchiolar smooth muscle;
2. reduction of bronchial secretion and inhibition of release of mast cell contents;
3. relaxation of uterine smooth muscle;
4. increase in heart rate, force of myocardial contraction, speed of impulse conduction and enhanced production of ectopic foci in the myocardium and automaticity in pacemaker tissue;
5. tremor;
6. vasodilatation in skeletal and myocardial muscle;
7. metabolic effects, e.g. increased glucose release by hepatocytes.

Adrenaline

This drug has mixed α- and β-agonist effects. It may be given subcutaneously in a dose of 0.1 ml of the 1 in 1000 Adrenaline Injection B.P. per minute up to a total of 1 ml in adults. The onset of action is rapid and was used in the treatment of an acute asthmatic attack. It has, however, been superseded by newer β-agonist drugs because of the risk of cardiac arrhythmias. However, it is recommended in acute anaphylaxis.

Ephedrine

This drug has effects similar to adrenaline, since it releases catecholamines from sympathetic nerves and adrenal medulla and also has some direct β-agonist activity. Because of its dependence upon catecholamine stores repeated doses become ineffective (tachyphylaxis).

Pharmacokinetics It is a phenylamine and less polar than catecholamines, resulting in better absorption from the gut. It is slowly metabolised by the liver and much is excreted unchanged by the kidneys; thus its effects are more prolonged than those of adrenaline, the $t_{1/2}$ being approximately 6 h. On repeated dosing there is no change in its disposition kinetics, demonstrating that tolerance is related to pharmacodynamic rather than pharmacokinetic factors.

Clinical uses It is given orally as ephedrine hydrochloride tablets B.P., ephedrine elixir. The usual dose is 15–60 mg, but patient sensitivity to ephedrine varies widely and repeated dosage produces tachyphylaxis (see above). The upper dosage limit is usually set by CNS side effects.

Adverse effects are those of catecholamines, and ephedrine has a relatively greater stimulatory effect on the CNS so that it produces anxiety, tachycardia, nausea and insomnia (or paradoxical drowsiness in some children). It can also provoke urinary retention in elderly men.

Isoprenaline

This drug has non-specific β-agonist properties and cardiac (β_1) properties are prominent.

Pharmacokinetics Isoprenaline is sulphated by enzymes in the gut wall and liver (first-pass effect) so that little enters the circulation if it is given orally. Sublingual administration avoids the gut first-pass effect and is of value. An effective method of administration is in an aerosol but the action is short lived. The maximum effect is reached in 5–10 min and lasts 1–2 h. Although most of an inhaled dose is swallowed, that part which reaches the lungs is rapidly taken up, and metabolised by O-methylation and sulphation. This constitutes a bronchial first-pass effect. Methoxyisoprenaline is formed—this has β-blocking activity and could therefore cause bronchoconstriction in asthmatics if large enough amounts accumulate.

Clinical uses
Oral
(i) sublingual tablets (10–20 mg)
(ii) sustained release preparation (Saventrine) containing 30 mg isoprenaline which is swallowed and used in the treatment of heart block. The dosage is large (90–840 mg daily) in order to overwhelm the hepatic first-pass metabolism. The efficacy of this preparation is variable.

Aerosols providing up to 0.4 mg isoprenaline sulphate/puff are most commonly used for asthma, e.g. Medihaler.

Intravenous isoprenaline is used in the highest tolerated dose to increase force and rate of cardiac contraction (2 mg is added to 500 ml saline and given initially at a rate of 0.2–0.4 μg/min) in cardiogenic shock.

Orciprenaline (Alupent) is a resorcinol derivative which is also a non-specific β-agonist having 10–40 times less activity than isoprenaline. It differs from isoprenaline in that it is not rapidly taken up by tissues prior to elimination, nor is it a substrate for catechol-O-methyl transferase or sulphatases. This results in a long half-life (about 6 h) and good absorption after oral administration.

Dangers of non-specific β-agonists

In the 1960s increasing mortality from asthma, especially among children and young adults, caused concern and a highly significant correlation was observed between the number of prescriptions for isoprenaline aerosols and mortality. The relationship between these phenomena is obscure. Possibly the excess mortality was due to inhaled isoprenaline precipitating a sudden cardiac arrhythmia in a heart sensitised by anoxia. It has been shown, however, that frequent aerosol use produces some resistance to the cardiac effects of isoprenaline due to the formation of the metabolite 3-O-methylisoprenaline, which is a weak β-antagonist. This could increase airways obstruction and clinical deterioration or else encourage further use of the inhaler. The amounts of this metabolite formed are small and another possibility is that prolonged use of any β-stimulant drug can produce receptor desensitisation, resulting in worsening airways obstruction due to loss of response to drugs and to endogenous sympathetic drive. Other possibilities are that the fluorocarbon propellant of the aerosol may have toxic effects or that a rebound bronchoconstriction could follow initial drug-induced bronchodilatation. None of these hypotheses has been fully substantiated. With the advent of more effective treatment the mortality of asthma is now declining again. This episode has given a great stimulus to the search for more selective β_2-stimulant drugs and to earlier therapeutic intervention in the evolution of an asthmatic attack. However small epidemics of asthma mortality still arise. Many physicians consider these to be due to undertreatment and delay in the administration of steroids in refractory asthma.

Selective β_2-stimulants

These drugs have some β_1-activity, but do not appear to lead to the dangerous cardiac complications which isoprenaline can cause when used in large doses.

Salbutamol (Ventolin)

Salbutamol given intravenously is as effective as intravenous isoprenaline as a bronchodilator but is 7–10 times less potent in increasing heart rate. It is therefore relatively β_2-selective.

Pharmacokinetics Salbutamol is not metabolised by catechol-O-methyl transferase, monoamine oxidase or sulphatase and is thus effective when given by mouth. When absorbed from the gut it undergoes hepatic first-pass conjugation to form a metabolite with negligible adrenergic activity which is excreted in the urine. Given intravenously salbutamol tends to remain unconjugated since it avoids the hepatic first pass. Most of the aerosol-administered drug is swallowed but that which is inhaled largely remains as free salbutamol in the blood suggesting that unlike isoprenaline it has no bronchial first-pass metabolism. The $t_{1/2}$ is about 2–4 h although the biological $t_{1/2}$ as measured by the decay in heart rate following termination of an intravenous infusion is only 15 min. A direct local action on the bronchi may be involved since there is a clear decrease in airways obstruction at a time when no drug can be detected in plasma.

Clinical uses

(i) Oral: 8–16 mg daily as tablets or sustained release spandets (8 mg)
(ii) Inhalation:
  (a) metered aerosol (100 μg/puff), dose 1–2 puffs up to 6 times daily;
  (b) aerosol administered by a nebuliser. 5 mg of salbutamol in sterile saline are given over 5–15 min. up to 6 hourly.
  (c) as dry powder. It has been found that whereas some 15 % of adults on aerosol inhalations may use these devices inefficiently despite careful instruction almost all patients can use a dry-powder inhaler correctly. A dry powder inhaler for salbutamol (Rotahaler) from which 400 μg gives a comparable degree of bronchodilatation to 200 μg salbutamol aerosol. The Rotacaps (100 and 200 μg) can be used in doses up to 800 μg 6 hourly.
(iii) i.m. injection: 500 μg 4 hourly.
(iv) i.v.: bolus of 250 μg followed by infusion of 5–20 μg/min.

The increase in FEV_1 after inhalation of 200 μg of salbutamol begins within 15 min, peaks at 1 h and persists beyond 4 h. Following intravenous injection of 100–300 μg over a period of 1 min the airways resistance in asthmatics usually falls to a minimum in 5–10 min although in severely affected patients it may be delayed by 30 min. Aerosol salbutamol has many advantages over oral and i.v. administration and there is some evidence to suggest that it produces a more prolonged bronchodilator effect with fewer side effects than an equivalent i.v. dose. In particular, raised plasma free fatty acids, triglycerides, glucose, insulin and cortisol are not observed after aerosol administration.

Adverse effects These are usually trivial, consisting mainly of tachycardia and tremor (30 %). Caution is essential when any β-adrenergic agonist is used intravenously. It is known that the other β-effects of salbutamol produce raised free fatty acid levels and increased insulin secretion, factors which experimentally are associated with the development of cardiac arrhythmias.

Potentiation of motor end plate transmission produces tremor when large therapeutic doses of β_2-agonists are used. This effect can show tachyphyllaxis and some patients who experience tremor with one drug may be unaffected by another β_2-stimulant. Night cramps in the legs are common and poorly recognised: they are better treated by reducing the dose of salbutamol than by quinine sulphate.

Terbutaline (Bricanyl) has twice the activity of isoprenaline on bronchial smooth muscle but only a quarter of its cardiac effects. Although conjugated by sulphation in the gut wall this is a relatively small effect compared with that for isoprenaline. This may explain why orally administered terbutaline, which is relatively poorly absorbed, is a more effective bronchodilator than isoprenaline which is completely absorbed. Terbutaline is a resorcinol derivative like orciprenaline and is thus not metabolised by monoamine oxidase or catechol-O-methyl transferase. It is therefore excreted unchanged in the urine when given i.v. and as the sulphate conjugate when given orally, illustrating the effect of the gastro-intestinal first-pass effect on patterns of drug metabolism. Terbutaline has a longer $t_{1/2}$ (3–4 h) than isoprenaline and may be given orally (2.5–5 mg 8 hourly), by injection or by inhalation. The Bricanyl inhaler delivers a metered dose of 0.25 mg per dose. As well as the usual small mouthpiece, a straight spacer (with an extended mouthpiece) and a 750 ml plastic cone spacer are available. These allow several inhalations to be made on each activation so that a higher fraction of each dose enters the lung—particularly in those patients with poor coordination. Another advantage of the spacer is that the aerosol enters the mouth at a lower speed and thus a smaller fraction strikes the posterior pharyngeal wall.

Ibuterol, a diester of terbutaline, is a pro-drug which is more efficiently absorbed than the parent compound and is then hydrolysed by blood and tissue esterases to the active drug.

Rimiterol (Pulmadil) belongs to a new chemical series, the aryl-2-piperidyl carbinols and has similar bronchodilator activity and β_2-selectivity to salbutamol when administered intravenously, although it has a shorter $t_{1/2}$. By aerosol it is equivalent to isoprenaline and, like isoprenaline, it is relatively inactive taken orally. These different potency ratios stem from the susceptibility of rimiterol to the same uptake and metabolic pathways as isoprenaline and illustrate the way in which different routes of administration can completely alter the pharmacological properties of a drug.

Rimiterol is available in a metered aerosol (0.2 mg per dose) and in a breath-actuated metered aerosol (0.2 mg per dose). A solution for a nebuliser is made by dissolving a 12.5 mg nebuliser capsule in 2.5 ml water.

Fenoterol (Berotec) is a β_2-selective agonist with a similar potency to salbutamol but with a longer $t_{1/2}$ (7 h), which may be advantageous. It is given as a metered aerosol (400 μg, as two puffs, two or three times daily).

Pirbuterol (Exirel) is a selective β_2-agonist with clinical properties similar to salbutamol. It is administered via a metered aerosol which delivers 0.2 mg per activation.

Phosphodiesterase inhibitors

Theophylline and its derivatives

These are the only drugs of this type in common therapeutic use. No drug in this group with any significant advantages over aminophylline has been synthesised. This is a mixture of theophylline and ethylene diamine. Theophylline is a powerful relaxant of smooth muscle and inhibits mediator release from mast cells because it raises intracellular cyclic AMP concentrations. In addition, theophylline increases the tone and contractility of the diaphragm and respiratory muscles. It is a weak diuretic and a weaker central stimulant than caffeine (another methylxanthine phosphodiesterase inhibitor) although it is this action which is partly responsible for the effectiveness of theophylline in terminating Cheyne–Stokes respiration.

Pharmacokinetics Theophylline is well absorbed from the small intestine and rectum, but i.v. administration is most effective in status asthmaticus. The volume of distribution is about 0.3–0.8 l/kg and at therapeutic concentrations 60 % is bound to plasma proteins. When the haematocrit is normal, the whole blood concentration is 55 % of the serum or plasma concentration, i.e. 10 μg/ml plasma is equivalent to 5.5 μg/ml in whole blood. It is at about this level of theophylline in the plasma that optimal therapeutic effects are obtained. Some bronchodilatation has been observed at plasma levels as low as 4–5 μg/ml. For resistant asthma 10–20 μg/ml plasma are necessary, but it is preferable not to exceed 10 μg/ml in children. In the plasma concentration range 25–70 μg/ml convulsions may occur.

The drug is largely metabolised in the liver—mainly to 3-methylxanthine—and only 10 % is excreted unchanged in the urine. Fixed-dose regimes may lead to high blood levels and toxicity in the presence of liver disease. Cigarette smoking accelerates metabolism and administration of nortriptyline and allopurinol impair it. The $t_{1/2}$ varies between 3 and 10 h making the design of a fixed-dosage regime to achieve a given therapeutic level difficult.

Clinical uses Aminophylline administered by aerosol is irritating and has no useful effect in treating bronchospasm. I.m. aminophylline is painful and absorption is variable: 500 mg i.m. produces little benefit in asthmatic subjects.

(i) Oral theophylline is obtainable in many different forms. For example, choline theophyllinate (Choledyl) is claimed to produce less gastric irritation than theophylline. However, there is a great variation in the bioavailability of different oral preparations; also the same preparation produces a wide range of blood levels in different patients. Sustained-release preparations of aminophylline are available which provide effective therapeutic levels for up to 12 h following a single dose and because of the slow release rate have a reduced incidence of gastrointestinal side effects. These include Slo-Phyllin (60, 125 and 250 mg), Theodur (200 and 300 mg), Uniphyllin (200 and 400 mg), Pro-Vent (300 mg), Phyllocontin Continus (225 mg) and Nuelin (125 mg). Oral theophylline is not extensively used by chest physicians in the management of asthma except in patients whose airways obstruction increases in the early hours of the morning (morning dippers).

(ii) Rectal aminophylline (as Aminophylline Suppositories B.P. containing 50, 100, 150 or 360 mg) is well absorbed and is an effective treatment for moderate attacks of bronchial asthma and for the control of dyspnoea and orthopnoea in left-ventricular failure. Suppositories can produce rectal irritation and rejection and accurate dosage in children is difficult. Because of this a solution of aminophylline may be used rectally. 300 mg aminophylline in 5 ml produces peak levels of about 5–6 μg/ml within 30–60 min which are maintained for about 4 h.

(iii) I.v. aminophylline usually produces rapid relief of asthmatic symptoms. It is given by single slow injection (250 to 500 mg over 5 minutes) or by a bolus followed by an infusion. The dose to produce a plasma level of 10 μg/ml is:

(a) 375 mg initially given over 20 min for moderately severe asthma (for large or small adults this dose should be adjusted to 5.6 mg/kg);

(b) a continuous infusion of 0.5 mg/kg/h to a maximum of 1.0 g in 24 h unless the dose is controlled by plasma estimations. It is mandatory to stop the infusion after 24 h unless plasma theophylline estimations are available. In patients with impaired liver function or heart failure the dose should be halved. It should also be reduced in the elderly. A solution of 250 mg of aminophylline can be diluted in 500 ml saline and given by infusion preferably using a pump.

It is essential to enquire about oral theophylline administration prior to intravenous injection. If the patient is receiving oral theophylline the plasma concentration should be measured and the dose modified accordingly.

Although synergism between β-adrenergic agonists and aminophylline has been demonstrated in vitro this does not seem to occur in patients where the effect of these combinations is additive. This may be advantageous in patients who experience unacceptable side effects from high doses of either drug alone but who may achieve comparable bronchodilatation without side effects from low doses of the combined agents.

Adverse effects are sometimes related to plasma levels and some toxic effects, in particular dyspepsia and sleep disturbances, can develop with low levels. Serial measurements of theophylline can be made on saliva in which the levels are about one half of those in plasma. Theophylline has a narrow margin of safety and guidance as to dosages should be by plasma or saliva levels, particularly if a therapeutic effect is not obtained or if toxicity is suspected. Some of the toxic effects resemble those of catecholamines since both drugs raise intracellular cyclic AMP levels. They include tachycardia, cardiac arrhythmias, hyperventilation and peptic ulceration. Theophylline crosses the blood–brain barrier and causes CNS stimulation resulting in insomnia, anxiety, agitation headache and fits. Nausea and vomiting are common and related both to stimulation of the medullary emetic centre and a local gastric effect.

Bronchodilators and arterial oxygen

Although treatment with bronchodilators causes an improvement in respiratory function, this may be preceded by a transient fall in arterial oxygen tension. The fall occurs both with β agonists and aminophylline and is believed to be due to vasodilation causing changes in ventilation/perfusion ratios in the lungs. Some clinicians believe, therefore, that oxygen should be given with these drugs in the treatment of status asthmaticus, although the fall in oxygen tension is rarely of importance in practice.

Corticosteroids

Anti-inflammatory glucocorticoids are effective in asthma.

Hydrocortisone (cortisol) may be given intravenously in emergency situations. Cortisol levels of about 100 μg/100 ml plasma (or above) appear to be necessary for optimal response. Following an initial loading dose of 4 mg/kg hydrocortisone hemisuccinate, no significant difference in blood levels or in response is observed in status asthmaticus if further doses are given by either intermittent intravenous injections of 3 mg/kg 3 hourly or by continuous infusion delivering 3 mg/kg 6 hourly. Plasma cortisol levels are maintained at about 130 μg/100 ml with either method of administration. The $t_{1/2}$ of hydrocortisone in the plasma is approximately 120 min and this is unaffected by previous steroid treatment. Although high cortisol levels are rapidly attained, subjective improvement is not experienced until after 1–4 h and objective improvement (rise in FEV_1 and FVC) does not begin until 6 h and is maximal at about 13 h after the start of treatment (see Fig. 13.2).

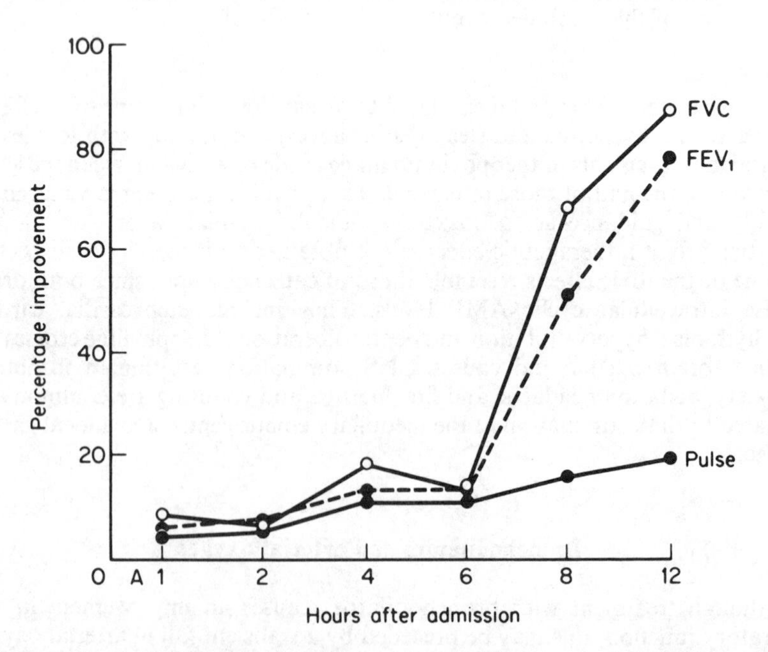

Fig. 13.2 Rate of improvement after starting treatment with hydrocortisone or tetracosactrin in 14 patients with severe acute asthma (From J. V. Collins *et al.*, *Quart. J. Med.*, **174,** 259 (1975)).

Corticotrophin or tetracosactrin (see p. 614) may be used in status asthmaticus instead of hydrocortisone. A single intramuscular injection of 1 mg tetracosactrin produces plasma cortisol levels of 50 μg/100 ml in about 3 h and peak levels of 90 μg/100 ml at 8–24 h. Subjective and objective improvement follows a similar time course to that observed with hydrocortisone treatment.

Prednisolone is (weight for weight) 4–5 times more powerful a glucocorticoid and anti-inflammatory agent than hydrocortisone but has the same mineralocorticoid activity. In asthma it may be given in a short course or as continuous oral therapy (see below). Used acutely in large doses (60–100 mg daily) urinary potassium loss may be considerable and plasma and urine potassium should be monitored. Oral potassium supplements should be administered to avoid the hazards of hypokalaemia on the hypoxic myocardium. With chronic dosage all the adverse effects of steroid administration may be encountered (see p. 640).

Inhaled steroids

Beclomethasone diproprionate (Becotide)
Betamethasone valerate (Bextosol)
Budenoside (Pulmicort)

These are fluorinated steroids which are inhaled as a metered aerosol. Halogenation renders molecules more polar, so reducing absorption through membranes (these steroids were orginally developed for topical use on the skin). They are extremely powerful anti-inflammatory agents and mainly exert a local action although systemic absorption occurs. About 10–20% enters the lungs, the rest being swallowed to be rapidly converted to inactive metabolites by the liver. Each single puff delivers a dose of 50 μg, and at the recommended daily dose of 400 μg produces no prolonged suppression of the pituitary–adrenal axis, although after cessation of treatment the blood cortisol concentration is suppressed for 48 h. Higher doses produce more prolonged depression of adrenal function.

Moniliasis of the pharynx (13% of patients) or larynx (5% of patients) may complicate this treatment. In this event the dose of inhaled steroid is reduced to 100–200 μg/day and amphotericin lozenges given.

When high doses of inhaled steroid are needed, it may be convenient to use aerosols delivering big doses at each actuation. Thus beclomethasone is given at a dose of 500 μg twice daily from a Becloforte inhaler and budenoside (as Pulmicort) is given at a dose of 200 μg twice daily. The Pulmicort metered aerosol canister can be used with a collapsible spacer or with the 750 ml plastic cone (Nebuhaler) which is also compatible with the Bricanyl canister.

Steroid aerosols can be used to reduce the daily dose of oral steroid required or even completely replace it. The approximate equiactive doses are 400 μg beclomethasone and 5 mg prednisolone. Worsening of the patient's condition when taking 400 μg beclomethasone daily usually means that a switch to oral prednisolone is necessary. Patients taking less than 15 mg prednisolone orally per day can often be completely controlled by aerosol steroids.

Mast-cell stabilisers

Sodium cromoglycate (Intal)

This drug does not prevent antigen–antibody combination, but if given before exposure to an antigen can prevent Types I and III allergic reactions. The drug acts by preventing histamine and leukotrienes release from sensitised mast cells. In addition, mast cell degranulation produced by non-immunological mechanisms is prevented by this drug. Sodium cromoglycate prevents mediator release by blocking calcium flow into mast cells and possibly by inhibiting phosphodiesterase and thus inactivates the contractile microfilamentary proteins necessary for degranulation. However the mode of action of this drug is not fully understood: there appear to be direct stabilising effects on the mast-cell membrane and actions on other cell types which antagonise the changes produced by released chemical mediators of the allergic response.

Pharmacokinetics It is poorly absorbed from the gut and is therefore given as an inhaled powder. The powder is mainly swallowed but some 10% reaches the alveoli where it is absorbed. Mast cells in the lungs (but not in the peripheral blood) are stabilised by the drug when given by this route.

Clinical uses It is administered by inhalation of a powder liberated from a 20 mg capsule (Spincap) and dispersed by devices containing an inspiration-driven propeller (Spinhaler) and by spinning of the punctured capsule in a plastic chamber (Halermatic). A metered aerosol is available delivering 5 mg or 1 mg per puff. The nebuliser solution contains 10 mg per ml. Cromoglycate produces no benefit during an asthmatic attack but taken regularly (e.g. 20–40 mg 6 hourly) will diminish the frequency of attacks of allergic asthma. In addition exercise-provoked attacks may be prevented. Bronchospasm due to chest infection is not affected. Spincaps of Intal Compound contain 20 mg of cromoglycate and 0.1 mg of isoprenaline sulphate. This mixture is not generally favoured by physicians, but has been found to be effective by asthmatic athletes when taken before exercise.

A good response to Sodium cromoglycate may allow a rapid reduction in the dose of steroid given. Presently there is no method to predict which patients will benefit from the drug and therefore all patients require a therapeutic trial although the necessary duration of such a trial is uncertain. Little is known of the individual variations in dosage requirements or whether there are differences in bronchial penetration.

Sodium cromoglycate is also used as nose drops and spray for perennial and allergic rhinitis and as eye drops in allergic conjunctivitis. Recently some improvement has been demonstrated when the drug is given orally in inflammatory bowel disease and in food allergy (see p. 824).

Adverse effects Cromoglycate is virtually non-toxic. The powder may produce bronchospasm and hoarseness. The former can be treated with an inhalation of salbutamol and the latter usually responds to a drink of water.

A limitation of Sodium cromoglycate in asthma is that since it is poorly absorbed from the gut it is inactive when taken orally. **Ketotifen (Zaditen)** is an oral agent used in the prophylaxis of asthma which prevents mediator release and blocks histamine receptors (H_1). Side effects include drowsiness and drying of salivary, bronchial and other secretions. These may be a disadvantage in treating asthma. At present ketotifen is not widely prescribed by chest physicians. The dose is 1 mg twice daily.

Anticholinergic drugs

There is increased parasympathetic activity in patients with reversible airways obstruction resulting in bronchoconstriction through the excessive effects of acetylcholine on muscarinic cholinergic receptors in the bronchi. The cholinergic system may be involved in bronchospasm induced by irritants such as cold air or sulphur dioxide. Atropine-like drugs thus cause bronchodilatation. They also reduce bronchial secretions and possibly inhibit the release of mediators from sensitised mast cells as well as interrupting vagal reflexes. Atropine has a bronchodilator action in some bronchitics but has little useful effect in asthma, partly because of its inspissating effect on sputum, and its use is precluded by side effects. However, some benefit may be produced in exercise-induced asthma.

Ipratropium (Atrovent)

This is isopropyl atropine which, although equipotent with atropine in its effects on inhibiting vagally mediated increases in heart rate, has a greater effect as a bronchodilator with decreased effect on sputum secretion. Its bronchodilator activity is similar to that of isoprenaline and salbutamol in some patients.

Pharmacokinetics It is administered by aerosol when plasma concentrations are some 1000 times lower than is necessary for the same degree of bronchodilatation when given systemically. When given in this way the plasma levels (which are very low) do not relate to the bronchodilator effect, indicating a local action on airways rather than a systemic effect. Ipratropium appears in the blood approximately 2 min after inhalation and the levels continue to rise for 1–3 h thereafter, because of swallowed drug absorbed from the gut. The plasma $t_{1/2}$ is 3–4 h and the drug is mainly excreted in the faeces and urine as metabolites and unchanged compound.

Clinical uses Ipratropium is given as 1–2 puffs (containing 20 μg) three or four times daily from a metered aerosol. It can be given via a nebuliser. For this the stock solution contains 0.25 mg per ml. As the latter is hypotonic, isotonic saline should be used as a diluent. The dose is 2 ml of Atrovent solution diluted with 2 ml of saline. In those patients who respond the onset of bronchodilatation with ipratropium is somewhat slower than with inhaled isoprenaline, but is more prolonged, and similar effects are found with terbutaline and salbutamol. The place of this drug in therapy is not yet decided. Its slower onset of action makes it more likely to be useful in maintenance therapy, especially in chronic bronchitis, rather than in the management of acute airways obstruction. It may be useful for patients with heart disease or thyrotoxicosis in whom sympathomimetics might be unsuitable. Its use is compatible with β-adrenergic agonists and such combinations may be synergistic, although this is not rigorously proven.

Adverse effects Blood pressure, pulse rate, intraocular tension, pupil size and salivary secretion are unaffected during the normal use of the drug but caution is advised in its use in patients with prostatic hypertrophy. Its only known contraindication is sensitivity to atropine.

Deptropine (Brontina) is similar to atropine. It is given as 1 mg tablets twice daily.

Brontisol is a metered aerosol which delivers deptropine citrate 0.1 mg and isoprenaline hydrochloride 0.15 mg per actuation. The maximum recommended dose is 8 puffs per day.

THE ROLE OF DRUGS IN THE MANAGEMENT OF CHRONIC ASTHMA AND BRONCHITIS

Chronic asthma

1. Bronchodilators are used in the treatment of chronic wheeziness and to stop acute episodes. The metered aerosols—particularly of salbutamol—have a powerful action, and with correct usage little enters the circulation. If the clinical state deteriorates such that the frequency of inhalations is rising, the physician must be contacted immediately.

The aerosols are particularly useful in treating an acute episode of breathlessness, but for more chronic wheeziness some physicians prefer oral therapy. In paediatric practice ephedrine is still used. Mixtures of small doses of ephedrine, theophylline and barbiturates are not favoured because there is no objective evidence of their efficacy. Naturally if a patient prefers such a preparation he should not be required to change.

2. All patients with asthma provoked by allergy, exercise or physical agents (e.g. cold air, sulphur dioxide), sufficient to need bronchodilator drugs should be given a trial of Sodium cromoglycate for at least 1 month. History and lung function tests before and after exercise are used to determine whether the drug is of sufficient value to continue. Some patients with intrinsic asthma respond to this drug.

3. Steroids are used in chronic asthma when:

(i) bronchodilators are not effective in allowing the patient normal activity and sleep;
(ii) repeated attacks interfere with work or school;
(iii) the growth of a child is impaired (however, it should be remembered that steroids themselves may suppress growth).

An inhaled steroid should be tried first in all patients requiring steroid treatment. The inhaled steroid should be tried for 2–3 weeks in doses up to beclomethasone 500 μg twice daily or budesonide 400 μg twice daily. Severely affected patients ($FEV_1 < 1.5$ l for adults) do not usually respond. Such patients frequently improve on oral prednisolone. Initially intermittent therapy is tried during an episode of repeated attacks of bronchospasm not responding to bronchodilators. During a chest infection 35–40 mg of prednisolone is given daily until a response is attained. The drug is then reduced by 5.0 mg every day.

There are patients for whom continuous steroid therapy is necessary—but they also need to increase the steroid dose during episodes of deterioration. If a patient eventually improves to such an extent that withdrawal of steroids can be tried, this should be done gradually (2.5 mg prednisolone/week). After complete withdrawal steroids will be required if an attack does not respond readily to bronchodilators.

Alternate day treatment with steroids may produce less adrenal and growth suppression than daily administration. ACTH and tetracosactrin do not affect linear growth and have the added advantage of producing no adrenal suppression. They are given by injection and this alone is considered sufficient disadvantage to detract from general use in adults.

4. Asthma associated with a chest infection may be treated with a tetracycline, cotrimoxazole or a broad-spectrum penicillin. Ideally it is preferable to anticipate the situation and give antibiotics to prevent a chest infection leading to a worsening of the asthma.

5. Hypnotics and sedatives should be used as little as possible and are contraindicated in the presence of respiratory failure and acute attacks.

Late-onset asthma This is often difficult to treat and long-term steroid treatment may be the only way to control the disease. Nevertheless bronchodilators and Sodium cromoglycate should be tried, particularly if sputum eosinophilia is present.

Management of severe refractory asthma (status asthmaticus)

1. Arrange for hospital admission. Before the ambulance arrives give 250 mg aminophylline intravenously over 5–10 minutes only if oral theophylline has not been taken recently. It is dangerous to give intravenous aminophylline to patients who have received theophylline within 24 hours. In addition, if the patient is not vomiting give 40 mg of prednisolone orally. If oral therapy is not possible 200 mg of hydrocortisone hemisuccinate is given intravenously instead.

2. Set up an intravenous infusion, initially 5% glucose. Avoidance and treatment of dehydration is mandatory to prevent sputum inspissation. If hydrocortisone has not been given before admission to hospital, a 200 mg bolus should be given intravenously. Because the half-life of hydrocortisone is short this must be followed by an intravenous infusion at the rate of 3 mg/kg/6 h or further boluses at four hourly intervals.

3. The steroids take up to 4 h for some subjective improvement and up to 6 h for the beginning of objective benefit. During this time bronchodilator drugs are given .

   (a) Salbutamol is given via a nebuliser. Air is driven through the solution at a flow rate of 6–8 litres per minute producing a mist of optimum particle size. 0.5–1.0 ml of Ventolin nebuliser solution (0.5% salbutamol) is diluted to 4.0 ml with sterile saline giving a dose of 2.5–5.0 mg of salbutamol. Inhalation may be repeated four hourly. Salbutamol may also be given by slow intravenous injection (4 μg/kg).

(b) An alternative is to give intravenous aminophylline provided the patient is not already receiving the drug. The dose is 5.0 mg/kg (usually 250–350 mg) given slowly over 10–15 min and may be followed by an infusion of 0.3 mg/kg over 24 h diluted in 500 ml of saline. Plasma levels are necessary if the drug is infused for more than 24 h.

4. (a) If the $p_aO_2 < 8.5$ kPa (< 65 mm Hg) and p_aCO_2 normal or low, give 65 % oxygen by MC mask, but if p_aCO_2, is raised, give 28 % oxygen by Ventimask.

(b) Failure to improve with this management, or a $p_aO_2 < 6.5$ kPa (< 50 mm Hg), a rising p_aCO_2, a pulse over 130/min and the presence of pulsus paradoxus requires intubation and intermittent positive-pressure ventilation. This is maintained for 24–48 h until the maximum effect of the steroids has been attained. During this time sedation with opioids is necessary to suppress the patient's own respiratory efforts and also to allow him to rest. Naturally opioids are absolutely contraindicated in asthma, unless assisted ventilation is being used.

5. Antibacterial chemotherapy is given routinely; suitable drugs include cotrimoxazole, amoxycillin or oxytetracycline, orally, although initially intravenous dosing will be required for some patients.

6. After 48 h of hydrocortisone treatment, the steroid is replaced by 80 mg prednisolone daily. This is progressively reduced and finally withdrawn 10 days after admission.

7. Initially the patient is exhausted and vigorous physiotherapy is inappropriate during the first few hours, but once improvement has occurred physiotherapy in conjunction with inhalation of bronchodilators is beneficial.

8. Reassuring the patient who is often very frightened during the early stages of acute severe asthma is humane and commonly improves the response to drug therapy.

Acute bronchitis

This condition commonly presents to general practitioners. There is often pressure from patients for the prescription of antibiotics and yet a randomised double-blind trial reveals that no benefit is obtained in otherwise fit patients presenting with cough and purulent sputum. In the absence of abnormal clinical findings it seems best to avoid antibiotics for this self-limiting condition.

Chronic bronchitis and emphysema

Chronic simple bronchitis is associated with chronic or recurrent increase in the volume of a mucoid bronchial secretion sufficient to cause expectoration. At this stage there need be no disability and measures such as giving up smoking and avoidance of air pollution may improve the prognosis. Simple hypersecretion may be complicated by infection or the development of airways obstruction. Bacterial infection is usually due to *Haemophilus influenzae* although pneumococci, staphylococci or occasionally coliforms may also be responsible. The commonly encountered acute bronchitic exacerbation is due to bacterial infection in only about one third of cases; in the rest other factors such as increased air pollution, environmental temperature changes, or viruses which do not respond to antibiotics, are presumably responsible. Mycoplasma infections may be responsible for some cases and these usually respond to tetracyclines or erythromycin. In practice it is usually assumed that the infection is bacterial or has become secondarily infected with bacteria and treatment is begun with antibiotics. The appropriate antibiotic is chosen from those drugs penetrating sputum, the decision being assisted by sputum culture:

(a) Ampicillin penetrates purulent more readily than mucoid sputum, possibly via active transport. Nevertheless 1 g 6 hourly is required to achieve bactericidal levels against *H. influenzae*.
(b) Amoxycillin produces sputum concentrations twice those from equivalent ampicillin dosage.
(c) Tetracyclines must be given in doses of 500 mg 6 hourly to achieve adequate sputum penetration. Doxycycline given as 200 mg initially followed by 100 mg daily penetrates well into sputum; it is also suitable for the older patient with renal insufficiency in whom other tetracyclines are contraindicated.
(d) Cotrimoxazole is often used and seems to be effective. Theoretically the synergistic action of its two components may be decreased since the sulphamethoxazole penetrates sputum poorly and the 1 : 20 ratio of trimethoprim : sulphamethoxazole achieved in the blood is reduced to 1 : 1, making a bacteriostatic action more likely (see Chapter 19).

It should be noted that cephalosporins play little part in the routine management of bronchitis since they penetrate sputum poorly and have minimal activity against *Haemophilus*. In the absence of respiratory disability, antibiotics alone may be sufficient treatment, but in cases of increased respiratory difficulty sputum retention may be responsible for failure to respond to treatment. Physiotherapy with rehydration if necessary, to ease expectoration, helps in patients with this problem. The use of mucolytic agents such as bromhexine has proved disappointing and the inhalation of steam (traditionally with added tinct. benz. co.) is probably of marginal benefit in most cases.

Prevention of acute exacerbations is difficult. It is widely accepted that stopping smoking and avoidance of climatic extremes are beneficial. Prevention of influenza by administration of influenza vaccines (or more controversially by amantadine) is also helpful. The evidence regarding antibiotic prophylaxis of exacerbations is confused. Overall it appears that continuous prophylaxis with tetracycline does not reduce the number of exacerbations in most bronchitics but may reduce their duration. Therefore for this group of more severely affected patients, prophylaxis with either a tetracycline or cotrimoxazole may be useful. Alternatively the patient may be given a supply of antibiotic to take at the first sign of infection. This has the benefit of reducing drug exposure (so limiting toxicity and emergence of bacterial resistance) and of allowing a number of different antibacterial agents to be used. Unfortunately neither prophylaxis nor early intensive therapy of infections appears to affect the rate of decline of ventilatory function.

Airways obstruction is invariably present in chronic bronchitis but is of variable severity. Bronchodilators, either β-adrenergic stimulants or aminophylline, are often used but frequently fail since much of the obstruction is irreversible. In some patients, however, there is a reversible element and a trial of these drugs is usually justified to assess whether benefit will be obtained. Similarly a therapeutic trial of corticosteroids (20 mg prednisolone twice daily for 2 weeks followed by a rapid reduction in dose if no benefit is obtained) may be used in more severe cases of airways obstruction unresponsive to conventional bronchodilators or where an allergic component is suspected to be important.

Intermittent use of oxygen at low concentration by patients at home is probably ineffective. Long-term oxygen therapy (15 h or so daily) in severely disabled bronchitics with pulmonary hypertension has been shown to decrease mortality and morbidity. The mortality of these patients is related to the degree of pulmonary hypertension which is increased by chronic anoxia. Relief of anoxia on a long-term basis by increasing (within safe limits) the concentration of inspired oxygen may reverse the obstruction in the pulmonary arteries and decrease pulmonary hypertension.

Almitrine is a new drug, as yet unavailable in the UK, which has a complex mode of action to increase ventilation via stimulation of peripheral chemoreceptors. It also affects the pulmonary vasculature and improves alveolar ventilation/perfusion matching. It may be given orally and possibly delays onset of cor pulmonale so that it could be an alternative to chronic oxygen therapy.

Respiratory failure

Respiratory failure is the result of a number of disorders of lung function in which gas exchange is impaired. This is defined as a p_aO_2 below 8 kPa (60 mm Hg) with or without a p_aCO_2 above 6.3 kPa (47 mm Hg).

1. A normal or lowered p_aCO_2 is characteristic of ventilation/perfusion inequality (as in pneumonia, left-ventricular failure, pulmonary fibrosis and shock lung).
2. A combination of hypoxaemia and hypercapnia (ventilatory failure) are associated with chronic airways obstruction (as in obstructive bronchitis, kyphoscoliosis and primary alveolar hypoventilation), drug overdosage depressing the respiratory centre, neurological disorders, e.g. Guillain–Barre syndrome.

1. The treatment of ventilation/perfusion inequality is that of the underlying lesion and in such cases there is no danger of precipitating carbon dioxide retention so that oxygen at high flow rate can be given (by nasal cannulae or by MC or Polymask). 'Shock lung' is treated by controlled ventilation, oxygenation and positive end expiratory pressure (PEEP).

2. Ventilatory failure is treated by:

(a) *Supportive measures:*

Physiotherapy—to encourage coughing to remove tracheobronchial secretions to encourage deep breathing to preserve potency of airways and prevent progressive closure due to shallow breathing.

Oxygen therapy improves tissue oxygenation but prolonged administration of high concentrations may depress respiration by removing the hypoxic respiratory drive. A small increase in the concentration of inspired oxygen to 24% using a Venturi-type mask is cautiously tried. If the p_aCO_2 does not increase or increases by only a small amount, say 0.66 kPa (the error of the estimation), and if the level of the consciousness of the patient is unimpaired, the inspired oxygen concentration is increased to 28%, and after further assessment to 35%. Low flow rates of oxygen should be continuous since severe hypoxia can develop if it is given intermittently. If oxygen produces respiratory depression, assisted ventilation is urgently needed.

Sedatives must not be used. Even benzodiazepines can produce fatal respiratory depression in patients with ventilatory failure.

(b) *Specific measures*:

Respiratory failure may be precipitated in chronic bronchitis by infection, fluid retention and bronchoconstriction. Antibacterial drugs such as oxytetracycline, amoxycillin, ampicillin or cotrimoxazole are used if the sputum has become purulent. In the presence of oedema, particularly with left-ventricular failure, a thiazide or high-ceiling diuretic is indicated. Bronchospasm may respond to 5 mg of salbutamol given 6 hourly in a nebuliser via a tight-fitting mask. If this fails to reduce bronchospasm, hydrocortisone (750–1250 mg/day) is infused intravenously.

If, despite the above treatment, p_aO_2 continues to fall and p_aCO_2 to rise and consciousness becomes impaired so that the patient fails to cough adequately, analeptics may be tried. These include nikethamide (1–4 mg of a 25% solution intravenously) or doxapram (35–100 mg intravenously). If these respiratory stimulants do not lead to a substantial improvement, endotracheal intubation and suction with controlled respiration should be considered.

ANALEPTICS

Analeptics are drugs which stimulate the CNS. Small doses produce respiratory and cardiovascular stimulation, but larger amounts are convulsant. The use of analeptics to counteract overdose of central depressant drugs is much less successful than intensive respiratory and circulatory supportive care, but their value in acute exacerbations of chronic lung disease and in other forms of respiratory failure has not yet been fully assessed.

Nikethamide (Coramine) A single intravenous injection has a short-lived effect (5–10 min) due to rapid redistribution in the body. Metabolism appears to be a slower process. Repeated doses readily produce toxicity (tachycardia, sneezing, itching, tremors, fever and convulsions). Deeply sedated patients do not respond to subconvulsive doses. Nikethamide fits may be followed by central depression which worsens the original condition for which it was used.

Doxapram (Dopram) is another non-specific central nervous system stimulant, and was originally used post-operatively to stimulate respiration and hasten arousal in patients recovering from general anaesthesia. The cough reflex was more rapidly restored, and this reduced the incidence of post-operative lung complications. In drug-induced respiratory depression, doxapram increases tidal volume (with a smaller increase in respiratory rate) resulting in a prompt rise in pO_2 and fall in pCO_2. In the treatment of hypnotic drug overdose, the need for assisted ventilation is not eliminated by analeptics and there is an increase in mortality from barbiturate overdose when these drugs are used.

The ratio of convulsant to respiratory stimulant dose is 70:1 compared with 15:1 for nikethamide, but large doses of doxapram produce general central nervous stimulation and adverse effects similar to those of nikethamide.

Doxapram (like other analeptics) is contraindicated in epilepsy, hypertension, cerebral oedema, hyperthyroidism and phaeochromocytoma and should not be used with monoamine oxidase inhibitors or sympathomimetic drugs.

Doxapram is given intravenously by continuous infusion or bolus injections of about 0.5–1.5 mg/kg hourly. The $t_{1/2}$ is 2.5–4.0 h and the CNS effects are related to plasma doxapram concentrations.

Analeptics in ventilatory failure

The standard treatment of ventilatory failure (carbon dioxide retention and hypoxia) with controlled administration of oxygen in low concentrations is usually successful. However, in some patients the administration of nikethamide may be useful in rousing a patient, enabling him to cough up retained secretions and to co-operate with physiotherapy.

Doxapram is possibly slightly more effective than nikethamide in treating patients with acute exacerbations of chronic bronchitis complicated by hypercapnia and hypoxia, probably because of its slightly more favourable therapeutic index. Doxapram is also effective (over short periods) in reversing the fall in pO_2 which may result from oxygen administration in these patients. There is, however, no convincing evidence that drugs of this type can produce prolonged benefit in patients with respiratory failure.

DRUGS AFFECTING COUGH

Cough suppressants

Cough is a normal physiological reflex which acts to keep the respiratory tract free from accumulated secretions and removes particulate matter. The reflex is usually initiated by irritation of the mucous membrane of the respiratory tract and coordinated by a cough centre in the medulla. Cough requires suppression when it distresses or exhausts the patient. Ideally treatment should not impair elimination of bronchopulmonary secretions. A number of antitussive drugs are available but critical evaluation of their efficacy is difficult. In volunteers cough can be produced by inhalation of irritants such as sulphur dioxide or citric acid and the suppression of cough by a drug estimated. An alternative technique to measure the concentration of ether in air which produces a single cough after inhalation: an effective antitussive should alter the cough-induction threshold. Subjective estimates of efficacy by patients are valueless since objective measurement by tape recording reveals that patients with chronic cough usually have little idea of the effects of drugs on their cough or of its spontaneous variation in intensity from day to day. Using such recording methods it has been possible to show dose-dependent efficacy for some cough suppressants.

Coughing to bring up sputum is an important mechanism to clear the airway and should not normally be suppressed except in a few circumstances such as intractable cough in carcinoma of the bronchus, and an unproductive cough interfering with sleep.

In many patients cough can be relieved by a bland demulcent syrup (e.g. Simple Linctus B.P.C.) containing no active drug.

Opiates (but not pethidine or related drugs) depress the medullary cough centre. Codeine linctus B.P.C. is most commonly used amongst the non-proprietaries. It has not been convincingly demonstrated that any of the alternatives of codeine such as pholcodeine, noscapine or dextromethorphan are superior. In intractable cough due to malignant invasion of the respiratory tract Linctus Diamorphine is sometimes effective. Coughing provides bronchial catharsis and clearance and logically cough suppressants are best avoided if the cough is productive. The reduction in respiratory drive associated with more powerful opiates may be hazardous in chronic bronchitis and asthma. It is doubtful if any of the more complex proprietary cough medicines so liberally prescribed have value other than as placebo or as a convenient way for the doctor to end the consultation with a prescription. It is sensible therefore only to use the cheapest of them.

Expectorants

Associated with chronic cough in many patients is a difficulty in clearing the chest of viscous sputum. A variety of mucolytic agents are available although there is little evidence of efficacy in most cases.

(a) Drugs increasing production of watery bronchial secretion by reflex stimulation of stomach and duodenum. These include sodium chloride given in a hot draught (Mist. Sod. Chlor. Co. B.P.), squill (Squill Opiate Linctus B.P.C.), ammonium chloride (Ammonium Chloride Mixture B.P.C.), ammonium bicarbonate (Ammonium and Ipecacuanha Mixture, B.P.C.). Iodides, creosotes, guiacols and other volatile oils are often included in proprietary mixtures. Some of these may act directly on bronchial secretory cells.

(b) Drugs reducing the viscosity of secretions by altering the nature of the organic components are also used. They are sometimes called mucolytics. **Bromhexine (Bisolvon)** is a synthetic derivative of an alkaloid which when taken orally can cause fragmentation of the mucopolysaccharide fibres, which contribute to sputum viscosity, possibly by the liberation of lysosomal enzymes from bronchial mucosa. The oral dose is 8–16 mg 6–8 hourly. **Acetylcysteine** and **Methylcysteine** are given by aerosol and have free sulphydryl groups which may split disulphide bonds in sputum proteins.

All of these drugs have been used in patients where extremely viscous sputum contributes to their respiratory distress, e.g. cystic fibrosis, chronic bronchitis.

It must be admitted, however, that these drugs are by and large ineffective.

A simple and often most effective method of improving expectoration is inhalation of steam. There is little evidence that the addition of a medicinal smell with Friars Balsam (Tinct. Benz. Co.) gives any advantage. In all cases rehydration, if necessary with intravenous fluids, will discourage increased sputum viscosity.

DRUG-INDUCED LUNG DISEASE

The lungs may be affected by drugs in several ways, although serious adverse pulmonary reactions to drugs are relatively uncommon.

Physical irritation by the powder of disodium cromoglycate and by the fumes of sulphur dioxide (used as a preservative in some foods and drinks) can precipitate bronchospasm in asthmatics.

Allergy to drugs of the immediate variety (Type I) is particularly common in atopic individuals. Specific reaginic antibodies (IgE) to drugs can produce disturbances ranging from mild wheezing to laryngeal oedema or anaphylactic shock. Delayed bronchospasm may be due to drug interactions involving IgG antibodies (Type III). Any drug may be responsible for allergic reactions, but antibiotics appear to be particularly powerful allergens.

In some asthmatics (particularly those with nasal polypi and late onset of respiratory symptoms) aspirin may increase airways obstruction. The mechanism for this is unknown, but interference with prostaglandin synthesis may be involved. In support of this, these patients may also suffer a reaction from other anti-inflammatory analgesics such as mefenamic acid and indomethacin. On the other hand, bronchospasm can also be caused in many of these individuals by dextropropoxyphene, pentazocine and tartrazine (a yellow colouring used in many foods and drugs).

Pharmacological actions β-blockers can produce severe prolonged and dangerous bronchospasm in asthma and hay fever sufferers. Parasympathomimetic drugs such as physostigmine can increase bronchial secretion and raise airways resistance.

Pulmonary eosinophilia presents as dyspnoea, cough and fever. The chest X-ray shows widespread patchy changing shadows and there is usually eosinophilia in the peripheral blood. The pathogenesis of the condition is not understood but the following drugs are known to produce this reaction:

aspirin	nitrofurantoin
imipramine	streptomycin
penicillin	P.A.S.
isoniazid	

Polyarteritis Polyarteritis nodosa is often drug induced, and thus may produce asthma and pulmonary eosinophilia. Sulphonamides are most often implicated in precipitating this reaction.

Systemic lupus erythematosus (S.L.E.) is drug induced in about one-fifth of cases. Examples of drugs which are known to precipitate S.L.E. are hydralazine, procainamide and practolol. The lungs can be involved by pleuritic reactions, pneumonia-like illness and impaired respiratory function due to small, stiff lungs. The clinical and serological components of this reaction usually (but not always) disappear on withdrawing the drug (see also p. 105).

Pulmonary fibrosis Some cytotoxic and other drugs can produce pulmonary oedema. This fluid may become organised and in this way pulmonary fibrosis develops. The drugs implicated include:

busulphan	methotrexate
bleomycin	gold salts
cyclophosphamide	nitrofurantoin

Chapter 14
DIURETICS AND DRUGS ACTING ON THE KIDNEYS

Diuretics are drugs which increase the rate of urine production by the kidneys. They achieve this by modifying renal function and it is therefore necessary to consider the mechanism of urine formation in order to understand their modes of action.

NORMAL PHYSIOLOGY

In a normal man with a glomerular filtration rate of 125 ml/min, 180 l of fluid containing 25 000 mmol of sodium are filtered daily although only 1–2 l of urine containing about 100 mmol of sodium are passed. Thus over 99% of filtrate and sodium is reabsorbed. Urine secretion is essentially a two-stage process:

(i) An ultrafiltrate of plasma is formed in the glomerulus which depends on the hydrostatic pressure of the arterial circulation. A marked fall in blood pressure stops filtration and results in anuria. The ultrafiltrate consists of all the components of the plasma except protein and lipids. Substances, including drugs, which are bound to protein will not be filtered through the glomerulus.

(ii) Reabsorption of water and electrolytes is achieved in the renal tubules by a number of energy-requiring processes and it is these processes that are modified by diuretics. The renal tubules may be divided into four zones with distinctive patterns of reabsorption (see Fig. 14.1).

Zone I At this site about 65% of the filtered sodium is reabsorbed by active transport along with an isosmotic volume of water. About two thirds of the accompanying anion is chloride and the rest largely bicarbonate. Filtered potassium is completely reabsorbed at this site.

Zone II Chloride ions are actively reabsorbed in the ascending limb of the loop of Henle, together with sodium (25% of filtered load) which moves passively. This area of the tubule is impermeable to water and so the concentration of sodium and chloride in the tubular fluid falls progressively. At the same time the concentration of sodium and chloride in the interstitial fluid of the renal papilla will rise and this is responsible for the generation of the sodium chloride component of the hypertonic medullary interstitium. It is the long loops of Henle of the juxtamedullary nephrons (20% of the total nephron population) which act as a counter-current multiplier system, with their associated vasa recta acting as counter-current exchangers that allow the production of hypertonic urine in the collecting ducts.

Zone III In the cortical segment of the ascending loop of Henle (the cortical diluting segment) sodium is absorbed (5% of filtered load) without water, rendering the tubular fluid hypotonic. Because this sodium is reabsorbed

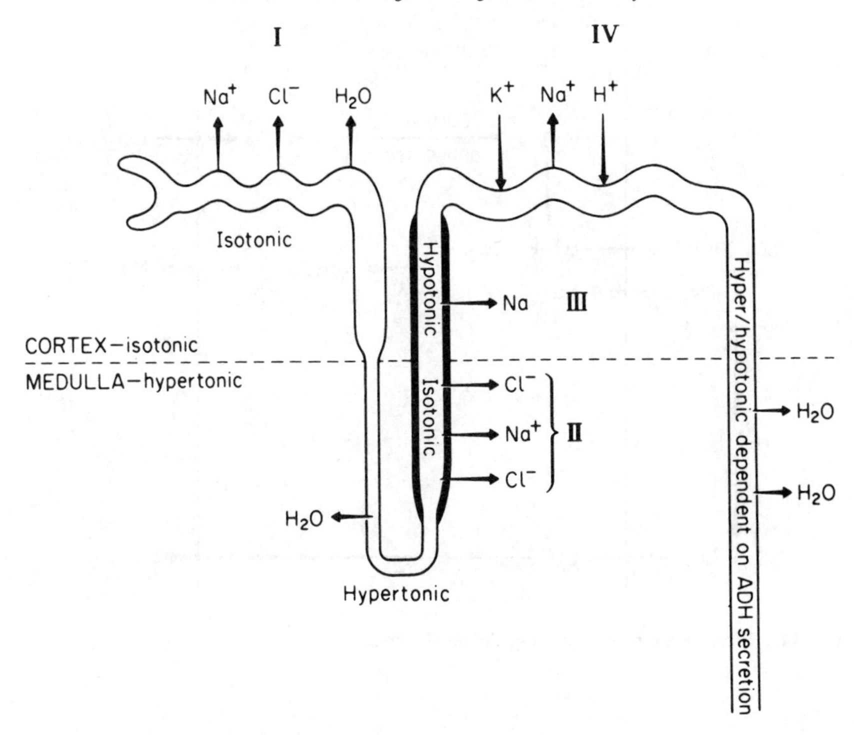

Fig. 14.1 Tubular sites of sodium and water reabsorption.

beyond the region which contributes to medullary hypertonicity (zone II), drugs inhibiting sodium reabsorption at zone III can diminish diluting capacity without affecting concentrating capacity.

Zone IV Some further sodium reabsorption occurs in this area of the distal convoluted tubule and collecting duct together with secretion of potassium and hydrogen ions and absorption of chloride. The secretion of potassium and hydrogen ions is in exchange for sodium and is determined by both aldosterone and the amount of sodium present at the excretion site (see Fig. 14.1). Any diuretic acting proximally to zone IV will allow delivery of increased amounts of sodium to this site and leads to increased exchange with potassium and thus increased potassium loss in the urine.

In this zone major reabsorption of water also occurs under the control of *antidiuretic hormone* (*ADH*) also known as arginine vasopressin (AVP). The tubules which are surrounded by hypertonic interstitial fluid are impermeable to water. In the presence of ADH they become permeable and water passes out of the tubule down the osmotic gradient into the medullary interstitium, resulting in hypertonic urine.

Renal regulation of acid–base balance

The kidney regulates acid-base balance by:

1. controlling the rate of tubular absorption of filtered bicarbonate ion;

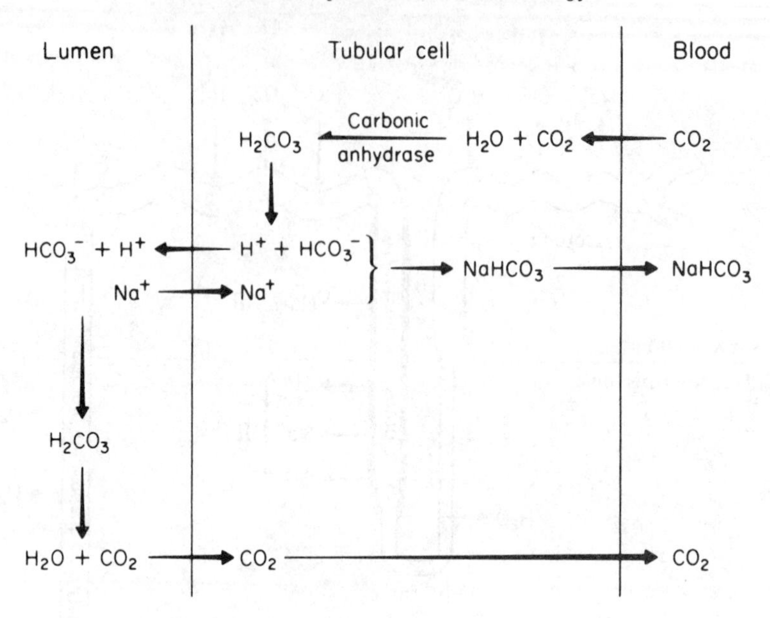

Fig. 14.2 Bicarbonate reabsorption in the renal tubule.

2. excretion of hydrogen ions with simultaneous regeneration of bicarbonate.

This process is illustrated in Fig. 14.2.

Carbonic acid is synthesised in tubular cells by the hydration of carbon dioxide in a reaction catalysed by carbonic anhydrase. Hydrogen ions formed by dissociation of this carbonic acid are then secreted into the lumen in exchange for sodium ions which are reabsorbed into the peritubular blood along with the bicarbonate ions formed from the dissociation of carbonic acid. In addition to contributing to bicarbonate ion reabsorption the secreted hydrogen ions also form the titratable acid of the urine and allow the excretion of ammonium ions.

Excretion of organic acids and bases

Many drugs are weak organic acids or bases and are excreted by active transport systems into the renal tubules, probably in the proximal tubule. Some drugs may be partially reabsorbed again from the tubules and this is dependent on nonionic diffusion. The tubular cells are permeable only to the nonionic fraction of the drug, so reabsorption is dependent on the pK_a of the drug and the pH of the urine. For example, salicylates are highly ionised in an alkaline solution: in the treatment of salicylate overdosage the urine is made alkaline so that the salicylate becomes highly ionised and there is little back diffusion.

Determining the site of action of diuretics in the renal tubule

Most diuretics act by preventing the reabsorption of sodium from tubular fluid. This leads to retention of water in the tubules and thus promotes a diuresis. There are several ways of determining the site of action of diuretics, but most of them are only applicable to animals and suffer the disadvantage that they may not be translated to the human situation as the dose used in experiments may be well above that used therapeutically.

1. *Micropuncture studies* In the experimental animal it is possible to cannulate a single tubule to remove samples of fluid and also to isolate a segment by introducing a drop of oil into the tubular lumen. This is the most precise way of assessing the effect of drugs on the composition of tubular fluid and their sites of action.

2. *Stop flow* This method is useful if the site of action of a drug is on the peripheral part of the nephron. The ureter is clamped for a while and then released and samples of urine are collected at intervals. Analysis of the samples gives some evidence of what happened when the urine was held in the tubular lumen. This method is of little use when the site of action is on the proximal part of the nephron.

3. *Effect of the drug on urine osmolality* This method is useful in that it is applicable to humans using therapeutic doses of drugs. It requires that the osmolality of the urine is measured under conditions of water diuresis and water deprivation:

(a) *Free-water clearance in water diuresis* The free-water clearance (C_{H_2O}) depends upon the amount of sodium presented to the sodium absorption sites in the ascending limb of the loop of Henle (zones II and III) and in the distal tubule (zone IV), provided these sites are functioning properly. If the drug acts in the proximal tubule (zone I) increased amounts of sodium and chloride will reach zones II and III, resulting in an increase in Na^+Cl^- reabsorption and increased free-water clearance. If the drug acts in zones II or III free water clearance will diminish as Na^+Cl^- would not be absorbed from the tubular fluid at these sites.

(b) *Free-water reabsorption in water deprivation* If a drug acts on zone II it will interfere with the Na^+Cl^- reabsorption and thus with the concentrating mechanism of the kidney. This will be reflected in a decrease in free-water reabsorption ($T^C_{H_2O}$) under conditions of water deprivation (see Table 14.1).

Table 14.1 Effect of agents acting at different sites in the nephron on water clearance and reabsorption

Site of action	C_{H_2O}—*free water clearance*	$T^C_{H_2O}$—*free water reabsorption*	*Other changes*
Proximal (zone I)	↑	↑	↑ Glucose ↑ Amino acids ↑ Bicarbonate
Loop (zone II)	↓	↓	0
Distal (zone III)	↓	0	↑ K^+

Examples:
Mannitol Increases free-water clearance suggesting an effect on proximal tubular reabsorption.
Frusemide Decreases free-water clearance and impairs free-water absorption suggesting an effect on the ascending limb (zone II) and possibly more distal sites.

4. *Changes in urine composition* An increase in urinary bicarbonate suggests that the diuretic is a carbonic anhydrase inhibitor which interferes with the excretion of hydrogen ions.

DIURETICS

Carbonic anhydrase inhibitors

Carbonic anhydrase is important in the reaction (see Fig. 14.2):

$$CO_2 + H_2O \underset{A}{\longrightarrow} H_2CO_3 \underset{B}{\longrightarrow} H^+ + HCO_3^-$$

Carbonic anhydrase catalyses stage A of the reaction but stage B is almost instantaneous and does not depend on enzyme action. This reaction occurs in many tissues including the kidney, the choroid plexus and the eye. As diuretics, carbonic anhydrase inhibitors are largely obsolete but their actions elsewhere in the body allow other therapeutic uses.

Acetazolamide (Diamox)

The drug is the carbonic anhydrase inhibitor most commonly used in clinical practice. Some other diuretics have some inhibiting effect on carbonic anhydrase but it is not an important part of their diuretic action.

Acetazolamide is a sulphonamide derivative which acts as a non-competitive inhibitor of carbonic anhydrase in zone IV and in the proximal tubule. In normal circumstances hydrogen ions are generated in the tubular cell by the action of carbonic anhydrase and exchanged with sodium in the tubular fluid. The hydrogen ions then combine with bicarbonate to become carbon dioxide and water which passes back into the tubular cell (see Fig. 14.2). The net result of this is to prevent bicarbonate loss in the urine. By inhibiting carbonic anhydrase, acetazolamide

(a) prevents the production of hydrogen ions in the tubular cell and thus prevents sodium–hydrogen ion exchange, so that sodium remains in the tubular fluid;
(b) allows excess bicarbonate to escape in the tubular fluid.

The excess sodium reaching the sodium–potassium exchange site in the distal tubule (zone IV) causes more potassium to be excreted into the urine. The result is an alkaline diuresis with loss of sodium, potassium and bicarbonate together with a developing metabolic acidosis.

The eye Acetazolamide inhibits carbonic anhydrase in the eye and thereby decreases the rate of secretion of the aqueous humour in the anterior chamber of the eye and lowers intraocular pressure.

The brain Carbonic anhydrase is present in the brain and acetazolamide has some anticonvulsant properties and other effects whose importance is not known. This drug reduces formation of CSF by carbonic anhydrase inhibition in the choroid plexus, and is therefore occasionally useful in the management of benign intracranial hypertension.

Pharmacokinetics Acetazolamide is well absorbed from the intestine and has a plasma half-life of about 3 h. It is excreted by the kidney. With repeated doses tolerance occurs because excretion of an alkaline urine results in metabolic acidosis with a compensatory increased respiratory loss of CO_2. This reduces the filtered plasma bicarbonate and eventually this falls so low that the tubular sodium can be exchanged for the relatively small amount of hydrogen ion available in the presence of carbonic anhydrase inhibition. Thus sodium and water diuresis ceases. It also activates the tubulo-glomerular feed-back thus reducing the GFR.

Clinical uses It is a weak diuretic and tolerance develops (see above) but this may be avoided by intermittent use so that plasma bicarbonate is restored before the next dose. Because of these problems it is rarely used as a diuretic but it can be used to produce an alkaline urine in the treatment of cysteine stones.

It is used in acute closed angle glaucoma in doses of 250 mg i.v. followed by 250 mg four times daily; in open angle glaucoma 125 mg three times daily is adequate.

In the lower dose range acetazolamide can be given for long periods but larger doses cause troublesome side effects (see below). Fortunately the change in acid–base status does not interfere with its action on aqueous formation. The effect of the drug lasts about 6 h. Sustained-release tablets (Sustets) allow twice daily dosing.

Adverse effects Hypersensitivity reactions and blood dyscrasias may occur. Prolonged use may lead to renal-stone formation which is thought to be due to the fall in urinary citrate caused by the drug since it is believed that citrate is a factor which helps to keep calcium in solution in the urine. The large doses used for glaucoma produce paraesthesiae, dyspepsia, muscular fatigue and dyspepsia.

Thiazides

The pharmacological actions of the drugs in this group are very similar, but they differ in their diuretic potency per unit weight of the drug, and to some degree in the duration of their action.

Originally derived by modification of the sulphonamide structure of carbonic anhydrase inhibitors, thiazides have a weak inhibitory effect on this enzyme in the proximal tubule. This results in increased bicarbonate and phosphate excretion. However, the primary diuretic action of the thiazides is to decrease sodium reabsorption in the cortical diluting segment (zone III) of the renal tubule, thus producing an increased excretion of sodium and water. The

Table 14.2 Summary of the effects of diuretics and other ions on sodium reabsorption in the nephron

Diuretic	*Glomerular filtration*	*Site of action on sodium reabsorption*				*Inhibition of reabsorption*				*% filtered Na excreted*
		I	II	III	IV	*Na*	*Cl*	*K*	*Ca*	
Thiazides	Probably ↓	Inhibited (minor effect)	0	Inhibited	0	+	+	+	−	5–10%
Loop e.g. frusemide	Possibly ↑	Inhibited (minor effect)	Inhibited	Inhibited	0	++	++	++	+	15–25%
Amiloride (triamterene)	0	0	0	0	Inhibited	+	(+)	−	0	5%
Spironolactone	0	0	0	0	Inhibited	+	(+)	−	0	3%
Osmotic	Possibly ↑	Inhibited	0	0	0	+	+	+	0	5–10%
Carbonic anhydrase inhibitors	↓	Inhibited	0	0	Inhibited (minor effect)	+	0	+	+	5%

+ = Decreased reabsorption (∴ increased urinary loss).
0 = No effect.
− = Increased reabsorption (∴ decreased urinary loss).

molecular basis for this action is unknown. The sodium is accompanied by the anions chloride and bicarbonate, and with the thiazides either may predominate, depending on the composition of the extracellular fluid. If the patient is alkalotic, the amount of bicarbonate in the urine increases, and conversely in acidosis urinary chloride excretion is enhanced. This is important as the thiazides do not tend to disturb the acid–base balance of the extracellular fluid. Because of their limited site of action thiazides are only moderately powerful diuretics and the maximum proportion of filtered sodium found in the urine with these drugs is about 8% (see 'High-ceiling diuretics').

The immediate result of the sodium and water loss induced by thiazides is a contraction of the extracellular space, but this later returns towards normal, although a small deficiency persists.

The increase in sodium in the tubular fluid allows increased sodium to reach the distal potassium–sodium exchange site (zone IV) , so considerable excretion of potassium occurs. Potassium loss is further enhanced by the weak carbonic anhydrase activity which results in a decrease of hydrogen ions in the tubular cells so that potassium is the main ion for exchange.

Thiazides also decrease urinary calcium excretion, but this rarely leads to hypercalcaemia. The mechanism of this effect of thiazides is unknown but appears to be renal since injection of a thiazide into one renal artery produces hypocalciuria from that kidney. Thiazides increase urinary magnesium loss, which may be clinically significant, since many patients in heart failure are already magnesium depleted due to secondary hyperaldosteronism. (See p. 510).

Thiazide diuretics have an important antihypertensive effect which appears to depend upon both a reduction in blood volume and a reduction in peripheral resistance. This latter effect is due to a direct vasodilator action in part dependent on an alteration in the electrolyte concentration or distribution in the vessel wall which reduces vascular responsiveness to pressor stimuli. This subject is further discussed on p. 423.

Pharmacokinetics Thiazides are given orally, the more lipid soluble being better absorbed and requiring smaller doses. The duration of action depends on water solubility and on protein binding. They are highly tissue and plasma protein bound (> 80%) and gain access to their renal site of action via the proximal tubular non-selective organic acid secretory mechanism. Because the active secretory pathway of the proximal tubule is non-specific, other organic acids such as probenecid or penicillin may compete for secretion. Probenecid in fact increases the sodium and water excretion produced by chlorothiazide and elevates chlorothiazide plasma levels. This increase is associated with a prolongation of diuresis rather than an increase in its intensity, suggesting that prolonged excretion of diuretic within the tubular fluid produces a greater overall effect. Thiazides competitively decrease penicillin secretion into the proximal tubule.

These drugs are variably metabolised, some quite considerably, e.g. bendrofluazide is 30% excreted unchanged in the urine and 70% is metabolised, whilst hydrochlorothiazide is 95% excreted unchanged. Some of the metabolites have stronger carbonic anhydrase inhibitory properties than the parent molecule.

Clinical uses Thiazides are usually given orally in the morning and they produce a diuresis through the day. Diuresis starts about 2 h after an oral dose and lasts for 8–20 h depending on the drug. They are not very powerful diuretics. They are used in:

1. Cardiac failure—they are useful when failure is not severe.
2. Hypertension—this is probably their main indication at present.
3. Oedema due to the nephrotic syndrome or cirrhosis of the liver–loop diuretics may well be required as thiazides are often ineffective.
4. Diabetes insipidus. Thiazides reduce the urinary volume in diabetes insipidus due to ADH deficiency and in the primary nephrogenic type.
5. In idiopathic hypercalciuria thiazides may lessen the tendency to urinary stone formation via their action to reduce urinary calcium excretion.

Table 14.3 shows some thiazides in common use. Except for some differences between the duration of action of this group of diuretics, there is little to choose between them. They do, however, differ somewhat in cost. In treating hypertension the lowest dose should be used as increasing the dose does not increase efficacy. Metolazone is particularly effective if added to a loop diuretic in the treatment of refractory oedema. It is expensive and for this reason should not be used as a routine thiazide or in the treatment of hypertension.

Adverse effects Except for potassium deficiency (see below) these are not commonly a problem.

1. Impaired glucose tolerance is produced by thiazides so that diabetic control may be altered. After six years of continuous thiazide therapy about 10% of patients have been found to develop a frankly diabetic type of glucose tolerance curve. The risk increases with age and degree of obesity or if the patient is a latent diabetic. The effect is probably dose related and usually reversible. Rarely the hyperosmotic non-ketotic diabetic syndrome is precipitated by treatment with thiazides or

Table 14.3 Some thiazide and related diuretics currently used in the UK

Approved name	*Proprietary name*	*Usual daily dose range (mg)*	*Approximate duration of action (h)*
*Chlorothiazide	Saluric	500–2000	10
*Hydrochlorothiazide	e.g. Hydrosaluric	25–100	10
*Bendrofluazide	e.g. Neo-Naclex	2.5–10	20
*Clopamide	Brinaldix	20–80	12–15
Mefruside	Baycaron	12.5–50	20–24
*Polythiazide	Nephril	1–4	24–30
*Cyclopenthiazide	Navidrex	0.25–1.0	12
*Chlorthalidone	Hygroton	50–200	48
*Hydroflumethiazide	Hydrenox	50	4–6
Metolazone	Metenix	2–50	18–25

* Suitable for treating hypertension.

frusemide. It may develop within a week or two of starting the drug. There may be no history of diabetes but subsequent control of diabetes is usually required.

2. Hyperuricaemia: competition with uric acid at the non-specific acid secretion site in the proximal tubule results in uric acid retention which, combined with a decreased extracellular fluid volume, causes a rise in plasma uric acid levels and may occasionally precipitate gout. Uricosuric agents (see p. 335) act more distally in the nephron to block reabsorption of uric acid. They are still effective during thiazide treatment, as is allopurinol.
3. Allergy and blood dyscrasias are rare but thrombocytopenia may occur from time to time.
4. Impotence has been reported in around 20% of males receiving long-term thiazide treatment for hypertension. The cause of this is not clear.

Interactions Thiazides reduce the excretion of lithium and therefore a reduced dose of lithium is required when these drugs are combined.

Xipamide (Diurexan)

This diuretic is similar in action to the thiazides. The plasma half-life is five to eight hours and the diuresis lasts about twelve hours. It has been used to treat hypertension in doses of 20 mg daily and as a diuretic in doses of 20–40 mg daily. Like other diuretics it causes uric acid retention and sometimes quite severe potassium depletion so that regular estimation of plasma potassium levels are advised.

High-ceiling or loop diuretics

These are the most potent agents currently available. They are designated high-ceiling diuretics because unlike the thiazides or other agents the dose–response curve is steep and by increasing the dose the maximal fractional sodium excretion (i.e. the fraction of sodium filtered at the glomerulus appearing in the urine) may reach 35% (see Fig. 14.3). They are called loop diuretics because they inhibit active chloride transport over the entire length of the thick ascending loop of Henle (zones II and III) and both dilution and concentration or urine are impaired. The increased delivery of sodium to zone IV results in potassium loss and alkalosis. There is usually complete reabsorption of filtered bicarbonate and hence a hypochloraemic, hypokalaemic alkalosis can develop during therapy. Frusemide and bumetanide but not ethacrynic acid have mild carbonic anhydrase inhibitory activity in the proximal tubule and when large doses are given of these drugs, an alkaline diuresis may occur, thus preventing metabolic alkalosis. These drugs also increase urinary calcium excretion (cf. thiazides) and the hypercalciuric effect of frusemide is exploited in the treatment of hypercalcaemia (see p. 676). Frusemide but not bumetanide also increases magnesium clearance. The molecular basis of the action of these drugs is not known but it appears that their action is exerted from the luminal side of the renal tubule and thus diuresis is dependent on tubular excretion. Present theories include:

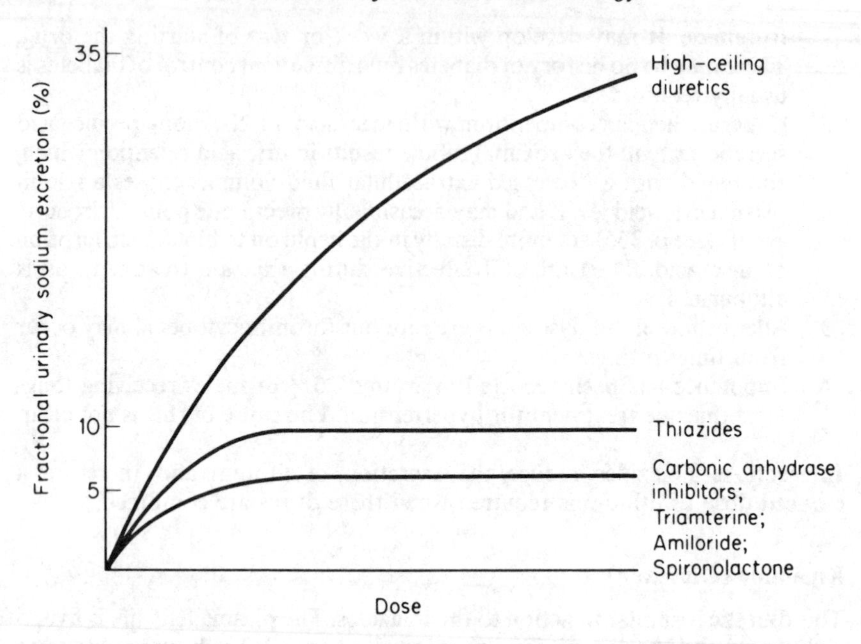

Fig. 14.3 Dose-response curves (diagrammatic) for diuretics.

1. Inhibition of $Cl^- HCO_3^-$ ATPase.
2. Inhibition of adenylate cyclase and possibly ADH.
3. Inhibition of Na^+, K^+ ATPase (unlikely).
4. Inhibition of prostaglandin action (unlikely).

Loop diuretics also inhibit the tubulo-glomerular feedback mechanism thus preventing the fall in GFR produced by some diuretics and which to some degree reduces their efficacy. An entirely separate action of loop diuretics is to increase the capacity of the vascular bed thus lowering left atrial filling pressure and improving the circulation in heart failure (see p. 368).

Frusemide (Lasix)

Frusemide is an anthranilic acid derivative which shares similarities with the thiazides.

Pharmacokinetics It is rapidly absorbed from the gut to the extent of 50–75%. It is 95% bound to the plasma protein and elimination is mainly via the kidneys, both filtration and tubular excretion being involved. After intravenous injection 77% of the dose has been excreted in the urine within 4 h and 80% at the end of 24 h. The remainder of the drug is metabolised or excreted in the faeces. The plasma $t_{1/2}$ is 1.5–3.5 h. In renal failure the $t_{1/2}$ is prolonged to 10 h or more but toxicity is unusual. In these circumstances the non-renal clearance increases and may account for up to 98% of total elimination, so that after a single dose nearly all the drug is eliminated by 24 h and accumulation is negligible. The relationship between plasma frusemide levels and diuretic response is complex, since it is the drug level in a tissue compartment which appears to govern diuresis. The range of response to a single dose of frusemide is wide and the response of an individual to a given dose may vary over a period of time. This is probably partially due to the fact that sodium depletion shifts the dose–response curve to the right (i.e. a larger dose is required to achieve a comparable sodium diuresis). The urinary frusemide concentration bears a relationship to the diuretic response.

Clinical uses Frusemide can be used orally to treat the oedema of heart failure, in doses usually between 20 and 120 mg daily. The diuresis begins about 30 min after oral dosage and lasts for about 6 h. Unlike the thiazides which lose effect below a glomerular filtration rate (GFR) of 15–20 ml/min, frusemide can produce some diuresis with a lower GFR when larger doses of 0.25–2.0 g daily may be required.

In patients with incipient acute renal failure, frusemide in doses of 250–500 mg i.v. will sometimes produce a diuresis and prevent the development of established failure. Frusemide is also given intramuscularly and intravenously in doses of 20–80 mg in the treatment of acute pulmonary oedema. Under these circumstances diuresis may commence 10 minutes after i.v. administration but relief of symptoms may even precede this and is believed to be due to the drug causing venodilation and thus lowering right ventricular filling pressure.

In refractory oedema frusemide has been administered by low-dose continuous infusion (4–16 mg/h) which allows a controlled but continuous diuresis without any adverse effects. The plasma levels of frusemide achieved by this method of administration are lower than those after a bolus dose and effective diuresis is achieved at levels below those at which extrarenal adverse effects of frusemide occur.

An alternative in refractory oedema is to combine frusemide (or bumetanide) with spironolactone or amiloride as this will decrease potassium loss and may augment the diuretic action of frusemide.

Although thiazides are the preferred diuretic in the treatment of hypertension, frusemide in an initial dose of 80 mg daily (increased as required), is sometimes effective when substituted for a thiazide in patients with resistant hypertension. It is particularly useful with impaired renal function.

Adverse effects

1. Frusemide in high doses can cause a massive diuresis: up to 35 % of the glomerular filtrate may be passed in the urine. This is followed by a rapid decrease in blood volume and in the extra-cellular fluid. Such acute hypovolaemia can be dangerous especially in those who are already debilitated. Single doses of frusemide have been shown to reduce the GFR, which may cause some slowing of the elimination of drugs which are excreted via the kidney, e.g. gentamicin. It does not appear, however, to alter the excretion rate of digoxin with which it is frequently combined.

2. Prolonged use can produce alkalosis (due to loss of chloride ions in the urine) and potassium deficiency which may predispose to digitalis toxicity.

3. Frusemide, like thiazides, may cause uric acid retention and may rarely produce acute gout.
4. Carbohydrate intolerance may occur as with thiazides.
5. Blood dyscrasias are rare.
6. Ototoxicity with hearing loss is rare and probably associated with excessively high peak plasma levels caused by too rapid intravenous injection. It is usually reversible.
7. The combination of frusemide with cephaloridine or an aminoglycoside is nephrotoxic and should be avoided.
8. The diuretic effect of frusemide may be reversed by indomethacin, salicylate and other NSAIAs.

Bumetanide (Burinex)

Bumetanide is a 3-aminobenzoic acid derivative. It has some structural similarity to frusemide in that it shares a sulphonyl group. Its actions on the kidney are very similar to those of frusemide, mainly inhibiting sodium and chloride reabsorption in the ascending limb of the loop of Henle. The resulting diuresis resembles that produced by frusemide but bumetanide causes slightly less potassium loss than frusemide. This could be related to the much weaker carbonic anhydrase inhibition produced by bumetanide. Its duration of action (4–6 h) is even shorter than that of frusemide (6–8 h). Bumetanide probably inhibits the same mechanisms as frusemide and their actions are not additive.

Pharmacokinetics It is almost completely and rapidly absorbed from the gut and circulates mainly (95%) bound to protein. Bumetanide is partly metabolised and partly excreted unchanged via the kidneys, some 65% of the dose being passed in the urine within 24 h. The plasma $t_{1/2}$ is 1.5 h. In renal failure, although excretion is greatly reduced, plasma levels still fall at normal rates. The reason for this is not known.

Clinical uses It may be used as a substitute for frusemide but is more powerful on a weight-for-weight basis (1 mg being equipotent with 40 mg frusemide at low to moderate doses but, because of non-parallelism of the dose–response curves of the two drugs, at high doses such as are used in chronic renal failure this ratio changes to 1 : 20). The oral dose is 1–4 mg, the intravenous dose is 0.5–2 mg. Its extremely short duration of effect may enable the timing of diuresis to be tailored to suit the life style of the patient, e.g. a dose taken in the early evening will not produce nocturia and may be used to prevent paroxysmal nocturnal dyspnoea.

Adverse effects are similar to those of frusemide but in addition muscle pain has been reported.

Ethacrynic acid (Edecrin)

Ethacrynic acid differs structurally from frusemide and possesses an unsaturated group capable of binding with tissue sulphydryl groups. It probably inhibits proximal tubular sodium reabsorption (zone I) to some degree as well as affecting the ascending loop of Henle like the other high-ceiling diuretics. The increased sodium load at zone IV results in increased urinary potassium loss. Urinary calcium loss is also enhanced (cf. thiazides and frusemide).

Pharmacokinetics Ethacrynic acid is rapidly absorbed from the gut. It is largely protein bound in the plasma and is partly excreted via the kidney and partly metabolised in the liver.

Clinical uses Ethacrynic acid is used in the same circumstances as frusemide. The clinical dose is 50–400 mg orally or 50 mg intravenously.

Adverse effects In addition to those of frusemide, ethacrynic acid more frequently causes gastro-intestinal disturbances (including haemorrhage, which is severe in 4.5% of patients receiving the drug) and occasionally deafness if large doses are given. It is rather more liable to produce side effects than frusemide and is therefore considerably less popular.

Potassium sparing diuretics

With most diuretics the increased urinary excretion of sodium ions is accompanied by increased excretion of potassium. This results from greater secretion of potassium at the sodium/potassium exchange site in the distal tubule (zone IV). In addition to a high concentration of sodium in the tubular fluid following the use of diuretics, hyperaldosteronism, which is often found in oedematous states, may augment potassium loss.

Potassium depletion can be troublesome in certain situations so that diuretics which do not cause potassium loss are useful. They are not very powerful, however, but they can be combined with other diuretics.

Amiloride (Midamor)

Amiloride probably prevents sodium diffusing into the tubular cells at distal tubular sites and thus prevents potassium exchange. There is no evidence that it has any effect on the renal action of aldosterone. If combined with a thiazide or high-ceiling diuretic it inhibits the loss of potassium caused by these drugs.

Pharmacokinetics Only 20% is absorbed after oral administration. It is not given intravenously since it can cause severe hypotension by this route, probably via histamine liberation. It is not metabolised and is excreted unchanged by the kidneys, the plasma $t_{1/2}$ being 6 h.

Clinical uses Amiloride is given in doses of 10–20 mg and the diuresis lasts about 24 h. It is frequently combined with the thiazides or loop diuretics to reduce potassium loss. It has a hypotensive action similar to the thiazides.

Adverse effects The main danger with this drug is potassium retention leading to dangerous hyperkalaemia. Plasma potassium and blood urea should be monitored as it may cause a fall in the glomerular filtration rate in patients with impaired renal function. Diabetics also seem especially prone to hyperkalaemia and in the elderly both hyperkalaemia and hyponatraemia may occur particularly if it is combined with a thiazide (i.e. Moduretic). Supplementary potassium should not normally be given. Serum uric acid levels may rise with amiloride treatment.

Triamterene (Dytac)

This is a substituted pteridine with only weak natriuretic properties, the maximum fractional excretion of sodium being less than 2%. It acts at the sodium–potassium exchange site (zone IV) in the distal tubule but not by aldosterone antagonism. It can be used like amiloride in conjunction with thiazides or loop-diuretics to potentiate their diuretic effect and to prevent hypokalaemic alkalosis.

Pharmacokinetics Absorption after oral administration is rapid (the drug is not used parenterally). It is rapidly metabolised, 90% of the drug circulating as metabolites, and both drug and metabolite appear in the urine and bile. The plasma $t_{1/2}$ is 1.5–2 h. Diuresis starts within 2 h of administration and is complete within 8–10 h.

Clinical uses As for amiloride. The dose is 100 mg twice daily.

Adverse effects As for amiloride.

Spironolactone (Aldactone)

Aldosterone promotes sodium retention and potassium loss by increasing the amount of sodium exchanged for potassium in the distal tubule. Excess loss of potassium results in metabolic alkalosis because hydrogen ions pass from the extracellular fluid into the cells to replace lost potassium, and thus the ratio of H^+/HCO_3^- in the extracellular fluid is decreased.

Spironolactone is structurally similar to aldosterone and competes with it at zone IV in the distal tubule. It has no intrinsic action on the receptors and is a competitive inhibitor. It is thus ineffective after adrenalectomy.

In normal subjects spironolactone has little diuretic effect, but in patients whose excess aldosterone production plays an important part in the genesis of their sodium retention and oedema, spironolactone increases sodium and water excretion and conserves potassium.

Pharmacokinetics It is rapidly metabolised after administration and unchanged spironolactone has not been detected in plasma or urine. The principal metabolite is *canrenone* which is also a mineralocorticoid antagonist and is probably the active metabolite mainly responsible for the diuretic effects of spironolactone, although other metabolites also contribute to the effect. The plasma $t_{1/2}$ of canrenone is about 10 h.

Clinical use Spironolactone is given orally. It has a weak action when given alone and is therefore combined with other diuretics in the treatment of refractory oedema, particularly that due to the nephrotic syndrome or cirrhosis of the liver. The dose is 25–50 mg three times daily. It is used occasionally to treat hypertension particularly when hyperaldosteronism is believed to be the cause. In these circumstances it may be combined with a thiazide diuretic. In general its potassium sparing effect is more useful than its hypotensive or diuretic action.

Adverse effects Hyperkalaemia may occur in patients with impaired renal function and spironolactone should be avoided in these cases. It is perhaps less likely to cause dangerous hyperkalaemia than amiloride or triamterine, since as the plasma potassium concentration increases, aldosterone secretion increases and the spironolactone effect diminishes. Nausea may be a problem. In women it has a weak androgenic action, producing hirsutism and menstrual irregularities, and gynaecomastia may develop in men, presumably because of its steroid structure resembling progesterone. It may also interfere with renal tubular secretion of digoxin and can cross-react in some digoxin immunoassays, again because of its structural resemblance to digoxin. The healing action of carbenoxolone on gastric ulcers is abolished.

Ataxia, mental confusion and drowsiness have occasionally been reported with administration of large doses.

Osmotic diuretics

Osmotic diuretics undergo glomerular filtration but are only very poorly reabsorbed from the renal tubular fluid. Their main diuretic action is exerted on the proximal tubule. This section of the tubule is freely permeable to water and under normal circumstances sodium is actively reabsorbed with an isosmotic quantity of water. However, the presence of another solute prevents some of the water being reabsorbed from the tubular fluid. As the proximal tubule is a major site of water reabsorption more water together with sodium passes through the loop of Henle to the distal tubule, where some sodium exchanges with potassium at zone IV. The result is an increase in urine volume with excretion of increased amounts of sodium and potassium. They also exert an effect by 'washing-out' the medullary osmotic gradient, resulting in less water absorption from the thin descending loop of Henle and collecting duct. An excellent example of an osmotic diuresis in clinical medicine is the diuresis followed by dehydration with sodium and potassium depletion which occurs in diabetic ketosis, where excess glucose in the renal tubule acts as an osmotic diuretic.

Mannitol

Mannitol is an alcohol. It is poorly absorbed from the intestine and must be given intravenously. It is not metabolised in the body but is filtered by the renal glomerulus and is not reabsorbed from the tubules, thus acting as an osmotic diuretic.

Clinical uses Osmotic diuretics may be used to increase urine flow to help eliminate a poison which is excreted via the kidneys and in impending acute renal failure. However, the use of osmotic diuretics in this situation has largely been replaced by loop diuretics.

It must be remembered that an infusion of mannitol will increase the plasma volume. This makes it unsuitable for the treatment of most causes of oedema including cardiac failure. Repeated infusions must not be given unless it produces a diuresis, as there will be gross expansion of the plasma volume which may cause heart failure and this will be difficult to relieve.

Mannitol is given intravenously as a 10% or 20% solution and a single infusion contains between 25 and 50 g. Infusion may be repeated if it produces a satisfactory diuresis.

Osmotic diuretics are also used in other circumstances, since because they do not enter cells or some anatomical areas, e.g. eye, brain, when given as a concentrated solution water leaves cells down the osmotic gradient. This 'dehydrating' action is used in two circumstances:

(a) Reduction of intraocular pressure preoperatively in closed-angle glaucoma. Urea (1.5 g/kg) intravenously or glycerol (1.5 g/kg orally) are used for this purpose as well as mannitol.
(b) Reduction of intracranial pressure in conditions such as head injury or brain tumour.

Other agents

1. Demeclocycline (see p. 722)

This drug inhibits adenyl cyclase in the renal medulla which responds to antidiuretic hormone and thereby produces a nephrogenic diabetes insipidus.

It has been used to treat water retention due to inappropriate production of antidiuretic hormone and in patients with resistant oedema complicating cirrhosis of the liver or cardiac failure. The dose is 1.2 g daily.

Side effects Demeclocycline may produce deterioration of renal function and increased loss of sodium in the urine. Electrolytes and renal function should therefore be monitored during treatment.

2. Combined diuretic preparations

The fixed combination of a thiazide or loop diuretic with a potassium sparing diuretic is sometimes useful. The main object of these combinations is to prevent potassium loss but the addition of the potassium sparing diuretic may increase the diuresis. They may suit patients with stable and well defined diuretic requirements. A number of combined preparations is available:

Hydrochlorothiazide 25 mg + triamterene 50 mg (Dyazide)
Hydrochlorothiazide 50 mg + amiloride 5.0 mg (Moduretic)
Benzthiazide 25 mg + triamterene 50 mg (Dytide)
Hydroflumethiazide 25 mg + spironolactone 50 mg (Aldactide)
Frusemide 40 mg + amiloride 5.0 mg (Frumil)

It is important that the prescriber does not overlook the actions of the constituents in these preparations. Both hyperkalaemia and sodium depletion can occur particularly in the elderly, in diabetics and in those with impaired renal function.

3. A number of other drugs possess diuretic properties but are rarely used for this purpose today. These include:

(a) **Organic mercurials** (e.g. mersalyl) which were once the only powerful diuretic agents available but have now been superseded by loop diuretics. They act by enzyme inhibition (probably by combination with sulphydryl groups) throughout the nephron. They do not cause significant potassium loss or hyperuricaemia but result in a hypochloraemic alkalosis. All effective mercurials require parenteral administration.

(b) **GFR raising agents** such as caffeine, theophylline and dopamine which work (in part) by efferent arteriolar dilatation and/or efferent arteriolar constriction. Dopamine additionally acts by redistributing intrarenal blood flow to cortical nephrons (see p. 383).

Diuretics and potassium deficiency

Most of the diuretics which have been described cause an increase in urinary potassium and might be expected to produce some degree of potassium depletion.

Over the last two decades there have been a number of investigations aimed at establishing the degree of depletion and methods of avoiding it, but the results have been conflicting. Much depends on the method used in assessing potassium deficiency.

In the adult the total body potassium amounts to about 3500 mmol and 90% of that is intracellular. The daily intake is about 60–80 mmol daily and a roughly similar amount is excreted in the urine. The plasma potassium represents only a small fraction (0.4%) of the total body potassium and unfortunately changes in plasma potassium concentration do not necessarily reflect total body or intracellular potassium. The latter can only be assessed by isotope exchange using ^{42}K, or by using a whole-body counter which estimates the natural isotope ^{40}K, both methods being outside the usual range of clinical investigation.

Diuretic treatment causes an initial fall of plasma potassium over 1–2 weeks, thereafter a new steady state is established. The average fall in plasma potassium is 0.6 mmol/l on a moderate dose of thiazide and 0.3 mmol/l on a moderate dose (40–80 g) of frusemide. In treating hypertensives with thiazide less than 10% have plasma potassium levels of less than 3.0 mmol/l. Patients with mild heart failure show similar changes and these changes rarely cause any symptoms.

There are, however, certain patients who are at risk of developing more serious hypokalaemia

(a) Those on high doses of diuretics. Hypokalaemia is continuously dose related.
(b) Those with a low potassium intake—elderly and impoverished.
(c) High aldosterone production, i.e. cirrhosis—when hypokalaemia may precipitate coma, nephrotic syndrome, severe cardiac failure.
(d) Concurrent potassium-losing treatment, i.e. steroids, carbenoxolone, chronic laxative use.

In addition even relatively mild potassium depletion will exacerbate the toxicity of digitalis and perhaps incur the risk of serious arrhythmias following myocardial infarction.

Against this rather confused background a practical approach is:

1. In hypertensive patients on small doses of diuretics and taking a full mixed diet potassium replacement is not usually required. The plasma potassium should be estimated after two months of treatment as a low level (< 3.0 mmol/l) may be found occasionally and replacement treatment is justified.
2. In congestive cardiac failure and the nephrotic syndrome the plasma potassium should be monitored regularly and replacements given as required. Patients on digitalis should receive replacements.
3. Patients with cirrhosis should receive replacements.
4. Patients on diuretics who develop cardiac arrhythmias or who have a myocardial infarct should have their plasma potassium levels kept above 4.5 mmol/l.
5. Patients with other risk factors should be monitored and given replacements as required.

Potassium replacement

There are two ways of replacing potassium

(a) *Potassium supplements* (Table 14.4) to be effective 30–50 mmol of potassium daily is required. Combined diuretic and potassium tablets are inadequate as they contain so little potassium (usually 7–8 mmol). It is necessary to give potassium either as an effervescent or slow-release preparation as potassium chloride tablets cause ulceration and stricture formation in the small bowel. The preparations in Table 14.4 cause nausea but only rarely small bowel ulceration.

Table 14.4 Some potassium supplements

Proprietary name	*Constituent*	*Potassium content*	*Presentation*
Kay-Cee-L	Potassium chloride 75 mg in 10 ml	1 mmol K/ml	Liquid
Kloref	Potassium bicarbonate 455 mg Potassium chloride 140 mg	6.7 mmol K/tab	Effervescent tab
Kloref-S	Potassium chloride 500 mg Potassium bicarbonate 1.35 g	20 mmol K/sachet	Sachet
Slow K	Potassium chloride 600 mg	8 mmol K/tab	Slow-release tab
Leo K	Potassium chloride 600 mg	8 mmol K/tab	Slow-release tab

The diet can be supplemented by foods with a high potassium content such as meat, milk, orange, sprouts, leeks, nuts, instant coffee and concentrated fruit juices.

(b) *Potassium sparing diuretics* An alternative is to combine a thiazide or loop diuretic with amiloride or spironolactone. This is more effective in maintaining body potassium in the normal range but it is more expensive than supplements (see p. 503).

Hyperkalaemia can develop both with potassium supplements and with potassium sparing diuretics. This is particularly liable to occur in patients with impaired renal function and in the elderly and regular estimations of plasma potassium are advised. In general supplementary potassium and potassium sparing diuretics should not be combined owing to the risk of hyperkalaemia.

Intravenous potassium

This is usually given in the form of potassium chloride and is used either to maintain body potassium in patients receiving intravenous feeding or to restore potassium levels in severely depleted patients. It is difficult to deal fully with the management of intravenous potassium because much depends on individual circumstances. There are, however, several general rules:

1. The main danger of intravenous potassium is hyperkalaemia, which can cause any type of arrhythmia, including cardiac arrest. A plasma level above 7.0 mmol/l is highly dangerous. Neuromuscular weakness progressing to flaccid quadriplegia and respiratory paralysis are rare manifestations of hyperkalaemia.
2. Potassium should be given by infusion and the maximum rate should not exceed 10 mmol/h unless there is severe depletion when 20 mmol/h can be given with plasma level and if possible ECG monitoring.
3. A 24 h infusion usually should not exceed 120 mmol unless there is severe depletion. It has been found that there is a circadian variation in response to potassium infusion and that increase in the plasma potassium level is higher (sometimes by as much as 40%) when the infusion is given at midnight than when it is administered at midday. This appears to be unrelated to changes in aldosterone secretion. The clinical implications of these observations have not yet been assessed but special caution may be necessary when potassium infusions are administered at night.
4. Plasma levels of potassium should be monitored regularly.
5. Great care is required if there is impaired renal function.
6. Potassium should not be combined with blood (because of the danger of haemolysis), mannitol, aminoacids or lipids (it may cause precipitation).

It should be recalled that in the experience of the Boston Collaborative Drug Surveillance Program, the administration of potassium was associated with an incidence of 12 adverse effects per 100 exposures.

Treatment of hyperkalaemia

The effects of an abnormal intracellular/extracellular K^+ ratio may be counteracted by:

(a) Calcium injection to antagonise the cardiac membrane effects of hyperkalaemia. 10–30 ml of 10 % calcium gluconate may be given over 5 min with electrocardiographic monitoring. Calcium ions decrease the membrane threshold potential, thereby widening the difference between threshold and membrane potentials and thus decreasing membrane excitability. The beneficial effects are transient, however, if hyperkalaemia is not also reduced by some other method.
(b) Glucose and insulin may be given to shift excess potassium into the cells. Over 30 min 200–500 ml of 10 % glucose is given accompanied by 10 units of soluble insulin. Over the course of an hour the plasma potassium may fall by 1–2 mmol/l and this persists for several hours.
(c) Sodium bicarbonate (100–150 mmol) given intravenously also shifts potassium into cells. This method is particularly valuable when acidosis is present but is also effective in patients with normal acid–base balance. The effect occurs within an hour of administration and persists for several hours thereafter.
(d) Ion-exchange resins such as Resonium A may be used. This is sodium polystyrene sulphonate which exchanges sodium for potassium. It is given as a retention enema (30 g) or by mouth (15 g, 3 or 4 times daily). Unlike the other methods detailed above this drug removes potassium from the body rather than altering its distribution. This effect usually begins about an hour after administration. In a few patients the sodium ion exchanged for potassium may lead to sodium overload and heart failure. For such cases a Calcium Resonium is available.

Diuretics and Magnesium Deficiency

Magnesium depletion with low plasma levels can occur with the use of loop diuretics but not with amiloride or spironolactone. Alcoholism, a diet low in magnesium and a soft water supply are said to be exacerbating factors. Magnesium and potassium may be linked under these circumstances and there is some evidence that correction of potassium deficiency is impeded by coexistent magnesium deficiency.

The most important clinical features of magnesium deficiency are increased cardiac excitability with ventricular arrhythmias and refractory atrial fibrillation. Digitalis toxicity is increased. Other symptoms are depression and muscle weakness. The serum magnesium level is usually below 0.7 mmol/l, but cellular depletion can exist with normal plasma levels. The deficiency can be corrected by giving magnesium sulphate as 2 ml of a 50 % solution (1 ml = 2 mmol Mg) i.m. but this may be painful, or it can be diluted and given as an intravenous infusion. The usual daily dose is 16 mmol Mg, modified in the light of the clinical condition. Magnesium sulphate can also be given orally in a dose of 2.5 g twice daily but it may cause diarrhoea.

TREATMENT OF OEDEMA

Oedema is excess fluid in the tissue spaces and is subsequent to an increase in the volume of the extracellular space. Sodium and its associated anions chloride and bicarbonate are the principal electrolytes of this space, and the volume of the extracellular space is directly related to the amount of sodium in the body. It follows, therefore, that although the development of oedema may be due to several disorders each with its own mechanisms, the most important factor is retention of sodium ion by the kidney. Treatment with diuretic drugs is aimed at reversing this process and encouraging the renal excretion of sodium and water.

Oedema occurs in three important diseases:

1. Cardiac failure

The causes of oedema in cardiac failure are complex. The fundamental defect is a reduced cardiac output providing an inadequate circulation. This stimulates a number of homeostatic mechanisms which promote sodium and water retention by the kidney. Unfortunately the ensuing increase in extracellular volume aggravates rather than relieves the condition and is responsible for the oedema.

Although there is an increase in both extracellular fluid (ECF) volume and total body sodium, the sensors in the intrathoracic vascular bed which control ECF volume behave as if this volume were reduced. The reason for this is not clear, but the result is that the kidney retains sodium and water and several mechanisms may be involved.

1. The glomerular filtration rate may be normal in mild heart failure but it falls as the degree of failure increases. The balance between filtration and reabsorption is disturbed so that a larger proportion of filtered sodium is reabsorbed by the tubule with resulting sodium retention.
2. The circulation through the kidney is altered so that juxta-medullary nephrons with greater sodium-retaining properties receive a higher proportion of the renal blood flow.
3. Late in cardiac failure, due to low cardiac output and hypovolaemia secondary to intensive use of diuretics, the renin–angiotensin system is activated, with the release of aldosterone which increases sodium reabsorption in the distal tubule (see p. 642).
4. There is certainly another factor involved, probably within the kidney itself and it is of major importance. It is sometimes called the third factor and may be a hormone. It is largely concerned with proximal tubular reabsorption of sodium.

In addition to renal factors, the rise in hydrostatic pressure in the capillaries causes fluid to be retained in the tissues by increasing the filtration pressure across the capillary wall.

In the early stages of cardiac failure sodium and water are retained in much the same proportions as isotonic saline so that there is no change in the plasma sodium concentration. Later in the disease, particularly if diuretics have been used extensively and the patient is severely ill, the plasma sodium may fall, although the oedema persists. This is due to inappropriate water retention and has several causes:

(a) The fall in GFR ensures that less sodium reaches the diluting sites for sodium reabsorption in the distal tubules (see p. 490). Thus the kidney is unable to generate enough dilute urine to prevent water retention (fall in free-water clearance).

(b) Both thiazides and high-ceiling diuretics interfere with the diluting mechanism of the kidney.

(c) There may be inappropriate production of ADH causing water retention. This is secondary to extracellular volume depletion and is probably mediated via volume receptors in the right atrium.

(d) Sodium ions may pass into cells, thus causing a fall in the extracellular sodium concentration (see 'Sick-Cell Syndrome' below).

Which of these factors is most important in heart failure is debated and it may well vary from patient to patient.

The other important electrolyte disturbance which may occur in heart failure is that potassium tends to replace sodium as the chief cation in the urine and this leads to potassium depletion. There are several reasons for this:

1. In advanced cardiac failure, although the total extracellular space is large, this consists of mainly fluid which is in the tissue spaces. The functional extracellular volume, including the blood volume, may be diminished and this is sensed by volume receptors which cause further stimulation of the renin–aldosterone axis with ensuing potassium loss.

2. Although a fall in GFR and avid reabsorption of sodium at the proximal sites in the renal tubule means that less sodium is presented at the sodium–potassium exchange site this is nearly all exchanged for potassium due to excess aldosterone.

3. Prolonged hypoxia and perhaps other metabolic disturbances which occur in chronic severe cardiac failure may interfere with the sodium–potassium pumps which maintain sodium and potassium gradients across the cell membranes. The result is a leakage of potassium into the extracellular space, and ultimate excretion by the kidneys, while sodium is lost from the extracellular space into the cells. This is sometimes called the 'Sick-Cell Syndrome'.

Treatment Cardiac oedema is treated by improving the function of the heart (see p. 368) and by diuretics and occasionally salt restriction. Thiazides are adequate for mild congestive failure, although small doses of high-ceiling diuretics are frequently used. In more severe congestive failure high-ceiling diuretics become essential. With these diuretics supplementary potassium will be required, or they may be combined with a potassium-retaining diuretic.

Although relief of oedema is the objective treating cardiac failure, it is important not to overtreat the patient as there is a risk of reducing the blood volume with subsequent activation of the homeostatic sodium-retaining and water-retaining systems, thus producing a vicious circle. Intermittent diuretic therapy may be useful because the days between diuretic administration allow the patient to make homeostatic adjustments to the altered electrolyte balance.

In acute left-ventricular failure with pulmonary oedema a rapid diuresis can be produced by giving frusemide 10–40 mg or bumetanide 0.5–1.0 mg intravenously.

In mild cases of hyponatraemia with oedema the fluid intake should be restricted to 750–1000 ml daily. More severe cases are difficult to treat unless the cardiac function can be improved. If facilities are available excess water can be removed by dialysis.

2. Nephrotic syndrome

The primary fault in this disorder is protein loss from the plasma through the glomeruli. The osmolality of the plasma falls and water passes from the circulation into the tissue spaces, producing oedema. In addition, the fall in blood volume stimulates the renin–aldosterone mechanism and leads to sodium retention and potassium loss by the kidney.

Treatment The most effective way of treating the nephrotic syndrome is to reverse the process by stopping the leakage of protein through the glomerulus. This can sometimes be achieved by giving corticosteroids or immunosuppressive drugs. In other types of nephrotic syndrome where treatment is only symptomatic, diuretics can play a part. Usually this treatment needs to be aggressive and a high-ceiling diuretic such as frusemide is combined with spironolactone, which is used to minimise the effects of the secondary hyperaldosteronism. Some patients become very oedematous and yet are hypovolaemic: in these cases powerful diuretics should only be used during an infusion of plasma or purified protein fraction.

3. Cirrhosis of the liver

Fluid retention in cirrhosis of the liver usually takes the form of ascites, the localisation of the fluid being due to obstruction of the portal vein, leading to exudation within the portal drainage area. Other important factors are the low level of plasma albumin due to failure of synthesis in the damaged liver, hyperaldosteronism due to stimulation of receptors sensing decreased circulatory volume and failure of the diseased liver to break down aldosterone and possibly antidiuretic hormone. Dependent oedema may also occur in this condition.

Treatment Diuretics should be used with care in treating oedema and ascites in cirrhosis of the liver as they may cause serious complications. Increased production of aldosterone is common and the use of thiazides or high-ceiling diuretics may lead to potassium depletion and alkalosis, which in cirrhosis is often associated with increasing confusion and ultimately coma. The effects of hypokalaemia and alkalosis are complex, but one result is the increased production of ammonia by the kidney which could be expected to contribute to the development of hepatic encephalopathy. A further factor in the development of coma may be an alteration in amino-acid metabolism. Diuretics increase protein catabolism and this is followed by an increase in the blood levels of aromatic amino acids which are normally metabolised by the liver, and to a fall in the branched chain amino acids. One result of this is an increased cerebral uptake of tryptophan which can precipitate encephalopathy. Amiloride or spironolactone can be used, but if these are not adequate, more powerful diuretics may be given with full potassium supplements. It is important to monitor plasma potassium levels. Salt-free albumin (25–50 g/day intravenously) given slowly may occasionally improve the response to diuretics.

DRUGS WHICH ALTER THE URINARY pH

Acidifying drugs

(a) **Ammonium chloride**

Ammonium chloride is given orally and after absorption the ammonium ion is converted to urea by the liver with the release of hydrogen and chloride ions. This produces an acidosis to which the kidney responds by excreting acid urine. There is also increased excretion of chloride ions together with a balancing cation (largely sodium) and water which results in a transient diuresis.

Clinical uses Ammonium chloride is occasionally used to produce an acid urine for experimental purposes or in treating renal infection in doses of 8–12 g daily. It is a gastric irritant and is given as enteric-coated tablets. The elimination of some basic drugs such as morphine and amphetamine is enhanced by acidification of the urine.

Adverse effects Ammonium chloride should not be given in hepatic failure as the toxic ammonium ion will not be converted to urea but will be released into the circulation and may precipitate encephalopathy. It will also exacerbate the acidosis of renal failure. It is a gastric irritant and causes nausea, vomiting and abdominal pain.

(b) **Vitamin C (ascorbic acid)**

Vitamin C given in large doses is largely excreted in the urine and will acidify it. It is less dangerous than ammonium chloride. A dose of at least 2.0 g daily is required (see p. 570).

If the urine is alkaline because of infection by a urea-splitting organism, such as *Proteus* which liberates free ammonia into the urine, then acidifying drugs cannot acidify the urine and should not be used since systemic acidosis may result if the dosage is increased.

Alkalinising drugs

Citrate and bicarbonate

These substances given as the sodium or potassium salts (e.g. potassium citrate mixture B.P.C.) tend to cause an alkalosis and this will produce an alkaline urine. They are given orally, the usual dose being 3 g 2 hourly for bicarbonate until the urine pH is 7 and 3–6 g every 4–6 h for the citrate. Potassium must be avoided in renal failure as retention of potassium ions may cause hyperkalaemia. In general these mixtures are nauseating and unpleasant to take: sodium bicarbonate is probably best tolerated.

Clinical uses Alkalinisation of the urine may be used to treat renal infection, to give symptomatic relief for the dysuria of 'cystitis', and to prevent the formation of uric acid stones. Alkalinisation may increase the efficacy of sulphonamides and aminoglycosides in the urine and discourages the growth of some bacteria, e.g. *E. coli.* The use of forced alkaline diuresis to increase urinary excretion of some drugs is discussed on p. 876.

DRUGS AND RENAL DISEASE

(A) Chemical agents can interfere with renal function in several ways. These include the production of acute tubular necrosis, acute interstitial nephropathy and ureteric obstruction.

1. **Acute tubular necrosis** resulting in acute renal failure can be caused by a wide range of substances which can act as nephro-toxins or as haemolysins. Nephrotoxins include:
   - metals (e.g. mercury, lithium, gold) and their compounds;
   - organic solvents (e.g. carbon tetrachloride, chloroform, tetrachloroethylene);
   - radiocontrast media (bunamiodol);
   - glycols (e.g. ethylene glycol);
   - antimicrobials (e.g. aminoglycosides, polymyxin B, colistin, amphotericin B, cephaloridine (especially with frusemide));
   - miscellaneous (e.g. methoxyflurane, EDTA, penicillamine, captopril, desferrioxamine, phenols, paraquat).

Substances which produce haemolysis may destroy normal red cells (arsine, potassium chlorate) or lyse only cells lacking G6PD (see p. 111). Acute haemolysis may lead to anuria.

2. **Acute interstitial nephropathy** is a form of acute renal failure, which is usually a consequence of bacterial infection. The condition is also occasionally seen in allergic drug reactions due to penicillin, methicillin, rifampicin and phenindione.

3. **Ureteric obstruction** can produce post-renal failure. This may be a result of periureteric fibrosis (e.g. due to methysergide, practolol) or blockage of the ureter with drug (e.g. sulphonamide) or by necrotic tissues (e.g. phenacetin-induced papillary necrosis).

4. **Chronic renal damage** by drugs can be due to ureteric obstruction, analgesic nephropathy (see p. 307), systemic lupus and nephrotic changes. Systemic lupus erythematosus may be induced by hydralazine, isoniazid, procainamide and the penicillins. The nephrotic syndrome can be produced by many agents:

sodium aurothiomalate	probenecid
D-penicillamine	tolbutamide
perchlorate	troxidone
phenindione	inorganic and organic mercury compounds

(B) Drugs in established renal failure can lead to an exacerbation of symptoms. Thus tranquillisers and hypnotics can precipitate the neurological crises of uraemia (such as fits or coma).

The tetracyclines not only aggravate uraemia by their anti-anabolic action on protein metabolism but rarely may cause cortical necrosis. Outdated, degraded tetracycline may damage the tubules producing a Fanconi syndrome. The excretion of many antibiotics is impaired and their toxicity is thus enhanced. The danger of ototoxicity and nephrotoxicity of the aminoglycosides is increased unless the size or frequency of the dose is adjusted according to blood levels. Kanamycin and neomycin may also cause proximal tubular damage. Amphotericin B commonly causes renal vasoconstriction. Nitrofurantoin should not be given in renal failure because of the increased likelihood of vomiting and peripheral neuropathy. Nalidixic acid and the penicillins are usually well excreted in renal insufficiency. The sulphonamides may be normally excreted but cotrimoxazole should be given less frequently in advanced disease and both drugs may occasionally cause irreversible deterioration in renal function.

Methods of adjusting drug regimes in renal failure based upon a knowledge of the altered kinetics in renal impairment are discussed in Chapter 5.

DRUGS AFFECTING THE URETERS AND BLADDER

Ureters

The sympathetic nerve supply to the ureters arises from the synaptic relay cells in the coeliac plexus. The parasympathetic supply has a contribution from both the vagus and the pelvic splanchnic nerves. It seems that the nerves supply only the blood vessels in the wall of the ureter. The ureteric muscle itself has no nerve supply and the waves of peristalsis which propel the urine down the ureter are an inherent property of the muscle fibres and probably arise in pacemakers in the lesser calyces. It follows that drugs which modify the autonomic system will not alter ureteric activity.

Drugs used in renal colic The pain of renal colic is due to a sudden rise in pressure in the renal pelvis and ureter and is associated with the peristaltic wave. Competitive acetylcholine inhibitors such as atropine do not prevent these contractions and so do not relieve the pain of renal colic although they are sometimes given for this purpose. This pain is best treated by morphine or by pethidine (the latter used for its analgesic rather than its antispasmodic properties).

The bladder

The bladder is supplied by sympathetic fibres from the hypogastric plexus, parasympathetic fibres from the pelvic splanchnic nerves, and somatic nerves. Micturition is a spinal reflex but can obviously be inhibited by higher centres. At the start of micturition parasympathetic impulses cause the detrusor muscle to contract. This distends the posterior part of the urethra and results in reflex relaxation of the external urethral sphincter. The bladder base, neck and proximal urethra is rich in α-adrenoreceptors whilst the bladder vault has largely β-receptors.

Drugs which affect micturition

1. Drugs to decrease bladder activity

Emepronium (Cetiprin) This is a quarternary ammonium compound which is an acetylcholine antagonist. It appears to be particularly effective in reducing cholinergic activity in the bladder, thus promoting bladder relaxation and reducing the frequency of micturition. It is used therapeutically for this purpose, especially in the elderly, the usual dose being 200 mg three times daily. 400 mg may be given before going to bed if nocturnal frequency is a problem.

Adverse effects If there is marked urinary obstruction emepronium may cause retention. Its parasympathetic blocking action can give rise to a dry mouth and may exacerbate glaucoma. Prolonged sucking of the tablets can cause oral and oesophageal ulceration and they should be swallowed with water. It does not enter the CNS and so central effects are not a problem (cf. atropine).

Other drugs with cholinergic blocking effects can cause urinary retention. These include the atropine group, the phenothiazines and the tricyclic antidepressants. The latter drugs by blocking noradrenaline reuptake promote α-adrenergic stimulation and imipramine in particular is used in enuresis (dose 25 mg nightly) to cause constriction of the bladder neck. Local anaesthetic properties may also contribute to this therapeutic effect. Beta-adrenergic agonists (ephedrine, salbutamol, terbutaline) are unlikely to cause retention if administered by inhalation but may do so when given intravenously or orally. They are of little benefit in treating incontinence.

Oxybutynin produces relaxation of smooth muscle by a direct action on the muscle fibre, it also has some acetylcholine-blocking effect but this is less important. In addition, it is a mild analgesic and also a local anaesthetic. It is used to relieve frequency, urgency and urge incontinence in patients with uninhibited and reflex neurogenic bladders.

Oxybutynin is given orally, the usual dose being 5.0 mg two or three times daily. Elimination is by hepatic metabolism.

Adverse effects are those associated with anticholinergic drugs: dry mouth, blurred vision, occasionally urinary retention and constipation. It should be avoided in patients with glaucoma. Allergies have been reported.

Flavoxate (Urispas) This is a tertiary amine with a selective papaverine-like action on smooth muscle where it inhibits phosphodiesterase and increases plasma levels of cyclic AMP. It also has some local anaesthetic properties and minor analgesic effects. The dose is 200 mg 8 hourly and it is used for the relief of dysuria, urgency, incontinence and nocturia but it is of doubtful efficacy. Adverse effects are uncommon but include diarrhoea, nausea, headache and blurred vision.

Bromocriptine (see p. 610) This decreases frequency, nocturia and urgency and increases the bladder capacity possibly by its dopamine antagonism. It should be given in incremental doses to avoid nausea and vomiting beginning with 1.25 mg daily for two days and slowly increasing to 2.5 mg twice daily.

2. **Drugs to increase bladder activity**

These should never be used in the presence of severe obstruction to outflow.

Cholinergic drugs These stimulate cholinergic receptors and probably the best known is **bethanechol (Myotonine)** which has fewer nicotinic effects and is more resistant to cholinesterase than carbachol. The oral dose is 5–30 mg up to four times daily.

Anticholinesterases such as **distigmine (Ubretid)** or pyridostigmine also have a parasympathomimetic action. Distigmine is given by i.m. injection (0.5 mg) or orally 5 mg daily.

Chapter 15
THE ALIMENTARY SYSTEM AND LIVER

PEPTIC ULCERATION

This is a disease of considerable economic consequence and has been estimated to affect around 10 % of the population of western countries.

Peptic ulceration of the mucosa of the digestive tract occurs in a number of clinical settings and is not a disorder with a unitary cause. Therefore it is unlikely that a single drug will provide the answer in all cases. The aetiology of ulceration is not understood but it is clear that there are two main factors to be considered:

(a) *acid–pepsin secretion*
(b) *mucosal resistance to attack by acid and pepsin*

Recent studies show that gastric and duodenal mucosa is protected against acid/peptic digestion by a mucus layer into which bicarbonate is secreted. Damaging agents such as salicylate, ethanol and bile reduce bicarbonate and mucus secretion and impair the protective function of this layer. A theory which integrates these facts into a coherent exploration of the genesis of peptic ulcers is presently unavailable.

Acute gastric ulceration is usually multiple and can present as bleeding or may be asymptomatic and detected only at endoscopy. It appears to bear little relationship to chronic peptic ulcer disease which is a different disorder. Chronic peptic ulcers are usually single and penetrate the muscularis mucosae. Chronic gastric ulcers are associated with normal or reduced acid secretion, suggesting that impaired mucosal resistance may be involved. Qualitative changes in gastric mucus, mucosal ischaemia, biliary reflux into the stomach and gastritis are also possible mechanisms. Duodenal ulcers are associated with excessive acid production in about 50 % of cases. Other mechanisms are presumably involved as in the remainder acid output is normal.

The aims and success of therapy for this condition may be evaluated at several levels:

1. *symptomatic relief*;
2. *promotion of ulcer healing*;
3. *prevention of recurrence once healing has occurred*;
4. *prevention of complications.*

The assessment of these outcomes is difficult for several reasons:

(a) Until the advent of fibre-optic endoscopy evaluation had to rely upon imprecise criteria. For gastric ulcers healing may be assessed by barium meal, although endoscopy is more reliable. Duodenal ulceration must be endoscopically evaluated since the radiological features of scarring, spasm and active ulceration are indistinguishable. Acute mucosal erosions often cannot be detected radiologically.

(b) Symptomatic relief does not correlate with ulcer healing or occurrence. In the case of gastric ulcers it is important to exclude a malignant ulcer. In the past a satisfactory response to treatment has been regarded as diagnostic of a benign ulcer. However, the complete healing of malignant ulcers has been described during treatment with cimetidine and there is no fundamental reason for believing that such spurious healing can occur only with this drug. Endoscopy, and if necessary biopsy, is the only effective method of excluding malignancy in suspicious cases.

(c) The natural history of chronic peptic ulceration is one of remission and relapse. Spontaneous fluctuations in severity can therefore confound treatment effects. Spontaneous cure usually occurs after a period of 5–10 years of activity.

(d) A substantial placebo response is common in peptic ulceration.

Thus conclusions as to the effects of treatment should be ideally based upon a carefully conducted double-blind control including placebo in an adequate number of patients which utilises endoscopic assessment of ulcer size.

At present 85% of peptic ulcers are managed medically, the remainder being treated surgically. It should be realised that at least as many patients consult their doctors for dyspepsia in which no ulcer can be found as attend with peptic ulcer. In these ulcer-negative dyspeptic cases careful follow-up has shown that up to 50% develop ulcers over 5 years.

Since ulcers are believed to arise from imbalance between 'damaging' intraluminal and 'protective' mucosal factors, specific therapy aims to restore this balance by either reducing acid secretion or peptic activity, or by enhancing mucosal resistance.

A. DRUGS REDUCING ACID/PEPSIN ACTIVITY

H_2 receptor antagonists

The actions of histamine are mediated by two classes of receptor:

H_1 receptors mediate vasodilatation, increased capillary permeability and the triple response, itch and contraction of smooth muscle and bronchi. Antagonised by drugs such as chlorpheniramine and terfenadine (see p. 825).

H_2 receptors mediate gastric acid secretion and are also present in human heart, blood vessels and uterus (and probably brain) although their function is not clearly defined. Cimetidine and ranitidine are the two competitive H_2-receptor antagonists in present clinical use although several others have been developed. Cimetidine is a histamine derivative with a modified side chain although the imidazole ring is present; ranitidine also has a side chain differing from histamine and in addition the nucleus is a furan.

The role of histamine in controlling gastric acid secretion remains controversial. Recent studies suggest the presence on the parietal cell of separate but interacting receptors for histamine, gastrin and acetylcholine which are histamine-dependent. H_2-receptor antagonists profoundly inhibit basal and nocturnal acid output as well as secretion stimulated by histamine, gastrin and vagal activity. This suggests that histamine is the final common mediator of all these stimuli (see Fig. 15.1). Given intravenously, they inhibit histamine or pentagastrin-stimulated acid output by about 90 % (Fig. 15.2): both the volume and acid output is decreased and with a lesser decrease in pepsin secretion.

Cimetidine (Tagamet)

Cimetidine inhibits basal and nocturnal secretion as well as the response to pentagastrin, insulin, caffeine and food (see Fig. 15.2). It may act non-competitively on pentagastrin-stimulated secretion, but whatever the mechanism it is remarkably effective and reduces gastric acid secretion to about 20 % within an hour of oral administration, although pepsin secretion is not inhibited quite as much. The other effects of H_2-receptor inhibition are not observed at the clinically obtained levels of cimetidine.

Pharmacokinetics Cimetidine is well absorbed (70–80 %) orally and is subject to a small hepatic first-pass effect. Intramuscular and intravenous injections produce equivalent blood levels. The plasma $t_{1/2}$ is 2 h. Elimination is mainly renal as the unchanged compound but some is excreted as metabolites, mainly the sulphoxide. Renal tubular secretion (by the non-specific base transport carrier) occurs and its renal clearance exceeds

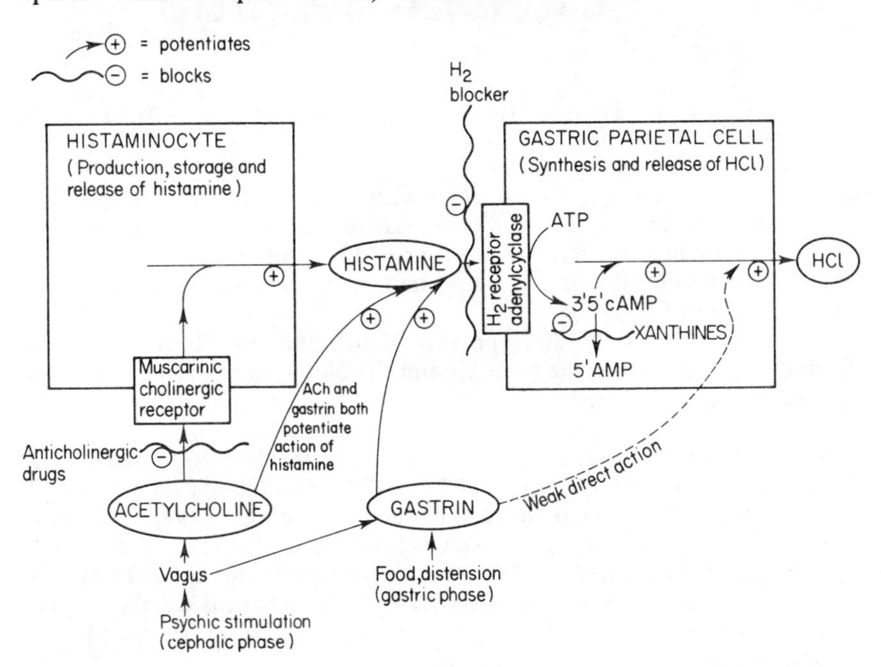

Fig. 15.1 Diagrammatic representation of the relationship between histaminocytes and parietal cells in the gastric mucosa.

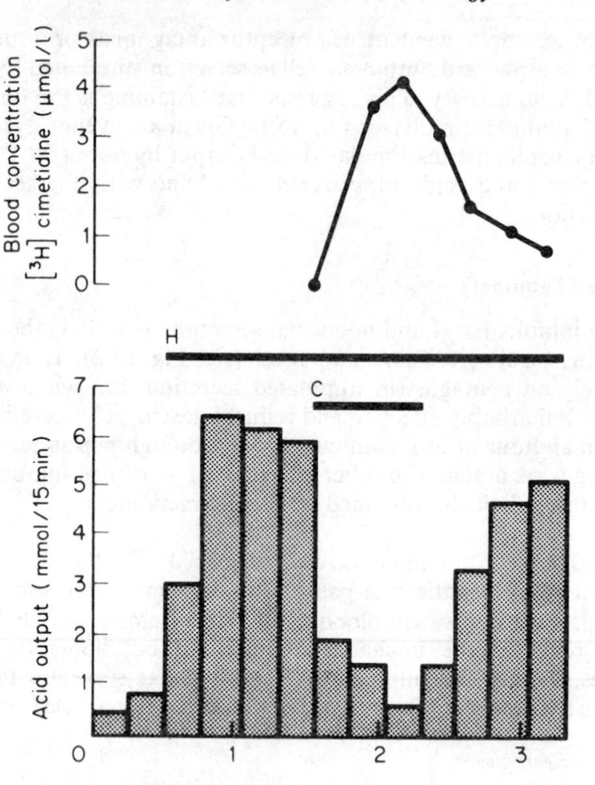

Fig. 15.2 Effect of intravenous cimetidine (C, 100 mg/h) on gastric-acid secretion stimulated maximally by histamine acid phosphate (H, 40 μg/kg/h) in a single subject (From W. L. Burland *et al.*, *Brit. J. Clin. Pharm.*, **6,** 481 (1975)).

glomerular filtration rate. Competition with renal creatinine secretion may explain the transient rise in serum creatinine that occurs during the first few weeks of cimetidine treatment. There is probably a minor excretory pathway into the gut which may become important in renal failure when the $t_{1/2}$ is prolonged up to 5 h.

Cimetidine is only 15–20% protein bound and may be removed by haemodialysis. It crosses the placenta and the blood–brain barrier, particularly in seriously ill, elderly patients.

Adverse effects Cimetidine has few adverse effects. Diarrhoea, rashes and dizziness, usually mild and transient have been reported. Although animal studies suggested that cimetidine does not enter the central nervous system, it has been detected in human cerebrospinal fluid. Patients with severe impairment of hepatic and renal clearance have high plasma cimetidine levels and under these circumstances, particularly if the patient is elderly, mental confusion has been reported. Such patients must therefore be treated with reduced doses.

Cimetidine given orally or by infusion can transiently increase serum prolactin levels but the significance of this is unknown. In animals an antiandrogenic effect has been demonstrated and *in vitro* it can weakly compete for androgen binding sites. In man no consistent effect on endocrine secretion has been found and although decreased libido and impotence have occasionally been reported during cimetidine treatment, there is no clear evidence of a causal relationship. Controlled studies have shown that earlier reports of reduced sperm counts associated with cimetidine administration were ill-founded. The only endocrine effect associated with chronic cimetidine administration is gynaecomastia which is reversible and appears with a frequency of 0.1–0.2%.

The role of H_2-receptors in the cardiovascular system is controversial and oral H_2-blockers have not been associated with cardiovascular effects. Rapid intravenous injection of cimetidine or ranitidine has rarely been associated with bradycardia, tachycardia, asystole or hypotension.

Drug interactions

1. Absorption of ketoconazole (which requires a low pH) is reduced. High doses of antacids can inhibit cimetidine absorption.
2. Metabolism of several drugs is reduced due to inhibition of cytochrome P_{450} by cimetidine which results in raised plasma drug concentrations. Interactions of potential clinical importance occur with:
   - Warfarin
   - Phenytoin
   - Theophylline
   - Lignocaine (cimetidine-induced reduction of hepatic blood flow is also a factor in this interaction)

   Other interactions of less certain clinical importance occur with:
   - Diazepam, chlordiazepoxide (but not oxazepam or lorazepam which undergo glucuronidation not oxidation)
   - Propranolol, labetalol
   - Metronidazole
   - Verapamil
   - Caffeine

   There is also evidence for raised levels of noradrenaline and reduced metabolism of endogenous aldosterone and cortisol during cimetidine treatment.
3. Renal excretion of procainamide is inhibited by cimetidine probably by competition for the non-specific basic drug transport system which secretes both procainamide and N-acetylprocainamide into the renal tubules.

Ranitidine (Zantac)

Ranitidine resembles cimetidine closely in its pharmacology although it is chemically distinct. It is 5–12 times (on a molar basis) as effective as cimetidine in inhibiting stimulated acid secretion in doses of one-fifth of those of cimetidine. This potential for usual doses of ranitidine to produce a greater inhibition of acid secretion may explain why ranitidine has been effective in some patients who have not responded to cimetidine.

Pharmacokinetics Ranitidine is well absorbed after oral administration but the bioavailability is only 50% suggesting an appreciable first-pass metabolism. Absorption is not affected by food ingestion. Like cimetidine, the half-life is about two hours and some 70% of the drug is excreted unchanged by the kidneys by tubular secretion and filtration. The plasma concentration producing 50% inhibition of gastric acid secretion is only one-fifth of the concentration of cimetidine which produces the same effect. A standard dose of ranitidine thus has a longer duration of action (about 6–8 h) since this concentration is exceeded for a longer period.

In geriatric patients the half-life is prolonged by about 50%, probably because of reduced renal excretion. In patients with liver disease the clearance is only slightly reduced and alteration in the dose is unnecessary. In severe renal failure (creatinine clearance < 20 ml/min), therapeutic levels can be achieved with half-doses of ranitidine (75 mg twice daily).

Adverse reactions There is less clinical experience as compared to cimetidine, but it produces a similar incidence of minor side effects. Unlike cimetidine, ranitidine does not bind to androgen receptors and impotence and gynaecomastia in patients on high doses has reversed when they were switched to ranitidine. Cardiovascular effects have been even more infrequently reported than with cimetidine. Small amounts of ranitidine penetrate the CNS and (like cimetidine) it can rarely cause mental confusion, mainly in the old and in patients with hepatic or renal impairment.

Drug interactions Ranitidine, perhaps because of its furan structure, apparently has lower affinity for cytochrome P_{450} than cimetidine. Interaction with warfarin has been demonstrated by some but not all studies probably because ranitidine is used in lower dosage than cimetidine. Although the metabolism of propranolol or diazepam is not altered, there is more evidence that the elimination of metoprolol and nifedipine are decreased.

Ranitidine absorption is inhibited by high doses of antacids although this may not be clinically important because of its high potency.

Clinical uses of H_2-blockers

1. *Duodenal ulcer* H_2-blockers achieve endoscopically verified healing of around 70% ulcers as compared to 30% healing in placebo-treated patients. It appears that at least 3–4 weeks of treatment are required to achieve these results although pain may be relieved within a few days. The usual course of treatment is cimetidine 400 mg twice daily after meals (this slows absorption but does not reduce bioavailability) or ranitidine 150 mg twice daily. Larger doses supplemented with other drugs may be used in resistant cases. Acid rebound after cessation of therapy does not occur when the drug is discontinued, although relapse may occur, often quite rapidly. Maintenance treatment with 400 mg cimetidine or 150 mg ranitidine at night reduces the relapse rate from 70–80% per year to about 20% but the required duration of such maintenance is unknown. If this maintenance dose is discontinued there is a risk of relapse. The question of whether an indefinitely prolonged course of therapy will be necessary is unresolved and partly depends upon the long-

term safety of H_2-blockers. Possibly where relapse is infrequent or mild, short courses of cimetidine may be best, with surgery reserved for the more troublesome relapse.

2. *Gastric ulcer* Rates of healing of around 75% have been reported together with rapid pain relief, although the associated chronic gastritis is unaffected. Cimetidine is probably more effective than carbenoxolone in this condition. Relapse may occur after stopping therapy. It is important to exclude carcinoma endoscopically since H_2-blockers can symptomatically improve malignant ulcers.

3. *Peptic oesophagitis* may be treated with 400 mg cimetidine four times a day with meals and at bed-time for 4–8 weeks, and produces considerable symptomatic improvement although endoscopic appearances may not improve so strikingly.

4. *Acute upper gastrointestinal haemorrhage and stress ulceration*, particularly in the absence of a focal lesion, is often controlled with cimetidine: the intravenous preparation is useful in these cases. It may also be given prophylactically in patients after major trauma or burns or in acute respiratory, hepatic or renal failure.

5. *Zollinger—Ellison syndrome* Cimetidine given in very large doses (up to 2 g/day) may control symptoms and heal ulcers.

6. *Replacement of pancreatic enzymes in steatorrhoea* due to pancreatic insufficiency is often unsatisfactory due to destruction of the enzymes by acid and pepsin. Cimetidine can improve bioavailability of these enzymes in such cases.

7. *In anaesthesia*, H_2-receptor blockers can be given before emergency surgery to prevent aspiration of acid gastric contents (Mendelson's syndrome).

H_2-blockers and gastric cancer

It has been suggested that chronic use of these drugs may produce gastric cancer. The hypothesis underlying this suggestion is that reduced gastric acidity could allow bacterial colonisation of the stomach by nitrate-reducing bacteria. These could produce nitrite from dietary nitrates and could form N-nitroso compounds with food amines. Some of these N-nitroso compounds are mutagenic to bacteria and resemble animal carcinogens. All of these steps could theoretically follow any anti-ulcer treatment and it is certainly the case that carcinoma of the gastric remnant has followed some ulcer operations and occurs in 0.5–20% of patients in several studies. Vagotomy, however, is not associated with this problem and similarly no causal link has been established between chronic administration of H_2-blocking drugs and gastric cancer in man or animals.

Proton pump inhibitors

Gastric acid secretion results from the activity of a hydrogen/potassium ATPase, an enzyme located at the acid-secretory face of the parietal cell and involved in the final step of proton secretion. This enzyme is relatively unique to the parietal cell and recently selective, long-acting inhibitors of this enzyme have become available for investigative use. One of these, omeprazole,has been shown to produce virtual anacidity in patients with Zollinger–Ellison syndrome and those with peptic ulcer disease resistant to other treatments. Their safety and general efficiency remain to be assessed, but further developments of this class of drug may be expected.

Antacids

Antacids produce prompt pain relief in the majority of patients. It has been the predominant view in the UK that antacids provide purely symptomatic relief, whereas in the USA there has been the opinion that they may produce healing in duodenal ulcer, although until recently there was no evidence to support this belief. Antacid therapy aims to raise intragastric pH, thereby reducing irritation by gastric acid and simultaneously inactivating pepsin. There are, however, several proteolytic enzymes in gastric secretions, some of which are active at a higher pH range than pepsin, so that this concept may be incorrect. Alkalis usually leave the stomach too quickly to be very effective and the doses given routinely usually produce only a transient reduction in gastric acidity lasting less than an hour, although pain relief lasts much longer. By continuous tablet sucking the patient with duodenal ulcer can maintain his intragastric pH near 3.0 throughout the waking hours, but to control nocturnal acid secretion an intragastric antacid drip is required. It is not easy therefore to explain why antacids relieve pain so regularly and reliably, why some patients prefer one particular antacid to another with apparently identical neutralising power or why the effect of one preparation may wane but another apparently equivalent preparation is effective.

Antacids react with gastric acid to form a neutral salt. They may be divided into:

(a) those with systemic actions which may alter the pH of the extracellular fluid, e.g.; sodium bicarbonate:
(b) those without systemic effect, e.g. magnesium trisilicate.

Clinical uses In practice the choice of antacid is not usually critical, although some have greater neutralising power (Table 15.1). Sodium bicarbonate is rapid in action but produces carbon dioxide by reacting with acid, so belching and distension often follow its use. It may produce systemic alkalosis, particularly if renal function is impaired. Calcium carbonate is also rapidly acting and produces carbon dioxide but alkalosis is unlikely. A danger is the absorption of excess calcium resulting in hypercalcaemia (*milk-alkali syndrome*) which also produces gastric hypersecretion. Magnesium salts (oxide, trisilicate, hydroxide) have a relatively slow action due to their insolubility and may produce diarrhoea. Aluminium salts (hydroxide, phosphate, glycinate) on the other hand are constipating. Aluminium ions are neurotoxic but only minimal absorption occurs from antacid formulations.

Large doses of aluminium or magnesium antacids taken at fixed intervals (30 ml, 1 and 3 h after meals and at bedtime) have been shown by trials in the

Table 15.1 Neutralising capacity (ml of 0.1 N HCl neutralised in vitro in 2 h at 37° C by 10 ml liquid antacid or 1 tablet) of some antacid preparations (Adapted from R. E. Barry and J. Ford, *Brit. Med. J.*, 1978, 1, 413.)

	Neutralising capacity
1. Liquid antacids	
Magnesium carbonate mixute B.P.C.	202
Magnesium hydroxide mixture B.P.C.	258
Magnesium trisilicate mixture B.P.C.	220
Aluminium hydroxide gel B.P.C.	255
Aludrox-SA	301
Maalox	233
Polycrol gel forte	230
Mylanta	200
2. Tablet antacids	
Magnesium trisilicate compound B.P.C.	45
Actal	84
Maalox	240
Nulacin	93
Polycrol forte	100

USA to reduce gastric acidity to a degree comparable to cimetidine, with comparable effect on duodenal ulcer healing and pain relief. Such doses are somewhat larger than the usual (10 ml as required) dosage used in the UK for symptomatic relief. Such large doses may, however, be associated with adverse effects due to alteration of bowel habit. The full regime requires an intensely obsessional patient to ensure complete compliance, and a suitcase in which to carry the drugs home. The low cost of antacids, however, makes them an attractive alternative to cimetidine.

Gastrointestinal bleeding associated with severe acute illness, e.g. respiratory failure, sepsis, renal failure, hypotension, may also be prevented in many cases by administration of antacids (preferably with control of pH to 3.5 or above as determined by pH paper). Patients who suffer haematemesis from peptic ulceration or erosions may also benefit from administration of antacids (often with cimetidine) during a trial of medical treatment.

Adverse effects Apart from systemic absorption and the effects on bowel habit these are relatively few. The presence of sodium should be remembered in patients on strict salt-free regimes to whom large amounts of antacids are given. In general the sodium content is too small to make any difference.

Drug interactions Magnesium and aluminium salts can bind other drugs, reducing the rate and extent of absorption of iron, tetracyclines, digoxin, indomethacin, cimetidine, ranitidine and levodopa, amongst others. In large doses used chronically, they can bind phosphate in the bowel, precipitating osteomalacia.

Anticholinergic drugs

These agents reduce gastric-acid secretion but also decrease gastric motility and possibly spasm produced by irritation from ulceration (hence they have been termed antispasmodics) although this latter concept may well be spurious. Cholinergic blockade interferes with both the direct cholinergic stimulation (vagus) of the parietal cells and the indirect cholinergic mechanism mediated via gastrin. The delayed gastric emptying and retention of food in the stomach could prolong the antral phase of secretion which could be a disadvantage of these drugs. Anticholinergic agents tend to decrease the volume of secretion rather than alter its composition so that the pH of the gastric juice produced is still low. In the presence of antacids (or food) this represents a smaller number of H^+ ions to be neutralised.

Historically atropine was the first to be used but a number of others such as dicyclomine (Merbentyl), poldine (Nacton) and propantheline (Pro-Banthine) followed although lack of specificity as inhibitors of gastric secretion limits their use. Subcellular studies suggest that there are different sub-classes of muscarinic receptors and organs differ in the density of these receptor groups. Progress has been made in the synthesis of more selective cholinergic antagonists and the first of these, *pirenzepine* (Gastrozepin) is now available. This is related to the tricyclic antidepressants but unlike this group of drugs it is strongly hydrophilic with poor penetration into the nervous system and so has no CNS side effects. It also binds more effectively to the subclass of muscarinic cholinergic receptors found in the gastric mucosa and exocrine glands rather than to those in the heart or smooth muscle. This results in effective inhibition of acid and pepsin secretion without significant anticholinergic effects elsewhere. It has a long half-life (12.5 h) allowing twice daily dosage and, because it does not penetrate the blood–brain barrier, has no CNS effects.

Clinical use In theory these drugs should be effective but clinical trials of the older anticholinergics have in general proved disappointing. They have been called a 'logical placebo' for peptic ulcer patients. It is usually stated that the traditional anticholinergics must be used in near toxic doses to inhibit secretion effectively. Since individual sensitivity is variable the optimum dose must be determined by dosage titration over several weeks and the final dose can be several times the manufacturer's recommended dose. When used as an adjunct to cimetidine, propantheline in low dosage (15 mg, 8 hourly) is as effective as near toxic doses. This may represent the best use of the older anticholinergics.

Pirenzepine, on the other hand, used as a single agent, has given healing rates for duodenal ulcer comparable to those of cimetidine. The dose for acute duodenal ulceration is 100 mg twice daily continued for 4–6 weeks to allow healing. In patients requiring longer-term therapy it can be given for up to 3 months but little experience of maintenance treatment exists.

Adverse effects These are predictable from their action on the parasympathetic nervous system:

(a) dryness of the mouth (decreased salivation);

(b) blurring of vision and photophobia (paralysis of accommodation and dilatation of the pupil); precipitation of glaucoma
(c) constipation;
(d) urinary retention and difficulty with micturition;
(e) tachycardia;
(f) occasionally impotence.

Contraindications include glaucoma, prostatic enlargement, coronary artery disease and pyloric stenosis. Anticholinergic drugs may alter the absorption pattern of other drugs if they are given concurrently (see Chapter 2).

Pirenzepine produces relatively few of the above effects because of its higher selectivity for the gastric mucosa but some patients may notice mild difficulty with accommodation and dry mouth.

B. DRUGS ENHANCING MUCOSAL RESISTANCE

Liquorice derivatives

There are at least three factors in liquorice root which influence ulcer symptoms and healing:

(a) a healing-rate factor;
(b) a spasmolytic agent;
(c) glycyrrhizinic acid.

Carbenoxolone (Biogastrone; Duogastrone)

This is synthesised from glycyrrhetinic acid (the aglycone of glycyrrhizinic acid). The mode of action is complex and it acts by increasing mucosal resistance without affecting acid secretion or motility: this is a local rather than a systemic effect. Its actions include:

(a) Enhanced mucus secretion, especially of that fraction adherent to and protective of the gastric mucosal cells. Changes also occur in the composition of the mucus with alteration in the balance of the various sugars incorporated into the mucopolysaccharides.
(b) Increased gastric epithelial cell life span by up to 50 % associated with reduced cell turnover.
(c) Decreased back-diffusion of hydrogen ion into the mucosa. It also prevents biliary reflux into the stomach which promotes back-diffusion of acid into the epithelium.
(d) Mild anti-pepsin action.

Pharmacokinetics Carbenoxolone is rapidly absorbed from the stomach since it is a weak acid which is highly lipid soluble in its non-ionised form. At levels above pH 2 the absorption of carbenoxolone falls and appreciable plasma levels are not found. Its absorption is therefore markedly reduced by antacids and anticholinergic drugs and it is best given one hour after meals when the acid stimulated by the meal maintains the drug in its non-ionic readily absorbed form. Given with food it may become bound to food protein which would slow absorption. Biliary obstruction is a contraindication to carbenoxolone since the bile is the major excretory route. Less than 1 % appears in the urine, the rest being eliminated in the faeces. The plasma $t_{1/2}$ is12–24 h. At therapeutic levels the drug is 99 % bound to plasma protein, 83 % to albumin, which has two distinct binding sites, the rest to plasma globulins. This binding is responsible for some drug interactions but also prevents the drug exerting its effect as an uncoupler of oxidative phosphorylation which would prevent its safe use in man.

Clinical uses

1. *Gastric ulcer* Introduced in 1962, carbenoxolone was the first drug demonstrated to have a healing effect on gastric ulcers. Used in doses of 100 mg 8 hourly after meals for 1 week, then 50 mg 8 hourly for 6 weeks or longer, it rapidly produces symptomatic relief, and healing occurs in 40–50 %.

2. *Duodenal ulcer* Carbenoxolone tablets have no effect on duodenal ulcer healing because it is absorbed from tl : stomach and exclusively excreted in the bile, thus bypassing the ulcer-bearing area of the duodenum. To overcome this problem a 'positioned-release' capsule has been designed, containing 50 mg carbenoxolone in a gelatine capsule partially denatured by formaldehyde treatment (Duogastrone). This capsule swells in the stomach and is broken up in the pyloric mill releasing its contents in the duodenum. The effects of carbenoxolone on duodenal ulcer are less impressive than the results in gastric ulceration, but some small (10–15 %) healing effect has been demonstrated.

3. *Aphthous ulceration*, and *periadenitis mucosae necrotica recurrens* may benefit from local carbenoxolone but controlled trials have not yet been performed.

Adverse effects Side effects are frequent and can be hazardous. Those particularly at risk are the elderly and patients with cardiac, renal and hepatic disease.

1. Sodium retention has been reported in up to 60 % of patients. Carbenoxolone displaces aldosterone from protein binding, thus potentiating its action. There may also be a direct renal action, since sodium retention occurs in patients after bilateral adrenalectomy. Headache, oedema, dyspnoea, cardiac failure, hypertension and epilepsy have all been reported in association with sodium retention. Blood pressure and weight should be monitored during therapy and a weight gain of more than 4–5 % or evidence of oedema are an indication to measure the plasma electrolytes.

Mild fluid retention can be corrected with a thiazide diuretic but spironolactone cannot be used since, although effective, it interferes with the ulcer-healing effects. Use of a diuretic adds further electrolyte complications to those already present in the carbenoxolone-treated patient.

2. Hypokalaemia occurs in 30–40 % of patients. This commonly presents with muscle weakness, myositis, myasthenia, myoglobinuria and peripheral neuropathy and a diagnosis of hyperaldosteronism or Guillain–Barré syndrome may be considered. The effect of hypokalaemia in patients on digoxin is potentially very serious and the plasma electrolytes must be checked weekly. Hypokalaemia is treated with potassium supplements (see p. 508).

Deglycyrrhizinated liquorice

Because of the electrolyte disturbances associated with carbenoxolone efforts have been made to produce a liquorice preparation with minimal side effects. Removal of glycyrrhizic acid produces deglycyrrhizinated liquorice (DGL) which contains the 'healing rate' factor and 'spasmolytic agent' and other substances. Caved-S tablets each contain 380 mg DGL and small amounts of bismuth subnitrate, frangula (a purgative) and mixed antacids. They are given as two tablets 8 hourly. These compounds are probably effective in the treatment of gastric ulcer but less so than carbenoxolone; their efficacy in duodenal ulceration is unproven. There are no serious side effects and DGL is probably suitable for use in patients in whom carbenoxolone is contraindicated.

Bismuth chelate (De-Nol)

Colloidal tripotassium dicitratobismuthate precipitates at acid pH to form a layer over the mucosal surface and ulcer base where it combines with the proteins of the ulcer exudate. This coat is protective against acid and pepsin digestion. It also stimulates mucus production and may chelate with pepsin thus speeding ulcer healing. Several studies show it to be as active as cimetidine in the healing of duodenal and gastric ulcers after 4–8 weeks of treatment.

Dose De-Nol elixir given as 5 ml diluted with 15 ml water 30 minutes before meals and 2 hours after the last meal of the day. This liquid has an ammoniacal, metallic taste and odour which is unacceptable to some patients, and chewing tablets (De-Noltab) can also be given, one tablet four times daily. Antacids or milk should not be taken with it since they may interfere with its action.

Adverse reactions Mainly trivial, consisting of blackening of the tongue, teeth and stools (causing confusion with melaena).

Bismuth is potentially neurotoxic and could cause encephalopathy. Urine bismuth levels rise with increasing oral dosage indicating some intestinal absorption. Although on usual doses the blood concentration remains well below the toxic threshold, this drug should not be used in renal failure or for maintenance treatment.

Sucralfate (Antepsin)

This is a basic aluminium salt of sucrose octasulphate which in the presence of acid becomes a sticky adherent paste which retains antacid efficacy. This material has an affinity for binding to the ulcer crater and thus exerts its acid neutralising properties locally at the ulcer site, unlike conventional antacid gels which form a diffusely distributed antacid dispersion. In addition it exerts antipepsin activity both by direct adsorption of pepsin and forming complexes with substrate proteins. In addition it absorbs bile salts and prevents their contact with the ulcer base. Sucralfate compares favourably with the results of cimetidine treatment of both gastric and duodenal ulcers and is equally effective in symptom relief.

Dose 1 g (1 tablet) 4 times daily for 4–6 weeks. Antacids may be given concurrently.

Adverse effects It is well tolerated but because it contains aluminium, constipation can occur and it should be used with caution in patients with renal impairment.

General management

1. *Bed rest* although no longer used for all patients, has been demonstrated to accelerate healing in gastric ulcers. No effect has been shown on healing of duodenal ulcers, although symptomatic improvement often occurs.
2. *Stopping smoking* has been proven to increase the healing rate of gastric ulcers. Giving up smoking may be more effective in the prevention of duodenal ulcer recurrence than cimetidine administration.
3. *Diet.* Traditionally this has been part of management but there is no evidence that the standard ulcer regimen influences the rate of healing of gastric or duodenal ulcers. Food is both an antacid (because of its content of amphoteric protein) and a stimulus to secretion. A meal usually neutralises the gastric contents for 30–60 min, after which the increased acid secretion predominates. The mean acidity of gastric contents sampled at half-hourly intervals in patients taking small sloppy meals ('gastric diet') is greater than when they take a normal diet, probably because the more liquid meals empty rapidly from the stomach. Patients with active ulcers are often more comfortable with frequent light meals which contribute to the neutralisation of gastric contents. Regular small 2 hourly feeds during the day produce more even buffering and lower total acidity of the gastric contents. Patients usually discover for themselves which foods upset them.
4. *Avoidance of 'ulcerogenic' drugs.* These include caffeine (as strong coffee or tea), alcohol, indomethacin, phenylbutazone, aspirin (paracetamol is a safe minor analgesic in these cases) and corticosteroids. There is some argument as to the exact role of such agents in the genesis of ulcers and their complications, but avoidance of these drugs seems prudent.

Drug-related gastric ulceration and haemorrhage

Whilst many drugs have given the clinical impression that they may produce gastric irritation, ulceration and bleeding, the evidence which incriminates them is mostly inadequate. Only five drugs have been objectively shown to cause gastric bleeding.

Aspirin used continuously as in the treatment of rheumatoid arthritis causes oozing from gastric erosions which may be multiple. The usual blood loss on aspirin is 3–6 ml/day but 10–15% of patients may lose more than 10 ml/day and develop anaemia. The Boston Collaborative Drug Surveillance Program (see p. 185) found that heavy aspirin use (4 or more days/week) was associated with gastric ulcer and major bleeding, but not with duodenal ulcer. Occasional aspirin use was not associated with peptic ulcers of any type. Annual hospital admissions for gastric ulcer and major haemorrhage were 10 and 15 per 100 000 heavy aspirin users respectively. In such individuals approximately 3% of all new peptic ulcers are due to aspirin: a small risk considering the frequent use of this drug. The old, the uraemic and the malnourished may be particularly susceptible. There are a few individuals who for unknown reasons repeatedly suffer severe bleeding when given aspirin.

The pathogenesis of peptic ulcers by aspirin is believed to occur as follows:

(a) *Action on bicarbonate/mucus protective layer* Unionised aspirin (low pH reduces drug ionisation) diffuses into the mucus layer and alters its composition. Gastric acid follows and neutralises the bicarbonate thus destroying the protective pH gradient (which may be near pH 7 at the cell surface).

(b) *Cellular effects of aspirin* Inhibition of cyclo-oxygenase inhibits formation of protective prostaglandin endoperoxides. ATP production also declines and active ion transport stops.

(c) *Intracellular damage* Acid floods into the cell and with aspirin causes further damage. Cell death releases histamine and vasodilatation, increased blood flow and capillary damage ensue with erosion and subsequent haemorrhage.

Similar effects probably occur with other *non-steroidal anti-inflammatory agents* although in general propionic and anthranilic acid derivatives (see p. 300) are safer than aspirin in this respect. They are contraindicated in patients with known active peptic ulceration. Even *paracetamol*, which does not cause erosions, has been epidemiologically associated with gastric ulcer: although aspirin sales in the UK have declined in the last decade, those of paracetamol have increased, as have hospital admissions for gastrointestinal bleeding.

Phenylbutazone unlike aspirin, rarely causes a slow loss of blood from the mucosa, and when bleeding occurs it is from radiologically demonstrable gastric ulcers which are often in unusual sites. This complication was estimated to occur in about 1 in 200 patients but this has not been the BCDSP experience. The ulcers heal when the drug is discontinued.

Indomethacin When originally administered in tablet form this drug caused serious gastric bleeding, but changing the formulation to powder in capsules reduced its incidence. In 1983 a controlled-release indomethacin tablet (Osmosin) which continuously released indomethacin by an osmotic pump principle as the tablet passed along the gut was withdrawn due to bleeding and perforation of the small bowel.

Ethanol In usual social amounts alcohol alone does not cause bleeding but increases the gastric bleeding due to aspirin. In chronic alcoholics gastric bleeding is a common problem and occurs from erosions, gastritis, chronic ulcers and occasionally oesophageal varices.

Ethacrynic acid was found by the BCDSP to produce major gastrointestinal bleeding in 4.5% of patients and this incidence was increased by concurrent administration of steroids or heparin.

Corticosteroids probably slightly increase the incidence of peptic ulcer and haemorrhage: the relative risk of such events is about doubled by steroids. This risk is dose-related and is probably increased by concurrent aspirin use.

Drugs producing gastric secretion

Direct stimulation of parietal cells is used to demonstrate achlorhydria which is typically histamine 'fast' in pernicious anaemia.

Pentagastrin is an active fragment of gastrin which, when given parenterally, has effects similar to gastrin and stimulates acid, pepsin and intrinsic factor secretion. The usual diagnostic dose is 6 μg/kg by subcutaneous injection. It may cause nausea, flushing, headache and hypotension, but these effects are rare. Repeated administration has produced hypersensitivity.

DRUGS USED FOR OESOPHAGEAL DISORDERS

Reflux oesophagitis is a common oesophageal problem: it may cause symptoms of heartburn and acid regurgitation and possibly dysphagia if a stricture forms as a result of ulceration. It is now known that the important factor determining the production of reflux is the lower oesophageal sphincter (LES) pressure, rather than the presence of a hiatus hernia, as was once thought (1 in 3 male adults have been shown to have an anatomical hiatus hernia).

Drugs which may be useful include:

1. *Metoclopramide (Maxolon)*—raises LES pressure.
2. *A mixture of alginate with antacids (Gaviscon)*—the alginate forms a viscous layer floating on the gastric contents. This reduces the amount of reflux. However, if the patient lies down the mixture migrates to the antrum and is thus ineffective. Mixtures such as Gaviscon have not been shown to be more effective than simple antacids.
3. *A mixture of a silicone with an antacid* (e.g. Asilone, which is dimethicone, aluminium hydroxide and sorbitol). These mixtures are supposed to lower surface tension and thus allow formation of large and easily expelled gas bubbles from the stomach without encouraging reflux. It is not clear why this helps in reflux: possibly the silicone coats the lower oesophagus and 'protects' it from acid/bile digestion.
4. Symptomatic relief may be obtained with *antacids*—with or without a *local anaesthetic*, e.g. Mucaine (oxethazine plus aluminium and magnesium hydroxides).
5. *Cimetidine* decreases gastric-acid production and produces symptomatic relief. However, evidence of healing (as proven by endoscopy) is lacking as yet.

Other measures which may be useful include:

(a) sleeping with the bed head raised—most damage to the oesophagus occurs at night when swallowing is much reduced and acid can remain in contact with the mucosa for long periods;
(b) avoidance of constricting clothing around the abdomen;
(c) avoid—large meals;
—alcohol and/or food before bed;
—smoking (lowers LES pressure) and coffee;
—aspirin and non-steroidal anti-inflammatory drugs;
(d) weight reduction.

Achalasia is usually treated by dilation or cardiomyotomy, but if the patient is unfit or unwilling drugs may help. Symptomatic control may be obtained from:

1. Sublingual isosorbide dinitrate 5 mg 15 minutes before meals releases spasm: glyceryl trinitrate acts too briefly to be clinical value.
2. Nifedipine, 10–20 mg sublingually before meals relaxes the cardia but may be associated with a higher incidence of side effects.
3. Hydralazine 75–200 mg/day orally has also been found effective in several small, uncontrolled studies.

INFLAMMATORY DISEASE OF THE COLON

The two commonly encountered diseases requiring special consideration are ulcerative colitis and Crohn's disease. The mediators of the inflammatory response in these diseases include kinins and prostaglandins. The latter stimulate adenyl cyclase activity which induces active ion secretion and thus diarrhoea. Synthesis of prostaglandin E_2, thromboxane A_2 and prostacyclin by the gut increases during disease activity but not during remission. Sulphasalazine inhibits prostaglandin E_2 synthesis but only its active metabolite 5-aminosalicylic acid inhibits that of thromboxane A_2 and prostacyclin. Prednisolone suppresses prostaglandin E_2 production whereas disodium cromoglycate inhibits prostacyclin and thromboxane synthesis. The role of prostaglandins in the pathogenesis of inflammatory bowel disease is, however, uncertain since flurbiprofen, a potent inhibitor of their synthesis is ineffective in colitis. Apart from correction of dehydration, nutritional and electrolyte imbalance and other non-specific treatment, the following drugs may be valuable:

1. **Corticosteroids** Prednisolone 21-phosphate or hydrocortisone given orally or intravenously are of proven value in treatment of acute colitis, or exacerbation of Crohn's disease. Topical therapy in the form of a rectal drip or enema of hydrocortisone or prednisolone is of value in milder attacks of ulcerative colitis. They are apparently less useful in Crohn's colitis. Systemic absorption of steroid may occur when it is given in this way. Synacthen and ACTH are useful for chronic management.

Steroids in doses which do not produce unacceptable side effects are useless in maintaining remission in ulcerative colitis. They may have some efficacy in this respect in Crohn's disease but their hazards are such that failure to maintain remission below 15 mg prednisolone/day necessitates adoption of alternative steroid sparing therapy such as azathioprine or even surgery.

2. **Sulphasalazine (Salazopyrin)** Sulphasalazine (salicylazosulphapyridine) is a combination of 5-aminosalicylic acid and sulphapyridine through an azo link. It is believed that it is the constituents of the molecule which are the active principles in treatment. The addition of bran or hydrophilic colloid in patients undergoing treatment with sulphasalazine increases remission rates in ulcerative colitis suggesting that the metabolites of sulphasalazine must be delivered to the lumen of the diseased distal colon to achieve

therapeutic effect. The faeces of patients with active ulcerative colitis contain excess prostaglandins and these are reduced to normal by sulphasalazine treatment. In vitro sulphasalazine and its 5-aminosalicylic acid moiety resemble aspirin in inhibiting prostaglandin synthesis.

Pharmacokinetics Sulphasalazine is relatively poorly absorbed and it is transported to the colon where the bacterial flora reductively split the azo link to liberate the active aminosalicylate moiety. This acts locally in the bowel and sulphasalazine largely acts as a carrier for the active compound to the colon. Patients with an ileostomy lack the appropriate gut flora and do not split sulphasalazine so that it has little place in their management. Sulphapyridine probably has little therapeutic effect although it is responsible for most of the adverse effects. Not surprisingly various other ways of administering 5-aminosalicylate, including the administration of enteric-coated capsules and enemas of the compound are being studied. Sulphasalazine kinetics may be summarised as shown in Fig 15.3. Sulphapyridine is a convenient marker of drug lysis which can be measured in plasma. Successful treatment of ulcerative

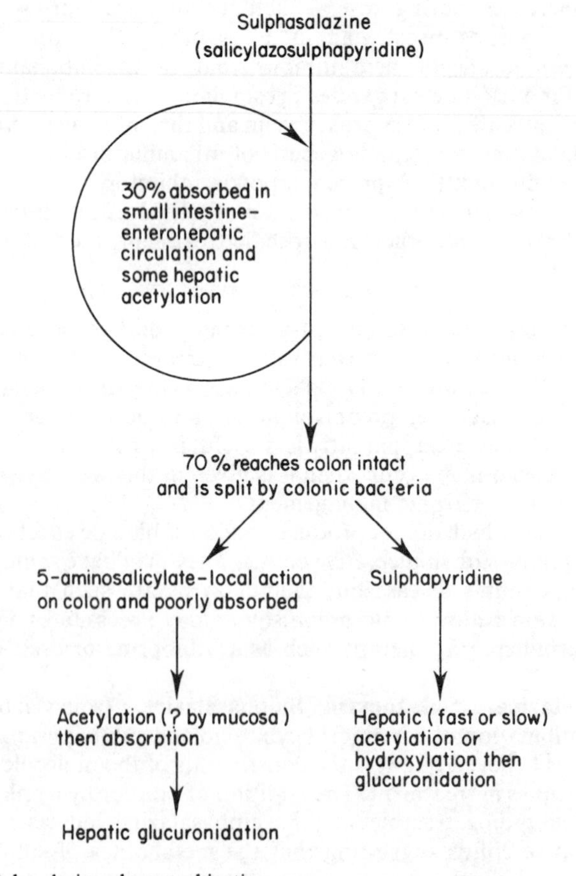

Fig. 15.3 Sulphasalazine pharmacokinetics.

colitis correlates approximately with a serum sulphapyridine concentration of 20 μg/ml: the levels of sulphonamide metabolites or unmetabolised sulphasalazine are irrelevant. The acetylator status of the patient (see p. 100) is therefore important in the interpretation of the plasma concentration.

Clinical uses Sulphasalazine is used solely for maintenance treatment of ulcerative colitis, where it is the only drug which has been shown to reduce significantly the number of relapses of ulcerative colitis. This effect persists for as long as the drug is taken. Rapid acetylators of sulphapyridine achieve therapeutic serum levels (20 μg/ml) when given 3–4 g sulphasalazine orally daily, but slow acetylators on this dose are likely to experience side effects because their serum level usually reaches 50 μg/ml on this dose. They usually require only 2.5–3 g/day. It is best tolerated by all patients if it is begun in a small dose of 0.5 g twice daily. Sulphasalazine does not help any but the mildest acute attacks and steroids are the treatment of choice.

Sulphasalazine is available as a suppository for use when disease is confined to the rectum or as an adjunct to oral treatment in total colitis. Enteric-coated tablets are also available.

Although effective in treatment of acute Crohn's disease, it does not maintain remission. It is not effective in patients with disease confined to the small bowel as would be predicted from its pharmacokinetics.

A recent survey has shown sulphasalazine has similar efficacy to penicillamine in active rheumatoid arthritis although it is much less toxic.

Adverse effects Nausea and vomiting may occur but sulphasalazine is generally well tolerated. All of the adverse effects associated with sulphonamides occur with sulphasalazine: they are more pronounced is slow acetylators. Toxic effects on the red cells are particularly common (70 %) and in some cases lead to haemolysis, anisocytosis and methaemoglobinaemia. These do not occur below doses of 1.5 g daily.

Temporary oligospermia with decreased sperm motility and infertility occurs in up to 70 % of males treated for over 3 years. Although sulphasalazine and its metabolites can cross the placenta it does not increase the incidence of kernicterus, probably because it binds at a different site on albumin from bilirubin.

3. Sodium cromoglycate (see p. 478) At least in some patients an immediate-type hypersensitivity reaction in the colon releases pharmacologically active mediators from mast cells and the consequent local tissue damage may play some part in tissue damage. Although this process is inhibited *in vitro* by disodium cromoglycate, the use of very large doses (as Nalcrom, 200 mg 6 hourly) has little effect in ulcerative colitis.

4. Immunosuppressive drugs such as azathioprine show only small benefit in ulcerative colitis and there are major risks associated with their use: chiefly bone-marrow depression in the short term and the threat of malignancy in the long term. In Crohn's disease they may be more useful particularly in preparation for surgical excision of disease which has formed a large inflammatory mass or as prophylaxis against recurrence.

5. Metronidazole (p. 727) has little effect in colitis or severe Crohn's disease but does reduce pain and encourage fistula healing in Crohn's disease of the perineum.

DRUGS USED IN THE TREATMENT OF CONSTIPATION

Bowel function and constipation

Under normal circumstances the rectum is empty and faecal material is stored in the descending and pelvic colon. Under the appropriate stimulation, which may include food or drink, certain surroundings and specific times of the day, the colon contracts and faeces enter the rectum. Sensors in the rectal wall are activated by the rise in pressure and also probably by tactile stimulus and this results in the 'call to stool'. If this is answered the rectum and distal portion of the colon are emptied by complex co-ordinated activity consisting of:

(a) colonic contraction;
(b) relaxation of the anal sphincter;
(c) voluntary elevation of the intra-abdominal pressure.

There is considerable variation among healthy people in the frequency of bowel evacuation and anything between 3 times weekly up to 3 times daily may be considered the normal range.

The term 'constipation' when used by patients describes what they consider to be abnormal bowel function and it is worth determining first whether indeed their bowels are behaving abnormally. The term may be used to describe infrequent bowel evacuation, or the evacuation of hard and often painful faecal masses which may be combined with difficulty in achieving full evacuation.

There are two main mechanisms which can lead to constipation:

1. *Decreased colonic activity* Causing the bowel contents to pass slowly through the colon and become dehydrated and hard and of small volume. Under these circumstances emptying of the colon into the rectum is infrequent and rectal stimulation is minimal. This may be due to a variety of factors:

(a) old age, immobility;
(b) low bulk diet, dehydration;
(c) metabolic disorders—hypercalcaemia, porphyria, myxoedema;
(d) depression, confusional states;
(e) various local conditions of the colon;
(f) drugs—tricyclic antidepressants, opiates, anticholinergic agents.

2. *Decreased sensitivity of the rectal sensors.* This usually occurs when the call to stool is neglected. After a while the stimulus dies away and the rectum becomes chronically full of faecal material. The condition is called *dyschezia.* It may occur in an acute form in patients who are too ill to appreciate or be able to respond to the call to stool or when bowel evacuation is painful, or in a chronic form in which for domestic or other reasons the patient has not the time or opportunity to open the bowels at the appropriate time.

LAXATIVES

The medical use of these agents has suffered an eclipse over the past few years although they are still widely used by the public. There is now a greater knowledge of intestinal pathophysiology and of outstanding importance is the finding that the fibre content of the diet has a marked regulatory action on gut transit time and motility and on defaecation performance.

As a general rule their use should be avoided. They are employed:

(i) if straining at stool will cause damage, e.g. post-operatively, in haemorrhoids, post-myocardial infarction.
(ii) in hepatocellular failure to reduce formation and/or absorption of neurotoxins produced in the bowel.
(iii) occasionally in drug-induced constipation.

1. Lubricants and stool softeners

These were believed to act by softening or lubricating the faeces but recent evidence suggests they act similarly to stimulant purgatives by inhibition of intestinal electrolyte transport probably mediated via an increase in mucosal cyclic AMP.

(a) **Liquid paraffin** Its habitual use is not without disadvantages:

(i) Prolonged use may interfere with absorption of fat-soluble substances and in particular the fat-soluble vitamins A, D and K.
(ii) Inhalation can occur into the lungs, causing lipid aspiration pneumonia. This is liable to occur with vomiting or with disorders of the lower oesophagus such as achalasia of the cardia.
(iii) Leakage of oil often occurs through the anus.
(iv) Mineral oil cannot be cleared from the tissues and can cause a chronic granuloma. If, therefore, as a result of surgery, paraffin leaks from the bowel into the tissues, a paraffinoma may develop.
(v) Repeated use may be related to the development of carcinoma of the large bowel.

In view of these side effects there is no indication to use liquid paraffin as a laxative.

(b) **Dioctyl sodium sulphosuccinate (DSS, Dioctyl)** This drug is a surface-active agent which acts on hard faecal masses and allows more water to penetrate the mass and thus soften it. The problem with substances of this type is that they increase the permeability of the gut wall and the long-term effects on intestinal function could be deleterious. Their use therefore should be confined to patients with faecal impaction and they should not be given over long periods.

Clinical use The usual dose is 100 mg three times daily by mouth.

2. Osmotic agents

These have been thought for many years to act by retaining fluid in the bowel by virtue of the osmotic activity of their unabsorbed ions. The increased bulk in the lumen would then stimulate peristalsis. However, 5 g magnesium sulphate would be isotonic in only 130 ml and acts within 1–2 hours, well before it could have reached the colon. It has thus been postulated that, because it can also contract the gall bladder, relax the sphincter of Oddi and increase gastric, intestinal and pancreatic enzyme secretion, it may act indirectly via cholecystokinin. The ions themselves may also have direct pharmacological effects on intestinal function. Although their complete action has not been elucidated it is clear that mechanisms other than osmotic effects account for their laxative properties.

Sodium sulphate (Glauber's salt) or **magnesium sulphate (Epsom salts)** are most commonly used. It should be remembered that a certain amount of magnesium may be absorbed and accumulation can occur in renal failure. There is little, if any, use for these saline purges apart from hepatocellular failure.

Lactulose (Duphalac) is a disaccharide. It passes through the small intestine unchanged but is broken down in the colon by carbohydrate fermenting bacteria to unabsorbed organic anions (largely acetic and lactic acids) which retain fluid in the gut lumen and also make the colonic contents more acid. This produces a laxative effect and also a good deal of gas formation. The place of lactulose in the management of constipation is limited but it has been useful in the management of patients with hepatic encephalopathy.

Clinical use For constipation the dose is 30 ml of Duphalac by mouth after breakfast. In liver failure larger doses are required, usually between 30 and 50 ml three times daily.

Lactulose should not be given in galactosaemia.

3. Bulk laxatives

(a) **Plant fibre** There have been many attempts to define dietary fibre. It is essentially that portion of the wall of plant cells which is resistant to digestion in the intestine. Its main constituents are:

(i) cellulose
(ii) hemicelluloses
(iii) pectins
(iv) lignins

The proportion of these constituents may vary depending on the source of the fibre and thus may alter its properties. The main effect of increasing the amount of fibre in the diet is to increase the bulk of the stools and to decrease bowel transit time; this is probably due to the ability of fibre to take up water and swell. It can also bind organic molecules including bile salts. Fibre does not increase the caloric content of the diet significantly.

Bran This contains about 30% of fibre and also has some starch and sugars, but its constitution varies considerably. Wholemeal bread contains about 2.5% of fibre and white bread contains about 0.2%.

There has been a great deal written about fibre and bran in recent years and much of it is conflicting. Its main uses are:

1. Constipation, particularly if combined with a spastic colon. By increasing the bulk of the intestinal contents, fibres slowly distend the wall of the colon and this causes an increase in useful propulsive contraction. The main result is a return of the large-bowel function towards normal. Similar results are obtained in diverticular disease in which there is colon over-activity associated with a high intraluminal pressure. Bran has been shown to reduce the intraluminal pressure and relieve symptoms.

2. Considerable interest is centred around the possibility that fibre might bind bile salts and thus increase their excretion. Although this has been demonstrated in animals, the position is less clear in man. There is also no evidence that fibre lowers plasma cholesterol in man. The effects of fibre in preventing large-bowel carcinoma, piles, appendicitis, coronary artery disease and varicose veins are still speculative.

Clinical uses The starting dose of bran is a dessertspoonful daily and this can be increased at weekly intervals until a satisfactory result is obtained. It may be mixed with food as it is difficult to swallow if taken neat.

Adverse effects Bran usually causes some flatulence which is dose related. Phytates in bran could theoretically bind calcium and zinc ions and this should be considered if its use in patients with calcium deficiency is contemplated.

(b) Other bulk purges Methylcellulose takes up water in the bowel and swells thus stimulating peristalsis. If for some reason bran is not satisfactory, it seems a reasonable substitute. There are a number of preparations available: Celevac, 1 teaspoonful twice daily with 300 ml of fluid, is usually adequate.

4. Chemical stimulants

These comprise a wide variety of drugs including some of great venerability such as calomel, jalap, aloes and podophyllum which are too toxic for current use. The idea that these drugs increase peristalsis by 'irritation' of the smooth muscle or intramural nerve plexuses is no longer tenable, especially as some like phenolphthalein are so non-irritant that they can be put into the eye with impunity. Current theories of their action suggest that they inhibit ionic flux out of the gut lumen possibly by inhibition of the Na^+ K^+ ATPase enzyme which is usually identified with the membrane-bound 'sodium-pump'. This is unlikely to be the only transport mechanism affected by these drugs and phenolphthalein for example is a powerful inhibitor of glucose transport (via a carrier mechanism which requires no energy) through erythrocyte membranes. Some of these drugs increase intestinal contraction *in vitro*, an effect blocked by topical application of lignocaine and attributed to an action on Auerbach's plexus.

(a) Castor oil This oily and unpleasant-tasting liquid is the triglyceride of ricinoleic acid. In the small intestine it is saponified to form sodium ricinoleate which is irritant to the wall of the small bowel. It hastens the passage of the intestinal contents and produces purgation in about 2 h. It is an effective, but now rarely used, aperient and repeated use can cause loss of fluid and electrolytes in the watery stools.

(b) Senna Senna in the form of pods or leaves has been used as a laxative for many years. The important constituents appear to be glycosides, which can be hydrolysed by colonic bacteria to the active principles sennoside A and sennoside B. Their main effect is to enhance the response of the colon to normal stimuli which underlines the importance of combining them with a high bulk diet so that there is an adequate physiological stimulus. It seems likely that senna acts directly on the intramucosal plexus of the gut wall and possibly also on electrolyte transport systems. The sennosides are absorbed in the small intestine and secreted into the colon, which explains why this drug takes about 8 h to produce an effect (therefore it should be given before sleep).

Clinical use Senna is best given as Senokot which contains sennosides A and B. The usual dose for an adult is between 2 and 4 tablets. It is usual to start with 2 tablets and increase until the required effect is obtained.

Adverse effects Griping and diarrhoea will occur if the dose is too large. When given to nursing mothers it enters the milk and many cause diarrhoea in the baby. Senna causes a yellow or red discolouration of the urine. Melanosis coli (a benign condition due to deposition of anthroquinone pigment derived from the drug) may also occur.

Co-danthramer (Dorbanex) has similar properties to senna.

(c) Bisacodyl is deacetylated in the gut and then absorbed undergoing transformation to the glucuronide in the liver. This is excreted in the bile and converted back to the deacetylated drug which acts on the colon. It thus has an enterohepatic absorption excretion cycle. It can be given as an enteric-coated tablet or as a suppository: in the latter form it presumably acts directly on the rectal mucosa, although systemic absorption may also occur.

Clinical use The usual dose is 10 mg of bisacodyl given at night, and the effect is seen in about 10 hours. The suppositories contain 10 mg of the drug and produce bowel evacuation in about half an hour.

Adverse effects Bisacodyl tablets are enteric coated and should not be chewed or given with antacids.

(d) Phenolphthalein was formerly widely used as a laxative, but at the present time it is less popular, although it is still an ingredient in a number of non-ethical preparations.

It is usually prescribed in the form of so-called white phenolphthalein, although there is a yellow preparation available which contains a number of impurities but is a more powerful laxative.

The exact mode of action of phenolphthalein is unknown. About 15% is absorbed from the small intestine and excreted by the liver in the bile. There is evidence that the active fraction is produced during metabolism in the liver and possibly by some further modification in the colon. Its main action is to stimulate increased activity in the large bowel and it usually takes 8–10 h to produce an effect. Because of hepatic recycling its action may be prolonged.

Clinical use The usual dose of phenolphthalein is 60 mg orally at night.

Adverse effects In about 4 % of people phenolphthalein produces a fixed drug eruption which takes the form of pink or purple macular plaques which may itch and burn. They leave a pigmented area on the skin which may last for many months. It may also produce a number of other rashes and a systemic lupus-like syndrome. An alkaline urine will be turned pink by phenolphthalein.

The management of constipation

When constipation occurs it is important first to exclude both local and systemic disease which may be responsible for the symptoms. This is particularly so when the change in bowel habit is of recent onset. It is important to remember the considerable variation in the normal frequency of bowel habit.

In general patients with constipation present in two ways:

1. Long-standing constipation in otherwise healthy people. This may be due to decreased colon motility or to dyschezia or a combination of both. It is usually sufficient to reassure the patient and to instruct them in the importance of re-establishing a regular bowel habit. This should be combined with an increased fluid intake and increased bulk in the diet. Bran is cheap and often satisfactory. As an alternative, non-absorbed bulk substances such as methylcellulose (Celevac) are helpful. In elderly subjects regular aperients are sometimes necessary. Senokot 2–4 tablets daily can be used.
2. Loaded colon or faecal impaction. Sometimes it is necessary to evacuate the bowel before it is possible to start re-education. This is particularly so in the elderly or those who are ill. In severe cases the impacted faeces can first be softened by olive oil retention enemas (150 ml of olive oil) repeated twice daily for a day or two. This can be followed by two glycerine suppositories or by an enema. If this fails the rectum will have to be evacuated digitally.

In less severe cases a laxative such as standardised senna (Senokot) 6 tablets twice daily combined with two glycerine suppositories should be adequate.

Laxative abuse

The continued use of laxatives, particularly in increasing doses, may lead to ill health.

(a) After prolonged use of chemical stimulant laxatives, the colon may become dilated and atonic with diminished activity. The cause of this is not clear but is perhaps due to damage to the intrinsic nerve plexus of the colon. The disorder of bowel motility may improve after withdrawing the laxative and using a high-residue diet.

(b) A group of subjects, largely women, take purgatives secretly. The reasons for this probably bear some relationship to disorders, such as anorexia nervosa, concerned with weight loss. It results in a complex of symptoms due to electrolyte loss from the bowel. These include:

Sodium depletion—postural hypotension, cramps, secondary hyperaldosteronism;

Potassium depletion—weakness, renal damage.
In addition there may be features suggestive of enteropathy and osteomalacia. Diagnosis and treatment are difficult but melanosis coli is a feature and may provide a diagnostic clue.

DIARRHOEA

Obviously treatment of the cause of diarrhoea is the best course, but in some circumstances this is impossible and symptomatic treatment is necessary. Two main types of drug action are employed.

A. **Drugs increasing intestinal transit time**

1. Opioids act directly on the gut and reduce peristalsis (see p. 317).

Codeine (p. 327) is widely used for this purpose in doses of 15–60 mg. **Morphine** is also given, usually as Kaolin and Morphine mixture B.P.C., which contains 700 μg of anhydrous morphine in every 10 ml dose.
Diphenoxylate is related to pethidine and also has structural similarities to anticholinergic drugs. It is usually prescribed as Lomotil (diphenoxylate 2.5 mg; atropine sulphate 0.025 mg). Diphenoxylate may cause drug dependence and euphoria. Overdose of Lomotil in children, which demonstrates features of both opioid and atropine intoxication, may be fatal.

2. Loperamide (Imodium) antagonises peristalsis, possibly by antagonising acetylcholine release in the intramural nerve plexus of the gut, although non-cholinergic effects may also be involved. It is poorly absorbed and probably acts directly on the bowel. The dose is 2 capsules (4 mg) initially followed by 2 mg after each loose stool up to a total dose of 16 mg/day. Adverse effects include dry mouth, dizziness, skin rashes and gastric disturbances.

B. **Drug increasing bulk and viscosity of gut contents**

These are usually satisfactory for milder cases of diarrhoea. Preparations include **Kaolin Compound Powder** B.P.C., which includes kaolin, (a natural form of aluminium silicate), sodium bicarbonate and magnesium carbonate (dose 2–10 g 4 hourly) and Chalk and Kaolin Mixture B.P.C.

Travellers' diarrhoea

This is a syndrome of acute watery diarrhoea lasting 1–3 days and associated with vomiting, abdominal cramps and other non-specific symptoms, resulting from infection by one of a number of enteropathogens, the most common being enterotoxigenic *Escherichia coli*. It has many geographical names: originally called gippy tummy by British troops in Egypt before 1914, it has subsequently been variously called Basrah belly, Hong Kong dog, Rangoon runs, Ho Chi Minhs, Aztec twostep and, for visitors to London, Thames Valley belly. In Mexico it is known simply as turista, which is sensible, since tourists are the most commonly affected because it probably reflects colonisation of the bowel by 'unfamiliar' organisms. Because of the variable nature of the pathogen there is no specific treatment. Prophylactic antibiotics (**neomycin**, **phthalylsulphathiazole** and **sulphatriad**, a mixture of sulphonamides) have been shown to decrease attack rates. Recently **doxycycline** has been shown to prevent most episodes of traveller's diarrhoea. Despite their effectiveness, there is a danger that widespread use might encourage bacterial antibiotic resistance. These drugs can also create problems for the traveller due to their side effects. Early treatment of diarrhoea with cotrimoxazole or trimethoprim alone will control 90 % of cases and this, with oral replacement of salts and water, is the presently preferred approach.

IRRITABLE BOWEL SYNDROME

This motility disorder of the gut probably affects some 10 % of the population to some degree. Although the symptoms are mostly colonic, patients with the syndrome have abnormal motility throughout the gut and this may be precipitated by dietary items such as alcohol or wheat flour. The important management principles are firstly to exclude a serious cause for the symptoms and to determine whether exclusion of certain foods or alcohol would be worthwhile. An increase in dietary fibre over the course of several weeks may also reduce symptoms. Drug treatment is symptomatic and often disappointing. Those in current vogue are:

1. Anticholinergic drugs such as **hyoscine butylbromine** (Buscopan) have been used for many years although evidence of efficacy is lacking. The oral use of better absorbed anticholinergics such as atropine is limited by side effects (see p. 528).
2. *Mebeverine* (Colofac) given as one tablet (135 mg) daily before meals directly relaxes intestinal smooth muscle without anticholinergic effects and there is limited controlled trial evidence of efficacy.
3. *Peppermint oil* also relaxes intestinal smooth muscle and is given in an enteric-coated capsule which releases its contents in the distal small bowel (Colpermin). It is given as one capsule (0.2 ml oil) before meals and some trials have shown efficacy.
4. Antidiarrhoeal drugs such as codeine, loperamide and diphenoxylate reduce the painless diarrhoea variant of the syndrome.
5. *Psychotropic drugs* such as neuroleptics and antidepressants with anticholinergic properties have also been effective in some patients. In general, however, they should be avoided for such a chronic and benign condition.

GALLSTONE DISSOLUTION

About 10 % of gallstones are purely cholesterol and 80 % of the remainder contain more than 70 % cholesterol. The outstanding biochemical abnormality in these patients is the secretion of bile which is saturated or supersaturated with cholesterol. At least two factors are responsible: increased cholesterol secretion and reduced bile-acid secretion associated with a smaller than normal bile-acid pool. Cholesterol is virtually insoluble in water. The relative concentrations of cholesterol, bile acid and phospholipid in bile determine whether cholesterol remains in solution or precipitates to form gallstones. The relationship between these components of bile is summarised by the phase diagram (see Fig. 15.4). The equilibrium solubility line defines the concentration above which cholesterol precipitates from solution. Patients with gallstones have been shown to produce lithogenic bile. Therefore drugs which influence cholesterol output from the liver into the bile may influence gallstone formation and, if the cholesterol concentration in bile falls low enough so that there is 'spare' cholesterol-carrying capacity, they may actually dissolve.

There is no evidence that any particular diet influences gall-bladder or gallstone disease. Low-fat diets are often recommended but their effectiveness remains to be established. High intake of dietary fibre (e.g. bran) reduces the cholesterol content of bile but insufficiently to produce gallstone dissolution. Dietary measures may well offer a means of reducing the re-formation of stones once drug treatment has been discontinued (see below). At present only one drug is widely used for dissolution treatment of gallstones, but further developments in this field may be confidently expected.

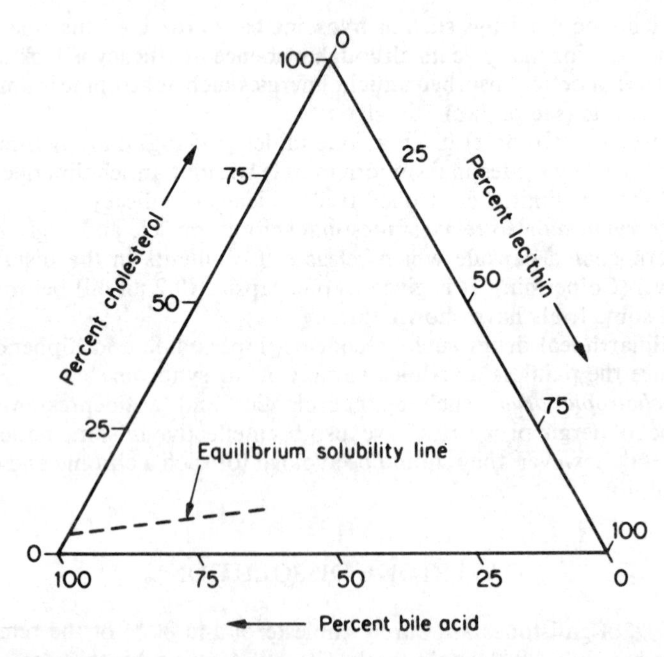

Fig. 15.4 Phase-equilibrium diagram for a model system of bile acids, cholesterol and lecithin. When cholesterol is present in concentrations above the equilibrium solubility line it will precipitate out of solution.

Chenodeoxycholic acid (Chendol; Chenofalk)

This is a bile acid derived semisynthetically from animal bile and is similar to that produced in the human liver, where it comprises 40% of the total bile acids. Its major action is to reduce cholesterol output into the bile. The hepatic synthesis of cholesterol is regulated by microsomal 3-hydroxy-3-methylglutaryl-coenzyme A (HMG-Co A) reductase, whereas the rate limiting enzyme for bile acid synthesis is 7α-hydroxylase (Fig. 15.5). Chenodeoxycholic acid inhibits HMG-Co A reductase to a greater extent than it inhibits 7α-hydroxylase. Probably of secondary importance is the expansion of the bile acid pool accompanying chenodeoxycholate administration. The fall in cholesterol secretion results in biliary unsaturation with respect to cholesterol and cholesterol may therefore dissolve from the surface of gallstones.

Pharmacokinetics Chenodeoxycholic acid is given orally and whilst there is a small amount of passive non-ionic absorption in the jejunum, the major absorption occurs by active transport in the terminal ileum. After returning to the liver, chenodeoxycholic acid completes its enterohepatic cycle by secretion into the bile conjugated with glycine or taurine. Intestinal bacterial action results in its transformation into the secondary bile acid lithocholic acid. Lithocholic acid is hepatotoxic in animals but not in man because in man it is either excreted in the stool or reabsorbed into the portal circulation and

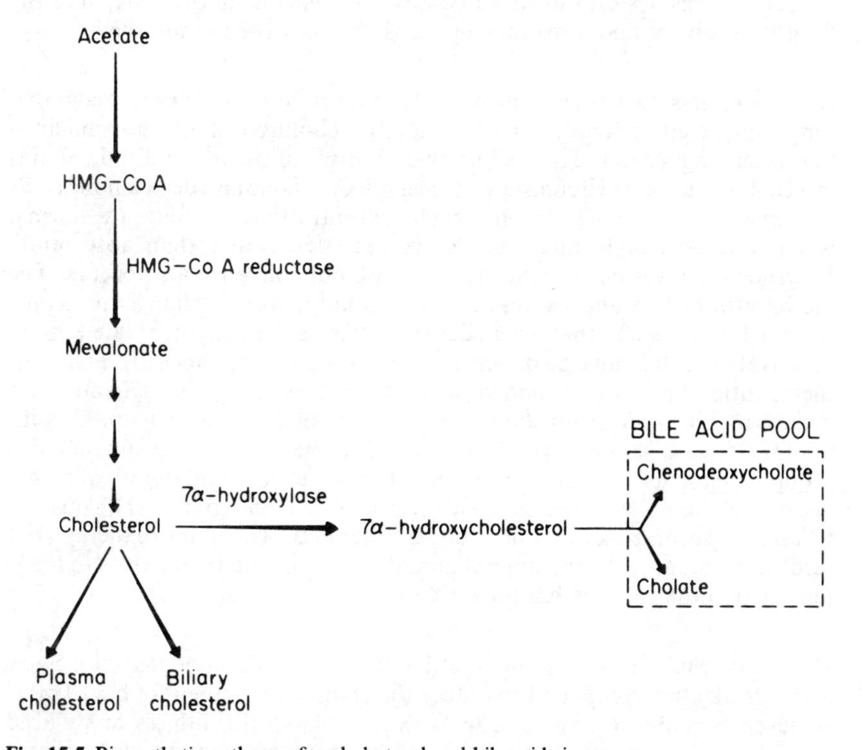

Fig. 15.5 Biosynthetic pathways for cholesterol and bile acids in man.

returned to the liver, where it is conjugated and most is additionally sulphated and excreted again into the bile. The sulphated compound is too water-soluble to be reabsorbed and therefore little lithocholic acid accumulates in the body. There is therefore little chance of hepatotoxicity due to lithocholic acid.

Clinical use Chenodeoxycholic acid is useful only for cholesterol stones and thus only radiolucent stones should be treated; a functioning gall-bladder which allows the stones to be bathed in unsaturated bile is also necessary. These two requirements mean that only about 20% of patients requiring cholecystectomy can benefit. Drug treatment cannot therefore replace surgery in most patients. A dose of 15 mg/kg daily is usually enough to keep the bile unsaturated but a few patients do not respond and need a larger dose, and this also increases side effects. Obese patients usually require up to 20 mg/kg/day. The effects are probably enhanced by giving the whole dose at bed-time and by a low cholesterol diet. The rate of dissolution (checked by repeat cholecystograms) is slow. Complete dissolution of a small stone (less than 5 mm diameter) usually takes 6–9 months, whereas most stones over 1 cm diameter require more than 2 years. A single large stone is presently unsuitable for treatment because dissolution rate is proportional to surface area. Chenodeoxycholate therapy does not cure the underlying abnormality and on stopping treatment the bile becomes supersaturated with cholesterol again and recurrence of stones has been reported. Thus prophylactic treatment is probably necessary and likely to be life-long. This is unfortunate since the drug is expensive and a maintenance dose has not been established.

Adverse effects Diarrhoea which is often intermittent is the only recognised symptomatic effect. This is almost certainly a choluretic diarrhoea similar to that occurring when the active bile acid absorption site in the distal ileum is resected. Under such circumstances, chenodeoxycholic and deoxycholic acids may reach the colon in sufficiently high concentrations to reverse the normal water and electrolyte flux and induce secretion rather than absorption. Diarrhoea is reversed by reducing the dose but tolerance also occurs. The mechanism of tolerance is unknown but could involve a change in colonic bacterial flora such that chenodeoxycholate is 7α-dehydroxylated more effectively to lithocholic acid, which does not induce diarrhoea. Tolerance of therapeutic doses of chenodeoxycholate is less likely in patients with decreased bile acid absorption in the distal small bowel, e.g. those with Crohn's disease or those who have undergone iliectomy. Unfortunately this group of patients also have an increased incidence of cholesterol gallstones because of their disordered bile-acid metabolism. Transient minor changes in transaminases and alkaline phosphatase occur at the beginning of therapy but resolve spontaneously and are not an indication to stop treatment. No long-term hepatotoxicity has been described.

Ursodeoxycholic acid (Destolit) is the 7β-epimer of chenodeoxycholic acid and acts like this compound to reduce the cholesterol content of bile. This is achieved by either a reduction in hepatic cholesterol synthesis or reduced cholesterol absorption or both. It is more efficient than chenodeoxycholic acid in achieving biliary cholesterol unsaturation and the usual dose is 8–10 mg/kg/day (600 mg).

It has fewer side effects than chenodeoxycholic acid: diarrhoea is rare as are changes in biochemical tests of liver function.

Rowachol This is a mixture of six plant monoterpenes (menthol, menthone, pinene, borneol, camphene and cineol). These essential oils reduce hepatic HMG-CoA reductase activity in animal studies. In man this proprietary mixture has given similar results to chenodeoxycholic acid therapy and may be used either alone or as an adjunct to chenodeoxycholic acid.

DRUGS AND THE LIVER

PRINCIPLES UNDERLYING DRUG TREATMENT OF HEPATIC ENCEPHALOPATHY AND LIVER FAILURE

In severe liver disease neuropsychiatric changes occur and can progress to coma. The mechanism which produces these changes is not established but it is known that in hepatic coma and pre-coma the blood ammonia concentration rises and encephalopathy usually occurs if the level exceeds 3.0–3.5 μg/ml. In many patients the progress of encephalopathy parallels the rise in blood ammonia. Orally administered nitrogenous compounds (e.g. protein, amino acids, ammonium chloride) yield ammonia in the gut, raise blood ammonia levels, and are associated with provocation of encephalopathy. The liver is the only organ which can extract ammonia from the blood and convert it to urea. It is suggested therefore that bacterial degradation products of nitrogenous material within the gut (which includes ammonia) enter the systemic circulation either because of a failure of the usual first-pass hepatic extraction mechanism (due to hepatocellular damage) or due to bypass of the hepatocytes by collateral circulation or intrahepatic shunting. One important source of ammonia is dietary protein and normally about 4 g of ammonia/day is produced by bacteria from protein in the gut. Another source is urea which undergoes an enterohepatic circulation and yields about 3.5 g/day of ammonia (see Fig. 15.6).

Ammonia is able to move bidirectionally across the large bowel wall into the blood by non-ionic diffusion down the concentration gradient to the more acidic side, where it is trapped by becoming ionised and thus unable to pass easily through lipid membranes. Thus ammonia usually passes into the blood from the colon because of the high intraluminal ammonia concentration and because of the alkalinity of its contents, whilst in the upper gut ammonia is secreted into the lumen down its concentration gradient.

Ammonia cannot be the only toxin involved since perhaps 20% of patients with encephalopathy have normal blood ammonia levels and methionine can provoke encephalopathy without causing a significant rise in blood ammonia. Furthermore, ammonia toxicity affects the cortex but not the brain stem, yet this is also involved in encephalopathy. Other hypotheses include:

(a) Intestinal bacterial decarboxylation produces hydroxyphenyl amines such as octopamine (from tyramine) which could replace the normal transmitters at nerve endings in the central and peripheral nervous systems,

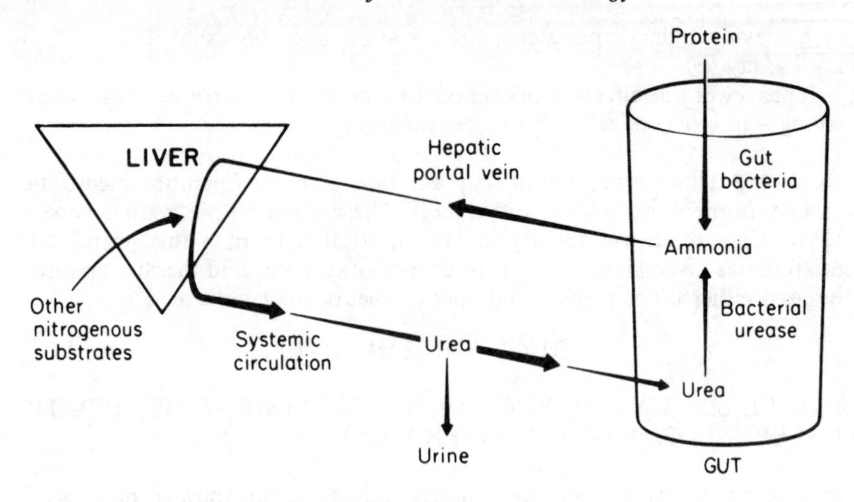

Fig. 15.6 Enterohepatic circulation of urea and ammonia.

thus acting as 'false transmitters' and changing the balance of inhibition and excitation of synapses.

(b) Changes in fatty acid metabolism increase plasma free fatty acids, some of which may have anaesthetic properties. In addition, these determine the availability of tryptophan to the brain and hence have an effect on 5-hydroxytryptamine turnover.

(c) Hepatic failure changes the distribution of free amino acids in the plasma. The aromatic amino acids (tyrosine, phenylalanine and tryptophan) increase since they are normally catabolised by the liver, whilst branched-chain amino acids (valine, leucine and isoleucine) which are catabolised by skeletal muscle decrease. The excess tryptophan may be converted in the brain into 5-hydroxytryptamine, which causes sleep. Branched-chain amino acids in some way control the entry of tryptophan into the brain and an experimental treatment of encephalopathy has included infusion of these amino acids or their keto precursors.

Treatment of hepatic encephalopathy includes measures to reverse these putative mechanisms:

1. Dietary protein restriction.
2. Emptying the lower bowel by enemas and purgatives which reduces the bacterial sources of ammonia.
3. Oral or rectal administration of non-absorbable antibiotics such as neomycin to reduce the bacterial population of the large bowel. 1–2 g of neomycin four times daily is often used: it should be remembered that a 2 g dose produces a blood level of about 1 μg/ml and that if the patient also has renal impairment this drug may accumulate and produce toxicity.
4. Oral lactulose 50–100 g/day may help chronic encephalopathy. This disaccharide is not a normal dietary constituent and man does not possess a lactulase, so that lactulose is neither digested nor absorbed but

reaches the colon unchanged where the bacterial flora splits it to lactate, acetate and other acid products. These possibly trap ammonia and other toxins within the lumen by ionic effects, but in addition act as a cathartic and reduce ammonia absorption by reducing colonic transit time.

5. Lactobacilli given freeze-dried (Enpac) can improve encephalopathy due to chronic liver failure, presumably by displacing colonic organisms which produce ammonia and other toxins but are not useful in acute failure.
6. Levodopa has an arousing effect in patients with acute hepatic coma, and in chronic hepatic encephalopathy a significant improvement may occur following levodopa therapy. At present such treatment is regarded as experimental.
7. Bleeding may occur due to interference with clotting factor synthesis. The prothrombin time indicates the extent of such problems. Vitamin K is given intramuscularly and fresh frozen plasma, platelets and fresh blood may be used as required. Cimetidine is often used to prevent gastric erosions and bleeding.
8. Sedation is avoided since patients with liver disease are extremely sensitive to such drugs. Chlorpromazine, although recommended by some, has been shown to produce deleterious electroencephalographic changes. Phenobarbitone (less dependent upon hepatic metabolism than most barbiturates) tends to be cumulative, particularly in renal failure which may complicate severe liver disease. If sedation is essential diazepam appears to be the safest available agent. The hazards of narcotic analgesics to the patient with acute or chronic liver disease cannot be stressed too strongly (see p. 320).

DRUG THERAPY OF PORTAL HYPERTENSION AND OESOPHAGEAL VARICES

Oesophageal varices form a collateral circulation in response to raised pressure in the portal system and are of clinical importance because of their tendency to bleed. Two-thirds of patients with varices die, and of these one-third die of the first bleed, one-third rebleed within six weeks and only one-third survive one year. Sclerotherapy and surgical shunt procedures remain the mainstay of treatment and drug therapy must be judged against these gloomy survival figures. Emergency treatment of bleeding varices may include the following drugs:

1. *Vasopressin* (see p. 616).
2. *Propranolol* given intravenously may arrest bleeding but has the disadvantage of producing cardiovascular effects in patients who are already haemodynamically unstable.
3. *Somatostatin*—an experimental treatment not yet validated.

Prevention of bleeding may be achieved by propranolol given orally in doses sufficient to slow the pulse by 25 %. It is believed to lower portal pressure by decreasing cardiac output, reducing splanchnic blood flow (via β_2-blockade on mesenteric arterioles) and decreasing hepatic artery flow (again via β_2-blockade) which produces a secondary fall in hepatic portal pressure. Despite initially encouraging results this treatment is not effective in all patients and does not reduce portal pressure in decompensated cirrhotics. This may result from higher circulating catecholamine levels known to exist in decompensated patients. These facts plus other unanswered questions such as long-term safety, optimum duration of treatment and safety of stopping therapy mean that for the present its use should be restricted to controlled trials.

DRUG-INDUCED JAUNDICE AND LIVER DAMAGE

The drugs most commonly reported as being associated with jaundice are shown in Table 15.2.

Table 15.2 Jaundice associated with drugs

Drugs	*Mechanism of jaundice*
Halothane	Hepatitis
Phenelzine, iproniazid, isocarboxazid	Hepatitis
Methyldopa	Hepatitis. Rarely haemolysis.
Chlorpromazine and phenothiazines	Stasis with hepatitis
Imipramine, amitriptyline, iprindole	Statis with hepatitis
Benzodiazepines	Stasis with hepatitis
Phenylbutazone, oxyphenbutazone, indomethacin	Stasis with hepatitis
Isoniazid	Hepatitis
PAS, rifampicin, ethambutol, pyrazinamide	Stasis with hepatitis
Tetracycline	Direct hepatocellular toxicity; fatty liver.
Erythromycin, ampicillin, sulphonamides, nitrofurantoin	Stasis with hepatitis
Chlorpropamide, tolbutamide	Stasis with hepatitis
Combined contraceptive pill	Pure cholestasis
Methotrexate	Cirrhosis
Oxyphenisatin	Chronic active hepatitis

The principal mechanisms of drug-induced jaundice may be grouped as follows:

1. haemolysis:
2. competition for binding of bilirubin to plasma proteins (e.g. sulphonamides, salicylates);
3. competition for binding of bilirubin to cell proteins (e.g. flavaspidic acid—the active principle of male fern extract, an anthelmintic);
4. competition for glucuronide-forming enzymes (e.g. novobiocin);
5. intrahepatic cholestasis due to competition for biliary canalicular excretory mechanisms (e.g. rifampicin);

6. intrahepatic cholestasis due to alterations in the canalicular membrane which could result in increased permeability so that water leaks out leaving concentrated bile in these tiny ducts (e.g. C_{17} alkyl testosterone derivatives, such as methyltestosterone and norethandrolone; oestrogens and progestogens of the pill);
7. diffuse hepatocellular damage (e.g. carbon tetrachloride).

Hypersensitivity (allergy) may account for some instances of drug-induced jaundice. It can be associated with other features such as rashes, fever, eosinophilia and arthralgia. The reaction is not dose-related, affects only a small number of patients taking the drug and is commoner after multiple exposures. Although usually occurring after a week or so of treatment, it can happen after weeks of drug administration. The drugs most frequently implicated are hydrazines, erythromycin estolate (not stearate) and phenothiazines. The principal types of hypersensitivity jaundice are:

(i) *Hepatitis-like reactions*: monoamine oxidase inhibitors of the hydrazine type (up to 20 % of patients may develop this reaction); isoniazid; α-methyldopa; oxyphenisatin (may develop after 1–2 years of regular administration of this laxative. It has now been withdrawn because of the danger of development of chronic active hepatitis). The hepatitic reactions to halothane and methoxyflurane probably also involve hypersensitivity.

(ii) *Cholestasis* (with a hepatitic component): chlorpromazine (0.5 % of patients); tricyclic antidepressants; benzodiazepines; phenylbutazone (0.3 % of patients—but the mortality rate is 20 %); oxyphenbutazone; indomethacin; sulphonamides; erythromycin estolate; nitrofurantoin; thiouracil; phenindione; chlorpropamide and tolbutamide.

Fatty liver The agents which produce liver injury may also cause accumulation of abnormal amounts of fat (mainly triglycerides) in parenchymal cells, including: e.g. carbon tetrachloride, tetrachloroethylene, trichloroethylene, ethyl alcohol, chloroform, *Amanita phalloides* alkaloids.

The basic mechanism appears to be a block in the release of hepatic triglyceride into the plasma. This is paralleled by a decrease in plasma lipoprotein concentration.

Drug-induced hepatic fibrosis may occur in patients treated with inorganic arsenicals (e.g. Fowler's solution for psoriasis) and in workers exposed to vinyl chloride. Angiosarcoma may develop in these patients which can metastasise, predominantly to the lungs.

Hepatic adenoma, usually a rare tumour, may develop in patients on oral contraceptives, the risk being increased 25 times in women on the pill for more than 5 years. There may also be a relationship between the pill and the malignant primary hepatoma since the incidence of this tumour is increased by chronic androgen administration.

Gallstones have an increased prevalence in patients on oral contraceptives (which increase the cholesterol content of bile). Clofibrate has also been shown to increase gallstone formation.

Drug interactions and hepatotoxicity Some liver toxins are produced by biotransformation. This may explain why enzyme-inducing agents such as phenobarbitone and DDT enhance the toxicity of carbon tetrachloride, paracetamol and chloroform. Conversely the toxic actions of these substances can be diminished by the coadministration of cysteine or methionine. This is because they injure the liver by depleting cellular stores of these substances which are normally protective. Isoniazid is first acetylated to acetyl isoniazid and then hydrolysed to acetyl hydrazine which is converted by cytochrome P_{450} to a reactive acylating metabolite which may cause liver damage in excess. Therefore rapid acetylators (see p. 100) are likely to develop isoniazid toxicity because they produce greater amounts of the toxic metabolite. Similarly enzyme induction encourages its formation and patients who are alcoholics or those treated with rifampicin also show a higher incidence of this complication. This drug reaction is unusual if para-aminosalicylic acid is combined with isoniazid, probably because this drug reduces the acetylation of isoniazid.

Veno-occlusive liver disease from the pyrrolizidine alkaloids in 'bush teas' is also due to metabolism to more toxic substances. Thus enzyme induction enhances toxicity.

In many interactions involving mutual potentiation of hepatotoxicity by the simultaneous administration of two toxins, the mechanism is not understood. However, individuals recovering from excessive alcohol ingestion are more susceptible to the liver-damaging effects of halogenated hydrocarbons.

DRUGS USED IN TREATMENT OF PANCREATIC DISEASE

Acute pancreatitis, although relatively rare, has a high mortality. A number of drugs have been advocated for its treatment but very few controlled trials of these have been made to prove efficacy.

1. Aprotinin (Trasylol) This is a polypeptide (58 amino acids) extracted from bovine lungs which acts as a proteolytic enzyme inhibitor. It is given as an intravenous bolus of 200 000 units followed by 800 000 units/day by infusion. The $t_{1/2}$ is approximately 2 h and it is metabolised to inactive peptides which are mostly excreted in the urine. A multicentre trial carried out by the MRC has failed to show that this drug affects mortality. It is uncertain whether the complication rate is altered. Aprotinin is expensive. It is well tolerated, although being a polypeptide it occasionally produces hypersensitivity and rarely anaphylaxis.

2. Glucagon reduces the volume and enzyme concentration of pancreatic juice. The MRC multicentre trial failed to demonstrate any benefit from glucagon.

3. Anticholinergic drugs which might be expected to block vagally mediated pancreatic secretion are useless in pancreatitis since the excess pancreatic enzyme release is not vagally mediated.

4. Corticosteroids have sometimes been advocated as part of treatment for 'shock'. There is no scientific basis for this practice and they could even be harmful.

Pancreatic insufficiency

Exocrine pancreatic insufficiency is an important cause of steatorrhoea. The pancreas has a large functional reserve and malabsorption does not usually occur until enzyme output is reduced to 10 % or less of normal. This type of malabsorption is usually treated by replacement therapy using pancreatic extracts usually of porcine origin. Unfortunately, although useful, these preparations rarely abolish steatorrhoea. A number of preparations (e.g. Cotazym, Pancrex) are available but the enzyme activity varies between preparations: one with a high lipase activity is most likely to reduce steatorrhoea. Unfortunately less than 10 % of the lipase activity and 25 % of the tryptic activity is recoverable from the duodenum regardless of the dose schedule. This limited effectiveness of oral enzymes is due to acid-peptic inactivation in the stomach and duodenum. Antacids fail to improve results when given with pancreatic enzymes, probably because they increase the volume of gastric secretion which dilutes ingested enzymes. This theoretically offsets the benefit derived from neutralisation of the acid and an increased gastric and duodenal pH. Cimetidine decreases both acidity and volume of secretion and has been demonstrated both to retard the inactivation of exogenous pancreatic enzymes and to improve steatorrhoea when given as an adjunct to these preparations.

Drugs associated with pancreatitis

This is a rare iatrogenic disease. The most commonly reported associations (although causality is sometimes difficult to attribute) have been:

Asparaginase	Oestrogens
Azathioprine	Pentamidine
Corticosteroids	Sodium valproate
Frusemide and thiazides	Sulphonamides and sulphasalazine
Methyldopa	Tetracycline

DRUGS MODIFYING APPETITE

ANORECTIC DRUGS

The commonest malnutrition in Western society is obesity. Obesity is a killing disease and it is presumably preventable since the obese are fat because they eat too much for their needs. The cure is ostensibly simple: they must eat less. In practice, however, treatment is much more difficult. Naturally a calorie controlled diet and sensible amounts of exercise are the essentials of treatment. Unfortunately the results of treating patients at weight-reduction clinics are disappointing: many patients default at an early stage, there is a high relapse rate and only a few achieve permanent weight loss. There has accordingly been a great deal of interest in the possibility of altering appetite pharmacologically so as to help the patient reduce his calorie intake. Unfortunately the causes of obesity are not understood. There is conflicting evidence concerning the relative role of overeating, lack of exercise and individual variation in the utilisation of food energy. One hypothesis is that lean people do not become obese when they overeat because their tissues preferentially liberate heat (in particular from brown fat). Despite this uncertainty, there is no doubt that starvation leads to weight loss. Therefore, research into drugs for obesity have concentrated on finding substances that inhibit appetite.

Social conditioning plays only a minor role in signalling normal satiety, but learned behaviour probably is important in determining the frequency of eating and whether food is taken between major meals. Stretch receptors in the stomach are stimulated by distention, but the main factors that terminate eating are humoral. Bombesin and somatostatin are two candidates for humoral satiety factors released by the stomach. The most important satiety factor released from the gastrointestinal tract beyond the stomach is cholecystokinin (CCK). A small peptide fragment of this (CCK-8) has been synthesised, and has been found to cause humans to reduce their food intake, possibly by acting on the appetite/satiety centre in the hypothalamus.

Since obesity does not have a statistically significant impact upon mortality until an individual is more than 30% over ideal weight, any treatment designed for people less than 30% above their desirable weight must be essentially risk-free. When drugs are used the patient must be told that they are being given with the specific purpose of helping him to follow his diet more strictly. Patients should never be allowed to believe that drugs will allow relaxation of diet. As a corollary, there is little point in persisting with drug therapy if there is no effect after sufficient trial has been made.

Amphetamine and related drugs (see p. 846)

Amphetamine was first shown to be anorectic in man in 1938 and since that time a number of congeners have been employed for this purpose. The site of action of these compounds appears to be in the hypothalamus, where they increase noradrenaline and dopamine levels by causing transmitter release and blocking re-uptake. Table 15.3 shows some commonly used members of this group.

Table 15.3 Amphetamine and congeners used as anorectics

Approved name	*Proprietary name*	*Daily dosage (mg)*
Amphetamine	Durophet	7.5–20
Diethylpropion	Tenuate, Apisate	225–300
Phentermine	Duromine, Ionamine	15–30
Fenfluramine	Ponderax	60–120
Mazindol	Teronac	2

The central effects of amphetamine, diethylpropion and phentermine are those of excitation, anxiety and tremor. There is a high incidence of dependence and abuse with amphetamine and it should never be used for obesity. Dependence has also been described for diethylpropion and it would be unwise to assume that it cannot occur with the others. Cardiovascular effects are frequently observed with these drugs, a dose-related increase in heart rate and blood pressure being the most common. Amphetamine increases plasma free fatty acids and glycerol.

Fenfluramine probably increases 5-HT rather than noradrenaline levels in the brain and it may have a peripheral effect by enhancing lipolysis and increasing glucose uptake in fat cells. Although related to amphetamine this drug is not metabolised to amphetamine but is present in the blood and excreted in the urine, partly as unchanged fenfluramine and partly as norfenfluramine, which also has anorectic properties. The anorectic effect is related to the plasma fenfluramine concentration and the long plasma $t_{1/2}$ accounts for its prolonged effects. Although qualitatively its cardiovascular effects are similar to amphetamine they are less marked. Both stimulation and more commonly depression of the central nervous system including drowsiness and dysphoria have been described. Habituation and dependence are rare, but withdrawal may cause subjective depression for several days. Nightmares may occur and it interferes with sleep EEG patterns. It has been described as a drug of dependence but not of abuse. Unlike amphetamine it causes diarrhoea. Acute confusional states may arise if given with a monoamine oxidase inhibitor, and it may potentiate the action of antihypertensive, antidiabetic, sedative and other anorectic drugs.

Mazindol appears to increase central dopamine levels but its effects closely resemble those of amphetamine, although it has no effect on plasma lipids. Its biochemical novelty does not appear to confer any superiority over other agents.

The long-term efficacy of all these agents has never been established, although double-blind trials against placebo have demonstrated a maintained reduction in body weight with up to 20 weeks of treatment. In clinically effective doses there is probably little to choose between these compounds in terms of effectiveness and duration of weight loss.

Bulk agents

Such substances as methylcellulose and guar gum acting as bulking agents in the diet are as harmless as they are ineffective.

Enthusiasts suggest that a high-fibre diet may help weight loss.

APPETITE STIMULATION

This is often difficult since patients with a poor appetite may have a debilitating systemic illness or an underlying psychiatric disorder. Only one drug has been objectively shown to increase appetite: **cyproheptadine** (**Periactin**). It has been used to increase the appetite of underweight patients with tuberculosis and may be effective in some cases of anorexia nervosa. The dose is 2–4 mg three or four times daily and weight is gained most rapidly during the first few weeks of therapy and is lost again when the drug is stopped. It may also have a place in treating Cushing's disease (see p. 615).

Weight gain occurs during treatment with some other drugs: chlorpromazine (but other phenothiazines or butyrophenones have not been shown to have this effect), amitriptyline, lithium, corticosteroids and ACTH, and the oral contraceptive pill.

ANTIEMETIC DRUGS

Complex processes underlie nausea and vomiting. Nausea (recognition of the desire to vomit) is associated with autonomic effects (sweating, tachycardia,

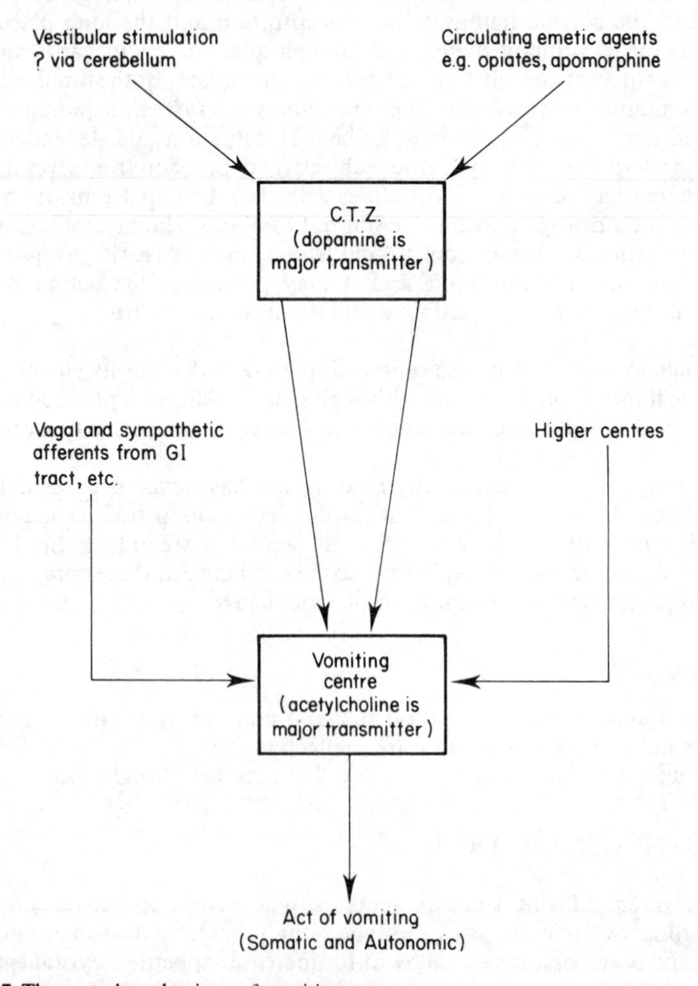

Fig. 15.7 The central mechanisms of vomiting.

pallor and profuse salivary secretion). Vomiting is preceded by the rhythmic muscular contractions of the 'respiratory' muscles of the abdomen (retching). Thus, unlike nausea, vomiting is a somatic rather than an autonomic function. Central coordination of these processes occurs in a group of cells in the dorsolateral reticular formation in the floor of the fourth ventricle of the medulla oblongata in close proximity to the cardiovascular and respiratory centres with which it has synaptic connections. This *vomiting centre* (Fig. 15.7) is not directly responsive to chemical emetic stimuli but is activated by one or more input circuits either within or outside the nervous system. The major efferent pathways from the vomiting centre are the phrenic nerve, visceral efferents of the vagus to stomach and oesophagus and the spinal nerves to the abdominal musculature.

One important receptor area for emetic stimuli within the CNS is the *chemoreceptor trigger zone* (CTZ). This is a group of neurones in the area postrema of the fourth ventricle which is sensitive to emetic stimuli such as radiation, bacterial toxins and uraemia. Associated with the CTZ neurones are astrocytes which are thought to release the neurotransmitter dopamine when the blood contains emetic drug molecules, e.g. nicotine, opioids, cardiac glycosides, nitrogen mustard. This dopamine excites CTZ neurones which in turn activate the vomiting centre and emesis.

Emetic stimuli originating in the pharynx, oesophagus and gut are transmitted to the vomiting centre via the vagus and glossopharyngeal nerves. Those from the vestibular organs (in travel sickness and Ménièré's disease) act indirectly upon the vomiting centre via the CTZ. A histamine pathway is apparently involved in labyrinthine vomiting. Naloxone, an opioid antagonist, can block the antiemetic effect of nabilone on the vomiting produced by apomorphine and nitrogen mustard in cats. This and other evidence suggests that opioid receptors may be involved in some centrally induced emesis involving higher centres. Drugs may act in more than one site to provoke emesis, e.g. nitrogen mustard (CTZ, cortex, gut), digitalis (CTZ and gut). Antiemetic drugs act in several sites also but are classified pharmacologically in Table 15.4.

Table 15.4 Pharmacological classification of antiemetics

Anticholinergics	
Antihistamines (H_1-blockers)	
Dopamine antagonists	
Cannabinoids	
Miscellaneous –	corticosteroids
	benzodiazepines
	trimethobenzamide

Antiemetics should only be used when the cause of nausea or vomiting is known lest the symptomatic relief produced should mask or delay treatment of a remediable or serious cause. Nausea and sickness during the first trimester of pregnancy will respond to most antiemetics but should rarely be treated with drugs because of the possible dangers (unquantifiable) of teratogenesis and present medical and public anxiety about such treatment.

1. Anticholinergics

These act partly by their anti-muscarinic action on the gut but also have some central action. *Hyoscine* is a well-tried remedy for motion sickness and is given as 1 mg of the hydrobromide (*scopolamine*) or in proprietary form as Kwells (0.3 mg/tablet). It is useful in single doses for short journeys but the anticholinergic side effects (dry mouth, blurred vision, drowsiness) are too troublesome for chronic use. The only practical uses are for motion sickness and in post-anaesthetic vomiting, where it should be remembered that the emetic action of morphine outlasts the antiemetic effect of a single dose of hyoscine because of the longer $t_{1/2}$ of the former.

2. Antihistamines (H_1 blockers)

These are most effective in motion sickness and labyrinthine disorders. They are also anticholinergic and this action may largely account for their antiemetic action. They include:

(i) Cyclizine (Marzine, Marezine) given either orally 50 mg or by injection but it is also effective in opiate-induced vomiting and has been given widely in pregnancy without any untoward effect on the foetus, although animal studies showed high doses to be teratogenic. The main side effects are drowsiness and a dry mouth.

(ii) Meclozine (Ancolan; Sea-Legs) is only given orally (150 mg) and has a deserved reputation for treating motion sickness. It has a low incidence of side effects, drowsiness being the main one, and is useful for prolonged use. It is also beneficial in vestibular disease, radiation sickness and in pregnancy.

(iii) Promethazine hydrochloride (Phenergan) 25–50 mg—relatively ineffective, causes drowsiness.

(iv) Promethazine chlorotheophyllinate (Avomine)—25 mg once daily. Allegedly less soporific. It is given for travel sickness and pregnancy vomiting.

(v) Betahistine (Serc) is used only in vestibular vomiting, the dose being 8–16 mg three times daily after meals.

(vi) Cinnarizine (Stugeron) is an antihistamine but may also have a specific sedative action on the labyrinth. It is effective in motion sickness and in vertigo. The dose is 30 mg three times daily orally.

3. Dopamine antagonists

(a) Metoclopramide (Maxolon) This derivative of procainamide has negligible cardiac and local anaesthetic effects, although it is a powerful antiemetic and has profound effects on the gut. Its main pharmacological properties are:

(i) Effects on the gastrointestinal tract including increased oesophageal sphincter and gastric tone and decreased stomach emptying time; enhanced pyloric activity; increased peristalsis of the duodenum with accelerated transit through the duodenum and jejunum. There is little effect on colonic motor activity, nor is there any effect on gastric secretion. These actions are blocked by anticholinergic drugs such as atropine but its actions are unaffected by ganglion-blocking drugs. The evidence suggests that it increases the amount of acetylcholine released at the postganglionic terminals. In the oesophagus it has been proposed that it also interferes with an intrinsic dopaminergic mechanism since its action at this site is blocked by levodopa.

(ii) Antiemetic effects—it prevents apomorphine-induced vomiting and is equipotent with prochlorperazine. It is a central dopaminergic antagonist and acts raising the threshold of the CTZ. It also decreases the sensitivity of the visceral nerves carrying impulses from the gut to the emetic centre. It is, however, relatively ineffective in motion sickness and other forms of centrally mediated vomiting, suggesting that the important effect in its antiemetic effects are those on the gut.

(iii) Although lacking antipsychotic properties it can produce extrapyramidal effects.

Pharmacokinetics Metoclopramide is well absorbed orally and may also be given by i.v. or i.m. injection. It undergoes metabolism by dealkylation and amide hydrolysis, about 75 % being excreted as metabolites in the urine. The plasma $t_{1/2}$ in man is 4 h.

Clinical uses

1. *Antiemetic* Trials have shown it to be effective for the following:

(i) postoperative vomiting;
(ii) radiation sickness (its use in patients with breast cancer may be contraindicated because it releases prolactin);
(iii) drug-induced nausea including that due to digitalis, antiparkinsonian drugs and antibiotics but is only effective in some patients taking cytotoxic drugs in large (2 mg/kg) doses.

Other causes of vomiting, e.g. gastritis, gastric carcinoma, vertigo and labyrinthine disorders have been suppressed in some uncontrolled studies. It appears less effective than promethazine and other standard treatments for motion sickness.

2. *Migraine* it improves absorption of paracetamol and aspirin and may be effective in removing other symptoms (see Fig. 9.11).

3. *Diagnostic radiology of the small intestine* is made easier by metoclopramide, which reduces the time required for the barium to reach the caecum and reduces the number of films required. It also prevents vomiting of barium by nauseated patients.

4. *Duodenal intubation* is facilitated, permitting rapid and successful biopsy of the small intestine. Endoscopy is also made easier and it may have a special place in emergency endoscopy.

5. Acceleration of gastric emptying and its antiemetic action make it useful in *emergency anaesthesia* (including in pregnancy) when clearance of gastric contents is necessary.

6. *Hiatus hernia symptoms* may be improved since it prevents nausea, regurgitation and reflux, epigastric burning and heartburn, although it is less successful in relieving flatulence and abdominal bloating.

The usual effective dose is 10 mg orally 3–4 times daily; i.m. or i.v. it is given 10 mg 1–3 times daily depending on the severity of the condition.

Adverse effects These are usually mild, transient and reversible:

1. Extrapyramidal effects (about 1% of patients) consist of dystonic effects such as oculogyric crises, trismus, torticollis and opisthotonus, but Parkinsonian features are absent. These effects are commoner in females and the young. They are abolished by benztropine or diazepam. Overdosage in infants, in whom the maximum dose is 0.5 mg/kg, has produced convulsions, hypertonia and irritability.
2. Other milder effects include dizziness, drowsiness, lassitude and bowel disturbances. Metoclopramide may increase lactation by releasing prolactin.
3. Drug interactions. Metoclopramide potentiates the extrapyramidal effects of phenothiazines and butyrophenones. Its effects on intestinal motility result in numerous alterations in drug absorption which include increased absorption of:

aspirin	tetracycline
paracetamol	pivampicillin
ethanol	levodopa

and decreased absorption of digoxin.

Domperidone (**Motilium**) is a dopamine receptor blocker similar to metoclopramide. It does not penetrate the blood–brain barrier and thus rarely causes sedation or extrapyramidal effects. The CTZ, however, lies functionally outside the barrier and thus domperidone is an effective antiemetic. The dose is 10–20 mg orally or by injection 4–8 hourly.

(b) Phenothiazines (see p. 243) These act particularly on the trigger zone although larger doses depress the vomiting centre as well. The following appear to have established uses as antiemetics:

(i) Chlorpromazine (Largactil) 25–50 mg orally or by injection; 100 mg by suppository – causes sedation.
(ii) Trifluoperazine (Stelazine) 2–6 mg/day orally or by injection – less sedative than chlorpromazine.
(iii) Prochlorperazine (Stemetil; Compazine) 5–25 mg orally; 12.5 mg by intramuscular injection; 25 mg by suppository.
(iv) Perphenazine (Fentazin) 2–5 mg.
(v) Thiethylperazine (Torecan) 10 mg.

These last three drugs are most effective against opioid and radiation-induced vomiting and sometimes are helpful in vestibular disturbances. They are least effective in motion sickness. All carry a risk of extrapyramidal disturbances, dyskinesia and restlessness. Perphenazine is probably the most soporific of this group.

(c) Butyrophenones (see p. 249) Droperidol is the most widely used member of the group as an antiemetic. It is given by intramuscular or intravenous injection in a dose of 2.5–10 mg. Its use is largely restricted to opioid-induced vomiting. Extrapyramidal effects and oculogyric crises are a particular risk.

4. Cannabinoids

Cannabis and its major constituent, delta-9-tetrahydrocannabinol (THC) have antiemetic properties and have been used to prevent vomiting after cytotoxic drugs. In an attempt to reduce side effects and increase efficacy, a number of analogues including **nabilone (Cesamet)**, levantradol and nonabine have been synthesised.

The site of action of these drugs is not known but an action on the cortical pathways affecting vomiting via descending pathways seems probable. There is some evidence that opioid pathways could be involved in these actions. There appears to be very little to choose between the members of the group both in terms of efficacy and side effects.

They are perhaps a little more effective than dopamine antagonists but do not entirely prevent vomiting.

Adverse effects are sedation, confusion, incoordination, dry mouth and hypotension. These are more prominent in older patients.

5. Miscellaneous agents

Large doses of corticosteroids have been found to exert some antiemetic action when used with the more emetic cytotoxic drugs. Their mode of action is not known but may include the suppression of prostaglandin synthesis.

Benzodiazepines given before treatment with cytotoxics reduces vomiting. Whether this is a specific antiemetic action or is due to reduced anxiety is unknown.

Chapter 16

VITAMINS AND THERAPEUTIC NUTRITIONAL DRUGS

THE VITAMINS

Man is unable to synthesise any vitamins except for vitamin D in the skin and nicotinamide from tryptophan. Vitamin deficiency may produce a recognisable syndrome and usually results from either

(a) inadequate dietary intake;
(b) increased demand e.g. pregnancy, growth;
(c) decreased absorption e.g. malabsorption syndrome.

Such deficiency states are frequently multiple, which accounts for the multivitamin preparations, e.g. Parenterovite (mixed vitamin B complex and vitamin C) which are often used clinically. Recognisable vitamin deficiencies are relatively rare in practice in the UK. It is suggested by some that subclinical deficiencies might impair the bodily functions before overt deficiency appears and that therefore routine vitamin supplements would be useful. There is no evidence to substantiate this view. Vitamins should therefore be employed as are other drugs—for specific indications; they are not in any sense tonics, although occasional use as a placebo may be justified.

Vitamins fall into two groups:

(i) *Water-soluble*: the B complex and C
(ii) *Fat-soluble*: A, D, E and K. The absorption of this group is particularly impaired in steatorrhoea since they are sequestered in the bowel lumen by solution in the fatty stool.

Vitamin A

The vitamin exists in several forms: retinol (vitamin A_1) is a primary alcohol and is present in the tissues of animals and sea-water fishes; 3-dehydroretinol (vitamin A_2) is present in fresh-water fishes; retinoic acid shares some but not all the actions of retinol; retinol ethers and esters also show retinol-type activity. The plant pigment carotene is pro-vitamin A and is readily converted into the vitamin in the body. Vitamin A has several physiological functions. It is essential for the integrity of epithelial cells, it stabilises membranes and is required for skeletal and soft-tissue growth. The mechanism for these actions may be that it acts as a cofactor in mucopolysaccharide synthesis, sulphate activation, hydroxysteroid dehydrogenation, cholesterol synthesis and microsomal drug-metabolising enzyme function. There is growing evidence that vitamin A may inhibit tumour formation and encourage the regression of epithelial tumours. Deficiency of retinol retards growth and development, causes night blindness, keratomalacia, dry eyes, lung disease and keratinisation and drying of the skin.

Dietary sources of vitamin A include eggs, fish liver oil, milk and vegetables. Margarine is artificially enriched with the vitamin.

Pharmacokinetics Retinol is well absorbed from the normal intestine. Amounts not greatly exceeding dietary needs are completely absorbed but large amounts escape in the faeces. Although bile enhances retinol absorption, aqueous suspensions of retinol are better absorbed than oily solutions. Vitamin A absorption is impaired in patients with steatorrhoea and under these circumstances water-miscible preparations of vitamin A can be administered orally and are absorbed better than oily preparations.

Absorption is by active transport in the intestinal wall. Esterified retinol reaches peak plasma levels 4 h after ingestion. About 100 μg/g is stored in the parenchymal and Kupffer cells of the liver. Vitamin E enhances vitamin A storage. In the plasma retinol released from the liver is bound to γ_1-globulin (retinol-binding protein).

The normal plasma concentration of vitamin A is 30–70 μg/100 ml. When a vitamin A deficient diet is taken, plasma concentrations are maintained for several months until the hepatic stores have been depleted. Clinical evidence of vitamin A lack appears when the plasma concentration falls below 20 μg/100 ml. Low plasma levels of vitamin A may be present in pregnancy, liver disease and kwashiorkor without a corresponding reduction in liver stores.

The placenta acts as a partial barrier to vitamin A, but the vitamin is present in milk. Unmetabolised vitamin A is not normally present in urine. Retinol is partly conjugated to a glucuronide and undergoes an enterohepatic circulation.

Carotene is also absorbed from the intestine in the presence of fat in the diet and bile. Absorption is greatly impaired in patients suffering from steatorrhoea. Carotene is converted to vitamin A by first-pass metabolism in the intestinal wall.

Clinical uses Vitamin A is mainly used to prevent and treat deficiency states. Dietary supplementation with halibut liver oil capsules B.P. (containing vitamin A 4000–5250 I.U. and vitamin D 450 I.U.) are used to prevent vitamin A deficiency. The normal adult daily requirement is about 5000 I.U., but during pregnancy this is estimated to be about 8000 I.U. Infants and growing children require about 4000 I.U. daily. Carotene, as a precursor of vitamin A, can replace the vitamin in the diet. One international unit (I.U.) corresponds to 0.34 μg of vitamin A and this is equivalent to 0.6 μg of carotene.

In clinical deficiency large doses are given. A recommended daily dose is 5000 I.U./kg. Thus 25 000–200 000 I.U. may be given daily. Although a single large intramuscular injection of retinol palmitate (30 000 μg of retinol) has been used in severe malnutrition, this should be followed by oral therapy. In vulnerable and malnourished communities intramuscular doses of 60 000–

120 000 μg of retinol should be given to children 6 monthly. Continuous dietary or injected supplementation of vitamin A may be necessary in steatorrhoea.

Retinoic acid is irritating when applied to the skin and is used in the treatment of acne to promote peeling. There is evidence that vitamin A accelerates the healing of wounds in normally nourished patients.

Large amounts of vitamin A have been given orally to patients with ichthyosis and other skin diseases.

Adverse effects Long-term ingestion of more than double the recommended daily intake of vitamin A can lead to toxicity. Excess of vitamin E protects against hypervitaminosis A.

Early signs of chronic hypervitaminosis include anorexia, irritability, vomiting, headache, itching and dry skin. Hepatosplenomegaly may ensue and eventually the intracranial pressure rises and in young infants the fontanelles bulge producing a clinical syndrome resembling a brain tumour. Tender hyperostoses develop on the skull and long bones. Retinoic acid is less hepatotoxic than retinol. Congenital abnormalities have been reported in infants following the mother taking large amounts of vitamin A during pregnancy.

Acute poisoning (as after eating polar bear liver) manifests as drowsiness, headache, vomiting and papilloedema. Desquamation of the skin may occur. Acute intoxication follows injection of more than 500 000 μg of vitamin A.

Derivatives of vitamin A (retinoids)

Etretinate (Tigason) is a derivative of retinoic acid. It produces desquamation (as does natural vitamin A) but at doses which do not raise the intracranial pressure or cause organ damage. Etretinate is remarkably effective in severe psoriasis (including pustular psoriasis) and in congenital ichthysiform dermatoses. The initial dose is 0.75–1 mg/kg daily taken orally in divided doses with food. Absorption is enhanced with fatty meals. Toxicity includes drying and peeling of the lips and skin, diffuse hair loss, mucosal drying, pruritus, headache and vomiting. The substance is teratogenic.

Isotretinoin (Roaccutane) is 13-cis-retinoic acid. It has a strikingly beneficial effect in severe refractory acne in doses which do not affect psoriasis and ichthyosis. The usual dose is 0.5–1 mg/kg daily for 8–16 weeks. Following the course of treatment prolonged remissions are frequently produced. Toxic effects are similar to those with etretinate.

Retinoids and cancer Retinoids have powerful effects on cell differentiation and proliferation and can inhibit or retard malignant transformation of cells *in vitro*. In animals they can prevent the action of carcinogens and there is limited epidemiological evidence that a person's retinoid status is a determinant of the risk of developing cancer. There are presently a number of trials (including one in which 20 000 male US doctors are taking either β-carotene or placebo for at least 5 years) which have been set up to determine whether dietary supplementation with retinoids can prevent cancer. In addition retinoids, either alone or in combination with established anti-cancer drugs, are being used to treat cancer. The results of all these studies are yet to be reported.

Thiamine (Vitamin B_1)

All plant and animal cells require thiamine for carbohydrate utilisation. Its most important role is as a coenzyme for decarboxylases. Thiamine deficiency leads to the various manifestations of beri-beri—including peripheral neuropathy and cardiac failure. Increased carbohydrate utilisation requires increased thiamine intake because this is consumed during carbohydrate metabolism. It is therefore useful to express thiamine needs in relation to the calorie intake (which is usually mainly related to carbohydrate consumption). Diets associated with beri-beri contain less than 0.3 mg thiamine/1000 kcal. If the diet provides more than 0.33 mg/1000 kcal the excess is excreted in the urine. Thus the recommended daily intake of 0.4 mg/1000 kcal provides a considerable safety margin. The body possesses little ability to store thiamine and if the vitamin is withdrawn from the diet, beri-beri will develop in a few weeks.

In a marginal diet deficiency is likely to occur if large amounts of refined cereal, refined sugar or alcohol are taken. Thiamine occurs in many plant and animal foods, e.g. yeast, pork. The outer coating of grains is rich in thiamine which is lost in the preparation of 'refined' foods such as white flour or polished rice.

Pharmacokinetics Absorption of thiamine is rapid and complete following intramuscular injection. Absorption from the intestine is limited to a maximum of 8–15 mg in one day. This can be achieved by taking 40 mg in divided doses. Thiamine is absorbed through the mucosa of the upper part of the small intestine by both active and passive mechanisms. The minimal daily requirement is 1 mg and this corresponds to the amount of thiamine which is metabolised. Thus at this level of intake, no unchanged vitamin is excreted. Once tissue stores are saturated and over 1 mg is ingested, some of the surplus is excreted in the urine as unchanged vitamin. The principal metabolite is pyrimidine.

Clinical use Prophylaxis or the treatment of deficiency are the only indications for thiamine administration. In the presence of thiamine deficiency, the parenteral route may be used. Up to 30 mg is injected i.m. or i.v. 8 hourly. Once the deficiency state has been corrected the oral route should be used, unless gastrointestinal disease interferes with ingestion or absorption of the vitamin. Thiamine hydrochloride tablets range from 3 to 300 mg but a generous oral dose is 5 mg daily.

Thiamine is used in the treatment of beri-beri and other states due to thiamine deficiency. These include alcoholic neuritis, Wernicke's encephalopathy, Korsakoff's psychosis and the neuritis of pregnancy.

Thiamine may also produce some improvement in subacute necrotising encephalomyelopathy. This is a genetically determined disease which is due to an inability of the brain to utilise thiamine.

Prophylactic use of thiamine is particularly indicated in chronic diarrhoeal states and following intestinal resections.

Adverse effects There have been reports of allergy to manufactured thiamine preparations, but this appears to be uncommon.

Riboflavin (Vitamin B_2)

Riboflavin is converted in the body into two essential coenzymes: flavine mononucleotide and flavine adenine dinucleotide. These are coenzymes for respiratory electron transport proteins. Riboflavin is present in significant amounts in yeast, green vegetables, liver, eggs and milk. The minimum daily requirement to prevent the signs of riboflavin deficiency is about 0.3 mg/1000 kcal.

Riboflavin deficiency is common in developing countries and occurs sporadically amongst the poor and in alcoholics in the UK. It rarely occurs in isolation from deficiencies of other B vitamins. Angular stomatitis and a sore throat are early findings and are followed by seborrhoeic dermatitis, itching and burning of the eyes with photophobia and corneal vascularisation. Late findings include a neuropathy and mild anaemia.

Pharmacokinetics Riboflavin is well absorbed via the small intestine. Absorption is impaired in patients with liver disease. Excellent absorption occurs from i.m. injections. Very little is stored in the tissues so when amounts in excess of daily requirements are taken the surplus appears unchanged in the urine. On an average diet only about 10% is excreted in the urine. The riboflavin in the faeces is probably due to bacterial synthesis in the large intestine. This is not absorbed.

Clinical use The only therapeutic application for riboflavin is in the prevention or treatment of deficiency. Riboflavin deficiency usually occurs with other dietary deficiencies but specific therapy consists of giving 5 mg of riboflavin orally daily.

Niacin (Nicotinic acid) and Nicotinamide

Niacin belongs to the B group of vitamins. Its vital metabolic role is as a component of nicotinamide adenine dinucleotide (NAD) and of nicotinamide adenine dinucleotide phosphate (NADP). It is thus essential in numerous hydrogen-transport steps within the cell including drug metabolism. Deficiency of the vitamin leads to pellagra. Because niacin is utilised in energy-yielding processes from food, as with thiamine, the dietary requirements are expressed in terms of calorific value of the diet. Also, niacin can be formed in the body from tryptophan, 60 mg of the amino acid yielding 1 mg of niacin. To cover this, 'niacin equivalents' are used to describe the pellagra-preventing properties of a diet. Pellagra may develop on diets containing less than 5.0 mg niacin equivalents/1000 kcal. When 5.5 mg niacin equivalents/1000 kcal are taken, large amounts of nicotinamide are excreted in the urine. The recommended dietary intake includes an added safety margin to account for individual variation and is 6.6 niacin equivalents/1000 kcal. Niacin occurs in significant amounts in yeast, rice, liver and other meats.

Both niacin and nicotinamide are well absorbed via the intestine and from parenteral sites of administration. These substances are distributed to all tissues. When the usual dietary amounts of niacin or nicotinamide are administered, a high proportion is excreted as N-methyl nicotinamide, nicotinuric acid, N-methyl-2-pyridone-5-carboxamide and N-methyl-4-pyridone-3-carboxamide. When increased doses are administered, a higher proportion of unchanged vitamin is excreted.

Clinical use

1. The least disputed use of niacin and nicotinic acid is in the treatment and prevention of pellagra. In the acute disease the oral dose of niacin is 50 mg up to 10 times daily. If oral treatment is not possible, intravenous injections of 25 mg are given two or three times daily. Because in the west the commonest causes of pellagra are gastrointestinal disease or alcoholism, multiple vitamin deficiency states may coexist and require treatment simultaneously. The response in acute pellagra is rapid and the swelling and soreness of the tongue, mental state and diarrhoea greatly improve within 24 h. The skin changes respond more slowly.

2. Nicotinamide is also used to lower raised blood lipids (see p. 577) and as a vasodilator in peripheral vascular and cerebrovascular disease (see p. 463). Nicotinyl alcohol may also be administered for peripheral vascular disease. It is metabolised to the active substance nicotinic acid.

Adverse effects In replacement therapy for pellagra toxicity is uncommon. Large doses can produce flushing, generalised vasodilatation (with syncope, nausea and vomiting) and itching. Some patients taking the high doses necessary for the treatment of hyperlipidaemia may exhibit impaired glucose tolerance and aggravation of hyperuricaemia.

Pyridoxine (Vitamin B_6)

Pyridoxine is one of the three forms of naturally occurring vitamin B_6. The other two forms are pyridoxal and pyridoxamine. All three forms are converted in the body into pyridoxal phosphate, which is an essential cofactor in several metabolic reactions including decarboxylation, transamination, racemisation and various other steps in amino acid metabolism. The minimal daily requirements is 1.25 mg per day/100 g of dietary protein. Pyridoxine is present in significant amounts in wheat germ, yeast, bran, rice and liver. Deficiency of the vitamin can produce glossitis, seborrhoea, fits, peripheral neuropathy and anaemia. Isoniazid prevents the activation of pyridoxal to pyridoxal phosphate by inhibiting the enzyme pyridoxal kinase. Pyridoxine hydrochloride tablets (10–50 mg) may be given to patients receiving isoniazid to prevent the development of peripheral neuropathy due to lack of vitamin B_6.

Pyridoxine is sometimes used for nausea and vomiting in pregnancy and in the treatment of radiation sickness after radiotherapy: its efficacy is unproven.

Megadoses of pyridoxine (> 2 g daily for more than 2 months) have produced ataxia and sensory neuropathy.

Vitamin B_{12} and Folic Acid (see Chapter 17)

Vitamin C (ascorbic acid)

Vitamin C is essential to man who, like the monkey and guinea pig, cannot synthesise it from glucose. Dietary lack of vitamin C ultimately results in scurvy.

Ascorbic acid is concerned in several metabolic processes, including collagen biosynthesis, steroid metabolism, electron transport chain function, activation of folic acid and in the cytochrome P_{450} system of drug metabolism. There is evidence that patients with liver disease and vitamin C deficiency have impaired drug metabolism. Ascorbic acid is present in large quantities in citrus fruits, tomatoes and green vegetables in general.

Pharmacokinetics Ascorbic acid is well absorbed following oral administration. In the presence of vomiting or malabsorption the sodium salt can be given by intramuscular or intravenous injection. Ascorbic acid is mainly metabolised by oxidation (to dehydroascorbic acid) and to 2,3-diketogulonic acid and oxalic acid. Normally about 40% of urinary oxalate is derived from ascorbic acid. When the body stores of ascorbic acid are saturated some ingested vitamin is excreted in the urine unchanged. Excretion is by both glomerular filtration and tubular secretion. Plasma clearance of ascorbic acid is greatly reduced in scorbutic patients.

Feedback control of vitamin C metabolism exists: the amount of vitamin oxidised is reduced when the body stores become depleted. However, a minimal amount of ascorbic acid (1.4–1.8 mg/kg) is oxidised or excreted daily and this represents the nutritional requirement for the vitamin.

Nutritional status for vitamin C in a patient can be assessed by measuring plasma and urinary concentrations of the vitamin. These do show wide variation and a more constant and reliable index is the intracellular leucocyte concentration. Daily intakes of 40–100 mg of vitamin C give plasma levels of 0.4–1 mg/100 ml when the tissues are saturated. Plasma levels of 0.4 mg/100 ml correspond to leucocyte levels of 20 $\mu g/10^8$ cells. When the daily intake is less than 40 mg tissue saturation falls. A daily intake of 10–15 mg results in approximately 50% of tissue saturation.

Plasma concentration of ascorbic acid falls with age, but leucocyte concentration does not. Smokers exhibit both low plasma and low leucocyte levels. Supplementary ascorbic acid is indicated when plasma levels are below 0.4 mg/100 ml in the elderly patient and below 0.7 mg/100 ml in the younger and the leucocyte level is below 15 $\mu g/10^8$ cells.

Clinical use

1. The main use of ascorbic acid is in the prophylaxis and treatment of scurvy. Normal dietary requirements are usually less than 70 mg daily. However, during infections the needs may double. Daily ingestion of 120 mg will meet the highest requirements in non-scorbutic individuals. In fully developed scurvy, 1 g daily is given until body stores have been replenished, i.e. when the total body pool is 20 mg/kg. Some clinicians recognise subclinical scurvy. This is said to occur with a dietary intake of less than 40 mg of vitamin C.

2. Ascorbic acid increases the absorption of orally administered iron. It is unlikely that in practice the vitamin need be given with iron.

3. The reducing property of ascorbate may be used in the treatment of methaemoglobinaemia. However, methylene blue is more effective.

4. Large amounts of ascorbic acid (0.5–2 g daily) are ingested by some individuals to reduce their susceptibility to the common cold and similar

respiratory illnesses. Clinical trials have indicated a small degree of protection. Nevertheless such doses of ascorbic acid may predispose to oxalate renal calculi.

5. In normally nourished patients ascorbic acid does not accelerate wound healing. In scorbutic patients wound healing is delayed and this is restored to normal by administration of ascorbic acid.

Adverse effects

1. Ascorbic acid is generally non-toxic. However, administration of 4 g daily raises the excretion of oxalate by 12 mg and a daily intake of 9 g results in a 68 mg increase in oxalate excretion. Such large doses of the vitamin have resulted in calcium oxalate urolithiasis.
2. Cholestyramine may reduce the absorption of ascorbic acid.
3. Ascorbic acid deficiency can result in a macrocytic anaemia due to block of the conversion of folic acid to folinic acid. Paradoxically the administration of folic acid to a patient lacking both substances may precipitate overt ascorbate deficiency.

Vitamin D (see p. 671)

Vitamin E (Tocopherol)

This is present in wheat-germ oil and many foods. Deficiency in animals causes abortion in females and degeneration of the germinal epithelium of the testes in males. In man no known deficiency syndrome exists. In an experiment in which volunteers took a diet containing only one third of the normal vitamin E content, over 8 years there were no effects apart from a minor reduction in erythrocyte survival time, although the blood levels of vitamin E fell by 80 %. Feeding large amounts of polyunsaturated fatty acids increases vitamin E requirements. Vitamin E appears to protect the erythrocyte against haemolysis and possibly acts as an anti-oxidant and detoxicates naturally generated carcinogens. It has been suggested that if this were so then ingestion of low cholesterol, high polyunsaturated fatty acid diets could be associated in the long term with an increased incidence of cancer. There is no evidence to substantiate this hypothesis. Despite lack of knowledge of its functions vitamin E is widely consumed as part of the multiple vitamin therapies taken by some enthusiasts. This represents an uncritical approach to therapy: fortunately large doses of the vitamin are harmless.

Vitamin K (see p. 595)

DRUG THERAPY IN HYPERLIPOPROTEINAEMIA

The pathogenesis of atherosclerosis is not understood but there is evidence that the lipid in atheromatous plaques enters the blood-vessel wall from the plasma. Thus control of blood lipids might be expected to affect the development of atheroscelerosis. Although such measures are carried out in practice, the elimination of other risk factors such as hypertension, lack of exercise and smoking are also very important, as is the management of diseases which predispose to arterial disease, such as diabetes mellitus.

The distribution of cholesterol and the lipoprotein fractions are of great importance. The plasma lipoproteins are formed in the liver and may be divided into the main classes shown in Table 16.1.

Table 16.1 Classification of plasma lipoprotein fractions

Fraction	*Protein* %	*Cholesterol (free and esterified)* %	*Triglyceride* %	*Phospholipid* %
High-density lipoprotein (HDL) α-lipoprotein	45	21	8	26
Low-density lipoprotein (LDL) β-lipoprotein	21	51	10	18
Very low-density lipoprotein (VLDL) pre β-lipoprotein	1	21	54	9

Prospective studies have shown that a low HDL cholesterol in relation to total plasma cholesterol is a more reliable predictor of coronary disease than a raised total cholesterol or triglycerides. Conversely a raised HDL fraction appears to have some protective function in preventing the development of coronary artery disease. Individuals with familial hyperalphalipoproteinaemia are known to have an above-average life expectancy ('longevity syndrome'). These observations may also explain the relative immunity of pre-menopausal women to coronary disease since they have HDL concentrations 30–60% higher than males of the same age.

HDL levels are increased by exercise, weight loss and in those living on fish diets. Regular alcohol intake, chlorinated hydrocarbon pesticides, phenobarbitone and phenytoin may also raise HDL levels, the link between these drugs being hepatic enzyme induction. Nicotinic acid and clofibrate have similar effects on HDL synthesis.

Although the site and mechanism of hepatic HDL synthesis are unknown it is probable that smooth endoplasmic reticulum is the site of secretory protein synthesis. The clinical significance and possible therapeutic exploitation of these observations is presently under investigation.

Evidence is now appearing that correction of blood lipids in patients with hypercholesterolaemia can induce regression of atherosclerosis as measured by radiographic techniques. Lowering tissue cholesterol will raise HDL cholesterol levels as this represents mobilised cholesterol from tissue deposits into the plasma. Thus, a drug such as clofibrate which depletes tissue cholesterol pools and raises HDL may theoretically be more useful than a resin such as cholestyramine which lowers total serum cholesterol but has no significant action on tissue pools of cholesterol.

In practice, the initial measure in controlling blood lipids is diet. Even when this has not been successful on its own and drug therapy is employed, dietary measures should be continued.

Cholestyramine (Questran)

This is a basic anion-exchange resin containing quaternary ammonium groups capable of exchanging chloride for bile salt anions. It is not absorbed from the intestine and binds to bile acids, disrupting micelles, thereby inhibiting the reabsorption of bile salts and cholesterol into their enterohepatic cycle. The cholestyramine and bound bile salts pass out in the faeces so that faecal excretion of bile salts and cholesterol is increased.

This lowers plasma cholesterol in two ways:

(a) A larger proportion of cholesterol synthesised by the liver is converted into bile salts and less enters the circulation as cholesterol and its esters.
(b) Since bile acids inhibit the rate-limiting 7-hydroxylation step in cholesterol metabolism the decreased absorption of bile salts increases the oxidative removal of cholesterol.

However, because cholesterol itself exerts a negative feedback inhibition on the enzyme β-hydroxyl β-methylglutaryl coenzyme A reductase which is concerned with cholesterol synthesis, lowering plasma cholesterol levels removes this inhibition and accelerates cholesterol production. Therefore removal of cholesterol can accelerate cholesterol synthesis and in some patients this can compensate for the loss of cholesterol. As this increase in cholesterol output by the liver does not appear in plasma β-lipoprotein, it may account for increases in tissue pools of cholesterol which have been observed in patients treated with cholestyramine. It may therefore be advantageous to administer drugs which block cholesterol (and triglyceride) synthesis with bile-acid-binding resins. Examples of such synergistic combinations are cholestyramine with nicotinic acid and DEAE-Sephadex with clofibrate.

Clinical uses

1. Type IIa hyperlipoproteinaemia: with cholestyramine alone serum cholesterol levels are usually reduced by 20–40 % within 3–6 weeks. The serum triglyceride level may transiently be initially elevated. Cholestyramine is taken as a flavoured suspension in water in a dose of 8–16 g 8 hourly immediately before meals. The palatability may be increased by giving it with lemonade or other drinks.

2. Diarrhoea due to ileal resection or Crohn's disease affecting absorption of bile salts in the terminal ileum is due to the unabsorbed bile salts irritating the colon to produce catharsis. Cholestyramine in divided doses of 16 g/day has been shown to help this condition by absorbing the excess bile acids.

3. Diarrhoea after vagotomy or in diabetic autonomic neuropathy affecting the vagal fibres controlling gall-bladder function occurs due to the release of large amounts of bile salts into the small intestine, swamping its reabsorptive capacity and producing colonic catharsis. This may be counteracted by cholestyramine.

4. Pruritis in partial biliary obstruction.

Table 16.2 Treatment of hyperlipoproteinaemia

Frederickson type	*Lipoprotein increased*	*Cholesterol*	*Triglyceride*	*Coronary heart disease risk*	*Diet*	*Drugs*
I	Chylomicra Minor ↑ VLDL	+	+++	Low	Low fat (< 30 g/day) High carbohydrate	None
IIa	LDL	+++	±	Very high	Low cholesterol/ Low saturated fat	Cholestyramine Probucol d-thyroxine Nicotinic acid
IIb	LDL VLDL	+++	+++	Very high	Weight reduction Low cholesterol/ Low saturated fat	Cholestyramine Probucol Clofibrate d-thyroxine Nicotinic acid
III	Abnormal lipoprotein 'floating β'	++	++	High	Weight reduction Low cholesterol Low carbohydrate	Clofibrate Probucol Cholestyramine Nicotinic acid
IV	VLDL	±	++	High	Weight reduction Low carbohydrate Alcohol restriction	Clofibrate Nicotinic acid
V	VLDL Chylomicra	+	+++	Low	Weight reduction High protein/low fat/ Low carbohydrate No alcohol	Clofibrate Nicotinic acid

Key: ± Normal/slight increase; + Slight increase; ++ Moderate increase; +++ Greatly increased.

Adverse effects Since cholestyramine is unabsorbed the major side effects are limited to the gut and consist of bloating, excessive flatus and constipation, which affects 20–25 % of patients. Usually constipation can be controlled with a stool softener such as dioctyl sodium sulphosuccinate.

Absorption of vitamins D, K, folic acid, phenylbutazone, thiazides, antibiotics, warfarin, thyroxine and cardiac glycosides may be impaired. The absorption of clofibrate is unaffected.

Colestipol (Colestid)

This is a resin with similar properties to cholestyramine.

Dextrothyroxine

L-thyroxine lowers serum cholesterol and LDL levels by increasing steroid metabolism and faecal excretion. Cholesterol biosynthesis is increased to a smaller extent. Dextrothyroxine has the same action but less cardiac effects than L-thyroxine. It has been used in children when bulky resins cannot be readily taken. Dextrothyroxine is usually given with propranolol.

The starting dose for an adult is 2 mg daily, slowly increasing up to 2–4 mg twice daily.

Dextrothyroxine is contraindicated in patients with ischaemic heart disease and with cardiac arrhythmias. Because of the excessive mortality in such patients, the use of dextrothyroxine is at present very restricted. Dextrothyroxine potentiates the action of cardiac glycosides and anticoagulants.

Clofibrate (Atromid-S)

Cholesterol synthesis by the liver is inhibited by clofibrate at two defined enzyme steps, the most significant being the inhibition of the reaction of acetyl coenzyme A and mevalonate. In addition the excretion of neutral sterols is enhanced. VLDL is more rapidly removed from the circulation resulting in a fall in plasma concentration of about 20–25 %, but LDL levels fall by only 4–10 %. The HDL concentration rises, presumably due to mobilisation of tissue cholesterol which is incorporated into HDL. As a result of these changes, there is a modest overall fall in total plasma cholesterol of around 6 %.

Pharmacokinetics Clofibrate is completely absorbed from the intestine. It circulates in the form of the free acid, p-chlorophenoxyisobutyric acid (CPIB), which is highly bound to albumin. This binding is saturable and at high therapeutic plasma levels the proportion of unbound drug increases (see Fig. 16.1) so that drug clearance increases. Due to this inconstant binding it is impossible to predict steady-state levels from the kinetics of a single dose. The $t_{1/2}$ is approximately 10–25 h. CPIB is completely excreted in the urine, 60 % as the glucuronide.

Clinical use Clofibrate is given orally in a dose of 0.5–1 g twice daily. Recent studies have caused the place of clofibrate in therapy to be reconsidered since it

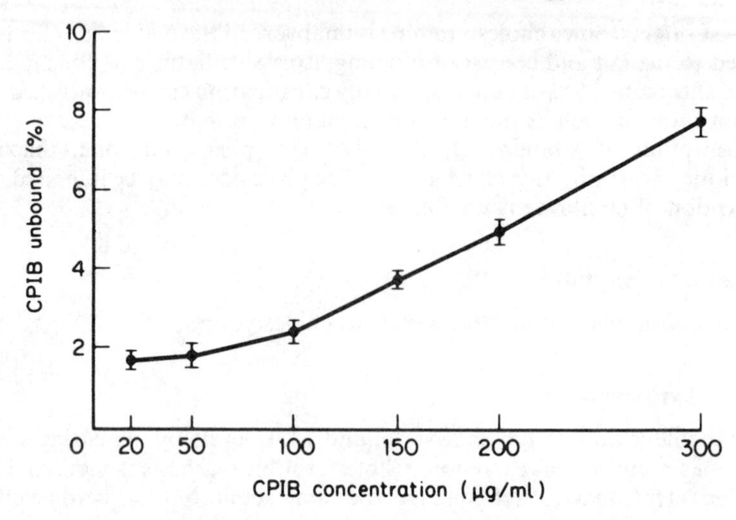

Fig. 16.1 Relationships of unbound CPIB to total plasma concentration (From R. Gugler and J. Hartlapp, *Clin. Pharm. Ther.*, **24**, 432 (1978)).

produces only modest falls in cholesterol and has significant toxicity. It has a limited place in the management of gross hypercholesterolaemia and in the prevention of pancreatitis in massive hypertriglyceridaemia.

Adverse effects The Coronary Drug Project in the USA, a prospective clinical trial of a number of drugs in ischaemic heart disease, identified a hitherto unsuspected incidence of serious adverse effects. These were an increased frequency of common medical conditions which would be difficult to detect without the employment of careful trials:

(i) Gall-bladder disease and gallstones: a threefold excess of cholecystectomies occurred amongst treated patients possibly related to mobilisation of cholesterol from the body and secretion of lithogenic bile.
(ii) Non-fatal pulmonary emboli and thrombophlebitis.
(iii) Arrhythmias, particularly ventricular.

About 5% of patients suffer gastrointestinal upset when clofibrate treatment is begun.

Clofibrate is highly protein bound in the plasma and may potentiate the action of oral anticoagulants by displacement from albumin-binding sites. It also interferes with thyroxine binding to thyroid hormone binding globulin.

Bezafibrate

This is structurally related to clofibrate. It lowers total cholesterol and triglycerides, mainly lowering LDL whilst HDL cholesterol may be raised.

It is highly protein bound and is mainly excreted by the kidneys.

Clinical uses like clofibrate, it produces a fall of about 20 % in cholesterol in Types IIa and IIb hyperlipidaemia. The dose is 200 mg 8 hourly.

Adverse effects These include abdominal bloating and rarely impotence and myositis. Drug interactions occur due to its high protein binding and it potentiates oral anticoagulant action.

Probucol (Lurselle)

This is unrelated to other hypolipidaemic drugs and lowers serum cholesterol by inhibition of its dietary absorption and hepatic synthesis. It also increases faecal loss of bile acids.

Given in doses of 500 mg twice daily, it is used with diet in hypercholesterolaemia. It should not be used during pregnancy nor in nursing mothers (it is secreted in milk). Although usually well tolerated, 10 % of patients have self-limiting diarrhoea.

Nicotinic acid

In large doses (3–6 g daily in divided doses) this rapidly decreases serum triglyceride levels by 30–50 % and in some patients reduces blood cholesterol by 15–20 %. The mechanisms of action appear to be:

(i) inhibition of triglyceride lipase, resulting in reduced release of free fatty acids and a block in triglyceride synthesis by the liver;
(ii) reduction in the rate of synthesis of LDL in patients with type IIa hyperlipoproteinaemia.

Clinical use Reductions in blood lipids occur in all types of hyperlipoproteinaemia apart from type I. Increases in HDL also occur. Perhaps the most firmly established indication for nicotinic acid in this context is the treatment of homozygous familial hypercholesterolaemia (IIa) when optimum dietary and resin therapy have not restored plasma lipids to normal. Nicotinic acid is used concurrently with these other measures. Reductions in blood cholesterol are usually modest when nicotinic acid is used alone, apart from type III hyperlipoproteinaemia.

Adverse effects Dose-related toxic effects are prominent because of the large doses of nicotinic acid required. These include: itch and flushing (tolerance may occur if the dose is slowly increased from 0.25 g 8 hourly); diarrhoea; dyspepsia; cholestatic jaundice; raised serum aminotransferase; hyperuricaemia with gout and hyperpigmentation.

Chapter 17
DRUGS ACTING ON THE BLOOD

HAEMATINICS

Iron

Although iron is the most abundant heavy metal in the earth's crust, anaemia due to iron deficiency is prevalent throughout the world. Iron plays a vital role in the body—it is present in haemoglobin, myoglobin, enzymes (such as cytochromes, catalase and peroxidase) and stored in the reticuloendothelial system and bone marrow. In an adult the total body iron is 3.5–4.5 g of which 70 % is incorporated in haemoglobin, 5 % in myoglobin and 0.2 % in enzymes. Most of the remaining iron (1–1.5 g, i.e. approximately 25 %) is stored as ferritin or haemosiderin. In addition, about 2 % (80 mg) lies in the 'labile iron pool' and about 0.08 % (3 mg) is active transport iron which is bound to the specific iron-binding protein transferrin.

Pharmacokinetics Absorption is the main mechanism controlling total body iron which remains remarkably constant in healthy individuals despite variations in diet, erythropoietic activity and iron stores. Iron absorption occurs in the small intestine and is influenced by many factors.

1. *Form of iron*

(a) Inorganic ferrous iron is better absorbed than ferric iron.

(b) Absorption of iron from the diet depends on the source of the iron. Most dietary iron exists as non-heme iron and is poorly absorbed (5 % approximately) mainly because it is combined with phosphates and phytates (in cereals) which prevent absorption. Heme iron is well absorbed (20–40 %) but is often deficient from the diet of poorer people and vegetarians.

(c) Absorption of iron from orally administered iron salts is poor—around 10 %, and is reduced by concomitant administration of cereals and other bulky foods.

2. *Factors increasing absorption*

(a) Vitamin C (ascorbic acid) facilitates iron absorption, and iron-deficiency anaemia commonly accompanies vitamin C deficiency. Combined preparations are available but the therapeutic advantage is minimal in iron-deficiency states, so long as an adequate dose of elemental iron is given (see below).

(b) Alcohol increases ferric but not ferrous iron absorption and there is an association between alcohol abuse and iron overload (haemosiderosis).

3. *Gastrointestinal tract* Gastric acid enhances absorption of iron from some foods. Intrinsic factor may potentiate the absorption of iron as well as

vitamin B_{12}. Thus iron deficiency may occur in pernicious anaemia and after operations such as partial gastrectomy.

4. *Drugs* Tetracycline given concurrently chelates iron and there is mutual malabsorption.

Disposition of iron

Iron in the gut becomes bound to a protein (known as mucosal transferrin) in the gut lumen and is transported across the mucosa where it becomes assimilated into the total body iron pool. In plasma iron is transported by the protein transferrin (molecular weight 76 000–80 000), each molecule of which can bind 2 atoms of iron. This protein gives up its iron complement to red cell precursors in active bone marrow. When red cells are broken down in the marrow at the end of their life span, macrophages bind the iron atoms released which are then taken up again by transferrin. About four-fifths of total body iron exchange normally takes place through this cycle (see Fig. 17.1).

The main storage form of iron is the ferritin molecule. This protein is shaped as a hollow sphere and iron atoms are stored in the cavity inside. Ferritin is found principally in the liver. Aggregates of ferritin molecules which have a very high iron content are called haemosiderin, and accumulate when hepatic iron stores are high.

Placental passage of iron At term 4.5 mg of iron is the average daily net flow across the placenta from mother to fetus. At this stage of pregnancy 90 % of maternal plasma iron turnover is directed towards the fetus. Thus a pregnant woman during the last trimester requires 5.0 mg iron daily (see p. 587).

Iron deficiency In iron-deficient states, the serum iron (normally 14–31 μmol/l in males and 11–29 μmol/l in females) falls only when stores have

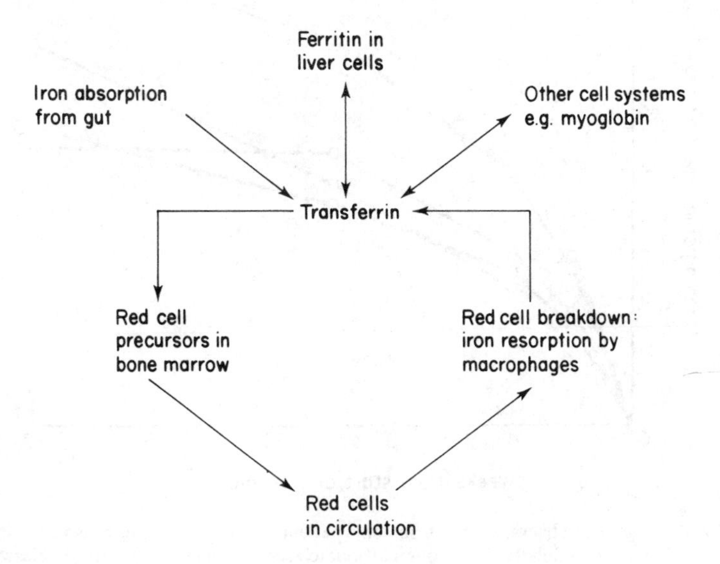

Fig. 17.1 Iron metabolism.

become considerably depleted. The total amount of transferrin determines the total iron binding capacity (TIBC) of plasma, and is normally 54–80 μmol/h.

Transferrin saturation (i.e. plasma iron divided by TIBC) is normally 20–50 % and this provides the most clinically useful index of iron status. In iron-deficiency states, TIBC rises in addition to the fall in plasma iron and when transferrin saturation falls to less than 16 % basal erythropoeisis starts to decline.

Iron deficiency is the commonest cause of anaemia and although predictably it is commoner in third world countries, even in developed countries its incidence is appreciable, e.g. in one study 8 % of menstruating women in north west America were found to have mild iron-deficiency anaemia. The cause of iron deficiency is most often multi-factorial, e.g. poor diet may be combined with excessive demands on stores (pregnancy, chronic blood loss, lactation), reduced stores (premature birth) or defective absorption (achlorhydria, surgery to the GI tract, hookworm infestation).

Although treatment of iron deficiency is often relatively simple, its cause must always be determined so that the underlying condition can be treated.

Oral iron

The majority of patients with iron deficiency can be given simple oral preparations. A total daily dose of 100–200 mg of elemental iron should stimulate a reticulocyte response after 5 days (which lasts about 10 days) and the haemoglobin concentration will start to rise at 0.1–0.2 g/dl/day until an optimum level is reached (in 8–10 weeks in moderate anaemia, see Fig. 17.2).

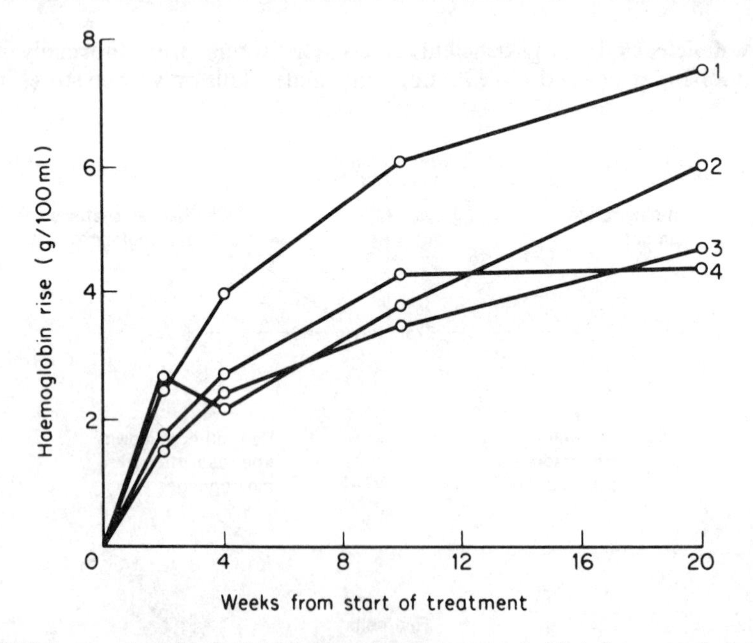

Fig. 17.2 Average rise in haemoglobin in anaemic patients treated with: 1, ferrous succinate/succinic acid; 2, ferrous sulphate 3, ferrous carbonate/ascorbic acid; 4, sustained release iron preparation. (From M. C. G. Israëls and T. A. Cook, *Lancet*, **2**, 654 (1965)).

Occasionally the marrow response is delayed for up to 10 days. Treatment is continued for 3 to 6 months after haemoglobin levels have entered the normal range in order to replace iron stores.

Failure to respond may be due to a number of reasons:

(i) wrong diagnosis (i.e. iron deficiency is not the primary cause of the anaemia);
(ii) failure of patient compliance;
(iii) continued blood loss;
(iv) malabsorption, e.g. coeliac disease, post-gastrectomy.

There are over 70 iron-containing oral preparations but many of these are combined preparations containing vitamins as well as iron. None of these combinations carries an advantage over iron salts alone except for those containing folic acid which are used prophylactically in pregnancy. Slow-release preparations of iron may be unreliably absorbed from the upper small intestine (where iron uptake is at its most efficient) and are not recommended.

For most patients, treatment should start with a simple preparation such as ferrous sulphate (200 mg t.d.s.) or ferrous fumarate (200 mg t.d.s.) or ferrous gluconate (600 mg t.d.s.). These and other inexpensive simple preparations are shown in Table 17.1.

Side effects of oral iron include nausea, epigastric pain, heartburn, constipation and diarrhoea. No preparation has been shown to be less irritating than any other (when equivalent doses of elemental iron are given) but patients with ulcerative colitis and those with colostomies often suffer particularly severely from these side effects. Although iron is best absorbed in the fasting state, gastric irritation may be reduced by recommending that it is taken after food.

Parenteral iron

Oral iron is effective, easily administered and cheap. Parenteral iron is also effective but can be associated with serious side effects and is expensive.

The rate of rise in haemoglobin is the same following parenteral iron and oral iron because the rate-limiting factor is the capacity of the marrow to produce red cells. The only advantages of parenteral iron are that the iron stores are rapidly and completely replenished and there is no doubt about compliance.

The relative indications for parenteral iron are:

(i) malabsorption;
(ii) genuine intolerance to oral iron preparations;
(iii) when continued blood loss is not preventable and large doses of iron cannot be readily given by mouth;
(iv) failure of patient compliance;
(v) when great demands are to be made on a patient's stores—as in an anaemic pregnant woman just before term.

The parenteral iron preparations available are iron dextran and iron sorbitol citric acid.

Table 17.1 Oral iron preparations

Name	*Total amount (mg)*	*Iron content (mg)*	*Daily dose of iron (mg)*	*Cost of one day's treatment relative to ferrous sulphate*
Ferrous sulphate B.P.	200/tablet	60/tablet	180 adult	1.0
Ferrous fumarate B.P.	200/tablet	65/tablet	195 adult	2.8
Ferrous gluconate B.P.	300/tablet	35/tablet	210 adult	4.0
Ferrous succinate B.P.	100/tablet	35/tablet	210 adult	6.2
Ferrous sulphate mixture paediatric B.P.C.	60/5 ml	12/5 ml	9–18 premature infant	12.6
Ferrous fumarate mixture B.P.C.	140/5 ml	45/5 ml	9–18 premature infant	2.2
Ferrous gluconate (Ferlucon elixir)	250/5 ml	29/5 ml	7–15 premature infant	2.0
Ferrous succinate (Ferromyn elixir)	105/5 ml	37/5 ml	7–15 premature infant	3.0

Iron dextran (Imferon) is a stable complex of ferrous hydroxide and dextran with a molecular weight of 180 000. The solution for injection contains 50 mg/ml.

Pharmacokinetics Iron dextran is usually given by deep intramuscular injection and excites a local tissue reaction with the eventual formation of dense fibrous tissue. The injected iron slowly leaves the site of injection via lymphatics (50% leaves within 72 hours, and thereafter removal occurs at a much slower rate). It is ingested by macrophages and stored as ferritin molecules in the reticuloendothelial system. From here it is released into the plasma where it is transported linked to transferrin to the bone marrow. The release of iron is so slow that transferrin does not become saturated, but concurrent oral iron therapy should be stopped.

Clinical use The total dose of iron required is first calculated. Tables based on body weight and haemoglobin level are provided with each pack of ampoules, alternatively the following formula can be used:

$$\text{mg of iron required} = (15 - \text{patient's Hb in g}) \times \text{body wt in kg} \times 3$$

Treatment is started with a test dose of 0.5 ml i.m. Thereafter 2.5 ml i.m. may be given at intervals until the total dose required has been given. In patients with a history of allergy a graded series of injections is recommended, e.g. 0.5 ml, 1.0 ml, 1.5 ml, then 2.0 ml until the course is completed.

Adverse effects Even after taking the advised precaution of injecting iron dextran intramuscularly, along a Z-track, grey-brown staining of the skin often occurs. This lasts several months. Systemic reactions are rare. They include fever, headache, sensations of heat, vomiting, arthralgia, regional lymph-node enlargement, urticaria, bronchospasm and anaphylaxis. It is wise to give concurrent antihistamines if the patient has a history of allergic disorder.

In rats and mice repeated very large doses of iron dextran have produced sarcomas at the site of injection. There is no evidence that this occurs in man.

Failure to respond may be a result of abnormal reticuloendothelial function. For example in active rheumatoid arthritis there may be a hypochromic anaemia in the presence of adequate marrow iron stores. These patients have a relative block at the point of release of iron in macrophages to plasma transferrin. They do *not* respond to oral or parenteral iron.

Intravenous iron dextran may be given to patients requiring parenteral iron who have a small muscle mass, a disorder of haemostasis contraindicating i.m. injections, or who cannot tolerate i.m. injections. The initial solution (50 mg/ml) is diluted in 0.9% saline or 5% dextrose to give a final concentration of 500 mg/250 ml. A small test dose is first infused (5 drops/minute for 10 minutes). The patient is carefully observed both during and for 5–10 minutes after this, during which time any anaphylactic reactions would be expected to occur. If this is without incident, the total dose infusion may then be given over a period of 6–8 hours, with supervision continuing for 1 hour after completion of the infusion.

Iron sorbitol citric acid (Jectofer) This preparation may only be given intramuscularly and, again, deep injections should be given to minimise staining of the skin. It is not a homogeneous compound, having a molecular weight between 3000 and 4000. It diffuses more readily from the site of injection than iron dextran and, as a result, up to 40% may be lost in the urine. Peak concentrations often with complete transferrin saturation occur at 2–8 hours. Of the retained iron, 30% is immediately available for haem synthesis and the rest is stored.

Side effects include a metallic taste in the mouth and a tendency to exacerbate pre-existing urinary tract infections (probably related to high levels of free iron in saliva and urine respectively). Occasionally allergic reactions resulting in cardiovascular collapse are seen which may be related to the toxic effects of free iron in the circulation. If the patient is concurrently taking oral iron, a proportion of the transferrin binding sites will already be occupied and this may further elevate the free iron levels when iron sorbitol is given thus exacerbating toxicity. To minimise this risk, oral iron should be stopped at least 3 days before iron sorbitol is administered, and the i.m. injections (of not more than 100 mg each) should be given at intervals of at least 24 hours, with no more than 3 injections weeky.

Vitamin B_{12}

Vitamin B_{12} consists of a nucleotide linked to four pyrrol rings (similar to a porphyrin) with a cobalt atom attached. Attached to the cobalt atom may be cyanide (**cyanocobalamin**), hydroxyl (**hydroxocobalamin**), methyl (**methylcobalamin**) or a 5′-deoxyadenoxyl group. These forms are interconvertible, cyanocobalamin spontaneously forming hydroxocobalamin on exposure to light. Vitamin B_{12} in nature is produced only by bacterial synthesis and none is present in plants. Rich sources are liver, kidney and heart, and moderate amounts are found in other meats, fish and eggs.

Vitamin B_{12} is needed for normal erythropoiesis and for the maturation of other cell types. However, its precise role in cellular growth is not understood, although it is required for certain biochemical reactions such as the isomerisation of methylmalonyl coenzyme A to succinyl coenzyme A, and the conversion of homocysteine into methionine (which also utilises 5-methyltetrahydrofolate). Vitamin B_{12} is also involved in the control of active folate metabolism, thus both substances are required for intracellular nucleotide synthesis.

Deficiency of vitamin B_{12} leads to a macrocytic anaemia with megaloblastic erythropoiesis in the bone marrow, and may be accompanied by neurological disorders which include peripheral neuropathy, subacute combined degeneration of the spinal cord, dementia and optic neuritis.

Pharmacokinetics The normal total body stores of B_{12} are about 3 mg and following total gastrectomy (which abolishes B_{12} absorption) the effects of malabsorption do not occur for 3–5 years. Thus the daily loss is 2–4 μg which results mainly from metabolic breakdown. Normally absorption from the diet is very efficient and the daily requirement is 3–5 μg.

Absorption of vitamin B_{12} requires secretion of intrinsic factor from the gastric parietal cells (which also produce gastric acid). Intrinsic factor is a glycoprotein of molecular weight approximately 55 000 and it forms a stable complex with vitamin B_{12} in the presence of acid. The complex passes down the small intestine and is absorbed at specific receptor sites in the terminal ileum, in the presence of a neutral pH and calcium ions.

Absorption is slow, starting 4 hours after ingestion, with a peak at 8–12 h and continuing for up to 24 h. Very small amounts (approximately 1 %) of an oral dose are absorbed by passive diffusion, and although B_{12} is synthesised by colonic bacteria it is not appreciably absorbed because it has bypassed the active absorption mechanism.

In pernicious anaemia, parietal cells are destroyed by an autoimmune reaction and thus intrinsic factor is not produced, resulting in B_{12} deficiency.

Vitamin B_{12} is transported by two plasma proteins, transcobalamins I and II (TCI and TCII). TCII is a beta-globulin and acts as a transport protein collecting B_{12} from the ileal cells and transporting it to the liver. TCI is an alpha-globulin which carries most of the body's B_{12} and this complex is probably the storage form of the vitamin.

The normal range of plasma vitamin B_{12} levels is 170–900 ng/l. Values below this must be present for a diagnosis of vitamin B_{12} deficiency to be made, but low levels are found in other conditions such as pregnancy and simple atrophic gastritis, where total body B_{12} deficiency is *not* present.

The main excretion route of B_{12} is into the bile but an enterohepatic circulation results in most of this being reabsorbed via the intrinsic-factor mechanism. Unbound B_{12} is excreted by glomerular filtration, but this is of minor importance.

Clinical uses Replacement therapy is required in B_{12} deficiency which may be:

1. Nutritional (rare, usually only found in vegans).
2. Gastric malabsorption (pernicious anaemia, total or partial gastrectomy).
3. Intestinal malabsorption (jejunal diverticulae, strictures, anastomoses or fistulae; Crohn's disease, irradiation damage, *Diphyllobothrium latum* infection).

In purely nutritional deficiency replacement therapy may be given orally. In these cases commercially available preparations containing doses far in excess of those actually required (5 μg daily) are usually given, e.g. 50 μg daily.

When B_{12} deficiency is due to malabsorption, replacements are given by intramuscular injection. Two parenteral forms are available, cyanocobalamin and hydroxocobalamin, but the latter is preferred as it is retained more efficiently, e.g. only 10–20 % of a 1 mg injection of cyanocobalamin is retained compared to 70 % of 1 mg of hydroxocobalamin.

The recommended dose of hydroxocobalamin is 250 μg monthly or 1000 μg every 2 months. Contrary to popular belief, larger doses are unnecessary in subacute combined degeneration of the cord.

A peak in the reticulocyte response is seen 5 days after commencing treatment. Following treatment a high incidence (up to 10 %) of sudden death has been observed – the mechanism is obscure but may be due to the sudden fall in plasma potassium (on average 1 mEq/l) in patients with pre-existing hypokalaemia. This may provoke fatal cardiac arrhythmias, and thus potassium deficiency must be corrected and drugs such as digoxin given with care to patients undergoing this therapy.

Iron-deficiency anaemia may be uncovered several months after remission of megaloblastic anaemia, and iron therapy will be needed as well.

Patients with B_{12} deficiency due to malabsorption are likely to require life-long replacement therapy; they should be given an adequate explanation of this, and preferably should carry a card with an up-to-date record of their B_{12} therapy.

Tobacco amblyopia Vitamin B_{12} deficiency makes patients unduly sensitive to retinal damage by tobacco. Optic neuritis occurs in tobacco amblyopia (and may also be seen in pernicious anaemia in non-smokers). The administration of hydroxocobalamin to patients with tobacco amblyopia restores the blood picture to normal but usually does not improve visual acuity.

Folic acid

This is made up of a pteridine linked to glutamic acid via para-aminobenzoic acid. It is present in a wide variety of plant and animal tissues, the richest sources being liver, yeast and green vegetables. The major dietary form is as polyglutamate conjugates with up to seven additional glutamate residues being attached to the glutamate of folic acid. These are split off by α-carboxypeptides in intestinal juice and serum.

Folic acid is required for normal erythropoiesis. As with vitamin B_{12} a deficiency of folic acid results in a megaloblastic anaemia and abnormalities in other cell types. The role of folate in cell metabolism results from its ability to transfer groups containing single carbon atoms in biochemical reactions. These include the methylation of deoxyuridylic acid to form thymidylic acid and other reactions in purine and pyrimidine synthesis. A key reaction in folate metabolism is its reduction to various forms of tetrahydrofolate by dihydrofolate reductase. It is this enzyme which is inhibited by drugs such as methotrexate, pyrimethamine and trimethoprim in different organisms.

Pharmacokinetics Orally administered folate is mainly absorbed in the proximal small intestine within 5–20 min of ingestion. There appears to be a specific absorptive mechanism as patients are known with specific defects in folate absorption. During the absorptive process folic acid is initially formylated and then methylated before entering the portal blood.

About one third of the total body folate (70 mg) is stored in the liver (which normally contains 7 μg/g).

The requirements and losses are such that when no folate enters the body the stores last for about 4 months. Thus folate deficiency develops more rapidly than vitamin B_{12} deficiency. As with vitamin B_{12} the faeces contain folate which has been synthesised by colonic bacteria, but this occurs too low in the gut for absorption into the portal blood.

The normal range for serum folate is 4–20 μg/l but values may be falsely elevated by haemolysis and the red cell folate concentration (normal range 140–450 μg/l) is more reliable.

Clinical uses Folate deficiency may be:

1. Nutritional (children, old age, alcoholism);
2. Malabsorption (coeliac syndromes, sprue, specific malabsorption, diseases of the small intestine);
3. Excessive utilisation (pregnancy, chronic haemolytic anaemias, malignant disease, chronic inflammatory diseases);
4. Drugs (phenytoin, phenobarbitone, primidone, nitrofurantoin).

The normal requirement for folic acid is about 200 μg daily. In established folate deficiency large doses (5–15 mg p.o. daily) are given. If the patient is unable to take the drug by mouth, it may be given intravenously. Patients with severe malabsorption may be deficient in both folic acid and vitamin B_{12}, and the administration of folic acid alone may precipitate acute vitamin B_{12} deficiency neuropathy. These patients require careful evaluation and replacement of *both* vitamins concurrently if indicated.

Patients taking long-term anticonvulsants commonly have macrocytic red cells and the majority have no detectable folate deficiency. A few patients, however, develop a megaloblastic anaemia due to folate deficiency, the cause of which is complex but is partly due to interference with DNA synthesis by these drugs, and their ability to induce hepatic enzymes which increase folate breakdown. Treatment involves the addition of folic acid 5 mg daily to the anticonvulsant regimen.

Iron and folic acid therapy in pregnancy

Pregnancy imposes a substantial increase in demand on maternal stores of iron and folic acid. A net gain of around 500–600 mg of elemental iron is required for each pregnancy to accommodate the requirements of the growing fetus together with the expansion of the maternal red cell mass, and most women are iron-depleted by the end of the pregnancy if they do not receive supplements. Requirements for folic acid also increase two- to three-fold and deficiency in pregnancy may lead to prematurity and to the birth of infants who are of low birth weight for their gestational age.

In the United Kingdom the usual practice is to give iron and folic acid supplements throughout pregnancy. Tablets containing 100 mg of elemental iron and 200–500 μg of folic acid are available to be taken once daily, and these have substantially removed the problem of anaemia in pregnancy.

Therapy for aplastic anaemia

Aplastic anaemia is a rare syndrome characterised by pancytopenia associated with the replacement of normal cellular bone marrow by fat, there is no evidence of malignancy and no proliferation of reticulin. Some cases are congenital (usually Fanconi's anaemia) but many are idiosyncratic although in 50% of these an aetiological agent (a virus, chemical or drug) can be implicated. Certain drugs have a particularly strong association with aplastic anaemia, and these include phenylbutazone, oxyphenbutazone, amidopyrine and chloramphenicol. They should be avoided for this reason unless there is a specific clinical indication, for although cases of aplastic anaemia are very rare, they are not uncommonly fatal.

Treatment Support with transfusions (of red cells and platelets) and appropriate antibiotics prior to bone marrow transplantation from a histocompatible donor has become the therapy of choice in recent years for young patients.

For those who are unsuitable for this treatment *anabolic steroids* may reduce the requirement for transfusions. Two 17-alpha alkyl derivatives of testosterone have been used: oxymetholone and stanozolol.

Oxymetholone (Anaprolon)

High doses (1–2 mg/kg daily) have been used and it may take 3 months to see any benefit. Their use should not continue unless a response is seen as the side effects are considerable.

Adverse effects

1. Cholestatic jaundice and, rarely (with prolonged use), hepatocellular carcinoma. They should not be used in patients with pre-existing liver disease.
2. Virilisation of children and adult females.
3. Premature closure of the epiphyses in children.
4. Fluid retention.

Stanozolol (Stromba)

The recommended dose is 50 mg every 2–3 weeks by deep intramuscular injection. The side effects are similar to oxymetholone.

Danazol (Danol) (see p. 614)

This is also a 17-alpha alkyl derivative of testosterone but is an anabolic steroid with mild androgenic side effects.

It was originally introduced for the treatment of fibrocystic disease of the breast and endometriosis (see p. 622), but has recently been shown to be of benefit in α_1*-antitrypsin deficiency*, *idiopathic thrombocytopenic purpura* (ITP) and in two types of *haemophilia*.

ITP is a disorder in which platelets react with an autoantibody and are destroyed by macrophages. Splenectomy may diminish antibody production and lead to a remission but in those for whom this is inappropriate or ineffective, danazol may lead to sustained elevation of platelet counts. The exact mechanism of action is unknown but may be due to effects on T-cell function or to its ability to bind to steroid-binding globulin thus displacing active hormones which may then be available for uptake by other tissues.

There are also some early reports that danazol is able to reduce requirements for clotting factor infusions in patients with classical haemophilia (factor VIII deficiency) and Christmas disease (factor IX deficiency).

Clinical use Doses of 400–800 mg/day by mouth in divided doses have been used for some time in endometriosis, and similar doses have been used in the treatment of ITP.

Side effects are due to the mild androgenic effect and thus include acne, hirsutism and fluid retention. These are only occasionally severe, and if so, this may be an indication to withdraw the drug. Cholestatic jaundice has not been a problem with this drug. It must not be given in pregnancy.

ANTICOAGULANTS

Injury to the vessel wall, stasis of blood and activation of platelets lead to thrombosis. Anticoagulants interfere with the process of clotting which is only part of the complex series of events producing thrombosis. Clotting takes place via a chain reaction of activation of a number of clotting factors; the purpose of this cascade of activation is to amplify a small initial change in a single factor to produce splitting of large numbers of fibrinogen molecules to give a fibrin clot. The process is activated either by contact with collagen or other material or more physiologically by the release of thromboplastin from traumatised tissue (Fig. 17.3). A thrombus formed *in vivo* however (clotting is an *in vitro* phenomenon) consists of a platelet head, which is the initial aggregated mass of

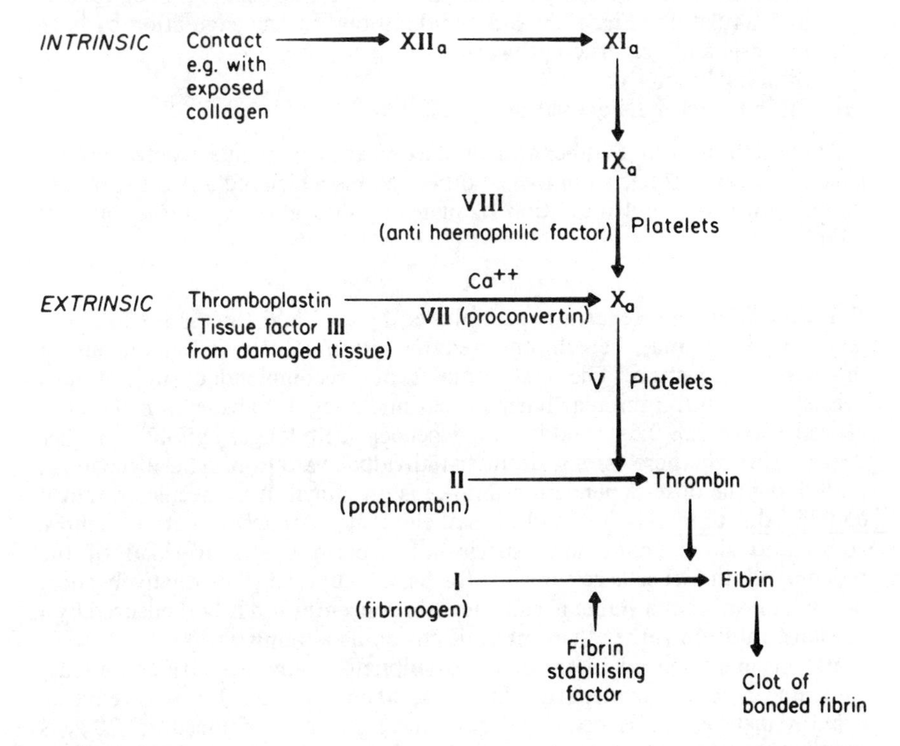

Fig. 17.3 Simplified clotting factor cascade. ('a' indicates activation of appropriate clotting factor).

platelets, and a fibrin tail which is formed secondary to platelet aggregation. Conventional anticoagulants largely fail to interfere with the important part played by platelets in thrombosis and do not affect the formation of the initial platelet aggregate. They are therefore only a partial answer to the clinical problems posed by thrombosis.

Heparin

This is a highly sulphated acidic mucopolysaccharide (M.W. 6000–20 000). It is prepared commercially from ox lung and intestinal mucosa although originally discovered by McLean (whilst he was still a medical student at the Johns Hopkins Hospital) in heart, liver and lung tissue. It is usually prescribed in international units, one unit keeping 1 ml of blood fluid for 1 h and 1 mg being equivalent to 120 units. The anticoagulant activity of heparin is caused by its interaction with proteins, particularly the blood-clotting factors. It exerts an action at several points in the clotting cascade:

(a) It acts as an antithrombin but only in the presence of a plasma 'heparin cofactor' known as antithrombin III. This inhibits conversion of fibrinogen to fibrin and prolongs the whole blood-clotting time.
(b) Inhibition of activated factor X activity, again the presence of antithrombin III is necessary for this action. Factor X_a occupies a central role in coagulation (Fig. 17.3) and its inhibition blocks coagulation by both intrinsic and extrinsic pathways.
(c) Inhibits factor IX_a.
(d) Inhibits factor IX activation by XI_a.

These actions mean that heparin, unlike oral anticoagulants, is active *in vitro* as well as *in vivo*. It has a number of other actions which include activation of lipoprotein lipase and inhibition of platelet aggregation by fibrin (but not ADP).

Pharmacokinetics Heparin is precipitated by acid and thus is ineffective if given orally. It may be administered by intramuscular, subcutaneous or intravenous injection. The first route is not recommended since it may predispose to intramuscular haematomas and irregular absorption. The $t_{1/2}$ varies between 0.5–2.5 h. and is dose-dependent with longer half-life at higher doses although there is a wide inter-individual variation. The mechanism underlying the dose-dependent clearance is unknown. It is speculated that it could be due to metabolite inhibition of elimination or accumulation of more active and slowly eliminated species of heparin or to overload of the reticuloendothelial cells responsible for heparin uptake. This relatively short half-life means that a stable plasma heparin concentration is best ensured by a constant infusion rather than intermittent bolus administration.

80% is metabolised in the liver to sulphates, oligosaccharides and desulphated heparin (uroheparin). In shock, when liver blood flow is reduced, heparin metabolism is decreased with increased risk of bleeding. 20% is excreted unchanged by the kidney. Heparin does not cross the placental barrier or enter milk.

Clinical use

1. *Full anticoagulation*

(a) Take blood for baseline clotting studies.
(b) Give a loading dose of 5000 units of heparin i.v. followed by an i.v. infusion of 1500 units per hour (in saline), e.g. via a syringe pump.
(c) Re-check the clotting studies approximately three hours later. Aim for values two to three times the baseline.

Indications for full heparinisation

(a) Immediate induction of anticoagulation in a patient known or suspected to have a deep venous thrombosis or pulmonary embolus. Oral anticoagulants are started at the same time and thus heparin can usually be discontinued once these have established their effect (usually about 72 hours).
(b) Acute arterial obstruction to a limb (although thrombolytics may be more effective—see p. 602.
(c) Crescendo angina—to prevent infarction.
(d) Disseminated intravascular coagulation. Heparin is only used if the patient continues to deteriorate despite adequate resuscitative measures and a continuing decline in the fibrinogen level with bleeding after 4 packs of fresh frozen plasma. Its use requires experience and meticulous laboratory control.
NB. Heparin is also used to prime haemodialysis and extracorporeal circulation circuits.

2. *Low dose heparin* This refers to administration of 5000 units 8–12 hourly subcutaneously as prophylaxis against deep venous thrombosis. At this dose its major activity is against factor X_a with the other factors being relatively unaffected. Ultra-low dose heparin refers to continuous infusions of 1 unit/kg/hour intravenously.

The clinical situations where prophylaxis may be indicated include:

(a) Major surgery. At least 30% of patients develop a deep vein thrombosis after major surgery (as verified by ^{125}I fibrinogen scans). Those at particularly high risk are the obese, the elderly, those with previous or family histories of deep vein thrombosis, those with disseminated malignancy and patients undergoing pelvic or hip surgery. There *is an increased incidence of minor bleeding* with this treatment, e.g. wound haematomas. Subcutaneous heparin is started immediately pre-operatively and continued until the patient is ambulant.
(b) Post-myocardial infarction.
(c) Post-partum.
(d) Patients with polycythaemia or other hypercoagulable states.

Adverse effects

1. Bleeding. This is the chief side effect and one of the commonest drug-induced adverse effects in hospital patients, as shown in the Boston Collaborative Drug Surveillance Program (see p. 185). Its management is described below.

2. Osteoporosis and vertebral collapse: with chronic dosage of over 10 000 units daily this rarely occurs. It has been reported in pregnancy at lower doses.
3. Alopecia } these are very rare.
4. Thrombocytopenia }

Management of dangerous bleeding with heparin

1. Protamine sulphate. This is given as a slow intravenous injection: rapid injection has caused anaphylactoid reactions. It is of no value if it is more than 3 hours since heparin was administered.
   (i) If it is 1–3 hours since heparin was stopped, give 0.5 mg protamine per 100 units of heparin.
   (ii) If it is < 1 hour since heparin was stopped, give 1.0 mg protamine per 100 units of heparin.
2. If bleeding is very severe or continuous despite protamine, give fresh frozen plasma (FFP) or fresh whole blood.

Control of heparin therapy Before starting anticoagulant treatment of any type it is wise to obtain control figures for the various anticoagulant factors (clotting screen). Heparin affects all stages of blood coagulation and tests of both extrinsic (prothrombin time) and intrinsic (partial thromboplastin time) pathways reflect its action. The most sensitive part of the coagulation system is the thrombin–fibrinogen reaction which can be monitored by the thrombin time. The whole-blood coagulation time is altered but rather inconvenient to monitor regularly. There is no effect on bleeding time. The usual effects of heparin therapy are as follows:

Test	*Normal*	*Heparin therapy*
Clotting time (Lee–White)	10 min	30 + min
Activated partial thromboplastin time (Kaolin–Cephalin time)	35 s	90 + s
Thrombin time	10–12 s	60 s

If heparin is given for 48 h in conjunction with oral anticoagulants until the latter become effective, many users do not measure the effect on coagulation unless there is some special reason. If, however, heparin treatment is prolonged it is important to prevent heparin accumulation. If the drug is given intermittently a coagulation test should be carried out before each dose of heparin to ensure satisfactory heparin clearance. If heparin is given by continuous infusion, then the coagulation test should be measured at least once daily and the dose adjusted according to results.

Oral anticoagulants

The commonly used oral anticoagulants belong to one of two groups of compounds:

1. Derivatives of 4-hydroxycoumarin, e.g. **warfarin, bishydroxycoumarin**.
2. Derivatives of indan 1:3 dione, e.g. **phenindione**.

Pharmacology Oral anticoagulants prevent the synthesis of clotting factors II, VII, IX and X which are dependent upon vitamin K for synthesis.

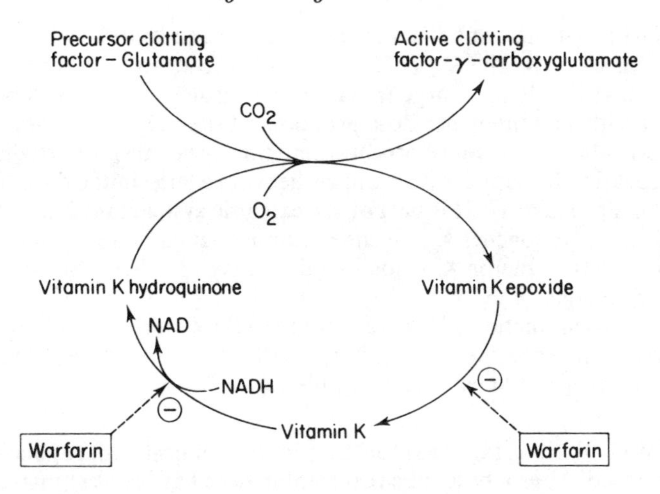

Fig. 17.4 Proposed mechanism of action of warfarin.

Functional forms of these factors contain residues of γ-carboxyglutamic acid. This is formed by carboxylation of a glutamate residue in the peptide chain of the inactive precursor. This is a vitamin K-dependent process and is accomplished by the recycling of vitamin K (Fig. 17.4). This cycle is interrupted by warfarin. The γ-carboxyglutamate residues bind calcium and wounds which expose phospholipid-rich surfaces bind prothrombin and other vitamin K factors via these calcium ion bridges. After warfarin treatment partially carboxylated inactive forms of these clotting factors which are unable to bind calcium accumulate in the blood.

Pharmacokinetics Following oral administration warfarin absorption is almost complete and maximum plasma concentrations are reached within 2–8 h. Approximately 97 % is bound solely to plasma albumin but it can cross the placental barrier. The mean $t_{1/2}$ is about 44 h but there is a 12-fold variation in $t_{1/2}$ between individuals. Metabolism involves hydroxylation followed by conjugation and excretion into the gut in the bile. Deconjugation and reabsorption occur to complete the enterohepatic cycle. The basal rate of metabolism is inherited and the $t_{1/2}$ is the same in identical twins and different in fraternal twins, i.e. it is under polygenic control (see Chapter 4). A hereditary pattern of warfarin resistance probably due to an abnormal receptor site for warfarin has been described. The aged are relatively more sensitive to warfarin than the young and require a smaller maintenance dose. This is correlated with reduction in plasma albumin levels but there is no alteration in the binding or overall kinetics of warfarin. Possible explanations are an altered sensitivity of the clotting-factor system to the drug in the old or a relative deficiency of vitamin K due to deficient intake or altered kinetics.

The plasma drug level is not clinically useful since this cannot be directly related to effect: it can be shown that decrease in rate of prothrombin synthesis is proportional to the logarithm of the coumarin level. Since these drugs act by inhibiting synthesis of active vitamin K-dependent clotting factors anticoagulation must await the catabolism of these factors and so the peak effect is not achieved for 24–36 h. The $t_{1/2}$s of the factors involved are II, 60 h; VII, 6 h, IX, 20 h and X, 40 h. Giving a large initial dose of drug as opposed to beginning treatment with a maintenance dose produces a faster depression of factor VII (the fastest catabolised). Since prothrombin time measures, in part, this factor, the therapeutic effect appears to occur earlier with a large initial dose. This may be in error since factor VII is part of the extrinsic system and is not therefore involved in thrombogenesis. The chronic anticoagulant effect is most closely related to levels of factor X. A loading dose may not therefore produce any clinical advantage.

The pharmacokinetics of bishydroxycoumarin elimination are apparently dose-dependent since the $t_{1/2}$ increases with increasing dose. Phenindione kinetics however are linear and resemble those of warfarin.

Clinical uses Various regimens for the initiation of oral anticoagulation have been proposed. After a baseline prothrombin time has been estimated, one of the simplest schemes is to give warfarin 10 mg/day for 3 days although a loading dose of 6 mg/day for 3 days is more appropriate for those patients who are likely to be particularly sensitive to warfarin, i.e. the elderly and debilitated, post-major surgery, those with intercurrent heart failure, liver disease or severe diarrhoea.

The prothrombin time (PT) is then repeated on the morning of the fourth day and the maintenance dose is estimated. If heparin is being infused concurrently, it should be stopped 3 hours before blood is taken as heparin itself will have some effect on the PT. If the PT is in the therapeutic range (i.e. 2–3 times control) then heparin may be discontinued permanently. There is a wide variation in the maintenance dose of warfarin due to the variability in drug elimination, the average daily dose is 6 mg, range 1–20 mg. (Tablets are available in 1 mg—buff coloured, 3 mg—blue, and 5 mg—pink, sizes.) For phenindione the equivalent doses are a load of 200–400 mg over the first 3 days and a maintenance dose of 25–200 mg (average 100 mg).

There is little evidence that abrupt cessation of oral anticoagulant therapy results in a rebound hypercoagulable state. It is therefore unnecessary to taper off the dose. The long $t_{1/2}$s of these drugs ensure that suddenly stopping the drug does not produce a sudden fall in the plasma drug level.

Indications for oral anticoagulation

1. *Deep vein thrombosis and pulmonary embolism* There is good evidence that recurrence may be prevented if oral anticoagulants are continued for at least 3 months (although some evidence suggests that 6 months is more preferable) after a single episode of deep vein thrombosis and for at least 6 months after a single episode of pulmonary embolism. Recurrent deep vein thrombosis probably requires life-long anticoagulation, and similarly recurrent pulmonary embolism with the attendant risk of secondary pulmonary hypertension may also be an indication for life-long treatment.

2. *Atrial fibrillation* There is substantial evidence that the morbidity from embolism may be reduced in atrial fibrillation associated with many conditions including mitral stenosis, thyrotoxicosis, chronic sino-atrial disease, congestive cardiomyopathy and ischaemic heart disease.

There is also good evidence that moderate to severe mitral stenosis (where there will be left atrial dilatation) in sinus rhythm also carries a substantial risk of embolism which can be reduced by anticoagulants. There is no good evidence yet that patients with asymptomatic mitral valve prolapse in sinus rhythm should be anticoagulated.

3. *Following cardiac surgery* Patients receiving prosthetic valve replacements should have life-long anticoagulation but this does not apply to those receiving tissue valves or undergoing coronary artery bypass grafting unless there is a complicating arrhythmia.

There is as yet no substantial evidence that anticoagulation should be instituted routinely for patients post-myocardial infarction, with peripheral vascular disease, or primary pulmonary hypertension, or for prophylaxis against cerebrovascular embolism in patients who have had transient ischaemic attacks.

There are a number of contraindications to anticoagulant therapy, which are divided into absolute and relative.

1. *Absolute*

(a) active bleeding from gastrointestinal, respiratory or genito-urinary tracts, e.g. peptic ulceration, active lung disease, ulcerative colitis;
(b) blood dyscrasias with haemorrhagic diathesis;
(c) dissecting aneurysm of the aorta;
(d) surgery of CNS or eye;
(e) space-occupying CNS lesion.

2. *Relative*

(a) history of potential bleeding lesion;
(b) severe hypertension;
(c) severe diabetes;
(d) chronic alcoholism;
(e) pregnancy;
(f) hepatic or renal insufficiency;
(g) lack of sufficient intelligence or co-operation on the part of the patient.

Adverse effects Coumarins are the safer of the two groups although anticoagulation is by no means a completely safe procedure and these drugs have a relatively poor therapeutic index.

1. Haemorrhage This is the chief adverse reaction and it may be serious in the short term in 10% of patients suffering this complication. The incidence depends on the degree of control, and it increases with prolongation of the prothrombin time but is unaffected by age. Intercurrent diseases such as diarrhoea (reducing vitamin K absorption) and cardiac failure, increase the risk of bleeding.

   Vitamin K_1 (5–25 mg) is an effective antidote for both warfarin and phenindione. It must be given intravenously slowly over 3–5 minutes to avoid dysphoric reactions and hypotension, or orally by which route it is rapidly absorbed. Control of bleeding is usually achieved within 6 hours although the prothrombin time takes 12–36 h to return to normal. If anticoagulant therapy needs to be continued, only 5 mg vitamin K_1 is given since the larger doses saturate the body and make the patient resistant to oral anticoagulants for 2–3 weeks. If bleeding occurs fresh frozen plasma will be required to replace deficient clotting factors. Fresh whole blood may be required to replace deficient clotting factors and correct hypovolaemia.

2. Drug interactions—see below.
3. Specific side effects of the coumarins:
   (a) alopecia;
   (b) skin rashes;
   (c) teratogenesis and abortion (see p. 600).
4. Specific side effects of the phenindiones:
   (a) interference with iodine uptake by the thyroid;
   (b) uricosuria and renal tubular damage;
   (c) hepatitis;
   (d) agranulocytosis;
   (e) dermatitis;
   (f) secreted into breast milk (unlike warfarin)
   (g) metabolites may colour the urine pink or orange (distinguished from blood by adding a few drops of acetic acid when it fades).

Phenindiones, in contrast to warfarin, are secreted into breast milk and since neonates are deficient in coagulation factors until several days after birth because of liver immaturity, there is a danger of neonatal haemorrhage. Phenindiones should be avoided therefore in the puerperium, but warfarin appears safe.

Drug interactions Numerous drug interactions occur with oral anticoagulants which are of practical importance. These are summarised in Table 17.2.

Displacement of coumarins from protein binding by competing drugs such as aspirin (see Chapter 1) produces major changes in drug effect because of the relatively small apparent volume of distribution of these drugs. Until recently it was thought that the major effect of phenylbutazone was exerted via this process. Certainly competition between warfarin and phenylbutazone for binding to plasma albumin can be demonstrated *in vitro*. The mechanism underlying this interaction turns out to be more interesting, and is concerned with the racemic nature of commercial warfarin which is a mixture of R- and S-warfarin. In many respects R- and S-warfarin are different drugs, for S-warfarin is 3–4 times more potent than R-warfarin. The S-isomer is metabolised more rapidly than the R-form and the principal metabolic product is 7-hydroxy-warfarin, in contrast to the warfarin alcohol formed by R-warfarin. If phenylbutazone were acting to displace warfarin from albumin binding, the $t_{1/2}$ of warfarin should be reduced (see Chapter 1). This is not observed but it has been found that the formation of 7-hydroxy-warfarin is reduced by phenylbutazone and studies of the effect of phenylbutazone on the elimination of R- and S-warfarin revealed the situation shown in Fig. 17.5. Phenylbutazone increases the plasma clearance of R-warfarin approximately twofold but decreases S-warfarin clearance. Paradoxically, the clearance of racemic warfarin appears to be unchanged, however, since the decrease in S-

Table 17.2 Drug interactions with oral anticoagulants

	Mechanism	Drugs involved	
1.	*Enhanced anticoagulant effect*		
A.	Inhibition of hepatic metabolism of anticoagulant	Alcohol Amiodarone Chloramphenicol Cimetidine Colchicine Dextropropoxyphene Influenza vaccine	Metronidazole MAOI Phenylbutazone Sulphinpyrazone Sulphonamides Tetracyclines
B.	Reduced Vitamin K absorption	Oral neomycin Liquid paraffin	
C.	Reduced plasma triglycerides carrying Vitamin K	Clofibrate	
D.	Drugs with intrinsic potential to cause GI ulceration	Aspirin and all the NSAIDs (although to variable extent, naproxen, ibuprofen said to be safer)	
E.	Displacement of oral anticoagulant from plasma protein binding	Chloral (trichloroacetic acid metabolite) Ethacrynic acid	
F.	Unknown mechanism	Chloroquine Danazol	Miconazole Ketoconazole
2.	*Reduced anticoagulant effect*		
A.	Induction of hepatic enzymes metabolising oral anticoagulant	Barbiturates Griseofulvin	Carbamazepine Rifampicin
B.	Administration of vitamin K in occult form	Some enteral feeding preparations e.g. Complan, Flexical, Triosorbon	

warfarin clearance masks the increased R-warfarin clearance. However, the relative amount of the more powerfully anticoagulant S-warfarin is now increased and hence the anticoagulant potency of the racemic mixture is apparently enhanced.

There is a danger that the uncritical extrapolation of experimental data may lead to unnecessary restrictions on prescribing drugs to patients on warfarin. For example, although it is true that broad-spectrum antibiotics inhibit bacterial vitamin K synthesis in the gut, in practice most of the vitamin K we absorb comes from the diet, and a clinically significant interaction of the penicillins and cephalosporins with warfarin is rare. The parenteral aminoglycosides do not interact with warfarin although oral neomycin must be avoided as it produces a malabsorption state leading to reduced vitamin K absorption. Phenytoin may increase the free warfarin concentration by protein binding displacement but this is offset by its hepatic enzyme inducing effect and in

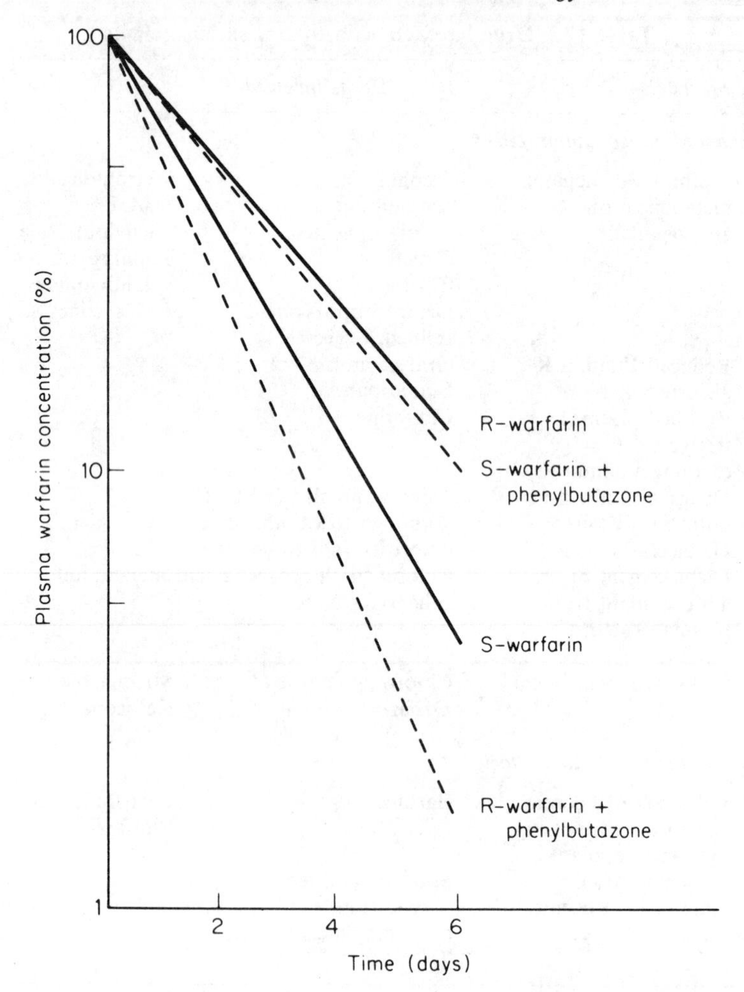

Fig. 17.5 Single doses of R- and S-warfarin were administered before and after 100 mg phenylbutazone three times daily for 10 days. The concentrations of the isomers are expressed as a percentage of the extrapolated initial plasma concentration. (From R. J. Lewis *et al.*, *J. Clin Invest.*, **53,** 1067 (1974).)

practice it rarely causes problems in patients taking warfarin. Table 17.3 shows those drugs unlikely to show clinically significant interactions with warfarin.

Control of oral anticoagulant therapy This is usually done by measurement of the prothrombin time, a test of the extrinsic pathway. This is however sensitive to depression of factor V, which is not a result of oral anticoagulant therapy, and insensitive to depression of factor IX, which is. The test measures the clotting time of citrated plasma when calcium and an extrinsic thromboplastin are added. The variability of this thromboplastin gives widely different results between laboratories and a correction is made using the standard

Table 17.3 Drugs unlikely to react with warfarin

(The following drugs can usually be given safely to patients on warfarin therapy.
However, caution is always necessary when altering the drug treatment of a patient taking anticoagulants.)

Analgesic/anti-inflammatory drugs	—ibuprofen*, indomethacin*, naproxen*, paracetamol
Antiarrhythmic drugs	—atropine, disopyramide, lignocaine
Antibacterial drugs	—aminoglycosides (parenteral), cephalosporins, fusidic acid, penicillins
Anticonvulsant drugs	—ethosuximide, phenytoin, sodium valproate
Antihypertensive drugs	—hydralazine, methyldopa, prazosin
Beta-adrenoceptor blockers	—water-soluble drugs (e.g. atenolol) preferred
Bronchodilator drugs	—aminophylline, salbutamol, terbutaline
Drugs for gastrointestinal diseases	—antacids (conventional doses), carbenoxolone, ranitidine, most laxatives
Drugs for heart failure	—frusemide, thiazides
Hypnotics and anxiolytics	—benzodiazepines
Hypoglycaemic drugs	—no major effect with biguanides or sulphonylureas
Oral contraceptives	—'progesterone-only'

* Care needed with all non-steroidal anti-inflammatory analgesics due to the increased risk of GI bleeding.
(Reproduced with kind permission of the authors from *Adverse Drug Reaction Bulletin*, 1983, (no. 183), 382.)

British Comparative Thromboplastin to give the British Corrected Ratio (BCR). Some thromboplastins are relatively insensitive to lowering of factor X and consequently may lead to overdosage unless correction is made. The therapeutic range is a prolongation of the prothrombin time by a factor of two or three. The prothrombin time must be performed within a few hours of blood collection and is unsuitable for samples sent by post.

The Thrombotest contains cephalin and gives a longer and thus more sensitive clotting time than the usual prothrombin time method. It is more sensitive to factor IX deficiency. The results are expressed as the percentage of normal of clotting factors and the therapeutic range is 7–15%.

Once oral anticoagulant control is established, laboratory monitoring is required on an outpatient basis every 4–12 weeks.

Anticoagulants in pregnancy

Warfarin crosses the placenta and when taken throughout pregnancy will result in complications in about one-third of cases: 16% of fetuses will be spontaneously aborted or stillborn, 10% will have post-partum complications (usually due to bleeding) and 7% will suffer teratogenic effects.

The problem is that in any case there is an increased risk of embolism in pregnancy, and women at risk (e.g. those with prosthetic heart valves) must continue to be anticoagulated.

The commonest teratogenic effect of warfarin is a defect in ossification which can lead to optic atrophy, deafness, nasal bone hypoplasia and limb deformities in affected fetuses. This occurs if warfarin is taken between the 6th and 9th weeks of gestation and most damaged fetuses are spontaneously aborted. Other problems include fetal haemorrhage *in utero* which can lead to CNS damage, and placental separation due to retroplacental bleeding.

Heparin does not cross the placenta but has not been convincingly shown to prevent arterial thromboembolism in pregnancy. In addition its long-term use may cause osteoporosis, alopecia and retroplacental bleeding resulting in fetal death. One practical scheme for the management of pregnancy in women on anticoagulants would be to warn the patient to seek medical advice as soon as she thinks she may be pregnant. If this is confirmed and it is within the first 9 weeks then it may be best to change to subcutaneous heparin until this critical period for teratogenesis has passed. The patient should then switch back to warfarin with very careful control to avoid overdosage with its attendant risk of bleeding.

The patient should be admitted to hospital at 36 weeks and should be changed to intravenous heparin before the onset of labour. The heparin is reversed with protamine before delivery, but heparin together with warfarin is restarted immediately post-partum and continued until the full effect of warfarin is re-established. If labour starts suddenly in a patient still receiving warfarin, she should be given fresh frozen plasma and the baby given vitamin K_1.

Ancrod (Arvin)

This is a glycoprotein (M.W. 30 000) extracted from the venom of the Malayan pit viper. It is a proteolytic enzyme which acts as an anticoagulant by directly destroying fibrinogen. It does not cleave fibrinogen in the same way as thrombin, since a different residue is left and the fibrin stabilising factor (factor XIII) is not activated, so that an unstable fibrin is formed which is removed by the reticuloendothelial system.

It is given by slow intravenous injection of 1–3 units (0.5–1.5 mg)/kg initially over 2–12 h followed by a maintenance dose of 2 units (1 mg)/kg 12-hourly. It is weakly antigenic, and hypersensitivity and acquired resistance have been reported. Microangiopathic haemolytic anaemia has also been described, but spontaneous haemorrhage is rare. The effect of treatment is monitored by measurement of the fibrinogen level. When the drug is discontinued the fibrinogen level returns to normal over several days; rebound hypercoagulation does not occur. A specific antivenom is available for treatment of acute defibrination. The therapeutic role of Ancrod is not defined: it has been used to treat central retinal-vein thrombosis, priapism, sickle-cell crisis and deep-vein thrombosis.

Drugs affecting the fibrinolytic system

Control of thrombus formation and prevention of intravascular coagulation is as important as the formation of stable clots at sites of vascular injury. Fibrinolysis is effected by plasmin, an enzyme whose proteolytic activity is not confined to fibrin. This system is as closely controlled as that of clotting by a number of activating and inhibiting factors (see Fig. 17.6).

The coagulation system may be constantly active in laying down fibrin to seal endothelial deficiencies and the fibrinolytic system in removing fibrin deposits to ensure vascular patency. It is possible to lyse thrombus by administration of plasminogen activators such as urokinase and streptokinase.

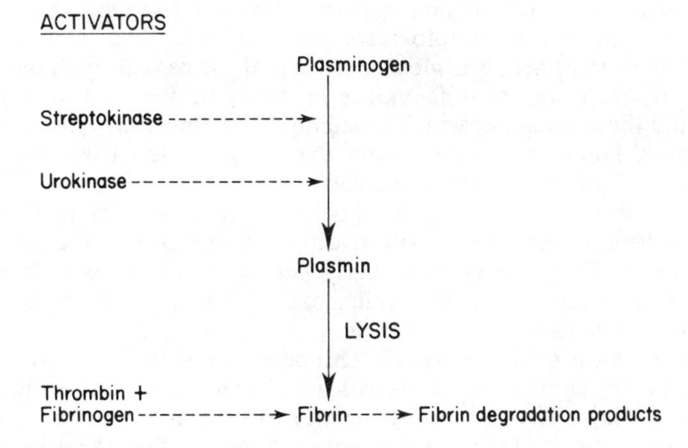

Fig. 17.6 The fibrinolytic system.

Table 17.4 Properties of streptokinase and urokinase

	Streptokinase	*Urokinase*
Source	Cultures of Group C beta-haemolytic streptococci	Human urine; human fetal kidney tissue culture
$t_{1/2}$	10–12 min	11–16 min
Antigenicity	Yes	No
Stability	Room temperature	4°C

Thrombolytic agents

The two commonly used agents in clinical practice are streptokinase and urokinase. Some of their properties are compared in Table 17.4.

Mechanisms of action Streptokinase is an indirect plasminogen activator. It initially combines with plasminogen in equimolar amounts to form a streptokinase–plasminogen complex which then activates the fibrinolytic mechanism by converting free plasminogen into plasmin. The streptokinase–plasminogen complex is also progressively converted into the streptokinase–plasmin form which can also activate plasmin.

Streptokinase is a foreign protein and thus antigenic. As antibodies to streptococci are very common in man, a variable amount of streptokinase is initially needed to neutralise these antibodies and hence an adequate loading dose is required prior to a continuous infusion.

Urokinase is a direct activator and can stimulate plasmin formation without first forming an activator complex. As it is a protein derived from man, it is not antigenic.

Clinical indications

1. *Pulmonary embolus* Two large studies in the USA in patients with angiographically proven pulmonary emboli showed faster and more complete resolution with either streptokinase or urokinase than with heparin. Thrombolytic treatment was most effective in those patients with the largest emboli and there was no difference in mortality between the thrombolytic group and those given heparin. Thrombolytic treatment may also minimise the chronic pulmonary hypertension that may develop from incomplete resolution of multiple pulmonary emboli.

2. *Deep venous thrombosis* Thrombolytics produce faster resolution of clots than heparin and are more effective in the preservation of the function of venous valves. They may be particularly valuable when clot extends into the more proximal veins of the leg, which leads to a higher risk of subsequent pulmonary embolism.

3. *Peripheral arterial thrombosis* Thrombolytics have been shown to be effective in the majority of patients with acute arterial thrombi, ie. present for less than 10 days. They may either be infused systemically or into the local arterial circulation. There is no evidence, however, that these agents are effective in patients with chronic peripheral arterial disease.

4. *Acute myocardial infarction* Systemic infusion of streptokinase or urokinase has been shown to lead to angiographic resolution of occluded coronary vessels in several small series but the results of larger well-controlled trials are awaited.

Intracoronary infusion of thrombolytics has been shown effectively to lyse thrombi provided treatment is started within six hours of the onset of symptoms. The best results are obtained in patients who are also given subcutaneous heparin which may protect the reperfused vessel against recurrent thrombosis.

5. *Other indications* Local instillation of thrombolytics into occluded shunts (e.g. in renal dialysis patients) or occluded intravascular lines (e.g. central venous catheters) is effective in restoring patency in a substantial proportion of cases.

There is no evidence as yet that these drugs are effective in the treatment of cerebrovascular events due to emboli.

Clinical use

Streptokinase Treatment is commenced with a loading dose of 250 000 i.u. (via a constant infusion pump) followed by a maintenance infusion of 100 000 i.u./h for up to 72 hours.

Occasionally patients have relatively high titres of streptococcal antibodies and theoretically require higher loading doses. However, in practice with the schedule recommended above, this is not a problem. Because of its antigenicity, streptokinase should generally not be used for one year after a course of therapy, and urokinase may be used instead.

Urokinase The loading dose is 4400 i.u./kg over 10 minutes followed by 4400 i.u./kg/h as a maintenance infusion for 12 hours. Note that urokinase is much more expensive than streptokinase.

Laboratory monitoring The thrombin time may be measured before and 4 hours after therapy commences. It should be prolonged to two to four times control. If not, a further loading dose should be given. When the infusion is stopped, the thrombin time must fall to less than twice the control value before a heparin infusion is started.

In practice strict control is probably unnecessary when standard doses are given, provided there is close clinical observation to detect signs of bleeding.

Complications of thrombolytic therapy

1. *Bleeding* This is the commonest complication, and is severe enough to discontinue therapy in up to 25% of patients. It may be minimised by observing the following guidelines:

(a) Minimise the number of venepunctures taken and physical handling of the patient generally (thus avoid intramuscular injections and intra-arterial sampling).
(b) No non-steroidal anti-inflammatory drugs or anticoagulants should be given concurrently.

Management of bleeding during thrombolytic therapy As the half-life of these agents is very short, lytic activity stops very shortly after the infusion is discontinued. If bleeding is severe, then replacement with whole blood (fresh if possible), fresh frozen plasma or cryoprecipitate may be required and *epsilon aminocaproic acid* (EACA) may be used which competitively antagonises plasminogen. It is given as a loading dose of 5 g, either intravenously (over 30 minutes to avoid hypotension) or orally (as it is well absorbed) followed by 1.25 g hourly. Apart from hypotension, other side effects include nausea, diarrhoea and dizziness.

Persistent oozing from venepuncture sites during thrombolytic therapy may be stopped by compression with a pledget of cotton wool soaked in EACA.

2. *Allergic reactions* These occur in up to 15% of patients treated with streptokinase but are very rare with urokinase. They include urticaria, itching, flushing, headaches and occasionally bronchospasm and hypotension. They may be minimised by giving 100 mg of hydrocortisone intravenously at the start of therapy and 12 hourly thereafter.

3. *Pyrexia* This occurs in 33% of patients given streptokinase and is again reduced with prophylactic hydrocortisone.

Contraindications These may be divided into absolute and relative:

(a) *Absolute*
1. Active internal bleeding.
2. A recent (i.e. less than 2 months previously) cerebrovascular accident or cerebral neoplasm.

(b) *Relative*
1. Major surgery, trauma or invasive procedures performed within the previous 10 days.
2. Pregnancy and within 10 days post-partum.
3. Uncontrolled severe hypertension.
4. Uncontrolled anticoagulation defects.
5. Post-cardiopulmonary resuscitation with rib fractures.
6. Medical conditions pre-disposing to bleeding, e.g. bronchiectasis, severe liver or renal failure.

Inhibitors of fibrinolysis

A number of haemorrhagic conditions may be due to excess fibrinolytic activity, e.g. menorrhagia may result from fibrinolysis within the endometrium; haematuria following prostatectomy may be due to the unopposed action of the urokinase released during operation; acute gastric erosions are associated with fibrinolysis and bleeding. A number of drugs which inhibit the system are known, the most widely used being:

1. Epsilon Aminocaproic acid (EACA) At low concentrations it competitively antagonises plasminogen activation, higher concentrations *in vitro* inhibit plasmin activity itself. It is rapidly absorbed orally and rapidly excreted unchanged in the urine. It is given as a loading dose of 5 g followed by 1.25 g hourly either orally or by intravenous infusion. The loading dose should be given over 30 min to avoid hypotension. The theoretical hazard of inducing widespread thrombosis is remote and the main side effects reported include hypotension, dizziness, diarrhoea, abdominal discomfort and nausea. It has been shown to reduce blood loss in menorrhagia and after prostatectomy.

2. Tranexamic acid This is aminomethyl cyclohexane carboxylic acid and is a powerful inhibitor of plasminogen activation, being almost ten times more potent than EACA. It has been shown to be effective in arresting haemorrhage from acute gastric erosions and peptic ulcer. Recent trials suggest that these drugs, tranexamic acid in particular, may reduce the incidence of rebleeding in the acute phase of subarachnoid haemorrhage. It is less toxic than EACA, the main adverse effect being diarrhoea.

DRUGS MODIFYING PLATELET FUNCTION

The commonest cause of death in western countries is thromboembolic vascular disease and recent research has provided important insights into the possible role of platelets in these events. In particular, attention has focused on prostaglandins, which are produced not only by platelets and in the endothelial cells lining blood vessel walls, but also are involved in reproduction and parturition, and in inflammation.

Prostaglandins (PGs) are fatty acids which share a basic structure consisting of a cyclopentane ring and two unsaturated side chains. The substitutions on the cyclopentane ring define the type of prostaglandin (e.g. PGH, PGG) and the number of unsaturated bonds in the side chains defines the class of prostaglandin (e.g. PGH_2, PGI_3). Figure 17.7 briefly summarises the way in which the important vascular PGs are produced.

The theory of Moncada and Vane proposes that cyclic endoperoxides in platelets are converted into the pro-aggregatory thromboxane A_2, whereas in endothelial cells lining blood vessel walls they are converted into the anti-aggregatory compound PGI_2 (known as prostacyclin or epoprostenol). Normally these two pathways are in balance such that platelet aggregation is prevented. If damage to the endothelial cells occurs, then the platelet thromboxane pathway predominates and aggregation occurs, so that a platelet plug forms at the site of injury, and potential blood loss is also reduced by vasoconstriction.

In atheroma there is evidence suggesting that prostacyclin synthesis is locally impaired, and it is possible that this allows production of platelet thrombi at these sites. This may lead to occlusion of affected vessels in the coronary, cerebral or peripheral limb circulations, which may be either transient (possibly triggering arrhythmias or transient ischaemic attacks) or permanent, leading to distal tissue infarction.

These theories have led to extensive research into drugs which might alter platelet function and reduce thromboembolism.

Antiplatelet drugs

1. Aspirin (see also p. 292) Aspirin inhibits prostaglandin synthesis by irreversibly acetylating the enzyme cyclo-oxygenase. Both on theoretical

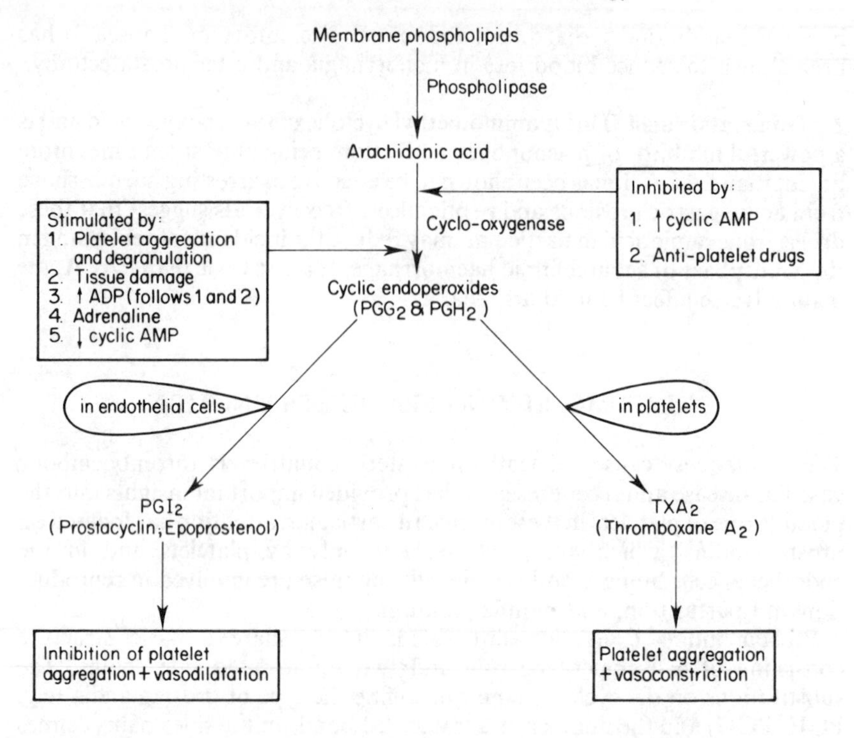

Fig. 17.7 Role of prostanoids in platelet function.

grounds and from observations *in vivo*, this may be expected to lead to an undesirable situation in which the beneficial effect of inhibiting platelet thromboxane production is counterbalanced by an undesirable inhibition of prostacyclin production in endothelial cells. However, as platelets have no nuclei and are unable to synthesise new protein, recovery of endothelial cell prostacyclin production would be expected to occur faster than thromboxane production by new platelets. It has been claimed that a low dose of aspirin given at suitable intervals (e.g. 40 mg daily) is able to produce this differential effect, but there is no general consensus on the ideal dose schedule.

2. Sulphinpyrazone (Anturan) (see p. 336) This is a uricosuric drug related to phenylbutazone which competitively inhibits cyclo-oxygenase. It thus has a similar mechanism of action to aspirin but its competitive action means that it is only an effective inhibitor of thrombosis for as long as it is present in the circulation. The $t_{1/2}$ is 2 hours and doses of 200 mg 8 hourly are required which are usually well tolerated, although some patients experience dyspepsia and peptic ulceration may occur. (All the non-steroidal anti-inflammatory group of drugs can inhibit prostaglandin production and theoretically they could all be used as antiplatelet drugs.)

Inhibition of platelet aggregation persists for a much longer period than the presence of sulphinpyrazone in the plasma would suggest. Recently a sulphide metabolite with a half-life in man of 10–20 hours has been described. This is a more potent inhibitor of platelet aggregation than sulphinpyrazone and it is probably responsible for most of the effects of the drug *in vivo*. There is some evidence that its formation is non-linear with disproportionately higher concentrations of sulphide being formed with increasing doses of sulphinpyrazone.

3. Dipyridamole (Persantin) This drug was originally used as a coronary vasodilator but controlled trials later showed it to be ineffective. However, it is a phosphodiesterase inhibitor and increases platelet cyclic AMP levels (as does prostacyclin) thus inhibiting platelet aggregation. The dose is 400 mg daily and this may occasionally cause headache, nausea and vomiting.

Use of antiplatelet drugs

1. *Prevention of re-infarction after a first myocardial infarction.* Several large double-blind studies have now been completed which have addressed this question. Five of the six studies which have looked at aspirin have found trends in favour of aspirin, with 10–15% reductions in mortality in the aspirin-treated groups. The addition of dipyridamole may produce a small additional benefit but sulphinpyrazone has not been shown to be effective. In view of the far more convincing data showing the benefits of certain β-blockers in this group of patients, current evidence does NOT favour the use of anti-platelet drugs in these patients.

2. *Prevention of stroke after transient ischaemic attacks* A large trial evaluating aspirin at two dose levels in these patients is currently under way in Britain as previous smaller studies have suggested that this drug is effective in preventing strokes and transient ischaemic attacks.

3. *Peripheral vascular disease* There is no convincing evidence that these drugs are of benefit.

4. *Cardiac surgery*

(a) The addition of dipyridamole to warfarin after prosthetic valve replacement has been shown to reduce the incidence of embolic events.

(b) Coronary bypass grafts. Dipyridamole (75 mg t.d.s.) begun 2 days before operation and aspirin (325 mg t.d.s.) started 7 hours post-operatively (and continued for at least one year) have been shown to reduce vein graft occlusion at least a year after surgery.

5. *Arteriovenous shunts* The incidence of thrombi is reduced in dialysis patients with these shunts who are given antiplatelet drugs, but arteriovenous fistulae are now preferred for access in these patients so this is rarely a clinical problem.

6. *Thrombocythaemia and patients with recurrent thrombosis* Although controlled evidence does not exist in these rare conditions, antiplatelet drugs are reported to be effective.

Newer agents

Prostacyclin, Epoprostenol This prostaglandin is now available for clinical use. It is inactive orally, and has a very short half-life (about 2 minutes) at physiological pH, so it is given by continuous intravenous infusion.

The main indications for its use are:

(a) Cardiopulmonary bypass and charcoal haemoperfusion: prostacyclin reduces platelet aggregation when blood is exposed to artificial surfaces thus reducing the incidence of thrombocytopenia and microangiopathy associated with these procedures.
(b) Renal dialysis: prostacyclin may be used as an alternative to heparin in patients at high risk of bleeding in whom heparin may be dangerous.
(c) Other circumstances in which prostacyclin has been used include thrombotic thrombocytopenic purpura, unstable angina, severe peripheral vascular disease and pulmonary hypertension. As yet this drug cannot be recommended in these conditions.

Side-effects Most patients experience headache and facial flushing; severe bradycardia and hypotension may occur and require immediate reduction or cessation of the infusion.

Dazoxiben There has been intensive research directed at finding drugs which could selectively inhibit thromboxane synthetase without affecting prostacyclin production. Imidazole was the first such compound, but it is toxic in man. However, one of its derivatives, dazoxiben, is now undergoing clinical trials. It has no obvious efficacy in stable angina, but may be of use in unstable angina and peripheral vascular disease, particularly Raynaud's syndrome. It may be given orally and is well absorbed. It is not associated with any adverse cardiovascular side effects.

Dextrans

These are high-molecular-weight glucose polymers which reduce platelet adhesiveness and aggregation. Two types are available: dextran 40 (molecular weight 40 000) and dextran 70 (molecular weight 70 000) and they are provided as solutions for intravenous infusion. They may be used in the post-operative period to prevent venous thromboembolism but daily infusions of 0.5–1.0 l are required. Problems encountered in their use include interference with cross-matching of blood, and the risk of circulatory overload, precluding their use in patients with cardiac or renal failure. These solutions are also used for volume replacement in patients who have undergone venesection, and in resuscitation, e.g. following acute haemorrhage. However, it must be noted that they have a $t_{1/2}$ of 4–6 hours, so their intravascular volume expanding effect will be only temporary.

Chapter 18
ENDOCRINE SYSTEM

THE PITUITARY

ANTERIOR PITUITARY HORMONES

Growth Hormone (GH; Somatotrophin)

Somatotrophin is a protein of molecular weight 27 000 which consists of 191 amino acids. The rate of secretion varies during the day. The normal output over 24 h is about 1.4 mg. When released into the circulation aggregates and prohormones of somatotrophin are called growth hormones (GH). Secretion is stimulated by hypoglycaemia, fasting and stress, α- and β-adrenergic, dopaminergic and serotoninergic agonists. The serotoninergic pathway is involved in the stimulation of somatotrophin release during slow wave sleep. Secretion is inhibited by glucose, protein and corticosteroid administration. Control of release is modulated by adrenergic, cholinergic and dopaminergic neurotransmitters. Thus L-dopa and methylamphetamine produce a rise in GH levels. The release of GH following hypoglycaemia is inhibited by α-adrenergic blockers and potentiated by β-blockers. The hypothalamus secretes both a growth-hormone release inhibiting hormone (somatostatin) and probably a growth-hormone releasing factor (GHRF). *Somatostatin*, a tetradecapeptide, has been synthesised and also inhibits insulin, glucagon and gastrin secretion. GH itself promotes protein synthesis and synergises with insulin causing amino acid uptake by cells. However, its effect on skeletal growth is mediated by somatomedin (a small peptide synthesised in the liver, secretion of which depends upon GH).

GH deficiency is a cause of growth retardation. Treatment by GH derived from human pituitary glands has ceased due to possible transmission of Jakob-Creutzfeldt dementia. It is replaced by **Somatrem**, a genetically engineered drug. Injections should begin early, before puberty, and continue until growth ceases. The dose is variable but 0.5 i.u./kg i.m. weekly is common. No benefit occurs after epiphyseal fusion so that it is important that in children with hypopituitarism, replacement therapy with gonadotrophin or sex hormones is delayed until maximum growth has been achieved.

GH is used to treat children with dwarfism due to hypothalamic disease. In the future synthetic GHRF may be preferable to GH which, because of its source from autopsy material, is in very short supply.

GH oversecretion produces gigantism and acromegaly. An agent which selectively inhibits GH secretion and is satisfactory for clinical use has not been found. Bromocriptine in doses of 5–30 mg/day (q.v.) is probably the best drug therapy presently available: it suppresses prolactin as well as GH but has little effect on other pituitary functions. The size of the pituitary fossa must be assessed repeatedly in order to detect further growth of the pituitary.

Somatostatin is effective in lowering GH levels in acromegalics but has to be given by continuous intravenous infusion and has widespread effects on other hormones. Irradiation and surgery are alternative modes of treatment.

Prolactin

This is present in the human pituitary in an amount roughly $\frac{1}{100}$ that of growth hormone. The structure of the hormone has recently been elucidated and it has structural resemblances to somatotrophin presumably both arose from a common ancestral molecule early in vertebrate evolution. It has a molecular weight of 25 000 and contains 170 amino acids. It has a wide variety of actions:

(a) *Mammotropic*—in animals it is essential for normal development and maturation of the mammary gland.

(b) *Lactogenic*—during human pregnancy prolactin secretion is high and the levels rise steadily towards term. Under the combined stimulus of oestrogens, prolactin, progesterone and probably insulin and cortisol, milk formation occurs. Placental lactogen also adds to the pituitary prolactin effect. Oestrogens antagonise prolactin's effect on milk secretion so that lactation begins when oestrogen levels fall post-partum. This explains why oestrogens can suppress lactation. The action of prolactin in initiating and maintaining lactation in females is the only established physiological function of prolactin.

(c) *Behavioural*—serum prolactin rises in a number of altered psychic states in man, e.g. stress, sleep, orgasm and the administration of tranquillisers. There is little evidence that prolactin plays a causative role in mental disorders.

Hyperprolactinaemia may lead to impotence, hypogonadism and gynaecomastia in men and cause galactorrhoea or amenorrhoea in women.

Prolactin release is under inhibitory control by the hypothalamus which releases a prolactin inhibitory factor (which is dopamine) into the portal vessels. This may be the main inhibitory mechanism and explains why dopamine antagonists such as phenothiazines, butyrophenones and metoclopramide, and dopamine-depleting agents like methyldopa and reserpine increase prolactin secretion. There is a good correlation between the prolactin-elevating potency and both antidopaminergic and antipsychotic properties. Thus prolactin measurements may serve as an objective index of the activity of these drugs and may be useful in screening. L-dopa, apomorphine and other dopamine agonists decrease prolactin secretion. The most extensively investigated of these drugs is bromocriptine.

Bromocriptine (2-brom-α-ergocryptine; Parlodel)

This semi-synthetic ergot derivative has dopamine receptor agonist properties. Because of this action on the pituitary and hypothalamus, bromocriptine acts like prolactin inhibitory factor (PIF) and stimulates inhibitory dopamine receptors, thus inhibiting prolactin secretion. In normal subjects it produces a small increase in GH secretion, but in acromegaly it paradoxically suppresses GH release, possibly due to abnormal pituitary dopamine receptors, although hypothalamic factors may also be involved.

Pharmacokinetics Bromocriptine is administered orally and 90% is absorbed via the small intestine. Bromocriptine is metabolised in the liver and excretion is predominantly via the bile. It has a long $t_{1/2}$ of 66 h. Raised prolactin and GH levels fall within a few hours of starting treatment, but the length of this action appears to vary with the original level of the circulating hormone.

Clinical uses

(a) *Puerperal lactation* can be suppressed by giving bromocriptine in a single dose of 2.5 mg initially followed by 2.5 mg b.d. for two weeks. Breast tenderness and engorgement after cessation of treatment should be treated with bromocriptine 2.5 mg daily for 1 week. Bromocriptine appears to be more effective than oestrogen therapy and can be given even when suckling has commenced.

(b) *Hyperprolactinaemia* is an important factor in male and female hypogonadism and appears to account for 13% of cases of secondary amenorrhoea. Alternatively hyperprolactinaemia may present as infertility with normal menstruation. Nevertheless galactorrhoea occurs in only 30% of these patients: galactorrhoea on its own is rarely due to hyperprolactinaemia. In men hyperprolactinaemia most commonly presents as impotence with or without decreased volume of seminal ejaculate. Galactorrhoea occurs in less than one third of these male patients and gynaecomastia is uncommon. The influence of prolactin on gonadal function is not understood, but bromocriptine is often highly successful in the treatment of impaired sex function with hyperprolactinaemia (Fig. 18.1). The dose needed is usually 2.5–7.5 mg twice daily. Fertility and cyclical ovarian function is usually restored within 2 months, but up to 6 months' treatment may be required. Malformations have not been reported. Nevertheless if pregnancy occurs the drug should be immediately stopped. Multiple ovulations (as occur with gonadotrophins and clomiphene) have not been reported.

If a pituitary tumour is the primary cause of the hyperprolactinaemia (acidophil adenoma producing pressure on the hypothalamus or a chromophobe adenoma with prolactinoma function), the tumour may enlarge during pregnancy. Thus visual fields should be carefully measured during bromocriptine therapy for infertility.

(c) *Hyperprolactinaemic syndromes* may also be associated with *hypothyroidism* and with *drug therapy*. In hypothyroidism, simple replacement therapy corrects the condition. Drug therapy (in particular phenothiazines, butyrophenones, metoclopramide, oral contraceptives and methyldopa) may produce galactorrhoea, which usually ceases when the drug is stopped. If the condition persists, bromocriptine may reverse it, but a pituitary tumour should also be looked for. When a drug such as a neuroleptic cannot be withdrawn, concurrent administration of bromocriptine may suppress galactorrhoea.

(d) Bromocriptine provides an effective medical treatment for *acromegaly* and successfully improves the hypogonadism which occurs in many of these patients. It is possible that the drug not only suppresses the secretion of GH and prolactin, but may also suppress somatomedin production by the liver and other peripheral responses to GH.

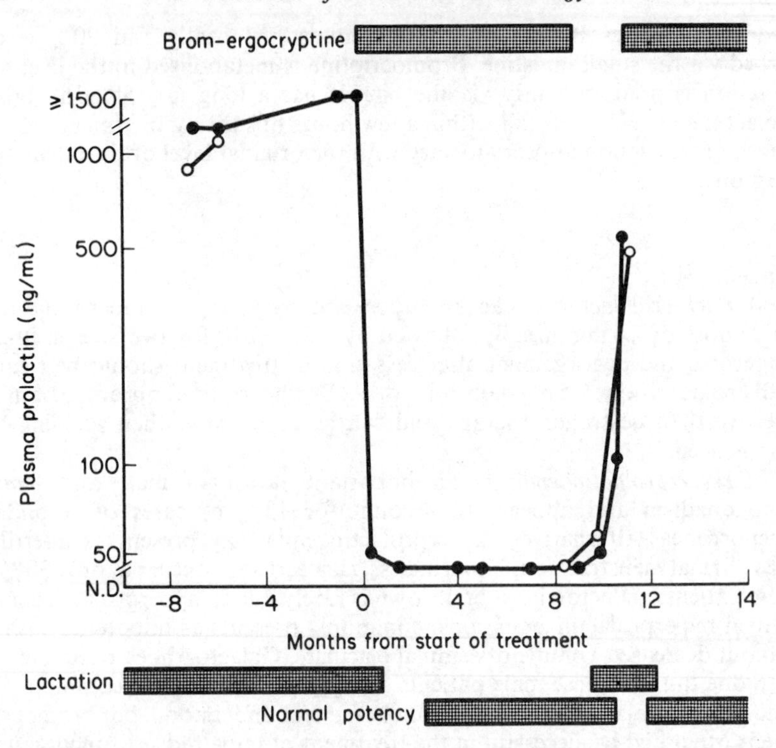

Fig. 18.1 Plasma prolactin concentrations measured by bioassay (●) and radioimmunoassay (O) in a man with galactorrhoea and impotence during treatment with bromocriptine (From G. M. Besser *et al., Brit. Med. J.*, **3,** 669 (1972). Reproduced by permission of the Editor.)

Pituitary-gland growth and possibly tumour size are suppressed with improvement of visual fields.

A dose of 5 mg bromocriptine 6 hourly in acromegalic patients suppresses GH levels within 2 h of the first dose with a maximum effect at 4 h. On this regime there is considerable clinical improvement, with abolition of excessive sweating, reduction in soft tissue swelling and improvement of glucose tolerance.

(e) Bromocriptine is an effective mode of therapy in 80% of patients with *Parkinsonism*, although large doses may be needed (up to 100 mg daily in divided doses). Its action on the on – off phenomenon is not known (see p.261). It only rarely produces additional benefit in patients on full doses of levodopa. Like this drug it is least effective in postencephalitic patients, and patients unresponsive to levodopa derive no benefit from bromocriptine.

Adverse effects with low doses (2.5–12.5 mg daily) the only toxic effect commonly encountered is constipation. Occasionally unexpected postural hypotension may occur with the initial dose of bromocriptine which is reminiscent of the 'first-dose' effect seen with prazosin (q.v.). Higher doses may produce nausea and vomiting. If the dosage is raised slowly (2.5 mg every three days to the required level) the patient may become accustomed to higher doses.

However, continuous high doses (over 20 mg daily) may lead to the following toxic actions: nasal congestion, dry mouth, metallic taste, vascular spasm, cramps in the legs, pains in extremities, dystonic reactions, visual hallucinations, cardiac arrhythmias, and alcohol intolerance.

Gonadotrophins

The human pituitary secretes follicle-stimulating hormone (FSH) and luteinising hormone (LH). FSH is a glycoprotein (M.W. 30 000) which in females controls development of the primary ovarian follicle, stimulates granulosa cell proliferation and increases oestrogen production whilst in males it increases spermatogenesis. LH is also a glycoprotein (M.W. 30 000) which induces ovulation, stimulates thecal oestrogen production and initiates and maintains the corpus luteum in females. In males LH stimulates androgen synthesis by Leydig cells, thus having a secondary role in the maturation of spermatocytes and the development of secondary sex characteristics.

Human menopausal urinary gonadotrophin (HMG, Pergonal) and human chorionic gonadotrophin (HCG) are prepared commercially. They have a number of uses:

(a) Primary or secondary amenorrhoea may result from lack of gonadotrophin secretion. This is only infrequently due to obvious pituitary or hypothalamic disease. Ovulation and hence fertility may be restored using a combination of gonadotrophins contained in HMG and HCG (mainly LH). Their use requires skill and experience. Usually HMG is given for 8 days followed by a large dose of HCG on the 10th day. The total dose of FSH is increased each month until ovulation occurs as shown by a rise in urinary oestrogens and pregnanediol. Multiple ovulation with the danger of multiple pregnancy is the main problem.
(b) Sequential treatment with HMG and HCG is used for the polycystic ovary syndrome.
(c) Gonadotrophins may correct defective spermatogenesis in secondary testicular failure, and also be used to differentiate primary and secondary testicular failure.
(d) 1500 units intramuscularly thrice weekly of HCG for 6 weeks may be used to treat undescended testes.

Clomiphene (Clomid) is an antioestrogen which blocks oestrogen receptors in the hypothalamus. Thus feedback inhibition by oestrogen is blocked and gonadotrophin secretion is stimulated.

Clomiphene is used to treat subfertility in the female by inducing ovulation but multiple ovulation may occur resulting in multiple births. It has replaced partial or wedge resection of the ovary in the polycystic ovary syndrome. For this indication it is given in doses of 50–200 mg daily for 5 days in each cycle. The drug inhibits lactation.

Clomiphene in doses of 3 mg/kg/day for 7–10 days can assist in the diagnosis of secondary hypogonadism: if the hypothalamus is intact then the release of LH and FSH will be increased. No increase occurs in hypothalamic or pituitary disease.

Danazol (Danol) inhibits gonadotrophin secretion. It reduces breast size in gynaecomastia in the male and in precocious pubery in the female. Danazol is also used in endometriosis and fibrocystic mastitis. There is no evidence of long-term suppression of the hypothalamic–pituitary gonadal axis following its withdrawal. It may cause fluid retention (see also page 588).

Gonadorelin (gonadotrophin-releasing hormone) is a FSH/LH releasing factor, produced in the hypothalamus. It is used in a single i.v. dose to assess anterior pituitary reserve in patients with suspected impairment.

Adrenocorticotrophic hormone (ACTH; Corticotrophin)

This is a straight-chain polypeptide of 39 amino acid residues (M.W. 4500). It has been completely synthesised and it is structurally similar to melanocyte-stimulating hormone which accounts for their overlapping properties. Its release from the pituitary is mediated by corticotrophin-releasing factors (CRF) synthesised in the hypothalamus and secreted into the local portal circulation. These hypothalamic centres are controlled by brainstem and suprahypothalamic centres and respond to the circulating ACTH and cortisol levels and stressful stimuli. There is a diurnal rhythm to corticotrophin secretion with high secretion rates in the later part of the night and early morning and low levels towards midnight. Superimposed upon this underlying rhythm are bursts of corticotrophin release each lasting 1–2 h. The fate of corticotrophin is incompletely known, but tissue uptake is mainly responsible for its short plasma $t_{1/2}$ of about 10 min.

Corticotrophin stimulates synthesis and release of corticosteroids (mainly cortisol) and to a lesser extent androgens and oestrogens from the adrenal cortex. There is only a minor effect on aldosterone production which is not dependent upon corticotrophin for synthesis.

Corticotrophin used in the UK is from pig pituitary glands and is rendered long acting with gelatin (Acthar Gel) or zinc (Corticotrophin-Zn) for intramuscular injection. A synthetic analogue containing only the first 24 amino acids of natural corticotrophin is available as **tetracosactrin (Synacthen, Cortrosyn).** These are the only amino acids associated with biological activity, and the remaining 15 which are species specific are associated with antigenic activity. Thus although generalised allergic reactions can occur with corticotrophin or tetracosactrin they are less common with the latter. The $t_{1/2}$ of tetracosactrin (15 min) is slightly longer than that of corticotrophin, but otherwise its properties are identical. Both may produce painful local reactions around the intramuscular injection site.

The indications and adverse reactions are largely those of corticosteroids (q.v.). The degree of stimulation to the adrenal cortex from corticotrophin or tetracosactrin is unpredictable. The hormone may be absorbed to a variable degree from the injection site, destroyed locally or in the blood by proteolytic enzymes, and there are great variations in the responsiveness of the adrenal cortex. Corticotrophin is particularly liable to produce acne, skin pigmentation, increased bruising, sodium retention and hypertension as compared with corticosteroids.

Since corticotrophin stimulates the adrenals to produce mainly hydrocortisone, it cannot be used to obtain a selective anti-inflammatory effect. This outpouring of hydrocortisone is mainly responsible for the sodium retention and heart failure which can occur with ACTH treatment. The output of the adrenals is limited in practice to about four times the resting output so that the maximal effect is limited; this is not the case with exogenous steroids. Since corticotrophin also stimulates release of androgens (hence the higher incidence of acne) and oestrogens in addition to corticosteroids, there is theoretically less liability to osteoporosis, although this is unproven. In children, linear growth, which may be retarded by corticosteroids due to their antagonism of GH and their anti-anabolic effects on protein metabolism, is much less affected by corticotrophin.

The effect on the adrenal cortex is also different from corticosteroids since administration of corticotrophin causes hypertrophy rather than the atrophy produced by corticosteroids. The increased secretion of endogenous corticosteroid following repeated corticotrophin injection suppresses the release of CRF from the hypothalamus and corticotrophin from the pituitary thus attenuating the natural response to stress, albeit in a different fashion from exogenous corticosteroids. Corticotrophin will not therefore restore suppressed pituitary–adrenal function after withdrawal of chronic steroid therapy since the limiting factor in this case is the pituitary and/or hypothalamus, not the adrenal cortex. Similarly, attempts to use it to prevent adrenal-axis suppression during steroid therapy are unsuccessful. Intermittent corticotrophin administration results in less suppression of the hypothalamic pituitary axis than continuous daily treatment. Patients who are currently receiving or have in the past year been treated with corticotrophin or tetracosactrin should be carefully observed during operations and in the post-operative period for signs of adrenal insufficiency. They may also require steroid supplements during severe infection or other stress.

Corticotrophin and tetracosactrin must be given by injection and are rarely required more frequently than 2 or 3 times weekly as the depot preparation for maintenance therapy, the usual doses being 40–80 I.U. and 0.5–1 mg respectively. Since corticotrophin acts indirectly and the response may be variable its use cannot be recommended for acute emergencies like status asthmaticus although it is suitable for maintenance treatment in chronic asthma.

Cyproheptadine (Periactin)

This drug is a powerful antagonist of histamine, serotonin and acetylcholine. It has proved disappointing as an antihistamine but two other potential uses have emerged:

1. It is an appetite stimulant, leading to increase in weight. It probably acts by modifying serotonin activity in the hypothalamus.
2. Serotonin is probably involved in the secretion of CRF and thus in the activation of the adrenal cortex by corticotrophin. In Cushing's disease there is evidence of deranged regulation of corticotrophin release and cyproheptadine has been reported as producing remissions in about two-thirds of patients with this disorder.

Adverse effects are largely due to its anticholinergic action and include drowsiness, dry mouth, urinary retention and glaucoma. Increased appetite and weight gain may be a disadvantage in treating Cushing's disease.

POSTERIOR PITUITARY HORMONES

Vasopressin (antidiuretic hormone; ADH) and oxytocin are peptide hormones synthesised in the anterior hypothalamic nuclei and transported along nerve fibres to the posterior lobe of the pituitary for storage and subsequent release (neurosecretion).

Vasopressin; Argipressin (synthetic vasopressin)

Two forms exist—arginine vasopressin (in man and most other mammals) and lysine vasopressin in the pig and hippopotamus. This hormone contains 8 amino acid residues. It is released into the circulation by several stimuli, in particular increased plasma osmotic pressure, decreased blood volume, drugs (e.g. morphine, nicotine) and physical or emotional stress. Vasopressin acts on the distal tubules and collecting ducts of the kidney and increases water reabsorption.

Vasopressin can be administered by intravenous, subcutaneous or intramuscular injection or by nasal insufflation. The hormone is destroyed by trypsin when given orally. In the blood vasopressin is largely unbound and has a short half-life (15 min in man) because of inactivation by the liver and kidneys. The urinary clearance is 5–10% of the glomerular filtration rate.

Arginine vasopressin (Argipressin) is effective in the treatment of cranial diabetes insipidus. In this condition the action of a single injection lasts 3–5 h. However, injections of vasopressin tannate (Pitressin tannate) in oil have a more prolonged action but are no longer available. Vasopressin can also be administered in the form of snuff but this preparation is not recommended as it may cause rhinitis, bronchospasm and pulmonary fibrosis.

Intravenous vasopressin is used for the initial emergency arrest of bleeding from oesophageal varices in portal hypertension since the splanchnic vasoconstriction that it produces leads to decreased portal blood flow. It is given in a dose of 20 units diluted with 200 ml 5% dextrose and infused over 20 min. In this dose abdominal colic, bowel evacuation and facial pallor occur. If these effects are absent it is probable that the vasopressin is inactive and a new pack should be tried. Portal pressure falls within 3 min of injection, is maximally depressed at 15 min and remains low for an hour. Vasopressin infusions may be given 2-hourly but efficacy decreases with repeated use. Reduced hepatic blood flow may impair circulation to functioning liver cells and in some centres selective infusion of vasopressin into the mesenteric artery, which preserves hepatic arterial flow is used. Because of its vasoconstrictor action the dose must be reduced in patients with a history of angina and in hypertension.

Synthetic lysine vasopressin (LVP) can be given as a nasal spray for mild diabetes insipidus but its effects are too short-lasting to be useful in severe cases. It has advantages over pituitary snuff in that it does not result in local or pulmonary hypersensitivity phenomena. Each metered dose delivers 5 units. 10 units are administered to each nostril twice or more times daily. The plasma $t_{1/2}$ is 15 min and its fate is similar to that of natural vasopressin.

Desmopressin (DDAVP) is a synthetic long-acting analogue of vasopressin which is also administered nasally. It is effective for 12–24 h having a plasma $t_{1/2}$ of 75 min due to slow metabolic clearance, which may be due to the presence of D-arginine isomer in position 8 in its structure. DDAVP has full antidiuretic potency but unlike vasopressin does not significantly raise blood pressure or contract smooth muscle. Thus pallor, colic, bronchospasm, coronary artery or uterine spasm do not occur. DDAVP is at present the drug of choice for cranial diabetes insipidus. The usual effective dose is 10–20 μg (0.1–0.2 ml of nasal solution) intranasally or 1–2 μg intramuscularly once or twice daily.

Other drugs in diabetes insipidus

Chlorpropamide increases renal sensitivity to vasopressin and carbamazepine increases vasopressin secretion. Either drug may be used as oral therapy in mild cranial diabetes insipidus when some functioning pituitary tissue remains. The thiazide diuretics are also used in the treatment of nephrogenic diabetes insipidus. The mechanism of this drug action is not known but free water clearance is reduced.

Felypressin (octapressin; PLV-11)

This is a phenylalanine-2, lysine-8-vasopressin. It has mainly vasoconstrictor activity and is used to delay the absorption and dissipation of local anaesthetic injections. It does not produce the cardiac stimulating effects which adrenaline may have when used in equieffective amounts with local anaesthetics.

Oxytocin

This hormone has a similar octapeptide structure to vasopressin. It produces contractions of the smooth muscle of the fundus of the uterus and of the mammary-gland ducts. It is reflexly released from the pituitary following suckling and by emotional stimuli. Its role in the initiation of labour is not completely established. There is no known disease state of over- or under-production of this hormone.

When given orally the hormone is destroyed by trypsin. It is effective by any parenteral route and can be absorbed from the buccal and nasal mucosae. Like vasopressin, oxytocin has a short plasma $t_{1/2}$ (5–10 min), mainly because of tissue inactivation, but a small amount is excreted via the kidney bound to a larger protein molecule. Oxytocin injection (Pitocin) contains 10 units/ml. It is usually given intravenously or intramuscularly. To initiate labour at term it may be infused at a rate of 5–20 milliunits/min. A nasal spray (containing 40 units/ml) or buccal tablets (200 units each) are usually less successful and because of irregular absorption carry a higher risk of uterine rupture and fetal asphyxia. Since there is in addition a wide variation in uterine sensitivity, these effects may follow a comparatively small dose of oxytocin given by injection. Water retention and intoxication and occasionally hypertension may follow large doses.

Oxytocin or synthetic oxytocin (**Syntocinon**) which is pure and uncontaminated by vasopressin is occasionally given to control post-partum haemorrhage (dose 2–5 units i.m. or i.v.) but more usually **Syntometrine** is used. This is a proprietary mixture containing 5 units of synthetic oxytocin and 500 μg ergometrine maleate in 1 ml. It therefore combines the sustained oxytocic action of oxytocin with the more rapid effect of ergometrine.

A retrospective study has shown a small but significant increase in the incidence of neonatal jaundice following maternal oxytocin infusion. This is probably not of clinical significance.

THE TESTIS

Testosterone

The principal hormone of the testis is testosterone which is secreted by the interstitial (Leydig) cells passing from the testis in the blood and lymphatics and circulating in the blood 95 % bound to a plasma globulin. The plasma level is variable but should exceed 10 nmol/l (350 ng/100 ml) in adult males. The nuclei of cells in the target tissues convert testosterone into the more active androgen dihydrotestosterone. Both testosterone and dihydrotestosterone are inactivated in the liver. Androgens have a wide range of activities, the most important of which are:

development of male secondary sex characteristics;
nitrogen retention, growth and bone maturation, muscle development;
temporal recession of hair line;
sebum secretion;
spermatogenesis and seminal fluid formation.

Testicular function is controlled by the anterior pituitary:

(a) Follicle-stimulating hormone (FSH) acts on the seminiferous tubules and promotes spermatogenesis.
(b) Luteinising hormone (LH) stimulates testosterone production.

The release of FSH and LH by the pituitary is in turn mediated by the hypothalamus via gonadotrophin-releasing hormone (GRH).

Table 18.1 lists some of the androgen preparations used therapeutically.

Pharmacokinetics Although testosterone is readily absorbed orally, like the naturally occurring oestrogens, a considerable first-pass metabolism occurs in the liver. It can also be administered sublingually, although advantage is rarely taken of this. Testosterone in oil is well absorbed from intramuscular injection sites but is also rapidly metabolised. The esters of testosterone are much less polar and are therefore more slowly released from oily depot injections and can be used for prolonged effect (see Table 18.1). Inactivation of testosterone takes place in the liver. The chief metabolites are androsterone and etiochola-

Table 18.1 Androgens used in therapeutics

Androgen	*Proprietary name*	*Administration*
Testosterone propionate in waxy base	Testoral	10–30 mg/day sublingually in divided doses
Testosterone propionate	Virormone	100 mg i.m. three times a week
Testosterone oenanthate in oil	Primotestone Depot	250 mg i.m. every 2–4 weeks
Testosterone esters in oil (propionate 30 mg phenylpropionate 60 mg; isocaproate 60 mg; decanoate 100 mg)	Sustanon 250	250 mg i.m. 1 or 2 times monthly
Fluoxymesterone	Ultandren	5–15 mg/day orally in divided doses
Mesterolone	Pro-Viron	100 mg orally daily
Less virilising preparations	*(Anabolic steroids)*	
Nandrolone phenylpropionate B.P. inj.	Durabolin	25–50 mg weekly by i.m. injection
Nandrolone decanoate	Deca-Durabolin	25–50 mg i.m. every 3 weeks
Methandienone	Dianabol	5–10 mg daily orally for men 2.5 mg daily for women
Norethandrolone	Nilevar	10–30 mg daily

nolone which are mainly excreted in the urine. About 6% of administered testosterone appears in the faeces having undergone enterohepatic circulation.

Clinical uses

1. Replacement therapy for primary or secondary (due to gonadotrophin deficiency) hypogonadism rarely reverses sterility but improves secondary sex characteristics and libido. Subcutaneous implants of testosterone are often absorbed erratically but a dose of 4–6 implants of 100 mg can be effective for up to 6 months. Replacement therapy is best achieved by intramuscular injection of testosterone esters in oil (250 mg of *Sustanon 250*). They are usually needed at 2–3 week intervals to control symptoms.
2. Delayed puberty, if due to gonadal deficiency, can be treated by testosterone esters. *Sustanon* 100 mg monthly by injection is satisfactory. If, however, it results from gonadotrophin deficiency, replacement of FSH and LH will be required.
3. Anabolic effects may be helpful in a few circumstances, e.g. osteoporosis, renal failure, following severe burns or other injuries. There is no evidence to justify their indiscriminate use to accelerate convalescence or post-operative recovery. The less virilising preparations are used as anabolic steroids.
4. Hypoplastic anaemia and the anaemia of neoplastic disease and renal failure are said to respond sometimes (see p. 587).

5. 20–30% oestrogen-dependent metastases of breast cancer in pre-menopausal patients shrink and become less painful with large androgen doses (see p. 810).
6. Itch in jaundice can be relieved. N.B. methyltestosterone should not be used since it may cause a cholestatic jaundice.

Adverse effects Virilisation in women and increased libido in men are predictable effects.

In women, acne, growth of facial hair and deepening of the voice are common undesirable features produced by androgens. Other masculinising effects and menstrual irregularities can also develop.

In the male, excessive masculinisation can result in frequent erections and aggressive behaviour.

Young children may undergo premature fusion of epiphyses or other abnormal growth phenomena.

Other adverse effects include jaundice, particularly of cholestatic type; because of this complication methyltestosterone is no longer prescribed. Impotence and azoospermia occur following prolonged use due to inhibition of gonadotrophin secretion. In patients treated for malignant disease with androgens, hypercalcaemia, which may be severe, is produced by an unknown mechanism. Salt and water retention is unusual with androgens, cf. oestrogens.

Cyproterone (Androcur) is an anti-androgen with progestagenic activity. It acts by competing with testosterone for target organ receptors, blocking testosterone (and oestrogen) synthesis and its progestagenic activity blocks the rise in gonadotrophins which would normally follow decreased plasma testosterone levels. When given as the acetate ester in daily doses of 100–200 mg to men suffering from unacceptable sexual deviations, it produces suppression of sexual activity in 10–14 days. The daily dosage should always be divided owing to its poor absorption (10–50% of dose) and rapid metabolism. On cessation of treatment the effect passes off in 14 days. It may also be useful in precocious puberty. The chief adverse effects are: inhibition of spermatogenesis (which usually returns to normal 6 months after cessation of treatment); gynaecomastia (20% of patients treated) and tiredness and lassitude (which make it dangerous if patients are allowed to drive vehicles). It is important that the fully informed consent of the patient to treatment with this agent be obtained in view of its effects on sexual behaviour and fertility.

THE OVARY

Three main hormones are secreted by the ovary: oestradiol-17β, oestrone and progesterone. In addition small amounts of androgens are produced. The oestrogens are physiologically concerned with the development of the secondary sex characteristics in the female such as breast development, female distribution of fat and proliferation of the endometrium. Progesterone acts on the endometrium to render it receptive to the fertilised zygote and thus allow implantation to take place. It also causes the mid-cycle rise in basal body temperature.

The pituitary gonadotrophins, follicle-stimulating hormone (FSH) and luteinising hormone (LH) control ovarian steroid secretion. Oestrogens exert a feedback control on both LH and FSH, whereas progesterone probably has little effect on gonadotrophin secretion. The hypothalamus secretes the gonadotrophin-releasing hormone (LH/FSH RH) which stimulates the anterior pituitary to release LH or FSH. FSH stimulates maturation of the ovarian follicle and release of oestrogens, whilst LH stimulates progesterone release from the corpus luteum, and in mid-cycle the sudden rise in LH causes ovulation.

Oestrogens

Pharmacokinetics Absorption of oestrogens is rapid via the skin or mucous membranes. In fact the rate of urinary excretion of oestrogens is similar if the hormones are given orally or intravenously.

Synthetic derivatives such as ethinyl oestradiol and diethylstilboestrol are also well absorbed when given by mouth.

The most potent natural oestrogen is oestradiol-17β. It is largely oxidised to oestrone and then hydrated to produce oestriol. The three oestrogens are metabolised in the liver and excreted as glucuronide and sulphate conjugates in bile and urine. Estimation of urinary oestrogen excretion provides a measure of ovarian function.

The synthetic oestrogen diethylstilboestrol is as potent as oestradiol but has a longer action because it is metabolised more slowly. Another highly active synthetic oestrogen is ethinyl oestradiol. This also has a prolonged action because of slow hepatic metabolism, the $t_{1/2}$ being about 25 h.

Adverse effects Oestrogens are commonly nauseating and may cause headaches. In males gynaecomastia is a dose-dependent effect. Withdrawal uterine haemorrhage may occur 2–3 days after stopping oestrogen treatment. Salt and water retention with oedema, hypertension and exacerbation of heart failure occur with large doses. Thromboembolism (see below) may occur. Oestrogens are carcinogenic in some animals and there is some evidence suggesting a sevenfold increase in the risk of developing endometrial carcinoma following exogenous oestrogen given alone continuously (i.e. this risk does not apply to the oral contraceptive pill). It has also been shown that many of the mothers of girls developing the rare vaginal adenocarcinoma in their teens had been treated with stilboestrol during pregnancy.

Clinical use

1. Oral contraception (see below).

2. Replacement therapy in hypofunctioning ovarian syndromes, e.g. 1 mg stilboestrol daily for 20 days and repeated after 10 days, or, if withdrawal bleeding occurs, after 5 days. The contraceptive pill can also be used. Replacement hormone therapy at the menopause is controversial but may be needed if climacteric symptoms do not respond to simpler measures. The lowest effective dose of oestrogen should be used for the shortest possible time. The aim is to gradually reduce the oestrogen dose so that the body becomes accustomed to waning ovarian function: the use of high doses of oestrogen

prevents this. Oestrogens have been shown to be effective in preventing post-menopausal osteoporosis for as long as the oestrogen treatment is maintained. Replacement therapy should start with ethinyl oestradiol (10 μg/day) or oestradiol valerate (1 mg/day) given for three weeks out of four. In addition norethisterone acetate (5 mg/day) should be given for the last five days of the course of oestrogen. The object of giving a progestogen is to ensure shedding of the endometrium and thus to reduce the risk of endometrial carcinoma. Any intermenstrual bleeding or other suspicious symptom must be fully investigated to exclude uterine carcinoma. Senile vaginitis may be treated by local or systemic oestrogen therapy.

3. Suppression of lactation: oestrogens do not themselves suppress lactation but reduce breast congestion. They have to be given early in the puerperium to be effective. Firm binding of the breasts and analgesics or bromocriptine are preferable in view of the dangers of thromboembolism. Diuretics, although commonly used, are in general not of much benefit.

4. Dysfunctional uterine bleeding.

5. Dysmenorrhoea.

6. Neoplastic disease: androgen-dependent prostatic carcinoma and 30–40% of breast-cancer patients who are at least five years post-menopausal respond to oestrogen (see p. 808).

Progesterone and progestogens

Pharmacological effects of large doses of progestogens include suppression of ovulation, inhibition of uterine contractility and of sodium excretion, and negative nitrogen balance.

Pharmacokinetics Progesterone itself is not well absorbed from the gut because of first-pass hepatic metabolism. It is more effective when injected intramuscularly or administered sublingually. It is excreted in the urine as pregnanediol and pregnanolone. Norethisterone, a synthetic progestogen component of many oral contraceptives, is rapidly absorbed orally and has a $t_{1/2}$ of 7.5–8 h.

Clinical uses are gynaecological and details are beyond the scope of this book.

1. metropathia haemorrhagica;
2. endometriosis;
3. dysmenorrhoea;
4. threatened or habitual abortion;
5. amenorrhoea—with oestrogen in cyclic dosage may be useful in some cases;
6. contraception;
7. carcinoma of the endometrium.

A number of preparations are used for these purposes. **Norethindrone** has some androgenic effect and should not be used in threatened abortion because of its masculinising effect on the fetus. **Dydrogesterone** has neither oestrogenic nor androgenic effects and is 20 times more active weight for weight than progesterone. The use of large doses of progestogens in combination with

Table 18.2 Some contraceptive pills available in the UK

Proprietary name	*Oestrogen*	*Progestogen*
Intermediate oestrogen combined contraceptive pills		
Anovlar 21	ethinyloestradiol 50 μg	norethisterone acetate 4 mg
Eugynon 50	ethinyloestradiol 50 μg	norgestrel 500 μg
Gynovlar 21	ethinyloestradiol 50 μg	norethisterone acetate 3 μg
Minilyn	ethinyloestradiol 50 μg	lynoestrenol 2.5 mg
Minovlar	ethinyloestradiol 50 μg	norethisterone acetate 1 mg
Norlestrin	ethinyloestradiol 50 μg	norethisterone acetate 2.5 mg
Orlest 21	ethinyloestradiol 50 μg	norethisterone acetate 1 mg
Ovran	ethinyloestradiol 50 μg	levonorgestrel 250 μg
Ovulen 50	ethinyloestradiol 50 μg	ethynodiol diacetate 1 mg
Norinyl-1	mestranol 50 μg	norethisterone 1 mg
Ortho-novin 1/50	mestranol 50 μg	norethisterone 1 mg
Low oestrogen, biphasic and triphasic combined contraceptive pills		
Binovum	ethinyloestradiol 35 μg ethinyloestradiol 35 μg	norethisterone 0.5 mg for 7 days norethisterone 1 mg for 14 days
Brevinor	ethinyloestradiol 35 μg	norethisterone 500 μg
Norimin	ethinyloestradiol 35 μg	norethisterone 1 mg
Ovysmen	ethinyloestradiol 35 μg	norethisterone 500 μg
Conova 30	ethinyloestradiol 30 μg	ethynodiol diacetate 2 mg
Eugynon 30	ethinyloestradiol 30 μg	levonorgestrel 250 μg
Logynon	ethinyloestradiol 30 μg ethinyloestradiol 40 μg ethinyloestradiol 30 μg	levonorgestrel 50 μg for 6 days levonorgestrel 75 μg for 5 days levonorgestrel 125 μg for 10 days
Marvelon	ethinyloestradiol 30 μg	desogestrel 150 μg
Microgynon 30	ethinyloestradiol 30 μg	levonorgestrel 150 μg
Ovran 30	ethinyloestradiol 30 μg	levonorgestrel 250 μg
Ovranette	ethinyloestradiol 30 μg	levonorgestrel 150 μg
Trinordiol	ethinyloestradiol 30 μg ethinyloestradiol 40 μg ethinyloestradiol 30 μg	levonorgestrel 50 μg for 6 days levonorgestrel 75 μg for 5 days levonorgestrel 125 μg for 10 days
Loestrin 20	ethinyloestradiol 20 μg	norethisterone acetate 1 mg
Progestogen-only contraceptives		
Femulen	—	ethynodiol diacetate 500 μg
Micronor, Noriday	—	norethisterone 350 μg
Microval, Norgeston	—	levonorgestrel 30 μg
Neogest	—	norgestrel 75 μg

oestrogen (e.g. norethisterone 10 mg and ethinyloestradiol 50 μg) as a pregnancy test has been linked with congenital malformation if the patient happens to be pregnant, and it is therefore dangerous. Progestogens may produce masculinisation of the fetus if given during pregnancy.

The oral contraceptive pill

Since the original pilot trials in Puerto Rico 25 years ago proved that steroid oral contraception was feasible the use of this method has been increasing. Presently perhaps 20 million women throughout the world use contraceptive steroid pills and this technique remains the most consistently effective contraceptive method.

The oestrogens used in the pill are ethinyloestradiol and its 3-methyl ester mestranol. The latter has a pharmacological potency of about 60% of that of ethinyloestradiol in animals but they are probably equipotent in man. Their main contraceptive action is to suppress ovulation by interfering with gonadotrophin release by the pituitary via their action on the hypothalamus. This prevents the mid-cycle rise in LH which triggers ovulation. Whereas other oestrogens like stilboestrol also suppress ovulation for a few cycles they may fail to do so when used over a long time. Ethinyloestradiol and mestranol seem to be different in that no pituitary 'break-through' ovulation is likely to occur. The progestogens used are 19-nortestosterone derivatives: norethynodrel, norethisterone, lynoestrenol, norgestrel and ethynodiol acetate. Nortestosterone derivatives are metabolised to a small extent to oestrogenic metabolites which may account for their anti-ovulatory effect. Progestogens have two main actions:

(i) A pseudodecidual (pseudopregnant) change is produced in the endometrium which discourages implantation of the zygote.
(ii) A direct action on cervical mucus is produced making it impenetrable to sperm.

The endocrine effects of the combined oral contraceptive include:

(a) absence of normal pre-menstrual rise and mid-cycle peaks of LH and FSH and loss of rise of progesterone plasma levels in the luteal phase;
(b) increased hepatic synthesis of carrier proteins, e.g. thyroid-binding globulin, caeruloplasmin (causing a green tinge to the plasma), transferrin;
(c) reduced carbohydrate tolerance;
(d) raised erythrocyte sedimentation rate;
(e) decreased albumin and haptoglobulin synthesis.

Combined oestrogen–progestogen pill

It is taken daily for 21 consecutive days, the initial cycle being commenced on the fifth day of the menstrual cycle. Medication is then stopped for 7 days and withdrawal of oestrogen produces uterine bleeding some 2–3 days after the last pill. The pill is restarted again after 7 drug-free days and bleeding ceases.

Originally oestrogen doses in excess of 50 μg/day were used but the risk of thromboembolism has made it desirable to reduce oestrogen levels as low as possible. Deep-vein thrombosis is uncommon with 50 μg pills. Further oestrogen reduction must be balanced against the risk of unwanted pregnancy which increases as the oestrogen dose is reduced. The situation with the 30 μg pill is uncertain in terms of mortality or serious adverse effects but epidemiological observations suggest a decrease in cardiovascular and neoplastic complications.

The **triphasic** (e.g. Trinordiol) and **biphasic** pill preparations (e.g. Binovum) mimic more closely the normal hormone cycle. The triphasic formulation produces a mid-cycle peak of oestrogen and a progressive rise in progestogen followed by a fall in both before menstruation.

There are distinct effects associated with each of the components and some women may be suited by a pill with greater progestogenic effects which may reduce menorrhagia or dysmenorrhoea but may find that a pill having predominantly oestrogenic effects produces ankle oedema and nausea. To a certain extent these effects will depend upon the pre-existing hormonal status of the woman. The side effects associated with different types of ovarian steroid are shown in Table 18.3. Many of these attributions are speculative and may be incorrect. The overall acceptability of the combined pill is around 80 %: minor side effects can often be controlled by a change in formulation.

Adverse effects There is no doubt that apart from minor discomforts there are some important effects related to the use of oral contraceptives containing oestrogen and progestogen. Users have an increased risk of 1 per 5000 per year of dying from cardiovascular disease, this risk being concentrated in women over 35 years of age, especially if they smoke cigarettes and have used oral contraceptives for five years or more continuously. There are a number of elements in this increased cardiovascular mortality:

(i) Myocardial infarction: the pill acts synergistically with other risk factors such as smoking, age, hypertension, diabetes, obesity, hyperlipoproteinaemia and reduction of HDL.

Table 18.3 Side effects associated with different types of ovarian steroid

Oestrogen	*Progestogen*	*Both*
Breakthrough bleeding	Acne	Depression
Carbohydrate intolerance	Hirsutism	Hypertension
Cerebral arterial thrombosis	Reduced libido	Irregular bleeding
Cervical erosion	Vaginal dryness	Post-pill amenorrhoea
Cloasma	Migraine during pill-free days	
Cholestatic jaundice		
Menstrual cramps		
Migraine		
Myocardial infarction		
Oedema		
Vaginal discharge		
Vaginal candidiasis		
Venous thrombosis		

(ii) Cerebral arterial thrombosis is increased 6- to 8-fold.

(iii) Increased blood pressure is common with the pill but in about 5% of patients this elevation extends into the pathological range after a variable interval. Thus the blood pressure should be monitored at each visit by the patient. When medication is stopped the blood pressure usually falls to normal levels after a variable interval of up to one year.

(iv) Venous thrombosis and thromboembolism are commoner in users of oral contraceptives: the mortality rate per 100 000 women between the ages of 35 and 44 years is 3.9 as compared to 0.5 for non-users. This risk is only about one third as great among women with blood group O, i.e. it demonstrates a pharmacogenetic variation. This risk must be seen in the context of a risk of 58 per 100 000 of dying during pregnancy in this age group, the risk due to thromboembolism alone during pregnancy at this age being 2.3 per 100 000. The failure rates of other contraceptive methods suggest that the thromboembolic hazards may be balanced by the risks of an unwanted pregnancy (see Tables 18.4 and 18.5).

(v) Mesenteric artery thrombosis and small-bowel ischaemia.

These cardiovascular adverse effects appear to be related to the oestrogen component.

Jaundice similar to that of pregnancy cholestasis can occur, usually in the first few cycles. Recovery is rapid on drug withdrawal. Patients should always be questioned about pregnancy jaundice and severe pruritis occurring late in pregnancy since these may recur on the pill. Infectious hepatitis occurring within 6 months of the planned starting date of the pill is a contraindication to its use. Depression may also be related to oestrogen-induced alterations of tryptophan metabolism and pyridoxine 50 mg daily may help. A pill formulation containing pyridoxine has been undergoing clinical trial.

Oral contraceptives may affect migraine in a number of ways:

(a) precipitation of attacks in the previously unaffected;
(b) exacerbation of previously existing migraine;
(c) alter the pattern of attacks, in particular, focal neurological features may appear;
(d) occasionally the incidence of attacks may decrease or they may even be abolished whilst the patient is on the pill.

Table 18.4 Mortality related to contraceptive methods

Deaths attibutable to contraceptive methods plus those due to pregnancies (per 100 woman years)

	Age, 20–34 years	*35–44 years*
'Pill'	0.002–0.004	0.02
I.U.D.	0.002–0.004	0.002
Occlusive devices	0.002–0.004	0.002

Table 18.5 Morbidity with contraceptives

Method of contraception	*Excess of admissions to hospital (per 100 woman years)*	*Pregnancies (per 100 woman years)*	*Full term*	*Spontaneous abortion*	*Ectopic*	*Terminations*
'Pill'	Stroke 0.035 Venous thrombosis and embolus 0.07 Myocardial infarction 0.01	0.36	0.2	0.045	0.01	0.094
I.U.D.	Uterine perforations 0.05 Pelvic inflammatory disease 0.2	2.0	0.495	0.755	0.12	0.605
Occlusive devices	Nil	5.0	3.045	0.64	0.02	1.295

Other important adverse effects include an increased incidence of gall-stones. Endometrial and cervical cancer is increased. The latter appears to be related to long periods of pill use starting in early adult life. It is possible that prolonged sexual activity and not medication is the important aetiological link with cervical cancer. There is controversy about the effect of the oestrogen and progestogen content of the pill and the incidence of breast cancer. At present it appears that the early use of the pill for prolonged periods may increase the risk of breast cancer and that there is suggestive evidence that the use of moderately high oestrogen (50 μg) pills may also be associated with a raised incidence of this tumour. The situation with regard to the progestogen content is at present unproven. The rare vascular adenoma of the liver appears to be more frequent in pill users. There is a decreased incidence of benign breast lesions and functional ovarian cysts. Diabetes mellitus may be precipitated by the pill. Amenorrhoea is not unusual (about 5%) after discontinuing the pill but is rarely prolonged and although there may be temporary impairment of fertility after stopping the pill, permanent sterility is unlikely, full fertility being regained in about 40 months.

Absolute contraindications to the pill:

- phlebitis and thromboembolism
- arterial disease
- hyperlipidaemia
- heart disease
- hypertension of any degree greater than mild (> 100 mm Hg diastolic)
- severe liver disease
- cancer of breast or uterus
- porphyria
- pregnancy

Relative contraindications:

- age (> 35 years)
- amenorrhoea
- asthma
- cholelithiasis
- depression
- diabetes mellitus
- epilepsy
- fibroids
- migraine
- multiple sclerosis
- obesity
- severe varicose veins
- otosclerosis

Drug interactions

1. Oral anticoagulants: oral contraceptive steroids increase plasma levels of factor VII and can interfere with the efficacy of oral anticoagulants.
2. Antidepressant therapy becomes less effective in the presence of oral contraceptives despite the inhibition of metabolism of some tricylics by contraceptive steroids.
3. Antihypertensive therapy is adversely affected by oral contraceptives which increase renin substrate and produce a raised blood pressure.
4. Antidiabetic therapy is impaired by oral contraceptives which may be diabetogenic in some women.

It should be remembered that some enzyme inducers can decrease the plasma levels of contraceptive steroids, thus decreasing the effectiveness of the pill. Break-through bleeding and/or unwanted pregnancy have been described after phenobarbitone, phenytoin, chloramphenicol and rifampicin. Oral contraceptive steroids undergo enterohepatic circulation and conjugated steroid in bile is broken down in the gut by bacteria to the parent steroid, and subsequently reabsorbed. Antibiotic treatment with, e.g., ampicillin, neomycin, which alters the colonic bacterial populations, has been shown to increase their faecal excretion and decrease plasma levels resulting in decreased effectiveness.

Low-dose progestogen only preparations

These may be useful if oestrogen-containing pills are poorly tolerated or contraindicated. The contraceptive effectiveness is reduced since ovulation is suppressed in only approximately 40 % of women and the major contraceptive effect is on the cervical mucus and endometrium. Pregnancy rates are of the same order as with the intra-uterine contraceptive device or barrier methods (approximately 1.5–2 per 100 women per year—cf. 0.3 per 100 women per year for the combined preparation). This pill is taken continuously throughout the menstrual cycle which may be convenient for some patients. They can be used in the puerperium since they do not interfere with lactation nor does the progestogen pass into breast milk in significant amounts. As yet there is no evidence of any serious adverse effects and the main problems are:

(a) irregular menstrual bleeding, which can be heavy. This often settles down after a few cycles;
(b) breast tenderness;
(c) skin flushing, a rash similar to acne or merely skin roughness;
(d) headache and migraine have been reported.

Depot progesterone injections

A single intramuscular injection of 150 mg medroxyprogesterone acetate (Depot-Provera) may provide contraception for 3 months with a failure rate of 0.25/100 women per year. The side effects are essentially similar to those of low-dose progestogen-only preparations. Long-term use is not advisable since after 2 years treatment up to 40 % of women develop amenorrhoea and infertility so that pregnancy is unlikely for 9–12 months after the last injection.

Other methods of contraception

Postcoital contraception The risk of pregnancy ensuing from a single unprotected intercourse is around 1 in 30. The 'morning-after' pill is the commonest form of post-coital contraception presently in use and consists of two doses each of ethinyloestradiol 100 μg and levonorgestrel 500 μg (e.g. as two tablets of Ovran or Eugynon 50) given 12 hours apart within 72 hours of unprotected intercourse. The failure rate of this method is 0–3 % but up to 50 % of women experience nausea and vomiting (if one of the doses is vomited within 3 hours of ingestion it should be repeated). If this method fails most patients request termination: should a woman wish to continue her pregnancy she should be warned that the possibility of fetal damage cannot be excluded although there is little evidence for its occurrence.

Male oral contraception is also being pursued. The most likely method will probably be analogous to the combined pill for women, i.e. suppression of gonadotrophin output with exogenous testosterone replacement. This could be achieved by, e.g., a mixture of ethinyloestradiol and methyltestosterone. Other substances have been found which will have a direct effect on the testis to suppress spermatogenesis although their safety is not established.

Intrauterine chemical release The frequency of side effects and lower efficacy as compared to the pill of the intrauterine contraceptive device has prompted the development of devices to release contraceptive agents directly into the uterine cavity. The release of metallic copper from devices such as the Cu-T and Cu-7 may produce a number of effects since the endometrial exudation of leucocytes evoked is probably directly embryotoxic: the copper ion may interact with -SH groups in sperm, changes may occur in cervical mucus to make it impenetrable to sperm, or the uterus and tubes may be stimulated, thus resulting in too rapid a passage of the zygote into the uterus so that implantation is unsuccessful. Progesterone release to alter the endometrium directly has also been used and appears an effective contraceptive, which probably acts by producing a decidual change in the endometrium with glandular atrophy. These devices have had to be withdrawn from the UK since there is an unacceptable probability of ectopic pregnancy. They indicate, however, the possible direction for further research.

Ergot and its derivatives

This topic may be conveniently discussed here since one of the main uses of ergometrine is in obstetrics.

Ergot is a fungus, *Claviceps purpurea*, which parasitises rye. It contains a number of potent pharmacological agents which include the ergot alkaloids, many of which are lysergic acid derivatives. The important alkaloids are ergotamine, ergometrine (ergonovine) and ergotoxin (which is itself a mixture of three alkaloids). They have three major actions each to varying degree:

(a) smooth-muscle stimulation producing vasoconstriction and uterine contraction;
(b) blockade of α-adrenoceptors;
(c) CNS effects producing hypotension and nausea.

Ergotamine is used in the treatment of migraine (q.v.) It has a very slow action on the uterus even when given intravenously.

Ergometrine is a powerful oxytocic but the vasoconstrictor effects are less marked and it has no α-blocking properties. The uterus is sensitive at all times but especially so in late pregnancy. Ergometrine is used in the third stage of labour to decrease postpartum haemorrhage. It is given intramuscularly (with or without hyaluronidase) or intravenously in doses of 0.3–0.5 mg, and is effective for at least 3 h. It is also well absorbed by mouth when 0.5–1 mg is given twice daily for incomplete abortion.

The action of ergometrine differs from that of oxytocin:

(a) oxytocin produces slow contractions with full relaxation between, whilst ergometrine produces faster contractions superimposed upon a tonic contraction. For this reason ergometrine is unsuitable for induction of labour.
(b) given intramuscularly, oxytocin acts within 1–2 min, although the contraction is brief, but ergometrine takes 5 min to act. This delay can be fatal in post-partum haemorrhage and so the preparation **Syntometrine** (ergotamine 0.5 mg plus oxytocin 5 I.U.) is preferred for midwives, who do not administer drugs intravenously in the UK.

Hypertension lasting hours or even days after ergometrine administration may particularly occur in toxaemic patients, in whom the drug should be used with care.

Ergot poisoning is now extremely rare in Europe. In acute poisoning there may be vomiting, diarrhoea, headache, convulsions, paraesthesiae and gangrene of the fingers, toes, nose or ears (St Anthony's fire).

PROSTAGLANDINS

There are at least twenty naturally occurring postaglandins which are 20-carbon unsaturated fatty acids containing a 5-carbon (cyclopentane) ring. They are widely distributed throughout the body since they are synthesised by virtually every tissue. Their release is promoted by various means, including hormones (e.g. angiotensin II, bradykinin), mechanical damage or stretch, decreased oxygen tension and nerve stimulation. Since, there is no mechanism for prostaglandin storage, release reflects *de novo* biosynthesis. Prostaglandins are formed by the enzymatic oxygenation of the polyunsaturated fatty acids arachidonic acid and dihomo-γ-linolenic acid which form prostaglandins of series 1 and 2 respectively, which thus determines the degree of unsaturation. Prostaglandins (PGs) are also identified by letters A, B, F, E etc. which refer to the state of the cyclopentane ring. Prior to prostaglandin synthesis (see Fig. 18.2) the unsaturated fatty acids must be released from binding to phospholipid or triglyceride by activation of lipases (e.g. phospholipase A_2). The released fatty acid is acted upon by an enzyme cyclo-oxygenase with the incorporation of oxygen to form the cyclic endoperoxides, PGG_2 and PGH_2, which themselves have considerable biological activity and contract smooth muscle and cause platelet aggregation. They also serve as intermediates for synthesis of other prostaglandins. Each tissue may have different synthetic enzymes which require PGG_2 or PGH_2 as substrate but which produce different products. Little, if any, prostaglandin is found in arterial blood, largely because of efficient pulmonary destruction so that prostaglandins may be regarded as local tissue hormones synthesised at or near their site of action.

Prostaglandins are an extremely potent group of compounds and have a broad range of activities which vary within the group but include:

1. stimulation of the pregnant uterus;
2. inhibition of gastric acid secretion;
3. bronchial relaxation;

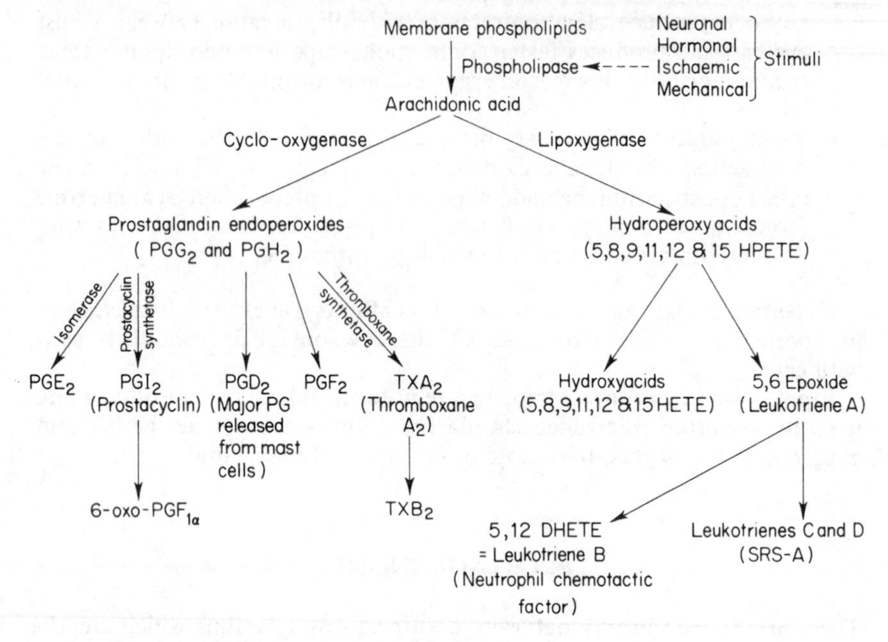

Fig. 18.2 Some pathways of prostaglandin synthesis.

4. vasodilator and hypotensive activity, including control of blood flow through the renal medulla;
5. natriuresis;
6. inhibition of platelet aggregation;
7. lipid mobilisation;
8. mediation of some phases of inflammation;
9. contraction of the iris.

Prostaglandins have therefore numerous roles in normal tissues. In reproduction, they affect the smooth muscle of the female genital tract, causing rhythmical contraction and aiding sperm transport. These effects are mediated by seminal prostaglandins acting locally and via the circulation following vaginal absorption. It has been noted that 70% of infertile males have decreased semen prostaglandin levels. Prostaglandin $F_{2\alpha}$($PGF_{2\alpha}$) is present in menstrual fluid, and it is thought that high levels may result in uterine spasm and dysmenorrhoea, thus giving a rational basis to the use of prostaglandin synthetase inhibitors such as indomethacin and aspirin in this condition. Prostaglandins also have a role in labour and changes in prostaglandin levels in the blood correlate well with changes in intra-uterine pressure. It is suggested that oestrogen from the placenta may trigger prostaglandin synthesis and release to initiate labour. This mechanism may also be initiated by injection of hypertonic saline, artificial rupture of the membranes or insertion of a catheter into the uterus, thus representing a final common pathway. Prostaglandins have found several uses in therapeutics:

(a) Induction of pre-term labour, e.g. for intrauterine fetal death, hydatidiform mole, or to induce abortion by either **Dinoprost**, i.e. prostaglandin $F_{2\alpha}$ (Prostin F2alpha) or **Dinoprostone**, i.e. prostaglandin E_2 (Prostin E2). These may be given intravenously or by extra-amniotic instillation. Extra-amniotic dinoprostone may also be used to 'prime' the cervix prior to vacuum termination of pregnancy. Intra-amniotic instillation can only be used after 14–16 weeks gestation. Dinoprostone may be given orally or by vaginal tablet as well. Their action may be augmented by concurrent administration of oxytocin. Prostaglandins are not used to induce labour at term as excessive uterine action is easily provoked with resulting fetal harm. This powerful activity is of value in pre-term induction although uterine rupture remains a possible but rare outcome.

Adverse effects include dose-related nausea, vomiting, dizziness, headache, fever and reversible leucocytosis. Given intravenously they produce a high incidence of thrombophlebitis.

Caution is required if the patient has glaucoma or asthma because of prostaglandin effects on iris and bronchi.

(b) Maintenance of patency of the ductus arteriosus in neonates with congenital heart disease. In the fetus about 90% of the right ventricular output bypasses the lungs via the ductus arteriosus. Prostaglandins like PGE_1 and PGE_2 relax the ductus thus indomethacin may be used to close a postnatally patent ductus. Infants with congenital lesions such as coarctation, transposition of the great vessels or obstructive right heart disease may be treated palliatively with **alprostadil**, i.e. prostaglandin E_1 (Prostin VR) during resuscitation pending corrective surgery. It cannot be used chronically as weakening of the ductus and pulmonary artery occurs.

DRUGS AFFECTING SEXUAL FUNCTION

The complex interplay between physiological and psychological factors which determines sexual desire and performance makes it difficult to assess the influence of drugs on sexual function. In the male the nervous basis for coitus is a spinal reflex and the act can occur in the absence of sensation following section of the spinal cord. Stimulation of sacral parasympathetic nerves results in erection whilst the sympathetic nervous supply abolishes it by vasoconstriction of the vessels supplying the corpus spongeosum and corpora cavernosa. The sympathetic supply to the smooth muscle of the vasa deferentia, seminal vesicles and prostate is responsible for co-ordinating ejaculation. Thus any drugs which affect the autonomic supply to the sex organs may interfere with sexual function. These include:

phenothiazines, e.g. chlorpromazine, thioridazine,
butyrophenones, e.g. haloperidol, benperidol;
centrally acting antihypertensive agents such as reserpine,
clonidine and methyldopa (but β-blockers do not often interfere with male sexual function);
adrenergic neurone blockers, e.g. guanethidine, bethanidine and debrisoquine;
tricyclic antidepressants, e.g. clomipramine, protriptyline, imipramine.

The most common effect is interference with ejaculation although secondary impotence may occur via psychogenic mechanisms. Isolated erectile impotence has been described following excessive exposure to anticholinesterase herbicides and pesticides. Thiazides used in treating hypertension cause impotence in about 20% of patients.

Drugs decreasing sexual desire probably act via central depressant effects and include:

antihypertensive agents: clonidine, methyldopa, reserpine;
alcohol;
butyrophenones: the use of benperidol in this context is indicated on p. 250,
oral contraceptives;
oestrogen therapy in males;
anti-androgens, e.g. cyproterone (see p. 620).

The existence of *aphrodisiac drugs* which increase libido is probably a myth, although there is a market for such agents. The use of cocaine, amphetamine or yohimbine as sexual stimulants, as well as more traditional mixtures, have their devotees, but their medical use in the treatment of impotence is disappointing. Cannabis enjoys a reputation for enhancing sexual enjoyment and desire. The reason for this is not clear but it may be due to a general release of inhibition. In fact, continual smoking of cannabis lowers male serum testosterone levels. An anxiolytic agent, e.g. diazepam, in a small dose may be helpful if anxiety over performance is at the root of the problem. A few cases of reduced libido and impotence in males and females are associated with hyperprolactinaemia and in such cases bromocriptine (5–10 mg/day) may restore potency.

Androgenic hormones probably play a role in both male and female in arousability and arousal.

Certain peptide hormones–for example LHRH–can produce sexual readiness in female rats. In man and animals LHRH potentiates the behavioural effects of levodopa.

Dopamine may be another endogenous substance required for sexual activity. Increased libido has been reported in patients suffering from Parkinson's disease treated with levodopa.

THE ADRENAL CORTEX

The adrenal cortex normally secretes:

1. glucocorticoids: principally cortisol (hydrocortisone) and small amounts of corticosterone;
2. mineralocorticoids: principally aldosterone and small amounts of desoxycorticosterone;
3. androgens in small amounts, e.g. testosterone, androsterone;
4. other steroids in very small amounts, e.g. oestrogens, progesterone.

1. Glucocorticoids

Cortisol (Hydrocortisone)

Even though cortisol is classed as a glucocorticoid, it has considerable mineralocorticoid activity (see Table 18.6). In the normal human the

Table 18.6 Relative potencies of corticosteroids and mineralocorticoids

Compound	*Relative potency* *Anti-inflammatory*	*Mineralocorticoid*	*Equivalent doses for anti-inflammatory effect (mg)*
Cortisol (Hydrocortisone)	1	1	80
Cortisone	0.8	1	100
Prednisolone and prednisone	4	0.8	20
Methylprednisolone	5	0.5	16
Triamcinolone	4	0	20
Dexamethasone	25	0	2
Betamethasone	25	0	2
Aldosterone	0	1000*	—
Fludrocortisone	15	500	—

* Injected—other preparations as oral doses

physiological role of cortisol is not known, but its salt-conserving properties could be of importance, particularly in view of the fall in blood pressure, dehydration and loss of sodium which occurs when cortisol is not secreted. The glucocorticoid properties of steroids require the presence of an α-ketol side chain at carbon 17, as in the molecule of cortisol. At physiological levels cortisol plays a very minor role (at the most) in controlling blood glucose. At much higher concentrations, cortisol raises blood glucose because of enhancement of gluconeogenesis, and diabetes may be precipitated. In very high doses (such as 1 g or more) cortisol acts as a vasoconstrictor. This may be a direct action on the arteriolar wall, but could be because of its ability to inhibit the removal of noradrenaline by non-neuronal cells (uptake$_2$). The actions of cortisol and the effects of its over-secretion (Cushing's syndrome) and undersecretion (Addison's disease) appear in Table 18.7.

Pharmacokinetics The synthesis of cortisol by the adrenals is controlled via cyclic AMP by pituitary corticotrophin (ACTH). The release of corticotrophin is stimulated by a peptide produced by the hypothalamus, the corticotrophin-releasing factor (CRF), which travels in the portal circulation from hypothalamus to anterior pituitary. There is a feedback regulatory control by cortisol which inhibits both corticotrophin and CRF production. The diurnal variation in cortisol blood levels reflects alterations in corticotrophin release. Secretion rate of corticosteroids rises with age to a maximum at about 30 and then declines. It is higher in men than in women and subject to increase by many stimuli since it is part of the bodily response to environmental stress.

The rate of secretion of cortisol is not constant during the day. The maximum blood level is reached at about 8.00 a.m. and the minimum about midnight. The normal plasma concentration is 170–720 nmol/l (6–26 μg/100 ml) at 9.00 a.m. and at midnight less than 220 nmol/l (8 μg/100 ml). The half-life of cortisol in the circulation is about 110 min, although the $t_{1/2}$ of its biological effects is approximately 8–12 h. In patients

Table 18.7 Actions of cortisol and consequences of under and over-secretion

	Actions	*Deficiency*	*Excess*
Carbohydrate, protein and fat metabolism	Enhances gluconeogenesis; antagonises insulin hyperglycaemia ± diabetes mellitus; centripetal fat disposition; hypertriglyceridaemia; hypercholesterolaemia; decreased protein synthesis e.g. diminished skin collagen	Hypoglycaemia, loss of weight	Cushing's syndrome: weight gain, increase in trunk fat, moon face, skin striae, bruising, atrophy, wasting of limb muscles.
Water and salt metabolism	Inhibits fluid shift from extracellular to intracellular compartment; antagonises vasopressin action on kidney; increases vasopressin destruction and decreases its production. Sodium and water retention, potassium loss.	Loss of weight, hypovolaemia, hyponatraemia	Oedema, thirst, polyuria. Hypertension. Muscular weakness.
Haematological	Lowers lymphocyte and eosinophil counts; increases RBC, platelets and clotting tendency.		Florid complexion and polycythaemia.
Alimentary	Increased production of gastric acid and pepsin.	Anorexia and nausea	Dyspepsia; aggravation of peptic ulcer.
CVS	Sensitises arterioles to catecholamines; enhances production of angiotensinogen } —hypertension Fall in high-density lipoprotein with increased total cholesterol.	Hypotension, fainting	Hypertension, atherosclerosis

Table 18.7 (continued)

	Actions	*Deficiency*	*Excess*
Skeletal	Decreased production of cartilage and bone; osteoporosis; anti-vitamin D; increased renal loss of calcium; renal calculi formation.		Backache due to osteoporosis, renal calculi, dwarfing in children (also anti-GH effect).
Nervous system	Altered neuronal excitability. Inhibition of $uptake_2$ of catecholamines.		Depression and other psychiatric changes.
Anti-inflammatory	Reduces formation of fluid and cellular exudate; reduces fibrous tissue repair.		Increased spread of and proneness to infections.
Immunological	Large doses lyse lymphocytes and plasma cells (transient release of immunoglobulin)		Reduced lymphocyte mass, diminished immunoglobulin production.
Feedback	Inhibits release of ACTH and MSH.	Pigmentation of skin and mucosa	

with cirrhosis of the liver the plasma $t_{1/2}$ is lengthened up to 300 min, and in thyrotoxicosis it may be reduced to 60 min.

More than 95% of plasma cortisol is protein bound, mainly to an α-globulin termed transcortin (CBG) which has a much higher affinity for cortisol than albumin, although the total capacity of the latter for cortisol is greater since it is present in larger amounts. With high cortisol levels plasma binding becomes saturated and the percentage of free cortisol may rise to 25% of the total. Cirrhosis reduces cortisol binding whilst pregnancy increases it. Steroid dosage should be reduced in patients with hypoalbuminaemia, since adverse effects are correlated with this measurement presumably due to increased amounts of circulating free drug. Corticosteroid binding globulin (CBG) also shows circadian fluctuation with maximum binding occurring at midnight and minimum binding at 8.00 a.m. This diurnal variation disappears after prednisolone treatment, which also depresses the absolute binding capacity. Theoretically the pharmacological effect of administering single doses of cortisol or prednisolone to normal subjects should vary since diurnal alterations in protein binding change the amount of free, and thus active, drug present. The biological effect of cortisol may be delayed and, following a single intravenous injection for a condition such as status asthmaticus, the maximum effect is not attained until 5 h, although a definite response is apparent at 1 h.

Cortisol is metabolised mainly by the liver and kidney and the metabolites excreted in the urine as '17-hydroxycorticoids' or '17-ketogenic steroids' depending upon the laboratory method used.

Clinical uses Cortisol is given intravenously for rapid effect in emergency as hydrocortisone sodium succinate injection B.P. Hydrocortisone acetate injection B.P. is an insoluble suspension which can be used intramuscularly for prolonged effect or injected into joints.

Cortisone has a similar structure to cortisol, but has a keto group instead of a hydroxyl group on C^{11}. It is pharmacologically inactive but is converted to cortisol by the liver. Thus cortisone is unsuitable for topical use, but parenterally it has been given instead of cortisol. However, absorption from the intestine can be inefficient, and some patients with liver disease may fail to activate the substance. Cortisone has a $t_{1/2}$ of 30 min.

Prednisolone

This drug is a semi-synthetic analogue of cortisol in which a double bond has been inserted between the first and second carbons of the A ring. Weight for weight it produces less sodium and water retention and potassium loss than cortisol, but is about four times more active as a glucocorticoid and anti-inflammatory agent. Thus, although the drug carries a diminished risk of producing sodium retention and hypertension, there are still toxic effects associated with glucocorticoid activity which are dose dependent and correlated with plasma levels. The $t_{1/2}$ of prednisolone is 2.5–3 h and it binds to CBG. It is administered orally, by injection, or (in inflammatory bowel disease) by enema. In the latter case systemic absorption may occur which is comparable to the same dose given orally. Prednisolone retention enemas may thus exert a systemic effect. Enteric-coated prednisolone preparations (e.g. Deltacortril) are also available. Although the bioavailability relative to the uncoated preparation is identical, the evidence that their administration produces less gastric irritation than conventional preparations is largely unsubstantiated.

Prednisone is derived from cortisone by the insertion of a double bond between carbons 1 and 2 of the A ring. It undergoes conversion to prednisolone in the liver by hydroxylation. There is individual variation in this activation step, and this provides a good reason for ceasing its use. Also, prednisolone is cheaper than prednisone.

6 α-methyl prednisolone (Medrone) is slightly more potent than prednisolone.

Triamcinolone (Ledercort) is 9-α-fluoro, hydroxy prednisolone and is similar to prednisolone in action but even more powerfully anti-inflammatory. In addition to exhibiting the toxic effects of prednisolone, its administration is particularly associated with flushes, sweating and muscular weakness. On stopping the drug, arthritis may appear.

Dexamethasone (Decadron) is 9-α-fluoro-16-α-methyl prednisolone and is powerfully anti-inflammatory. The presence of a methyl group on carbon 16 neutralises the salt-retaining influence of the 9-α-fluoro group, and enhances the glucocorticoid effects of the molecule. It has no advantages over prednisolone and does not exhibit the peculiar toxic effects seen with triamcinolone. Dexamethasone therapy is sometimes associated with a sustained negative calcium balance.

Betamethasone (Betnelan; Betnesol) has a methyl group on carbon 16 in the β-position. It has no advantages over prednisolone.

The choice between these alternative drugs is often immaterial, although some patients experience fewer side effects with one particular preparation as compared to another. For replacement therapy cortisol or cortisone are usually used because of their sodium-retaining properties. For anti-inflammatory activity prednisolone is probably the most widely used in the UK.

Adverse effects

1. Rapid withdrawal after prolonged steroid administration may result in acute adrenal insufficiency. Gradual withdrawal is less hazardous, but even in patients who have been taken off steroids, for 1–2 years afterwards a stressful situation (such as trauma, surgery, infection, emotional crises or status asthmaticus) may precipitate an acute adrenal crisis and necessitate the administration of large amounts of steroids, electrolytes, glucose and water. Less dangerous corticosteroid withdrawal features include malaise, fever, arthralgia, myalgia, pseudo-tumour cerebri (raised intracranial pressure and papilloedema).

These effects arise because exogenous corticosteroids, by increasing plasma corticosteroid level, suppress CRF release by the hypothalamus which in turn depresses corticotrophin secretion. As a consequence of minimal or zero corticotrophin secretion over a long time, physiological and anatomical atrophy of the adrenal cortex occurs as well as of the hypothalamic–pituitary axis. Usually the adrenal cortex takes longer to recover full activity while corticotrophin secretion becomes normal within weeks of steroid withdrawal. Full restoration of the hypothalamic—pituitary—adrenal axis may take 9 months to a year. Suppression is unusual if the daily dose of prednisolone is less than 5 mg or its equivalent. The rate at which patients can be weaned off their steroids depends in part on their underlying condition and also on the dose and duration of therapy. Provided there is no exacerbation of disease the daily dose may be reduced by 2.5–5.0 mg weekly until reduction reaches 5 mg prednisolone per day. This is converted to a once daily dose and reduced by 1 mg at a time depending upon symptoms and the plasma cortisol level. This should reach 276 nmol/l(10 μg/100 ml) in an early-morning sample before it is reasonable to completely withdraw the steroid.

2. Intercurrent illness in patients receiving corticosteroids increases the steroid requirements and may produce the clinical picture of acute adrenal failure. With moderate illness it is sufficient to double the dose of whichever steroid is being used. It is not usually necessary, however, to give more than 40 mg of prednisolone or its equivalent daily.

In severely ill patients, particularly when vomiting or electrolyte loss is a problem, it is best to give parenteral cortisol (hydrocortisone hemisuccinate) 100 mg 6 hourly.

3. Complications due to chronic administration of steroids (iatrogenic Cushing's syndrome—see also Table 18.7). These usually only develop on 7.5 mg/day of prednisolone or its equivalent.

(a) General appearance: Cushingoid.
(b) Effects on inflammation: steroids decrease the inflammatory and immune responses and resistance to infection is reduced. Symptoms and signs of acute infection are suppressed, although the spread of infection is enhanced. It follows therefore that patients on steroids who develop an infection require vigorous treatment with the appropriate antibiotic. Steroids also increase susceptibility to opportunistic infection with fungi or other organisms. Old tuberculous lesions may reactivate and such lesions should be carefully watched in patients on chronic steroid treatment: occasionally it may be necessary to give antituberculous cover with isoniazid and rifampicin.
(c) Electrolyte balance may be altered and some salt and water retention is usual. Potassium loss and hypokalaemia can be severe if steroids are combined with a diuretic.
(d) Hypertension can also accompany steroid usage.
(e) Diabetes mellitus may be exacerbated and its control be made more difficult by steroids. They may also precipitate diabetes in those with a genetic predisposition to this condition.
(f) Osteoporosis develops, particularly with high dosage. Vertebral wedge fractures are common.
(g) Peptic ulceration: although steroids rarely cause ulcers to develop de novo, they can delay healing, exacerbate haemorrhage and mask the symptoms and signs of perforation.

(h) Mental changes: anxiety, elation, sleeplessness and depression may develop. Occasionally a schizophrenic episode can be precipitated. Special care is therefore required in patients with a history of mental illness.
(i) The eye: posterior capsular cataracts have been reported. Locally applied steroids may encourage the spread of infection and for this reason they should never be used in active herpes simplex infections (dendritic ulcer). The pharmacogenetically controlled response of intra-ocular pressure to steroids is discussed on p. 112.
(j) Proximal myopathy is particularly liable to develop with the fluorinated steroids triamcinolone, betamethasone and dexamethasone.
(k) Linear growth. Steroids suppress the production and action of growth hormone. Prolonged use in childhood leads to stunting.
(l) Teratogenesis: there is no clear evidence that in man steroids taken by the mother can affect the fetus.
(m) Necrosis of bone.

Alternate day steroid therapy may produce less pituitary adrenal suppression with fewer side effects (particularly linear growth in children) than daily treatment without loss of efficacy. These claims have yet to be completely proven. In patients on single daily doses of steroids it may be better to give the dose in the early morning since this minimises the normal increase in endogenous steroid levels. An evening dose produces suppression of the hypothalamus and pituitary at a time when suppression by endogenous steroids is minimal since plasma steroid levels are low, and thus may prevent the morning rise in steroid secretion. High doses given in the evening may cause wakefulness.

Cushing's syndrome results from excess cortisol secretion by the adrenal cortex. Excessive corticotrophin production (due to a pituitary tumour or over-production of the hypothalamic corticotrophin-releasing factor) or the production of a corticotrophin-like peptide from tumours elsewhere in the body (ectopic ACTH syndrome). More commonly it results from the therapeutic administration of glucocorticoids when they are used as anti-inflammatory or immunosuppressive agents.

Some of the presenting symptoms are shown in Table 18.7. The urinary free cortisol is raised above 1000 nmol/day (360 μg/day) in men or 776 nmol/day (280 μg/day) in women. The plasma cortisol is not suppressed by dexamethasone.

Treatment of Cushing's syndrome of pituitary origin is difficult. The success rate of pituitary irradiation is only about 20% and takes several months to take effect. However, if external proton-beam irradiation is available, this has a 60% cure rate. The implantation of ^{90}yttrium or ^{198}gold seeds has a similarly high success rate, but there is a high morbidity: 50% of patients develop hypogonadism. Perhaps the ideal treatment is a local removal of a pituitary tumour—if this can be found—with minimal disturbance to the rest of the gland. However, such direct surgical treatment is not often possible and the delay of onset of the effects of conventional irradiation to the pituitary is too hazardous in an ill, hypertensive patient. Bilateral adrenalectomy alone will produce rapid reversal of the Cushing's syndrome of pituitary origin, but this can be followed by an increase in corticotrophin secretion, skin pigmentation and enlargement of the pituitary (Nelson's syndrome). Because of these problems many centres used to treat Cushing's syndrome of pituitary origin by bilateral adrenalectomy preceded by pituitary irradiation. Replacement treatment (as for Addison's disease) was required. However, this treatment is becoming much less favoured. When other types of treatment have not been completely successful bromocriptine or cyproheptadine may be used as supplementary measures.

Metyrapone is a drug which blocks cortisol synthesis by the adrenal cortex and can be given during the interval (which may be several years) between pituitary irradiation and diminution in pituitary function. The dose for this purpose is between 250 mg three times daily and 1 g four times daily. The dose is adjusted until the plasma cortisol levels fall within the range 330–80 nmol/l.

Metyrapone is also used to test the ability of the anterior pituitary to product ACTH, since corticotrophin plasma levels should increase after inhibition of cortisol synthesis, so producing a rise in urinary 17-oxogenic (-ketogenic) steroid excretion. For short-term treatment **aminoglutethimide** (250 mg, 8 hourly) will inhibit cortisol synthesis. This is used in severe Cushing's syndrome prior to operation.

Cushing's syndrome of adrenal origin If this is due to an adenoma it is treated by excision. As in phaeochromocytoma, in 10% of patients the tumour is bilateral. The tumours can be located using radiolabelled cholesterol. Administration of metyrapone for 3 months before the operation reduces the surgical risks because of improvement of the polycythaemia, hypertension, diabetes, heart failure and hypokalaemia.

Adrenal carcinomas can be treated similarly and the patients prepared with metyrapone. Following removal of a carcinoma of the adrenal, the Cushing's state may not be completely eradicated. For this metyrapone 500–750 mg 6 hourly or aminoglutethimide 250 mg 6–8 hourly may be used.

Mitotane (o-p-DDT) may be used if the tumour recurs, or if metastases develop. The drug is given in slowly increasing doses—but the amount given is usually limited because of nausea and vomiting. Mitotane diminishes cortisol secretion and inhibits adrenal cortical-cell growth. Pulmonary metastases may also regress.

2. Mineralocorticoids

Aldosterone

This is the main mineralocorticoid secreted by the adrenal cortex. It has no glucocorticoid activity but is about 1000 times more active as a mineralocorticoid compared with cortisol.

ACTH has transient stimulatory action on aldosterone production, but the main factors which control this are plasma sodium and potassium concentrations and plasma angiotensin II levels (see Fig. 18.3). Pituitary failure,

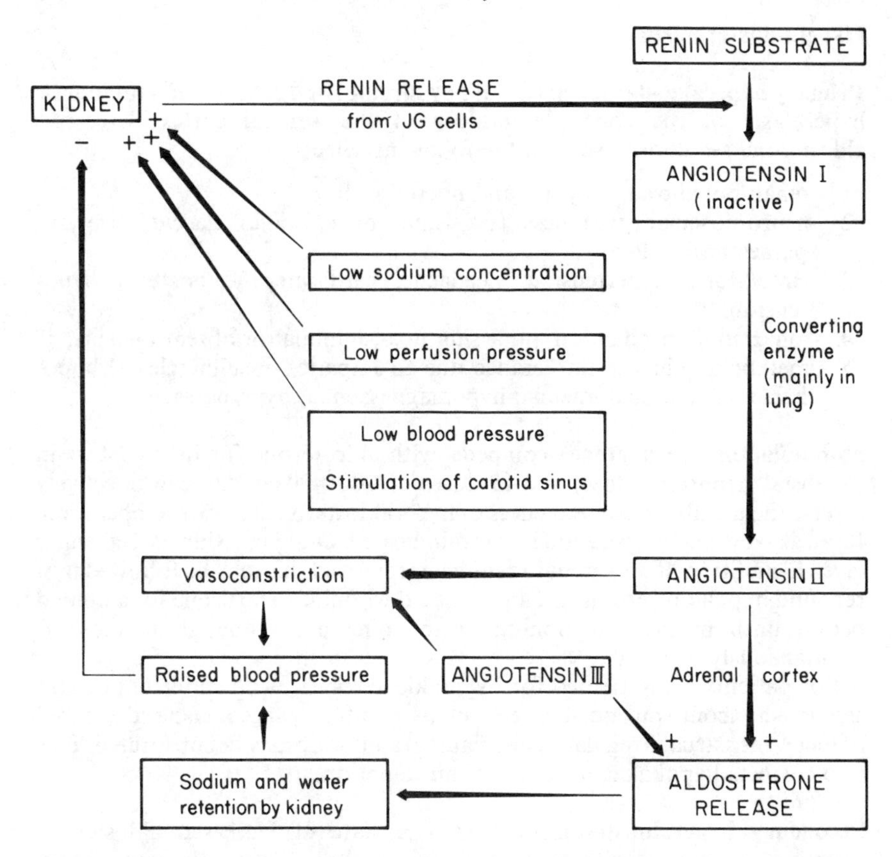

Fig. 18.3 Inter-relationships of renin, angiotensin and aldosterone.

producing a total absence of corticotrophin, allows aldosterone production to continue, even though cortisol is no longer released.

Aldosterone acts at site IV of the renal tubules and also on the gut and sweat glands to conserve sodium and enhance potassium and hydrogen ion loss. Continued administration produces elevated plasma sodium and chloride levels with a rise in extracellular fluid volume. After about 2 weeks sodium and water retention cease by an escape mechanism (which is not understood) although renal and gastrointestinal potassium excretion do not show this escape. Patients with adrenal tumours secreting aldosterone show this escape mechanism whilst those with secondary hyperaldosteronism do not and are therefore oedematous.

Absence of aldosterone results in sodium loss, potassium retention, reduction in the volume of extracellular fluid and poor peripheral tissue perfusion.

Aldosterone undergoes a large hepatic first-pass metabolism and cannot therefore be given orally. The plasma half-life after injection is about 50 min.

Hyperaldosteronism

Primary hyperaldosteronism (Conn's syndrome) is due to either a tumour or hyperplasia of the zona glomerulosa of the adrenal cortex. Excessive aldosterone secretion results in the following effects:

1. renal: polydipsia, polyuria and nocturia;
2. neuromuscular: weakness (persistent or episodic), flaccid paralysis, paraesthesiae, tetany;
3. circulatory: hypertension, headache, cardiomegaly, postural hypotension;
4. ionic: sodium retention, potassium loss, minimal or absent oedema;
5. metabolic: glucose intolerance due to impaired insulin release, hypokalaemia, hypochloraemia, hypomagnesaemia, hypernatraemia.

Spironolactone (Aldactone) competes with aldosterone for its receptors in the distal nephron (site 4) and in doses of 100–400 mg/day can effectively reverse the metabolic consequences of hyperaldosteronism prior to operation. It can also be used if operation is contraindicated. Oral potassium is frequently given in addition. If an adrenal adenoma is removed this may be followed by a rebound hypoaldosteronism. This is treated with fludrocortisone for a limited period until normal functioning of the remaining zona glomerulosa is spontaneously restored.

For patients being treated for hyperaldosteronism who suffer unpleasant side effects from spironolactone (such as painful gynaecomastia, decreased potency, menstrual irregularity and nausea) amiloride may be substituted. This also corrects hypokalaemia and sodium retention.

Secondary hyperaldosteronism This is a state of increased aldosterone secretion associated with increased plasma renin levels. Excessive renin secretion by the kidney is most commonly due to renal disease, cirrhosis of the liver, some cases of low output cardiac failure and accelerated hypertension.

Spironolactone raises the plasma potassium and contributes to the loss of salt and water, but in addition more powerful natriuretic agents, such as frusemide, may be required. These alone may not lower the blood pressure but hypotensive drugs will be effective once sodium excretion has been enhanced.

Fludrocortisone (9-α fluorohydrocortisone)

This is a remarkably active substance. On a weight-to-weight basis it is 15 times more powerful as a glucocorticoid and 500 times more powerful as a mineralocorticoid compared with cortisol. It is used for its salt-retaining properties, but when given in doses of 0.2 mg or so daily its glucocorticoid effects make it necessary to reduce the dose of cortisol. Its plasma $t_{1/2}$ is about 90 min but this is prolonged in some patients with liver disease, myxoedema, pregnancy and oedema.

Clinical uses of corticosteroids

1. *Replacement therapy in chronic hypoadrenalism* (*Addison's disease*) Since the physiological hormone can be given it is usual to give cortisol (hydro-

cortisone) 20 mg each morning and 10 mg each evening, thus mimicking the normal diurnal rhythm. The tablets should be taken orally with food to minimise gastric effects. The precise oral dose which each patient needs is found by measuring the cortisol concentrations in the plasma at various times during the day; the following values are satisfactory:

peak after morning dose:	690–966 nmol/l (25–35 μg/100 ml)
before evening dose:	165–276 nmol/l (6–10 μg/100 ml)
peak after evening dose:	not more than 690 nmol/l (25 μg/100 ml).

Cortisone acetate 25 mg each morning and 12.5 mg each evening is a reasonable alternative.

More severely affected patients will require aldosterone replacement and many physicians routinely give mineralocorticoids. Fludrocortisone is the drug of choice starting with a daily dose of 0.05 mg daily and increasing if necessary to a dose of 0.1–0.2 mg daily. Signs of overdosage are those of sodium retention, i.e. oedema, headache, hypertension and arthralgia, and potassium depletion, i.e., muscle weakness, and hypokalaemic alkalosis. Alternative mineralocorticoids are:

(a) Deoxycortone pivalate: 25–100 mg by intramuscular injection of the microcrystalline suspension every 3–4 weeks which ensures good compliance.
(b) Deoxycortone acetate: 2.5–5 mg subcutaneously or intramuscularly every alternate day or daily. This drug is very poorly absorbed orally and so must be injected.

Intercurrent illness will increase the cortisol requirements. With mild illness, doubling the dose of oral cortisol is sufficient, but parenteral hydrocortisone will be necessary if diarrhoea and vomiting develops.

Surgery in patients with Addison's disease requires 100 mg hydrocortisone hemisuccinate given 6 hourly by injection. This should be started 2 h before the operation and continued until recovery has occurred and oral feeding resumed.

2. *Treatment of acute hypoadrenalism* In addition to large quantities of salt, glucose and water, e.g. 2–4 l of i.v. isotonic saline dextrose, 100 mg cortisol (hydrocortisone hemisuccinate) are given intravenously every 6 h over the first 24 h. Occasionally more is needed to maintain the blood pressure. After the initial electrolyte imbalance has been corrected a daily dose of oral cortisol 20 mg 6 hourly is started and modified as required. Whilst the daily dose is above 60 mg daily there is usually sufficient mineralocorticoid action but at doses below this a mineralocorticoid may be required. Thus a daily dose of 20–30 mg of cortisol is supplemented by 0.05–0.2 mg of fludrocortisone.

3. *Congenital adrenal hyperplasia* is due to a failure of cortisol synthesis by the adrenal cortical cells. This is most commonly the result of a genetic deficiency of the enzyme 21-hydroxylase. The low plasma cortisol enhances ACTH release and excessive amounts of circulating ACTH produce adrenal cortical hyperplasia and increase steroid synthesis up to the level of the biochemical block. Since cortisol cannot be made because of the block at the 21-hydroxylation step, its precursors build up and are converted to androgenic steroids. Girls are virilised and boys have precocious sexual development due

Table 18.8 Topically administered steroids

Topically administered steroid preparations are most usefully classified according to their efficacy as anti-inflammatory agents.

Anti-inflammatory properties	*Steroid preparations*
Most active	clobetasol propionate 0.05 %
	fluocinolone acetonide 0.2 %
	halcinonide 0.1 %
Very active	fluocinolone acetonide 0.025 %
	betamethasone valerate 0.1 %
	triamcinolone acetonide 0.1 %
	fluocinonide 0.05 %
	diflucortolone valerate 0.1 %
	beclomethasone dipropionate 0.025 %
	desonide 0.05 %
	fluclorolone acetonide 0.025 %
	hydrocortisone butyrate 0.1 %
Moderately active	flurandrenolone 0.0125 %
	fluocinolone acetonide 0.01 %
	fluocortolone hexanoate 0.1 %
	with fluocortolone pivalate 0.1 %
	clobetasone butyrate 0.05 %
	flumethasone pivalate 0.02 %
Weak	hydrocortisone 0.1–2.5 %
	flurandrenolone 0.05 %
	methylprednisolone 0.25 %

to the excess of androgens, but they also have inadequate glucocorticoid secretion and lose sodium. They are treated with added salt and fludrocortisone and with a glucocorticoid which (apart from its other actions) inhibits the excessive secretion of corticotrophin.

4. *Immunosuppression*, e.g. renal transplantation, systemic lupus erythematosus (see p. 819).
5. *Suppression of inflammation*, e.g. rheumatoid arthritis, asthma.

Details of these uses of steroids will be found in textbooks of medicine. All patients taking corticotrophin or corticosteroids either for substitution therapy or for pharmacological effect should carry a card stating their diagnosis and treatment and the dose of the drug.

An important use of these drugs which is less commonly discussed by general physicians is their *topical use on the skin*:

Optimal absorption (about 3–10 %) into the skin of the steroid occurs from a vehicle of soft white paraffin. Lotions and creams allow less release of the steroid from the base and a lower proportion penetrating the skin. Absorption is increased by warming the skin, increasing its hydration, polythene occlusion and disruption of the horny layer by disease. The weakest preparation which will produce improvement in the condition should be used. Weak preparations may be effective in the eczemas whilst more potent preparations are usually needed in psoriasis. The most effective steroids are necessary for lichen planus and discoid lupus erythematosus. Topical steroids are not effective in urticaria and dermatitis herpetiformis. They are contraindicated in skin infections and in rosacea.

Adverse effects Local: atrophy of dermis and epidermis; telangiectasia; purpura; striae; bacterial, fungal and viral infection.

Systemic: temporary suppression of pituitary adrenal axis; this does not usually persist after stopping the steroid, but long-term steroid application can impair growth of children.

THE ADRENAL MEDULLA

This part of the adrenal secretes the catecholamines adrenaline and noradrenaline. Secretion is not under pituitary control but is stimulated by sympathetic nerves. Unlike the cortex it is not essential for life, but tumours can appear in this tissue, and may secrete pharmacologically active substances. A highly malignant tumour of infancy, the *neuroblastoma*, may secrete catecholamines. Another type of tumour which may arise in the adrenal medulla is the *phaeochromocytoma*. The tumour is rare, but is of importance because it is a treatable cause of hypertension. About 10% of these tumours are malignant, 10% are bilateral, and 10% arise from chromaffin tissue outside the adrenal. Catecholamine secretion from these tumours may produce hypertensive or hypotensive attacks, cardiac arrhythmias or prolonged hypertension. Such crises occur spontaneously or as a result of abdominal operations, investigatory procedures or during labour. Extra-adrenal phaeochromocytomas secrete largely noradrenaline as do metastases of adrenal tumours. If adrenaline is secreted in excess it is usually from an adrenal site, whereas malignant phaeochromocytomas tend to secrete large amounts of dopamine. It is possible to estimate these catecholamines in the blood and such estimations made at different sites during aortic catheterisation may help in localising a phaeochromocytoma. It is more usual to estimate the metabolites of the amines. These are hydroxymethoxymandelic acid (vanillylmandelic acid or VMA), metadrenaline and normetadrenaline. Table 18.9 gives the normal urinary excretion of these substances.

Table 18.9 Normal 24 hour excretion of catecholamine metabolites

	Daily total	*Total expressed per µmole or mmole of creatinine*
Total metanephrines (metadrenaline and normetadrenaline)	5.5 µmol (1.0 mg)	450 µmol/µmol
Hydroxymethoxymandelic acid (VMA)	35 µmol (7.0 mg)	2.5 µmol/mmol

The treatment of phaeochromocytoma is always surgical removal.

Drug treatment can ameliorate or prevent attacks of hypertension and cardiac arrhythmias due to phaeochromocytoma. For this a combination of an α-blocker (such as phenoxybenzamine, 10–20 mg orally, 8 hourly) and a β-blocker (such as propranolol, 40–80 mg orally, 8 hourly) is used. Such a combination of an α- and β-blocker may result in hypotension, and careful initial adjustment of the doses of the two drugs should be carried out in hospital. β-blockers must not be used alone as they may cause a rise in blood pressure due to unopposed α-adrenergic stimulation. Drugs possessing both α- and β-blocking activity may replace combined drug therapy but the only drug of this type which is available at present is labetalol and this possesses relatively weak α-blocking properties. Hypotensive attacks due to a phaeochromocytoma are treated with a β-blocker alone. Prolonged exposure of the heart to catecholamines may produce a cardiomyopathy when β-blockers may precipitate cardiac failure.

Prior to surgical removal of a phaeochromocytoma, oral propranolol and intravenous or oral phenoxybenzamine are given for about 5 days. This not only helps to prevent a hypertensive attack during manipulation of the tumour, but restores a normal plasma volume in these patients by relieving their generalised vasoconstriction. Such a restoration of the blood volume diminishes the hypotensive reaction which often occurs after removal of the tumour. If hypertension is precipitated by handling the tumour at operation, this can be treated with a short-acting α-blocker such as phentolamine 5 mg intravenously. An alternative pre-operative regime is to give α-methyl tyrosine (2.5–3.5 mg daily) which inhibits catecholamine synthesis. It is also effective in suppressing secretion from inoperable tumours and metastases.

DIABETES MELLITUS

The objective of therapy is to maintain glucose levels as normal as possible throughout the day without producing hypoglycaemia or severely restricting the patient's life. This is achieved by one or more of the following regimes:

(a) diet;
(b) diet plus insulin;
(c) diet plus oral hypoglycaemic drugs.

By maintaining blood glucose levels below 8 mmol/l and limiting glycosuria to less than 20 g daily, polyuria, polydipsia, dehydration, and weight loss can usually be avoided. In a few 'brittle' diabetics even those modest aims may not be achieved without considerable sacrifice and difficulty for the patient and it may be necessary to accept some glycosuria and moderate hyperglycaemia. A pre-requisite of all treatment, but particularly in a life-long, demanding treatment schedule such as is required for diabetes, is patient education. The attainment of a full understanding of the disease and its treatment plus an appropriate psychological and family adjustment should be a major goal of education.

1. Diet in diabetes

The calorie needs of the diabetic depend upon the sex, age, activity and body weight. If the patient is obese, the calorie intake should be restricted so that weight is gradually lost. The aim is to achieve ideal weight and then to maintain it by prescription of adequate calories. The daily basal needs may be roughly calculated by multiplying the ideal weight in pounds by 10 if the patient is inactive, 15 if he has a sedentary occupation or 20 if he is engaged in manual labour or during the growth years. Normal people have considerable latitude in the timing and calorie value of meals, but in diabetics with abnormal insulin secretion or who are dependent upon exogenous insulin, the calorie intake must be distributed so as to match the pattern of insulin activity. A common way to distribute daily calories is to give 2/7th at each of three meals and the remaining 1/7th at bedtime. This may need modification for individual patients, e.g. a snack at mid-afternoon may relieve the hypoglycaemia which often occurs at this time in patients taking intermediate-acting insulins. The carbohydrate content of the diabetic's diet approximates that of normal persons, i.e. 40% of the total calories. The important difference is in the nature of the carbohydrate, since simple sugars should be restricted because they are rapidly absorbed and cause postprandial hyperglycaemia and hypertriglyceridaemia. They are replaced by polysaccharides which are broken down to simple sugars by digestion and absorbed more slowly. Protein calories usually constitute 20% of the diet and protein sources containing unsaturated rather than saturated fat, e.g. skimmed milk, poultry, fish and vegetable protein should be prescribed. The remainder of the calories are obtained from fats which should restrict saturated fats and cholesterol.

To design a diet based on these allowances, it is necessary to use the facts that 1 g of carbohydrate yields 4 calories, 1 g of protein 4 calories and 1 g of fat 9 calories. Thus supposing the patient's ideal body weight is 160 lb (73 kg) and he has a sedentary occupation, the daily calorie intake should be $160 \times 15 = 2400$ calories. The carbohydrate intake will supply $2400 \times 0.40 = 960$ calories which is equivalent to $960 \div 4 = 240$ g. Similarly proteins supply $2400 \times 0.20 = 480$ calories, i.e. $480 \div 4 = 120$ g are needed and fats supply $2400 \times 0.40 = 960$ calories, i.e. $960 \div 9 = 107$ g. These weights may be translated to actual items of diet via the so-called exchange system in which an exchange unit of food comprises fixed weights of carbohydrate, protein, fat or combination thereof. Patients can then choose an appropriate dietary item from a list of exchanges which add up to the allowance for that particular meal.

The traditional dietary carbohydrate restriction with extra calories provided by fats is now thought to be a contributory factor in the formation of atheroma in diabetics. Preliminary studies have shown that both triglyceride and cholesterol levels may be reduced on an isocaloric diet with only 20% of the calories from fat and 60% from carbohydrate without deterioration in the blood-sugar control. The long-term effect of such diets is unknown, but it is possible that in the future more of the diabetic's diet will comprise carbohydrate than hitherto. The type of fat eaten should contain a high percentage of polyunsaturated lipids, the cholesterol intake should be severely limited and the fibre intake increased. A fibre-rich diet reduces the peak plasma glucose after meals and may reduce the dose of insulin required. Not all fibres possess these properties. Wheat bran does not influence glucose or lipid absorption but pectins and guar gum flatten the glucose absorption curve and lower blood cholesterol presumably by influencing lipid absorption. It appears that viscous non-absorbed carbohydrates such as these act by delaying gastric emptying and inhibiting sugar absorption from the intestine by providing a diffusion barrier in the lumen. Pulses such as beans and lentils also have the property of flattening the glucose absorption curve.

The mechanism of action of diet is not completely clear, but one interesting concept results from the observation that in obese diabetics with high circulating insulin levels the tissue insensitivity to insulin effect is associated with a reduction in the number of insulin receptors on the surface of peripheral tissue cells. Restriction of food, exercise and weight loss result in an increase in the number of receptor sites and therefore greater insulin sensitivity and a fall in blood glucose. The regulatory mechanisms controlling insulin receptors are not understood.

2. Insulin

Pharmacology Insulin is synthesised in the microsomal fraction of the β-cells of the Islets of Langerhans in the pancreas as a single long-chain polypeptide. This precursor molecule is proinsulin, which is shortened by proteolysis in the Golgi complex of β-cells to a double-chained molecule consisting of a 21 amino acid A-chain connected to a 30 amino acid B-chain which is insulin. The superfluous connecting C-chain, proinsulin and insulin are all released into the blood but only insulin has biological activity. The C-chain can, however, be used as an index of insulin secretion. Proinsulin may be degraded by the kidney but not other tissues to insulin. Insulin secretion is triggered by many stimuli, including carbohydrate (glucose, fructose, mannose), free fatty acids, amino acids, increased intracellular cyclic AMP (and thus by aminophylline and isoprenaline) and hormones (glucagon, ACTH, thyroxine, growth hormone, secretin, gastrin, pancreozymin, oestrogens and placental lactogen). Inhibitors of insulin secretion include insulin itself, somatostatin, adrenaline and other α-adrenergic agonists, β-adrenergic blockers and diazoxide.

Insulin acts via receptors on the cell membrane at three main points:

(a) activation of insulin-dependent glucose transport processes (in adipose tissue and muscle)
(b) inhibition of adenyl cyclase-dependent processes (lipolysis, proteolysis, glycogenolysis)
(c) intracellular accumulation of potassium and phosphate which may be linked to glucose transport in some tissues.

Secondary effects include increased cellular amino acid uptake, increased DNA and RNA synthesis and increased oxidative phosphorylation.

Pharmacokinetics Insulin is broken down in the gut and by the liver and therefore must be given by injection. The $t_{1/2}$ is 3–5 min. It is metabolised to the inactive A and B peptide chains largely by hepatic insulinase (insulin glutathione transhydrogenase) which breaks the disulphide bridges between A and B chains. Insulin from the pancreas is mainly released into the portal circulation and passes to the liver where up to 60% may be degraded before reaching the systemic circulation (first-pass metabolism). There is no evidence that diabetes ever results from increased hepatic destruction of insulin. Indeed, in severe cirrhosis the liver fails to inactivate insulin with consequent increased plasma insulin levels and sometimes hypoglycaemia. Many types of insulin preparations are available which differ in their pharmacokinetics of absorption and thus duration of action. They are extracted from either ox or pig pancreas and more recently human insulin has become available. The properties of some commonly used varieties are summarised in Table 18.10.

Choice of insulin *Soluble insulin* is a simple solution of insulin and is the only type suitable for intravenous use although it is also rapidly absorbed after subcutaneous injection. Insulin injection B.P. is acid and may cause pain and local reactions at injection sites: it has been largely superseded by neutral soluble insulins. Soluble insulin is essential in the treatment of ketoacidosis and other emergencies but its short action makes it unsuitable for use as a single daily dose in the long-term management of diabetes since relapse into hyperglycaemia occurs before the next injection is due. Increasing the dose to prolong duration of activity is effective but may result in prolonged hypoglycaemia. Soluble insulin is often successful if given two or three times daily when the total requirement exceeds 40 units daily. When the effect wanes before the next dose is due a longer-acting insulin with a later onset, e.g. isophane insulin, can be added.

Protamine zinc insulin (PZI) contains excess protamine which converts any soluble insulin which may be added to it into the long-acting form. It is sometimes given in a single daily injection with soluble insulin, but the long duration of PZI results in accumulation, with the risk of profound hypoglycaemia at night. PZI is not recommended.

Isophane insulin possesses all the advantages but none of the disadvantages of PZI. It does not contain excess protamine and can thus be used with soluble insulin without unpredictable results. It is often given twice daily in combination with soluble insulin so that it reaches its peak of activity at 3–4 p.m. and 3–4 a.m. The small dose of soluble insulin controls hyperglycaemia just after the injection. The chief danger is of a hypoglycaemic reaction in the early hours of the morning.

Biphasic insulins Soluble and isophane insulins form stable mixtures and formulations of highly purified porcine insulin in ratios of 50:50 (Initard) and 30:70 (Mixtard) are available. A mixture of highly purified soluble pig insulin (25%) and highly purified isophane ox insulin (75%) is called Rapitard MC but this often has too little soluble insulin for some patients who become hyperglycaemic on this mixture. Mixtard given twice daily is a useful regime for severe diabetics and avoids the inconvenience and inaccuracy of mixed injections from separate bottles of soluble and isophane insulin especially for patients with poor sight. Human versions of Isotard and Mixtard are available.

Insulin zinc suspensions exist in both amorphous and crystalline forms. The amorphous form is more rapidly absorbed from the injection site than the crystalline form because of its larger surface area. Thus semilente, which is amorphous, has a shorter action than ultralente which is crystalline. Lente is a mixture of amorphous and crystalline insulins in the ratio of 3:7 and has an

Table 18.10 Insulin Preparations

Type of Preparation	*Examples*	*Peak Activity (h)*	*Duration of activity (h)*
1. *Short acting*			
Acid soluble	Insulin injection B.P. (Ox)	2–4	6–18
Neutral soluble	Neusulin (Ox); Actrapid MC (Pig) Human Actrapid (emp); Humulin S (crb)		
2. *Intermediate acting*			
Isophane	Hypurin (Ox); Insulatard (Pig); Human Insulatard (emp); Humulin I (crb)	6–12	12–24
Biphasic	Rapitard MC (Ox); Mixtard (Pig); Human Initard (emp); Human Mixtard (emp)	3–8	16–22
Insulin zinc suspension			
– Semilente (amorphous)	Semitard MC (Pig)	4–8	12–16
– Mixed	Monotard MC (Pig); Human Monotard (emp)	6–14	16–22
3. *Long acting*			
Insulin zinc suspension			
– Lente (Mixed)	Hypurin Lente (Ox); Lentard MC (Ox and Pig)	6–14	18–30
– Ultralente (Crystalline)	Ultratard (Ox)	10–24	24–36
Protamine zinc insulin	Hypurin Protamine Zinc (Ox)	10–20	24–36

action of intermediate duration. Though effective in many cases of average severity its fixed composition limits its usefulness.

Many diabetics have insulin-binding antibodies in their blood and it is now clear that these are a response to impurities in the older insulin preparations. *Highly purified insulins* will in the next few years replace the older forms which are purified by repeated crystallisation and thus contain impurities like proinsulin, somatostatin, glucagon, vasoactive intestinal polypeptide and other pancreatic proteins. Monocomponent (MC) insulins are purified by anion-exchange chromatography and contain very little other than insulin. Nevertheless, bovine and pig insulins differ from human insulin by three and one amino acids respectively so that bovine insulin is intrinsically more antigenic than the others. It is therefore logical to use pig or human insulin rather than the bovine or mixed pig/bovine varieties. The daily requirement of such insulins may be 10–20% lower than for less pure conventional insulins. The main indications for the highly purified insulins are patients with insulin resistance due to antibodies, those with allergic reactions to conventional insulin, patients with local fat dystrophy and pregnant diabetics. Although insulin does not cross the placenta, IgG which may contain anti-insulin antibodies can do so and may contribute to the pancreatic β-cell hyperplasia which occurs in the infants of diabetic mothers so that MC insulins are indicated in pregnancy.

Human insulin is available from two sources:

(a) Pork insulin differs from human insulin by one amino acid. This alanine at position 30 on the B chain may be chemically changed to threonine to form human insulin (enzymically modified porcine; emp). Available preparations are: human Actrapid (neutral soluble insulin), human Monotard (insulin zinc suspension) and human Isophane (Protophane).

(b) Recombinant DNA techniques using *E. coli* allow complete synthesis of human A and B chains which are then combined to give human insulin (chain recombinant bacterial; crb). Preparations available are Humulin S (soluble insulin), Humulin I (Isophane insulin) and Humulin Zn (crystalline insulin zinc suspension).

Pharmacokinetic studies of human insulin generally have shown no differences from porcine insulin and there seems to be no important difference in blood glucose control when compared with that during treatment using animal insulins. Most diabetics who are well stabilised on an established insulin regimen are best advised to continue on that regimen, but diabetics newly diagnosed, or receiving insulin for the first time, or under certain conditions (e.g. pregnancy) should be started on human insulin. Although there are minute contaminants of porcine protein in one form and *E. coli* in the other these are not significant. When very rarely antibodies do form to injected human insulin (it is 50% less antigenic than pig insulin) they do so because:

(a) The injected insulin has become denatured either in the ampoule or the subcutaneous site.

(b) The insulin is injected subcutaneously rather than into the portal circulation as occurs naturally from the pancreas.

Insulin preparations are available in various concentrations and it is important to specify which of these is to be dispensed. Soluble insulin is available as 20, 40, 80 and 320 units/ml and the intermediate- and long-acting preparations as 40 and 80 units/ml. In the USA, Europe and the UK a 100 unit/ml concentration used with a suitably calibrated syringe replaces all these other concentrations and clear some of the confusion which exists because of the multiplicity of preparations available.

Clinical uses Diabetics with absolute insulin deficiency must be treated with exogenous insulin. Such patients are often under 30, below average weight, prone to ketosis and markedly hyperglycaemic even when fasting. Insulin is also required for symptomatic maturity onset diabetics in whom diet or oral hypoglycaemic drugs fail. It is also used in acute diabetic emergencies such as ketoacidosis, during pregnancy, post-operatively and severe intercurrent infections.

Patients are stabilised on an appropriate insulin dosage as judged by urinary and blood glucose measurements whilst they are active. A combination of a short- and medium-acting insulin (e.g. soluble and isophane insulins; Actrapid and Monotard) injected twice daily is commonly used. The short acting insulin of the morning dose controls hyperglycaemia after breakfast while the medium-acting insulin reaches its peak action after lunch. Insulin action after dinner and during the night is similarly provided by the short- and medium-acting components of the evening dose. When starting a diabetic on a two-dose regime it is helpful to divide the daily dose into two thirds to be given before breakfast and one third to be given before the evening meal. If the patient is engaged in hard physical work the morning dose of insulin is reduced slightly to prevent exercise-induced hypoglycaemia. Older patients who often require a smaller insulin dose can often be controlled with a single dose of a long-acting insulin. The dose is determined by monitoring the urinary sugar level at the time when the insulin is expected to be maximally active. If this is done it is relatively safe to increase the dose to improve glycosuria without the risk of hypoglycaemia at other times. The following factors may prevent successful control:

1. failure to adhere to diet;
2. infection, e.g. urinary tract infection, tonsillitis, pneumonia;
3. chronic renal failure provoking hypoglycaemic reactions;
4. violent exercise;
5. insulin resistance;
6. pregnancy;
7. drugs, e.g. oral contraceptives, corticosteroids, thiazide diuretics;
8. endocrine disorder: thyrotoxicosis, Cushing's syndrome, phaeochromocytoma.

Glucose tolerance deteriorates and ketosis may occur after vascular accidents, in particular myocardial infarction.

Dose adjustment may be facilitated by home glucose monitoring of capillary blood using enzyme impregnated test strips or reflectance meters.

Continuous subcutaneous insulin infusion using battery-powered portable pumps which may be programmed to match dietary glucose intake with increased insulin delivery are still experimental. They are indicated when traditional insulin treatment has failed in pregnancy, with painful diabetic neuropathy or in cases where unstable diabetes produces disabling hypoglycaemic attacks.

Special problems requiring insulin treatment

(a) *Intercurrent infections* Even the common cold may upset the equilibrium of good control. Insulin requirements may increase by up to a third and the patient must be instructed accordingly. The dose will need to be promptly reduced when the infection has cleared. Vomiting which precludes taking the normal diet often causes patients to stop insulin for fear of hypoglycaemia. Since vomiting rapidly produces ketosis there is little danger of hypoglycaemia but it may result in ketoacidosis. Patients may be managed with soluble insulin on a sliding scale giving 4 hourly doses as judged by the results of urine and/or blood testing in accordance with the scheme shown in Table 18.11.

(b) *Surgery* Patients having elective surgery should be admitted to hospital 48 hours before operation and if they are on long acting insulins, should be changed to a regime of three times daily soluble insulin. Patients receiving oral hypoglycaemic agents should be changed to insulin control if they have proved difficult to control with oral agents.

During surgery it is easiest to infuse 3 units of soluble insulin hourly together with glucose, 6 g per hour. The infusion rates may be modified to produce a blood glucose level of 6–8 mmol/l. This is continued until oral feeding and intermittent soluble insulin control can be resumed. A similar regime is suitable for emergency operations but frequent measurements of blood glucose levels are required. Patients with very mild diabetes can be managed without insulin but the blood glucose level must be regularly checked in the post-operative period.

Previous regimes which utilised sliding scales (Table 18.11) can be used but control is less satisfactory with this method.

(c) *Ketoacidosis.* The metabolic changes in this condition resemble those of starvation but in fact the opposite is true and there is an increased availability of glucose and ketones which are energy-rich substrates. Increased glycogenolysis and gluconeogenesis in the liver result in hyperglycaemia,

Table 18.11 Four hourly sliding scale of soluble insulin for emergency situations

Urinary Glucose (%)	Ketones	*Blood glucose or Dextrostix reading* (mg %)	(mmol/l)	*Dose of soluble insulin (units)*
2	+++	250+	14+	24
2	+	250+	14+	20
2	0	250+	14+	16
1–2	0	175	9.8	12
½–1	0	175	9.8	8
¼–½	0	125	7.0	4
0	0	<90	<5.5	0

which in turn leads to osmotic diuresis, electrolyte depletion and dehydration. Hypokalaemia is particularly common since in the face of an osmotic diuresis potassium conservation is less efficient than that of sodium. Increased breakdown of muscle releases glucogenic amino acids which are taken up by the liver and converted to glucose. Fat is mobilised from adipose tissue releasing glycerol (converted to glucose by the liver) and free fatty acids which result in excessive production of ketone bodies: acetone, acetoacetate and β-hydroxybutyrate. Increased release of ketogenic amino acids from proteolysis also contributes to formation of ketone bodies. These are neutralised by plasma bicarbonate leading to a fall in bicarbonate, the formation of excess carbon dioxide, acidosis and hyperventilation. Hyperglycaemia gives rise to an osmotic diuresis with loss of electrolytes and water which, coupled with intracellular dehydration, produces shock. There are therefore a number of abnormalities which require correction:

(i) *Insulin deficiency* Traditionally insulin has been given in large amounts in this condition but recently it has been shown that it can be treated effectively by much smaller quantities. The aim is to achieve an effective insulin concentration of 20–200 μunits/ml as quickly as possible. This may be done by giving an intravenous insulin infusion at a rate of 0.1 unit/kg/h with a syringe pump until there is no ketosis (judged by blood pH, standard bicarbonate and blood Ketostix reaction) and until the blood glucose is below 17 mmol/l (300 mg/100 ml). The blood glucose usually falls at a rate of 75–100 mg/100 ml/h. (Fig. 18.4). If ketones have not cleared at this blood glucose level the infusion is slowed to 0.05 units/kg/h and 4 g of glucose/unit of insulin added to prevent hypoglycaemia, thus allowing continuation of the insulin until metabolic normality is restored. Intramuscular insulin may be given instead, which requires no special apparatus using a 20 unit loading dose followed by 5 units hourly. Subcutaneous injections are absorbed slowly, particularly in shocked patients, and cannot be used in this situation.

(ii) *Fluids* to reverse dehydration are important and 0.9% saline (0.45% saline if plasma sodium is over 155 mmol/l) is used. An approximate guide is 1.5–2 l over the first 2 h, 2 l over the next 4 h and 2 l over the next 6 h. When blood glucose falls to below 17 mmol/l (300 mg/100 ml), 5% glucose is given in place of saline. Potassium must be replaced, and if the urinary output is satisfactory and the plasma potassium low, 20–40 mmol/h can be given, the rate of replacement being judged by frequent measurements of plasma potassium.

(iii) *Acidosis* is often treated with bicarbonate. Recently this procedure has been reconsidered. The acidosis is due to acetoacetate and β-hydroxybutyrate which, when insulin is given, can be metabolised by the Krebs cycle to regenerate bicarbonate, so that there is less reason to give exogenous bicarbonate in ketoacidosis than in metabolic acidosis from other causes. Raising blood pH with bicarbonate may also cause decrease in CSF pH since the blood–brain barrier is more permeable to carbon dioxide than to bicarbonate. If bicarbonate administration raises blood pH the stimulus to hyperventilation decreases and the blood pCO_2 rises, allowing carbon dioxide to cross into the brain and worsening the state of consciousness. Acidosis, by shifting the haemoglobin dissociation curve to the right, may be beneficial since this enhances oxygen release in the tissues. Presently accepted indi-

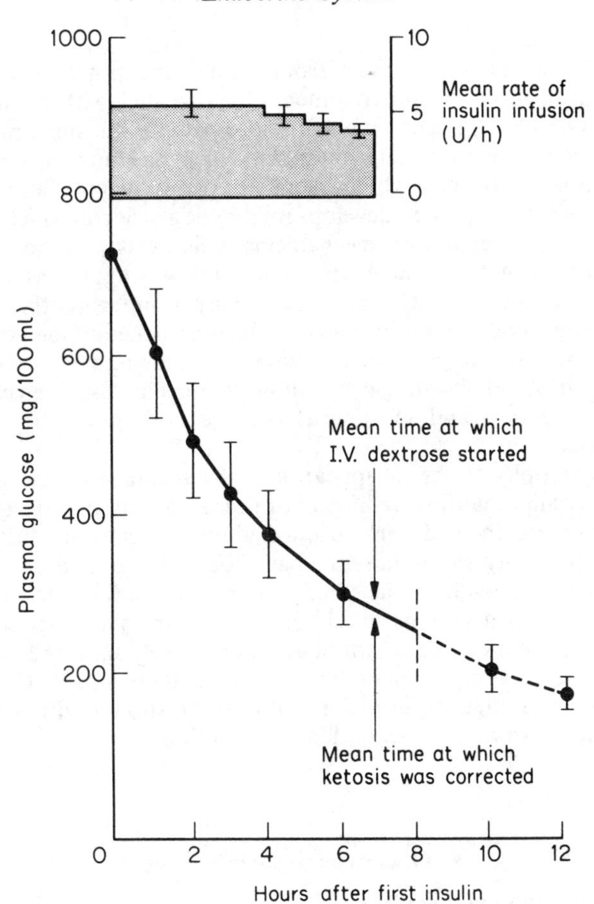

Fig. 18.4 Mean plasma glucose in 13 ketoacidotic patients treated with low dose continuous insulin infusion (From P. F. Semple *et al.*, *Brit. Med. J.*, **2** 694 (1974). Reproduced by permission of the Editor.)

cations for bicarbonate are stricter than formerly—an arterial pH below 7.0 or plasma bicarbonate below 5 mmol/l—since at these levels myocardial contractility is decreased, arrhythmias occur and respiration is depressed. Bicarbonate is given at a dosage of approximately 2 mmol/kg.

(iv) *Other measures* include aspiration of the stomach (gastric stasis with inhalation of vomit can be fatal) and treatment of the cause of coma. Thus antibiotics are given if infection is the precipitating cause.

(d) *Hyperosmolar non-ketotic coma* Less insulin is required in this situation since the blood pH is normal and insulin sensitivity is retained. Fluid loss is repleted using 0.45 % saline and large amounts of intravenous potassium are often required. There is a case for prophylactic anticoagulants, since the incidence of thrombotic episodes is high.

Adverse reactions

1. Hypoglycaemia is the most troublesome and potentially dangerous complication of insulin treatment. It is treated with an intravenous injection of 50% glucose in unconscious patients but sugar may be given orally in those with milder symptoms. Glucagon (1 mg i.m.) may be used.
2. Insulin-induced post-hypoglycaemic hyperglycaemia (Somogyi effect) occurs when the patient develops mild hypoglycaemia which induces an overshoot of regulatory mechanisms which elevate blood sugar (adrenaline, growth hormone, corticosteroids, glucagon). Ketonuria may result and the unsuspecting physician may misinterpret the situation as requiring increased insulin, thus producing further hypoglycaemia. The syndrome may be prevented by slowly decreasing insulin dosage.
3. Local or systemic allergic reactions to insulin. Skin sensitivity with itching, redness and swelling at the injection site is the commonest reaction.
4. Lipodystrophy is the disappearance of subcutaneous fat or the formation of lipomatous swellings at or near injection sites. Atrophy is now rare: perhaps the wider use of purified insulins prevents this condition which probably has an immune basis. Fatty tumours occur if repeated injections are made at the same site and they still occur with purified insulins. Thus injections should be made in areas not exposed socially.
5. Insulin resistance due to antibodies is relatively unusual. It is defined arbitrarily as a requirement of more than 200 units daily. Changing the patient to a highly purified insulin preparation is often successful, although a small dose should be used initially.

3. Oral hypoglycaemic drugs

These fall into two major groups:

(a) sulphonylureas;
(b) biguanides.

Sulphonylureas

The hypoglycaemic effect of these drugs depends upon the presence of functioning β-cells and *in vitro* they stimulate insulin release from isolated islets of Langerhans. Sulphonylureas, like glucose, initiate action potential discharge in islet cells which results in insulin release. Acute administration either orally or intravenously results in a fall in blood sugar accompanied by a rise in plasma insulin. Thus, even in normal subjects, these drugs may produce hypoglycaemia. While the acute effects are presumably due to insulin release, it is less certain that the effects of chronic administration are similarly mediated, for this results in plasma insulin levels below those observed before treatment, although glucose tolerance remains unchanged. One explanation might be an alteration in sensitivity of the β-cells so that nearly normal insulin levels are achieved following a lesser hyperglycaemic stimulus. The more appropriate insulin secretion restores glucose tolerance towards normal. Alternatively sulphonylureas may produce extrapancreatic changes, particularly in the liver, which result in reduced glucose production and increased glucose uptake following a glucose load. Such changes may result from an increase in membrane insulin receptors. Sulphonylurea therapy could therefore improve the glucose tolerance test without correcting the impaired glucose utilisation of the peripheral tissues.

The drugs differ in their effect on water excretion. Chlorpropamide has been employed as an antidiuretic agent in the treatment of patients with diabetes insipidus who have some residual hormone. It may cause dilutional hyponatraemia in some diabetics. It probably acts both by stimulating antidiuretic hormone release and by potentiating its action on the kidney. Tolbutamide has similar but less marked activity, whereas acetohexamide and glibenclamide appear to be diuretic.

Pharmacokinetics These drugs are all well absorbed orally and the chief differences between them lie in their relative potency and metabolism (Table 18.12). Tolbutamide is the most rapidly metabolised of the group and requires 8 or 6 hourly administration, whilst chlorpropamide which is cleared from the body mainly by renal excretion, is given only once daily. Because of its long half-life the steady-state blood levels are reached after 7 days, and this is clinically important since the dose should not be increased at more frequent intervals. Renal failure prolongs the action of chlorpropamide and many physicians prefer to use tolbutamide in the elderly, for this has no danger of accumulation with reduced renal function. Acetohexamide undergoes hepatic metabolism to 1-hydroxyhexamide, which is $2\frac{1}{2}$ times as potent a hypoglycaemic agent as acetohexamide. Since hydroxyhexamide is excreted by the kidney, renal failure prolongs the action of this compound. Glibenclamide is extremely potent and has a moderately long duration of activity so that it should be used with care. Gliquidone shows a rapid α-phase after which the blood levels fall to a low and ineffective level thereby terminating its action. It thus has a relatively short action compared to the other oral hypoglycaemics and does not accumulate. It is almost completely metabolised and 95% of the metabolites are eliminated in the bile. It can be used in renal failure without dosage modification.

A recent study measuring serum tolbutamide and chlorpropamide concentrations in diabetics attending an outpatient clinic showed wide variation in blood levels, some of which is doubtless related to poor compliance. The conclusion of this work was, however, that the levels observed were far from optimal and that monitoring of blood levels in this situation might possibly improve efficacy.

Clinical uses These drugs are used for maturity onset diabetics who have not responded to diet alone and who show no tendency to ketosis. The place of these drugs in other types of patient is limited. They are sometimes useful in controlling difficult ('brittle') insulin-dependent diabetics, in whom they tend to smooth out the characteristic fluctuations in blood sugar. In a few patients a short period of amelioration follows stabilisation on insulin, in which case insulin may be withdrawn and a sulphonylurea substituted. Such patients nearly always relapse and finally require insulin so that oral therapy can only be used when the patient is closely supervised by experienced physicians. Whenever oral hypoglycaemic agents are used it is necessary to stress to a

Table 18.12 Pharmacokinetic properties of some sulphonylureas

Drug	*Metabolism and elimination*	$t_{1/2}$ (*h*)	*Daily dose range*	*Duration of action* (*h*)
Tolbutamide (Rastinon)	Oxidised in liver, excreted in urine	4–5	0.5–3.0 g in divided doses	6–12
Chlorpropamide (Diabinese)	Minimal metabolism, primarily excreted unchanged in urine	36	0.1–0.5 g in single daily dose	60
Acetohexamide (Dimelor)	60% reduced in liver to active hydroxyhexamide which is actively secreted by renal tubules	6–8	0.25–2.5 g as one or two daily doses	12–24
Glibenclamide (Daonil, Euglucon)	95% metabolism to inactive hydroxylated metabolites excreted in urine and bile	5–8	2.5–20 mg as one or two daily doses	12
Glibornuride (Glutril)	95% metabolism to numerous inactive metabolites	5–12	12.5–75 mg as one or two daily doses	16
Glipizide (Glibenese)	85% metabolism to several inactive hydroxylated metabolites	2.5–4	2.5–30 mg, doses below 10 mg given as single daily dose	6–10
Gliquidone (Glurenorm)	95% metabolism. Metabolites undergo 95% biliary excretion. 5% renal excretion.	1.5 (α-phase)	45–180 mg daily in divided doses before meals.	2–4 (α-phase determines duration of action).

patient that such drugs are prescribed in addition to dietary treatment and not in its place.

Adverse effects The chief danger of these drugs is hypoglycaemia, which may result in coma and irreversible neurological damage. Chlorpropamide, the longest-acting agent, is responsible for over half the reported cases.

Tolbutamide is associated with adverse reactions in about 3% of patients, chiefly allergic skin reactions, gastrointestinal upsets, transient (cholestatic) jaundice, haemopoietic changes and hypothyroidism. The other drugs have similar effects. Chlorpropamide produces adverse reactions with a frequency of about 6%. Because of its antidiuretic effects, dilutional hyponatraemia and water intoxication are well-recognised complications of chlorpropamide; thus diabetics with heart failure or renal disease should not receive this drug.

Drug interactions Oral hypoglycaemic drugs are, as a group, highly prone to produce dangerous adverse effects due to interaction with other drugs.

Monoamine oxidase inhibitors, although they do not alter the $t_{1/2}$ of sulphonylureas, potentiate their activity by an unknown mechanism. Drugs which are highly protein bound, e.g. clofibrate, phenylbutazone, displace sulphonylureas from protein binding (see Chapter 1). Specific interactions occur as follows:

(a) *Tolbutamide*

(i) Phenylbutazone, sulphaphenazole and bishydroxycoumarin inhibit its oxidation and so prolong its action.

(ii) Alcohol enhances the hypoglycaemic effect and may produce a mild disulfiram type of reaction (see p. 855). Chronic alcoholism diminishes the hypoglycaemic effect, probably due to more rapid metabolism of the drug.

(b) *Chlorpropamide*

(i) Alcohol produces facial flushing and light-headedness sometimes associated with dyspnoea in up to a third of patients. It has been suggested that this tendency is inherited as an autosomal dominant trait, but this is disputed as is the assertion that diabetic retinopathy is commoner and often severe in diabetics who do not flush with alcohol and chlorpropamide.

(ii) Aspirin interferes with urinary chlorpropamide excretion and so increases the chlorpropamide plasma level. At high aspirin intake such as is used in rheumatic fever or rheumatoid arthritis this effect, coupled with the direct stimulation of muscle glucose uptake produced by aspirin, can produce clinically significant hypoglycaemia.

A number of drugs can antagonise the hypoglycaemic effects of sulphonylureas by virtue of their intrinsic impairment of glucose tolerance. Such drugs include corticosteroids, thiazide diuretics, frusemide, oral contraceptives, large doses of thyroxin and nicotinic acid.

Biguanides: Metformin

The mechanism whereby these drugs produce hypoglycaemia remains uncertain. They have no effect in normal individuals and, unlike sulphonylureas, do not depend upon insulin for their actions since they are effective in pancreatectomised animals. The two main hypotheses about their action are:

(a) Reduced glucose absorption from the gut occurs, which explains why the oral but not the intravenous glucose tolerance test is improved. Absorption of vitamin B_{12} is also reduced.
(b) Facilitation of glucose entry into tissues by a non-insulin responsive mechanism, thus increasing glucose uptake by peripheral tissues. There is some evidence to suggest that biguanides suppress oxidative glucose metabolism and enhance anaerobic glycolysis, producing increased plasma lactate and pyruvate levels.

Administration of biguanides is associated with anorexia and weight loss, which may also contribute to their beneficial effects on diabetics. Phenformin has also been shown to increase fibrinolytic activity and to decrease platelet adhesiveness.

Pharmacokinetics Metformin (Glucophage) has a duration of action of 18–12 h and is excreted, virtually unchanged, in the urine. The usual dose is 0.5–3 g given as 1–3 divided doses.

Clinical uses Metformin is used in maturity-onset diabetics without a tendency to ketosis in whom dietary carbohydrate restriction has not controlled the hyperglycaemia or glycosuria. Its main use is in the overweight patient because its anorectic effect may aid weight reduction. Treatment of such patients with sulphonylureas may lead to weight gain as a result of stimulation of insulin release. Metformin may also exert an additive effect in patients uncontrolled by sulphonylureas alone. It may also help in the stabilisation of blood-sugar fluctuations in 'brittle' insulin-dependent diabetics.

Adverse effects Metformin affects the gastrointestinal tract causing nausea, a metallic taste in the mouth, anorexia, vomiting and intermittent diarrhoea which occur upon initial drug administration. About 3% of patients cannot tolerate this drug even in small doses because of these effects.

An uncommon, but severe, toxic effect is the occurrence of lactic acidosis which has a mortality in excess of 60%. This presents with the features of a metabolic acidosis (drowsiness or coma, abdominal pain, vomiting and hyperventilation) often with shock. Treatment is by reversal of hypoxia and circulatory collapse, infusion of sodium bicarbonate and peritoneal dialysis or haemodialysis to alleviate sodium overloading and to remove the drug. Phenformin (an earlier biguanide) was more frequently associated with this problem than metformin. The occurrence of lactic acidosis cannot be predicted and has occurred as long as 4 years after beginning treatment. Patients at special risk are alcoholics and those with renal, hepatic or cardiac failure, and biguanides should be avoided for these groups. These drugs should always be withdrawn when patients suffer serious intercurrent illness, especially myocardial infarction and conditions associated with hypotension or reduced renal function.

Drug interactions are unusual with biguanides. Other hypoglycaemic agents like salicylates and sulphonylureas potentiate their action. Alcohol may precipitate lactic acidosis.

Efficacy of oral antidiabetic agents

About 60% of symptomatic maturity-onset diabetics achieve satisfactory control with these agents, the remainder cannot be controlled with drugs (primary failure). Subsequent failure, after initially adequate control (secondary failure) may be as high as one quarter of the patients per year. Probably the greatest continuous success rate is in the asymptomatic maturity-onset group of patients who are often as well controlled by diet as drugs. There is no evidence that treatment of this group with oral agents either restores to normal or prevents the deterioration of glucose tolerance.

The results of the University Groups Diabetes Program (UGDP) in the USA have contributed to the controversy surrounding the use of these drugs. The objectives of this study were to evaluate the efficacy of treatment in the prevention of vascular complications by a long-term multicentre trial. Maturity-onset non-insulin dependent diabetics were treated with either:

(a) diet and placebo;
(b) diet and tolbutamide 1.5 g daily;
(c) diet and phenformin 100 mg daily;
(d) diet and a standard dose of insulin;
(e) diet and a variable dose of insulin.

After 8½ years the study concluded that the combination of diet and tolbutamide or diet and phenformin were no more effective than diet and placebo in prolonging life. The finding of excess cardiovascular mortality in the groups treated with hypoglycaemic drugs prompted the FDA to propose restricted use for these drugs. Other prospective studies concerning the cardiovascular effects of these drugs have not confirmed the UGDP findings and after consideration the British Diabetic Association has not felt the need to alter its opinion as to the uses of these drugs.

The efficacy of treatment in diabetes mellitus

Diabetes is associated with progressive vascular disease leading to incapacity and decreased longevity. With the discovery of insulin it was hoped that both short- and long-term complications of diabetes would be prevented. This hope does not at present appear to have been realised. There is no convincing evidence, experimental or clinical, that insulin or hypoglycaemic drug therapy, as currently applied, alters the course of diabetic microangiopathy. The UGDP data, referred to above, failed to demonstrate prolongation of life in treated as compared to placebo groups of patients. This does not mean that there are no benefits of treatment for, apart from preventing ketoacidosis, the control of polyuria, polydipsia and weight loss is certainly desirable. Control of hyperglycaemia may benefit patients with vulvovaginitis, balanitis, frequent infections and some of the neuropathies of diabetes. It is thus prudent to strive for the best possible control of blood glucose, but this should not be at the risk of frequent hypoglycaemia, which is the commonest complication of treatment and which may be lethal.

THYROID

The thyroid secretes thyroxine (T4) and tri-iodothyronine (T3) and calcitonin. The release of T3 and T4 is controlled by the pituitary hormone thyrotrophin (thyroid-stimulating hormone: TSH). Secretion of TSH by the anterior pituitary is stimulated by the hypothalamic peptide thyrotrophin-releasing hormone (TRH).

TSH increases the vascularity, cellularity and size of the thyroid and accelerates synthesis and release of the thyroid hormones. Circulating T3 and T4 produce negative-feedback inhibition of TSH production acting at pituitary and hypothalamic levels.

Iodine The thyroid gland selectively concentrates iodine from plasma iodide. Dietary iodide normally amounts to 100–200 μg per day and is absorbed from the stomach and small intestine by an active process. Following uptake into the thyroid, iodide is oxidised to iodine—and from this a series of iodinated tyrosine compounds are made—including T3 and T4. Amongst its actions TSH stimulates concentration of iodine in the thyroid and iodisation of tyrosine residues. Iodine is used therapeutically to treat those cases of simple non-toxic goitre due to iodine deficiency. In this condition administration of oral potassium iodide 3 mg daily will prevent further enlargement of the gland but does not usually cause a reduction in size. Iodised salt is used to prevent this type of goitre particularly in areas where the diet is iodine deficient.

For a patient with thyrotoxicosis about to undergo subtotal thyroidectomy, pre-operative treatment with iodide (60 mg potassium iodide orally per day in divided doses) in combination with carbimazole or propylthiouracil reduces the vascularity of the gland and prevents thyroid crisis by reducing the release of T3 and T4 by the gland. This action of iodine in inhibiting thyroid hormone release is maintained for only 1–2 weeks, probably because the iodide-concentrating mechanism is also impaired. Similarly in the treatment of a thyroid crisis potassium iodide is given in addition to β-blockers, carbimazole and other therapy. Excessive infusion of iodine or iodide for long periods can in itself produce a goitre.

Thyroxine and Tri-iodothyronine

Actions and pharmacokinetics The normal range of serum T4 concentration is 50–100 μg/l and this comprises about 80% of the circulating thyroid hormone activity since the usual range of serum T3 is 1–1.6 μg/1.99.95% of T4 is bound to the thyroid-binding globulin (TBG) whilst only 99.5% of T3 is bound. Thus the concentration of free T4 is only 4–5 times that of free T3. However, the potency of T3 is greater, so that the physiological activity of the two hormones present in the circulation is similar. Drugs such as phenytoin, salicylates and phenylbutazone may reduce TBG binding capacity, thereby interfering with the results of diagnostic tests based upon this function.

The main functions of these hormones are:

1. stimulation of metabolism resulting in a raised basal metabolic rate, increased protein synthesis;
2. promotion of normal growth and maturation, particularly of the CNS and skeleton;
3. possibly sensitisation to the effects of catecholamines. This hypothesis neatly explains many of the features of thyrotoxicosis, e.g. tachycardia, hyperactive reflexes, but careful evaluation of the evidence has recently suggested that the case is unproven.

Thyroid hormones are absorbed from the gut. The effects of T4 are not usually detectable before 24 h and maximal activity is attained at about 7–10 days after commencement of treatment. T3 produces effects within 6 h and peak activity is reached within 24 h. It is therefore preferred for the urgent treatment of myxoedema coma. The $t_{1/2}$ of T4 is 6–7 days and that for T3 is 2 days or less. It therefore makes little sense to administer thyroid hormone more frequently than once a day.

The liver conjugates thyroid hormones and they undergo an enterohepatic circulation. Some (20%) T4 is converted to the more active T3 in the tissues.

Clinical uses L-thyroxine is used in the treatment of uncomplicated hypothyroidism. The starting dose for an adult is 0.05 mg daily, increasing the dose by 0.05 mg every 1–4 weeks until the patient has responded optimally clinically and the TSH level has fallen to the normal range. The optimal maintenance dose is usually 0.1–0.2 mg 1-thyroxine daily. Excessive dosage or too rapid an increase in dose may precipitate cardiac complications, particularly in patients with overt ischaemic heart disease. If angina pectoris limits the dose of thyroxine, the addition of a β-blocker such as propranolol will allow further increments in thyroxine dosage.

Cretinism is treated similarly but thyroxine must be given as early as possible, preferably within the first three weeks of life and increased to the highest tolerated dose.

In myxoedema coma (in addition to other therapy such as intramuscular hydrocortisone) the more rapid action of tri-iodothyronine (Liothyronine B.P.) is useful since the action of thyroxine is too slow. It is given in doses of up to 100 μg 12-hourly intramuscularly and at the same time maintenance therapy is commenced with thyroxine 0.05 mg given orally (or if necessary by a gastric tube). Liothyronine is also used diagnostically to detect borderline hyperthyroidism, since in normal subjects a dose of 120 μg daily for one week will suppress thyroid radioiodine uptake. This has no effect in hyperthyroidism.

Apart from primary thyroid hypofunction, hypothyroidism may result from hypopituitarism. This is also treated with oral thyroxine in the usual doses. Corticosteroid replacement must be started first, otherwise acute adrenal insufficiency will be precipitated.

Some simple non-toxic goitres due to iodine deficiency which have not responded satisfactorily to iodine, may reduce in size with 1-thyroxine treatment 0.1–0.25 mg/day. Goitres due to a genetic lack of thyroid enzymes may also respond to thyroxine.

Adverse effects of the thyroid hormones relate to their physiological functions. Rapid increases in thyroxin dose in hypothyroidism can lead to sudden death. This may be due to the precipitation of ventricular fibrillation. Angina, myocardial infarction, tachycardia and congestive cardiac failure can be precipitated. A common sign of excessive dosage is the production of diarrhoea. Tremor, restlessness, heat intolerance and other features of hyperthyroidism are dose dependent toxic effects of these hormones.

Thyrotrophin-releasing hormone (TRH)—Protirelin

TRH is a simple tripeptide (glu-his-pro) which is produced in the hypothalamus and is responsible for TSH release. It is useful in diagnosis and may be given intravenously or orally: the presence of ring structures hinders access of digestive enzymes to the amide bonds linking the amino acids. When it is given to normal people by i.v. injection there is a dose-related release of TSH. In primary hypothyroidism an exaggerated and prolonged TSH release occurs without change in T4 or T3 concentrations. In secondary cases there is a greatly attenuated TSH response. It may also be used to indicate pituitary TSH reserve in pituitary disease, although in acromegaly the response is often impaired, possibly due to the autonomous nodular goitre sometimes associated with acromegaly.

Thyroid-stimulating hormone (TSH)

This is the most important regulator of thyroid function which binds to thyroid follicular cells and activates adenyl cyclase resulting in increased cyclic 3′, 5′-AMP. This then stimulates iodine trapping, iodothyronine synthesis and release of thyroid hormones. TSH is secreted by basophil cells in the adenohypophysis. It comprises two conjoined polypeptide chains; the α-chain is identical to the α-chain of LH and FSH, and the β-chain confers biological specificity. Like TRH it may be used to distinguish primary and secondary hypothyroidism: and injection of 10 I.U. bovine TSH will cause a rise in radioiodine or technetium (^{99}Tc) uptake by the thyroid in patients with hypopituitarism, but no rise occurs in those with primary thyroid failure. The test is useful in patients on treatment with thyroid hormone who will have a negligible uptake regardless of whether they are hypothyroid due to suppression of endogenous TSH secretion by exogenous T4.

Antithyroid Drugs

The most important of these are carbimazole, propylthiouracil and potassium perchlorate.

Graves' disease is associated with an immunoglobulin which competes with TSH for binding to its receptor and which when bound can stimulate adenyl cyclase to release thyroid hormones. This substance may be similar to or identical with the so-called long-acting thyroid stimulator (LATS). This is an immunoglobulin and its production may cease as the autoimmune process spontaneously regresses. Preliminary evidence suggests that in thyrotoxic patients treated with antithyroid drugs disappearance of LATS indicates that remission will persist when drugs are discontinued.

Carbimazole (Neomercazole)

This drug is hydrolysed to methimazole in plasma and it is not possible to demonstrate the presence of carbimazole in the thyroid, although methimazole is present. Thus carbimazole acts by way of its active metabolite methimazole which acts as a substrate for peroxidase and is itself iodinated and degraded within the thyroid thus diverting oxidised iodine away from thyroglobulin thereby decreasing thyroid hormone biosynthesis. It also prevents T3 and T4 synthesis by interfering with tyrosine iodination and the coupling of iodotyrosines, but does not affect the mechanism of secretion. Thus hormone release diminishes after a latent period during which time the thyroid becomes depleted of hormone. There is some evidence that these drugs may also suppress the immune process causing thyrotoxicosis.

Pharmacokinetics Carbimazole is rapidly absorbed after oral administration and hydrolysed to its active metabolite methimazole which is rapidly concentrated in the thyroid within minutes of administration. Methimazole has an apparent volume of distribution equivalent to body water and the half-life varies according to thyroid status, being 9.3, 6.9 and 13.6 h in euthyroid, hyperthyroid and hypothyroid subjects respectively. It is metabolised in the liver and thyroid.

Clinical uses Carbimazole is used in the treatment of hyperthyroidism, particularly in children under 18 years and in pregnant women. It is usually recommended that initially 10 mg is given 8 hourly; however, a single daily dose of drug has been shown to be equally effective and probably improves compliance. The duration of action of antithyroid drugs, as might be surmised from their mechanism of action, does not correlate well with plasma levels, but rather with the size of dose administered and the intrathyroid drug concentration. A response is clinically discernible after about one month and the patient may be euthyroid after 2–4 months. The dose of carbimazole is then reduced to a maintenance regime of 10–20 mg daily. Treatment is maintained for 1–2 years and the drug is then gradually withdrawn. Recently evidence has been presented that shorter courses of therapy to induce euthyroidism followed by drug withdrawal will produce equally good results. If relapse occurs during drug withdrawal, the dose is again raised until clinical improvement is restored. If dosage adjustment proves difficult, smoother control may be obtained by giving thyroxine 0.1–0.2 mg/day together with carbimazole 20–30 mg/day.

In therapeutic use carbimazole is a relatively non-toxic drug. Nausea, some loss of hair and rashes occasionally develop. Drug fever, leucopenia and arthralgia are very rare.

Propylthiouracil has similar actions, uses and toxic effects to carbimazole. As with the latter, dangerous leucopenia may develop but is very rare.

The initial total daily dose is 300 mg and the maintenance dose is 50–100 mg. The scheme of attaining a euthyroid state with a large dose of drug and then reducing the dose to maintain this is carried out as with carbimazole.

Propylthiouracil is absorbed rapidly from the intestine, but like carbimazole, single doses produce only transient (3–6 h) inhibition of thyroid function. The plasma $t_{1/2}$ is 2 h. The antithyroid drugs cross the placenta and are found in milk so that the child of an affected mother may be born with a goitre which may persist during suckling. Propylthiouracil is less likely than carbimazole to produce this problem since it is more highly protein bound and is ionised at pH 7.4. This reduces its passage across the placenta or into milk.

Potassium perchlorate is an alternative drug used in the treatment of hyperthyroidism. It prevents the trapping and concentration of iodine in the thyroid. 800 mg is given daily for 2–3 months, then this is reduced to 100–200 mg daily for 2–3 years.

The drug rarely produces aplastic anaemia and therefore is only used in patients who have not been able to tolerate carbimazole and propylthiouracil.

The place of β-adrenergic blockers in treatment of thyrotoxicosis

β-blockers reduce the resting tachycardia, relieve the subjective feelings of anxiety and sweating, reduce tremor and prolong the hyperactive reflexes of thyrotoxic patients. They also have an action in blocking the conversion of T4 and T3 in the tissues. This effect seems to be a general property of β-blockade and is irrespective of β-specificity or intrinsic sympathomimetic activity. They may therefore be used for control of symptoms during therapy with antithyroid drugs, or in the control of thyroid crisis. They are also used as a rapid preparation for surgery when the patient may be operated upon after only 10–14 days of high-dose propranolol therapy. The gland is less friable, firmer and less likely to tear than after conventional preparation with antithyroid drugs. It must be recognised that patients treated with β-blockers are not euthyroid and therefore inadequate treatment or omission of a dose may provoke a thyroid crisis in the post-operative period. β-blockers do not affect uptake of radioactive iodine as do conventional antithyroid drugs and they have also been used as adjunctive therapy to radio-iodine. Accurate assessment of the effects of the radioactive therapy may be made via thyroid function tests without the confounding effects of concurrent antithyroid drug therapy.

Propranolol has been suggested as an alternative drug for the management of hyperthyroidism during pregnancy. This may not be ideal, however, since in one double-blind trial the respiration of offspring of women receiving propranolol was more depressed at birth than those on placebo. Another study has reported intra-uterine growth retardation following propranolol therapy. Thus propranolol cannot be regarded as the primary agent for long-term treatment of hyperthyroidism in pregnancy.

Thyroid crisis is a severe, and usually sudden, exacerbation of hyperthyroidism with hyperpyrexia, tachycardia, vomiting, dehydration, hyperkinesis and shock which may arise spontaneously, post-operatively following radio-iodine therapy or be associated with infection. The mortality is around 20% and urgent treatment is required with:

(a) β-blockers (i.v. propranolol 1–2 mg is usually used and repeated according to the response in the heart rate) to control tachycardia and tremor;
(b) fluids and cooling to combat dehydration and hyperthermia;

(c) antithyroid drugs to reduce hormone synthesis followed by iodides to slow secretion (200 mg propylthiouracil every 4 h by nasogastric tube);
(d) diuretics, digoxin, oxygen and steroids for shock and cardiac failure;
(e) in more severe cases 1 g of potassium iodide is given i.v. every 8 h for three doses.

Radioactive iodine is an effective oral treatment for thyrotoxicosis and causes no discomfort to the patient. The chief problem is the calculation of the dose required to render the patient euthyroid: too large a dose will produce hypothyroidism. This complication increases with the length of follow-up so that about 7% of patients require thyroxine after 5 years with an additional 1% of patients becoming hypothyroid each year thereafter. The usually employed isotope is ^{131}I with a $t_{1/2}$ of 8 days; there is no increased incidence of leukaemia, thyroid or other malignancy after its use, but it is advisable to avoid its use in children or young women to avoid any possible risk of genetic damage. ^{125}I with a longer $t_{1/2}$ (60 days) and a lower energy radiation has also been employed. Due to the shorter range of its radiation the radiobiological effects are largely concentrated at the apex of the follicle cell adjacent to the colloid, so that damage to the cell nucleus is avoided. This may reduce the risk of late hypothyroidism.

Some authorities use higher doses of radio-iodine which renders the patient euthyroid in 2–4 weeks. T4 replacement is started after 4–6 weeks and continued for life.

Eye signs of thyrotoxicosis usually resolve with treatment of the thyroid disorder. 5% guanethidine eye drops may improve the appearance of the eyes and orbital oedema can be reduced by using diuretics. Failure of visual acuity necessitates a 48 h trial of prednisolone 60 mg daily. If this fails then treatment is changed to dexamethasone 20 mg/day. Surgical decompression is required if steroid treatment is not successful.

Treatment of hyperthyroidism

The three alternative methods used in the management of hyperthyroidism are antithyroid drugs, radioactive iodine and partial thyroidectomy. The principal indications for these different treatments are:

Antithyroid drugs:	treatment of choice in	children under 18 years
		pregnant women (controlling the dose with measurements of T3 and T4 levels)
		small toxic goitre
	may also be used in	adults
		recurrence after drugs, ^{131}I or operation
		co-existing disease

Partial thyroidectomy:	treatment of choice in	adults 18–45 years large goitre severe disease possibility of malignancy recurrence after drug treatment
Radio iodine:	treatment of choice in	adults over 45 years in recurrence after operation or radio iodine coexisting illness (such as rheumatic heart disease)
	contraindicated in	pregnancy children and young adults

PARATHYROID HORMONE (PARATHORMONE), VITAMIN D AND CALCIUM METABOLISM

Plasma calcium is normally maintained within a narrow range by parathyroid hormone (PTH), vitamin D and calcitonin. PTH is a peptide containing 84 amino acids: the structure of bovine and porcine hormones is known and that of man has been nearly completely elucidated. Like other secreted polypeptide hormones it is synthesised as a larger polypeptide which is reduced in size prior to release into the blood. These precursors do not appear in the circulation and there is probably little intact hormone in the peripheral blood, the hormone being rapidly metabolised by liver and kidney so that a heterogeneous collection of inactive PTH fragments are found in plasma. Plasma calcium concentration is the major factor controlling PTH secretion, a reduction stimulating PTH release. Acute hypomagnesaemia elevates PTH levels but prolonged magnesium depletion impairs secretion. This may result from a requirement for magnesium ion by parathyroid adenylate cyclase, since PTH release by hypocalcaemia is mediated by cyclic AMP. PTH raises blood calcium and lowers blood phosphate levels.

PTH acts on kidney and bone. Both effects are mediated by stimulation of tissue adenyl cyclase with elevation of cyclic AMP. PTH causes phosphaturia and increased renal tubular reabsorption of calcium, which in association with the mobilisation of calcium from bone results in the elevation of the plasma calcium level. The actions on bone include stimulation of osteoclastic activity, formation of new osteoclasts from osteoprogenitor cells and the transient depression of osteoblastic activity. PTH also plays a role in the regulation of vitamin D metabolism. The increased gut absorption of calcium previously attributed to PTH may in fact be an indirect effect of the increased production of 1, 25-dihydroxycholecalciferol.

Although PTH (in parathyroid extract) is used in the investigation and short-term treatment of hypoparathyroidism, it has no place in long-term management of the condition. In the diagnosis of pseudohypoparathyroidism PTH is administered as a single test dose (200 units intravenously). In this condition there is end organ resistance to the hormone, so the plasma calcium does not rise and there is no increase in the urinary phosphate or cyclic AMP concentrations.

Vitamin D (Calciferol)

The metabolic pathway of vitamin D is diagrammatically shown in Fig. 18.5. Vitamin D_3 is synthesised in the skin by the action of ultraviolet light on 7-dehydrocholesterol and absorbed from food in the upper gut. It is fat soluble and therefore bile is necessary for absorption. Like other fat-soluble vitamins its absorption is reduced by liquid paraffin which dissolves it and sequesters it in the gut lumen.

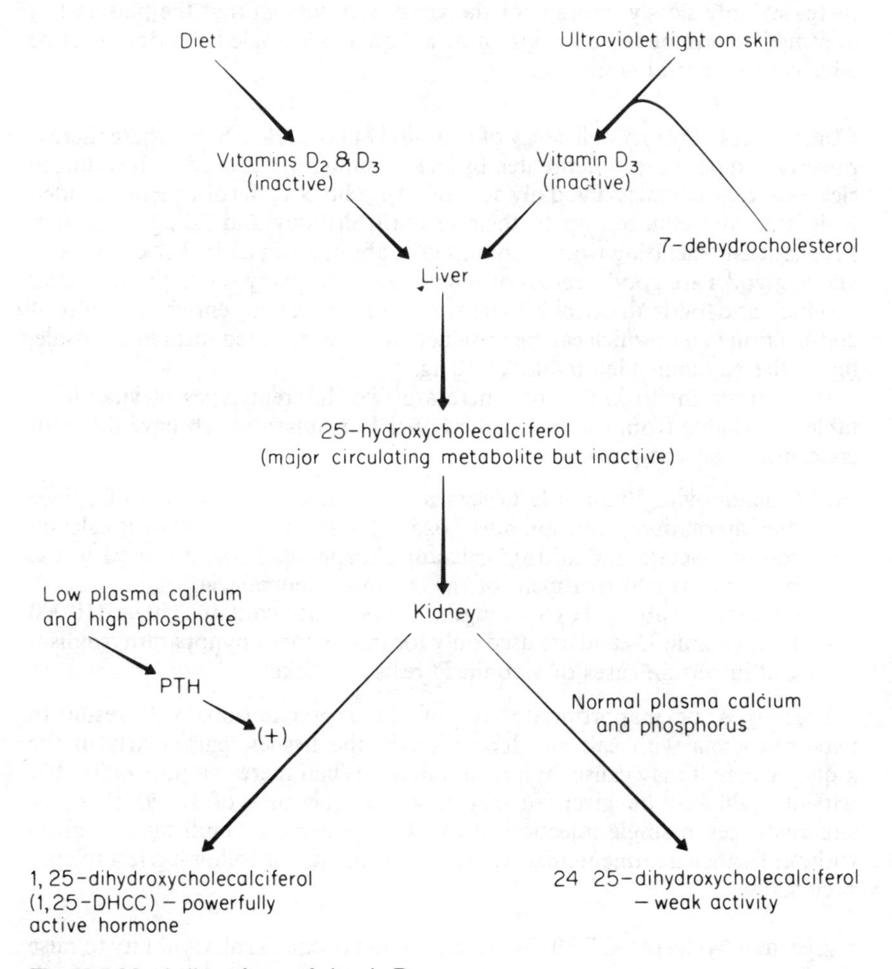

Fig. 18.5 Metabolic pathway of vitamin D.

Renal 1-α-hydroxylase is activated by PTH and inhibited by phosphate, thus controlling the amount of active 1,25-dihydroxycholecalciferol produced. This enzyme is also suppressed by 1,25-DHCC itself. 1,25-DHCC is effectively a hormone in that it is synthesised in the kidney and acts on the intestine to increase formation of a calcium-binding protein which augments intestinal calcium absorption. Vitamin D itself is biologically inactive and is simply a precursor of this hormone so that its claims to being a vitamin are dubious. Enzyme induction, particularly due to antiepileptic and hypnotic drugs, causes rapid metabolism and wasting of calciferol and thus can result in osteomalacia and rickets. 1,25-DHCC mobilises calcium from bone; presumably the purpose of this is to provide calcium for synthesis of new bone mineral and there is some evidence for the participation of a form of vitamin D other than, 1,25-DHCC in mineralisation. The action on the kidney is to stimulate calcium reabsorption, although this is a minor effect. The maximum anti-rachitic effect of cholecalciferol is delayed for several weeks and the plasma calcium similarly increases only slowly. Storage of the vitamin occurs so that the plasma $t_{1/2}$ does not determine the duration of its action and a single large dose may be effective for several weeks.

Clinical uses. Dietary deficiency of vitamin D in the UK occurs where there is poverty and poor diet accentuated by lack of sunlight, e.g. purdah. It results in rickets and osteomalacia. A daily dose of 10 μg cholecalciferol is recommended in infants and children up to their seventh birthday and 2.5 μg thereafter. Pregnant and lactating women should take about 20 μg daily. Milk, liver, fish and egg yolks are good sources of the vitamin and many foods (infant cereal products and foods, dried milk, margarine) are additionally enriched. A dose of cod-liver oil (5 ml), which can be provided in a concentrated form in a capsule, meets the recommended intake of 10 μg.

It is important to know that there are two different types of vitamin D tablets available from the British National Formulary which have different concentrations and purposes:

1. Calcium with Vitamin D tablets B.P.C. contain 12.5 μg (500 I.U. since one international unit contains 0.025 μg) vitamin D_2 with 450 mg calcium sodium lactate and 150 mg calcium phosphate. These are used in the prophylaxis and treatment of rickets and osteomalacia.
2. Calciferol Tablets High-strength, 10 000 units contain 250 μg (10 000 I.U.) vitamin D_2 and are used only for treatment of hypoparathyroidism and in certain cases of vitamin D resistant rickets.

Prolonged or inappropriate use of these preparations will result in hypercalcaemia with calcium deposition in the tissues, particularly in the kidney where it may cause fatal renal failure. When there is a possibility that patients will not be given further treatment because of social or other circumstances, a single injection of calciferol (7.5 mg in 1 ml) may be given without further treatment apart from arrangements for follow-up lest relapse occurs.

Dihydrotachysterol (A.T.10) is closely related to calciferol. Its ability to raise the plasma calcium concentration is about equal to that of calciferol, although it may act more rapidly and its antirachitic potency is less. It is given orally in an oily solution in a dose of 1–2 mg or up to 8 mg in emergency. Regular plasma calcium estimations are required since it may, like calciferol, produce hypercalcaemia. The maintenance dose is 0.25–1.5 mg weekly.

Adverse effects Hypercalcaemia is the main problem. It is therefore dangerous to administer more than 0.25 mg for more than three months unless the patient has vitamin D resistance. Idiopathic infantile hypercalcaemia has been attributed to excessive dietary intake from fortified foods. The Medicines Commission has recommended that no proprietary medicine containing more than 10 μg cholecalciferol be freely available to the public.

1-α-hydroxycholecalciferol (one-alpha)

This metabolite is now available for oral administration. It rapidly undergoes hepatic hydroxylation to 1,25-DHCC. Its main uses appear to be in:

(a) Renal rickets, where chronic renal failure leads to impaired 1,25-DHCC synthesis resulting in calcium malabsorption and hypocalcaemia with phosphate retention leading to secondary elevation of PTH levels. These result in the bony changes of osteomalacia and hyperparathyroidism. 1-α-HCC is given in a dose of 1 μg daily (together with phosphate-binding agents) and this produces a satisfactory symptomatic and biochemical response. Possibly prophylactic treatment in patients with renal failure may prevent the development of the syndrome.

(b) Hypoparathyroidism is usually treated with vitamin D in large doses but the response is slow, and unpredictable episodes of hypercalcaemia occur. This relative resistance to vitamin D is due to deficient 1,25-DHCC production secondary to PTH deficiency or hyperphosphataemia.

1-α-HCC (3–5 μg) plus calcium supplements correct plasma calcium levels within a matter of days and normocalcaemia may be maintained with smaller doses within a relatively narrow dosage range. Pre-operative administration in patients with hyperparathyroidism may prevent post-operative hypocalcaemia.

(c) Vitamin D resistant rickets.

(d) Nutritional and malabsorptive rickets may also be treated with small doses (0.5–1 μg) of 1-α-HCC instead of conventional vitamin D.

The main adverse reaction is hypercalcaemia and regular plasma calcium determinations are essential. It is more likely to occur in renal failure than in osteomalacia. An advantage of using 1-α-hydroxycholecalciferol is that vitamin D intoxication is rapidly reversed when the drug is withdrawn, whereas reversal may take several weeks with the older vitamin D compounds.

1,25-dihydroxycholecalciferol or calcitriol (Rocaltrol) is now available for the treatment of the above. Like 1-α-HCC it has a shorter biological half-life and less variable action than calciferol. Calcitriol is the treatment of choice for pseudohypoparathyroidism.

Calcium

Calcium lactate or gluconate is used in conjunction with calciferol in the treatment of rickets and osteomalacia and in hypocalcaemic tetany. In emergency it is given as calcium gluconate injection B.P. (10% solution) 10–20 ml being given intravenously over 5–10 min every 2–4 h. It must not be given intramuscularly since it is painful and can cause necrosis. Given intravenously it can be toxic due to its cardiac effects which mimic and potentiate those of digitalis. The place of calcium supplements in the treatment of osteoporosis is not established but it is justified to supplement the diet if the intake is below 1400 mg (35 mmol) daily. Sandocal calcium is an effervescent preparation which is easy to take and contains 400 mg (10 mmol) calcium per tablet. The dose is 2–5 tablets daily.

Calcitonin

This hormone is a polypeptide containing 32 amino acids (M.W. 3600) and is secreted by thyroid parafollicular cells and by the parathyroid glands. Acting via alterations in intracellular cyclic AMP it lowers plasma calcium and phosphate levels and antagonises the effects of parathormone on bone. These actions are produced by:

(a) A major effect on bone via a slowing of osteoclastic resorption, leading to a reduced release of calcium, phosphorus and hydroxyproline. The magnitude of the fall in plasma calcium levels depends upon the initial bone turnover and where this is high, e.g. in Paget's disease or thyrotoxicosis, the fall may be large. In normal adults the fall in plasma calcium is often unimpressive. Osteoblastic activity is increased.

(b) A minor renal effect promoting phosphate, calcium and sodium excretion.

(c) Calcitonin inhibits 1-hydroxylase and hence blocks the activation of vitamin D. The end result is a reduction in intestinal absorption of calcium.

Porcine calcitonin (Calcitare) and Salcatonin (Calsynar) Synthetic calcitonin is used therapeutically: the structures corresponding to porcine, salmon and human calcitonin being used. The dosage of the calcitonins is presently expressed inconveniently in MRC units based upon a rat bioassay not directly applicable to man, whose sensitivity to the hormone differs from rodents. Soon prescription will be by weight (100 MRC units human and porcine calcitonin = 1 mg; 100 MRC units salmon calcitonin = 0.025 mg). Calcitonin is given by intravenous or intramuscular injection. Porcine and salmon calcitonin may induce antibody formation but this is rarely present in high enough titre to interfere with treatment (cf. insulin antibodies).

Clinical uses

1. Paget's disease of bone: The two main indications for calcitonin treatment are bone pain and hypercalcaemia. Patients vary in their response, but pain relief should occur within 2 months of beginning treatment (50–100 MRC units of salmon calcitonin thrice weekly usually results in a fall

in plasma calcium, phosphate and alkaline phosphatase with reduced urinary hydroxyproline excretion). Treatment may be withdrawn in many cases after a few months without relapse although in active disease, cardiac failure or neurological compression, maintenance treatment may be needed. It is not known whether prolonged therapy can prevent deformity developing. Theoretically complete healing of bone disease could be achieved, although possibly this might take as many years as the disease took to develop.

2. Hypercalcaemia due to malignancy, vitamin D intoxication, infantile hypercalcaemia or immobilisation of patients with Paget's disease all respond to calcitonin. It may be useful in the preparation of patients with severe hyperparathyroidism for surgery but has no place in the long-term management of this condition. It has no useful clinical effect on osteoporosis. For hypercalcaemia doses of 4 units/kg/day may be used and in emergencies higher doses of 8 units/kg/h have been given intravenously with impunity.

Adverse effects Pain at the injection site; nausea (countered by giving the injection with an anti-emetic before going to bed); flushing of the face (20–30 %).

Etidronate (Didronel)

This is a diphosphonate and structurally resembles pyrophosphate except that the two phosphorus atoms are linked by carbon rather than oxygen. This renders such compounds very stable: no enzyme is known which degrades them. Etidronate modifies the crystal growth of calcium hydroxyapatite by chemical adsorption to the crystal surface. This high affinity for calcium phosphate has been exploited in their use for nuclear bone scanning as a complex of ^{99m}Tc (a γ-emitter) with ethane hydroxydiphosphonic acid. This is used to identify areas of increased skeletal turnover, particularly Paget's disease and bony metastases. Etidronate inhibits bone resorption and formation thereby reducing the accelerated bone turnover of Paget's disease, returns the histological bone pattern towards normal, lowers the associated elevated biochemical indices of the disease and relieves symptoms.

Pharmacokinetics It is given orally but is poorly (1–5 %) absorbed; food and antacids further reduce absorption. It disappears from the blood extremely rapidly into bone where its effects persist. Within 24 hours about 50 % of the absorbed dose is excreted unchanged in the urine, the remainder is excreted over many weeks.

Clinical use It is started at low dosage (5 mg/kg/day) over 6 months when many patients achieve remission for 3 to 24 months when a further course may be given on relapse. Use for longer than 6 months at a time does not prolong remission. Higher doses (up to 20 mg/kg/day) should be used only if lower doses fail or if rapid control of disease, e.g. with high output cardiac failure, is needed. Etidronate is effective when calcitonin has failed (and vice versa) and they may be used in conjunction. It is indicated for treatment of patients with bone pain (which responds well) or if there is extensive involvement of the skull or spine with possible danger of irreversible neurological damage or when a weight-bearing bone is involved. Stress fractures in long bones contraindicate its use.

Oral etidronate is more convenient than calcitonin and cheaper: it may become the drug of first choice in the future for Paget's disease.

Adverse effects It is well tolerated and at low doses there is only a low incidence of gastrointestinal complaints (diarrhoea, nausea).

Hyperphosphataemia occurs with high doses but is probably harmless.

A few patients (5%) have noted exacerbation of bone pain at Pagetoid sites during treatment with high doses.

There are no known drug interactions apart from reduction of its absorption by antacids.

Other treatments of Paget's disease

1. *Fluoride* A reduction in serum alkaline phosphatase and urinary hydroxyproline excretion has been reported following administration of sodium fluoride. Bone pain is reduced but the high doses required make skeletal fluorosis and fluoride intoxication a possible hazard.

2. *Cytotoxic drugs* Mithramycin and actinomycin D have been used. They act directly upon osteoclasts to inhibit bone resorption. The use of such toxic agents may not be desirable in a non-fatal condition such as Paget's disease.

Treatment of hypercalcaemia

Hypercalcaemia may be a life-threatening emergency and is produced by numerous pathological mechanisms ranging from bony destruction by tumour to hyperparathyroidism. Management divides into:

A. General

1. maintenance of hydration; and replacement of sodium.
2. avoidance of dietary calcium and vitamin D;
3. correction of acidosis;
4. avoidance of immobilisation.

B. Specific

1. Increasing calcium excretion:

(a) Frusemide 100 mg given orally every 1–2 h increases urinary calcium loss. Since hypercalcaemia is associated with polyuria and vomiting which produce dehydration, particular care is necessary to replete fluid loss. In addition potassium and magnesium losses must be compensated (the latter may be replaced empirically by giving 15 mg magnesium sulphate intramuscularly every hour).

(b) Sodium sulphate given intravenously as isotonic solution (3.85%) giving 2–3 l every 12 h. This enhances calcium excretion by increased delivery of sodium to the distal tubule plus formation of a non-resorbable calcium–sodium sulphate complex. The complications of this therapy are hypernatraemia (which makes it unsuitable for use in hypertension and heart or renal failure) and hypomagnesaemia.

(c) Infusion up to 3 l daily of 0.9% saline also increases renal calcium loss.

2. Decreasing bone resorption:

(a) Corticosteroids: 200 mg hydrocortisone or equivalent daily has an unpredictable effect on hypercalcaemia. The effect is slow and they may be ineffective in malignancy although they can be helpful in sarcoidosis and myeloma.

(b) Mithramycin given intravenously in a dose of 15 μg/kg over half an hour on four successive days is sometimes useful. Its main action is probably to decrease osteoclast activity. Nausea and vomiting are common complications and rarely a bleeding disorder and disturbance of liver function occurs.

(c) Calcitonin (see above).

3. Sequestration of calcium using phosphates given orally as a neutral phosphate mixture or intravenously (81 mmol disodium phosphate and 19 mmol monopotassium phosphate in 1 l of 5% dextrose). This produces a prompt, dose-dependent fall in urinary calcium excretion. The fall in plasma calcium level is directly proportional to the magnitude by which the calcium phosphate solubility product is exceeded, the calcium being deposited in bone and soft tissues. Plasma phosphate rises, and so this treatment is contraindicated by renal failure, but falls within 36 h whilst the plasma calcium level remains depressed for some 10 days after a single dose. Although soft-tissue calcification is a theoretical hazard, this has never been substantiated and the long-term risks are unknown.

It is important to treat the cause of the hypercalcaemia since the benefit of any other therapy will otherwise be short-lived.

Chapter 19
CHEMOTHERAPY OF INFECTIONS

ANTI-BACTERIAL DRUGS

Despite intensive study and the introduction of many new agents over nearly 50 years, the use of these drugs remains largely empirical.

The choice of an appropriate antibacterial drug should be based upon a bacteriological diagnosis with, if possible, determination of the drug sensitivity of the organism. If this is unavailable, then a provisional diagnosis based upon the clinical features of the case should be made. Fortunately there is often a good correspondence between accurate clinical diagnosis and the likely pathogen and its response to therapy. Local knowledge of the frequency of resistances to given antibiotics in the hospital or community may be a useful guide.

The site of the infection is sometimes relevant, because although the blood concentration may be an indication of tissue levels, this is not always the case. For example, only ampicillin, amoxycillin, rifampicin and some cephalosporins are secreted in high concentrations in the bile and are also active against biliary pathogens. Only antibiotics which are un-ionised at pH 6.4 can enter prostatic tissue and only trimethoprim, erythromycin, clindamycin and chloramphenicol comply with this constraint. Some drugs, e.g. nitrofurantoin, only attain useful concentration in the urine and so are not useful for tissue infections. Entry of anti-infective agents into the CSF (see Table 19.1) is particularly important, since the attainment of adequate concentrations of antibacterial substances in this fluid probably determines the success of therapy in meningitis. Some antibiotics, notably penicillins, achieve higher levels in the CSF when the meninges are inflamed. The penicillins are actively

Table 19.1 Penetration of anti-infective agents into CSF

Good penetration (approximately 50% plasma levels)	*Moderate penetration (approximately 20% plasma levels)*	*Poor penetration*
Chloramphenicol	Minocycline, Doxycycline	Tetracyline
Sulphonamides	Ampicillin	All aminoglycosides
Trimethoprim	Lincomycin	Penicillins (except ampicillin)
Isoniazid	Cephaloridine	Clindamycin
Pyrazinamide	Rifampicin	Some cephalosporins
Some cephalosporins		Colistin
		Polymyxin B

transported out of the CSF by the choroid plexus and in the presence of inflammation this active secretory process is impaired and the antibiotic builds up to higher levels in the CSF.

The least toxic of alternative drugs should be chosen and it should be compatible with concurrent treatment. Appropriate adjustment must be made for renal or liver failure and in some cases such organ dysfunction will preclude the choice of a particular drug, as may pregnancy or allergy. The cost of the drug either to the patient or society, whilst it should not be a final arbiter, must also be kept in mind.

It is usual to distinguish in antibacterial chemotherapy between antibiotics and other chemotherapeutic substances. The former are natural compounds manufactured by living micro-organisms and can either kill or inhibit the growth of other micro-organisms. The latter are synthesised *in vitro*. The distinction is somewhat blurred since nowadays many antibiotics are modified by chemical manipulation to produce substances not found in nature, whilst chloramphenicol, originally from a micro-organism, is now synthesised commercially de novo.

Table 19.2 Classification of antibacterials

Bactericidal	*Bacteriostatic*
penicillins	sulphonamides
cephalosporins	chloramphenicol
aminoglycosides	tetracyclines
cotrimoxazole	erythromycin
isoniazid	trimethoprim
	lincomycin and clindamycin
	para-aminosalicylic acid

A distinction is often drawn between bactericidal and bacteriostatic drugs (Table 19.2). Bactericidal drugs actively kill bacteria. Bacteriostatic drugs merely prevent the growth of the organisms, the final elimination depending largely on the body defences. Thus, if these defences are inadequate or if drug administration is discontinued prematurely, the bacterial population may increase again and a relapse occur.

This distinction is relative and bacteriostatic drugs may become bactericidal at high concentrations or after very long exposure of organisms to drug. It is also necessary to define the laboratory conditions of growth very precisely to demonstrate these properties, e.g. the bactericidal effect of aminoglycosides becomes bacteriostatic if the medium becomes acid. Thus the effects of these drugs may be bacteriostatic in pus or acid urine. It should not be thought that bacteriostatic drugs are in any sense less potent than bactericidal drugs. Thus, for example, chloramphenicol is the treatment of choice in typhoid and erythromycin in Legionnaire's disease, both of these potentially lethal infections responding to bacteriostatic drugs. In clinical practice the distinction is rarely important, apart from the special cases of treatment in patients with depressed defence mechanisms or in whom the phagocytic or immune response is impaired, e.g. bacterial endocarditis, streptococcal carrier state, chronic osteomyelitis. Under these circumstances a bactericidal drug should be chosen. Antibiotic combinations are used in four main situations:

(a) to achieve broad antimicrobial activity in critically ill patients with an undefined infection;
(b) to treat mixed bacterial infections where no single antibiotic would affect all the bacteria present;
(c) to prevent emergence of resistance;
(d) to achieve an additive or synergistic effect.

Drug combinations

It is believed by some that combinations of bactericidal drugs are either synergistic or additive and combinations of bacteriostatic drugs are additive. Combinations of bactericidal and bacteriostatic drugs may be synergistic, additive or antagonistic. This can be demonstrated *in vitro* by construction of an isobologram (Fig. 19.1).

There is both clinical and *in vitro* evidence that under some circumstances chloramphenicol may antagonise the action of penicillin, possibly by inhibiting the autolytic bacterial enzyme responsible for cell death after inhibition of bacterial cell-wall synthesis by penicillin. There is also evidence that in pneumococcal meningitis the mortality rate is increased if tetracycline

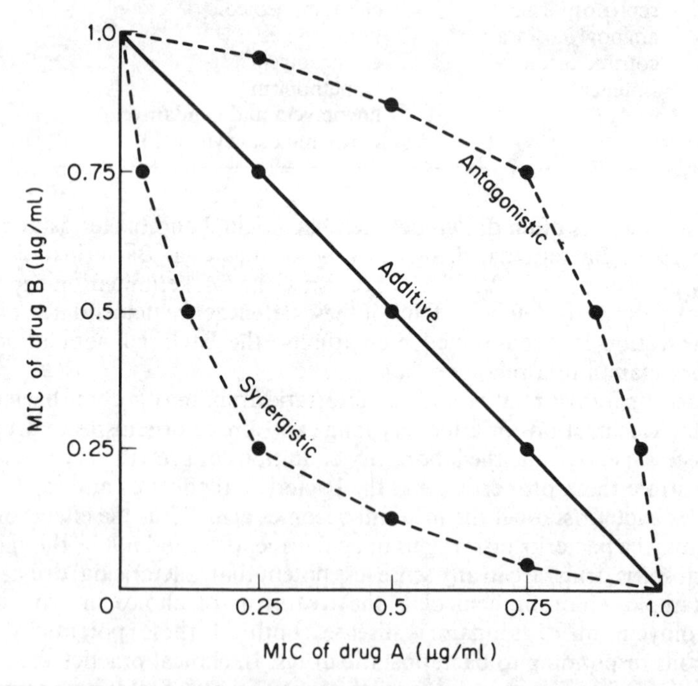

Fig. 19.1 Isobolograms for two antibiotics A and B against a single organism demonstrating synergism, addition or antagonism. The MIC for one of the pair is determined in the presence of several fixed concentrations of the other.

is given in addition to penicillin. There is no adequate evidence, however, to suggest antagonism of aminoglycosides by tetracycline or lincomycin. Probably only in conditions in which penicillin penetrates poorly to infected foci, e.g. in bacterial endocarditis or meningitis, is it susceptible to antagonism by bacteriostatic drugs.

In general bactericidal drugs may be preferred where possible, because they are less likely to leave residual 'persistent' organisms and may be more rapidly effective than bacteriostatic drugs.

Resistant organisms

The resistance of bacterial populations to antimicrobial agents is constantly changing and can become a serious clinical problem, particularly if the resistant strain supplants the sensitive, thus rendering a previously useful drug inactive. The evolution of drug resistance arises either by:

(a) Selection of naturally resistant strains existing within the bacterial population by elimination of the sensitive strain by therapy or environmental contamination. Thus the incidence of drug resistance is related to the prescription of that drug (Fig. 19.2). Hospitals are particularly likely to promote the proliferation of resistant organisms.

(b) Spontaneous mutation followed by selection and multiplication of the resistant strain.

(c) Transfer of resistance between organisms can occur either by transfer of naked DNA (transformation), by conjugation with direct cell-to-cell transfer of extrachromosomal DNA (so-called R factors), or by passage of the information by bacteriophage (transduction). In this way transfer of genetic information concerning drug resistance (which may be to a group of antibiotics) may occur between species.

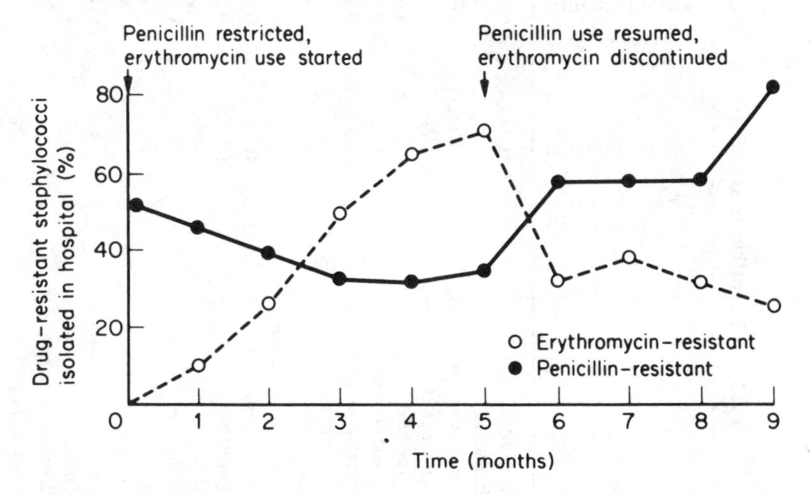

Fig. 19.2 Emergence of staphylococcal resistance in a hospital population and its relationship to antibiotic usage (From data of M. H. Lepper *et al.*, *J. Lab. Clin. Med.*, **42,** 832 (1953).)

Table 19.3 Antibiotic sensitivities of common isolates (minimum inhibitory concentrations in μg/ml; R = Resistant)

	Benzylpenicillin	Ampicillin	Cloxacillin	Piperacillin	Cephalexin	Cefotaxime	Cephradine	Erythromycin
Staph. aureus	0.03	0.06	0.1	32	2	2	2–4	0.1
Staph. aureus (penicillinase producing)	R	R	0.25	R	8	2–4	16–32	0.1
Strep. pyogenes	0.01	0.03	0.06	< 8	0.5	0.12	0.01	0.03
Strep. faecalis	2	1–2	32	32	R	R	64	0.5
Strep. pneumoniae	0.01	0.06	0.25		2	0.12	1	0.03
Clostridium welchii	0.1	0.25	1	8		0.5	2	2
Mycobacterium tuberculosis	R	R	R	R	R	R	R	R
Neisseria gonorrhoeae	0.01	0.03–1	0.5		0.25–4	0.015	0.5	0.06
Neisseria meningitidis	0.03	0.06	0.5	< 8	0.5–4	0.01	1	0.5
H. influenzae	0.5–2	0.25	16	< 8	8–64	0.03	4.8	1–8
E. coli	16–R	8	R	32	8	0.25	8–16	8–R
Klebsiella spp.	R	4–R	R	64	4–R	0.25	8–16	R
Proteus spp.	32	4	R	1	8	0.1	8–16	R
Proteus spp. (penicillinase producing)	R	R	R	8	8	1	8–16	R
Salmonella spp.	2–16	1–8	R	128	1–4	0.25	4–16	64–R
Pseudomonas aeruginosa	R	R	R	4	R	R	R	R
Bacteroides fragilis	8–R	16–32	32	2	32	64	16–32	1–4

Table 19.3 (continued)

	Clindamycin	Fusidic acid	Tetracycline	Chloramphenicol	Streptomycin	Gentamicin	Sulphadimidine	Metronidazole
Staph. aureus	0.06–1	0.06	0.1	4–8	2	0.06–1	16–32	**R**
Staph. aureus (penicillinase producing)	0.01–1	0.06	0.1	4–8	2	0.06–1	16–32	**R**
Strep. pyogenes	0.01–0.25	4–8	0.25	2	32	8–16	1–64	**R**
Strep. faecalis	0.1–32	4	0.5	2	32–64	4–16	100	250
Strep. pneumoniae	0.03–1	8	0.25	2	64	16–32	4–64	**R**
Clostridium welchii	0.03–1	0.25	0.03–0.25	4	**R**	**R**	8–32	1.25
Mycobacterium tuberculosis	**R**	64	8–16	32	1	4	**R**	**R**
Neisseria gonorrhoeae	0.03–4	0.05	1	1	4	1–2	16–128	**R**
Neisseria meningitidis		0.1	1	1	1	2	0.5–8	**R**
H. influenzae	2–32	8	1	0.5	2–4	0.1–0.5	8–16	**R**
E. coli	**R**	**R**	1	2–8	4	1–4	16–64	**R**
Klebsiella spp.	**R**	**R**	0.5	1–**R**	1–**R**	0.5	64–128	125
Proteus spp.	**R**	**R**	32–64	4–16	4–8	0.5–8	> 128	**R**
Proteus spp. (penicillinase producing)	**R**	**R**	32–64	4–16	4–8	0.5–8	> 128	**R**
Salmonella spp.	**R**	**R**		2	2–8	0.25–1	32–> 128	500–**R**
Pseudomonas aeruginosa	**R**	**R**	32–**R**	**R**	16–64	1–8	> 128	**R**
Bacteroides fragilis	0.1–1	1–**R**	0.5–2	8	**R**	**R**	**R**	0.6

The prescriber can minimise bacterial resistance by:

1. avoidance of unnecessary prescription of antimicrobials;
2. use of antimicrobials in adequate dosage for an adequate duration since inadequacy in these respects can promote resistance;
3. restriction of certain drugs, e.g. amikacin, for specific clinical and bacteriological indications.
4. use of drug combinations.

The mechanisms of drug resistance may broadly be divided into:

(a) Inactivation of the antimicrobial agent either by disruption of its chemical structure (e.g. penicillinase) or by addition of a modifying group which inactivates the drug (e.g. chloramphenicol, inactivated by acetylation).
(b) Restriction of entry of drug into the bacterium by altered permeability, e.g. methicillin, sulphonamide, tetracycline.
(c) Modification of the bacterial target. This may take the form of an enzyme with reduced affinity for an inhibitor (e.g. sulphonamide), or an altered organelle with reduced drug-binding properties (e.g. erythromycin and bacterial ribosomes).

In vitro and in vivo sensitivities

The usual estimate of sensitivity of an organism to a given drug is based upon an *in vitro* test in which the minimum inhibitory concentration of the drug is determined. It should be stressed that this is not necessarily analogous to the *in vivo* situation, since it is carried out with the organisms grown in specified and usually optimum conditions in the presence of a constant drug concentration. *In vivo* the situation is more complicated and the efficacy of an antimicrobial drug depends upon its ability to penetrate areas of infection. Regions in which blood flow is reduced are known to respond poorly to antimicrobial treatment. Thus in osteomyelitis, penetration of cephalothin and lincomycin has been shown to be negligible into sequestrated bone although the enveloping new bone (involucrum) is entered by these drugs. Similarly severe renal disease reduces renal parenchymal and urinary levels of antibiotics. Many antibiotics are protein bound and because only unbound drug is an effective chemotherapeutic agent, highly bound drugs may produce higher plasma drug levels (because their apparent volume of distribution is smaller) which may not necessarily be more effective. It is also important to realise that although intermittent bolus injections may produce intermittent spikes in plasma drug concentration, because of the damping effect of a compartmental system the concentration–time profile in the tissues where the drug is active may be sustained. Furthermore, effective levels may be present at some local site when no drug is detectable in the plasma. These factors must be borne in mind when considering the best mode of drug administration. Few studies have been carried out which convincingly demonstrate the superiority of intermittent high doses of antibiotics as opposed to continuous low doses. In animal studies the duration of exposure to penicillin in streptococcal infection appeared to be the most critical factor rather than the magnitude of the blood levels. Such information may not be relevant to clinical problems and no information is available for drugs acting by other mechanisms on bacteria. The effects of antibiotics depend presumably not only upon their pharmacokinetic behaviour in plasma but also upon their pharmacodynamic behaviour on bacteria and on local factors governing their tissue distribution.

Table 19.3 gives some representative minimum inhibitory concentrations for a number of organisms in the presence of a range of antimicrobial agents. It may be useful

(a) to observe the pattern of resistance of organisms to a given drug;
(b) to observe the spectrum of activity of the various drugs;
(c) to relate the pharmacokinetic information detailed in this chapter under the various drugs to the inhibitory concentrations for various organisms.

The prophylactic use of antibiotics

There are a limited number of occasions when it is justifiable to use antibiotics to prevent infection. In general the narrowest spectrum antibiotic which is suitable should be used. The following are satisfactory:

Medical condition	*Prophylaxis*
Meningococcal contacts:	Rifampicin 600 mg twice daily for 2 days.
Whooping cough contacts:	Erythromycin 40 mg/kg daily for 5 days.
Following rheumatic fever:	Phenoxymethylpenicillin 250 mg twice daily.
Prior to dental extraction, deep scaling or periodontal surgery in those at risk of infective endocarditis:	Amoxycillin 3.0 g orally one hour before operation. If penicillin-sensitive, erythromycin 1.5 g 1 h before operation +500 mg 6 h later.
In gastrointestinal or genital urinary surgery for those at risk of infective endocarditis	Ampicillin 1.0 g +gentamicin 120 mg both i.m. 1 h before the procedure followed by 500 mg of amoxycillin orally 6 h later.
Recurrent urinary infections:	Adults—trimethoprim 100 mg at night; nitrofurantoin 100 mg at night (avoid if renal function is impaired). Children—trimethoprim 2.5 mg/kg single dose at night.
Preoperative	
Large bowel surgery:	Metronidazole 1.0 g suppository +gentamicin 60–100 mg i.v. with premedication and then 8 hourly for 24 h.
Acute appendicitis:	Metronidazole 1.0 g suppository 2 h before operation and 8 hourly until oral medication can be started.
Biliary surgery:	Ampicillin 500 mg +gentamicin 60–100 mg with premedication or cephazolin 500 mg with premedication and then 8 hourly for 24–48 h. Not required in clean and elective cases.

Limb amputation for ischaemia:	Flucloxacillin 500 mg i.v. metronidazole 1.0 g suppository + ampicillin 500 mg i.v. repeated 8 hourly for 48–72 h.
Hip replacement:	Ampicillin 500 mg + flucloxacillin 500 mg with premedication and continued orally for 2–5 days.

ANTIBACTERIAL THERAPY

The choice of an appropriate antibiotic will depend on:

1. The infecting organism and its sensitivity to antibacterial agents as determined by an informed guess or by isolation and culture.
2. The site of infection.
3. The route of administration and toxicity of the antibiotics available.
4. Cost.

There will obviously be differences of opinion as to the best antibiotic to use in a given set of circumstances and the summary in Table 19.4 is for guidance and is by no means definitive. All treatments are oral and for adults unless otherwise stated.

For dose of aminoglycosides see under individual drugs.

Table 19.4 Summary of antibacterial therapy

Clinical conditions	*Likely causative organism(s)*	*Suggested treatment*
A. RESPIRATORY TRACT INFECTIONS		
Pharyngitis Tonsillitis Scarlet fever	Viruses *Strep. pyogenes*	Many *Strep. pyogenes* are resistant to tetracycline. Most infections are viral and require symptomatic treatment only. If treatment is required: *1st Choice:* Penicillin V 250–500 mg 6 hourly or benzylpenicillin 600 mg i.v. or i.m. 6 hourly if seriously ill/vomiting. *Alternative:* Erythromycin 500 mg 6 hourly.
Acute otitis media Sinusitis	*Strep. pyogenes* *H. influenzae* *Strep. pneumoniae*	Do not use tetracycline. *1st Choice:* Amoxycillin 250 mg 8 hourly. *Alternative:* Erythromycin 500 mg 6 hourly.

Table 19.4 (continued)

Clinical conditions	*Likely causative organism(s)*	*Suggested treatment*
Acute bronchitis in healthy adults	Viruses *H. influenzae* *Strep. pneumoniae*	Mild cases, usually viral, require symptomatic treatment only. Severe cases with purulent sputum: *1st Choice:* Amoxycillin 250 mg 8 hourly *Alternative:* Cotrimoxazole two tabs 12 hourly.
Acute on chronic bronchitis	*H. influenzae* *Strep. pneumoniae*	*1st Choice:* Amoxycillin 250 mg 8 hourly or cotrimoxazole two tabs 12 hourly. *Alternative:* Tetracycline 500 mg 6 hourly (if renal function is impaired doxycycline) or erythromycin 500 mg 6 hourly.
Acute epiglottitis in children	*H. influenzae*	*1st Choice:* Chloramphenicol initially i.v. treatment may be required.
Pneumonia—classical lobar	*Strep. pneumoniae*	*1st Choice:* Benzylpenicillin 600 mg i.v. 6 hourly. *Alternative:* Erythromycin 500 mg 6 hourly (i.v. for first 48 hours). Some strains of *Strep. pneumoniae* are tetracycline resistant.
Other pneumonias 'Broncho-pneumonia'	*Strep. pneumoniae* *H. influenzae* *Staph. aureus* and others	Many possible regimes. Usually start treatment with amoxycillin 500 mg 8 hourly plus flucloxacillin 500 mg 6 hourly. Add gentamicin i.v. in severely ill patients.
Pneumonia—post-influenza	Beware *Staph. aureus* *Strep. pneumonia* *H. influenzae*	If definitely staphylococcal flucloxacillin 500 mg i.v. 6 hourly plus sodium fusidate 500 mg i.v. 8 hourly. Otherwise flucloxacillin 500 mg i.v. 6 hourly plus gentamicin i.v. plus ampicillin 500 mg i.v. 6 hourly.
Pneumonia—primary atypical (penicillin resistant)	*Mycoplasma pneumoniae* *Chlam. psittaci* *Coxiella burnetii*	*1st Choice:* Erythromycin 500 mg 6 hourly. *Alternative:* Tetracycline 500 mg 6 hourly (if renal function is impaired doxycycline). Avoid tetracycline in pregnancy and children under 12

Table 19.4 (continued)

Clinical conditions	*Likely causative organism(s)*	*Suggested treatment*
Legionnaires' disease	*Legionella pneumophila*	*1st Choice:* Erythromycin up to 1 g i.v. 6 hourly and rifampicin 600 mg orally (i.v. if seriously ill) daily for 3 days.
Pneumonia in the immunosuppressed	Wide variety of organisms including gram-negative organisms, anaerobes and fungi	Initially gentamicin i.v. plus ampicillin 500 mg i.v. 6 hourly plus flucloxacillin 500 mg i.v. 6 hourly plus metronidazole 400 mg orally 8 hourly. Add cotrimoxazole one quarter of an adult tablet/kg/day in two divided doses if pneumocystis is suspected
Aspiration pneumonia	Mouth organisms including anaerobes	Amoxycillin 500 mg 8 hourly plus metronidazole 400 mg 8 hourly Some authorities recommend steroids, particularly in presence of airflow obstruction
	B. URINARY TRACT INFECTIONS	
Acute cystitis arising outside hospital in adults.	*E. coli* *Staph. saprophyticus* *Strep. faecalis* Other organisms (uncommon)	*1st Choice:* Trimethoprim 200 mg 12 hourly. *Alternative:* Amoxycillin 250 mg 8 hourly. In pregnancy amoxycillin or sulphamethizole are preferred. Avoid trimethoprim in first 3 months of pregnancy and sulphamethizole in last month.
Sulphamethizole		
Acute pyelonephritis (adults)	As above	As above. In severely ill patients add gentamicin i.v.
Prophylaxis against urinary tract infection (adults)	As above	*1st Choice:* Trimethoprim 100 mg at night
Hospital acquired and chronic urinary infection in adults	Variety of organisms, often multiply resistant	Requires consultation with microbiologist. Often difficult to eradicate. With indwelling catheters use chlorhexidine 0.02% bladder washout twice daily.
Urinary tract infection in children	*E. coli*	

Table 19.4 (continued)

Clinical conditions	*Likely causative organism(s)*	*Suggested treatment*
(a) Acute attack		*1st Choice:* Trimethoprim or amoxycillin *Alternative:* If severe requires consultation with microbiologist. Give ampicillin i.v. plus gentamicin i.v. until sensitivities are known.
(b) Prophylaxis		*1st Choice:* Trimethoprim 2.5 mg/kg as a single dose at night. *Alternative:* Cefadroxil 125 mg at night (rarely necessary).
C. SEVERE SYSTEMIC INFECTIONS (SEPTICAEMIA)		
Severe systemic infection —causative organism unknown	Many possibilities	Initial choice of antibiotics depends on the clinical condition and the pathogen background of the hospital. Later cultures may help.
Immunocompetent or immunosuppressed but no recent antibiotic treatment		Gentamicin i.v. plus ampicillin 500 mg i.v. 6 hourly (erythromycin if penicillin sensitive) plus metronidazole 400 mg orally 8 hourly (or 1 g rectally). Add flucloxacillin 500 mg i.v. 6 hourly if *Staph.* is suspected.
Immunosuppressed and seriously ill for whom the above treatment has failed or for those patients who have recently relapsed		The antibiotic regime will usually include an aminoglycoside plus a ureidopenicillin or one of the newer cephalosporins plus metronidazole. A typical initial regime would be gentamicin (or amikacin) plus piperacillin (or azlocillin if pseudomonas is suspected) plus metronidazole. For these patients close collaboration with the microbiology department is necessary. Many of the antibiotics used are very expensive.
Severe infection with gram-negative organisms.	*E. coli* *Proteus* *Klebsiella*	*1st Choice:* Ampicillin 500 mg i.v. 6 hourly plus gentamicin i.v. *Alternative:* For gentamicin-resistant *Klebsiella* cefuroxime 1.5 g i.v. 8 hourly plus amikacin i.v.

Table 19.4 (continued)

Clinical conditions	*Likely causative organism(s)*	*Suggested treatment*
	Pseudomonas	Take advice of microbiologist.
Severe infection with gram-positive organisms	*Staph. aureus*	Flucloxacillin 500 mg i.v. 6 hourly plus sodium fusidate 500 mg i.v. 8 hourly (erythromycin may be substituted for flucloxacillin in penicillin sensitive patients).
	Strep. pyogenes	*1st Choice:* Benzylpenicillin 600 mg i.v. 6 hourly *Alternative:* Erythromycin 500 mg i.v. 6 hourly
	Cl. welchii	*1st Choice:* Benzylpenicillin 600 mg i.v. 6 hourly. *Alternative:* Metronidazole 400 mg 8 hourly orally (or 1 g rectally) in penicillin allergy.

D. INFECTIVE ENDOCARDITIS

Bacteriological diagnosis is impossible once antibiotics have been given. Three sets of blood cultures must be taken BEFORE treatment is started.
The management of endocarditis requires expert laboratory advice as detailed sensitivity tests and serum assays are necessary. Intravenous therapy is recommended initially.

Treatment	*Strep. viridans* and related organisms	*1st Choice:* Benzylpenicillin 1.2 g i.v. 6 hourly for 6 weeks and i.v. gentamicin for 2 weeks. *Suitable Alternative:* Benzylpenicillin 1.2 g i.v. 6 hourly for two weeks followed by amoxycillin 500 mg 8 hourly orally for 4 weeks. If penicillin reaction develops erythromycin can be substituted.
	Strep. faecalis and related organisms	Benzylpenicillin or ampicillin i.v. plus gentamicin i.v. for 6 weeks.
	Other organisms	Seek laboratory advice.

E. OSTEOMYELITIS

Osteomyelitis	*Staph. aureus*	Prolonged treatment necessary, seek expert advice.

Table 19.4 (continued)

Clinical conditions	*Likely causative organism(s)*	*Suggested treatment*
		1st Choice: Initially flucloxacillin 500 mg i.v. 6 hourly plus sodium fusidate 500 mg i.v. 8 hourly. *Alternative:* Initially erythromycin 500 mg i.v. 6 hourly plus sodium fusidate 500 mg i.v. 8 hourly.
Osteomyelitis in children under 5 years	May be *H. influenzae* *Staph. aureus*	*1st Choice:* Amoxycillin plus flucloxacillin.
F. WOUND, SOFT TISSUE, SKIN AND SUPERFICIAL INFECTIONS		
Serious wound infection	Many possibilities including *Staph. aureus* *Strep. pyogenes* Anaerobic organisms (Coliforms) etc.	Before culture results available. *1st Choice:* Benzylpenicillin 600 mg i.m. or i.v. 6 hourly plus flucloxacillin 500 mg i.v. 6 hourly plus metronidazole 400 mg orally 8 hourly if anaerobes suspected. *Alternative:* Substitute erythromycin 500 mg i.v. 6 hourly for benzylpenicillin. Superficial wounds may require local antiseptic treatment only.
Erysipelas and cellulitis	*Strep. pyogenes*	*1st Choice:* Benzylpenicillin 600 mg i.m. or i.v. 6 hourly. *Alternative:* Erythromycin 500 mg i.v. 6 hourly.
Impetigo	*Staph. aureus and/or Strep. pyogenes*	*1st Choice:* Flucloxacillin 500 mg 6 hourly. *Alternative:* Erythromycin 500 mg 6 hourly. Avoid local antibiotics due to risk of sensitisation.
Boils	*Staph. aureus*	*1st Choice:* Flucloxacillin 500 mg 6 hourly plus sodium fusidate 500 mg 8 hourly. *Alternative:* Erythromycin 500 mg 6 hourly plus sodium fusidate 500 mg 8 hourly.

Table 19.4 (continued)

Clinical conditions	*Likely causative organism(s)*	*Suggested treatment*
G. GASTROINTESTINAL INFECTIONS AND ENTERIC FEVER		
Gastro-enteritis	*Salmonella* *Shigella*	No antibacterial treatment unless evidence of systemic spread or patient severely ill. Antibacterials prolong duration of carrier state in *Salmonella* infections. Maintain electrolyte and fluid balance.
	Campylobacter	Erythromycin 500 mg 6 hourly (only with prolonged symptoms).
Pseudomembranous enterocolitis (antibiotic associated)	Toxin of *Clostridium difficile*	Vancomycin 125 mg ORALLY 6 hourly for 5 days. Stop other antibiotics. A repeat course may be necessary.
Oral candidiasis.	*Candida*	Remove dentures (disinfect with sodium hypochlorite).
(a) Acute; adults		Nystatin 100 000 unit pastilles sucked (or 1 ml suspension) 6 hourly *or* amphotericin lozenges 10 mg sucked 6 hourly. Treat for 7 days.
(b) Chronic; adults		Nystatin as above *or* amphotericin lozenges 10 mg as above *or* miconazole oral gel 5 ml 6 hourly. Treat for 4 weeks.
(c) Acute; children		Miconazole oral gel; under 2 years 2.5 ml 12 hourly; 2–6 years 5 ml 12 hourly; over 6 years 5 ml 6 hourly. Hold in mouth as long as possible. Treat for 7 days.
Oesophageal and intestinal candidiasis	*Candida*	Amphotericin lozenges 10 mg 4 hourly. Or more effective, but more expensive, ketoconazole 200–400 mg orally daily.
Enteric fever	*Salmonella typhi* *Salmonella paratyphi* b, a and c	*1st Choice:* Chloramphenicol 500 mg 6 hourly. *Alternative:* Cotrimoxazole 2 tabs 12 hourly or amoxycillin. Do not treat carriers with chloramphenicol.
Acute cholecystitis	Coliforms *Strep. faecalis*	*1st Choice:* Ampicillin 500 mg i.v. 6 hourly plus gentamicin i.v.

Table 19.4 (continued)

Clinical conditions	*Likely causative organism(s)*	*Suggested treatment*
		Alternative: Cefuroxime 750 mg i.v. 8 hourly. Modify treatment if necessary when sensitivities are known.
H. BACTERIAL MENINGITIS		
Bacterial meningitis in adults and children (excluding neonates)	*N. meningitis*	Adults: Benzylpenicillin 1.2 g i.v. 4 hourly.
	Strep. pneumoniae	Adults: Benzylpenicillin 2.4 g i.v. 4 hourly. Children: 150 mg/kg/day given 4 hourly.
	H. influenzae	Adults: Chloramphenicol 1 g i.v. initially then 500 mg orally or i.v. 6 hourly.
	Before culture or smear results are known	*1st Choice:* Benzylpenicillin 1.2 g i.v. 4 hourly plus chloramphenicol 1 g initially i.v. then 500 mg i.v. or orally 6 hourly. *Alternatives:* Cefuroxime or cefotaxime in full doses are effective in the above types of bacterial meningitis. In penicillin-sensitive patients chloramphenicol alone.
Bacterial meningitis in neonates	Coliforms. Group B Streptococci Enterococci *Salmonella* *Listeria* etc.	Infants up to 3 weeks: *1st Choice:* Gentamicin i.v. and intrathecally plus benzylpenicillin i.v. *Alternative:* Cefotaxime (seek expert advice).

Sulphonamides

The sulphonamides are synthetic aromatic sulphanilamide derivatives. As antibacterial agents they have been largely replaced by the antibiotics, but they still retain certain useful clinical applications. They all act by interfering with folic acid synthesis from p-aminobenzoic acid (PABA) by competing with PABA for binding to tetrahydroxypteridine.

The sulphonamides all have a similar spectrum of activity, which includes:

Gram-positive organisms

Streptococcus viridans, pyogenes and *pneumoniae* but not *faecalis*.
Staphylococcus pyogenes (some strains)
Clostridia
Bacillus anthracis

Gram-negative organisms

All the enterobacteria such as *E. coli*, *Proteus*, *Salmonella*, *Klebsiella*, *Shigella* were originally sensitive: many have now acquired resistance.
Haemophilus influenzae (some strains)
Pseudomonas aeruginosa (some strains)
Pathogenic Neisseria (*gonococcus* and *meningococcus*)
but resistant strains are now common.

Other organisms

Nocardia
Actinomyces
Chlamydia
Plasmodium
Toxoplasma

The minimum inhibitory concentration for the various sulphonamides is different for each organism. Some examples are shown in Table 19.5 Thus sulphadiazine which is favoured in the USA for treating carriers of meningococcus is seen to be a better choice than sulphadimidine which is often used in the UK.

Table 19.5 Mean minimum inhibitory concentrations for some sulphonamides

	MIC (μg/ml)				
Drug	*Strep. pneumoniae*	*Staph. aureus*	*Meningococcus*	*E. coli*	*Proteus mirabilis*
Sulphadimidine	8	64	2	32	16
Sulphadiazine	16	32	0.25	8	16
Sulphamethoxazole	16	8	0.25	4	8

Resistance to these drugs can develop either by alterations in the target enzyme with decreased affinity for the sulphonamide relative to para-aminobenzoic acid or by decreased bacterial permeability to sulphonamide. Hospital strains of *Staphylococcus*, *Proteus* and *E. coli* are more likely to be resistant than organisms encountered in domiciliary practice. Resistant strains of gonococci have been known for many years, but resistant strains of meningococci only appeared in the 1960s.

The sulphonamides are bacteriostatic, but do not antagonise the bactericidal effect of penicillins. The combination of a sulphonamide with trimethoprim (as in cotrimoxazole) is bactericidal.

Pharmacokinetics The soluble sulphonamides are well absorbed from the intestine. After a dose of 2 g peak levels of about 100 μg/ml are reached in 2–4 h. The sodium salt of sulphadiazine can be given intravenously and sodium sulphadimidine can be injected intramuscularly. The plasma $t_{1/2}$s vary (see Table 19.6). Suphonamides may be divided into:

Table 19.6 Properties of some sulphonamides

Approved name	*Proprietary name*	$t_{1/2}(h)$	*Protein binding (%)*	*Dosage*	*Remarks*
Sulphamethizole	Urolucosil	1.2–2.6	85	100–200 mg 3–4 hourly	Urinary infection only
Sulphamethoxazole	Component of cotrimoxazole	7–14	68	See under cotrimoxazole	
Sulphadimidine		7–13	79	3 g initially up to 6 g daily in divided doses	General purpose Injection available
Sulphadiazine	Component of 'triple sulpha' mixture	14–25	45	3 g initially then up to 4 g daily	Injection for meningitis
Sulphamethoxypyridazine	Lederkyn, Midicel	24–48	92	1 g initially then 500 mg daily	
Sulphadoxine	Component of Fansidar	150	95		Used for malaria in combination (see p. 755)

(a) *Well-absorbed with short $t_{1/2}$* These include such general-purpose drugs as sulphadimidine and those with shorter $t_{1/2}$s such as sulphamethizole. These latter drugs have higher renal clearance so that high urinary concentrations of free drug result, although plasma concentrations suitable for the treatment of tissue infections (including renal tissue) may not be attained. These are used solely for urinary infections and the short $t_{1/2}$ requires dosage 4 hourly.

(b) *Well absorbed with long $t_{1/2}$* Highly protein bound, renally excreted with substantial tubular reabsorption. Sulphamethoxypyridazine is the only one now in use.

(c) *Poorly absorbed sulphonamides* Only 5–10% of these drugs are absorbed (thus making systemic toxicity possible) and most of the orally administered drug remains in the gut. Examples are phthalylsulphathiazole and succinylsulphathiazole, both of which hydrolyse to sulphathiazole.

(d) *Topically applied sulphonamides* Sulphacetamide is used in the eye, and marfanil, which is structurally different from other sulphonamides and is not cross-allergenic with them, has been employed for prophylaxis of infections in burns.

Plasma-protein binding varies between sulphonamides (Table 19.6). It is not true that the long-acting sulphonamides are necessarily more protein bound than short-acting ones and therefore less effective. Sulphonamides which are not highly bound enter the CSF at a concentration of 30–80% of the plasma level (sulphonamides must never be given intrathecally). Hypoalbuminaemia reduces protein binding, and displacement of the drugs from their binding sites occurs by oral anticoagulants, hypoglycaemic sulphonylureas and anti-inflammatory analgesics.

Sulphonamides undergo acetylation and conjugation with glucuronide in the liver. Acetylated sulphonamides are inactive, more protein bound, undergo more rapid renal clearance and are less soluble in water than sulphonamides. This can produce renal problems (see below). Acetylation of some sulphonamides, e.g. sulphadimidine, is subject to pharmacogenetic variation and individuals with slow acetylation phenotype derive more benefit and less toxicity from such sulphonamides than rapid acetylators. Slow acetylators may acetylate as little as 10% of the dose of sulphonamide compared to 60–70% by rapid acetylators. Sulphonamides are filtered at the glomerulus but some may undergo tubular reabsorption, tubular secretion or both reabsorption and secretion, these factors influencing the $t_{1/2}$. The urinary pH affects the renal clearance of all sulphonamides and their metabolites, being increased by alkalinisation. The lower the pKa (most lie between 5 and 7) the greater the reduction in tubular reabsorption (see Chapter 1). Elimination is therefore slower at night when acid urine is produced.

Renal impairment has a variable effect on sulphonamide kinetics, depending upon the renal handling of the drug. Hepatic insufficiency impairs metabolism and conjugation and excretion is reduced because unconjugated sulphonamide is less rapidly excreted.

Clinical uses Currently the main use of sulphonamides is the treatment of uncomplicated urinary tract infections and in prophylaxis of recurrent infections. i.v. sulphadiazine is now only rarely used (with benzylpenicillin) in the treatment of meningococcal meningitis since sulphonamide-resistant meningococci are common.

Sulphonamides are not now used in the treatment of gut infections or for the pre-operative sterilisation of the intestine. These drugs are used for the treatment of nocardiosis and (with pyrimethamine) for toxoplasmosis. Local treatment with sulphacetamide is still employed for infective conjunctivitis—particularly in the newborn and for chlamydial infections, although bacterial conjunctivitis is mainly treated with local chloramphenicol.

Mafenide is used as a local application to burns. It is not inactivated by p-aminobenzoic acid in tissue fluid. Mafenide is active against a wide range of organisms including *Pseudomonas aeruginosa*. Sulphapyridine in low doses over prolonged periods may control dermatitis herpetiformis.

Adverse effects With currently used sulphonamides methaemoglobinaemia, nausea, headache and dizziness are uncommon. Serious toxic effects are: renal damage, allergy, haematological changes, agranulocytosis, haemolytic anaemia.

The sulphonamides vary in their solubility and sulphadiazine, having a low solubility, is more likely to precipitate in the kidneys or ureters. The acetyl derivative is even less soluble and carries a greater risk of crystalluria. An early sign of this complication is haematuria, but anuria may rapidly follow. Renal blockage by sulphonamides can be prevented by using soluble sulphonamides such as sulphafurazole, by increasing the fluid intake and alkalinising the urine.

About 1% of patients taking sulphonamides develop an allergic rash. This is usually morbilliform, but may also be urticarial and is frequently accompanied by fever. There is complete cross allergenicity within the group. The Stevens–Johnson syndrome is a form of erythema multiforme with a high mortality rate. It is rare and most often associated with highly protein-bound long-acting drugs.

Haematological changes due to sulphonamides are rare but they can produce haemolytic anaemia in patients with glucose 6-phosphate dehydrogenase deficiency (see p. 111) and very rarely bone-marrow depression.

Although jaundice due to liver damage is rare, in the newborn sulphonamides can displace bilirubin from protein-binding sites and produce kernicterus. Even when taken by the mother before delivery, enough can enter the fetus to produce this complication post-natally.

Trimethoprim (Trimopan; Ipral)

Trimethoprim is a synthetic aromatic base which competitively inhibits bacterial dihydrofolate reductase and therefore interferes with conversion of dihydrofolate into the biochemically active tetrahydrofolate. Trimethoprim has an affinity for the bacterial enzyme which is 50 000 times that for human dihydrofolate reductase (Fig. 19.3). It is bacteriostatic against a similarly wide spectrum of Gram-negative and positive organisms to the sulphonamides, although it is several times more active than those drugs against most strains, the MICs ranging from 0.2 to 2 μg/ml for common pathogens. Trimethoprim

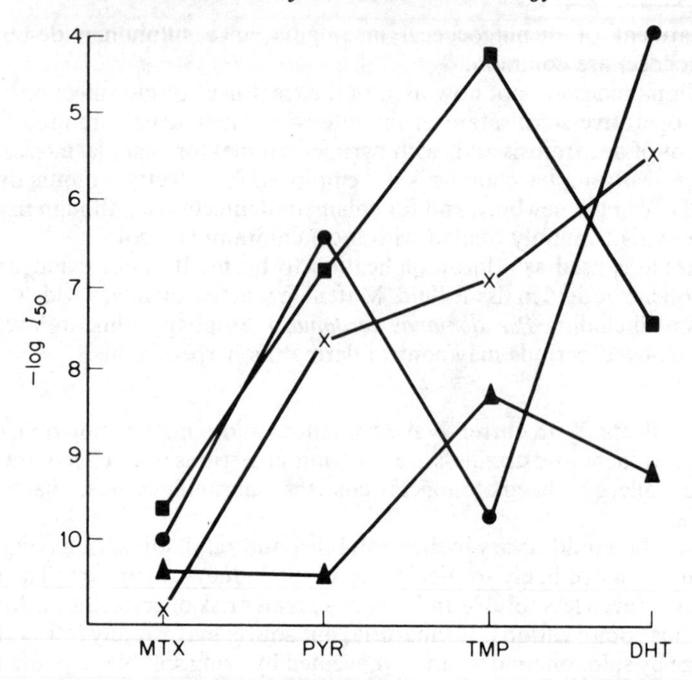

Fig. 19.3 Concentrations of inhibitors (MTX – methotrexate; PYR – pyrimethamine; TMP – trimethoprim; DHT – an experimental triazine DHFR inhibitor) expressed in moles/litre to produce 50% inhibition of dihydrofolate reductase (DHFR) from man (■); *E. coli* (●); *Plasmodium* (▲) and a trypanosome (x). (From G. H. Hitchings, *Postgrad. Med. J.*, **45,** 8 (suppl.) (1969).)

resistance is at present uncommon and is gained by bacterial acquisition of a different dihydrofolate reductase which will not bind trimethoprim.

Pharmacokinetics Trimethoprim is almost completely absorbed from the gut. After a dose of 100 mg a peak plasma level of 0.9–1.2 μg/ml is reached after $1\frac{1}{2}$–$3\frac{1}{2}$ h. About 45% is protein bound. The plasma $t_{1/2}$ is 6–12 h and more than 90% of the drug is excreted unchanged in the urine. High concentrations of active drug are present in the urine: usually 50–100 μg/ml.

Clinical use Trimethoprim is used only for urinary infections, the dose for an acute attack being 200 mg twice daily and for prophylaxis 100 mg nocte.

Adverse effects are uncommon: Nausea, vomiting and diarrhoea occasionally occur. Folate deficiency is rarely produced—usually in patients with low folate stores.

Cotrimoxazole (Septrin, Bactrim)

Addition of a sulphonamide to trimethoprim produces considerable potentiation as shown by the isobologram (see Fig. 19.1) and Table 19.7.

Table 19.7 Potentiation of effect of trimethoprim by addition of sulphonamide

× 2–8 *Potentiation*	× 16–64 *Potentiation*
Staph. aureus	*N. gonorrhoeae*
Strep. pyogenes	*Proteus mirabilis*
Strep. pneumoniae	
H. influenzae	
E. coli	
Klebsiella spp.	
Salmonella spp.	
Shigella spp.	

The degree of potentiation depends upon the ratio of sulphonamide to trimethoprim and is maximal when in the ratio of the respective MICs for the drugs for a particular organism. For a range of common pathogens this is usually about 20 : 1, sulphonamide : trimethoprim. For cotrimoxazole, sulphamethoxazole was chosen as the sulphonamide component because it has a similar $t_{1/2}$ to trimethoprim, although the distribution of the two drugs in the body differs, since trimethoprim is present in higher concentrations in the tissues than in the blood. Tablets of cotrimoxazole contain 400 mg sulphamethoxazole and 80 mg trimethoprim, this 5 : 1 ratio attaining the optimum 20 : 1 ratio in the blood following distribution of the drugs in the body. The $t_{1/2}$ of the components is about 10 h, so that steady state is not achieved for some 60–70 h on the recommended dosage of 2 tablets twice daily. In tissue or respiratory infections a loading dose of 4 tablets might be more rational in order to attain effective plasma and tissue levels more rapidly.

Apart from potentiation, another benefit of using the combined drugs is that lower doses of each may be given, thus reducing the incidence of side effects. When both drugs are given together the effect may be bactericidal. Although it is unknown how this effect is achieved, one factor may be the sequential blockade of tetrahydrofolate synthesis by the two components (Fig. 19.4).

This sequential effect may also be responsible for slowing the development of resistance in organisms sensitive to both sulphonamide and trimethoprim. However, when an organism is originally resistant to sulphonamides, resistance to trimethoprim may occur during cotrimoxazole treatment. With trimethoprim-sensitive but sulphonamide-resistant bacteria, no synergy occurs between the drugs, although resistance to sulphonamide or trimethoprim does not prevent successful treatment with cotrimoxazole.

Clinical uses (see Table 19.8) Cotrimoxazole is widely used in clinical practice (Table 19.8), most commonly for urinary and respiratory infections, the usual dose being two tablets twice daily. It can be given intramuscularly 960 mg (3 ml of i.m. preparation) 12 hourly or by intravenous infusion (expensive!). It has also been used successfully in low dosage (one tablet at night or on alternate nights) over long periods in the control of chronic bacteriuria.

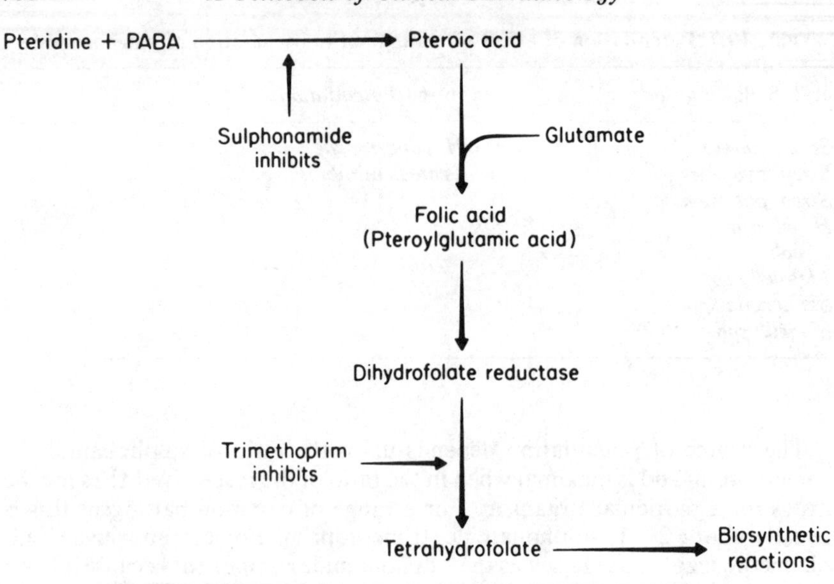

Fig. 19.4 Synthesis of tetrahydrofolate and effects of sulphonamides and trimethoprim.

Table 19.8 Clinical indications for cotrimoxazole

A. *First line drug*
1. Urinary tract infections
2. Respiratory tract infections
3. Prostatitis
4. Pneumocystis (high dose required)

B. *Second line drug*
1. Enteric fever
   (a) Acute typhoid and carrier state
   (b) Paratyphoid
2. Gonorrhoea
3. Cholera
4. Brucellosis
5. Toxoplasmosis
6. Nocardiosis (high dose required)

Cotrimoxazole should not be used in severe renal impairment (clearance < 15 ml/min) and in reduced dosage with clearances of 15–30 ml/min. Occasionally in these cases it causes a deterioration of renal function.

Adverse effects The toxicity of cotrimoxazole can be that of each component or of the components acting together to produce an adverse effect. Despite interference with folate metabolism at two sites. haematological adverse reactions are rare. Those reported include aplastic anaemia, agranulocytosis, thrombocytopenia and megaloblastic anaemia. Patients with borderline folate deficiency (e.g. those on anticonvulsant therapy or in pregnancy) are at greater risk of developing the later complication.

Antifolate compounds are known teratogens (see p. 148) and although this combination has been used without hazard in pregnancy, it should be avoided in this circumstance if possible.

Patients with AIDS frequently develop fever, malaise, rashes and cytopenia when being treated with high doses of cotrimoxazole for pneumocystis.

The presence of sulphonamide in the mixture should always be remembered because patients sensitive to this component will suffer adverse effects.

Dapsone and Solapsone

These sulphones are related to sulphonamides but are more effective than these drugs in the treatment of leprosy. The mode of action may be similar to sulphonamides since para-aminobenzoic acid antagonises their bacteriostatic effect. Dapsone is also used (as are some sulphonamides such as sulphapyridine) in the treatment of dermatitis herpetiformis, although this is not an infection and the mechanism of action of these drugs is unknown. Dapsone is well absorbed from the gastro-intestinal tract and distributes throughout the tissues. The $t_{1/2}$ is approximately 20 h and 70–80% is excreted in the urine free or as metabolites, although biliary secretion with an enterohepatic circulation also occurs. It is metabolised, like sulphonamides, by polymorphic acetylation (q.v.), slow acetylators having a higher risk of haematological abnormalities.

The main adverse effect is allergic dermatitis, but agranulocytosis, methaemoglobinaemia and haemolytic anaemia (in glucose 6-phosphate dehydrogenase-deficient subjects) also occur.

Leprosy treatment is lengthy, even after 5 years one half of lepromatous patients have positive smears. Dapsone may also have a prophylactic effect against leprosy.

β-Lactam antibiotics

This is the largest group of antibiotics. It has the common feature of a four-membered β-lactam ring in the nucleus (Fig. 19.5). On this common basic structure a number of distinct families of antibiotics have been and are being produced:

All the β-lactam antibiotics produce their antibacterial effect by interfering with bacterial cell wall synthesis.

Unfortunately the β-lactam ring can be broken and the antibiotic inactivated by a series of enzymes called β-lactamases. These enzymes can be produced by a variety of gram-positive and gram-negative bacteria. The genetic coding for their production is usually transmitted by plasmids. By substituting in the side chain it has proved possible to produce penicillins which are resistant to β-lactamase produced by gram-positive but not gram-negative organisms. Many of the newer cephalosporins and other recent β-lactam introductions however are resistant to β-lactamases, even those produced by gram-negative organisms.

Table 19.9 Uses and dosage of some penicillins

Approved name	*Proprietary name*	*Main indication*	*Adult dosage*
Benzylpenicillin	—	Serious infections requiring parenteral administration e.g. bacterial endocarditis; meningitis	Variable 0.3–12 g (0.5–20 megaunits) daily in divided doses or infusion.
Procaine penicillin	—	Depot preparation	300–900 mg i.m. daily
Phenoxymethylpenicillin	—	General-purpose oral drug	250 mg 6 hourly
Flucloxacillin	Floxapen	Staphylococcal infection	250 mg 6 hourly oral or i.m.
Ampicillin	Penbritin	Gram-negative infections of urinary and respiratory tract, otitis media	250–500 mg 6 hourly oral, i.v. or i.m.
Amoxycillin	Amoxil	As ampicillin	250 mg 8 hourly oral, i.v. or i.m.
Piperacillin	Pipril	Serious infections with Gram-negative organisms	100–300 mg/kg daily
Azlocillin	Securopen	particularly *Pseudomonas* infections.	2–5 g 8 hourly
Carfecillin	Uticillin	Certain lower urinary tract infections	0.5–1 g 8 hourly oral
Pivmecillinam	Selexid	Ampicillin-resistant urinary tract infections	200–400 mg 6–8 hourly oral

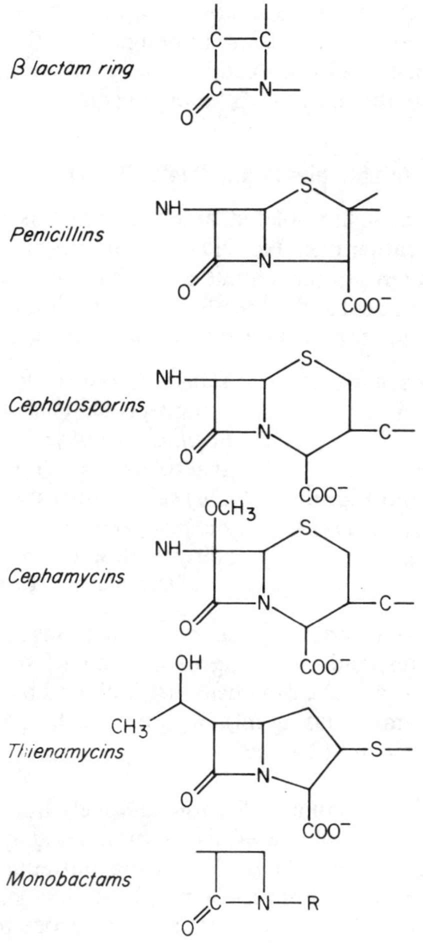

β lactam ring

Penicillins

Cephalosporins

Cephamycins

Thienamycins

Monobactams

Fig. 19.5 Beta-lactam structures.

An alternative method of dealing with the problem of enzyme degradation of the antibiotic is to combine it with a β-lactamase inhibitor. This has been done with:

amoxycillin + clavulanic acid (Augmentin)
ampicillin + sulbactam

This has proved successful in trials and is a method potentially capable of extension to other β-lactam antibiotics. The penicillin nucleus, produced by the mould *Penicillium notatum*, consists of fused thiazolidine and lactam rings. A range of antimicrobial penicillins can be made by adding different side chains to this nucleus. Penicillins act by preventing cross-linkage formation in the mucopeptide backbone of the bacterial cell wall and the bacteria therefore cannot survive osmotic and mechanical injuries. In addition, inhibition of enzymes responsible for formation of the septum across a dividing organism results in inhibition of cell division, although the cell continues to elongate, producing a filamentous form. Autolytic bacterial enzymes are also partially responsible for the dissolution of the organisms.

Benzylpenicillin (soluble penicillin, Penicillin G)

This was the first penicillin isolated, and it still remains one of the most useful antibiotics. It is a rather unstable acid and is used clinically as the more stable sodium or potassium salt (crystalline penicillin). Benzylpenicillin is 60–70% destroyed by gastric acid and is therefore usually administered parenterally. It is the drug of choice for the treatment of infections with:

- group A β-haemolytic streptococci
- pneumococci
- meningococci
- gonococci—most strains
- *Streptococcus viridans*—most strains
- *Staphylococcus pyogenes** (non-penicillinase producing)
- *Bacillus anthracis*
- anaerobes, including *Clostridium welchii*
- *Corynebacterium diphtheriae*
- *Actinomycetes spp.*
- spirochaetes, *T. pallidum*, *L. icterohaemorrhagiae*

The dosage of penicillins is often expressed in terms of the international unit (I.U.) which corresponds to 0.6 μg of a standard sodium benzylpenicillin preparation. Most sensitive organisms are inhibited by concentrations of the order of 0.06 unit/ml (0.035 μg/ml), but some, such as *Strep. faecalis*, require as much as 3.5 units/ml (2 μg/ml).

Pharmacokinetics Penicillin is distributed widely but unevenly throughout the body, the apparent volume of distribution being approximately 50% of body weight. The $t_{1/2}$ is 30 min. Following intramuscular injection peak plasma levels are reached within 15–30 min. After an injection of 300 000 units, the peak is normally about 8 units/ml and this drops to 0.5 units/ml at 2 h. Diabetic patients absorb penicillin poorly from intramuscular and subcutaneous sites. About 65% is bound to plasma albumin. The drug does not readily enter the cerebrospinal fluid, but inflammation of the meninges or fever greatly facilitates penetration into the cerebrospinal fluid. Injection of penicillin (usually 10 000 to 20 000 units) into the subarachnoid space produces an immediate high concentration in the cerebrospinal fluid, which falls rapidly at first and then more slowly over 24 h.

Only a small fraction of administered penicillin is metabolised by the tissues. The small amount of 6-aminopenicillanic acid in the urine is due to bacterial breakdown in the gut and its subsequent absorption and renal excretion. 60–90% of penicillin is excreted in the urine unchanged within 6 h of administration. A small amount is excreted in the bile. Anuria prolongs the $t_{1/2}$ to about 10 h. This results in high blood levels and up to 10% compensatory

* 90% of *Staphylococcus pyogenes* found in hospitals are penicillinase producers and thus resistant.

inactivation per hour by the liver. Combined renal failure and impaired hepatic function increases the $t_{1/2}$ to 30 h, although isolated hepatic dysfunction is without effect on penicillin pharmacokinetics. As 90 % is normally excreted by the renal tubules, a reduction in GFR does not greatly impair excretion. The presence of other organic acids (e.g. probenecid, which interferes with tubular acid transport) impairs renal penicillin excretion. In addition to affecting renal secretion of the penicillins, probenecid also decreases their apparent volume of distribution, presumably due to limitation of the accessibility of some outer tissue compartments to penicillin. Thus there is a greater amount of penicillin confined to the central compartment (which includes plasma). It is now rarely used to prolong the $t_{1/2}$ of penicillin.

Table 19.10 Clinical indications for benzylpenicillin or phenoxymethylpenicillin

1. Lancefield group A streptococcal infections, e.g. erysipelas, scarlet fever
2. Prophylaxis of rheumatic fever
3. Bacterial endocarditis due to sensitive *Strep. viridans*
4. Lobar pneumonia, i.e. *Strep. pneumoniae*
5. Infections due to non-penicillinase producing staphylococci
6. Acute otitis media in adults, i.e. not due to *H. influenzae*
7. Meningococcal infections
8. Puerperal sepsis
9. Tetanus and gas gangrene
10. Syphilis and yaws (long-acting penicillin preparation, e.g. procaine or benzathine penicillin used)
11. Gonorrhoea
12. Diphtheria
13. Anthrax
14. Actinomycosis

Adverse effects Penicillin is of low toxicity but in high concentrations it can produce an encephalopathy manifesting as convulsions, coma, neurological sequelae or death. This may occur if over 50 000 units are given intrathecally or following intramuscular administration of a standard dose in a patient with anuria. A large intravenous dose may provoke fits in patients with renal insufficiency. Haemolytic anaemia is a rare complication of high doses. Hypersensitivity is the commonest toxic effect of all penicillins and may manifest as:

A. Immediate anaphylactic reactions. These are rare, but fatal in about 10 % of patients. The incidence is around 1 in 100 000 administrations, and parenteral penicillin is responsible in most cases, although oral penicillins may also produce this effect.
B. Serum sickness. This manifests as fever, malaise, urticaria, rashes, arthralgia and angioneurotic oedema or erythema nodosum is seen in up to 5 % of patients occasionally accompanied by leucopenia. Rarely, fatal exfoliative dermatitis or the Stevens–Johnson syndrome occurs. Usually these reactions happen about a week or ten days after beginning penicillin but accelerated reactions (within 48 h) are described in previously sensitised individuals.

The major antigen from penicillin is the penicilloyl group although the breakdown products, penicillamine and penicilloic acid, can also be involved. These substances act as haptens either combining with large tissue molecules or forming polymers.

In addition to the reactions described above which are probably true allergies, maculopapular rashes are common with ampicillin, particularly in patients with infective mononucleosis or chronic lymphocytic leukaemia. It is thought that in this reaction other mechanisms are involved.

A careful history (and up to 10% of the population give a positive history) is the best prevention. Laboratory and skin tests may be unreliable as predictors of penicillin allergy. In patients with a history of a penicillin reaction alternative drugs such as erythromycin or clindamycin may be used. Cephalosporins show cross-reactions in penicillin-sensitive patients in about 10% of patients.

Prolongation of penicillin blood level

1. **Probenecid** in a daily dose of about 2 g blocks tubular secretion of penicillin, and may double and prolong penicillin blood levels (see above). Dyspepsia and rashes are not uncommon with this drug.

2. **Procaine penicillin G** is an equimolecular mixture of procaine and benzylpenicillin, and is injected intramuscularly as a slowly dissolving crystalline suspension. This produces a peak plasma level at 1–3 h and usual doses (300 000 units) remain effective for up to 48 h. Rarely signs of procaine intoxication (which includes convulsions, hypotension and psychosis) may appear.

3. **Benzathine penicillin G** gives detectable blood levels for more than 3 weeks. A single intramuscular injection of 1.2 million units produces a plasma concentration of about 0.15 units/ml on the first day, 0.03 units/ml on the 14th day and 0.003 units/ml on the 23rd day. It is therefore useful for prophylaxis (e.g. yaws) rather than treatment of acute infections.

Orally active alternatives to benzylpenicillin

Benzylpenicillin is largely destroyed in the stomach but about 30% of an oral dose is absorbed by the small intestine. In young infants and the elderly, more is absorbed because of low gastric acidity. A group of acid-stable orally active penicillins, the phenoxypenicillins, has been developed. These have much the same properties as benzylpenicillins, including inactivation by penicillinase, but are slightly less effective against susceptible organisms.

Phenoxymethylpenicillin (Penicillin V) is acid-stable and absorbed from the upper part of the small intestine, absorption being enhanced by food. It has an identical antibacterial spectrum to benzylpenicillin, but whilst the sensitivity of staphylococci and streptococci is similar to both drugs, penicillin V is inferior to benzylpenicillin for any Gram-negative infection, including the gonococcus. **Phenethicillin** is similar to phenoxymethylpenicillin but is better absorbed.

Table 19.11 Some properties of orally active penicillins

Drug	*Protein binding (%)*	*Blood level of free drug at 1 h after 250 mg in μg/ml*	*Activity factor concn. of free drug/MIC*	
			Staph.	*Strep.*
Phenoxymethyl-penicillin	81.8	0.36	6.0	24
Phenethicillin	76.4	0.64	10.7	21.3

The last column of Table 19.11 shows the free concentration of antibiotic relative to the minimum inhibitory concentration for staphylococci (where phenethicillin appears to be most active) and for streptococci (where phenoxymethylpenicillin is most effective).

Oral penicillins provide a convenient treatment for less severe streptococcal, staphylococcal and pneumococcal infections or those which have responded to initial parenteral penicillin. They are also used in prophylaxis of streptococcal infections in patients who have had rheumatic fever.

Penicillinase-resistant penicillins

Some staphylococci are resistant to benzylpenicillin because they produce a penicillinase which disrupts the β-lactam ring. In penicillinase-resistant penicillins the access of this enzyme to the β-lactam is hindered by the molecular geometry of the drug. These are all semi-synthetic penicillins and include methicillin and the isoxazolyl penicillins such as cloxacillin, flucloxacillin and oxacillin.

1. Cloxacillin (Orbenin) is acid stable and so absorbed after oral administration. It can also be given parenterally. Absorption from the gut is incomplete (usually 30–50 %). When given orally on an empty stomach, 1 g of cloxacillin produces a peak level of 5–10 μg/ml plasma in 1 h. The MIC against staphylococci of both cloxacillin and flucloxacillin is 0.25 μg/ml.

2. Flucloxacillin (Floxapen) is similar to cloxacillin but better absorbed by mouth, giving approximately double the plasma levels produced by equivalent doses of cloxacillin. Both drugs are highly protein bound (94 %), so that the higher levels attained by flucloxacillin make it dose for dose the more effective of the two drugs. The $t_{1/2}$ is 0.8 h. Elimination is partly renal and partly hepatic. Reduced dosage is not necessary with impaired renal function.

3. Methicillin (Celbenin) is destroyed by gastric acid and has to be given by injection. It can occasionally cause interstitial nephritis and is now rarely used.

Complete cross-resistance exists between these three penicillinase-resistant penicillins.

Although effective against penicillinase-producing staphylococci, it must be stressed that these penicillins are far less effective against other bacterial species than benzylpenicillin. Their use is therefore confined to the penicillinase-producing staphylococci (which includes about 90% of hospital-acquired staphylococcal infections). Therefore any serious infection such as septic arthritis, lung abscess, or acute osteomyelitis should be treated with one of these drugs, and in serious infections they should be given by injection as absorption is variable.

Broad-spectrum penicillins

The low degree of activity of benzylpenicillin against most Gram-negative organisms (except gonococci and meningococci) stimulated the production of the broad-spectrum penicillins. However, these are all inactivated by penicillinase.

1. Ampicillin (Penbritin)

Ampicillin diffuses into Gram-negative bacteria more readily than benzylpenicillin and its spectrum includes many strains of *E. coli*, *Proteus mirabilis*, *Strep. faecalis*, *H. influenzae* and *Salmonella*. Coliforms, and more recently *H. influenzae*, may develop resistance, and indiscriminate use has played a part in this change. It is destroyed by staphylococcal penicillinase. Its main uses are in chest and urinary tract infections, otitis media and meningitis (see Table 19.12). Ampicillin has little place in the treatment of acute typhoid, but may eradicate the carrier state because of high drug levels in the bile. This drug should be used with discrimination for urinary tract infections because of the rapid increase in the incidence of resistant *E. coli*.

Table 19.12 Clinical indications for broad-spectrum penicillins

A. *Treatment of first choice*
1. Acute and chronic bronchitis and bronchopneumonia
2. Acute otitis media in young children (i.e. *H. influenzae* is likely pathogen)
3. Biliary tract infections (*E. coli* and *Strep. faecalis*)
4. Prevention of bacterial endocarditis (amoxycillin)

B. *Treatment of second line*
1. Enteric fever when chloramphenicol or cotrimoxazole unsuitable
2. Urinary tract infections when cotrimoxazole is contraindicated

Pharmacokinetics It is amphoteric and therefore ionised at all pHs, resulting in poor and slow oral absorption. The presence of food in the stomach delays absorption further. The $t_{1/2}$ is $1\text{–}1\frac{1}{2}$ h and it distributes into about 40% of body weight. An oral dose of 0.5 g produces peak levels of about 3 μg/ml in 2 h. The drug is detectable in the plasma for only about 4 h. About 25% of an oral dose and 70% of a parenteral dose appears in the urine within 6 h. Ampicillin appears in the bile and undergoes enterohepatic circulation. Ampicillin is usually given in doses of 250–500 mg six hourly. It can also be given by i.m. or i.v. injection.

Adverse effects Rashes with ampicillin are common (7% incidence) and often develop later than with benzylpenicillin, sometimes appearing 3–6 days after the drug is stopped. Rashes are commoner in patients suffering from glandular fever or lymphatic leukaemia or those receiving allopurinol. They may be urticarial as are other penicillin rashes but are more commonly erythematous.

Gastrointestinal disturbances (usually diarrhoea) occur in about 5% of patients on ampicillin.

2. Ampicillin pro-drugs: Talampicillin, Bacampicillin and Pivampicillin

These esters of ampicillin are hydrolysed in the intestinal mucosa and portal system to ampicillin. Esterification masks one of the polar groups of ampicillin so that there is a pH range at which the drug is un-ionised and so better absorbed (90%) than ampicillin. The serum levels are approximately twice those from an equivalent dose of ampicillin and absorption is less influenced by food. A consequence of better absorption is said to be a lower incidence of gastrointestinal side effects. The whole of the absorbed dose is excreted as ampicillin in the urine. These drugs can only be used orally since they may be toxic if given parenterally, and the unhydrolysed drugs have no antibacterial activity. They are expensive.

3. Amoxycillin (Amoxil)

This has a different structure to ampicillin and a slightly different mode of action since it inhibits side-wall synthesis by bacteria-producing lysis, whereas ampicillin inhibits end-wall synthesis producing filamentous forms. It shares the same spectrum as ampicillin but is more active against *Strep. faecalis* and *Salmonella spp.* The important difference is that it is better absorbed than ampicillin. When an oral dose of 250 mg is given, average peak levels of 4 μg/ml plasma are reached in 2 h. The $t_{1/2}$ of amoxycillin and protein binding (20%) are the same as for ampicillin, but because of more complete absorption amoxycillin can be detected in the blood for twice as long. After an oral dose, 60% is excreted unchanged in the urine. The drug also penetrates bronchial secretions more effectively than ampicillin.

Amoxycillin frequently produces rashes in patients suffering from infectious mononucleosis similar to those seen during ampicillin treatment. The incidence of gastrointestinal side effects with amoxycillin is 70% less than with ampicillin.

Amoxycillin is given orally in doses of 250 mg eight hourly. In severe infections this can be increased to 500 mg six hourly. To prevent bacterial endocarditis 3.0 g can be given orally 1 hour before operation. To treat simple urinary infection 3.0 g can be given followed in 12 h by a further 3.0 g. In purulent lung infection (i.e. bronchiectasis) 3.0 g 12-hourly has proved useful.

4. Mecillinam and Pivmecillinam (Selexid)

Mecillinam is a member of the amidinopenicillins, in which there is an amidino group at the 6 position instead of an amino group. It is not, therefore, a true penicillin, although it acts on the bacterial cell wall. It has a totally different spectrum of activity, being highly active against Gram-negative organisms but much less active against Gram-positive species. Thus *E. coli* (including many ampicillin-resistant strains), *Klebsiella*, *Shigella* and *Salmonella* species are sensitive but *Pseudomonas aeruginosa*, *Neisseria* and *Haemophilus* are resistant. Mecillinam can be destroyed by some but not all strains producing β-lactamase. The $t_{1/2}$ is 1.5 h and it is only 5–10% protein bound. It is eliminated in the urine, so that dosage adjustment is required in renal failure. It is useful in urinary tract infections. Mecillinam can only be given parenterally and the pro-drug pivmecillinam (the pivaloyl ester) is available for oral use. This is well absorbed from the gut and hydrolysed to pivalic acid, formaldehyde (which is oxidised to formic acid mainly by erythrocytes) and mecillinam. Pivmecillinam itself is microbiologically inactive but is toxic if injected into animals so that the preliminary hydrolysis in the gut is essential. The dose of pivmecillinam is 200 mg 6 or 8 hourly in urinary tract infections and 1.2–2.4 g daily for Salmonella infections. Adverse effects are uncommon and consist mainly of anorexia, nausea, vomiting and indigestion. It should be avoided in patients with penicillin or cephalosporin hypersensitivity since it has a β-lactam ring and cross-reaction is possible. Its safety in pregnancy has not been established.

5. β-Lactamase inhibitors

Bacterial resistance to the penicillins including ampicillin, amoxycillin and the antipseudomonal agents and some cephalosporins is commonly due to bacterial production of β-lactamase, an enzyme which hydrolyses the β-lactam ring of these antibiotics and renders them inactive.

Substances are now available which inhibit β-lactamase activity. There are however, many different β-lactamases and not all of them can be inactivated in this way.

Augmentin is a mixture of amoxycillin and clavulanic acid. The addition of this β-lactamase inhibitor results in amoxycillin being effective against most strains of penicillin/amoxycillin resistant *Staph. aureus* and resistant strains of *H. influenzae*, *Kl. aerogenes*, *N. gonorrhoeae*, *Bacteroides spp* and many resistant strains of *E. coli*. It is not effective against penicillin resistant *Strep. pneumoniae*. The main use for Augmentin will probably be for respiratory and urinary infections due to a resistant organism.

Pharmacokinetics A tablet of Augmentin contains 250 mg of amoxycillin and 125 mg of clavulanic acid. Both drugs reach peak plasma levels about one hour after oral administration and both have a $t_{1/2}$ of 1 h. Clavenulate is partly excreted in the urine but about 30% of the drug is metabolised. Tissue penetration is good but only low concentrations reach the CSF.

Adverse effects Nausea and occasional vomiting and diarrhoea. Otherwise as for ampicillin/amoxycillin.

Sulbactam/Ampicillin is a similar combination with much the same antibacterial spectrum. Sulbactam has the same absorption and elimination characteristics as ampicillin and its clinical usage would be similar to augmentin.

6. Broad spectrum antipseudomonal penicillins

Azlocillin   Piperacillin
Carbenicillin   Ticarcillin
Mezlocillin

These are broad spectrum semi-synthetic penicillins. Some like azlocillin belong to the class of ureidopenicillins. They are mainly used for treating *Pseudomonas aeruginosa* and other Gram-negative infections.

All these drugs possess similar Gram-positive and -negative spectra and have modest activity against *Bacteroides spp.* All are, however, susceptible to inactivation by β-lactamases and as a result some strains of *Staph. aureus*, *Haemophilus influenzae*, *E. coli* and *B. fragilis* are resistant. Table 19.13 compares their efficacy against a number of Gram-negative organisms. It should be remembered, however, that comparative tables depend to some degree on the populations of organism which are examined. The main characteristics of these drugs are given in Table 19.14. They are largely excreted via the kidney and reduced dose is required with impaired renal function.

Table 19.13

	Azlocillin	*Carbenicillin*	*Mezlocillin*	*Piperacillin*	*Ticarcillin*
Ps. aeruginosa	++	+	+	++	+
E. coli	−	+	+	+	+
Klebsiella	+	−	+	+	−
B. fragilis	+	+	+	+	+
Proteus spp.	++	++	++	++	++
Serratia spp.	−	+	+	++	+
Strep. faecalis	++	++	++	++	++

Key: ++ Highly active against most strains
+ Active against some, but not all, strains
− Inactive or poorly active

Table 19.14

Drug	*Daily dose by injection*	$t_{1/2}$	*Sodium content of daily dose*
Azlocillin	15 g daily at 8 hrly intervals.	1 h	15 g = 33 mmol
Carbenicillin	30 g daily at 4 hrly intervals	1 h	30 g = 163 mmol
Mezlocillin	15–20 g daily at 6–8 hrly intervals	1 h	20 g = 37 mmol
Piperacillin	4 g every 4–6 hours	1 h	16 g = 32 mmol
Ticarcillin	15–20 g daily at 4–8 hrly intervals	1.4 h	20 g = 107 mmol

Indications These penicillins should be reserved for treatment of severe systemic infections, usually by Gram-negative organisms, particularly *Pseudomonas*. They should not be used as general purpose broad-spectrum antibiotics or to treat staphylococcal infections.

Azlocillin is perhaps the most effective against *Pseudomonas* infection and piperacillin has the best overall activity against Gram-negative infections. Carbenicillin has now been superseded.

They can be combined with an aminoglycoside and the combination may be synergistic. However, they should not be mixed in the same container as an aminoglycoside since inactivation will occur.

They have also been used in combination with cephalosporins but this is more controversial. They are expensive drugs.

Adverse effects There is cross-sensitivity with other penicillins and sometimes with cephalosporins. Occasionally gastrointestinal disturbance and transient neutropenia occurs.

7. Pro-drug esters of carbenicillin

Carfecillin can be used when an oral preparation is required for urinary infections since other anti-pseudomonal penicillins are absorbed from the gut. Following a dose of 1 g carfecillin the peak plasma level does not exceed 10 μg/ml and gastrointestinal intolerance limits the oral dose so that the plasma levels which can be achieved are too low to treat systemic infections, although the urinary concentration is sufficient for treatment of susceptible pathogens. The need for this drug is thus confined to urinary infections with sensitive *Pseudomonas* or *Proteus* species. It should never be used indiscriminately for any urinary infection because this could lead to increased resistance in the bacterial population not only to carbenicillin but also to ampicillin and related compounds.

The cephalosporins

The cephalosporins are more widely used in the USA than in the UK. Until recently they were rarely considered as the antibiotic of first choice and even now their use is relatively limited.

In spite of this, there are now large numbers of these antibiotics available and it is useful to divide them into *first*, *second* and *third* generation cephalosporins. The later introductions are less toxic, more stable to β-lactamases and their range of activity in terms of Gram-negative organisms has been extended. However, many of them are less effective against Gram-positive organisms than the older drugs. It is perhaps worth noting that no cephalosporin shows useful activity against *Strep. faecalis*.

Against their widespread use is the fact that most of them have to be given parenterally and the newer ones are expensive.

The antimicrobial range of these groups differs and each generation will therefore be considered separately.

Cross sensitivity with penicillins

About 10% of patients who are allergic to penicillin will also react to first-generation cephalosporins. However, this figure is very much lower with the second and third generation drugs, which are thus not completely contraindicated in patients with a history of anaphylaxis after penicillin.

First generation

The early cephalosporins have been largely superseded either by other types of antibiotic which are less expensive, easier to give and at least as effective, or by the new cephalosporins. Their main characteristics are given in Table 19.15.

Table 19.15 Antibacterial activity of first and second generation cephalosporins

			Second generation	
	First generation	*Cefuroxime*	*Cephamandole*	*Cefoxitin*
Staph. aureus	++	++	++	+
β-lactamase stability	+	++	+	++
Strep. pyogenes	++	++	++	++
Strep. pneumonii	++	++	+	++
Strep. faecalis	–	–	–	–
H. influenzae	+	++	++	+
Neisseria	+	++	+	++
Ps. aeruginosa	–	–	–	–
B. fragilis	–	–	–	+
E. coli	++	++	++	++
Proteus	+	++	++	++

Key: ++ = Highly active
+ = Strain variability or generally low sensitivity
– = Inactive or poorly active

The group includes:

Cephaloridine (Ceporin) Dose: 0.5–1.0 g every 8–12 h i.v. or i.m. $t_{1/2}$: approx. 2 h. Largely excreted by the kidney. Large doses can produce renal damage and the risk is increased if it is combined with frusemide or gentamicin. It penetrates well into tissues but poorly into CSF.

Cephalothin (Keflin) has a short half-life (0.5 h) and low activity. There is little indication for its use.

Cephazolin (Kefzol) has $t_{1/2}$ of 1.8 h and is 80% protien bound in the plasma. Unlike most cephalosporins there is some biliary excretion and it has been

Table 19.16 Third generation cephalosporins

Drug	*Staph. aureus*	*β-lactamase stability*	*Strep. faecalis*	*H. influenzae*	*Ps.*† *aeruginosa (% susceptible)*	*B. fragilis*	*Entero-bacteriaceae*	*Elimination*	*% Protein bound*	*Dose by injection*	*Remarks*
Cefotaxime (Claforan)	+	++	−	++	+(58)	+	++	Liver and renal $t_{1/2}$ 1 h. Active metabolite $t_{1/2}$ 2 h	40	1–3 g 8 or 12 hrly	Good all round activity. Dose only needs reduction in severe renal failure.
Latamoxef (Moxalactam)	+	++	−	++	+(56)	++	+	Renal; $t_{1/2}$ 2 h	40	0.5–2 g 8 or 12 hrly	*Good activity against Gram −ve organisms but poor against Gram +ve, particularly pneumococci. May cause leucopenia and thrombocytopenia. platelet dysfunction and hypoprothrombinaemia. Vitamin K recommended, esp. in elderly. Antabuse-like reaction with alcohol.
Cefsulodin (Monaspor)	+	++	−	−	++(93)	−	−	Renal $t_{1/2} = 1.5$ h	35	0.5–1 g 8 or 12 hrly	High activity against pseudomonas, including many resistant strains.

Table 19.16 (continued)

Drug	*Staph. aureus*	*β-lactamase stability*	*Strep. faecalis*	*H. influenzae*	*Ps.*† *aeruginosa* (% *susceptible*)	*B. fragilis*	*Entero-bacteriaceae*	*Elimination*	% *Protein bound*	*Dose by injection*	*Remarks*
Cefoperazone	+	+	−	++	++(89)	+	++	Renal (30%) and biliary $t_{1/2}$ 2 h	90	1–2 g 12 hrly	Fair range of activity; antabuse-like effect with alcohol.
Ceftazidime (Fortum)	+	++	−	++	++(88)	+	++	Renal	15	1–2 g 8 hrly	High activity against *Pseudomonas*, poor against Gram +ve organisms.
Cephotetan	+	++	−	+	−	++	++	Renal $t_{1/2}$ 3.5 h	80	1 g twice daily	Active against *B. fragilis*.
Ceftizoxime (Ceftizox)	+	++	−	++	−	+	+	Renal $t_{1/2}$ 1.4 h	30	1–3 g 8–12 hrly	Similar to cefotaxime. Reduce dose with renal impairment.

† NOTE: Figures for other antibiotics: Tobramycin 95%
Amikacin 96%
Piperacillin 87%
Azlocillin 92%

* Hypoprothrombinaemia has been reported with some of these drugs, particularly with latamoxef. It occurs more frequently in the elderly and malnourished. Patients at risk should be given vitamin K.

Key: ++ Slightly active.
\+ Active against some strains.
− Inactive or poorly active.

used effectively to prevent infection in biliary surgery. Renal toxicity is low. The dose is 0.25–0.5 g 6 hourly.

Cephradine (Velosef; Eskacef) can be given orally or by injection in doses of 0.5–1.0 g 6 hourly. The $t_{1/2}$ is 0.7 h and it is 15 % protein bound. It is relatively stable to β-lactamase and is occasionally used in renal infections, gonorrhoea and to cover orthopaedic operations.

Second generation

These show a definite advance on the older cephalosporins. They are more resistant to β-lactamases, they are effective against streptococci, staphylococci and *Haemophilus influenzae* including ampicillin-resistant strains and against many strains of enterobacteria.

Cefuroxime (Zinacef) is given by injection. The $t_{1/2}$ is 70 min and it is 30 % protein bound. It is excreted by the kidneys. It is the most generally useful of this generation and may indeed be preferred to third-generation cephalosporins in some circumstances. Cefuroxime can be used for infection by sensitive organisms but there are often cheaper and equally effective substitutes.

Penetration into the CSF is good and it has been used very effectively for the treatment of bacterial meningitis (i.e. meningococcal, pneumococcal and *H. influenzae*). It is used prophylactically before biliary surgery in high-risk patients and as a single intramuscular injection (1.5 g) in penicillin-resistant gonorrhoea.

The usual dose is 0.75–2 g 8 hourly and in meningitis the higher dose should be used.

Cefamandole (Kefadol) is similar to cefuroxime but is a little less effective against pneumococci and gonococci and is rather less stable to β-lactamases. The $t_{1/2}$ is 35 minutes and it is 70 % protein bound. It is largely renally excreted. The dose is 0.5–1.5 g 6 hourly by injection.

Cefoxitin (Mefoxin) is a cephamycin (see p. 703). Its main attribute is activity against *B. fragilis* and therefore theoretically it would have a place in treating surgical sepsis but it is expensive and only moderately potent.

The $t_{1/2}$ is 40 min and the dose is 2.0 g 8 hourly by injection. It is largely excreted by the kidney.

Third generation

This group is characterised by an extended range of activity against Gram-negative organisms (some being effective against *Ps. aeruginosa*) and high β-lactamase stability. They are not in general as active against Gram-positive organisms as the older cephalosporins. The main characteristics of the group are given in Table 19.16.

These cephalosporins are expensive and require parenteral administration and there are cheaper and just as effective drugs for the treatment of most common infections. There appear at the moment to be a few situations where their use may be considered.

(a) In the treatment of severe infections (septicaemia etc.) particularly when the infecting organism is not known and the patient's immunity is compromised or they are penicillin sensitive. Whether these agents should be used alone or in combination with an aminoglycoside or more debatably with a ureidopenicillin is not settled. If they are used alone, their relative weakness against Gram-positive organisms should be remembered and cefuroxime might be preferred if a Gram-positive infection seems likely. They also vary considerably in their effectiveness against *Ps. aeruginosa* and *B. fragilis* and this may influence choice.

(b) In the treatment of meningitis, particularly in the neonate. This type of meningitis is usually caused by a Gram-negative organism. Penetration of these cephalosporins into the CSF is good and there are already a number of reports of the successful use of latamoxef and cefotaxime in this situation. Intrathecal injection is not required and response to a single agent looks promising.

Other possible uses for this group of cephalosporins are in hepatobiliary infections or in abdominal sepsis. If, however, it is likely that *Pseudomonas* is involved, an aminoglycoside or ureidopenicillin, e.g. piperacillin, should be added to the regime.

Many of the group are effective against penicillinase producing *N. gonorrhoeae* but not against *Chlamydia* and cost would have to be taken into account if their routine use were considered for gonococcal infection.

The newer cephalosporins are highly active against ampicillin-resistant *H. influenzae* and are useful in severe infection with this organism. Nearly all of them are excreted in the urine (see Table 19.15) and can be used for resistant renal infections although there are usually more suitable alternatives.

Cephalosporins used prophylactically

Cephalosporins are sometimes given before surgery, particularly in the USA, e.g. prior to biliary surgery (see under cefuroxime) and cardiac valve replacement. For bowel surgery metronidazole with an aminoglycoside is probably better unless there are problems with renal function. Cephalosporins have little place in medical prophylaxis.

Oral cephalosporins

There are four oral cephalosporins at present available, they resemble the first-generation cephalosporins in their antibacterial activity. Their main characteristics are given in Table 19.17. They can be used in infections caused by sensitive organisms but there are often cheaper and equally effective substitutes. The newest introduction, cefadroxil, is probably the most useful owing to its rather slower elimination so that only twice daily dosing is required.

Table 19.17 Characteristics of oral cephalosporins

	Staph. aureus	*H. influenzae*	*Entero-bacteriaceae*	*Ps. aeruginosa*	*B. fragilis*	*Elimination*	$t_{1/2}$	*Dose*
Cephalexin (Ceporex, Keflex)*	++	+	+	–	–	Renal	50 min	50 mg 6 hrly
Cephradine Velosef)	++	+	+	–	–	Renal	50 min	500 mg 6 hrly
Cefaclor (Distachlor)	++	++	+	–	–	Partially renal	45 min	250–500 mg 8 hrly
Cefadroxil	++	+	+	–	–	Renal	1.5 h	500 mg 12 hrly

* Can also be given by injection.

Key: ++ Highly active.
+ Active against some strains.
– Inactive or poorly active.

Thienamycin N-formimidoyl (Imipasin)

Thienamycin is the first of a new series of β-lactam antibiotics. It is produced by *Streptomyces cortleya.*

It has a very wide range of antibacterial activity being effective against most Gram-positive organisms including *Staph. aureus* and epidermis and most Gram-negative organisms including *Pseudomonas spp.* and *Bacteroides spp.* It is stable against β-lactamases.

Pharmacokinetics Thienamycin has a plasma half-life of about 1 hour. It is excreted via the kidneys and broken down by a dihydropeptidase probably in the renal tubule. This means that the urinary levels of the drug are much lower than would be expected from the renal clearance. It is therefore given combined with *cilastatin* which is a dihydropeptidase inhibitor. Although the plasma concentrations of the antibiotic given alone or in combination with the inhibitor are similar, the urinary concentration of thienamycin are much higher with the combined preparation.

Clinical use Clinical experience with this drug is limited. The dose schedule is 250–500 mg 6 hourly intravenously and it has proved successful in a wide range of infections.

Adverse effects Animal toxicity studies show that in very high doses thienamycin is nephrotoxic—this is prevented by co-administration of cilastatin and has not been reported in man.

Monobactams

Aztreonam (Azactam)

Aztreonam is a β-lactam antibiotic but has a single ring in the nucleus rather than the two rings found in the penicillins or cephalosporins.

It is highly effective against a wide range of Gram-negative organisms including *Pseudomonas* and *Serratia* but has little effective action against Gram-positive organisms and anaerobes.

Pharmacokinetics Aztreonam is excreted via the kidney with an elimination half-life of 1.7 hours. Reduced dose would be required with impaired renal function.

Clinical use The usual dose is 1.0 g i.v. two to four times daily. Clinical experience is limited but it has been used with success in a variety of infections caused by Gram-negative organisms.

Adverse effects are not common but include rashes, nausea and vomiting, and occasionally hypoprothrombinaemia.

The tetracyclines

This was the first group of broad-spectrum bacteriostatic antibiotics to be discovered. The members of the group are all related structurally. The earlier tetracyclines are tetracycline, chlortetracycline and oxytetracycline. Their range of activity is broad and covers Gram-positive and negative bacteria, Rickettsiae, *Treponema pallidum*, mycoplasmas and the Chlamydiae, e.g. the psittacosis and lymphogranuloma venereum organisms. These three antibiotics are products of different species of *Streptomyces*. They inhibit protein synthesis in bacterial ribosomes and also have an anti-anabolic action on protein metabolism in animal cells. An increasing proportion of pathogens are showing resistance to the tetracyclines (particularly coliforms, streptococci, pneumococci and staphylococci) which results from diminished permeability to the drugs.

Pharmaokinetics Tetracyclines can be given orally, intravenously, intramuscularly and by local application. Absorption occurs from the stomach and intestines but for most is variable and incomplete, partly due to the low solubility of tetracyclines and partly to binding Ca^{2+}, Al^{3+}, Fe^{2+} and Mg^{2+} in food or drugs in the alimentary tract. Gastrointestinal upset is least with the most completely absorbed members of the group (minocycline, doxycycline). After an oral dose the blood levels show a slow rise, a prolonged plateau and a slow fall due to prolonged absorption, high protein binding and an enterohepatic circulation of these drugs. After a 250 mg dose the plasma level peaks in the range 2–4 μg/ml.

The plasma $t_{1/2}$ is 6–9 h. Body tissues and cavities are well penetrated but CSF levels are about 10–20 % of plasma levels at best. Tetracycline itself hardly penetrates into CSF but doxycycline and minocycline produce CSF levels of 20–25 % the plasma level. The tetracyclines are laid down in growing bones and teeth, probably because of their chelating action with Ca^{2+}.

50 % of an intravenous dose appears in the urine and much of the remainder is excreted in the bile and enters an enterohepatic circulation. After an oral dose 30 % is excreted in the urine: the difference is due to incomplete intestinal absorption.

Clinical uses See Table 19.18. Because of unpredictable bacterial resistance they are unlikely to be first choices in hospital-acquired infections. Their bacteriostatic effect makes them unsuitable for use in patients having defective natural resistance. Many strains of *Strep. pyogenes* are resistant and they are not therefore useful in streptococcal soft-tissue infection or tonsillitis. They may be valuable in amoebic colitis—perhaps by reducing secondary bacterial infection. Tetracycline is used in low doses (250 mg twice daily) over long periods in the treatment of acne. Its mode of action in this disorder is not clear. It considerably reduces the population of *Prop. acnes* and to a lesser extent that of staphylococci although here the evidence is conflicting. Other possibilities are an anti-inflammatory action or reduction by enzyme inhibition of the irritant free fatty acids in the skin. Small differences exist between the tetracyclines (Tables 19.19 and 19.20) but these are rarely important. Cross-resistance exists between all of them except minocycline, which can be effective against tetracycline-resistant staphylococci and *H. influenzae*. The original tetracyclines (Table 19.19) remain the cheapest. Intravenous tetracyclines should be used only when they are the sole drugs of first choice in life-threatening infection because of their increased toxicity.

Table 19.18 Clinical indications for the tetracyclines

A. *First-line choice*
1. Acute exacerbations of chronic bronchitis
2. Non-specific urethritis
3. Mycoplasma pneumonia (primary atypical pneumonia)
4. Rickettsial infections, e.g. typhus
5. Pustular acne (prolonged treatment required)
6. Brucellosis (combined with streptomycin)
7. Lymphogranuloma venereum
8. Pulmonary infections with *Coxiella burneti* (Q fever) or the psittacosis agent.
9. Trachoma and inclusion body conjunctivitis
10. Cholera
11. Relapsing fever
12. Chlamydial infections
13. Tropical sprue

B. *Second-line choice*
1. Syphilis (in penicillin-sensitive patients it may be a first choice)
2. Actinomycosis
3. Anthrax
4. Meningococcal carriers (minocycline is excreted in tears and can eradicate sulphonamide-resistant organisms)

Table 19.19 Properties of the older tetracyclines

Drug (proprietary name)	$t_{1/2}$ *(h)*	*Plasma protein binding %*	*% absorbed orally*	*Comparison of peak blood levels after oral dosing*
Chlortetracycline (Aureomycin)	5–6	45	60	Lowest
Oxytetracycline (Terramycin)	8–10	20	65	Intermediate
Tetracycline (Achromycin)	7–9	25	75	Highest*

The usual adult oral dose of these drugs is 250 mg 8 hourly which may be doubled for severe infections.
In acne the dose is 250 mg twice daily orally.
The i.v. dose is 500 mg 12 hourly infused over 60 min.
*The i.m. dose is 100 mg 4–8 hourly. The i.m. preparation contains 40 mg procaine/vial.

Adverse effects Gastrointestinal effects include nausea, vomiting and diarrhoea. These are at least in part due to superinfection of the gut with *Candida*, *Pseudomonas* or *Proteus*. Less common and much more dangerous is the development of staphylococcal enterocolitis which occurs most commonly in post-operative patients and may have a mortality rate of 50%. Yellow and brown staining of the teeth can occur if the mother takes a tetracycline starting at the 5th month of pregnancy or if the child is given the drug up to the seventh year. Doxycycline which binds calcium less avidly is said to produce least effect on the teeth.

Table 19.20 Properties of some newer tetracyclines

Drug (proprietary name)	*Pharmacokinetics*	*Special features*	*Special toxicity*	*Adult dose*
Desmethylchlortetracycline (Ledermycin)	Moderate GI absorption (66%). Slow excretion, $t_{1/2}$ 10–17 h. Can be given 12 hourly. High protein binding (36–90%).	High stability. High antibacterial activity. Attains high blood levels. Used in inappropriate ADH secretion.	GI upsets. Photosensitivity. Especially prone to cause tooth discolouration in children.	300 mg 12 hourly. In inappropriate ADH secretion up to 300 mg 6 hourly.
Lymecycline (Tetralysal)	Highly soluble and well absorbed orally. Given orally, i.m. and i.v.	Probably less toxic than other tetracyclines given orally.		150 mg 6 hourly.
Clomocycline (Megaclor)	Soluble. Well absorbed from GI tract.	High antibacterial activity. Probably less absorbed into bone (because of instability).		170 mg 6 hourly.
Methacycline (Rondomycin)	$t_{1/2}$ 14–15 h. 75–90% protein binding.	Attains high blood levels. High antibacterial activity.		150 mg 8 hourly.
Doxycycline (Vibramycin)	Well absorbed from GI tract. GI & renal excretion. Can be given once a day. $t_{1/2}$ (15 h) unchanged in renal failure. Enters CSF moderately well (17% plasma levels).	Can be used in renal impairment because no anti-anabolic action and can be excreted into the gut. Less likely to stain teeth. May be useful prophylactic in traveller's diarrhoea.	Moderate photosensitiser.	200 mg initially then 100 mg 12 hourly.
Minocycline (Minocin)	Completely absorbed from GI tract. Long $t_{1/2}$ (13–18 h). 70–75% protein binding. Enters CSF moderately well (25% plasma levels).	Active against staphylococci resistant to tetracycline and anaerobes. Treatment of meningococcal carriers. Relatively little photosensitising effect.	Light-headness (?central effect). Vestibular toxicity.	200 mg initially then 100 mg 12 hourly.

In patients with renal failure most tetracyclines may produce clinical and biochemical deterioration and therefore should not be used for this condition. Doxycycline may, however, be used in such patients since it has no anti-anabolic effect and is excreted via the GI tract rather than the kidneys.

Tetracyclines given in excessive doses parenterally as well as orally can produce fatty degeneration of the liver. A total intravenous dose of 1 g/day is adequate for most purposes and should rarely be exceeded.

Benign intracranial hypertension has been described in infants and rarely in older children and adults. The mechanism is unknown.

Photosensitivity occasionally occurs and is particularly pronounced with desmethylchlortetracycline and doxycycline. This limits their use in tropical areas.

Chloramphenicol

Chloramphenicol was discovered a short time before chlortetracycline, these being the first broad-spectrum antibiotics to be discovered. Chloramphenicol was isolated from *Streptomyces venezuelae*, but is now manufactured synthetically. Unlike other antibiotics it is not produced by the fungus in the presence of other organisms but only in a sterile environment. This poses the problem of its role in fungal metabolism. Structurally it is a simple derivative of nitrobenzene. Chloramphenicol acts on bacterial 70S ribosomes and inhibits peptidyltransferase, thereby blocking protein synthesis. It can also inhibit the function of animal mitochondrial 70S ribosomes.

Chloramphenicol is bacteriostatic against a wide range of Gram-positive and -negative organisms including *Salmonellae*, *Haemophilus influenzae* and *Bordetella pertussis*, *Chlamydia*, *Brucella abortus*, *Escherichia coli*, *Streptococci* and *Staphylococci* also are sensitive to the drug. The MIC varies from about 0.5 μg/ml for *H. influenzae* and *B. pertussis* to 50 μg/ml or more for *Proteus* and *Pseudomonas*. Resistance to chloramphenicol may be due to bacterial production of an inactivating enzyme such as chloramphenicol acetylase. This property is transmitted between bacteria by R factors.

Pharmacokinetics The drug is well absorbed from the intestine, but large particle size may impair absorption. After a dose of 1 g in an adult, peak levels of 8–13 μg/ml are reached in 2–5 h and the $t_{1/2}$ is 1.5–3 h. In neonates, peak levels are attained later (6–12 h) and the $t_{1/2}$ is extended to 24–48 h because the immature liver has reduced levels of glucuronyl transferase, an enzyme required for chloramphenicol conjugation.

Fine suspensions of chloramphenicol can be given intramuscularly and the sodium succinate salt can be injected subcutaneously, intramuscularly or intravenously. The levels attained are similar to those after oral administration, but absorption from the intramuscular site is slower.

The drug is 60% bound to plasma proteins and penetrates better than any antibiotic into the tissues. Chloramphenicol enters the eye, fetus, saliva and sputum. The levels in the CSF are 30–50% those of the plasma.

It is mainly metabolised by reduction or by conjugation to glucuronide. Induction of the liver microsomal enzyme systems (e.g. with barbiturates) lowers blood chloramphenicol levels. Conversely chloramphenicol itself depresses microsomal function and may impair metabolism of phenytoin and tolbutamide, thereby increasing their action.

90% is excreted in the urine but only 10% is as unchanged chloramphenicol, although this is usually sufficient to be effective in treating urinary infections. About 3% undergoes biliary excretion, mostly as conjugated chloramphenicol, and enters an enterohepatic circulation: it is therefore useful in typhoid and other biliary infections.

Clinical uses Chloramphenicol should only be used for serious infections in which other drugs are not as effective. Accepted indications are typhoid and other serious *Salmonella* infections. The usual dose is 1.5–3 g/day in divided doses. Many paediatricians use chloramphenicol in the treatment of *H. influenzae* meningitis. It is used topically for eye infections. Used as an eye ointment, chloramphenicol penetrates into the aqueous humour. Epiglottitis.

Adverse effects Toxicity testing in animals did not reveal any harmful potential, but in man several significant toxic effects occur. These include:

sore mouth, nausea, diarrhoea
marrow aplasia and haemopoietic toxicity
grey syndrome
encephalopathy
optic neuritis.

Marrow aplasia is rare but usually fatal. The estimated incidence is about 1 in 40 000: aplastic anaemia is 10 times more common following chloramphenicol treatment than in the untreated. To place the risks of chloramphenicol treatment in perspective it should be noted that this is also the risk of fatal thromboembolism from the oral contraceptive in middle-aged women. Aplasia may follow only a small dose or even very rarely chloramphenicol eye drops and may develop after a latent period of up to a year. It may follow parenteral as well as oral administration. Usually the cellular elements of the marrow are totally inhibited and patients present with pallor, purpura and infections. Isolated granulocytopenia is unusual. A more common toxicity, probably unrelated to aplasia, is the dose-related, reversible depression of red- and white-cell production. This occurs when plasma chloramphenicol levels exceed 25 μg/ml and may be related to the inhibition of mitochondrial ferrochelatase and protein synthesis by chloramphenicol.

The grey syndrome consists of abdominal distension, vomiting, lethargy, anorexia, hypothermia, pallor and circulatory collapse in newborn (particularly low birthweight) babies given large doses of chloramphenicol. Doses of 100 mg/kg/day and above can produce blood levels of 170 μg/ml in infants with functional immaturity of the kidneys and liver. In doses of less than 25 mg/kg chloramphenicol is safe in babies of less than one month old. This syndrome results from the relatively inefficient metabolism of chloramphenicol by neonates whose hepatic chloramphenicol–glucuronyl transferase (a different enzyme from bilirubin–glucuronyl transferase) activity is lower than in adults. The resulting delay in drug elimination produces high circulating plasma levels of chloramphenicol, which are toxic to mammalian cells, possibly via inhibition of mitochondrial protein synthesis.

Lincomycin (Lincocin)

This is yet another antibiotic produced by a soil streptomyces. It is mainly active against Gram-positive organisms, with MIC of 0.05–0.5 μg/ml for many strains of *Staph. pyogenes*, β-haemolytic streptococci and pneumococci. Higher concentrations may be required for *Strep. viridans*, and *Strep. faecalis* is frequently resistant. Other sensitive organisms include mycoplasma, bacteroides and anaerobic cocci. Lincomycin inhibits bacterial protein synthesis by binding to bacterial ribosomes at the same site as erythromycin (which displaces it from ribosomes so that it is unwise to use these two drugs in combination). This binding apparently inhibits peptidyltransferase and may cause premature detachment of ribosomes from mRNA.

Cross resistance may occur with macrolides and lincomycin resistance is gained by ribosomal mutations, particularly by staphylococci, during treatment.

Pharmacokinetics Lincomycin is well, but not completely absorbed from the gut; 4 h after an oral dose of 500 mg, peak levels of 2–7 μg/ml are reached. The plasma $t_{1/2}$ is 4–6 h. The usual dose is 250–500 mg 6 hourly. Food in the stomach delays and diminishes the peak levels. After an intramuscular injection of 600 mg, peak levels of 8–18 μg/ml are reached within 1–2 h. Lincomycin readily enters tissues, including bone, apart from the CSF in which it attains relatively low concentrations except in meningitis, where 40% of the blood level is attained. The volume of distribution is approximately 50% of body weight. Although less than 30% is excreted unchanged in the urine, high and persistent blood levels occur in renal failure. Much of the drug appears to be inactivated in the liver and lincomycin metabolism is deranged in hepatic failure.

Clinical uses The use of lincomycin is being superseded by clindamycin in the UK, since the indications are largely identical (Table 19.21).

Table 19.21 Clinical indications for lincomycin and clindamycin

A. *First-line choice*	B. *Second-line choice*
1. Staphylococcal infections particularly osteomyelitis (methicillin resistant strains usually sensitive)	1. In place of a penicillin for penicillin sensitive patients
2. Bacteroides and other anaerobic infections	2. Actinomycosis

Adverse effects See clindamycin below.

Clindamycin (Dalacin C)

Clindamycin is 7-chloro-7-deoxylincomycin hydrochloride and has properties similar to lincomycin. The main differences are greater effectiveness against

Gram-positive cocci and bacteroides with some activity against *Haemophilus influenzae*. High blood levels result from better intestinal absorption and the failure of food to reduce absorption. The $t_{1/2}$ is 4 h, similar to lincomycin, but the volume of distribution is about double that of lincomycin.

Clinical uses of these two drugs are shown in Table 19.21. The usual doses are 150–450 mg 6 hourly orally or 600–1200 mg daily i.m. or i.v.

Adverse effects Abdominal discomfort, diarrhoea and occasional rashes have been reported with this drug but it is relatively well tolerated. The major side effect is *pseudomembranous enterocolitis*, although the incidence of this is not established, being variously estimated from 1 in 50 000 to 1 in 10. The likely cause is that antibiotic treatment suppresses many of the gut organisms and allows overgrowth by others which include *Clostridium difficile*, an organism which is present only in some individuals. This bacterium produces an enterotoxin with a necrotising effect on colonic mucosa. The treatment of this complication, which can be fatal, is either to eradicate the clostridium with vancomycin or metronidazole or to give the resin cholestyramine which binds the toxin, thereby inactivating it.

The Macrolides

Macrolides form a group of antibiotics which have in common a lactone ring to which is attached sugar molecules. They have similar pharmacological properties and include erythromycin, oleandomycin and spiramycin. Macrolides inhibit protein synthesis by bacterial ribosomes, probably by interfering with translocation of the growing peptide chain from one side of the ribosome to the other. They will not attach to human ribosomes.

Erythromycin

This is the most effective of the macrolides and has a similar spectrum of activity to benzylpenicillin. Of particular importance are β-haemolytic streptococci, *Staphylococcus pyogenes*, *Neisseria*, *H. influenzae*, some *E. coli* (but most enterobacteria are resistant) and *Mycoplasma pneumoniae* (not *M. hominis*). It is bacteriostatic in low concentrations but can be bactericidal at high concentrations. Resistance is rarely seen during short-term treatment but may arise during prolonged administration. Cross resistance, which is probably plasmid-borne, does not necessarily extend to other macrolides.

Pharmacokinetics Erythromycin base is destroyed by gastric acid. Acid-resistant salts such as the stearate or estolate produce effective plasma levels after oral administration, although the bioavailability from the estolate is spuriously high since much of the drug exists in the blood as the bacteriologically inactive estolate rather than active erythromycin. Thus 2–4 h after an oral dose of 250 mg of the estolate, peak levels of free erythromycin plus estolate of approximately 1.4 μg/ml are reached, whilst after 250 mg of the stearate the average peak is approximately 0.4 μg/ml, but this is entirely erythromycin base. This emphasises the importance of using specific assays for plasma drug estimation. With the exception of the estolate, food usually reduces the absorption of erythromycin. Erythromycin ethyl succinate is available for i.m. injection, and the lactobionate is suitable for i.v. injection but is painful given i.m.

The $t_{1/2}$ is 1.5–3 h and the volume of distribution is around 0.5 l/kg body weight. Erythromycin is well distributed throughout the body apart from the CNS which is penetrated only when the meninges are inflamed. Most of the drug is metabolised by demethylation and urinary levels of free drug are low. As renal excretion is not the main elimination route there is no significant accumulation in uraemia.

Clinical uses of the drug are shown in Table 19.22. The usual dose is 500 mg 6 hourly which may be increased with serious infections.

Table 19.22 Indications for erythromycin

A. *First-line choice*	B. *Second-line choice*
1. Alternative to a penicillin in penicillin sensitive patient	1. Rheumatic fever prophylaxis
2. Alternative to a tetracycline in mycoplasma pneumoniae	2. Chronic bronchitis
3. Pertussis	3. Otitis media
4. Diphtheria – especially in treatment of the carrier state	4. Penicillin-resistant staphylococcal infections
5. Legionnaire's disease	5. Chronic prostatitis
6. Chlamydial pelvic infection in pregnancy	
7. Campylobacter enteritis	

Adverse effects Erythromycin is one of the safer antibiotics, gastrointestinal disturbances and allergy being the commonest (5–10%) adverse reactions. Erythromycin estolate when administered for longer than 14 days can produce a hepatitis-like syndrome which seems to be due to cholestasis rather than cell necrosis. This is reversible and has never been fatal. Some clinicians never use the estolate since hepatitis is not seen with other erythromycin salts.

Metronidazole (Flagyl)

This is a synthetic heterocyclic nitro derivative of simple structure. It is active only against bacteria and protozoa with primarily anaerobic metabolism. The MICs against some representative organisms are:

Trichomonas vaginalis	1–5 μg/ml
Entamoeba histolytica	1 μg/ml
Balantidium coli	2 μg/ml
Clostridium welchii	4 μg/ml
Anaerobic *streptococci; Clostridium tetani*	< 1 μg/ml
Bacteroides fragilis	1 μg/ml
Bacteroides spp	1 μg/ml
Fusobacterium	1 μg/ml

It has no action on *Candida, Aspergillus, E. coli* or *Strep. pyogenes.*

Although it enters aerobic organisms it is only in anaerobic microorganisms that it is biochemically reduced to an active derivative which binds to DNA and inhibits further nucleic acid synthesis. It may also inhibit pyruvate and phosphate metabolism by inhibiting a hydrogenase occurring in Clostridia and other anaerobes.

Pharmacokinetics Metronidazole is usually well absorbed orally but occasionally poor absorption causes therapeutic failure, and suppository (0.5 and 1 g) and intravenous formulations are available. The plasma $t_{1/2}$ is 6–8 h and a single 200 mg oral dose produces a mean peak plasma level of 5 μg/ml at 1–2 h, falling to 1 μg/ml after 24 h. Single doses of 1 g and 2.4 g produce peak levels of about 26 and 45 μg/ml respectively. About one half of the plasma concentration has been measured in amoebic abscess pus. Similar levels to those in plasma appear in milk, but in the suckling infant blood levels are low. The drug is also present in the saliva. 15–60 % is excreted in the urine in the first 24 h after a single oral dose. The usual intravenous dose is 500 mg 8 hourly infused in isotonic saline over 20 min. Rectal absorption is also satisfactory, a 1 g suppository producing peak plasma levels of 10 μg/ml at about 4 h. 60–70 % of the drug is excreted unchanged, but renal failure does not usually affect plasma levels or necessitate dosage adjustment. The rest is metabolised to an acid oxidation product and a glucuronide. Sometimes an azometabolite colours the urine brownish-red.

Clinical uses

1. *T. vaginalis* genital infections. 200 mg 8 hourly for 7 days cures infections in 87 % of females (95 % are cured if both sexual partners are treated).
2. Acute ulcerative gingivitis due to anaerobic fusiforms and spirochaetes: pain and tenderness is relieved within 12 h of starting treatment. Optimum results are observed with a dose of 200 mg 8 hourly for 5 days.
3. *Giardia lamblia* infestations can be treated with a large single daily dose, 2.0 g, for 3 days.
4. Acute amoebic dysentery in susceptible individuals is treated with 800 mg 8 hourly for 5 days.

   Invasive amoebic intestinal infections, amoebic hepatitis, amoebic abscess in the liver and other organs and symptomless amoebic cyst passers are treated with 400 mg 8 hourly for 5 days. Such regimes cure over 90 % of patients.
5. Anaerobic infections due to *Bacteroides fragilis*, fusobacteria, clostridia, anaerobic streptococci and eubacteria, amongst others, may occur after gastrointestinal or gynaecological surgery. Metronidazole is one of the few antibacterials which is effective against anaerobes. Alternatives are clindamycin or latamoxef. Metronidazole can be used prophylactically and is given as a 1.0 g suppository at the time of the premedication and repeated eight hourly to prevent post-operative infection. It can also be given orally in doses of 400 mg orally or 500 mg i.v. eight hourly for developed infections.
6. Pseudomembranous colitis (caused by *Clostridium difficile*) 250 mg four times daily orally for 10 days.

7. Tropical ulcer (caused by Vincent's organisms).
8. Guinea worm infestations (dracontiasis): 25 mg/kg/day in divided doses for 10 days.
9. *Dracunculus medinensis* infestations: 200 mg 8 hourly for 7 days.

Adverse effects Metallic taste, furred tongue, nausea, vomiting, diarrhoea, drowsiness, headache, rashes, pruritus, and mild, reversible leucopenia during treatment. Rarely hypotension is produced and the dose of hypotensive drugs may have to be reduced.

It is thus a relatively safe drug although when used in large doses over several months a few cases of severe and sometimes irreversible peripheral neuropathy have occurred. Although bacterial and animal test systems suggest some mutagenic potential (its use is not sanctioned for infections other than trichomonas in the USA) there is no evidence for any of these effects in man. It would be unfortunate if this drug were withdrawn on the basis of such tenuous, and possibly irrelevant, evidence when it has proved by clinical usage to be of great therapeutic value.

Drug interactions:

1. It has an antabuse-like effect and patients should be cautioned about taking alcohol.
2. Metronidazole potentiates the effects of racemic and S(−) warfarin but not R(+) warfarin (q.v.) and careful adjustment of warfarin dosage is thus necessary.

Tinidazole (Fasigyn)

Tinidazole is another nitroimidazole which is effective against protozoa and anaerobes including *B. fragilis* and *spp,* Fusobacterium spp. and *Clostridium perfringens*; it is very similar to metronidazole.

The prophylactic dose is 2.0 g orally, given once only and the therapeutic dose is 2.0 g followed by 1.0 g once daily.

It is well absorbed from the intestinal tract, the $t_{1/2}$ is 12–14 hours, hence the once daily dosage. Tissue penetration is good and CSF concentration adequate. Tinidazole is cleared from the body largely by metabolism but there is a high concentration of the drug in the urine.

A preparation is available for intravenous infusion.

Adverse effects and interactions Similar to metronidazole.

The Aminoglycosides

These antibiotics are derived (and in some cases semisynthesised) from different species of *Streptomyces* or *Micromonospora.* The family includes streptomycin, gentamicin, kanamycin, tobramycin, amikacin, netilmicin, capreomycin, neomycin and framycetin. They act on bacterial, but not human, ribosomes by preventing the formation of the normal complex required to initiate protein synthesis. They are effective against a wide range of Gram-negative organisms and against staphylococci but are ineffective against streptococci including pneumococci and anaerobes. They are used for serious acute septic infection except streptomycin and capreomycin which are used mainly in treating tuberculosis and spectinomycin which is reserved for penicillin-resistant gonorrhoea. They have the following common properties:

(a) poor intestinal absorption (they are charged molecules) and they are administered parenterally;

(b) low protein binding (20–30%);

(c) excretion unchanged by kidneys;

(d) dose-related toxicity (Table 19.23) including:

(i) VIIIth cranial nerve: both auditory and vestibular divisions are affected but streptomycin, tobramycin and gentamicin predominantly affect the vestibular branch more commonly than neomycin, kanamycin and amikacin. These effects are often irreversible and aggravated by concurrent therapy with frusemide or ethacrynic acid.

Table 19.23 Comparative toxicity of aminoglucosides (toxicity %) in prospective clinical trials (After Kahlmeter and Dahlayer. *J. Antimicrob. Chemother.*, **13** Suppl A, (1984).)

	Renal	*Cochlear*	*Vestibular*
Gentamicin	14	8.3	3.2
Tobramycin	12.9	6.1	3.5
Netilmicin	8.7	2.4	1.4
Amikacin	9.4	13.9	2.8

(ii) Nephrotoxicity (all except streptomycin) affects up to 15% of patients but is usually mild and reversible. It is dose related and tends to develop later on in therapy (after the first week). The incidence is increased by concurrent administration of cephalosporins, frusemide or pre-existing renal disease. The lesion occurs in the proximal tubule and is associated with rises in serum urea and creatinine and the appearance of casts in the urine. Dosage adjustment in impaired renal function is necessary for these drugs and this is often aided by measurements of plasma drug level (see Chapter 5). The size or frequency of the dose must also be reduced in older patients. Neomycin is the most nephrotoxic of the group and even the small amount absorbed from the intestine can accumulate to toxic levels in renal disease.

Fear of renal or ototoxicity should never prevent the administration of adequate doses of these drugs: patients for whom aminoglycosides are indicated are usually seriously ill.

(iii) Neuromuscular blockade, potentiated by curare-like drugs, is rare.

(e) The aminoglycosides are bactericidal but bacterial resistance can be rapidly acquired and is partly mediated by the R-factors transmitted between bacteria of different species. Resistance can occur by the development of ribosomes which do not bind aminoglycosides or by acquisition of inactivating enzymes or by reduced permeability to the drug. Aminoglycosides possibly enter bacteria by transport on the carrier system naturally utilised by spermine and the potentiation of aminoglycoside action by penicillin may result from the effects of the latter drug on the bacterial cell wall increasing aminoglycoside entry. There are variations both between and within hospitals in the incidence and pattern of aminoglycoside resistance, so that it is necessary to be aware of these local patterns in using these drugs.

Streptomycin

This drug is produced by *Streptomyces griseus.* The MIC for many strains of *M. tuberculosis* is 0.5 μg/ml and for *Strep. faecalis* ranges from 64 to more than 256 μg/ml.

Pharmacokinetics Streptomycin is usually injected intramuscularly. Following a dose of 1 g peak levels of 25–50 μg/ml are attained in $\frac{1}{2}$–$1\frac{1}{2}$ h and the plasma $t_{1/2}$ is about $2\frac{1}{2}$ h. In patients over 40 years the dose of 0.75 g recommended for these patients gives a peak of 26–58 μg/ml and the $t_{1/2}$ is prolonged up to 9 h. Higher levels develop in ambulatory patients than those at rest.

Penetration of the blood–brain barrier is poor but some drug enters the brain and CSF if the meninges are inflamed. Tuberculous cavities and peritoneal fluid are penetrated, and levels in pleural fluid are the same as in plasma. The drug is excreted by glomerular filtration and 30–90% appears in the urine over 24 h. The rest is retained or metabolised. High concentrations are present in urine—up to 1 mg/ml after 1 g i.m.

Clinical uses The main use of streptomycin is in tuberculosis and it is combined with tetracycline in the treatment of brucellosis. Streptomycin combined with benzylpenicillin exhibits synergism against *Strep. faecalis* but resistant strains have appeared and it is no longer the preferred combination for infective endocarditis caused by this organism. Resistance to other Gram-negative bacilli also develops easily.

Adverse effects Allergy to streptomycin is common and handling of the drug can cause contact dermatitis. Rashes and drug fever occur in 5% of patients and usually appear in the first 6 weeks of treatment. Less frequently lymphadenopathy, hepatosplenomegaly, impaired liver function, encephalopathy, proteinuria, eosinophilia, exfoliative dermatitis and transient lung shadows are produced.

Injected streptomycin is often painful. Several hours afterwards there may develop paraesthesiae, mild vertigo, ataxia, headache and malaise. Severe vertigo frequently results from a daily dose of 2 g but is less common with 0.5–1 g/day. Deafness can also result and has even been detected in children born of mothers given streptomycin during pregnancy since streptomycin crosses the placenta. There is no correlation between VIII nerve damage and peak levels but the risk is correlated with total dosage and labyrinthine injury is associated with plasma levels above 3 μg/ml 24 h after administration of streptomycin (i.e. it is related to the 'trough' plasma concentration).

Gentamicin

This antibiotic is a product of *Micromonospora purpurea.* It is effective against many strains of *Pseudomonas aeruginosa* and a wide range of other Gram-negative pathogens including *E. coli*, *Proteus* spp., *Klebsiella* spp., other Gram-negative organisms and *Staphylococcus aureus*. Streptococci including *Strep. pneumoniae* are resistant however. The MIC for staphylococci is approximately 0.25 μg/ml but for enterococci may be up to 50 μg/ml. There are various estimates of the MIC for *Ps. aeruginosa*, 1–8 μg/ml being usually quoted.

Resistance to gentamicin of normally sensitive strains is still uncommon, but resistance by *Pseudomonas* is increasing. The R factor which is responsible directs the production of an enzyme which inactivates the drug by adenylation with ATP or acetylation by acetyl Co A.

Pharmacokinetics Although absorption from the gut is very poor, in patients with renal failure sufficient may accumulate in the body to produce toxic effects. Gentamicin is usually given intramuscularly or intravenously. From the intramuscular site absorption is rapid and peak levels are achieved in less than 1 h. The plasma $t_{1/2}$ is 120 min and for the MIC against *Pseudomonas* to be attained the plasma gentamicin level 1 h after i.m. injection should lie between 6–10 μg/ml (Table 19.24). This is attained in about 70% of patients by an initial dose of 2 mg/kg based on lean body weight. This dose is then given every 8 h if renal function is normal and adjusted appropriately if it is not (see p. 129). Trough plasma levels, i.e. the level present immediately before the next dose, are the best guide to cumulation and probably to toxicity since levels above 4 μg/ml are associated with ototoxicity.

Table 19.24 Therapeutic blood levels of aminoglucosides

	Ideal peak range (30 *min after i.v. or* 60 *min after i.m. injection*) (*mg/l*)	*Trough* (*immediately before injection*) (*mg/l*)
Gentamicin	5–10	below 2
Tobramycin	5–10	below 2
Amikacin	15–30	below 4
Netilmicin	5–12	below 3

Blood levels must be interpreted in the clinical context.

Gentamicin is excreted via the kidneys and 80% appears in the urine, typically at a concentration of 20–200 μg/ml. Excretion is impaired in the newborn and the elderly. Only 30% is protein bound and the drug is distributed to the fetus and other tissues, but the concentration is low in the bile and CSF. Intrathecal therapy may be necessary for Gram-negative bacillary meningitis. Use in renal failure is considered on p. 129.

Clinical uses include serious coliform infections, *Pseudomonas* infections (including septicaemia), Gram-negative septicaemia (often in combination with other antibiotics) and occasionally in severe staphylococcal infections when other drugs cannot be used. It is now the treatment of choice combined with benzylpenicillin for streptococcal endocarditis. Locally it has been applied to the skin, to eradicate nasal carriers of staphylococci, to treat otitis media and orally to suppress bowel flora.

Adverse effects The commonest affects vestibular function. The damage is usually permanent and may produce ataxia, especially at night, although visual cues can allow patients to achieve good balance. Deafness due to gentamicin is relatively uncommon.

Other aminoglycosides

Most of the other aminoglycosides are used in the same general circumstances as gentamicin and their characteristics are shown in Table 19.25.

Tobramycin is very active against *Pseudomonas* but less active than gentamicin against some other Gram-negative organisms.

Netilmicin is similar to gentamicin but there is some evidence that it is less oto- and nephrotoxic.

Amikacin is the most effective of the group with least resistant strains. It is very expensive.

Spectinomycin (Trobicin) is an aminocyclitol with a broad range of activity including Gram-positive and -negative organisms. In man its clinical use has been abandoned except for the treatment of infections by penicillin-resistant gonococci. The resistance to penicillin that gonococci have acquired over the past 30 years has gradually increased so that now 30 times the originally effective dose is advised (4 800 000 units of benzylpenicillin) in conjunction with probenecid. This resistance is relatively non-specific, since it involves decreased permeability to antibiotic and such strains are often resistant to most other antibiotics apart from spectinomycin. Since late 1975 strains of penicillinase-producing gonococci have been isolated worldwide. This R-factor mediated resistance, unlike the relatively resistant chromosomal mutants which evolved previously, cannot be overcome by increasing the dose of penicillin still further. Spectinomycin (2 g i.m.) is recommended for such cases and produces a cure of 95% in both sexes. It is not reliably effective in pharyngeal gonococcal infections and has no effect on concomitant syphilis. The dose is 2 g i.m. in males and 4 g i.m. in females.

Fusidic Acid (Fucidin)

This is a steroid antibiotic produced by *Fusidum coccineum*. Although chemically related to cephalosporin P, it acts not on the cell wall but on bacterial protein synthesis at the translocation step. Thus no cross-resistance occurs between fusidic acid and cephalosporins or penicillins. Clinically its antibacterial use is confined to staphylococci (including penicillinase-producing and methicillin-resistant strains). Streptococci are much less sensitive, but Gram-positive bacteria such as *Corynebacterium diphtheriae* and

Table 19.25 Aminoglycosides

Drug (*Proprietary name*)	*Dosage*	*Special features*	*Toxicity*	*Uses*
Amikacin (Amikin)	7.5 mg/kg i.m. or i.v. twice daily $t_{1/2} = 2$ h. MIC 2 μg/ml *Proteus spp.* MIC 6 μg/ml *Pseudomonas aeruginosa*	Semi-synthetic derivative of kanamycin, relatively resistant to enzyme inactivation compared to gentamicin and tobramycin	Mainly high-tone deafness.	Resistant Gram-negative infections especially *Pseudomonas* and *Klebsiella*. An alternative for gentamicin-resistant strains. Can also be given IT, IP.
Tobramycin (Nebcin)	50–80 mg i.m. 8 hourly. Kinetics similar to streptomycin. $t_{1/2} = 2$ h	Active against some *Pseudomonas* strains resistant to gentamicin	Vestibular toxicity	*Pseudomonas* infections as alternative to gentamicin (but cross-resistance with gentamicin is frequent)
Netilmicin (Netillin)	6 mg/kg daily in 2 or 3 divided doses	Similar to gentamicin	Probably less oto- and nephrotoxic than gentamicin	Alternative to gentamicin
Capreomycin	1 g i.m./day	Only active against mycobacteria	Eosinophilia and drug fever (no cross resistance with streptomycin)	Tuberculosis only.

Neomycin	Not now used systemically because of deafness 4 g/day orally	Mixture of neomycins B and C	Sensitisation if used topically. Topical use (skin or ear) may produce irreversible deafness.	Topical for staphylococcal and Gram-negative infections. Gut sterilisation in liver disease. Inhalation
Framycetin	Not now used systemically. 2–4 g/day orally	Could be neomycin B or similar to it	Local sensitisation	Mainly gut sterilisation and topical application
Paromomycin	Not used systemically. 1–2 g/day orally	Effective against *Entamoeba Histolytica*, (probably also *Taenia*)		Intestinal infections, amoebicide, anthelmintic
Vancomycin (Vancocin)	1 g i.v. 12 hourly maintains therapeutic level of 10 μg/ml $t_{1/2}$ = 4–6 h	Activity against Gram-positive organisms of main interest clinically especially for *Staphylococcus*, resistant to other drugs.	Deafness Local venous thrombosis	Septicaemia complicated by endocarditis due to *Staph.* or *Strep.* Enterocolitis due to *Staph.* or *Clostridium*

IP = intraperitoneal
IT = intrathecal

Clostridium tetani are highly sensitive. Apart from the *Neisseria spp.* all Gram-negative organisms are insensitive.

Pharmacokinetics The MIC for *Staph. pyogenes* (0.07 μg/ml) is easily achieved by an oral dose of 500 mg which gives a peak level of approximately 25 μg/ml within 3 h. The $t_{1/2}$ is 4–6 h. Penetration is good except into the CSF and therapeutic levels occur in most organs including bone. There is good penetration into pus. Very little of the drug is excreted in the urine so that accumulation in renal failure is not a problem. Metabolism, probably in the liver, to inactive products amounts for most of the dose.

Clinical uses It is given orally or intravenously in a dose of 500 mg 6 hourly or applied locally to the skin. It is reserved for severe staphylococcal infections and is a useful alternative drug for penicillin-sensitive subjects. Resistance occurs rather easily and many authorities advise that it should be combined with another anti-staphylococcal agent.

Adverse effects It is relatively non-toxic and mild gastrointestinal upsets and rashes are the most frequently reported adverse reactions. Jaundice may rarely occur particularly with intravenous administration. Despite its steroid structure, in normal usage steroid metabolic effects are negligible.

Vancomycin (Vancocin)

Vancomycin is obtained from *Streptomyces orientalis*. It is effective against Gram-positive organisms, in particular *Staph. pyogenes* (including strains resistant to benzylpenicillin and methicillin) and streptococci. The MIC for *Staph. pyogenes* is 0.16–1.8 g/ml, and for *Strep. viridans* is 0.30–2.5 μg/ml. It acts by inhibiting the synthesis of the cell wall of bacteria but the mechanism differs from that of penicillins and cephalosporins and so cross resistance does not occur.

Pharmacokinetics Vancomycin is not absorbed from the gut and is given intravenously. It enters pleural and ascitic fluid but does not enter the cerebrospinal fluid in therapeutic concentrations unless the meninges are inflamed. It is about 10% protein bound in the plasma. After a single intravenous injection, a therapeutic blood level is maintained for around six hours when the serum level after a 1.0 g dose is around 2.5 μg/ml. About 90% of the intravenous dose is excreted in the urine and with impaired renal function accumulation occurs.

Clinical use Vancomycin is reserved for infections with resistant Gram-positive organisms. Owing to its toxicity it is very much a second-line antibiotic. It should be considered in infective endocarditis due to streptococci or staphylococci resistant to more usual antibiotics and has been recommended to cover dental procedures in patients with cardiac valve disease where other antibiotics could not be used.

The usual adult dose is 1.0 g twice daily. Owing to its irritant properties, it should be infused in 200 ml of 5% dextrose solution over thirty minutes. In dental procedures the dose is 1.0 g infused over thirty minutes one hour before treatment followed by erythromycin 500 mg four times daily for 2 days. With impaired renal function the dose should be reduced and blood levels should be monitored and kept between 2.5–25 μg/ml.

It is also used in staphylococcal enteritis and pseudomembranous colitis in a dose of 250 mg in water orally six hourly.

Adverse effects Vancomycin is irritant and may produce venous thrombosis at the infusion site. High blood levels (> 50 μg/ml) are ototoxic and cause deafness. Other effects include proteinuria, skin rashes and fever.

Drugs used solely for urinary infections

Nitrofurantoin (Furadantin)

This is one of several nitrofurans with antibacterial properties (others are nitrofurazone, used topically for skin infections and furazolidone given orally, for gastrointestinal infections and 'travellers' diarrhoea'). It is effective against many Gram-negative urinary tract pathogens such as *E. coli* and *Klebsiella spp.* but *Proteus spp.* are often, and *Pseudomonas aeruginosa* always, resistant. It is thought to act by inhibiting acetyl-coenzyme A synthesis, thereby blocking bacterial carbohydrate metabolism. This inhibition may extend to human nervous tissues, causing polyneuritis.

The MICs of sensitive bacterial species are usually less than 35 μg/ml and urinary concentrations of at least 100 μg/ml are attained after the usual therapeutic dose of 200–400 mg/day. Orally or parenterally administered nitrofurantoin does not produce therapeutic plasma concentrations in the absence of renal failure. The $t_{1/2}$ is 1 h. Only about one third of the dose appears unchanged in the urine, the rest undergoes hepatic metabolism.

Adverse effects Nausea and vomiting are common and limit the usefulness of nitrofurantoin. Nausea appears to be centrally mediated, for it occurs after i.v. administration and is possibly associated with the rate of absorption of the drug. Modification of the crystal size to a macrocrystalline form (Macrodantin) which is more slowly absorbed without reduction in the total amount of drug absorbed (and thus therapeutic effect) may reduce this side effect.

Nitrofurantoin produces hypersensitivity reactions in about 5% of patients, and this may include eosinophilia, fever, rashes, asthma and rarely anaphylaxis. Haemolytic anaemia can occur in patients with glucose-6-phosphate dehydrogenase deficiency. Peripheral neuropathy (which is often progressive, sensory and motor) may be irreversible and is usually seen in patients with renal failure who develop toxic blood levels of the drug. Newborn and premature infants and the elderly are also at risk of this serious adverse effect. The pulmonary side effects have been mentioned in Chapter 13. Other rare adverse reactions include cholestatic jaundice, megaloblastic anaemia (structurally this drug resembles phenytoin) and bone-marrow depression.

Nalidixic acid (Negram)

This synthetic chemotherapeutic agent is unrelated to other antibacterials and inhibits bacterial DNA replication. Most Gram-negative organisms (except *Pseudomonas aeruginosa* and *Bacteroides spp.*) are sensitive to 10 μg/ml but Gram-positive organisms are resistant. Resistance is relatively easily acquired by sensitive species. Nalidixic acid is well absorbed orally and the usual dose of 1 g 6 hourly gives peak plasma levels of 25 μg/ml. It is 93% protein bound and the $t_{1/2}$ is 1–1.5 h. It therefore differs from nitrofurantoin in that therapeutic serum levels are attained, although it is not used for systemic infections. Nalidixic acid is metablised to hydroxynalidixic acid, which also has antibacterial activity. Both are conjugated in the liver to inactive glucuronides, which are excreted in the urine. The urinary concentration of active nalidixic acid is in the range 25–250 μg/ml after an oral dose of 1 g. Although there is little accumulation of nalidixic acid in moderate renal failure, in severe renal failure the glucuronides accumulate and may produce toxicity. Nalidixic acid is relatively non-toxic. Gastrointestinal upset, rashes, visual disturbances, epilepsy, intracranial hypertension and haemolytic anaemia the latter (especially in patients with glucose-6-phosphate dehydrogenase deficiency) have all been reported, but are rare.

Methenamine mandelate; methenamine hippurate These substances release methenamine which in acid urine is split to yield formaldehyde which kills all bacteria. However, urea-splitting organisms such as *Proteus spp.* will prevent urinary acidification, so inhibiting formaldehyde liberation. It is often necessary, even in the absence of urea-splitters, to administer acidifying agents. Resistance cannot be acquired to formaldehyde.

The drugs are well absorbed from the gut (usual dose 1 g 6 hourly) but formaldehyde is fortunately not liberated in the blood. They are contraindicated in renal failure because too little is excreted in the urine to be effective and the additional acid load may be dangerous. With normal renal function, however, over 90% of a dose is excreted within 24 h and antibacterial efficacy is maintained for at least 6 h. Methenamine salts are well tolerated. Formaldehyde can occasionally cause urinary tract irritation and some patients develop gastrointestinal side effects such as nausea, vomiting and diarrhoea. Their use is now infrequent, antibiotics usually being preferred for the treatment of urinary infections. They are still useful in chronic urinary tract infections.

Drugs employed in the treatment of tuberculosis

Isoniazid (Isonicotinic acid hydrazide; INH)

This is one of the most important agents for the treatment of tuberculosis. It is bactericidal only to *Mycobacterium tuberculosis* with an MIC of about 0.2 μg/ml. It acts only on growing bacteria, possibly by interference with the synthesis of mycolic acid, a constituent of the bacterial wall. Resistance is readily developed to INH by tubercle bacilli.

Pharmacokinetics It is readily absorbed from the gut, diffuses well into the body tissues, including the CSF, and penetrates into macrophages so that it is effective against intracellular tubercle bacilli. It undergoes genetically controlled polymorphic acetylation in the liver (see Chapter 4). The proportion of a given population characterised as fast or slow acetylators depends upon the group's ethnic make-up, a high percentage of fast acetylators being found in Japanese and Eskimo populations. In European populations 40–45% are rapid acetylators. A $t_{1/2}$ of less than 80 min is found in fast acetylators and one of greater than 140 min is seen in slow acetylators. 50–70% of the drug is excreted in the urine within 24 h as metabolite or free drug, and although impaired renal function is not usually a problem, abnormally high and potentially toxic levels may be reached in slow acetylators with renal impairment.

Clinical uses In tuberculosis a daily dose of 5 mg/kg for adults and 6 mg/kg for children is usually employed. A higher dose of 15 mg/kg is used in twice weekly regimes. High doses are also used in tuberculous meningitis. An injectable preparation is available for patients unable to take oral drugs. INH has often been given in a mixture with ethambutol (Mynah) or rifampicin (Rifinah) or PAS (e.g. Pasinah) to increase compliance and prevent inadvertent monotherapy with a single drug which might encourage the emergence of resistant strains.

Adverse effects Toxic effects are uncommon with the usual dosage of 200–300 mg/day but are more frequent in slow acetylators. The commonest effects are restlessness, insomnia and muscle twitching. More serious is a peripheral neuropathy which is reversed or prevented by pyridoxine (vitamin B_6) administration (10 mg daily is adequate). 1% of patients treated may develop a clinically significant hepatitis which rarely produces hepatic necrosis. It is possible that acetylisoniazid is responsible for this effect, since enzyme inducers such as rifampicin result in higher binding of the acetyl metabolite in the liver and are associated with increased toxicity.

Rifampicin (Rifadin; Rimactane)

Rifampicin is a derivative of rifamycin which is produced by *Streptomyces mediterranei* which is effective against several bacterial species including *Staphylococcus pyogenes*, *Neisseria gonorrhoea* and *meningitidis* and *Mycobacterium tuberculosis*. The bacilli are inhibited at concentrations well below 0.5 μg/ml. It acts by inhibiting bacterial RNA polymerase and because of its high lipid solubility it diffuses easily through cell membranes to kill intracellular bacteria.

Pharmacokinetics Absorption from the gut is almost complete but is impaired or at least delayed by food. Absorption is also impaired by concurrent PAS treatment. Peak levels of about 10 μg/ml plasma are reached 3 h after a single oral dose of 600 mg and significant levels persist for 12 h. The $t_{1/2}$ is $1\frac{1}{2}$–5 h. Renal insufficiency does not significantly raise the plasma levels of the drug. 85–90% of the drug is protein bound in plasma but rifampicin penetrates well into most tissues, cavities and exudates, although relatively little enters the brain and CSF. It is metabolised by deacetylation and is excreted mainly in the bile: less than 10% appears unchanged in the urine. The drug and its metabolite are actively secreted into the bile and undergo a prolonged enterohepatic circulation. Higher plasma levels and a longer $t_{1/2}$ follow administration of probenecid and toxicity is increased by biliary obstruction or impaired liver function.

Clinical uses In the primary treatment of tuberculosis, the drug is used with at least one other anti-tuberculous drug. Rifampicin alone predisposes to the proliferation of resistant strains. The dose is 600 mg once daily before meals. It is also used in the treatment of nasopharyngeal meningococcal carriers since it is present in the saliva, the dose being 600 mg twice daily for two days. In Legionnaire's disease 600 mg daily may be given (see p. 688).

Adverse effects The use of large doses (as in intermittent therapy) produces toxic effects in about one third of patients. Within a few hours flu-like symptoms—flushing, rashes, abdominal pain and respiratory symptoms—develop. Smaller daily doses do not often produce alimentary symptoms or rashes. The drug is hepatotoxic and it is important to measure pre- and intra-treatment serum aminotransferases. Serious liver damage is uncommon but minor histological changes and rises in aminotransferase are common and in the absence of jaundice are not an indication for stopping treatment. Rashes and thrombocytopenia are rare but potentially serious toxic effects. Rifampicin markedly induces hepatic microsomal activity and can accelerate the metabolism of corticosteroids, anticoagulants and oestrogens. In women who have hitherto used the contraceptive pill, the method of contraception should be changed.

Rifampicin turns the urine and tears pink—which may be a useful guide to compliance with therapy.

Ethambutol (Myambutol)

This is the d-isomer of ethylenediimino dibutanol. It inhibits about 75% of strains of *M. tuberculosis* at a concentration of 1 μg/ml. Other organisms are completely resistant. Resistance to ethambutol develops slowly and the drug inhibits strains which are resistant to INH or streptomycin.

Pharmacokinetics The drug is well absorbed (75–80%) by the intestine, and a single dose of 25 mg/kg gives a peak plasma level of 5 μg/ml at 2–4 h. The plasma $t_{1/2}$ is 5–6 h. The drug is concentrated in the red cells and this provides a depot for entry into the plasma. About 80% is excreted unchanged in the urine and 15% is excreted as an aldehyde or dicarboxylate. Ethambutol is contraindicated in renal dysfunction, as very high blood levels may be attained.

Adverse effects In high dosage (25 mg/kg) for prolonged periods there is a 10% risk of producing retrobulbar neuritis with scotomata and loss of visual acuity. The first signs are blurring of vision and loss of red–green perception. Withdrawal of the drug is usually followed by recovery. Doses of 15 mg/kg daily rarely produce ocular complications and higher doses (25 mg/kg) should be reserved for retreatment or tuberculosis meningitis. Testing of colour vision and visual fields should precede treatment and the patient should be regularly examined for visual disturbances.

High doses may also produce:

rashes, pruritus
joint pains
nausea, abdominal pain
confusion, hallucinations, peripheral neuropathy.

Ethambutol is one of the main agents used in the primary therapy of tuberculosis and has virtually replaced PAS.

Para-aminosalicylic acid (PAS)

This is a relatively weak antituberculous drug which has been used in combination therapy to inhibit the development of resistant strains of the tubercle bacillus to other concurrently used drugs.

PAS is an analogue of p-aminobenzoic acid and acts in a similar way to the sulphonamides. It is bacteriostatic to most strains of *M. tuberculosis* at a concentration of 1 μg/ml, but PAS-resistant strains may only be inhibited at several hundred times this concentration.

Pharmacokinetics PAS is well absorbed from the intestine. When a single oral dose of 4 g is given, peak levels of 75 μg/ml are reached in $1\frac{1}{2}$–2 h. The plasma $t_{1/2}$ is short (1 h). PAS may inhibit the absorption of rifampicin and the two drugs should not be given simultaneously. High concentrations are reached in pleural fluid and caseous lesions, but penetration into the CSF is poor.

80% of the drug is excreted in the urine, 50% as the acetyl form, but genetic polymorphism of acetylation of PAS has not been demonstrated. Excretion is greatly impaired in patients with renal dysfunction and the drug should not be used in such individuals.

Adverse effects PAS interferes with iodine metabolism and produces goitre and myxoedema. This can be treated with thyroxine without stopping PAS therapy.

Allergy to PAS commonly develops (5–10% patients). The large amounts required (10–12 g/day in single or divided doses) frequently cause nausea, vomiting, abdominal discomfort and diarrhoea. These tend to diminish after the first week of treatment. Other serious reactions which occur less commonly include syndromes which resemble hepatitis, encephalitis, and infectious mononucleosis.

The use of PAS is now decreasing because less toxic and more effective drugs have become available.

Pyrazinamide (Zinamide) is a powerful drug which is well tolerated in a dose of 30 mg/kg (maximum 2.5 g). It crosses the blood–brain barrier to achieve therapeutic CSF levels and is therefore a drug of first choice in tuberculous meningitis and is now being used by some authorities as the fourth drug in combination régimes. It may cause hyperuricaemia and precipitate an acute attack of gout. Pre-treatment plasma aminotransferase must be measured, as about 5% of patients develop hepatotoxicity so that repeated measurements must be made during treatment. It should be avoided if there is a history of alcohol abuse and treatment should not be continued for more than two months.

The management of pulmonary tuberculosis

In the mid-1950s, daily PAS, INH and streptomycin (PAS and INH given up to four times daily) for two years was shown to be highly effective therapy for tuberculosis. Sanatorium treatment, regular monthly radiographs and monthly sputum culture and sensitivity tests were routine accompaniments to drug treatment. There were many indications for surgery. In addition, a regular 3–6 monthly follow-up lasted several years.

More recently it has been found that constant inhibitory concentrations of drugs are not essential, and single pulses can inhibit bacterial replication for several days. Thus twice-weekly regimes can be used. Whereas 10 years ago about 3000 administrations of drug were required to cure tuberculosis, in some present regimes only 100 doses are necessary for cure.

Controlled clinical trials have failed to confirm benefit from bed rest, hospitalisation or any other component of the sanatorium regime. Repeated radiography has been relegated to a minor role, but sputum testing remains the most important way of assessing treatment. Surprisingly the presence or absence of drug-resistant bacilli has little value in predicting the response to a particular drug treatment. A much more important cause of relapse is a failure of compliance to regular drug administration. The use of lung resection (and other surgical procedures) in patients with residual radiographic signs has greatly declined because of the high success rate in these patients using chemotherapy alone. Long-term follow-up has also been found to be unnecessary because of the low relapse rate after chemotherapy.

In the UK the following plan of treatment is usually routinely employed:

1. Rifampicin 10 mg/kg once daily before food
   Isoniazid 5 mg/kg once daily
   Ethambutol 15 mg/kg once daily or streptomycin 0.75–1 g/day.

After 8 weeks treatment, it is usual to stop ethambutol and continue rifampicin and isoniazid for a further 7 months. Treatment may have to be modified depending on the clinical response, the sensitivity of the organism and the development of adverse effects. With this regime the sputum should be free of tubercle bacilli in a week.

Some authorities would use pyrazinamide 20–30 mg/kg daily for the first two months of treatment and given with the other three drugs, it reduces the course of treatment to six months.

In severely ill patients or those where rapid reduction in the size of the lesion is desirable (i.e. if it is causing pressure effects), corticosteroids should be combined with the antibiotics for the first 2 months of treatment and then withdrawn slowly.

2. If patients cannot be relied upon to take their drugs regularly, they are treated in hospital or as outpatients. Twice weekly supervised outpatient

treatment consists of streptomycin 1 g with INH 15 mg/kg, or rifampicin with INH.

3. If there is a relapse after previous treatment, the drugs of the previous regime are not used if resistance has been shown to have developed. Alternative, but less effective and more toxic drugs are:

PAS	cycloserine
ethionamide	capreomycin
prothionamide	viomycin
	kanamycin

4. Open healed cavities are not now surgically resected unless they are superinfected with aspergillus or they bleed. Bronchial stenosis may require surgical treatment.

Tuberculous meningitis

Many of the problems in treating tuberculosis meningitis arise from the poor penetration of most antimicrobials into the cerebrospinal fluid.

Isoniazid is the most useful drug. It is highly effective and concentrations inhibitory to tubercle bacilli are obtained in the CSF. Streptomycin penetrates well only when the meninges are inflamed and therefore is only effective in the early stages of treatment. Intrathecal streptomycin has been widely used in the past but is now no longer considered necessary. Ethambutol is somewhat similar with satisfactory penetration in the acute stage of the disease, particularly with higher dosage levels. Rifampicin penetrates poorly into the CSF, presumably because of the high protein-bound fraction in the plasma and the concentration in the CSF only just reaches the MIC for tubercle bacilli. Pyrazinamide penetrates quite well.

There is at present no optimal regime for treating meningeal infection. The following is suggested as satisfactory:

Isoniazid 10 mg/kg + pyridoxine 20 mg daily
Rifampicin 10 mg/kg daily
Pyrazinamide 30 mg/kg daily

After two months this should be followed by isoniazid and rifampicin for at least a further 8 months.

Steroids (dexamethasone 2.0 mg/kg) are sometimes used in the initial stages of treatment.

Primary tuberculosis is treated with one drug alone—usually INH.

Corticosteroids These are not often used in tuberculosis but may assist in:

resolution of large lymph nodes;
suppression of severe drug allergy;
advanced pleural effusions;
patients likely to die before chemotherapy can be effective;
tuberculous meningitis to reduce the formation of meningeal adhesions which could result in permanent neurological deficit.

Short-treatment regimes

Work in East Africa and Hong Kong has shown that courses of chemotherapy lasting 6 months can be effective, particularly using streptomycin, INH and rifamipicin or streptomycin, INH and pyrazinamide. A higher bacteriological relapse rate occurs with streptomycin, INH and thiacetazone and with streptomycin and INH alone (22–29% compared with 3–8% for standard therapy). With all regimes most relapses occurred in the first 6 months after the end of treatment.

Perhaps the most effective of the experimental short-treatment schemes is an initial intensive phase of 4 drugs (streptomycin, INH, rifampicin and pyrazinamide) followed by twice-weekly streptomycin, INH and rifampicin for the continuation phase, the total treatment time being 6 months. There is some evidence that daily therapy in the continuation phase may allow a further reduction in total treatment time. Reduction in the total number of doses as well as their frequency appears possible and a recent trial has shown the effectiveness of the following scheme:

(a) Daily treatment with streptomycin, INH and rifampicin for 2 weeks, followed by:

(b) Rifampicin 600 or 900 mg for a 70 kg adult and INH 15 mg/kg, once or twice weekly for 6 months.

Drugs for retreatment of tuberculosis

Although the detection of resistant bacilli before or during primary treatment is not of great value in predicting the outcome of an initial course of treatment, once a patient has relapsed after a completed course of therapy, careful planning is necessary. The previous drugs used should be known and current bacterial sensitivity found. If the organisms are still sensitive to the original drugs, then a more fully supervised and prolonged therapy with these drugs should be carried out. If bacterial resistance has arisen then the alternative drugs are used. These include the following.

Capreomycin (Capastat) is an effective drug, but like other aminoglycosides, can produce nephrotoxicity and ototoxicity with high plasma levels. A daily intramuscular dose of 15 mg/kg does not usually produce harmful effects. Nevertheless blood levels should be monitored. Hypokalaemia, hypocalcaemia and hypomagnesaemia can complicate capreomycin therapy and may require treatment.

Ethionamide (Trescatyl) and **prothionamide (Trevintix)** may both produce considerable nausea after oral administration. These drugs should therefore be given as a single daily dose in the late evening with a sedative. Other toxic effects include liver damage, neuropathy and mental disturbance.

Cycloserine is the most toxic of the second line drugs. In an effective therapeutic dose (1 g orally per day), epilepsy and toxic psychosis may be produced.

ANTIFUNGAL AGENTS

Fungi, like mammalian cells, are eukaryotic and possess nuclei, mitochondria and cell membranes containing sterols. None of these structures occur in bacteria which is one reason why antibacterial agents can act selectively. This similarity between fungal and mammalian cells militates against selective toxicity and antifungal drugs are in general more toxic than antibacterial agents.

The very success of antibacterial therapy has created ecological situations in which opportunistic fungal infections can arise. In addition, potent immunosuppressive and cytotoxic therapies have produced patients with seriously impaired immune defences, so that fungi which are non-pathogenic to healthy individuals can become pathogenic in these patients.

Amphotericin B (Fungilin; Fungizone)

Amphotericin is an antibiotic derived from *Streptomyces nodosus* which was isolated from soil collected in the Orinoco basin in Venezuela. It is a polyene macrolide with a hydroxylated hydrophilic surface on one side of the molecule and an unsaturated conjugated lipophilic surface on the other. It is insoluble in water but can be complexed to bile salts to give an unstable colloid which can be given intravenously.

Amphotericin binds to a sterol present in fungal cell membranes and increases their permeability, allowing leakage and loss of small molecules such as glucose, and essential ions including potassium, thus depressing metabolism. Amphotericin has higher affinity for the ergosterol of fungal membranes than for the cholesterol of mammalian membranes, thus permitting some selectivity, although it is likely that many of the adverse effects of amphotericin are due to a similar toxic effect on mammalian membranes.

The spectrum is effectively the widest of all antifungal drugs:

Blastomycosis dermatidis (causes N. American blastomycosis)
Histoplasma capsulatum (causes histoplasmosis)
Cryptococcus neoformans (causes cryptococcosis)
Candida spp. (local and systemic infections)
Coccidiodes immitis (causes coccidioidomycosis)
Sporotrichum schencki (causes sporotrichosis)

Nocardia and *Aspergillus spp.* are usually resistant.

Resistance is rarely gained by fungi during treatment. Some forms of infection, such as blastomycosis, often relapse and others, particularly coccidioidomycosis, are frequently impossible to cure.

Pharmacokinetics Amphotericin is poorly absorbed following oral and intramuscular administration; therefore for systemic mycoses it must be given by i.v. infusion or intrathecally. Given i.v. it distributes very unevenly throughout the body, levels in the CSF being only one fortieth of the plasma level. There may be selective concentration of drug in the reticuloendothelial system. The $t_{1/2}$ is 18–24 h. The drug is over 90 % protein bound, explaining the poor penetration into tissues. Only 5 % is excreted in the urine and elimination and protein binding are unaffected by renal failure.

Table 19.26 Antifungal agents

Drug	*Mode of action*	*Pharmacokinetics*	*Clinical usage*	*Adverse effects*
Clotrimazole (Canesten)	Increases permeability of fungal membrane (not a polyene but an imidazole). May inhibit peroxidases thus causing toxic peroxide accumulation	Poorly absorbed orally but cannot be given i.v. Metabolised in liver and induces hepatic enzymes	Vaginal candidiasis or trichomonas, ringworm. Vaginal tablets 200 mg nocte for 3 nights. 1% cream applied to skin for 2 weeks.	Gastrointestinal upset and hepatotoxicity if given systemically. Local application safe
Miconazole (Daktarin; Dermonistat)	As clotrimazole	As clotrimazole	Poor absorption so best used systemically 600 mg 8 hourly. Second-line treatment for systemic candidiasis. Also available as tablets or 2% cream (for ringworm) and candida.	Nausea, vomiting, rashes.
Ketoconazole (Nizoral)	As clotrimazole	Well absorbed orally unless given with H_2-blocker or antacid	Serious candidiasis, local and systemic mycoses. 200–400 mg daily with food	Nausea, rashes, diarrhoea, giddiness and *liver damage* (may be irreversible and progress when drug stopped). Do not use in pregnancy

Natamycin (Pimafucin)	Polyene antibiotic	Not absorbed orally	Locally for topical candidiasis as cream, vaginal tablets or inhalation	Local application safe
Tolnaftate (Tinaderm)	Unknown	Not absorbed orally	Local use only for dermatophytes in conjunction with griseofulvin. *Candida* is resistant	Local erythema
Povidone-iodine (Betadine)	Oxidising agent: (liberates iodine on to skin surface)	Only applied locally	Local use for candidiasis and dermatophytosis	Local erythema

Clinical use It is given as an intravenous infusion freshly prepared in 5% dextrose of pH above 4.2 over 4–6 h. A test dose of 1.0 mg should be given at least 6 hours before starting treatment. The initial dose is 5 mg daily in 500 ml of 5% dextrose which is increased daily by 5 mg to a dose of 0.5 mg/kg daily and continued for 6–12 weeks. Treatment on alternate days at 1.0 mg/kg may reduce toxicity. Amphotericin is also given intrathecally (0.5 mg thrice weekly) or topically as lozenges (10 mg 3 hourly) or suspension for oral or oesophageal and gastro-intestinal moniliasis respectively.

There is some evidence that effective therapy may be achieved by reduced doses and therefore lower toxicity if amphotericin is combined with 5-fluorocytosine as fluorocytosine increases penetration into the fungal cell. The dose of amphotericin should then be 0.3 mg/kg/day.

Adverse effects Common side effects during i.v. infusion are fever, chills, headache, nausea and vomiting, and the pulse and temperature should be monitored every 30 min so that the infusion can be halted if necessary.

Nephrotoxicity is almost invariable and results from vasoconstriction, impaired acid excretion (renal tubular acidosis), nephrocalcinosis and acute renal failure. Fortunately most of these lesions are reversible if detected early and the drug is discontinued.

A normochromic normocytic anaemia is also usual, but it is self-limited and reversible, being due to temporary marrow suppression.

It must be stressed that amphotericin should not be withheld in serious progressive infection caused by a sensitive fungus solely from fear of the possible side effects.

Nystatin (Nystan)

This is another polyene antifungal antibiotic isolated from a *Streptomyces sp.* with an identical mode of action to amphotericin. The spectrum is limited solely to fungi, but nystatin has a broad spectrum within this group. Unfortunately, its toxicity limits its use against all but cutaneous and mucocutaneous infections, especially those caused by *Candida spp.* which does not gain resistance to nystatin during therapy. Epidermophytes are not sensitive.

Pharmacokinetics Very little nystatin is absorbed from the gastrointestinal tract but it is extremely toxic if given by injection.

Clinical use As tablets, pastilles, lozenges or suspension it is given in doses of 100 000–500 000 units three times daily for oral or intestinal *Candida* infections. It is intensely bitter in taste, however, and many patients prefer amphotericin. Cutaneous infections are treated with ointment, vaginitis by suppositories and an aerosol has been used for pulmonary conditions.

Adverse effects No adverse effects result from the topical use of nystatin. Nausea and diarrhoea may follow large oral doses.

Griseofulvin (Grisovin; Fulcin)

This drug was isolated from *Penicillium griseofulvium* and its mode of action is obscure. Possibly, interference with fungal DNA replication results in the distorted hyphal growth which follows its application. Griseofulvin appears to be actively taken up by fungi. The spectrum is limited to the dermatophytes (ringworm fungi). Resistance is not a practical problem.

Pharmacokinetics Griseofulvin is nearly insoluble in water and is given as micronised particles, the absorption of which is facilitated by a fatty meal. The drug is slow in action because it must first be taken up in keratinised structures, which grow slowly, to reach the site of infection. Cell turnover time thus determines efficacy of treatment so that palmar and plantar skin requires at least eight weeks treatment, fingernails six months and toenails up to one year for eradicative treatment.

Griseofulvin is metabolised by the liver to inactive 6-demethylgriseofulvin, which is excreted in the urine. Inducing agents such as barbiturates enhance griseofulvin metabolism and griseofulvin itself, an inducing agent, interacts with coumarin anticoagulants to reduce their anticoagulant effect. Less than 1% free griseofulvin is renally excreted, so that it is used in usual doses in renal failure.

Clinical use As 0.5–1 g daily in two divided doses, with meals. It is useless applied topically. Treatment should be for 6 weeks in skin infections and up to 12 months for nail infections.

Adverse effects It is a safe drug but a minority of patients report headaches and mental dullness or inattention which restricts its use in some patients with demanding occupations. Occasionally diarrhoea or nausea follows its use. It has also caused skin rashes.

Its enzyme-inducing activity may aggravate acute intermittent porphyria and result in drug–drug interactions. It has a potentiating effect on alcohol.

Flucytosine (5-fluorocytosine; Alcobon)

Although originally synthesised as an antimetabolite it has little value as a cytotoxic agent. The precise mode of action is unknown but it is deaminated to 5-fluorouracil, a known antimetabolite which inhibits thymidylate synthetase thereby depressing DNA synthesis and is incorporated into RNA. Its relative specificity is due to the presence of cytosine deaminase in fungi. Flucytosine enters the fungus actively by permease enzymes. Amphotericin acts synergistically with it presumably by facilitating its entry.

Its spectrum is relatively restricted to *Cryptococcus neoformans*, *Candida albicans* and some other *Candida spp.*, *Torulopsis spp.* and *Cladosporum spp.* There are big differences in sensitivity between strains: 5–15% have innate resistance, and resistance is relatively easily acquired during therapy. Filamentous fungi, especially *Aspergillus*, are resistant to this drug.

Pharmacokinetics Flucytosine is well absorbed from the gut, peak levels of 75–90 μg/ml being attained on a dose of 50 mg/kg 6 hourly, and it penetrates adequately into the CSF and lung. It is largely excreted unchanged by glomerular filtration with less than 10% of the dose undergoing metabolism. The $t_{1/2}$ is 6 h and this is increased by renal failure.

Clinical use It can be used for systemic candidiasis and cryptococcosis, providing that the strain is sensitive. The optimal oral dose is 150 mg/kg/day in 6 hourly divided doses. For very ill patients an i.v. preparation is available. In attempts to limit the risk of acquired resistance it is used with amphotericin. It is far too valuable an agent for systemic infections to allow topical use because of the danger of widespread emergence of resistant *Candida*. It is also an expensive drug.

Adverse effects In contrast to amphotericin, flucytosine is a drug of relatively low toxicity. The main problems are gastrointestinal upsets, leucopenia and abnormalities of liver-function tests which should be monitored, but which do not appear to presage liver failure. At plasma concentrations below 100 μg/ml there is little danger of toxicity but at higher levels depression of bone marrow and hepatotoxicity can occur. Therapy in patients with decreased renal function should therefore be monitored by frequent plasma drug assays if these are available.

The effect of flucytosine is antagonised by concurrent administration of cytosine arabinoside.

ANTIVIRAL DRUGS

Antiviral chemotherapy is intrinsically more difficult than antibacterial therapy because:

(i) Viral replication is essentially intracellular so that drugs must penetrate into cells to be effective.

(ii) The process, although under control of the viral genome, predominantly involves metabolic processes of the host cells so that antiviral compounds must halt viral replication without affecting normal cellular functions.

(iii) Although viral replication begins almost immediately the host cell is penetrated, the clinical signs and symptoms of infection often appear after peak replication is over. These clinical manifestations often result from inflammatory and other processes mounted by the host in response to viral damage to tissues.

(iv) Many viral infections cannot be rapidly and specifically diagnosed with certainty using present diagnostic techniques, and therefore will be susceptible to chemotherapy only if a drug with a wide antiviral spectrum is available.

The main events in viral colonisation which might be susceptible to drug action are:

(a) Virus outside cells is susceptible to antibody attack but it has proved difficult to find drugs which are non-toxic yet can destroy viruses in this situation.

(b) Viral attachment to the cell surface probably involves a specific chemical reaction between the virus coat and the cell surface. Neuraminidase, an enzyme which destroys myxovirus receptors, including those on the cell surfaces, has an effect on experimental infections in animals.
(c) Penetration of the cell membrane can be prevented by amantadine in influenza.
(d) Uncoating of the virus with release of viral nucleic acid intracellularly.
(e) Viral nucleic acid acts as a template for new strands of nucleic acid which in turn direct the production of new viral components utilising the host cell's synthetic mechanisms. Most antiviral drugs in current use act at this stage of viral growth.
(f) Release of new viral particles.

At present the range of proven effective antiviral drugs is very limited.

Amantadine (Symmetrel)

This drug, used in the treatment of Parkinson's disease (see p. 262), was fortuitously discovered to have a prophylactic action in preventing the spread of influenza. Its usefulness is limited to influenza A: it is inactive on influenza B and only weakly active on influenza C and rubella. These are all RNA viruses. Its mode of action is unknown. Prophylaxis with amantadine has an advantage over immunisation in that the latter can be ineffective when a new antigenic variant arises in the community and spreads too rapidly for a killed virus vaccine to be prepared and administered. Prophylaxis by amantadine is possible in persons at risk, e.g. with severe lung or cardiac disease. It appears to be less effective during periods of antigenic variation than during periods of relative antigenic stability. The effectiveness of amantadine as treatment rather than prophylaxis when given during the first 48 h of illness is relatively slight: the fever is shortened by 24–30 h and headache and respiratory symptoms are reduced. The usual prophylactic dose is 200 mg daily, the compound is renally excreted with a $t_{1/2}$ of about 12 hours and precautions are needed when it is given to patients with renal failure.

Adverse effects with short-term use include dizziness, nervousness and headaches.

Rimantadine is similar to amantadine.

Methisazone (Marboran)

This is a substituted thiosemicarbazone derived from compounds originally developed as antituberculous drugs. It is active against pox viruses by inhibiting formation of viral structural proteins although viral DNA synthesis is unaffected. It has been used prophylactically in smallpox contacts in an oral dose of 1.5–3 g twice daily for 4 days. It should not be used, however, as a substitute for vaccination, which remains the most effective prophylactic. Given with vaccination it depresses the local reactions but may also impair the antibody response. Therefore it should not be used in this way. There may be a place for methisazone in the treatment of generalised vaccinia (eczema vaccinatum) and in progressive vaccinia (vaccinia gangrenosum). When untreated the latter is almost invariably fatal. Treatment with methisazone together with anti-vaccinial gamma-globulin halves the mortality rate. The usual dose is 50 mg/kg 6 hourly following a loading dose of 200 mg/kg. Anorexia, nausea and vomiting occur in about 80% of patients despite use of anti-emetics, and these effects are exacerbated by alcohol.

Idoxuridine (5-iodo-2-deoxyuridine; IDU)

IDU is an analogue of the DNA nucleotide thymidine and has been shown to inhibit the replication of certain DNA viruses, particularly herpes viruses. Likely mechanisms of action include incorporation of the drug into DNA and/or competitive inhibition of enzymes involved in nucleic acid synthesis. Because of this it is only relatively selective for viral nucleic acid synthesis and can cause toxic effects on mammalian bone marrow resulting in leucopenia and thrombocytopenia. Viral resistance to IDU is said to develop readily.

Idoxuridine is used in a number of situations:

(a) Herpetic keratitis: hourly drops of 0.1% IDU in saline encourage resolution of corneal ulcers providing a deep stromal reaction has not occurred. Prolonged use however may cause blepharitis, conjunctivitis and puctate lesions of the corneal epithelium.

(b) Herpes labialis: recurrent lesions may be aborted by treating the affected area with 5.0% IDU solution (Herpid) at the first sign of recurrence (usually a burning sensation in the affected skin precedes vesicle formation).

(c) Herpes zoster: applied topically as a 5% IDU solution in dimethyl sulphoxide (Herpid) it may hasten healing of the rash and possibly reduce the development of post-herpetic neuralgia. Dimethylsulphoxide enhances skin penetration but is an irritant and *must never be applied to the eye*. It is important to begin treatment as early as possible, preferably as the lesions are developing. It may be especially valuable in the elderly (in whom post-herpetic neuralgia is common) and those with immunological impairment (e.g. steroid or cytotoxic treatment).

BVDV is like idoxuridine, a halogenated pyrimidine. It is useful in herpes simplex (type I) and zoster and can be given orally or as a local ophthalmic preparation. Experience is limited but it appears less toxic than idoxuridine.

Adenine arabinoside (Vidarabine, Ara-A) has had some success in the treatment of herpes simplex encephalitis given intravenously in a dose of 15 mg/kg/day over 12 h for 10 days with less toxicity than Ara-C. Early diagnosis coupled with brain biopsy (to avoid unnecessary treatment of non-responsive encephalitides) is essential for good results. Clinical trials for systemic zoster affecting patients with immune suppression or deficiency have also been encouraging. Myelosuppression can occur and blood count monitoring is essential. It can cause gastrointestinal and CNS disturbances.

Ribarin is a broad spectrum antiviral agent with some action against several DNA (HSV 1 and 2, vaccinia) and RNA viruses. It may interfere with viral nucleic acid synthesis. It is absorbed orally with a $t_{1/2}$ of 24 hours. Clinical experience is limited but prolonged use can produce anaemia.

Interferons

These are glycoproteins secreted by cells brought into contact with viruses or foreign double-stranded DNA. They are non-antigenic and are active against a wide range of viruses, but unfortunately are relatively species specific since they protect only cells of the animal species in which they are manufactured. Thus it is necessary to produce human interferon to act on human cells. Interferons reversibly bind to receptors on the cell membrane which then activate intracellular enzymes that affect messenger-RNA translation and protein synthesis. The onset of these effects takes several hours but may persist for days. They also affect antibody synthesis, macrophage activation and T and NK (natural killer) cell cytotoxicity. The possibility of treating infections by stimulating endogenous interferon formation with substances derived from bacteria such as **helenine** and **statolon** or with synthetic macromolecules such as **polyinosine (poly I)** or **polycytosine (poly C)** has yet to reach effective clinical application.

Interferons belong to a class of hormone-like substances which are locally active regulatory glycoproteins, the so-called cytokines, which include erythropoietin, lymphotoxin, migration-inhibitory factor and epithelial-growth factor. Interferon production is triggered not only by viruses but also by tumour cells or previously encountered foreign antigens. There is increasing evidence that some interferons, such as those produced by T (suppressor) lymphocytes during immune responses are important in immune cell regulation. This being so, there is currently interest in assessing the effects of interferon in cancer chemotherapy. Intranasal interferon suppresses coryza.

Three main types of interferon with different structures, derivation and properties are recognised:

(i) *Interferon-alfa*: known previously as leucocyte or lymphoblastoid interferon. Subspecies of the human alfa gene produce variants designated by the addition of a number, e.g. interferon alfa-2, or in the case of a mixture of proteins, by N1, N2 etc. Two methods of commercial production have been developed to date and these are indicated by:

(rbe)—produced from bacteria (*E. coli*) genetically modified by recombinant DNA technology.

(lns)—produced from cultured lymphoblasts stimulated by Sendai virus.

Interferon alfa-2 may also differ in the amino acids at positions 23 and 24 and these are shown by the addition of a letter. Thus Alfa-2A has lys-his at these sites whilst Alfa-2B has arg-his. At present it is not certain whether these different molecules have different therapeutic properties.

(ii) *Interferon-beta*: from fibroblasts.

(iii) *Interferon-gamma*: formerly called ‘immune’ interferon as it is produced by lymphocytes in response to antigens and mitogens.

It is now possible to prepare large amounts of pure interferon by cloning of interferon genes into bacterial and yeast plasmids. Most clinical experience is with interferon-alpha. It has been given intravenously, intramuscularly or topically (nasal, vaginal, mucosal and eye) and does not penetrate the CSF. The half-life after intravenous injection is 2–3 hours. Toxicity is common but fever, malaise, chills and lymphocytopenia are reversible and tolerance may occur after a week or so. Rarer effects include alopecia, weight loss, fatigue and confusion.

Acyclovir (Zovirax)

This is a potent and selective inhibitor of herpes viruses (particularly herpes simplex). Its selective action results from its metabolism solely in infected cells to its monophosphate via a specific thymidine kinase coded by the virus but not the host genome. Subsequent conversion occurs to the di- and triphosphates, presumably by cellular kinases. The triphosphate of acyclovir inhibits viral DNA synthesis.

Pharmacokinetics The bioavailability after administration in man is only 20% after 200 mg orally and may be dose dependent. The $t_{1/2}$ is 3 hours. The drug penetrates widely and crosses the blood–brain barrier to give a concentration of approximately 50% of the plasma level. Plasma protein binding in man is around 20%. Clearance is largely renal and includes an element of tubular secretion. It is reduced if renal function is impaired.

Clinical uses

(a) Herpetic keratitis—3% ointment applied five times daily for up to 14 days accelerates healing and is probably the preferred treatment for this condition.

(b) Genital and labial herpes simplex. The efficacy of local application has not been impressive. In spite of its low bioavailability, 200 mg four hourly orally has been reported as accelerating healing in genital herpes. In larger doses (400 mg 5 times daily) it prevents infection in the immunosuppressed.

Table 19.27 Treatment of viral infections

Genital herpes	*Drug*
Severe with systemic symptoms	Intravenous (5 mg/kg 8 hourly for 5 days) or oral acyclovir (200 mg 5 times daily) for five days
Mild	Oral or topical acyclovir (5% cream applied 5 times daily)
Recurrent	No clear indications. Try oral acyclovir
Labial herpes	Povidone iodine twice daily for 4 days, or 5% idoxuridine 6 hourly for 4 days
Keratitic herpes	3% acyclovir ointment applied 5 times daily. Alternatively 0.1% IDU (*not* 'Herpid') hourly to begin with. Treatments must be continued for 3–5 days after healing has occurred.
Herpes zoster	IDU 5% in DMSO applied 6 hourly for 4 days. In severe cases substitute IDU 35%
Influenza A	Amantadine 100 mg orally twice daily
Prevention	
Cytomegalic virus	No proven effective agent

(c) In generalised herpes simplex or herpetic meningoencephalitis acyclovir can be given intravenously in doses of 5 mg/kg infused over 1 hour three times daily for 5 days. Reduced dosage is required with impaired renal function.

Adverse effects

(a) Reversible rise in plasma urea and creatinine
(b) Neurological disturbances
(c) Rashes
(d) Nausea and vomiting
(e) Increase in liver enzymes
(f) Contraindicated in pregnancy

ANTIMALARIALS

These may be divided into drugs used in the prophylaxis of malaria and those used to treat the disease.

1. Prophylaxis

Drugs used to prevent malaria are chosen mainly on the basis of local susceptibility patterns. The two main groups of malarial prophylactic drugs are 4-amino quinolines and dihydrofolate reductase inhibitors. Drug treatment must start one day before entering a malaria region, and continue for 4 weeks afterwards.

4-amino quinolines Chloroquine is used as a prophylactic in regions where falciparum Malaria is not resistant to it. The dose is 300 mg weekly. **Amodiaquine** (400 mg weekly) is also effective. There have been occasional reports of bone-marrow suppression from this drug.

Dihydrofolate reductase inhibitors. Pyrimethamine (25–50 mg weekly) is widely used. If pyrimethamine resistance is present, **proguanil** (200 mg daily) is also effective.

Prophylaxis of chloroquine-resistant falciparum malaria

One of the following schemes:
(i) Dapsone 25 mg with proguanil 200 mg daily.
(ii) Maloprim (12.5 mg pyrimethamine plus 100 mg dapsone) weekly.
(iii) Fansidar (sulphadoxine 0.5 g with pyrimethamine 25 mg) weekly. The plasma $t_{1/2}$ of both of these drugs is long: 96 h for pyrimethamine and 200 h for sulphadoxine. Fansidar occasionally causes the Stevens-Johnson syndrome and this adverse effect limits its use. At the time of writing its use is not recommended.

Prevention of malaria in pregnancy This is a difficult problem owing to the theoretical risk to the fetus by antimalarials. There is, however, no evidence

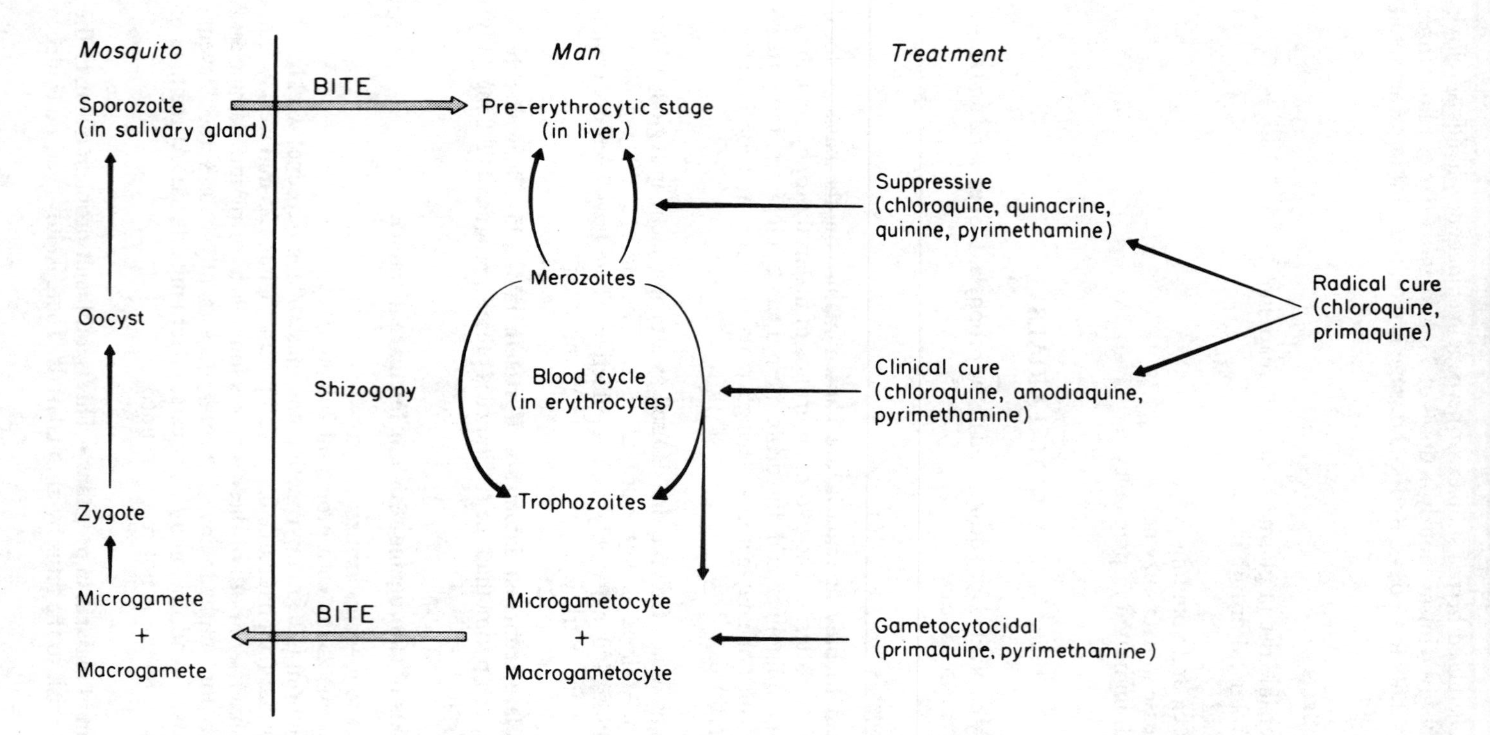

Fig. 19.6 Malaria cycle and type of drug treatment.

that chloroquine, proguanil, maloprim (pyrimethamine + dapsone) or Fansidar (pyrimethamine + sulphadoxine) cause fetal damage but it would be a resonable precaution to prescribe folinic acid during the first trimester if an antifolate (pyrimethamine) is used.

2. Drugs used in the treatment of an acute attack

(a) Chloroquine

This is one of the most widely used antimalarials, particularly against falciparum infections acquired in Africa, but even here partial resistance may exist.

Pharmacokinetics Chloroquine is rapidly and almost completely absorbed from the intestine. Approximately 50% is bound to plasma proteins and excretion is slow. The plasma $t_{1/2}$ is 120 h, but excretion is accelerated by acidifying the urine. High concentrations (relative to plasma) are found in all the tissues. 70% is excreted unchanged and the main metabolite is desethylchloroquine. Some metabolites are active antimalarials. As well as the usual oral route, the drug can also be given intramuscularly and intravenously.

Clinical uses

1. Malarial prophylaxis (suppression).
2. Acute malarial attack: In *vivax* malaria chloroquine is not radically curative, but terminates an acute attack even though relapses occur after treatment ceases. In *falciparum* malaria the drug is usually curative. The routine course of chloroquine is a total dose of 1.5 g (or 30 mg/kg) orally, given in divided doses: 600 mg initially, 300 mg after 6 h and then 300 mg daily for 2 days. Children receive a smaller dose—20 mg/kg. In areas where there is partial resistance to chloroquine, the course is extended for several days to a total of 50 mg/kg. In severe falciparum malaria which is chloroquine sensitive, 5–10 mg/kg of chloroquine is given intravenously every 12–24 h, each dose being administered over a 4 h period. In babies the dose is 5.0 mg/kg by slow intramuscular injection. If given intravenously it can cause encephalopathy.
3. Chloroquine is also used as an anti-inflammatory agent in rheumatoid arthritis and discoid lupus erythematosus. It may also be of some value in acute disseminated lupus erythematosus. Anti-inflammatory treatment given over long periods is prone to produce chloroquine retinopathy, unless dosage is restricted to < 4 mg/kg/day for 6 months.
4. Chloroquine is the drug of first choice in treating infestations with *Clonorchis sinensis* and is the drug of second choice for treating *Fasciola hepatica* and *Paragonimus* infestations. Chloroquine is effective in treating extra-intestinal amoebiasis and in giardiasis.
5. In large doses chloroquine is useful in the treatment of photoallergic reactions.

Adverse effects Malarial prophylaxis: nausea, dyspepsia.

Treatment of an acute malarial attack: mild headache, visual disturbances, pruritus, gastrointestinal upset.

Prolonged treatment with larger doses for diseases other than malaria may produce more serious toxic effects. These include a retinopathy characterised by loss of central visual acuity, macular pigmentation, and retinal artery constriction. Visual loss is not reversible on stopping the drug, but it does not progress.

Other toxic effects on prolonged administration are: lichenoid skin eruption; bleaching of hair; diminution of T waves in ECG; headache; weight loss; ototoxicity; cochleovestibular paresis acquired in fetal life.

Chloroquine and quinine are antagonistic and should not be used together.

(b) Quinine

This is the main alkaloid of the cinchona bark and is primarily used for the treatment of an acute attack of chloroquine-resistant falciparum malaria. However, it has a large number of actions on a number of cell types. It is toxic to bacteria, yeasts, protozoa and some spirochaetes. On animal tissues it has local anaesthetic and irritant effects.

Pharmacokinetics Almost complete absorption occurs in the upper part of the small intestine when quinine is given orally. Thus peak levels are similar following oral or intravenous administration, but are reached 1–3 h after ingestion. Absorption from intramuscular sites is poor and local tissue necrosis can result from subcutaneous injection.

The steady-state plasma levels show wide inter-individual variation. The plasma $t_{1/2}$ is 10 h, but is prolonged beyond this in severe falciparum malaria. Less than 5 % is excreted unaltered in the urine, the rest is metabolised in the liver, principally to hydroxy derivatives.

Adverse effects Large therapeutic doses of quinine give rise to cinchonism (as do large doses of salicylates and cinchophen). This consists of tinnitus, deafness, headaches, nausea and visual disturbances.

Other features of quinine toxicity are: abdominal pain, diarrhoea, rashes, fever, delirium, stimulation followed by depression of respiration, renal failure, haemolytic anaemia, purpura and hypoprothrombinaemia.

Some individuals may develop toxicity when exposed to small doses (idiosyncrasy). Intravenous quinine infusion can produce neurological toxicity: tremor of lips, and limbs, delirium, confusion, fits and coma.

Clinical uses

1. Quinine sulphate is the drug of choice in the treatment of an acute attack of *falciparum* malaria in areas where the parasite is known to be resistant to chloroquine. The usual course is 10 mg/kg orally given every 12 h for a total of four doses. To completely eradicate the disease this should be followed by three tablets of Fansidar (pyrimethamine 75 mg and sulphadoxine 1.5 g) given as a single dose.

2. For recrudescence of treated malaria or for severe falciparum malaria quinine is given intravenously by intermittent infusion in saline. The initial dose should be 10 mg/kg of quinine base infused over 4 h and repeated after 12 h. This interval is required because in the early stages of the disease the

plasma $t_{1/2}$ is prolonged. If there is evidence of liver or renal damage, the interval between infusions should be increased to at least 24 h. In children the dose should be reduced to 5 mg/kg. Four infusions are usually sufficient to control the infection.

3. Quinine may be effective in some patients with myotonia congenita and dystrophia myotonia in doses of 0.3–0.6 g 8 hourly.

4. Nocturnal cramps in ischaemic legs can be relieved by 0.2–0.3 g of quinine before going to bed.

(c) **Mefloquine** This drug, when used with quinine, may be effective in treating chloroquine-resistant falciparum malaria. Mefloquine causes transient abdominal pain, dizziness, nausea, vomiting and weakness in about 50% of patients.

3. Treatment of relapse

P. falciparum does not cause a relapsing illness after treating the acute attack with such schizontocides as chloroquine, because there is no persistent liver stage of the parasite.

Infections with *P. malariae* can cause recurrent attacks of fever for up to 30 years, but standard treatment with chloroquine eradicates the parasite.

Following treatment of an acute attack of *P. vivax* malaria with schizontocides, or a period of protection with prophylactic drugs, febrile illness can recur due to the establishment of liver stages of the parasite. Such relapsing illness is prevented (or treated) by eradicating the parasites in the liver with primaquine (see Table 19.28) 15 mg of the base (26.3 mg of the phosphate) is given daily for 2 weeks. Patients who lack G6PD in their erythrocytes can suffer an acute haemolytic episode from this drug (see p. 111). These individuals are given proguanil hydrochloride continuously (100 mg daily) for 3 years. This drug is a malarial suppressant and will allow time for the hepatic stages to die out naturally.

ANTI-TRYPANOSOMAL DRUGS

African sleeping sickness is caused by *Trypanosoma gambiense* and *Trypanosoma rhodesiense*. The insect vector is the *Glossina* (tsetse) fly. The drugs used in therapy include (Table 19.30):

(a) *Drugs active in blood and peripheral tissues:*

    suramin
    pentamidine
    melarsoprol and trimelarsan
(also: puromycin
    nitrofurazone)

(b) *Drugs active in the central nervous system:*

    tryparsamide
    melarsoprol and trimelarsan

Table 19.28 Drugs used in malarial relapse

Drug	*Pharmacokinetics*	*Toxicity*	*Actions*
Primaquine	Like other 8-aminoquinolines is well absorbed from intestine. Peak plasma concentration at 6 h. Most is metabolised.	Haemolysis in G6PD deficient patients. Mild abdominal discomfort. Mild anaemia. Methaemoglobinaemia. Leucopenia (rare)	Highly active against exoerythrocytic forms of *P. vivax* and *P. falciparum*. Powerful gametocidal activity against all human forms of the parasite
Proguanil (Paludrine)	Well absorbed from intestine. Peak plasma levels at 3 h. 60% excreted unchanged. 30% excreted as cycloguanil	Minor abdominal discomfort	Slow schizontocidal activity. Active against asexual erythrocytic forms of *P. vivax*. Active against exoerythrocytic forms of some stages of *P. falciparum*, but not *P. vivax*. Does not kill gametocytes, but renders them non-infective to mosquitoes

Table 19.29 Summary of the treatment of malaria

	Prophylactic	*P. falciparum* Severe	*P. falciparum* Ordinary	*P. vivax** *P. malariae* *P. ovale*
Chloroquine resistant areas (S.E. Asia and S. America)	Fansidar tabs 1 weekly Maloprim tabs 1 weekly	** Quinine iv 5–10 mg/kg over 4 h every 8 h for 4 doses followed by *** Fansidar.	Quinine orally 10 mg/kg 8 hourly for 6 doses followed by Fansidar a single dose of 3 tablets.	Chloroquine orally 600 mg followed in 6 hours by 300 mg then 300 mg daily for 2 days followed by Primaquine 7.5 mg b.d. for 14 days.
Chloroquine sensitive areas	Pyrimethamine 25 mg weekly Proguanil 100 mg daily Chloroquine 300 mg weekly	** Chloroquine iv 5–10 mg/kg over 4 h every 12–24 h	Chloroquine orally 600 mg followed in 6 h by 300 mg then 300 mg daily for 3–5 days	

+ Care in G6PD deficiency
* Resistant strains not a problem
** For babies give 5.0 mg/kg slowly i.m.
*** Tetracycline 250 mg 6 hourly for 7 days if Fansidar resistant.

Table 19.30 Drugs used in the treatment of African trypanosomiasis

Drug	*Administration*	*Pharmacokinetics*	*Toxicity*
Suramin (Antrypol)	Test dose 0.1–0.2 g i.v., then 24 h later 20 mg/kg on days 1, 3, 7, 14 and 21	After i.v. administration the drug persists in the plasma for up to 3 months due to tight plasma protein binding. Poor penetration into cells and into CSF. Very little is metabolised	Immediate: vomiting, shock, unconsciousness, colic, urticaria Late: rashes, parasthesiae
Pentamidine	3–4 mg base/kg i.m. daily for 10 days	Slow absorption from i.m. sites. Very brief half life in plasma. Firm binding to tissues	Dyspnoea, dizziness, tachycardia, headache, vomiting
Melarsoprol (Mel B)	3.6 mg/kg i.v. daily for 3 days, rest 1 week, then another 3 days treatment	Some penetration into CSF. Relatively rapid excretion—detected in plasma for a few days only	Encephalopathy Hypersensitivity
Trimelarsan (Specia; Mel W; Melarsonyl)	3–4 mg/kg i.m. (adults) 2 mg/kg i.m. (children) daily for 3 days, rest 2 weeks, then another 3 days treatment	Unknown	Toxicity similar to melarsoprol
Nitrofurazone	500 mg orally once daily for 2 days then thrice daily for 5–7 days	Unknown	Severe polyneuropathy. Haemolysis in G6PD deficient patients

Table 19.31 Anthelmintic and other anti-parasite drugs

Drug	*Administration*	*Special features*	*Toxicity*	*Clinical uses*
Diethyl-carbamazine citrate	*W. bancrofti and malayi:* 6–10 mg/kg/day for 21 days *Loa loa and O. volvulus:* 4 mg/kg 8 hourly for 10 days. Initial dose 1 mg/kg/day	Good absorption from intestine. Peak levels. 3 h, falls to zero levels in plasma at 24 h. Mainly excreted in urine as metabolite. Good penetration throughout body apart from fat	Allergic reactions to dead worms: fever, tachypnoea, tachycardia, hypotension, itching, cought, headache, malaise, joint pains	*W. bancrofti* Drug of *W. malayi* 1st choice. *Loa loa* Radical cure. *O. volvulus*: control only (suramin also used in combination) Effective against ascaris, but other drugs are better
Bephenium hydroxy-naphthoate	Adults: 5 g orally on an empty stomach. Children under 25 kg: 2.5 g. Single dose or daily dose for 4–7 days	Over 99% remains unabsorbed. Single dose effective in *A. duodenale* infections.	Mild nausea and diarrohea	*A. duodenale* Drug of *N. americanus* 1st choice (also effective against *Trichostrongylus orientalis* and *ascaris*)

Table 19.31 (continued)

Drugs	*Administration*	*Special features*	*Toxicity*	*Clinical uses*
Hycanthone	Single dose of 2.5–3 mg/kg i.m. Repeat in 1–3 months if necessary	Destroyed by gastric acid, but can be given as enteric coated tablet	Headache, weakness, abdominal discomfort, diarrhoea, anorexia, vomiting—common. Hepatic necrosis—rare. Contraindicated in non-schistosomal liver disease. Not to be used with phenothiazines	*S. haematobium* *S. mansoni* drug of 1st choice for mass treatment *S. japonicum*–not effective
Mebendazole	Single 100 mg oral dose for trichuriasis. 100 mg twice daily for 3 days for mixed infections	Useful in mixed infections e.g. hookworm, ascaris and trichiuris. Only 10% absorbed from intestine: this is decarboxylated and excreted in urine	Transient abdominal pain and diarrhoea	Drug of 1st choice in *T. trichiura*. Effective for ascaris, enterobiasis and hookworm
Antimony potassium tartrate (tartar emetic)	Usually given slowly i.v. as a 0.5% solution: test dose 8 ml then on alternate days increasing dose by 4 ml each dose till 28 ml daily reached.		Cough, vomiting, sudden death. Contraindicated in severe renal or hepatic disease	Effective against *S. japonicum*. Less toxic alternative treatment against *S. mansoni* and *S. haematobium*. May be valuable in treatment of granuloma inguinale and mycosis fungoides.

Table 19.31 (continued)

Drug	*Administration*	*Special features*	*Toxicity*	*Clinical uses*
Antimony sodium dimercapto-succinate (Stibocaptate)	5 × i.m. injections of a 10% solution at 3–7 day intervals. Total adult dose 30–50 mg/kg (max 2.5 g) Children under 20 kg given 40–60 mg/kg total		Rash, vomiting or pyrexia are indications to stop treatment. Contraindicated in bacterial & herpes infections	*S. mansoni* } as effective as *S. haematobium* } tartar emetic *S. japonicum*—partly effective
Stibophen	6.3% solution i.m. Initial test dose of 1.5–2 ml, 3.5 ml on 2nd day, 5.0 ml on 3rd day, then 6 further doses of 5 ml at 2–3 day intervals	Care to avoid i.v. injection	Vomiting, albuminuria, joint pain or fever are indications to stop treatment	Useful in all forms of schistosomiasis
Bithionol	30–50 mg/kg orally alternate days for 10–15 days		Diarrhoea Rashes	Trematodes, i.e. fascioliasis and paragonimiasis
Praziquantel	40 mg/kg single dose orally.		Nausea Abdominal pain	The best drug for schistosomiasis paragonimiasis.
Tetra-chloroethylene	Single dose 0.12 ml/kg (max. 5 ml) but best to repeat treatment at 4 and 8 days. Previously on low-fat diet. Drug given on empty stomach. Purgation not necessary. Ascaris should be treated first	Little is absorbed from gut, but enough to give CNS effects	Burning sensation in abdomen. Cramps and nausea. Headache, vertigo, inebriation	Effective against hookworm (*Necator* responds better than *Ancylostoma*)

Table 19.31 (continued)

Drug	*Administration*	*Special features*	*Toxicity*	*Clinical uses*
Niridazole	Daily dose of 25 mg/kg (max. 1.5 g) for 5–10 days	Well absorbed from gut over several hours. Considerable first-pass effect. Equally eliminated in urine and bile	Abdominal discomfort, nausea, dark urine, unpleasant body odour. Relative contraindications are epilepsy, psychosis and liver disease	Useful in schistosomiasis Also effective against *D. medinensis*
Niclosamide	Overnight fast then chew 2 g tablet (vanilla flavoured) and wash down with water. 0.5–1 g for children. Single dose, or (for *H. nana*) follow with 1 g daily for 6 days	Very little absorbed from the gut	Occasional gastro-intestinal disturbances. Viable ova remain in gut and can cause cysticerosis	Tapeworms: drug of 1st choice for *D. latum*, *H. nana and T. saginata.* (Drug of 2nd choice for this is paromomycin)
Piperazine	75 mg/kg (max. 4 g) daily for 2 days for ascaris. 65 mg/kg daily for 8 days for oxyuris—given to entire household. Unnecessary to fast or purge		Occasional mild gastrointestinal disturbances	Drug of 1st choice in ascariasis. Effective in oxyuris
Tetramisole	2.5–5.0 mg/kg single dose			Equally effective as piperazine in ascariasis
Levamisole	80 mg: 10–15 yrs 60 mg: 3–9 yrs 40 mg: < 3 yrs single dose		Occasional nausea. Bone marrow suppression	Effective in ascariasis

Table 19.31 (continued)

Drugs	*Administration*	*Special features*	*Toxicity*	*Clinical uses*
Pyrantel	Single dose of 11 mg/kg (max. 1 g)	Less than 15 % absorbed	Headache, dizziness	An agent of choice in ascariasis, Equally effective as bephenium against *Ancylostoma* and *Necator* hookworm
Viprynium pamoate	Single dose of 5 mg/kg (max. 350 mg). A second dose can be given 2 weeks later. Treat entire household	High cure rate with a single dose	Well tolerated. Occasional nausea and abdominal cramps	An effective alternative drug for oxyuris
Thia-bendazole	Oral administration of 25 mg/kg b.d. for 2 days (max. daily dose 3 g). No dieting or purgation necessary	90 % excreted in urine in 48 h. Peak blood levels at 1 h. Single day treatment for pinworms	Frequently produces nausea, dizziness, sedation, pruritus, headache. Should not drive or handle other dangerous machinery	Drug of 1st choice: *Dracunculus*. Drug of 2nd choice: hookworm Larvicidal for trichinella. Prevents development of ascaris eggs. Most useful in mixed infections with *Ascaris*, *Enterobius*, *Strongyloides* and *Trichiuris*.

Scheme of treatment

1. **Suramin** and **pentamidine** are both successful in treating bloodstream infections (with a normal CSF) of *T. gambiense*. In *T. rhodesiense* infections only suramin is effective. When CNS involvement has occurred, arsenical drugs are used. Advanced CNS disease caused by either parasite may respond to **melarsoprol**. **Trimelarsan** is effective only in *T. gambiense* infections.
2. Prophylaxis. A single 1 g injection of **suramin** protects an adult against both infections for 6–12 weeks. A single dose of 200–250 mg **Pentamidine** protects for 3–6 months against *T. gambiense*.
3. Treatment against *T. cruzi* infections (an American trypanosomiasis) is unsatisfactory. The effects of 8-aminoquinolines and nitrofurazone are being investigated in this disease.

Chapter 20
CANCER CHEMOTHERAPY

The management of a patient with malignant disease requires a multidisciplinary approach. In addition to the three principal treatment modalities of surgery, radiotherapy and chemotherapy (including immunotherapy) the importance of attending to psychiatric and social factors is increasingly being recognised.

Accurate staging (i.e. determining the extent of the disease) is an essential prerequisite of successful management. In those cases where localised disease is confirmed, cure may be possible with surgery or radiotherapy. In some cases chemotherapy may also be given on the supposition that widespread microscopic dissemination may have occurred (adjuvant therapy). If disease is widespread at presentation, systemic chemotherapy is more likely to be effective although radiotherapy or even surgery may be required for local disease control.

The use of drugs in treating cancer is based on the premise that malignant cells differ in some way from normal ones. Although the difference in behaviour between normal and malignant cells is all too obvious, and although there are quantitative differences in some metabolic processes, the basic change or changes which constitute malignancy are not known. It seems highly probable that there are derangements of the mechanisms which control cell replication and the synthesis of nucleotides and proteins. It may be that more than one defect is required to produce malignancy, and there may be several different ways in which these defects can be produced.

There is increasing evidence to implicate the insertion of foreign nucleic acid sequences into the host's genome (so-called oncogenes) in the genesis of certain malignant diseases.

At a practical therapeutic level, however, considerable progress has been made in recent years. A number of drugs which affect malignant cells (cytotoxic drugs) have been discovered, sometimes fortuitously, sometimes as a result of a reasoned approach. Most cytotoxic drugs interfere in different ways with the synthesis of DNA, RNA or with cell replication, with the result that cell death occurs or cell multiplication ceases. These effects are not confined to malignant cells and most cytotoxic agents depress normal cells, particularly those which are dividing rapidly in the bone marrow, gastro-intestinal tract, gonads, hair follicles and skin.

GENERAL PRINCIPLES IN THE USE OF CYTOTOXIC DRUGS

The number of cytotoxic drugs available has made possible the use of drug combinations. Because many of these drugs differ in their modes of action (see

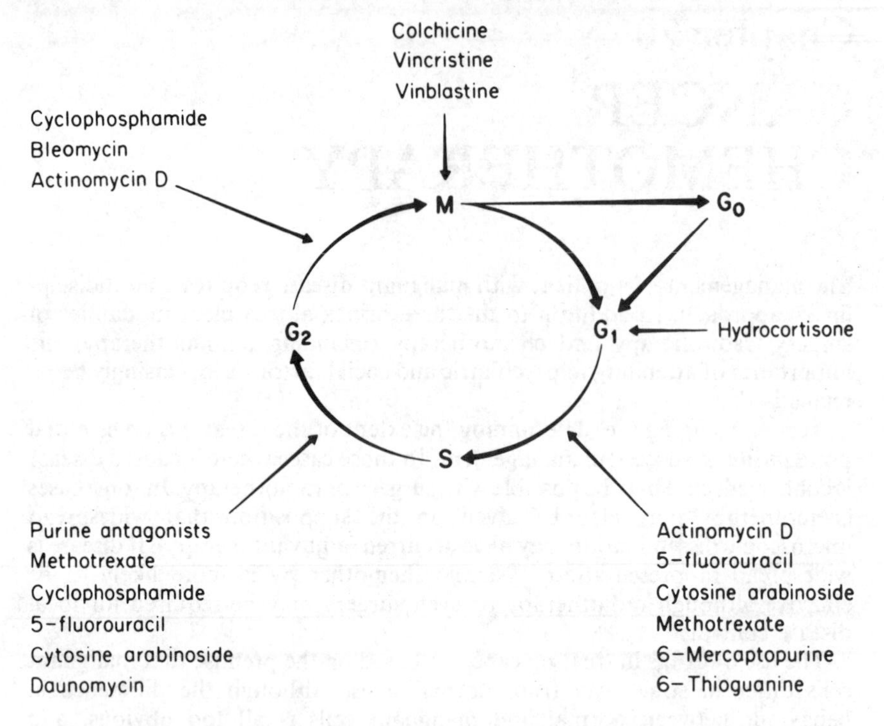

Fig. 20.1 The cell cycle and the phase specificity of some cytotoxic drugs.

below), by combining drugs it is possible to attack malignant cells in several ways at the same time. Originally this was done on an ad hoc basis: cocktails of drugs, each of which was known to have some action on a particular type of cancer, were given to the patient. By trial and error certain combinations were found to be effective and improvements in treatment were achieved. With increased understanding of drug action it is possible to combine these drugs more logically.

It is helpful at this stage to consider how the action of cytotoxic drugs is related to the cell cycle. Basic studies have distinguished the following phases in the cell cycle (see Fig. 20.1):

G_1 —pre-replicative phase involving operations preliminary to the S phase;
S —phase of DNA synthesis;
G_2 —post-replicative phase allowing preparation for cell division;
M —mitosis or cell division.

Cells which are not in any of the above phases are said to be in G_0. This quiescent phase includes those cells which are so differentiated that they will not undergo further division and those cells which can move into the cell-division cycle again in response to an appropriate stimulus.

In general, cytotoxic agents only affect cells in the proliferative phase since their action depends on interference with the synthesis or division of cellular material. They can be divided into two groups:

(a) *Cycle non-specific* This means that they act at all stages in the proliferating cell cycle but not on those in the G_0 (resting) phase. Because of this their dose–response curve follows first-order kinetics (i.e. cells are killed exponentially with increasing dosage).

The linear relationship between dose and log-response (see Fig. 20.2) may be exploited in the use of high-dose chemotherapy. Cytotoxic drugs are given at very high dose over a short period of time, thus rendering the bone marrow aplastic, but at the same time hopefully achieving a very high tumour cell kill. The ensuing period of intense myelosuppression requires intensive support with antibiotics, platelet transfusions etc. and in some cases re-infusion of either previously harvested autologous or allogenic bone marrow. Preliminary results in some tumours, e.g. leukaemias, lymphomas, have been encouraging. The drugs used in this therapy are those whose predominant toxic effects are on the bone marrow, as this is the only important normal tissue which can be supported and rescued. Agents used thus far include alkylating agents (e.g. cyclophosphamide, melphalan, CCNU, BCNU), etoposide and methotrexate (with folinic acid rescue).

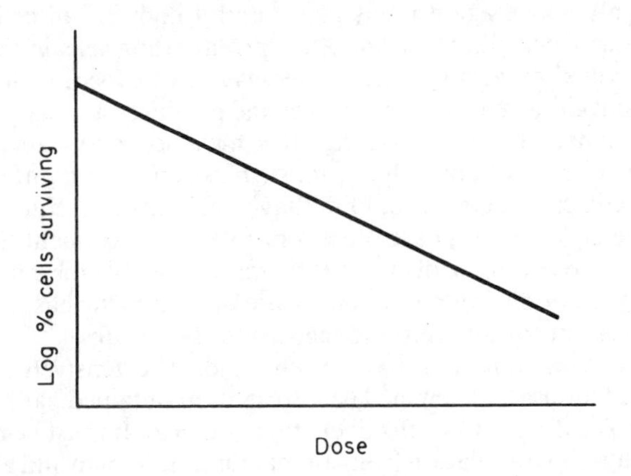

Fig. 20.2 Dose response curve for a cycle non-specific drug.

(b) *Phase specific* This means that they act only at a certain phase in the cell cycle. Therefore the more rapid the cell turnover the more effective they are. Their dose–response curve is initially exponential but at higher doses a maximum response is reached and the curve becomes asymptotic.

Table 20.1 classifies cytotoxic drugs according to their effect on the cell cycle but until the kinetic behaviour of human tumours can be adequately characterised in individual patients the value of this classification is limited. The distinction between cycle-nonspecific and phase-specific drugs, though fairly clear-cut in animal experiments, is probably over-simplified and presently of doubtful importance in treating human cancer.

By using combinations or sequences of drugs, attempts are being made to modify the cell cycle so as to increase therapeutic efficiency. For example, one drug can be given to 'fix' cells at a certain phase in the cycle; when a large number of cells have accumulated in this phase, a different drug can be given

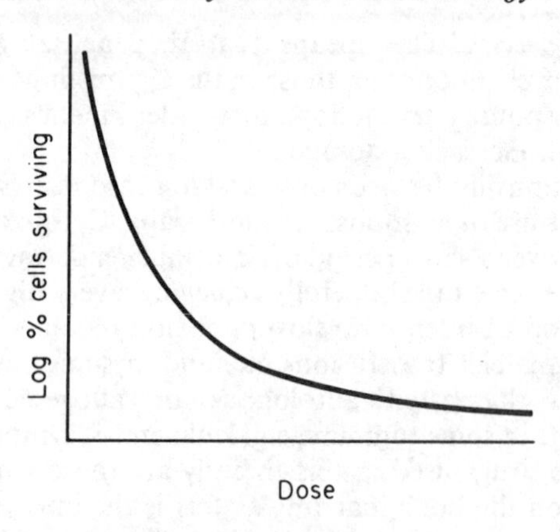

Fig. 20.3 Dose response for a phase-specific drug.

which is highly active against this phase and a high kill of cells should be achieved. Thus vinca alkaloids can block proliferating cells in mitosis where they can be killed by agents such as bleomycin. In experimental systems, a dose of bleomycin given 6 h after vinblastine produces an increased cell kill. There is circumstantial evidence that this may occur in human bronchial tumours. Despite this knowledge it must, however, be admitted that most attempts at clinical kinetic scheduling have been unsuccessful.

Cells in the G_0 (resting) phase present problems in treatment since they are not susceptible to cytotoxic drugs. It is therefore possible for a malignant cell to hide away and only emerge when cytotoxic treatment has been finished. This is one reason for giving prolonged courses of drugs.

Cell kinetics of tumours have been studied extensively in animals, particularly in mouse leukaemia. The information obtained has enabled us to deploy cytotoxic drugs more effectively than hitherto. It must be remembered that this requires extrapolation from animal tumour to man and although this

Table 20.1 Classification of cytotoxic drugs according to their effect on the cell cycle

Predominantly cycle non-specific	*Predominantly phase specific*
Nitrogen mustard	Methotrexate
Cyclophosphamide, Ifosfamide	6-mercaptopurine
Melphalan	6-thioguanine
Busulphan	5-fluorouracil
Thio-TEPA	5-FUDR
Chlorambucil	Cytosine arabinoside
CCNU, BCNU and methyl CCNU	Procarbazine
Dacarbazine (DTIC)	Hydroxyurea
Actinomycin D	Razoxane
Mitomycin C	Vinca alkaloids
Mitozantrone	VM 26
Doxorubicin, Daunomycin	Etoposide (VP 16–213)

has produced considerable advances, not all the animal findings can be translated to man. The main results of these studies are:

1. The natural history of cancer is much longer than it was once thought to be. Many tumour cells grow rapidly but this is not a uniform characteristic and their growth rates are varied and overlap with many normal tissues. Thus the length of cell cycle of a leukaemic blast cell is 50–80 h, but that of a carcinoma of the breast is 2–5 months. These may be compared with the 15–18 h of a polychromatophil normoblast and 1–2 months for epidermal cells. It has been calculated that the course of human myelomatosis takes 21 years from the appearance of the first malignant cell to the death of the patient. The clinical course of the disease is a relatively small proportion of the total course (Fig. 20.4). Studies in animals suggest that complete cure of cancer requires total eradication of all cancer cells. Therefore treatment will require to be prolonged beyond the point at which tumour is clinically evident if this aim is to be achieved.

In animal models it is found that a given dose of a drug kills a constant percentage of the cells in unit time and thus the number of cells present before therapy begins will determine the number of cells surviving after treatment. In lymphomas the percentage cell kill can be 90 % but for solid tumours it is often only 50 %. To take an extremely simplified example, and neglecting addition of cells by replication and any effect of host defence mechanisms, if 10^{11} cells are present in a clinically detectable solid tumour, approximately 40 courses of treatment with a cell-kill fraction of about 50 % would be necessary to eradicate the tumour. This could mean 4–5 years of therapy. Reduction of the tumour burden by preliminary surgery or radiotherapy before chemotherapy may be of value in this context.

2. The fraction of cells in a tumour which are dividing decreases as the mass of tumour increases; this is due to cells going into the G_0 (resting) phase, and means that the tumour is more susceptible to cytotoxic drugs when the mass is small, and when most cells are dividing. It becomes less easy to treat as its size increases. Death occurs in man when the malignant cell population reaches about 10^{12} (Fig. 20.4).

3. Cytotoxic drugs given in high doses for short repeated periods usually produce a higher kill of malignant cells than continuous low dosage schedules, because although drug toxicity is usually cumulative, the low kill of malignant cells achieved by low dosage can soon be replaced by proliferating surviving cells. The intermittent administration of large doses of cytotoxic agents allows the bone marrow to regenerate in the intervals between treatments (Fig. 20.5). Furthermore, intermittent doses are less immunosuppressant than continuous administration since immunologically competent lymphocytes are in the G_0 phase and so protected from injury during the action of the drug, but in the intervals are able to enter the cycle to form immunoblasts should an appropriate antigenic stimulus occur.

The superiority of intermittent dosage regimes is not absolute in human cancer and continued low dosage over long periods sometimes produces good results, perhaps because the turnover of cells in that particular tumour is slow.

4. Since every cancer cell has to be eliminated to produce a cure it becomes important to know when this aim has been achieved, since at that point medication can be stopped. As yet there are no practical methods for assessing

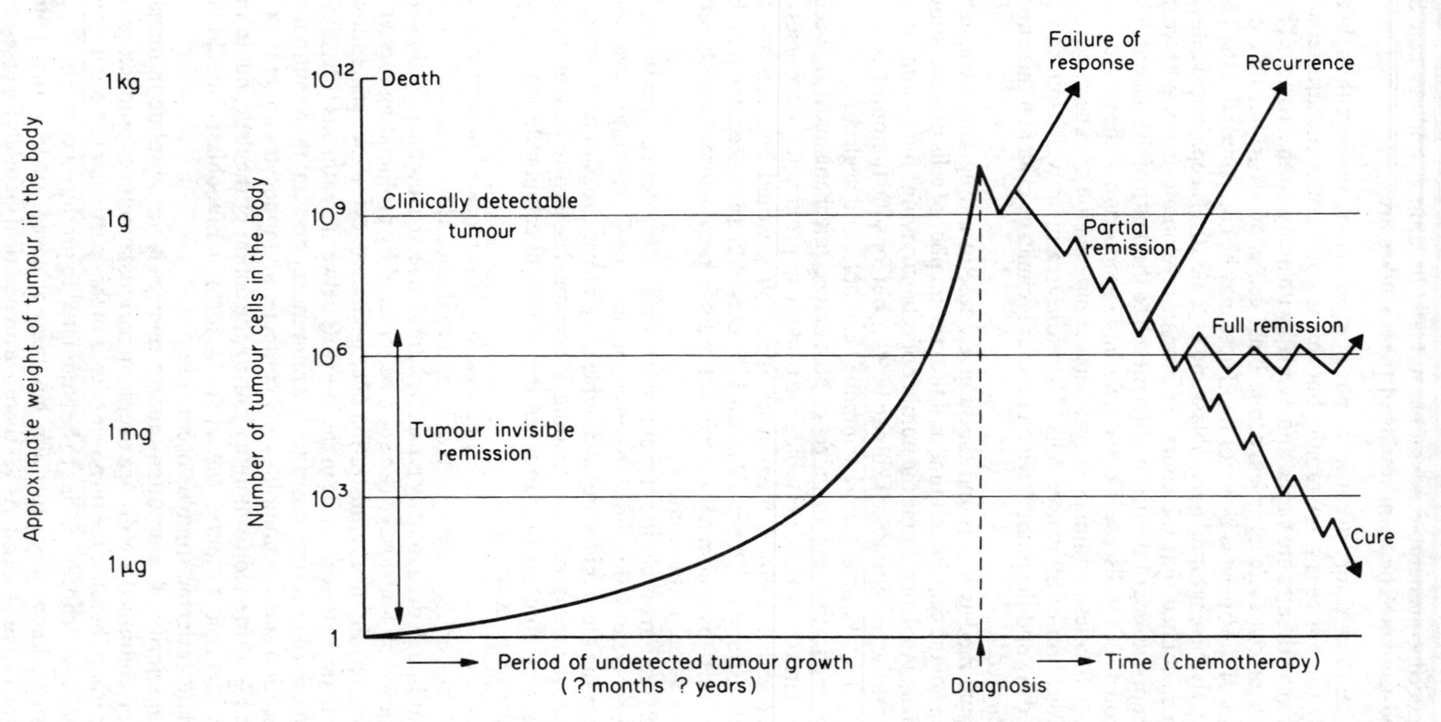

Fig. 20.4 Tumour growth and response to chemotherapy. The duration of undetected tumour growth has been shortened for diagrammatic representation: in most cases it is probably at least five times the length of the treatment phase.

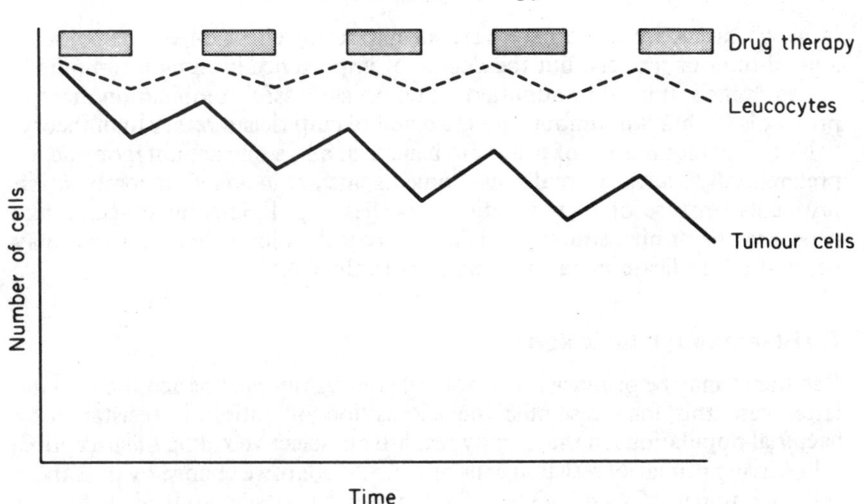

Fig. 20.5 Effect of intermittent therapy on bone marrow and tumour cells.

very small numbers of tumour cells. Tumour markers, e.g. myeloma protein, chorionic gonadotrophin, α-fetoprotein, can only detect of the order of 10^5–10^6 cells, and for many tumours no markers exist. It is possible that immune mechanisms may be able to cope with small numbers of malignant cells, so that it may not be necessary to kill every tumour cell with drugs. Nevertheless, the search for useful tumour-marker systems continues, since by this means more rational therapy will be possible. Because of the need to eradicate all the tumour it has become important to seek out and destroy neoplastic cells occurring in so-called *sanctuary sites*. Thus it was found that relapse of acute lymphatic leukaemia frequently occurred in the CNS, although it had been successfully eradicated from the marrow and other sites. Therefore irradiation of the brain and spinal cord accompanied by intrathecal administration of cytotoxic agents was added to the already rigorous protocol for this disease with a subsequent improvement in survival figures.

Combination chemotherapy

It is possible to devise combinations of drugs which have a different mechanism of action and provide greater benefit than the individual agents do alone. If the side effects of the components of the combination are different these will not be additive and the combination will not be more toxic than if the drugs were given singly. If they have different mechanisms of cytotoxic action there may be an increased tumour cell kill. They may also allow a more rapid host recovery and better selectivity with improved preferential killing of tumour cells. There are now a number of well-established combination therapies for human tumours (see below). A common procedure is to employ cycle non-specific drugs followed by phase-specific agents, since the former may reduce the non-proliferating cell pool which stimulates the survivors to enter mitosis when they can be killed by the phase-specific drug. The sequence in which drugs are given may have an important effect on the response in animal-tumour models, but the degree of importance in human tumours is undetermined. It must be admitted that most successful combination therapy protocols for human tumours are the result of empiricism rather than theory.

Not all combinations of drugs are beneficial and some are antagonistic, or preferentially attack normal cells. Some agents are included in combination protocols because of their kinetic properties, e.g. lipid-soluble agents like procarbazine or nitrosoureas, which can cross the blood–brain barrier, may be used to eradicate metastatic tumours in the CNS.

Resistance to cytotoxic agents

Resistance may be primary (i.e. a non-responsive tumour) or acquired. In the latter case this may resemble the acquisition of antibiotic resistance by bacterial populations in that it may result from selective killing of susceptible cells leaving primarily resistant cells or from an adaptive change by the cancer cell. A number of mechanisms of resistance have been studied in human tumours and these are summarised in Table 20.2.

Table 20.2 Acquired tumour resistance to cytotoxic agents

Mechanism	*Examples*
1. Reduced uptake of drug	Methotrexate; Daunorubicin.
2. Deletion of enzyme to activate drug	Cytosine arabinoside; 5-fluorouracil.
3. Increased detoxication of drug	6-mercaptopurine
4. Increased concentration of target enzyme	Methotrexate
5. Decreased requirement for specific metabolic product	Asparaginase
6. Increased utilisation of alternative pathway	Antimetabolites
7. Rapid repair of drug-induced lesion	Alkylating agents
8. Decreased number of receptors for drug	Hormones
9. Alteration in proliferation rate ? underlying mechanism	Myeloma, chronic myeloid leukaemia commonly terminate in a more aggressive phase (see Fig. 20.6).

The ability to predict the sensitivity of bacterial pathogens to antimicrobial substances in vitro produced a profound change in the efficacy of treatment in the infectious diseases. The development of analogous predictive tests has long been a priority in cancer research. They are particularly necessary since in contrast to antimicrobial drugs, cytotoxic agents are administered in doses which produce some degree of toxicity in most patients. Thus in treating metastatic colorectal cancer with fluorouracil the 80 % of patients who do not respond suffer toxicity effects as much as the 20 % of patients who benefit from treatment. In theory predictive toxicity tests could provide a considerable improvement in therapy particularly as patients with non-responsive tumours could be spared the toxic effects of these drugs. Unfortunately tests which are of clinical use do not yet exist. Recently promising results have been obtained using in vitro cultures of tumour stem cells. It is likely that with advances in cell culture techniques in vitro tumour colony assays will become a practical reality.

Adjuvant chemotherapy

About 75 % of patients with cancer die as a result of metastases rather than the primary tumour. These often arise in the pre-clinical course of a malignancy. Thus it would be unusual to detect a breast carcinoma clinically which was smaller than about 1 cm in diameter (this already contains 10^9 cells and has probably undergone some 30 divisions since the original malignant cell arose). Tumour cells may begin to escape into the lymphatic and blood circulation as soon as neovascularisation occurs when the tumour is less than 3 mm in diameter. It is obvious that the opportunity for systemic seeding is present long before most breast tumours are clinically apparent. Adjuvant chemotherapy aims to destroy these disseminated microfoci at a time when there is no clinical evidence of residual disease. It is thought that chemotherapeutic intervention could be more successful at this stage because:

(a) The total body tumour load is small and treatment is more likely to be effective with drugs possessing first-order cell-kill kinetics.
(b) Fewer cells in small tumours are in the G_0 phase, i.e. the cell-growth fraction is higher.

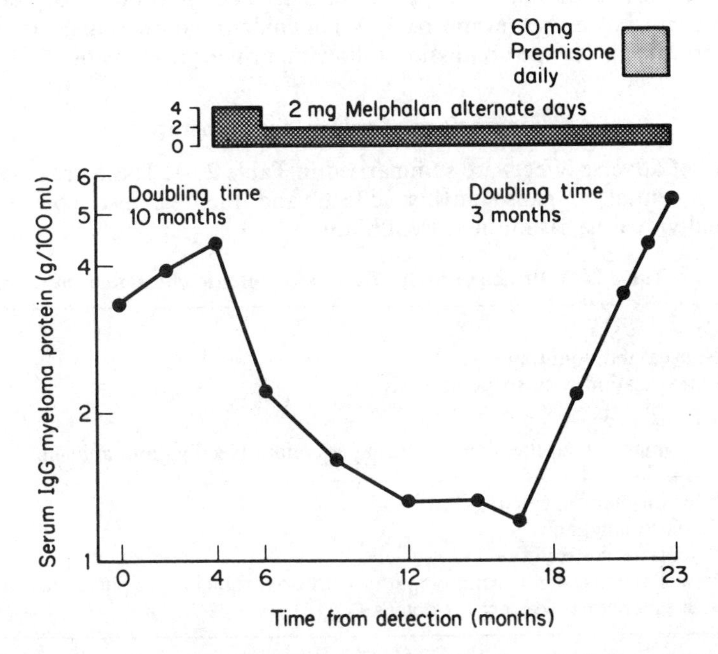

Fig. 20.6 Growth-rate relapse during treatment of mycloma as shown by the faster doubling rate of the serum paraprotein concentration (From J. R. Hobbs, *Brit. Med. J.*, **2,** 67 (1971). Reproduced by permission of the Editor.)

(c) Vascularisation of small tumours is greater and thus drug penetration is facilitated.
(d) Patients at this stage are less likely to be immunosuppressed so that intrinsic host factors may be operative. There is also less bone-marrow suppression and less likelihood of tumour infiltration into the marrow so that patients can tolerate chemotherapy better.

Against the possible benefits of eradicating early metastases must be set:

(a) The possibility that in treating a group of patients with putative metastases some patients who in fact do not have metastatic disease will be exposed to the toxic effects of chemotherapy.
(b) Adjuvant chemotherapy imposes the added burden of drug toxicity on patients who may already have undergone major surgery and/or radical radiotherapy
(c) Because of the danger of inducing second malignancies with cytotoxic drugs (see below), care must be used in employing potential carcinogens in patients whose primary neoplasm has a long natural history.
(d) Adjuvant chemotherapy may merely delay the development of metastatic disease, making this more difficult to treat when it does occur due to drug resistance. Overall survival is thus unaffected.

At present adjuvant chemotherapy is at an early stage of evaluation but encouraging results have been reported in some paediatric tumours (e.g. Wilm's tumour, Ewing's tumour, osteogenic sarcoma) and in breast cancer in adults. Adjuvant immunotherapy may also become important. For example, it has been shown that levamisole (q.v.) in epidermoid bronchial carcinoma may produce prolonged remission following primary treatment.

Complications of cancer chemotherapy

The chief adverse effects are summarised in Table 20.3. These drugs vary in their potential to cause adverse effects and there is also considerable interindividual variation in susceptibility.

Table 20.3 Principal toxic effects of cytotoxic chemotherapy

Immediate
1. Nausea and vomiting
2. Extravasation with tissue necrosis

Delayed
1. Bone-marrow suppression producing infection, bleeding and anaemia
2. Alopecia
3. Infertility/teratogenicity
4. Second malignancy
5. Psychiatric morbidity
6. Miscellaneous, e.g. cardiomyopathy with doxorubicin, peripheral neuropathy with vincristine (see text for details)

Nausea and vomiting with cytotoxic drugs Cytotoxic drugs vary in their emetogenic potential (see Table 20.4). This side effect is usually delayed for 1–

Table 20.4 Emetogenic potential of commonly used cytotoxic drugs

Severe	*Moderate*	*Rare*
Doxorubicin	BCNU, CCNU	Bleomycin
Cyclophosphamide	Mitomicin C	Cytarabine
Dacarbazine	Procarbazine	Vinca alkaloids
Mustine	Etoposide	Methotrexate
Cisplatin	Ifosfamide	5-fluorouracil
		Chlorambucil
		Mitozantrone

2 hours after drug administration and often lasts for 24–48 hours. The mechanisms by which these drugs induce vomiting include stimulation of the chemoreceptor trigger zone (in the floor of the fourth ventricle) and stimulation of peripheral receptors mediating gastric atony and cessation of peristalsis.

If vomiting is anticipated, it is kindest to use prophylactic antiemetics before treatment and to give the patient a supply of tablets to take as needed over the ensuing days. No treatment is entirely effective especially for cisplatin-induced vomiting. Drugs used for control of vomiting are discussed on p. 558. In addition, psychotherapy and hypnosis may be particularly effective for patients who vomit at the time of treatment or even in anticipation of it.

Extravasation with tissue necrosis may occur when one of the following drugs extravasate: doxorubicin, BCNU, mustine, vincristine, vinblastine, vindesine. It may cause sufficiently severe necrosis to require skin grafting.

Bone marrow suppression There appear to be two patterns of bone-marrow recovery (see Fig. 20.7), rapid and delayed. The usual pattern is of rapid recovery but chlorambucil, BCNU, CCNU and melphalan may cause prolonged myelosuppression (up to 8 weeks). Vincristine, bleomycin and corticosteroids rarely cause myelosuppression.

The main problems in myelosuppressed patients are bleeding, infection and anaemia which are readily treated. Severe thrombocytopenia (i.e. platelet count less than $20\,000 \times 10^9$/l) can be corrected by platelet transfusion.

Infection, the commonest life-threatening complication of chemotherapy, is often acquired from sources such as the patients own teeth or gastro-intestinal tract. Effective isolation can only be achieved in purpose-built units and even then this does not solve the problem of the patient's own bacteria despite the use of oral antibiotics such as neomycin to 'sterilise' the bowel. Classical signs of infection, e.g. pyrexia, may be absent in severely neutropenic patients and constant vigilance is required to detect and treat septicaemia before it becomes overwhelming. Broad-spectrum antibiotic treatment must be started before the results of cultures are available. A parenteral aminoglycoside with a penicillin (e.g. flucloxacillin) or cephalosporin (e.g. cepho-

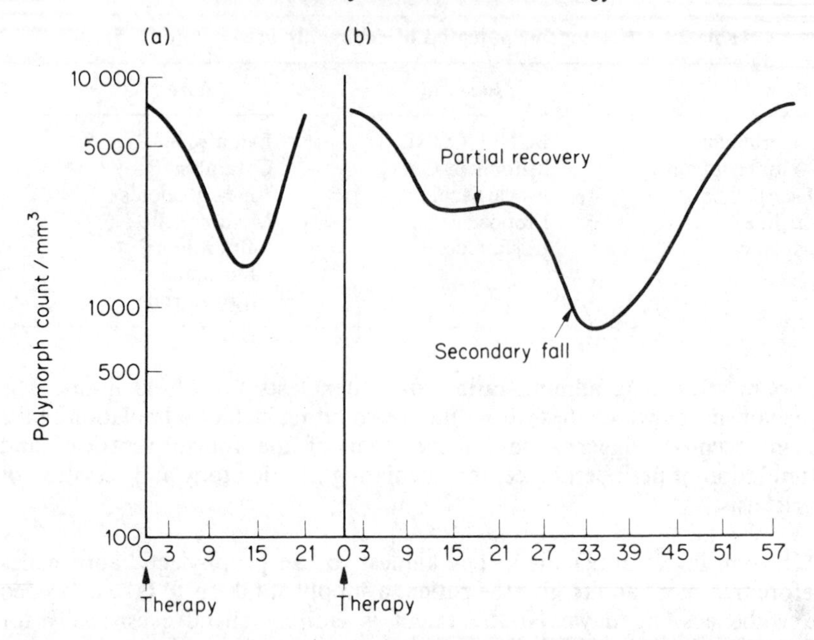

Fig. 20.7 Patterns of bone-marrow recovery following cytotoxic therapy (a) rapid (17–21 days) (b) delayed (initial fall 8–10 days, secondary minimum at 27–32 days, recovery 42–50 days) (After D. E. Bergasagel.)

taxime) which is active against β-lactamase producing organisms plus metronidazole provides suitable cover (see p. 689).

Opportunistic infections are a common problem in these patients. Oral candidiasis causing pain and dysphagia is best treated with oral nystatin suspension, amphotericin lozenges or oral ketoconazole. Systemic fungal infections are life-threatening and require prompt treatment with parenteral amphotericin B, possibly with flucytosine. *Pneumocystis carinii* is an opportunistic protozoan causing severe interstitial pneumonia. High-dose cotrimoxazole (4 tablets, 6 hourly) is the least toxic treatment but parenteral pentamidine may be needed in patients allergic to sulphonamides. Reactivation of pre-existing tuberculosis is another possible complication of immunosuppression.

Prophylactic treatment with cotrimoxazole (2 tablets, twice daily) and ketoconazole (200 mg orally daily) reduces the risk of serious infections in severely neutropenic patients and should be started when the neutrophil count falls below 500 × 10/l.

Alopecia is almost always severe with doxorubicin, ifosfamide and parenteral etoposide. It may be alleviated in the case of doxorubicin by cooling the scalp using ice-cold gel packs or ice caps. Some hair loss occurs with almost all cytotoxic agents.

Infertility and teratogenesis By the very nature of their action, cytotoxic drugs might be expected to impair fertility and to increase the incidence of fetal abnormalities.

Most women develop amenorrhoea if treated with cytotoxic drugs, however many resume normal menstruation when treatment is stopped and pregnancy is then possible. This is more common in younger women, and also probably related to the total doses of cytotoxic drugs given. Amenorrhoea is associated with low plasma oestrogen levels and high FSH and LH levels, suggesting a primary effect on the ovary.

In men, a full course of cytotoxic drugs usually produces azoospermia due to direct damage to the germinal epithelium of the testis. Alkylating agents are particularly harmful. Follow-up studies have shown that recovery can occur although it may be delayed for several years, and is most common after a short course of treatment with a single agent.

In prepubertial boys, cytotoxic drugs have definitely been associated with testicular damage, but the long-term outcome is unknown. Prepubertial girls are probably less prone to cytotoxic-induced ovarian damage.

Sperm storage prior to chemotherapy should be considered for males wishing to have children in the future. Both male and female patients must be strongly advised to take precautions against conception during chemotherapy as the reduction in fertility with these drugs is not universal. In addition, it is best to avoid conception for at least 6 months after completion of chemotherapy.

Second malignancy As many as 3–10% of patients treated for Hodgkin's disease (particularly those who received both chemotherapy and radiotherapy) develop a second malignancy: usually acute non-lymphocytic leukaemia. Similarly this malignancy is approximately 20 times more likely to develop in patients with ovarian carcinoma treated with alkylating agents with or without radiotherapy. This complication of treatment may become more commonly recognised as the number of patients surviving after successful cancer chemotherapy increases.

Summary

Cytotoxic drugs may be used in two ways in the treatment of cancer:

1. They are used when the disease has disseminated widely and is no longer amenable to eradication by surgery. If the cancer is very sensitive to drugs this may be successful, but cytotoxic drugs are not being used to the maximum advantage if the tumour cell mass is large.

It is conventional, although rarely feasible, to divide treatment into:

(a) Induction of remission: treatment until the patient is clinically disease-free. If no further treatment is given, however, the neoplasm will return in most patients.
(b) Consolidation and maintenance of remission often by the use of alternative drugs.
(c) Late-intensification: final intense form of therapy, often with phase-dependent drugs, aimed at killing the last surviving cells of the tumour.

2. Adjuvant therapy has been introduced more recently. Cytotoxic drugs are given when the cancer has apparently been destroyed by surgery or radiotherapy and its object is to eradicate seedling metastases which, being small in cell mass, should show maximum sensitivity to cytotoxic drugs.

The experimental background outlined above suggests that certain general principles should be applied when treating cancer with drugs.

(a) Cytotoxic drugs should usually be used in combination.
(b) Drugs should be given intermittently and in high doses.
(c) Treatment will usually need to be prolonged.
(d) The earlier in the disease (small tumour cell mass) treatment is started, the better the result.
(e) The toxicity of these drugs must be remembered and routine blood counts together with close clinical supervision are essential.

DRUGS USED IN CANCER CHEMOTHERAPY

For convenience, cytotoxic drugs may be divided into:

1. Alkylating agents
2. Antimetabolites
3. Vinca alkaloids
4. Antibiotics
5. Miscellaneous
6. Hormones

ALKYLATING AGENTS

These drugs cross-link mainly the guanine bases on opposing strands of DNA (see Fig. 20.8) by producing reactive intermediates containing positively charged carbonium ions which can form covalent bonds with the negatively charged DNA bases. The tightly bound DNA strands are then unable to separate and thus cannot act as templates for RNA production or form new DNA. Probably these agents also alkylate other cellular components such as enzymes and membranes: effects which contribute to their cytotoxicity. Alkylating agents are particularly effective when cells are dividing rapidly but they are not phase specific. They combine with DNA of both malignant and normal cells and thus damage not only the malignant cells but dividing normal cells, especially those of the bone marrow and the gastrointestinal tract (see Table 20.5).

The alkyl groupings on these drugs are highly reactive, so that although their most important action is on DNA they also combine with susceptible groups in cells and in tissue fluids.

Factors determining the selective toxicity of different alkylating agents have not been identified, although such selectivity exists. Thus while a tumour sensitive to one alkylating agent is usually sensitive to another, cross-resistance within the group does not necessarily occur. The pharmacokinetic properties of the different drugs are probably important in this respect. Thus

Table 20.5 Toxicity of alkylating agents at therapeutic dosage

Drug	*Nausea and vomiting*	*Granulocytopenia*	*Thrombocytopenia*	*Special toxicity*
Mustine	+++	+++	++++	Tissue necrosis if extravasated
Cyclophosphamide	++	+++	+	Alopecia (10–20%) Chemical cystitis (reduced by mesna) Mucosal ulceration Impaired water excretion Interstitial pulmonary fibrosis
Ifosfamide	++	++	+	Chemical cystitis (reduced by mesna) Alopecia Hypotension (if rapidly infused)
Chlorambucil	+	++	++++	Marrow suppression may be prolonged
Melphalan	0	+++	+++	Chemical cystitis (very rare)
Busulphan	0	++++	+++	Skin pigmentation Interstitial pulmonary fibrosis Amenorrhoea Gynaecomastia (rare)

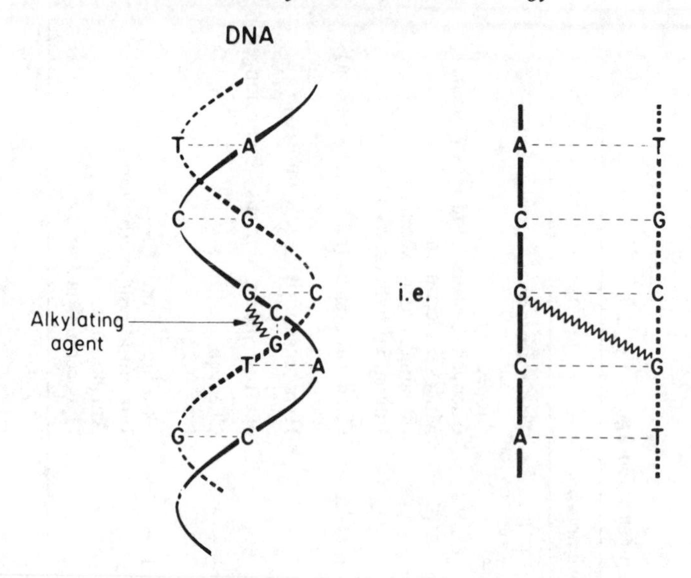

Fig. 20.8 Mechanism of intramolecular bridging of DNA by alkylating agents (A = adenine; C = cytosine; G = guanine; T = thymidine).

whilst most alkylating agents passively diffuse into cells, mustine is actively transported by some cells which may influence the selectivity of this agent.

Mustine (Mechlorethamine; Nitrogen mustard)

In solution mustine forms highly reactive ethyleneimmonium ions which make mustine a very irritant substance. Following i.v. injection the plasma half-life is short, probably about half an hour. The disappearance of the active compound is largely due to combination with the thiol groups of tissue protein.

Clinical use Mustine is unstable in solution and must be given immediately it is made up. It is preferable to set up an intravenous infusion of saline and give the drug slowly over 2–3 min into the drip tubing. This minimises the risk of local thrombosis and highly irritant extravasation into surrounding tissues. About 4 h after injection most patients become nauseated and vomit. The reason for this is unknown: presumably it depends on some central action, although the delay argues against direct stimulation of the vomiting centre. Anti-emetics, such as chlorpromazine, or sedatives help but do not always prevent this unpleasant side effect.

The dose and frequency depend upon the schedule being used. Mustine is usually combined with other cytotoxic drugs and the dose is 6.0 mg/m^2 body area weekly. It can also be given into the pleural cavity to prevent recurrent malignant effusion following removal of most of the effusion by aspiration. The usual dose is 15–20 mg. However, this drug is not recommended for chemical pleurodesis as it usually causes severe pain and other agents (e.g. *Corynebacterium parvum*, tetracycline) are as effective and less painful.

Mustine acts rapidly and if it is effective the tumour mass will begin to shrink within a week. This will be combined with other evidence of regression of the cancer such as disappearance of fever. It is now only used to treat Hodgkin's disease in combination with other drugs.

Adverse effects The most important toxic effect is bone-marrow depression with leucopenia and thrombocytopenia. This usually reaches its maximum depression with leucopenia and thrombocytopenia. This usually reaches its maximum 10–14 days after giving the drug and returns to normal by three weeks. It also causes severe vomiting.

Cyclophosphamide (Endoxana)

Cyclophosphamide itself is not cytotoxic but requires activation *in vivo*. It was originally synthesised with the object of improving the therapeutic index of alkylating agents. Since tumour cells show elevated phosphoramidase and phosphorylase activity it was hoped that alkylating metabolites would be more rapidly released from an inactive phosphoramide precursor in neoplastic tissue. It is now well established that the effectiveness of cyclophosphamide does not arise from enzymic cleavage of the phosphoramide ring within tumour cells but that activation occurs mainly in the liver with the active metabolites reaching the tumour cells via the circulation.

Pharmacokinetics The drug is metabolised in the liver with the production of a number of cytotoxic alkylating substances. It can be given intravenously or orally and is well absorbed from the intestine. The main metabolites are probably as shown in Fig. 20.9.

Although the most important metabolite in terms of cytotoxicity is not known, it is probably phosphoramide mustard. Aldophosphamide may act as a systemically transported precursor of this cytotoxic agent to the tumour.

The plasma half-life of cyclophosphamide is variable and ranges between 3 and 12 hours. When given repeatedly it becomes shorter on successive days: it is also shorter in children than in adults. There is a moderate (25 %) first-pass effect after oral administration. Plasma-protein binding is in the region of 10 % but is higher for some of the metabolites. Enzyme-inducing drugs appear to increase the rate of metabolism in animals but whether this effect is of significance in man is not known. The concurrent use of steroids does not appear to alter metabolism.

Cyclophosphamide and its metabolites are excreted in the urine. The clearance of unchanged cyclophosphamide is 11 ml/min (i.e. much lower than the amount filtered) and therefore tubular reabsorption of this lipid-soluble molecule must occur. This process of renal recycling ensures that most of the administered dose (80–90 %) undergoes metabolism. Renal excretion of acrolein is the cause of the non-infective ('chemical') cystitis which often accompanies cyclophosphamide administration.

Clinical uses Cyclophosphamide can be given orally or intravenously. Large doses can be nauseating and should be given intravenously. There are several regimes in current use which include cyclophosphamide (see p. 812); rarely it

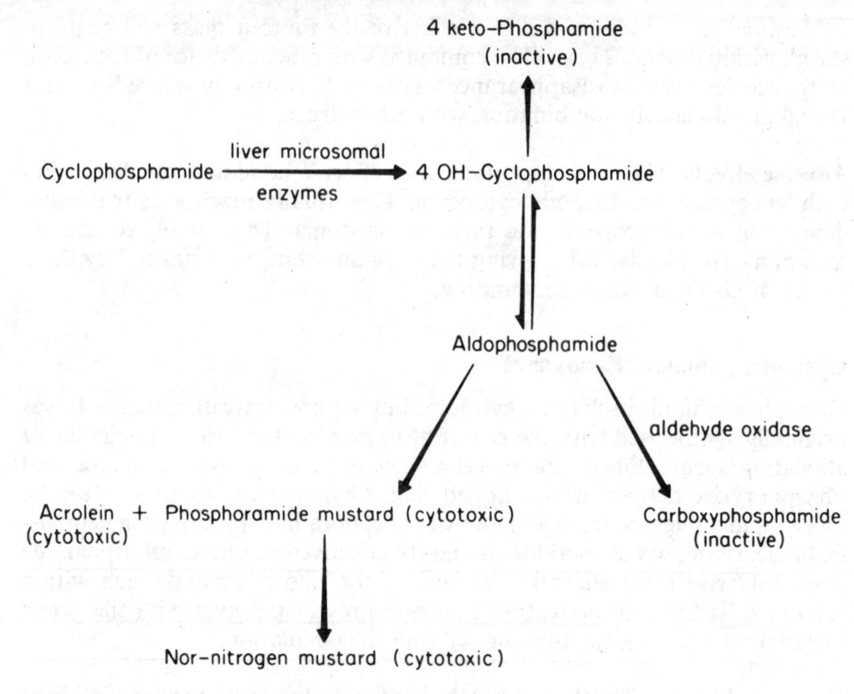

Fig. 20.9 Probable major metabolic pathways of cyclophosphamide.

may be used as the sole therapeutic agent. As a single agent it is often used in doses of 50–150 mg orally daily for varying periods. In combinations, doses of 400–600 mg/m^2 are commonly used whilst in high dose chemotherapy, e.g. to prepare patients with acute leukaemia and aplastic anaemia for allogeneic bone marrow transplantation, doses of 45–60 mg/kg/day for 2–3 days are employed.

Cyclophosphamide is most useful in the treatment of various lymphomas and leukaemias and in myelomatosis, but it has some effect in other cancers. Cyclophosphamide is also used as an immunosuppressive drug (see p. 817).

Adverse effects

1. Bone-marrow depression with least effect on platelets.
2. Hair loss is common with large doses but full recovery, sometimes even before stopping the drug, is the rule.
3. Sterile haemorrhagic cystitis results from chronic inflammation which leads to fibrosis and telangiectasia of the bladder wall due to toxic concentrations of acrolein in the urine. Chronic administration of cyclophosphamide may be associated with increased risk of developing bladder cancer. Urotoxicity (and probably the risk of cancer) is controlled by the use of mesna (see below) with diuresis (alkalinisation of the urine theoretically increases acrolein formation).
4. Impairment of water excretion may result in water intoxication, inappropriately concentrated urine, hyponatraemia and weight gain. Despite

superficial resemblances this syndrome does not appear to be due to inappropriate antidiuretic hormone secretion but may result from a toxic effect on the distal renal tubules. In renal failure there may be increased plasma levels of active metabolites and thus increased toxicity.

5. Rare adverse effects include myocardial damage, pulmonary fibrosis and hypoglycaemia (with enhancement of the effects of sulphonylureas).

Ifosfamide (Mitoxana)

Ifosfamide is an isomer of cyclophosphamide. It has no cytotoxic activity itself but is metabolised in the liver to a number of cytotoxic metabolites. Some of these differ from those obtained from cyclophosphamide but include acrolein and so ifosfamide produces severe renal and bladder toxicity although it has less myelosuppressive effect than cyclophosphamide.

Ifosfamide has been used with some benefit in a variety of cancers including those of the testis, lung, cervix and ovary; soft tissue sarcomas, osteosarcomas and lymphomas.

Pharmacokinetics The half-life of ifosfamide is shorter than that of cyclophosphamide at 3–7 hours and also shows time-dependence, i.e. it becomes shorter if the drug is used on successive days, thus reflecting a faster production of cytotoxic metabolites. Like cyclophosphamide, most of the drug is metabolised: only 15% undergoing renal elimination.

Clinical uses Ifosfamide is given intravenously. The use of mesna to protect kidneys and bladder has allowed the use of very high doses, e.g. 8 g/m^2 but more usual doses are of the order of 1–2 g/m^2. Ifosfamide is also used in combination with other agents such as etoposide and methotrexate.

Adverse effects The main toxicity is on the kidney, producing tubular damage, renal failure and on the bladder causing haematuria. This can be minimised by using mesna and maintaining a high urinary output.

Other side effects include nausea, depression of the bone marrow, hair loss and occasionally a confusional state.

Mesna (Uromitexan)

This is mercaptoethane sulphonate sodium and is used to protect the urinary tract against the irritant effects of the metabolites of cyclophosphamide and ifosfamide, and in particular acrolein. It does this by supplying sulphydryl groups to form a stable thio-ether with acrolein. It also reduces the decomposition rate of the 4-hydroxy metabolites of these drugs to acrolein by combining to form relatively stable compounds which are non-toxic to the urinary tract. This interaction with cyclophosphamide and ifosfamide metabolism occurs mainly in the kidney where dimesna (the oxidation product of mesna formed in the blood *in vivo*) is excreted and then reduced back to active mesna. Because mesna circulates in the body as dimesna and hardly penetrates the tissues there is no interference with the cytotoxic efficacy of these drugs and their pharmacokinetics are unaltered.

Clinical use Mesna is given by intravenous injection: an oral preparation will soon be available. Because it is excreted more rapidly (the $t_{1/2}$ is less than 30 min) than cyclophosphamide and ifosfamide it is essential that mesna is given at the commencement of treatment and that the maximum interval between doses is not more than 4 hours. The dose of mesna is usually 20% of the dose of the cytotoxic given immediately and repeated at 4 and 8 hours. Higher doses, e.g. 40%, given 4 times at 3 hourly intervals are used for patients at higher risk and children. The urine should be monitored for output, proteinuria and haematuria.

Adverse effects have not been observed at usual doses.

Chlorambucil (Leukeran)

In this drug the methyl group of mustine is replaced by a phenylbutyric group. As a result chlorambucil differs considerably from mustine. It is non-irritant and is well absorbed after oral administration. Peak plasma levels are reached in about one hour. The drug is largely metabolised ($t_{1/2}$ ~1 hour) and the major metabolite is phenylacetic acid mustard ($t_{1/2}$ ~2 hours).

Chlorambucil takes two to three weeks to produce its therapeutic effects, though this is to some degree dose dependent. It may be given over long periods. A useful regime is 6.0 mg/m² orally given for two weeks out of four and repeated as required. It can also be taken continuously in which case the dose is usually 2.0 mg daily. It can replace mustine in the MOPP regime for Hodgkin's disease.

Chlorambucil is most effective in chronic lymphatic leukaemia, where it is the drug of choice. It is also used in lymphomas, carcinoma of the ovary and as an immunosuppressant agent.

Immediate side effects are rare, but prolonged use causes depression of the bone marrow with leucopenia and thrombocytopenia which may last 6 weeks or sometimes longer.

Melphalan (Alkeran)

This is a phenylalanine derivative of mustine and since phenylalanine is a precursor of melanin was originally used to treat malignant melanoma. Subsequently it has been found useful in myeloma and a range of solid tumours.

The half-life of melphalan is short (0.5–1.5 hours) and reflects non-enzymic hydrolysis. Although only 10–15% of the drug undergoes renal excretion renal impairment may be associated with increased toxicity. Melphalan is often given orally but absorption from the gut is erratic, delayed and the bioavailability varies from less than 10 to about 60%. Intravenous injection may therefore be preferable.

Adverse effects are mainly related to bone-marrow depression.

Busulphan (Myleran)

This drug differs from the alkylating agents already described in that the active groups are methone sulphoxy radicles. It is well absorbed from the gut and extensively metabolised (only 1 % is excreted unchanged in the urine). The plasma $t_{1/2}$ is 2.5 hours. It is the drug of choice for treating chronic myeloid leukaemia. It suppresses only the myeloid cells and has no effect on the lymphoid series. The usual dose is 4.0 mg daily until the white-cell count is reduced to below 20 000/mm^3. Treatment may then be stopped and restarted when a relapse occurs, or the drug may be continued at a lower maintenance dose (1–2 mg/day) to keep the white-cell count between 10 000 and 20 000/mm^3. Busulphan is potentially highly toxic, and careful haematological control is required, as overdosage can cause irreversible bone-marrow depression.

Occasionally it gives rise to a fibrosing alveolitis of the lung. Pigmentation with hyponatraemia is rarely seen but may be confused with Addison's disease, although adrenal function is normal.

Nitrosoureas

These alkylate DNA although carbamoylation of proteins by isocyanates contributes to their actions.

Four nitrosoureas have come into general clinical use:

1. BCNU (1,3-bis(2-chloroethyl)-1-nitrosourea);
2. CCNU (1-(2-chloroethyl)--cyclohexyl-1-nitrosourea);
3. Methyl–CCNU (1-(2-chloroethyl)-3-(4-methycyclohexyl)-1-nitrosourea);
4. Streptozotocin.

BCNU, which is only given intravenously, has been most used in lymphomas, brain tumours and gastrointestinal carcinomas. CCNU and methyl-CCNU are absorbed after oral administration and have shown activity in malignant melanoma and squamous-cell carcinoma of the lung as well as in lymphomas.

Pharmacokinetics Nitrosoureas are both metabolised by the liver and undergo spontaneous decomposition. Their $t_{1/2}$ is of the order of 40–60 min. The interval to maximum toxicity is delayed in comparison to the onset of anti-tumour effects, suggesting the possibility that different metabolites could be responsible for these different effects. Their lipid solubility results in rapid and complete absorption following oral administration and allows penetration into the CNS explaining their activity against brain tumours.

Clinical uses CCNU is given orally as a single dose of 80–120 mg/m^2. Its maximum effect is not seen for several weeks and the dose is usually repeated at intervals of six to eight weeks. It is used in the treatment of lymphomas and may replace the alkylating agent in a multi-drug regime.

Adverse effects They cause nausea, venous pain after injection and produce delayed (nadir counts at 4–6 weeks) bone-marrow suppression, particularly affecting platelets. BCNU produces pulmonary fibrosis dependent upon the cumulative dose (upper limit 1.4 g/m^2), duration of treatment and pre-existing lung disease.

Streptozotocin is methyl nitrosourea derived from *Streptomyces achromogenes* which produces significant regression of some sarcomas. The principal side effects include nausea, vomiting, renal damage consisting of proteinuria, glycosuria and/or renal tubular acidosis. Significant bone-marrow suppression does not occur with doses used in tumour chemotherapy, but nearly one third of patients have raised serum transaminases and bilirubin.

This drug is used in combination with other cytotoxic agents. One schedule uses streptozotocin at a dose of 500 mg/m^2/day for 5 days every 3 weeks.

Dimethyltriazenoimidazolecarboxamide (DTIC; Dacarbazine)

DTIC is metabolised in the liver and produces a carbonium ion which arrests cell division at the G_2 phase. It is used in the treatment of melanomas and produces a regression in about 20% of patients. It is also used in Hodgkin's disease, combined with adriamycin, bleomycin and a vinca alkaloid (ABVD regime).

Pharmacokinetics and clinical use DTIC is poorly absorbed when taken orally, so it is given intravenously. The usual course is 250 mg/m^2 daily for 5 days and repeated every 4 weeks. However, nausea can be so severe that it may be given in combination as a single dose every 2–3 weeks and this is less troublesome to the patient. DTIC is unstable in solution, particularly in light, so it must be given immediately it is prepared. It is also very irritant so it should be given slowly into a fast-running drip.

Adverse effects Nausea and vomiting occur soon after the drug has been given. Depression of the myeloid series of cells appears after about 3 weeks. Other side effects include paraesthesiae, fever and diarrhoea.

ANTIMETABOLITES

Antimetabolites resemble metabolites used normally by cells. They may act by competing with physiological substrates for an enzyme and thus block an enzymic process or they may interfere with cell metabolism by becoming involved in other processes within the cell. It was hoped that they might block metabolic pathways which were unique to malignant cells, but this hope has not been fulfilled as the pathways which they block also occur in normal cells. They are usually phase specific as their action is in most instances confined to specific steps in the synthesis of nuclear material.

1. Folic acid antagonist

Methotrexate

Folic acid is required in the synthesis of thymidylic acid and purine nucleotides and so ultimately for the production of DNA (see Fig. 20.10). Methotrexate resembles folic acid and competes with it for the active site of the enzyme dihydrofolate reductase. The affinity of the drug for this site is

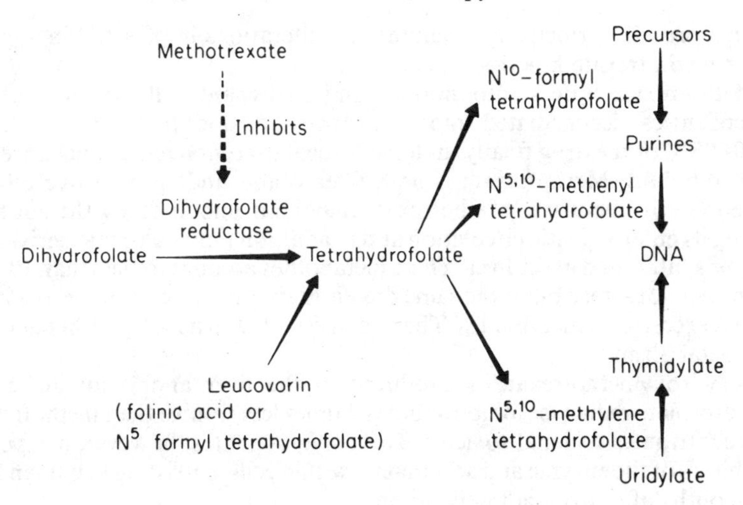

Fig. 20.10 Folate metabolism: effects of methotrexate and leucovorin.

100 000 times greater than that of dihydrofolate (Fig. 19.3). By blocking this step, methotrexate prevents nucleic acid synthesis which leads ultimately to cell death. It will be noted, however, that the administration of leucovorin (folinic acid) will circumvent the block and thus reverse the effect of methotrexate.

Pharmacokinetics Methotrexate can be given orally or by intravenous or intramuscular injection. The amount absorbed from the gut appears to depend upon a saturable transport process since small amounts (0.1 mg/kg) are rapidly and completely absorbed whilst larger doses of the order of 10 mg/kg are slowly and incompletely taken up. After intravenous injection methotrexate distributes in about 75% of body weight. Disappearance from plasma is best described by a three-compartment model since a triphasic decline in plasma concentration is observed. The initial-phase $t_{1/2}$ is 0.75 h; the second-phase $t_{1/2}$ is 2–3.5 h and is largely associated with renal elimination. The final phase (which begins 6–24 h after conventional doses and 30–48 h after high doses) is prolonged due to excretion via the bile and subsequent reabsorption from the gut, and has a $t_{1/2}$ of 10–12 h. This final-phase $t_{1/2}$ is important since the occurrence of gastrointestinal and bone-marrow toxicity is related to the plasma concentrations during this phase as well as to the peak concentrations achieved. The occurrence of this longer terminal-phase $t_{1/2}$ may explain the high incidence of toxicity in patients receiving chronic low-dose methotrexate therapy as compared to larger but more widely spaced single doses. Distribution of methotrexate into interstitial fluid spaces such as the CSF and pleural cavities is via passive diffusion and is slow, and it is usual to inject methotrexate directly into the CSF. When this is done drug may be slowly absorbed into the plasma and give prolonged cytotoxic levels with consequent toxicity. Thus a dose given into the CSF is potentially more toxic than the same dose given intravenously. 50–70% of the drug is bound to plasma protein (principally albumin) and alterations in plasma binding can affect methotrexate kinetics.

Methotrexate enters into normal and malignant cells via an energy-dependent carrier-mediated transport process, as does folate.

80–95% of the drug finally undergoes renal excretion either unchanged or as metabolites. Methotrexate is both filtered and undergoes active tubular secretion into the urine. Methotrexate may be metabolised by the gut flora during its enterohepatic circulation and in addition polyglutamate derivatives may be synthesised in the liver. These metabolites account for less than 10% of an intravenous dose but if the same dose is given orally, 35% of the absorbed dose is excreted as metabolites. This is consistent with a first-pass hepatic and gut metabolism.

7-Hydroxymethotrexate is produced in the liver and is an ineffective dihydrofolate reductase inhibitor but is 4 times less soluble than methotrexate and contributes to renal toxicity. The polyglutamates, however, are potent inhibitors of the enzyme and accumulate within cells, persisting in human liver for months after drug administration.

It has proved possible to derive a physiologically relevant tissue perfusion multicompartment model to describe methotrexate kinetics (see p. 35). As yet it is too complex to be of great clinical value, although eventually it may allow accurate prediction of methotrexate concentrations in tumour. It is believed that it is necessary to achieve plasma concentrations ranging from 1×10^{-4} to 1×10^{-3} M to produce sufficiently high methotrexate concentrations within the malignant cell to suppress tetrahydrofolate reductase adequately and to produce a cytotoxic effect.

Clinical uses Methotrexate is the drug of choice for chorioncarcinoma and for intrathecal therapy of malignancy. It is used in acute lymphatic leukaemia, lymphomas and several solid tumours including osteogenic sarcoma, epidermoid carcinoma of head and neck and some bronchial carcinomas. It has also been used as an immunosuppressant and occasionally to reduce the rapid cellular proliferation of severe psoriasis.

Methotrexate is used in several different regimes:

(a) Conventional dose: up to about 50 mg/m²/week does not require folinate rescue.
(b) Intermediate dose: up to 150 mg/m² by i.v. bolus injection does not require folinate rescue unless the patient has renal impairment but doses above this usually require folinate.
(c) High dose: 1–12 g/m² given intravenously over 1–6 hours always needs folinate rescue. This is an expensive procedure, presently there is no evidence that it is superior to conventional doses with the possible exception of non-Hodgkin's lymphoma and osteogenic sarcoma.

Methotrexate toxicity is determined by:

(i) a critical extracellular concentration for each target organ;
(ii) a critical duration of exposure which varies for each organ.

For bone marrow and the gut the critical plasma concentration is 2×10^{-8} M and the time factor is about 42 hours. Both factors must be exceeded for toxicity to occur in these organs. The severity of toxicity is proportional to the length of time that the critical concentration is exceeded and is independent of the amount by which it is exceeded.

Folinate (citrovorum factor; Leucovorin) rescue bypasses the enzyme block and reverses methotrexate toxicity. Malignant cells may be less able than normal cells to take up folinate thus introducing a degree of selectivity into the procedure. Rescue is normally commenced at 24 hours after methotrexate administration with oral or intravenous doses of 10–15 mg given at 6 hourly intervals for 4–8 doses. Folinate is continued until the plasma methotrexate concentration falls below 2×10^{-8} M. Monitoring plasma methotrexate levels has improved the safety of using this drug and allows identification of patients at special risk of toxicity (Fig. 20.11).

Intrathecal methotrexate is given in doses of 12 mg.

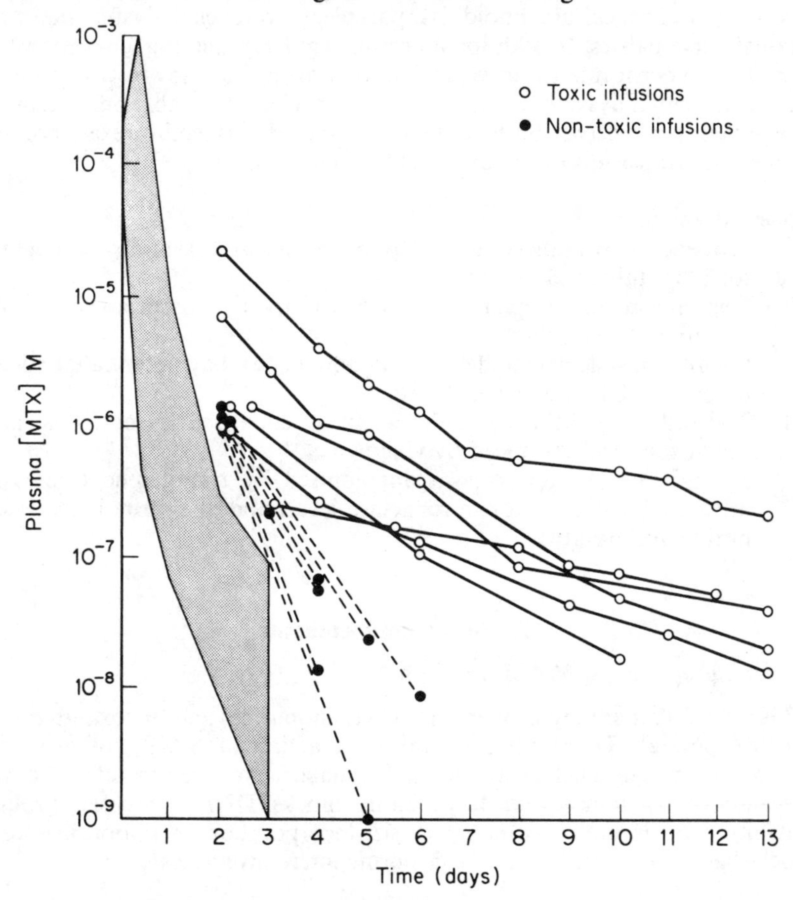

Fig. 20.11 Plasma methotrexate disappearance curves in patients receiving 50–250 mg/kg intravenous infusions. The profile for 14 patients who had no toxicity is included within the shaded area. Patients in whom evidence of myelosuppression developed had plasma levels as shown by the open circles. Six non-toxic patients with 48 h levels greater than 0.9 μM had the plasma levels shown by the solid circles (From R. G. Stoller *et al.*, Reprinted with permission from *New Eng. J. Med.*, **297**, 630 (1977).)

Adverse effects The principal effects are myelosuppression, nausea, vomiting, stomatitis and diarrhoea. Chronic low-dose administration (as for psoriasis) has been associated with hepatic fibrosis, interstitial pneumonitis and osteoporosis. With high-dose therapy renal dysfunction, acute vasculitis and seizures (which also occur more commonly when methotrexate is given intrathecally) may occur. Renal insufficiency poses problems since it interferes with methotrexate elimination and plasma methotrexate level monitoring is essential under these circumstances (see Fig. 20.11). Diuresis (> 3 l/day) with alkalinisation (pH > 7) of the urine reduces the incidence of nephrotoxicity: renal damage probably results from precipitation of methotrexate and 7-hydroxymethotrexate in the tubules.

Apart from convulsions, intrathecal administration is associated with neurotoxicity which includes a syndrome mimicking meningitis (which is probably a chemical arachnoiditis), paraplegia, cerebellar dysfunction and cranial nerve palsies. In addition a necrotising demyelinating leukoencephalopathy can occur months or years after treatment. This slowly progresses to severe dementia, dysarthria, ataxia and dysphagia. It probably only occurs if the patient has received both systemic and intrathecal methotrexate accompanied by irradiation of the brain and spinal cord.

Drug interactions

1. Probenecid and salicylate increase methotrexate toxicity by competing for renal tubular secretion.
2. Gentamicin and cisplatin increase toxicity by compromising renal excretion.
3. Phenytoin, salicylate and some sulphonamides may potentiate toxicity by protein binding displacement.
4. The cellular uptake of methotrexate is decreased by cortisone and prednisone and enhanced by vincristine.
5. Methotrexate action is also antagonised by triamterene (increases intracellular dihydrofolate reductase level) and allopurinol (increases purine availability).

2. Purine antimetabolite

6-mercaptopurine, 6-MP (Puri-Nethol)

This is a sulphur analogue of adenine (6-aminopurine) and hypoxanthine (6-hydroxypurine). The exact mechanism of action of 6-MP, following its conversion to ribonucleoside monophosphate, is still incompletely known because of its complexity. It probably blocks DNA synthesis through inhibition of de novo purine synthesis, incorporation of thiopurines into nucleic acids and interference with purine interconversions.

Pharmacokinetics It is only about 15% absorbed when given orally. The plasma $t_{1/2}$ in children is about 20 min but it is double this in adults. Although it is only 20% bound to plasma protein, the CSF levels are only 20% of those in the plasma. It is metabolised by xanthine oxidase and inhibition of this enzyme potentiates the action of 6-MP. About 20% of an intravenous dose of

6-MP is excreted in the urine within 6 h and renal impairment may therefore enhance its toxicity.

Clinical uses It is effective in the treatment of acute leukaemias, especially in children, and as an immunosuppressant (see Chapter 21). The usual oral dose is 2.5 mg/kg/day, administration may be continued for several weeks and if after 4 weeks there has been no response, the dose is increased to 5 mg/kg/day. It is usually given as part of a combination schedule.

Adverse effects The most important are leucopenia and thrombocytopenia. Nausea, vomiting and mild diarrhoea are uncommon but occur with high doses. Rarely renal calculi of the main metabolite thiouric acid occur.

Allopurinol inhibits xanthine oxidase and if these drugs are combined the dose of 6-MP should be reduced to one quarter to avoid toxicity.

3. Pyrimidine antimetabolites

Cytarabine; Cytosine arabinoside (Cytosar)

Cytarabine differs from naturally occurring deoxycytidine and cytidine in that arabinose replaces deoxyribose or ribose as the sugar moiety. It is converted into the triphosphate in the cell and this is the active cytotoxic compound (see Fig. 20.12). It is believed to inhibit DNA polymerase competitively and thus prevent DNA synthesis. Cytarabine is a cell-cycle phase-specific agent acting mainly in the late S-phase. Its effectiveness is directly proportional to the duration of exposure of cells to the drug. It is therefore necessary to use regimes which require continuous infusion of the drug or frequent intermittent injections.

Pharmacokinetics Cytarabine is metabolised by the widely distributed enzyme cytidine deaminase so that after intravenous injection it is rapidly metabolised by the liver to uracil arabinoside. The $t_{1/2,\beta}$ is 60–110 min and the kinetics are probably dose-dependent. It is rarely given orally because less than 20 % is absorbed due to intraluminal deamination in the gut. Although widely distributed in the body the CSF levels are only 40 % of those of the plasma even when the drug is given by continuous infusion. It is thus often given intrathecally. When given by this route it is only slowly deaminated and has a CSF half-life of 2–11 h. It is excreted unchanged exclusively by the kidney and dosage modification may be necessary in renal impairment.

Clinical use It is useful in acute leukaemia and lymphomas. The dose is 2–3 mg/kg every 24 h for up to 7 days as a single agent or in various combination schedules.

Adverse effects Toxic manifestations include nausea, vomiting, stomatitis and bone-marrow depression.

5-Fluorouracil; 5-FU

5-FU is activated by formation of the nucleotides (see Fig. 20.13):

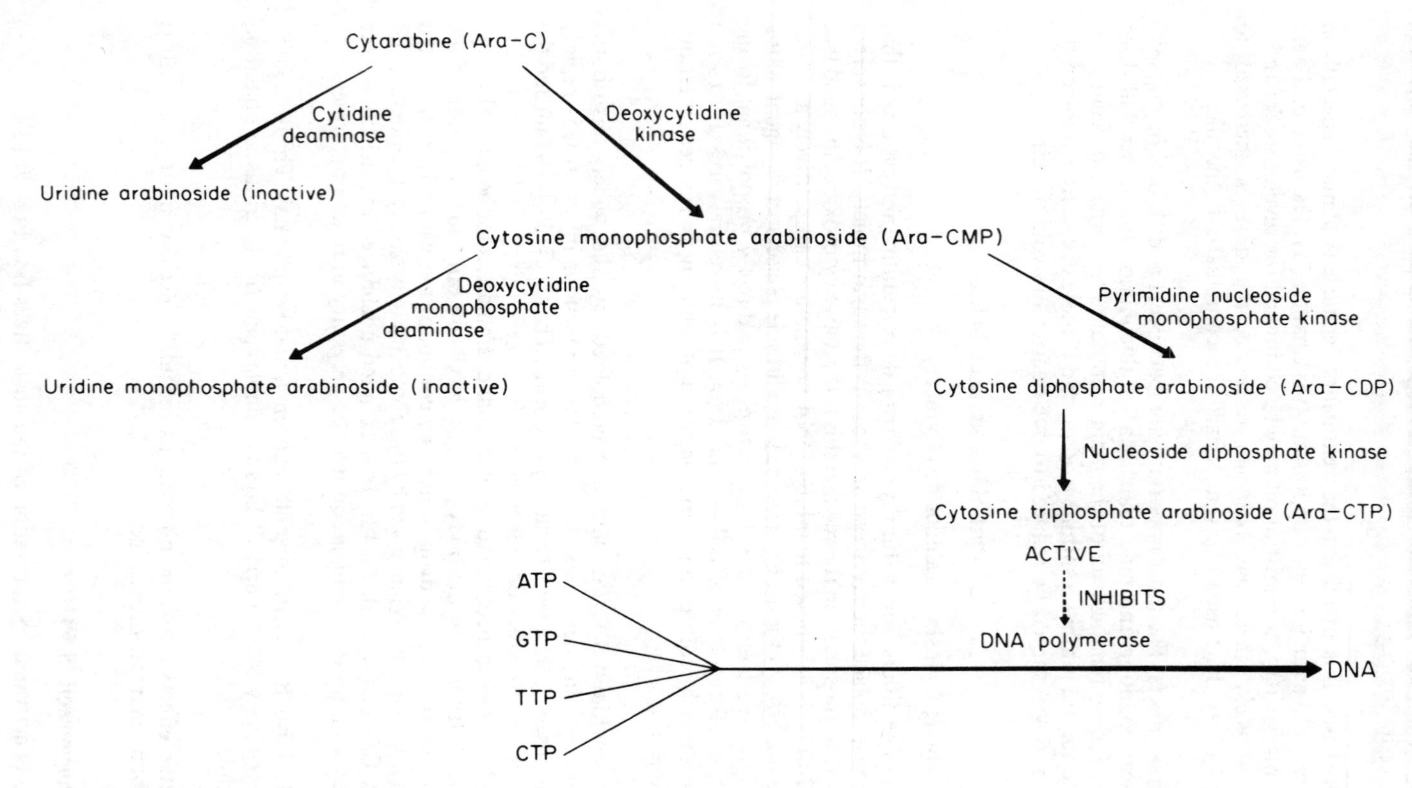

Fig. 20.12 Intracellular pathways of cytarabine metabolism.

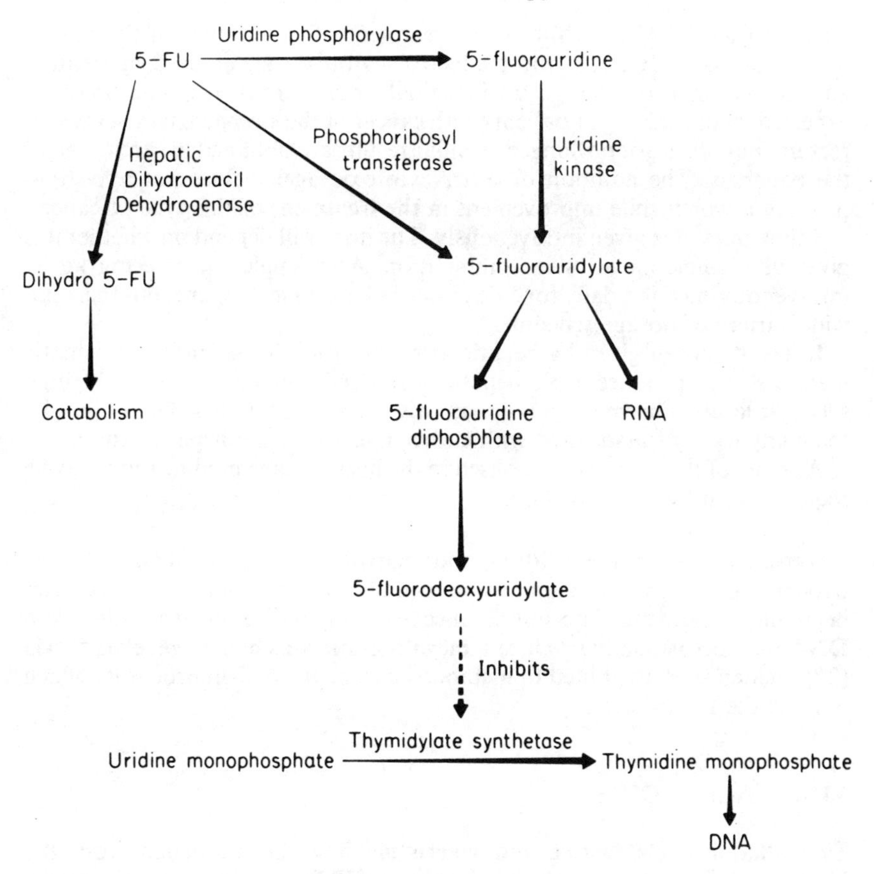

Fig. 20.13 Metabolism and activation of 5-FU.

(a) 5-fluorouridine monophosphate which is incorporated into RNA thereby altering its function.
(b) 5-fluorodeoxyuridylate which, in the presence of N^{5-10} methylene tetrahydrofolate, binds strongly to thymidylate synthetase and inhibits DNA synthesis. This is probably the most important cytotoxic effect of 5-FU.

Pharmacokinetics Whereas activation of 5-FU occurs in the target cell (and thus defines the specificity of the drug) inactivation occurs mainly in the liver (see Fig. 20.13). 5-FU is initially reduced and then cleared non-enzymatically to inactive products which are excreted in the urine. 5-FU is cleared rapidly from the plasma with a $t_{1/2}$ of 10–20 min. About 20% is excreted unchanged in the urine and the remainder is metabolised. The drug distributes in total body water and readily penetrates the CNS. 5-FU is usually given by injection since it is unreliably absorbed from the gut due to high hepatic first-pass metabolism.

Clinical uses 5-FU is useful in the treatment of carcinomas of the breast, ovary and skin. It is the most effective cytotoxic agent used in treating adenocarcinoma of the gastro-intestinal tract. Some response may be expected in about 30 % of patients with cancer of the stomach, large bowel or rectum, but life is not prolonged. Similar results are obtained in carcinoma of the pancreas. The addition of other cytotoxic agents does not appear to produce a worthwhile improvement in the treatment of this type of cancer.

5-fluorouracil is given intravenously. The dose will depend on whether it is given as a single agent or in combination. As a single agent 15 mg/kg by intravenous injection daily for 5 days would be a typical regime, but there is a wide variety of dosage schedules.

It has also been given by hepatic artery infusion in patients with hepatic metastases to produce high hepatic levels without correspondingly high systemic levels. This method is apparently successful but its value is offset by the complications associated with catheterisation of the hepatic artery.

As most of the drug is metabolised in the liver, dosage modification may be required with liver dysfunction.

Adverse effects Oral ulceration and diarrhoea occur in about 20% of patients. Bone-marrow suppression usually occurs about 14 days after beginning treatment. The interference with thymidine incorporation into DNA may occasionally produce a megaloblastic anaemia. Cerebellar ataxia (2% incidence) is attributed to metabolism to neurotoxic fluorocitrate which inhibits the Krebs' cycle.

VINCA ALKALOIDS

Two alkaloids, **vinblastine** and **vincristine** have been isolated from the Madagascan periwinkle plant. **Vindesine (Eldesine)** is a semi-synthetic modification of vinblastine. Despite their close structural relationship they differ in their clinical spectrum and toxicity (see Table 20.6).

These alkaloids bind to tubulin, the protein which forms the microtubules essential for spindle formation which separates the chromosomes at mitosis. The consequences of this binding are the crystallisation of tubulin and the dissolution of the spindle which halts mitosis. Although often called 'spindle-poisons' the vinca alkaloids have other actions on cell metabolism which include inhibition of nucleic acid and protein synthesis. Binding to micro-tubules concerned with neuronal growth may also explain their neurotoxicity.

Pharmacokinetics Vinca alkaloids are only given intravenously: they are poorly absorbed from the gut. They are extensively metabolised by the liver to largely unknown metabolites although the principal deacetylated metabolite of vinblastine is more active than vinblastine itself. They are largely excreted in the bile and have long terminal half-lives (vincristine, 85 hours; vinblastine and vindesine, 24 hours) so the dose should be reduced with hepatic impairment. Vincristine (and perhaps the others) exhibits non-linear pharma-cokinetics showing a disproportionate increase in area under the plasma concentration–time curve with dose. This may be because microtubules are

Table 20.6 Adverse effects of vinca alkaloids

	Vinblastine	*Vincristine*
Common	Leucopenia (dose-limiting effect usually occurring 4–7 days after administration)	Neurological toxicity (a) Motor: loss of tendon reflexes (often the earliest sign); weakness (b) Sensory: paraesthesiae; peripheral neuropathy; jaw pain (c) Autonomic: constipation; paralytic ileus (prostigmine may reverse this effect)
Less common	Neurological toxicity (as vincristine) Nausea and vomiting (20%) Alopecia (5–10%)	Leucopenia Convulsions, frequently associated with hypertension Alopecia (5–10%)

involved in biliary secretion and their dissolution by vinca alkaloids results in the drug inhibiting its own elimination.

Clinical uses vinblastine (Velbe) is used in the treatment of testicular cancer Hodgkin's disease. It is given in combination (see p. 813) at weekly intervals. The usual dose as a single agent is 0.1–0.15 mg/kg/week and in combinations is 6 mg/m^2 twice during each course.

Vincristine (Oncovin) is used in breast cancer lymphomas and also in the initial treatment of acute lymphoblastic leukaemia. It is usually given, in combination with other agents, in a dose of 1.4 mg/m^2 at monthly intervals.

Adverse effects The toxic effects of vincristine and vinblastine are strikingly different despite their structural similarity—see Table 20.6. Both drugs can produce a severe and prolonged inflammatory reaction if extravasation occurs. Vincristine can cause thrombocytosis and has been used in the treatment of idiopathic thrombocytopenic purpura. Depression of the bone marrow is much less with vincristine and this drug can be given to moderately leucopenic patients.

Vindesine has side-effects intermediate between vinblastine and vincristine.

PODOPHYLLOTOXIN DERIVATIVES

Podophyllin is extracted from the American mandrake or may apple: it is locally effective against warts. A number of derivatives of the active principle, podophyllotoxin have been investigated as antineoplastic drugs. One of these, **etoposide** (VP 16–213; Vepesid), is commercially available. Unlike vinca alkaloids they are not spindle poisons but produce DNA damage similar to that seen after radiation.

Pharmacokinetics Etoposide is given by i.v. injection or orally (bioavailability 50 %). It undergoes mainly hepatic metabolism and renal elimination is low. The $t_{1/2}$ is about 12 hours.

Clinical uses Etoposide is one of the most active drugs for small cell lung cancer and is also used in lymphomas, testicular teratomas and trophoblastic tumours.

Adverse effects Although relatively well tolerated, nausea and vomiting are common (especially after oral administration) as is alopecia.

Bone-marrow suppression is dose-dependent and reversible.

ANTIBIOTICS

1. The anthracyclines

These are some of the most widely used drugs for malignant disease. Present evidence indicates three main mechanisms of action:

(a) Intercalation between adjacent base pairs in DNA, thus inhibiting further nucleic acid synthesis and leading to fragmentation of DNA and inhibition of DNA repair.
(b) Membrane binding which alters membrane function. This may be responsible for the observed alteration in sodium and calcium concentrations seen in the myocardium and could be involved in the development of cardiomyopathy.
(c) Free-radical formation. This may also be involved in cardiotoxicity rather than tumour cell killing.

Daunorubicin and doxorubicin are the most widely used drugs in this group but many new analogues are undergoing clinical trial.

Doxorubicin (Adriamycin)

This red antibiotic is produced by the fungus *Streptomyces peucetius* (as is daunomycin). It is the most widely used drug of the anthracycline group with proven activity in acute leukaemia, lymphomas, sarcomas, and a wide range of carcinomas.

Pharmacokinetics Doxorubicin is given intravenously as less than 5 % of an oral dose is absorbed. The plasma concentration–time profile shows a triphasic decline with half-lives of 2–6 min, 0.5–2.5 h and 15–50 h respectively for the three phases. The volume of distribution is large reflecting extensive tissue uptake, the majority of the drug being located in cell nuclei. Hepatic extraction is high with 40 % of the dose appearing in the bile (40 % unchanged, 20 % as doxorubicinol and the remainder as other metabolites). Renal excretion accounts for less than 15 % of the dose. The major metabolite, doxorubicinol also has some antitumour activity.

Dose reduction is recommended in liver disease, although no relationship has been established between any liver function test, doxorubicin clearance and toxicity. A 50 % dose reduction is advised if plasma bilirubin is 20–50 μmol/l and a 75 % reduction if bilirubin > 50 μmol/l. Dose modification is not required in renal disease.

Despite widespread tissue distribution, doxorubicin does not enter the CNS. The usual dose schedule is 30–60 mg/m^2 (depending on other drugs concurrently administered) every 21 or 28 days.

Adverse effects

1. Bone marrow suppression with neutropenia and thrombocytopenia.
2. Alopecia occurs in nearly all patients but may be mitigated by scalp cooling.
3. Nausea and vomiting.
4. 'Radiation recall' reaction: this describes the ability of anthracyclines to exacerbate or reactivate dormant radiation dermatitis or pneumonitis weeks after cessation of radiotherapy.
5. Extravasation: If this occurs, severe tissue necrosis may result. The drug should never be injected into veins on the back of the hand as severe damage to nerves and tendons may result.

6. Cardiotoxicity: This is the major dose-limiting factor in long-term administration. There are two forms:
   (i) Acute: this occurs shortly after administration, with the development of various arrhythmias which are occasionally life-threatening, e.g. ventricular tachycardia, heart block. These acute effects do not predict the more severe chronic toxicity.
   (ii) Chronic: cardiomyopathy leading to death in up to 60% of those who develop signs of congestive cardiac failure. It is determined by the cumulative dose of doxorubicin administered with an incidence of less than 2% at total doses less than 400 mg/m², rising to over 20% at cumulative doses greater than 700 mg/m². Risk factors which increase the risk of cardiomyopathy and lower the cumulative dose at which this occurs include prior mediastinal irradiation, age (over 70 years) and cardiovascular disease, including coronary artery disease and hypertension.

Various agents have been used in an effort to protect against this complication: vitamin E, N-acetylcysteine (free-radical scavengers) can protect against acute toxicity but are not effective against cardiomyopathy. Digoxin has been effective in some studies but this has not been the universal experience.

Alteration of dose schedule, either by giving the drug on an intermittent weekly basis or as a prolonged continuous infusion has shown some promising early results. This reduces cardiotoxicity and allows administration of higher total doses of drug without loss of activity.

Daunorubicin (Daunomycin)

This is similar to doxorubicin, but its use is largely confined to the treatment of acute leukaemia. It penetrates peripheral tissues less effectively than doxorubicin which may account for its narrower range of activity. Its pharmacokinetics are similar to those of doxorubicin with extensive metabolism primarily to the less active daunorubicinol. The $t_{1/2}$ of daunorubicin is about 24 h.

The adverse effects of daunorubicin are almost identical to those of doxorubicin and include cardiotoxicity (recommended maximum cumulative dose is 500–600 mg/m²).

2. Mitozantrone (Novantrone)

This is a blue synthetic anthracenedione derivative. It is structurally similar to doxorubicin but lacks the amino-sugar moiety which may account for its reduced cardiotoxicity compared to the anthracyclines.

It has proven activity in advanced breast cancer and is probably effective in leukaemias and lymphomas. There is minimal cross-reactivity with doxorubicin.

Pharmacokinetics It is given intravenously and undergoes hepatic metabolism and biliary excretion with only 10% of the dose appearing in the urine. The terminal half-life is about 45 h.

Clinical use The usual dose is 12–14 mg/m^2 given every three weeks.

Adverse effects Compared with doxorubicin it has a low incidence of nausea and vomiting (usually only mild nausea) and extravasation does not cause serious tissue damage. Partial hair loss may occur but total alopecia is rare. Cardiotoxicity may occur but the incidence is much lower than with anthracyclines possibly because of structural differences and the lack of free-radical formation by this drug. To avoid cardiotoxicity, a maximum cumulative dose of 160 mg/m^2 is recommended, which should be cut to 120 mg/m^2 in patients previously treated with anthracyclines.

The major dose-limiting toxicity is bone-marrow suppression.

3. Actinomycin D, Dactinomycin (Cosmegen)

This antibiotic is derived from a species of *Streptomyces.* Its cytotoxicity results from intercalation and binding to double-stranded DNA, thus preventing action of RNA polymerase and thereby blocking RNA synthesis. DNA synthesis is blocked at higher concentrations *in vitro.*

Pharmacokinetics It is poorly absorbed from the gut. Because it causes severe local inflammation the only useful route of administration is by intravenous injection. It is very rapidly cleared after injection, little being detected in the blood after 2 min. It is widely distributed and may be taken up into some tissues by facilitated transport. It does not enter the brain. It is not metabolised, has a long tissue $t_{1/2}$ and 50 % is excreted unchanged in the bile over several days.

Clinical uses In combination schedules it cures the majority of patients with choriocarcinoma and combined with surgery and radiotherapy overall cure rates of 80 % may be obtained in patients with early Wilm's tumour. It can also be useful in rhabdomyosarcomas, Hodgkin's and non-Hodgkin's lymphomas and in testicular tumours. The commonly used dosage is 450 μg/m^2 over 5 days, in conjunction with other agents.

Adverse effects These are cumulative. Myelosuppression and mucous membrane ulceration are the dose-limiting side effects and alopecia is usually complete. Radiation may produce marked tissue reactions in patients previously treated with actinomycin, which may reflect the long tissue $t_{1/2}$ of the drug.

4. Bleomycin

This is a mixture of several polypeptide antibiotics synthesised by *Streptomyces verticillus*. Its mode of action is not well understood. It prevents thymidine incorporation into DNA and can also cause fragmentation of DNA, so that cells fail to progress through the G_2 and M phases of the cell cycle. Despite these effects on nucleic acid it has only minimal action on rapidly proliferating normal cells.

Pharmacokinetics Bleomycin disappears from plasma after intravenous injection with a half-life of about 9 h. Markedly prolonged elimination occurs in renal failure and is accompanied by increased toxicity, so that caution is required when bleomycin is given concurrently with nephrotoxic agents such as aminoglycoside antibiotics or high-dose methotrexate. It is metabolised to numerous fragments which are also excreted in the urine. In experimental tumours a correlation between bleomycin distribution and response has been demonstrated. Distribution is correlated with the presence or absence of peptidase activity (which inactivates the drug) and in man high drug concentrations occur in sensitive tumours in skin and lung. Thus the selectivity of action of this drug may be explained by its distribution.

Clinical uses Bleomycin is used in lymphomas, testicular carcinoma and various squamous-cell carcinomas. It is usually given intravenously (7.5–15 mg/m^2/day by continuous infusion or 5–15 mg/m^2 every week) or intramuscularly. If given by the latter route it should be combined with lignocaine as injection is painful.

Adverse effects As might be expected from the above, these affect the skin, mucous membranes and lungs. The skin may show hyperkeratosis, erythema and pigmentation. These changes may be associated with painful fingers and hands. Mouth ulceration can also be troublesome with high doses. The lungs can develop a diffuse interstitial fibrosis which can be fatal. It usually only occurs if the total cumulative dose exceeds 180 mg. It is also more liable to develop in the elderly and in those with already damaged lungs. Injection of the drug is usually followed in a few hours by shivering and by transient fever. The reason for this is unknown but it does not appear to be of any particular significance. Alopecia may also occur.

MISCELLANEOUS AGENTS

Procarbazine (Natulan)

Procarbazine is a hydrazine possessing some monoamine oxidase inhibiting properties. Its anti-tumour activity is believed to be dependent on its terminal methylhydrazine grouping which can undergo activation by microsomal enzymes, mainly in the liver, to various reactive free-radical metabolites which are cytotoxic.

The precise mode of action is unknown but it has several actions at cellular level:

1. It depresses DNA synthesis.
2. It combines with DNA, decreasing its viscosity and causing chromosome breaks.

Pharmacokinetics Procarbazine is rapidly and almost completely absorbed from the intestine, peak levels being obtained in 30–60 min. The $t_{1/2}$ of the parent compound in plasma is about 10 min. It is metabolised to a number of compounds which are excreted by the kidneys. Some of these compounds, particularly the hydrazines, may have cytotoxic activity. Procarbazine and its metabolites penetrate the blood–brain barrier.

Clinical uses

1. Hodgkin's disease It is part of the well-established MOPP regime (see p. 812) which produces complete remission in about 65% of patients.

2. Non-Hodgkin's lymphoma Procarbazine is less effective in this group, some benefit being obtained in 30–40% of patients.

It is not generally useful in other malignancies.

Procarbazine is given daily by mouth, usually for 2 weeks with other cytotoxic drugs. It is wise not to exceed 150 mg daily or myelosuppression may be a problem. The drug affects predominantly the neutrophils and platelets and maximum depression of the blood count occurs 10–14 days after dosing.

Adverse effects The major toxicity is dose-related haemopoietic suppression. Nausea and vomiting occur frequently after initial administration but are less prominent after repeated dosage.

Procarbazine is a weak monoamine oxidase inhibitor and the usual precautions are observed to avoid interaction (see p. 237). Such interactions appear in practice to be very rare and it is doubtful whether dietary restriction is really necessary, but care should be taken if CNS depressants, sympathomimetic agents or tricyclic antidepressants are used. Procarbazine also interacts with ethanol causing flushing and tachycardia. This is presumably due to interference with the oxidation of acetaldehyde (cf. disulfiram—an 'antabuse'-type of reaction).

Cisplatin (Cis-diaminedichloroplatinum)

This is an inorganic platinum (II) coordination complex in which two amine (NH_3) and two chlorine ligands occupy cis positions (the trans compound is inactive). Cytotoxicity results from selective inhibition of DNA synthesis by formation of intra- and inter-strand cross-links in the DNA molecule: a mechanism similar to that of alkylating agents.

Pharmacokinetics A biphasic plasma disappearance has been demonstrated: $t_{1/2,\alpha}$, 25–50 min and $t_{1/2,\beta}$, 60–73 h. Although initially rapidly excreted, over 50% is still retained by the body after 5 days and low urinary concentrations may be found up to one month after treatment. No preferential accumulation occurs in tumours but high concentrations occur in the ovary, testis and kidney.

Clinical uses Cisplatin is used in the treatment of a number of cancers. It is the most effective single agent in testicular teratomas but is usually given in combination with various other cytotoxic drugs. When combined with high dose bleomycin and vinblastine, a remission rate of 70% was achieved. In carcinoma of the ovary it can be combined with adriamycin and cyclophosphamide and appears more effective than a single alkylating agent. It has also been tried with some success in head and neck and bladder cancers.

Cisplatin is given intravenously either as a bolus or infusion in a number of cyclical regimes, often in combination with other cytotoxic agents. The usual dose is 50–100 mg/m^2 as a single dose or 15–20 mg/m^2 daily for 5 days every 3–4 weeks.

To minimise nephrotoxicity (see below) the patient must be fully hydrated and a urine flow of 200 ml/h maintained during treatment and for 6 hours afterwards. This is achieved by intravenous infusion combined with mannitol or frusemide.

Adverse effects Cisplatin may give rise to severe vomiting resistant to most antiemetics. It also causes myelosuppression.

The major and dose-limiting toxicity is renal. This is dose-related and is an acute distal tubular necrosis. Pre-hydration and diuresis reduce the immediate effects but cumulative and permanent damage may still occur. It is mandatory to perform creatinine clearances before and after each treatment. Clinically significant hypomagnesaemia has also occurred and it is usual to provide magnesium supplementation during infusion.

Up to 30% of patients develop ototoxicity: mostly in the frequency range above speech tones. Tinnitus may be associated with the deafness. Cisplatin irreversibly damages the organ of Corti and although the effects are not clearly dose-related they are cumulative. Audiometry should be carried out before, during and after treatment.

Peripheral neuropathy also occurs and can be disabling.

New platinum analogues The severe toxicity coupled with undoubted efficacy of cisplatin has stimulated the production of many analogues which are now in trial. Carboplatin (JM8) is presently the most promising and has almost no renal or ototoxicity, neuropathy is rare and vomiting, although common, is less severe than after cisplatin.

L-Asparaginase or Colaspase (Crasnitin)

The observation that guinea-pig serum had antitumour activity against some mouse tumours led to the identification of L-asparagine aminohydralase as the active agent in the serum. This enzyme is now produced from *E. coli* and has been given the approved name of colaspase. Its mode of action is unique in cancer chemotherapy and depends upon the inability of some tumour cells (unlike normal cells which possess L-asparagine synthetase) to synthesise the amino acid asparagine which is required for protein synthesis. Colaspase hydrolyses free plasma and tissue asparagine, thus depriving tumour cells of their exogenous source of this amino acid. In sensitive cells this results in immediate inhibition of protein synthesis and a delayed inhibition of nucleic acid synthesis.

Pharmacokinetics Colaspase cannot be administered orally since it is destroyed in the gut: it is therefore given intravenously, although it can be given intramuscularly. It is largely confined to the vascular space and penetrates extracellular fluid poorly so that it needs to be injected intrathecally if its action is directed towards tumour in the central nervous system. The $t_{1/2}$

depends upon the enzyme preparation and varies from 8 to 30 h. It is not excreted in any appreciable quantities in either urine or bile, and it is believed that it becomes sequestered in the reticulo-endothelial system and is slowly released from this site into the blood.

Clinical uses It is useful in acute leukaemias and acute transformation of chronic myeloid leukaemia. It is usually given by intravenous injection or infusion. This should be preceded by a test intracutaneous injection of 50 units which should be observed for an allergic reaction for 3 h before proceeding to the therapeutic dose. Dosage is 200 units/kg which, depending on response, may be increased to 1000 units/kg. This is usually given on 5 days per week for 2 or 3 weeks. Theoretically it should be an ideal cytotoxic agent: unfortunately in up to 65% of cases the tumour cells acquire asparagine synthetase.

Adverse effects Because of its unusual mode of action these do not include myelosuppression or alopecia but nausea, vomiting, pyrexia and anorexia are frequent. Since, it is a foreign protein, allergic reactions (chills, urticaria, anaphylaxis) may occur but a change in enzyme source may allow continued treatment. It can also produce insulin-responsive non-ketotic hyperglycaemia and alterations in liver function including hypoalbuminaemia and reduction in clotting factors.

Interferon (see p. 753)

There is now reasonable evidence that as a single agent alfa-interferon can produce useful remission in hairy cell leukaemia, low-grade non-Hodgkin's lymphoma, cutaneous T-cell lymphoma and some cases of chronic myeloid leukaemia. Responses in solid tumours are fewer and less dramatic. The availability of larger amounts of material and its use in combination with other drugs may improve future results.

HORMONES

Hormones may produce a remission in certain types of cancer. They do not eradicate the disease, it will recur sooner or later. They can sometimes alleviate symptoms over a long period and do not have the disadvantage of depressing the bone marrow. They are most effective in tumours arising from cells which are normally hormone dependent, namely the breast and prostate. They may also have some effect on lymphomas, hypernephromas, and adenocarcinomas of the body of the uterus.

There are several ways in which hormones can affect malignant cells:

(a) A hormone may have a direct cytotoxic action on the malignant cell. This is likely if cancer cells which are normally dependent on a specific hormone are exposed to high concentration of a hormone with the opposite effect. For example, the cells of the prostate are testosterone dependent, if a carcinoma arises from these cells, oestrogens in large doses will frequently be cytotoxic to the cancer.

(b) A hormone may suppress production of other hormones by a feedback mechanism. This will change the hormonal milieu surrounding the malignant cells and may suppress their activity.

In breast cancer, patients who respond to one form of endocrine therapy are more likely to respond to subsequent hormone treatment than those who fail to respond initially. Thus, sequencing one endocrine therapy after another may prolong survival and improve quality of life, often for several years.

Oestrogens

Oestrogens are used in treating two cancers which arise from cells that are partially hormone dependent.

(a) *Carcinoma of the prostate.* The cells of the prostate gland are androgen dependent and in the absence of androgens regression occurs in both normal and malignant tissue. This is best achieved by orchidectomy but oestrogens effectively block the production of androgens and a remission is obtained in about 60% of patients with advanced disease.

(b) *Carcinoma of the breast* Oestrogens will produce a remission in about 30% of women with widespread cancer, provided they are more than 5 years menopausal. In younger women oestrogens are not effective, indeed they may exacerbate the disease. It has been shown that, depending upon menstrual status, 40–85% of breast cancers possess specific oestrogen receptors. About 60% of receptor-positive tumours respond to oestrogens whereas only 10% of tumours lacking oestrogen receptors do so. The presence of oestrogen receptors is also correlated with the degree of differentiation of the tumours: the less well-differentiated ones are more likely to be oestrogen receptor negative and tend to recur sooner. In some studies, receptor-negative patients showed an increased response to chemotherapy rather than hormones. This correlation between lack of the oestrogen receptor and increased response rate to chemotherapy might explain the increased effectiveness of adjuvant chemotherapy in pre-menopausal women.

Clinical uses Oestrogens are usually given in large doses when treating cancer. In prostatic carcinoma the dose of diethylstilboestrol is sometimes as high as 5 mg three times daily, although it has now been demonstrated that 1 mg thrice daily is as effective and causes fewer cardiovascular complications. Controlled studies have not shown any difference in survival between treated patients and controls although the quality of life is improved. Survival is not impaired by delaying endocrine therapy until the patient is symptomatic and in view of the risks of therapy this approach is usually adopted.

In carcinoma of the breast, stilboestrol is given in doses of 5–15 mg three times daily. Remission is most frequently achieved in disease of skin and breast, metastases in bone, lung and liver respond less frequently. The mean duration of response is about a year, but a few patients remain in remission for longer periods.

Adverse effects The major disadvantage with oestrogen therapy is a high incidence of toxicity. Nausea, vomiting and anorexia occur in up to 60% of patients but often abate with continued treatment.

Fluid retention and heart failure may occasionally occur and there is an increased incidence of deep-vein thrombosis and cardiovascular accidents. Signs of feminisation occur in males (impotence, testicular atrophy, gynaecomastia). 5–10% of patients develop hypercalcaemia, which is an indication to stop the drug and increase the fluid intake.

Tamoxifen

This is an anti-oestrogen related to clomiphene. It has a complex, incompletely understood mechanism of action. It competes with naturally occurring oestrogen for binding to the cytoplasmic oestrogen receptor. The tamoxifen–receptor complex translocates to the nucleus in the same way as the normal oestrogen–receptor complex but once inside it remains there for a much longer time. This suppresses the replenishment of cytosol receptors which renders the cells less responsive to oestrogen effects.

Pharmacokinetics Tamoxifen is well absorbed orally and undergoes hepatic metabolism: the principal metabolite being desmethyltamoxifen which has comparable anti-oestrogen activity. The $t_{1/2}$s of tamoxifen and this metabolite are 4 and 9 days respectively after a single dose but with repeated dosing these are reversibly increased suggesting self-inhibition of metabolism.

Clinical use The conventional method of dosing is to give 20–40 mg/day in divided doses. The long $t_{1/2}$s of tamoxifen and its active metabolite may explain why clinical responses do not usually occur for some 6 weeks. A suggested loading dose of 100 mg/m^2 on day 1 followed by a maintenance dose of 20 mg/day is presently being evaluated.

Tamoxifen is effective in about 35% of postmenopausal patients and can be as effective as oophorectomy in premenopausal women. Response to tamoxifen may in fact predict response to oophorectomy. Breast and skin deposits most frequently respond but there is less effect on bone metastases and little response from liver deposits. Because of low toxicity tamoxifen is now the hormonal agent of first choice for breast cancer.

Adverse effects Tamoxifen is associated with minimal toxicity: less than 1% of patients have to be withdrawn from treatment. Mild nausea and vomiting, hypercalcaemia, weight gain, hot flushes, disease 'flare' and thrombocytopenia have all been reported.

Aminoglutethimide (Orimeten)

Originally introduced as an anticonvulsant it was withdrawn when found to cause adrenal suppression. It has been reintroduced for treatment of breast cancer and has two actions of importance:

(a) Inhibition of adrenal synthesis of oestrogens, glucocorticoids and mineralocorticoids by inhibition of the enzyme producing their common precursor, pregnenedione. A reflex rise in ACTH secondary to low circulating cortisol will override the adrenal blockade and so a glucocorticoid (e.g. hydrocortisone 20 mg twice daily) is given to prevent this.

(b) A second, more important effect is inhibition of tissue (fat, skin, muscle, carcinoma) aromatase which blocks conversion of androgens into oestrogens. Ovarian aromatase is resistant to such inhibition so aminoglutethimide is only useful in postmenopausal women. Similarly in normal men, a rise in LH overrides this action on the testis. Nevertheless, in castrated males, it could be useful in the management of prostatic cancer.

Pharmacokinetics As it is subject to polymorphic acetylation (see p. 100) to an inactive N-acetyl metabolite, fast acetylators have a $t_{1/2}$ of around 13 hours as compared to 20 hours in slow acetylators. This is not a major route of metabolism, more important is hepatic oxidation which is self-inducible so that on chronic dosing the half-life falls. Hepatic enzyme induction by aminoglutethimide may result in interactions with other drugs, e.g. warfarin.

Clinical use It is effective in about 30% of postmenopausal patients with best effects on skin and breast disease and although the response of bone metastases is higher than with tamoxifen, liver metastases rarely respond. Aminoglutethimide may be effective after tamoxifen has failed.

Conventionally given in doses of 1 g/day more recent studies show efficacy using 250 mg/day or less: at these doses the major effect is inhibition of the more sensitive aromatase.

Adverse effects Lethargy, nausea and dizziness are common on starting treatment although decline on chronic dosing (probably due to enzyme induction). 25% of patients develop an erythematous, itchy rash after about 10 days which fades on continued treatment. Overall 5–10% of patients cannot tolerate the drug.

Androgens

Androgens or anabolic steroids such as testosterone or fluoxymesterone are used in breast cancer in pre-menopausal women although oophorectomy is more effective. Remission is obtained in about 25% of patients. They presumably act by altering the hormonal environment of the tumour. Androgen receptors have been detected in 20–50% of breast cancers but insufficient evidence is available to correlate their presence with tumour response. Androgens produce no acute toxic effects, but on chronic administration fluid retention and virilisation occur commonly and hypercalcaemia and cholestatic jaundice may infrequently produce problems.

Progestogens

The endometrial cells normally mature under the influence of progestogens and some malignant cells arising from the endometrium may respond in the same way. About 30% of patients with disseminated adenocarcinoma of the body of the uterus will respond to a progestogen such as megestrol 20 mg twice daily.

Progestogens are also used in advanced breast cancer although their mechanism of action is uncertain. Progestogen bound to its receptor impairs regeneration of oestrogen receptors and also stimulates 17β-oestradiol dehydrogenase activity which breaks down intracellular oestrogen: these actions may deprive cancer cells of oestrogen effects. There is also a direct cytotoxic effect at very high doses.

Progestogens are also used in carcinoma of the kidney; a therapeutic response is rare and the reason for it is not known.

Most experience has been with medroxyprogesterone acetate (Farlutal; Provera) given in daily oral doses of 100–300 mg but recent studies using larger doses (1500 mg/day) have produced responses of over 40%. Other progestogens used are megestrol acetate (Megace), norethisterone acetate (SH 420) and hydroxyprogesterone (Primolut).

There are no important toxic effects of progestogens which occur during cancer chemotherapy.

Corticosteroids

Corticosteroids are cytotoxic to lymphoid cells and are used in combination with other cytotoxic agents in treating lymphomas, myeloma, and to induce a remission in acute lymphoblastic leukaemia. Their exact mode of action is not known but their effect is short-lived and treatment given for more than 2 weeks is unlikely to continue to be beneficial. Large doses of prednisolone 40–60 mg daily are used but side effects (see p. 636) are not usually troublesome as the drug is given in repeated short courses. Corticosteroids may also be of some benefit in carcinoma of the breast, perhaps by suppressing pituitary activity.

Luteinising Hormone Releasing Hormone (LHRH) analogues

Synthetic potent analogues of gonadotrophin releasing hormone have paradoxical effects on the pituitary which result in initial stimulation but subsequent inhibition of LH and FSH secretion. This in turn inhibits testicular secretion of testosterone and has proved effective in treating prostatic cancer (and also precocious puberty and as a potential contraceptive). A number of these compounds are now in trial. One, leuprolide is as effective as stilboestrol but with fewer side effects.

Ketoconazole (see p. 746)

High doses of this antifungal drug block synthesis of testicular testosterone and adrenal androgens (and other steroids). Experimentally this drug has given useful remissions in prostate cancer.

Combination Therapy

There are various combinations of cytotoxic drugs used in treating cancer, based to some degree on the principles which have been discussed. Those given below are merely examples. Figure 20.14 is a nomogram which is useful to determine dosage on the basis of body surface area.

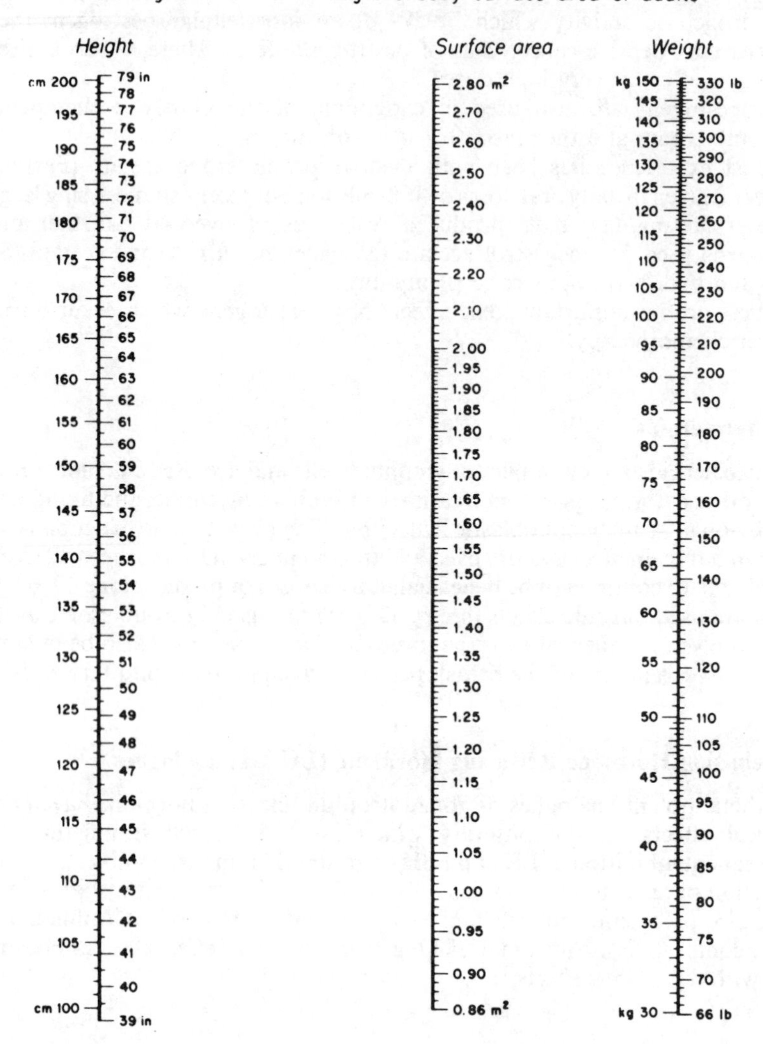

Fig. 20.14 Nomogram for calculating the body surface area of adults.

Hodgkin's Disease

MOPP: Mustine 6 mg/m² i.v. on days 1 and 8, *or*
Cyclophosphamide 600 mg/m² i.v. on days 1 and 8 *or*
Chlorambucil 6.0 mg/m² orally for 14 days, *together with*
Vincristine 1.5 mg i.v. on days 1 and 8
Procarbazine 100 mg orally daily on days 1–14
Prednisolone 40 mg orally daily on days 1–14.

The whole cycle is repeated after an interval of 2 weeks without drugs. In MVPP vinblastine 10 mg i.v. is substituted for vincristine, but a delay of 3–4 weeks is necessary because of greater bone marrow depression. These are the standard regimes for Hodgkin's disease and produce a remission in 70–80% of patients.

2nd Line Treatment for Hodgkin's Disease or in alternating cycles with MOPP

ABVD: Adriamycin 30 mg/m^2 i.v. day 1 (max total dose 500 mg/m^2)
Bleomycin 15 mg i.v. or i.m. day 1 (max total dose 180 mg)
Vincristine 1.5 mg i.v. day 1
DTIC 375 mg/m^2 day 1
Courses repeated every 3 weeks.

Non-Hodgkin's lymphomas

Well differentiated good prognosis type
Chlorambucil 6.0 mg/m^2 orally daily for 14 days every month
or

COP: Cyclophosphamide 600 mg/m^2 (max 1 g) i.v. on days 1 and 8
Vincristine 1.5 mg i.v. on days 1 and 8
Prednisolone 40 mg daily for 5 days
Cycle 3–4 weeks for 1 year or complete remission.

CHOP: Poorly differentiated poor prognosis type
Cyclophosphamide 400 mg/m^2 i.v. days 1 and 8
Doxorubicin 50 mg/m^2 i.v. day 1 only (max total dose 500 mg/m^2)
Vincristine 1.4 mg/m^2 i.v. days 1 and 8
Prednisolone 40 mg/m^2 daily for 5 days

Cycle: 3–4 weekly.

Acute lymphatic leukaemia (children)

Induction: Vincristine 1.4 mg/m^2 i.v. weekly
Prednisolone 40 mg/m^2 orally daily

Maintenance: 6-mercaptopurine 50 mg/m^2 orally daily
Methotrexate 20 mg/m^2 orally weekly

Some form of CNS prophylaxis by radiation or intrathecal methotrexate (12 mg intrathecally twice weekly for 5 doses) will be required. Methotrexate is often given via a chronically implanted Omeyer reservoir which allows direct injection into the cisterna magna via a subcutaneous reservoir.

Myeloma

Cyclophosphamide: 250 mg/m^2 daily for 3 days orally
Melphalan: 6 mg/m^2 daily for 3 days orally
Prednisolone: 40 mg daily for 3 days
with
Oral CCNU 50 mg/m^2 on day 4 *only*.

This course is repeated every 4 weeks for one year.

Advanced carcinoma of the breast

Cyclophosphamide	100 mg/m^2/d po × 14
Methotrexate	40 mg/m^2 i.v. d. 1 and 8
5-Fluorouracil	600 mg/m^2 i.v. d. 1 and 8
	Repeat every 28 days
Doxorubicin	60 mg/m^2 i.v. d. 1
Vincristine	1.4 mg/m^2 i.v. d. 1
	Repeat every 21 days

Chapter 21
ALLERGY AND IMMUNOSUPPRESSION

The introduction of a foreign substance (antigen) into the body may in certain circumstances provoke an immune reaction. For this to occur it is essential that the body recognises the antigen as 'non-self'. Antigens are usually large molecules with a molecular weight of over 5000. They are often multivalent and have a consistent charge and molecular profile. They may be proteins or large M. W. carbohydrates. It would appear that most antigens are first processed by macrophages before being passed to nearby lymphocytes. The immune response is initiated by the interaction of antigen with receptors on the surface of the lymphocytes, and the response may be of two types.

1. Humoral immunity with the production of circulating immunoglobulin by plasma cells which are derived from lymphocytes. In man these lymphocytes arise largely from the lymphoid tissue of the gastro-intestinal tract and are known as B cells. The humoral response occurs in two stages as follows:

(a) *Primary reactions*: These occur with the first exposure to the antigen. There is a small and short-lived rise in the antibody titre which consists largely of IgM.
(b) *Secondary reactions*: These occur with subsequent exposure to the antigen. The rise in antibody is greater and persists for a long period. The antibody consists mostly of IgG. The reaction requires the intervention of helper T cells as well as B lymphocytes.

2. Cellular immunity mediated by sensitised thymus-derived cells known as T-cells which act directly on the antigen by the production of lymphokines.

The immune response is an essential defence against invasion of the body by bacteria, viruses and other foreign material. However, it may be defective or disorganised and when this occurs it can produce a wide variety of diseases. The body has the latent potential to stimulate its immune system so that antibodies are produced against itself. Normally this situation is prevented by a number of suppression mechanisms. If these fail, which they do in certain circumstances, the so-called 'auto-immune' group of diseases may result. Deficiencies in the immune system are rarer but may be congenital or may result from the use of certain drugs, particularly cytotoxics and steroids.

Sometimes the immune response to an antigen may not only produce antibodies which damage the antigen but may also damage the body tissue; this is called hypersensitivity and may be of four types:

Type I An antigen/antibody combination occurs on the surface of the mast cells and releases pharmacologically active substances which include:

Histamine; slow reacting substance (SRS-A); eosinophil chemotactic factor (ECF); serotonin; bradykinin and other kinins and prostaglandins.

This type of reaction causes general anaphylaxis, allergic asthma, hay fever and some types of urticaria and is mediated by IgE antibodies.

Type II The antibody combines with an antigen in the cell membrane. The reaction often requires complement and results in cell lysis. An example of this type of reaction is haemolytic disease in the new-born where antibodies produced by a rhesus-negative mother against the rhesus factor on the red cells of the fetus, cross the placental barrier and cause haemolysis. It is mediated by IgM or IgG antibodies.

Type III (Arthus reaction) This is caused by circulating complexes of antigen/antibody formed in conditions of slight antigen excess, together with complement which can cause tissue destruction directly and also by attracting polymorph neutrophils to the site. This reaction is delayed and is maximum a few hours after exposure to the antigen. Serum sickness is a result of this type of response. It is mediated by IgM or IgG antibodies.

Type IV (Delayed cell-mediated hypersensitivity) is due to sensitised circulating lymphocytes of the T-cell type reacting to antigen. Most of the manifestations of the reaction are produced via lymphokines: soluble factors produced by these primed lymphocytes on contact with antigen which cause local inflammation, attract other lymphocytes and macrophages to the site, enhance phagocytosis and increase macrophage metabolism. This type of reaction takes place 1–2 days after secondary antigen exposure and is exemplified by contact dermatitis and organ-transplant rejection.

These complex expressions of the immune response are all essential for health. The problem of suppression of an unwanted component of this reaction is difficult. Ideally it should be highly selective and leave the rest of the immune mechanism intact. In practice two types of drug are used to try to achieve this.

(a) The whole immune system can be 'damped down' and rendered less efficient. This is usually done with drugs which are toxic to lymphocytes and thus reduces their number and perhaps also interferes with their immune function. This method has the disadvantage that suppression of immunity makes the body prone to infections, not only by bacteria but by viruses, yeasts and fungi.

(b) Attempts can be made to block the final chemical mediator of the immune reaction. This may be relatively successful when the mediator is known and susceptible to blockade, i.e. histamine in the Type I reaction, but for other types of immune response may be impossible.

It is also possible to manipulate the immune system by immunological methods and in some cases this may be the most appropriate way of obtaining selective depression of one facet of the immune response.

A. DRUGS WHICH DEPRESS THE IMMUNE REACTION (see Table 21.1)

Azathioprine (Imuran)

This drug is closely related to 6-mercaptopurine (6-MP), differing only in having an imidazole group added to the molecule. Its immunosuppressive properties and mechanism of action are virtually the same as those of 6-MP, but it appears to be the preferred drug for this purpose, possibly because its toxicity is marginally lower.

Azathioprine is an antimetabolite and therefore it is most effective on actively proliferating cells. It is metabolised to 6-MP in vivo. Like 6-MP it has little or no intrinsic activity but requires transformation to the ribonucleotide in the body which interferes with all stages of purine synthesis. It causes immunosuppression by inhibiting lymphocytes which would normally proliferate in response to stimulation by an antigen, and is thus only effective if given after an antigen. It inhibits delayed hypersensitivity (cell-mediated immunity) and those aspects of inflammation which depend on cell division. There is little evidence for any consistent effect on the normal humoral antibody response. The fact that its use is associated with an increased incidence of viral but not bacterial infections has been taken as evidence against any major effect on antibody production.

Clinical uses Azathioprine is used to prevent transplant rejection, the usual dose being 1 to 4.0 mg/kg/day orally. It has also been used with some success in the treatment of diseases in which auto-immunity may play a part, for example, systemic lupus erythematosus, chronic active hepatitis and some forms of the nephrotic syndrome. Due to its potential toxicity it is usually reserved for situations in which corticosteroids alone are inadequate.

Adverse effects Azathioprine is partly metabolised by xanthine oxidase. If it is given with a xanthine oxidase inhibitor such as allopurinol, accumulation and toxicity will occur. It can cause bone marrow suppression and its use requires regular blood counts.

Cyclophosphamide (Endoxana)

The cytotoxic action of cyclophosphamide is considered on p. 785. It produces immunosuppression by inhibiting cell proliferation. It appears to be most effective if given after an antigenic stimulation but has some effect if given in large doses before the antigen. Presumably this is because the active metabolites of cyclophosphamide combine with the DNA of the lymphocytes and its cytotoxic effect becomes apparent when the lymphocytes are stimulated to divide. It may appear to have a preferential effect on B-lymphocytes although it is in fact equally effective on both populations of cells when they have been stimulated into division by antigen. It can also reduce antibody production and depress cell-mediated immunity and the inflammatory reaction.

Table 21.1 The effect of immunosuppressive agents on various types of immune response

Type of immune response	*Suppressive agent*					
	Radiation	*Cytotoxic drugs*	*Corticosteroids*	*ALS*	*Anti-inflammatory drugs*	*Antihistamines*
Type I	+	+*	+ −	−	+ −	+
Type II	+	+*	+ −	−	+ −	−
Type III	+	+*	+	+ −	+ −	−
Type IV	−	+	+ −	+ +	+ −	−
Inflammation	−	+	+ +	+	+	+ −

* Only with large doses

Clinical uses Cyclophosphamide can be used to prevent graft rejection. It is also used in a variety of diseases in which disordered immunity is believed to be a causative factor. Perhaps its most important role in this context is in the treatment of the nephrotic syndrome with minimal change on microscopy, particularly in those patients who are resistant to steroids or when steroid toxicity is troublesome. It appears to be superior to azathioprine in this type of disease. It can also be used in the nephritis due to systemic lupus, Wegener's granulomatosis and rheumatoid disease. The usual dose is 3.0 mg/kg/day orally for 8 weeks.

Adverse effects See p. 786

Glucocorticosteroids (see p. 634)

Steroids are the most widely used immunosuppressive agents. They alter lymphocyte function and decrease the number of circulating lymphocytes either by a direct cell lysis or by redistributing lymphocytes throughout the body. The degree of lymphocytopenia is dose-dependent up to a point: high doses reduce lymphocyte numbers up to a maximum of 50–75 %. A decrease in the absolute number of both T and B lymphocytes occurs with T cells proportionately more affected. In animals these changes seem to be due at least in part to sequestration of lymphocytes in the bone marrow but in man the site of sequestration is unknown. Their main action is to depress cell-mediated immunity. They do not suppress antibody formation following antigenic stimulation but they may have some suppressive action on auto-antibodies.

Steroids have a marked anti-inflammatory effect and also decrease the release of pharmacologically active substances from mast cells in Type I hypersensitivity reactions. The release of lytic enzymes from the lysosomes of polymorphonuclear leucocytes is also prevented, possibly by their stabilising effect on membrane phospholipids. It is believed that this also contributes to the anti-inflammatory properties of steroids. Cortisol is more effective in suppressing type III hypersensitivity reactions (Arthus reaction) than cell-mediated type IV reactions (tuberculin reaction) in man possibly because of this effect on polymorph lysosomes, since polymorph tissue infiltration is a major feature of type III effects. Recently steroids have been shown to stimulate factors (macrocortin, lipomodulin) which inhibit phospholipase A_2 so reducing arachidonic acid release and subsequent formation of prostaglandins.

Clinical uses

(i) *Type I reactions* corticosteroids have been shown to be useful in allergic rhinitis, atopic dermatitis, status asthmaticus and acute anaphylaxis. In allergic rhinitis and atopic dermatitis the principal benefit probably arises from non-specific anti-inflammatory effects, including vascoconstriction and decreased vascular permeability, mediated in part by decreased histamine production and facilitation of β-adrenergic stimulation. In asthma the actions are more complex, involving anti-inflammatory effects reducing bronchorrhoea and bronchial oedema, relaxation of bronchial smooth muscle (either directly or more likely by facilitation of β-adrenergic effects) and inhibition of histamine and SRS-A mediated bronchoconstriction. Corticosteroids may also act to inhibit the specific immune phenomena occurring in asthma including lymphocyte infiltration of bronchial mucosa and the deposition of immune complexes in the basement membrane. In addition corticosteroids may decrease serum IgE concentrations.

(ii) *Type II reactions* Although steroids do not inhibit the normal humoral immune response, they are often effective in treating type II autoimmune diseases. They are the drugs of choice for pemphigus vulgaris and autoimmune haemolytic anaemia. In the latter they induce remission in about 80% of cases where warm-reacting antibodies are involved and about half of these will remain in long-term or permanent remission. Patients with positive indirectly reacting Coombs' tests (indicating free serum anti-red-cell antibody) are generally less responsive to steroids. Their mechanism of action in these conditions probably depends upon several factors, including (a) inhibition of auto-antibody production in some patients, (b) inhibition of erythrophagocytosis in the absence of any alteration in antibody titre and (c) decreased binding of autoantibody to red cells.

In pemphigus vulgaris there is a good correlation between depression of auto-antibody and clinical response, but this does not appear to be so clear in other diseases such as idiopathic thrombocytopenic purpura, where steroids may also be effective.

(iii) *Type III reactions* Steroids are widely used in immune complex diseases where their major effect is anti-inflammatory. They may produce symptomatic relief without altering the fundamental disease processes. Thus, in rheumatoid arthritis, although effective in controlling some features of the disease, the natural course of the disease will not be altered. However, in systemic lupus erythematosus, steroid therapy is often associated with decreases in antinuclear autoantibody titre and the frequency of LE cells, and there is some evidence that high doses may improve renal function and prolong survival in patients with renal involvement.

(iv) *Type IV reactions* Steroids are potent inhibitors of these reactions, being clinically used in prevention of graft rejection and contact dermatitis.

Adverse effects: These are considered on p. 639.

Antilymphocyte globulin (ALG)

This is prepared by injecting human lymphocytes into animals and raising antibodies in the usual way. Frequently T lymphocytes which are obtained from thymus tissue are used as they play a predominant part in graft rejection. The active immunoglobulin is largely in the IgG fraction and ALG is thus a complex biological product with inherent variability from batch to batch.

After injection ALG becomes attached to lymphocytes and is thus cleared from the circulation in about 6 h. Owing to the size of the molecule ALG is confined largely to the circulation and only low concentrations are found in the tissue fluids. This means that only circulating lymphocytes are exposed to a high concentration of ALG. In many circumstances there is a continuous exchange between tissue and circulating lymphocytes and ALG is thus able to exert an adequate effect. If, however, the active lymphocytes are confined to tissue—for example, around a graft during a rejection crisis—ALG is less effective.

Although ALG can produce cell lysis with the aid of complement, it is possible that at least some of its immunosuppressive effect is due to 'blinding' of the lymphocyte, which prevents it finding its target by blocking antigen recognition sites.

Animal data suggest that ALG has no direct inhibitory effect on B cells or humoral immunity, but in man some evidence of response and remission with disappearance of autoantibodies has occurred in both Type II and Type III autoimmune disease.

Clinical uses ALG reduces delayed hypersensitivity and prevents graft rejection and is particularly useful when rejection occurs soon after grafting. There have been no controlled trials concerning the efficacy of ALG in autoimmune disease, although it has been used on a sporadic basis.

Adverse effects Due to its method of production several adverse effects arise. At least 50% of patients treated with ALG raised in horses develop antibodies to horse IgG. This leads to poor absorption of ALG from i.m. injection and rapid clearance of ALG from the circulation resulting in decreased effectiveness. An immune response to ALG may also result in anaphylactoid symptoms, serum sickness and rarely immune complex glomerulonephritis. Another problem is specificity, since ALG frequently contains antibodies against non-lymphoid antigens such as red cells, platelets and kidney, which may produce toxic effects.

ALG is expensive, scarce and because of its inherent variability difficult to assess in terms of clinical effect.

Cyclosporin A

Cyclosporin A is a cyclic polypeptide extracted from fungi. It is a specific T lymphocyte suppressor with a unique effect on the primary but not the secondary immune response. Its main use is to prevent rejection after organ transplantation, bone marrow transplantation and in graft versus host disease. Its main advantage is that unlike many other immunosuppressives it does not interfere with bone marrow function.

Clinical use

Organ transplantation Regimes vary. Initially cyclosporin may be given in doses of 4.0 mg/kg/day i.v. but this is liable to produce renal failure and it is safer to start with 14 mg/kg/day orally reducing over three months to a maintenance dose of around 6 mg/kg/day. Estimation of the trough plasma levels of cyclosporin A should be kept between 300 and 100 ng/l. Opinions vary as to whether it should be combined with steroids. Results are superior to those obtained with azothioprine.

In graft versus host disease and bone marrow transplantation Initial intravenous treatment is used (3–5 mg/kg/day) followed by oral administration over a period of 6–9 months.

Adverse effects Nephrotoxicity is a serious problem. Serum creatinine and urea are higher in those receiving cyclosporin A. It is difficult to differentiate rejection from drug-induced renal damage and reduction of dosage together with careful control of plasma levels of cyclosporin A seem at present to be the only answer. Follow-up studies do, however, suggest that the deterioration in renal function is not progressive.

Other adverse effects are nausea, depression and general misery, impaired hepatic function, hirsutism, tremor and gum hypertrophy. Anaphylaxis may occur with intravenous administration. Although it was originally feared that the use of cyclosporin would result in a serious number of malignancies (mainly lymphoma) developing, careful control of dosage and the avoidance of undue immunosuppression has considerably reduced this risk.

General adverse effects of immunosuppression

The prolonged use of non-specific immunosuppressive drugs is associated with an appreciable incidence of adverse effects due to reduced immunity or drug induced damage to the nuclear structure of the cell.

(a) Increased susceptibility to infection Bacterial infections are common and require prompt treatment with the appropriate antibiotic. Tuberculosis may also occur and sometimes takes unusual forms.

Viral infections may be more severe than is usual and include the common herpes infection but occasionally such rarities as multifocal leukoencephalopathy caused by the JC virus.

Fungal and related infections are also common including *Candida albicans* which may be local or systemic, and *Pneumocystis carinii*.

(b) Sterility Azoospermia in men is particularly common with alkylating agents. In women there may be hormone failure leading to amenorrhoea.

(c) Teratogenicity Not so common as would be expected. It is wise not to attempt conception while on these drugs and to wait 12 weeks after stopping treatment which is the time required to clear abnormal sperm in the male.

(d) Carcinogenicity Immunosuppression is associated with an increased incidence of malignant disease. Early in treatment large cell diffuse lymphoma develops but with prolonged treatment other types of malignancy may appear. The incidence in transplant patients is about 1%.

Other drugs which may attenuate the immune response are:

Penicillamine (see p. 310)
Gold (see p. 309)
Chloroquine (see p. 312)

B. CHEMICAL MEDIATORS OF THE IMMUNE RESPONSE AND THEIR BLOCKADE

An alternative method of modifying the immune response is to block the release or action of chemical mediators which play an important part in certain immune reactions, especially Type I immunity.

There are several pharmacologically active mediators and their relative importance differs in different species. Histamine is one of the most important of these substances, although in man it is certainly not the only mediator involved.

Histamine

This is widely distributed in the body and is derived from the decarboxylation of histidine. It is particularly concentrated in mast cell granules. In tissues the highest concentrations are found in the lung, nasal mucous membrane, skin, stomach and duodenum. Histamine may be released by drugs, usually when given in large quantities intravenously: such drugs include curare, morphine, codeine, pethidine, atropine, hydralazine and some sympathomimetic amines. Little is known for certain about the physiological role of this potent amine: it may function as a local controller of vascular responses, particularly in the skin, where it is concerned with the responses to injury. There is also evidence of its involvement in neuronal transmission in the brain and ganglia. Its main functions seem to be the release of gastric acid (see p. 521) and as part mediator of the allergic response. There are two types of histamine receptors:

1. *H_1 receptors* Stimulation of these receptors produces the following effects in man:

Blood vessels Histamine causes dilatation of small arteries and capillaries, together with increased permeability, which leads to the formation of oedema. Large vessels also dilate and one result is the development of a histamine headache due to this effect on cerebral vessels. The resulting fall in peripheral resistance causes a fall in blood pressure and sometimes even a state of shock.

Histamine injected into the skin produces the characteristic triple response which consists, in order of appearance, of

(a) a localised red spot (due to capillary dilatation).
(b) a larger flush or flare (due to arteriolar dilatation via an axon-reflex mechanism).
(c) a wheal (localised oedema subsequent to increased vessel permeability).

Smooth muscle contraction is not so pronounced in man as in other mammals but bronchospasm may occur, especially in asthmatics.

Nerve endings Local injection of histamine causes itch and sometimes pain due to stimulation of peripheral nerves.

2. *H_2 receptors* are principally concerned with stimulation of gastric acid release (see p. 520). They may make a minor contribution to the vascular responses.

Hypersensitivity reactions involving histamine release

Anaphylactic shock (Acute anaphylaxis) In certain circumstances injection of an antigen is followed by production of antibodies in the IgE class. These antibodies coat mast cells and basophils and further exposure to the antigen results in rapid degranulation of the mast cells with the release of histamine and other substances such as leukotrienes. Clinically the patient presents a picture of shock and collapse with hypotension, bronchospasm and laryngeal oedema often accompanied by urticaria and flushing. A similar so-called anaphylactoid reaction may occur after the non-immunological release of mediators such as X-ray contrast media.

Atopy Some individuals with the so-called hereditary atopic diathesis have a propensity to develop local anaphylactic reactions if exposed to the appropriate antigens, causing hay fever, allergic asthma or urticaria. This is due to the antigen combining with mast-cell IgE in the mucosa of the respiratory tract or in the skin.

Serum sickness This is a Type III hypersensitivity reaction and is due to circulating complexes of antigen/antibody and complement. These complexes can release histamine and probably other vaso-active substances from mast cells.

BLOCKADE OF CHEMICAL MEDIATORS OF ALLERGY

Two possible therapeutic approaches to the management of allergic disease produced by mediators are (a) to block their release, (b) to block their effects.

Blockade of release of mediators

Sodium cromoglycate (see p. 478)

This agent was found to be effective in preventing bronchospasm when given to asthmatic subjects before challenge with an antigen. It is not a bronchodilator, nor does it block the actions of histamine, 5-HT or slow-reacting substance on smooth muscle. It was originally believed that its most important action was to prevent the release of pharmacologically active substances from mast cells when exposed to an antigen. It was believed to accomplish this by stabilising the mast cells, possibly by interfering with calcium ion entry, so that degranulation did not occur when the mast cells took part in a Type I antigen/antibody reaction. However it is now apparent that this is n_t sufficient explanation for its clinical effect.

In clinical studies it has been found that sodium cromoglycate is not only effective in early-onset asthma, in which allergic factors are important, but also in late-onset asthma, in which such factors are thought to play little part. This is rather difficult to explain; it is possible that in late-onset asthma, factors other than allergy may be responsible for mast-cell degranulation, but the stabilising effect of the drug is still effective.

Clinical uses Sodium cromoglycate is used to prevent attacks of asthma.

Attempts are being made to use the drug in other disorders where allergic factors may play a part. It can be given as a powder for nasal insufflation or as nasal drops for allergic rhinitis (Rynacrom). It is used prophylactically when the only adverse effects are occasional nasal irritation. It is also used as a 2%

solution in eye drops (Opticrom) for the treatment of hay fever conjunctivitis and vernal kerato-conjunctivitis.

β-agonists may also exert some of their anti-allergic action by blocking mediator release from mast cells, but have little demonstrable effect except in asthma.

Blockade of effects of mediators

Antihistamines

There are over 50 compounds which block the actions of histamine mediated via H_1 receptors; they do not, however, affect H_2 receptor stimulation. More recently specific H_2 receptor antagonists have been synthesised and are considered on p. 520.

H_1 receptor blockers These are competitive antagonists of histamine at H_1 receptors and are very similar in their general action. In man they are fairly effective in blocking the oedema and vascular response to histamine but not in relieving the state of shock. Although they will block the bronchoconstrictor action in vitro, they have little effect on bronchoconstriction which results from a hypersensitivity reaction such as allergic asthma, presumably because other mediators are also involved.

Two other actions of H_1 blockers are of some importance. Most have some central sedative action even in therapeutic doses and in some individuals this may be severe enough to interfere with everyday activities. Their simultaneous use with alcohol, barbiturates or other central depressant drug may produce synergistic effects. One antihistamine, phenindamine (Thephorin), is unusual in that it has excitatory properties in clinically used doses. With overdosage, however many of these drugs may show evidence of central excitation with seizures and hyperpyrexia.

Most of the group also have some anti-emetic action. It seems probable that this is associated with central acetylcholine-blocking properties which they possess; in this respect they are similar to two other important anti-emetic groups, i.e. hyoscine and related compounds and the phenothiazines. This action of antihistamines may also be responsible for their minor usefulness in treating Parkinson's disease, which is considered on p. 257. Their anti-cholinergic effects also result in drying of secretions (like atropine) which may have adverse effects in asthma by increasing the viscosity of secretions in the respiratory tract but may contribute to their efficacy in rhinitis.

There are a large number of antihistamines and a selection is given in Table 21.2. Their antihistaminic actions are similar when used in clinically appropriate dosage but they differ in duration of effect, degree of sedation and antiemetic potential.

Orphenadrine is used in the treatment of Parkinson's disease rather than for its antihistamine properties; the initial dose is 50 mg three times daily and increased as required.

Pharmacokinetics Antihistamines are rapidly and well absorbed from the intestine and are effective within about half an hour. They are metabolised in

Table 21.2 Properties of some H_1-antihistamines

Drug (*Properierietary name*)	*Duration of effect* (h)	*Degree of sedation*	*Anti-emetic action*	*Single dose* (mg)
Promethazine (Phenergan)	20	Marked	Some	10–25
Diphenhydramine (Benadryl)	6	Some	Little	50
Chlorpheniramine (Piriton)	4–6	Moderate	Little	4
Dimenhydrinate (Dramamine)	6	Some	Marked	50
Cyclizine (Marzine)	6	Some	Marked	50
Clemastine (Tavegil)	12	Some	Little	1
Triprolidine (Pro-Actidil)	24 (slow release)	Moderate	Little	10
Terfenadine (Triludan)	12	Nil	Little	60
Astemizole (Hismanol)	24	Nil	Little	10
Phenindamine (Thephorin)	6	May be stimulant	Little	25–30

the body and are largely cleared within about 6 h. Some, e.g. chlorpheniramine (Piriton) are available for intravenous administration in allergic emergencies.

There is no relationship between the antihistaminic potency of these compounds and their central depressant activity, e.g. chlorpheniramine produces less sedation than diphenhydramine at equivalent histamine-blocking doses. For the latter drug, however, a relationship has been demonstrated between blood levels and sedation, but there is no correlation with inhibition of the triple response produced by histamine injection.

Clinical uses Antihistamines are widely used to treat hypersensitivity reactions and are most effective in some types of urticaria and hay fever; they are not so useful for anaphylactic shock. They will help to clear the oedema which is occasionally dangerous in anaphylaxis, particularly if the larynx and pharynx are involved, but are rather slow to act, so adrenaline, which is more rapidly effective, should be used. They may be useful if given promptly and systemically in preventing excessive reactions to bee and wasp stings which both contain histamine and also trigger its release. Relief of itching is probably due to their sedative action rather than any specific anti-pruritic action. Local application as a cream is liable to lead to contact dermatitis.

They have not proved to be of much use in bronchial asthma, probably because other mediators are important.

Antihistamines can also be used for their central sedative actions, particularly in the prevention of sea or motion sickness, e.g. cyclizine, dimenhydrinate, but sleepiness may prove troublesome.

Antihistamines are also used, but are useless, in symptomatic treatment of the common cold. They are used in combination in various cough mixtures where their sedative action plays a major role.

Sedation is often a problem with antihistamines, particularly if they are taken regularly. Recently, however, several antihistamines have been introduced with little if any central effect (Table 21.2). They are more expensive but are indicated in those who find sedation a major problem.

Adrenaline is important as an effective antagonist of the acute anaphylactic reaction. Its rapid action may be life saving in general anaphylaxis due to insect venom allergy and reaction to drugs. The usual dose is 0.5 ml of a 1:1000 solution given intramuscularly. It acts by virtue of its α-antagonist activity which reverses vascular dilation and oedema and by its β_2-agonist activity producing bronchodilation. It may also reduce the release of mediator.

5-Hydroxytryptamine (5HT; Serotonin)

The most striking effect of 5HT is seen in patients with carcinoid tumours which release large amounts of 5-HT and other compounds such as histamine, kallikrein and prostaglandins.

It is synthesised in the body from tryptophan and has the following actions:

(a) It causes contraction of smooth muscle. In the gut this is responsible for the diarrhoea which is a feature of the carcinoid syndrome. It also contracts bronchial smooth muscle, resulting in the wheezing of the carcinoid syndrome.
(b) It has a mixed constricting and dilating effect on blood vessels. Patients with carcinoid may develop characteristic flushing, but whether this is entirely due to 5-HT is not known.
(c) 5-HT stimulates nerves if applied locally, producing severe pain.
(d) 5-HT is a transmitter in the central nervous system.
(e) Patients with carcinoid develop fibrosis of the endocardium with distortion and stenosis of the valves. It is not known whether this is due to 5-HT.

5-HT has no therapeutic use but it may be necessary to block its action in patients with carcinoid.

Drugs blocking 5-HT effects

Methysergide (Deseril) (see p. 283)
Methysergide blocks the action of 5-HT and is useful in controlling the diarrhoea of carcinoid syndrome. It is not so useful against other symptoms

and it is not used in the control of those manifestations of hypersensitivity which are due to the release of 5-HT. It is also useful as a prophylactic in migraine. The usual dose in carcinoid is 12–20 mg/day.

Adverse effects Methysergide may cause some dizziness and light-headedness when first used. Occasionally it causes such vasoconstriction as to seriously interfere with the peripheral circulation. Prolonged use may occasionally cause retroperitoneal fibrosis, and the drug should be given in courses which last for no more than 4 months with rest periods between them.

Cyproheptadine is an antihistamine with potent anti-5-HT properties. It is effective in some cases of urticaria and allergic rhinitis. It is further discussed on p. 615.

IMMUNE ENHANCEMENT

Adjuvants non-specifically augment the immune response when mixed with the antigen or injected into the same site. This is achieved in a variety of ways:

(a) The release of the antigen is slowed and thus exposure to it is prolonged.
(b) Various cells are attracted to the site of injection and the interaction between these cells is important in antibody formation.

There are a number of such substances, usually given as mixtures and often containing lipids, extracts of tubercle bacilli and various mineral salts.

Immunostimulants non-specifically enhance the immune response, examples being BCG or killed *Corynebacterium parvum*.

Levamisole Originally developed as an anthelmintic, this drug has been found to stimulate immune responses. In animal studies it is found that newborn rats given a lethal number of staphylococci on the third day of life will survive if they receive levamisole on the preceding three days. In addition a reduction in the number of metastases in animals injected with malignant cells and a reduction in the size of established tumours suggests that immune responses to tumours are also enhanced. The mechanism of action of the drug on immune mechanisms has not been established. It is believed to stimulate macrophages and T lymphocytes and restore depressed lymphocyte function. Its main use is in the management of immune-deficiency states associated with rheumatoid arthritis.

Adverse effects include agranulocytosis (particularly if given in ankylosing spondylitis) and rashes.

ALLERGIC REACTIONS TO DRUGS

Immune mechanisms are involved in a number of adverse effects caused by drugs. The development of allergy implies previous exposure to the drug or to some very closely related substance. Most drugs are of low molecular weight

(< 1000) and thus are not antigenic. They can, however, combine with substances of high molecular weight, usually proteins, and the conjugate thus formed is antigenic provided that the bond is covalent and irreversible. Weak and reversible bonding does not usually produce an antigenic conjugate. When a drug acts in this way it is said to be a *hapten*. Sometimes it is a metabolite of the drug which acts as the hapten and sometimes it is not the drug at all but some impurity introduced during manufacture. Rarely, as in the case of bovine insulin or porcine pituitary snuff, the molecule is a foreign protein and an immune response follows directly. It is important to remember that the development of antibodies to a drug does not necessarily mean that symptoms will ensue.

The factors which determine the development of allergy to a drug are not fully understood. Some drugs (e.g. penicillin) are more likely to cause allergic reactions than others and Type I reactions are more common in patients with a history of atopy. A correlation between allergic reactions involving IgE and HL-A serotypes has been reported and so genetic factors may also be important. There is also some evidence that they are more liable to occur in older people, although this may merely represent increased liability to drug exposure.

Types of Allergy (See Fig. 21.1.)

Drugs may cause a variety of allergic responses and sometimes a single drug can be responsible for more than one type of allergic response.

Type I (immediate anaphylactic) reaction (see p. 816) is due to the production of antibodies known to consist predominantly of class IgE. The antigen–antibody reaction on the surface of the mast cells causes degranulation of the cells with release of pharmacologically active substances. It occurs commonly with foreign serum or penicillin but may also occur with streptomycin and some local anaesthetics. With penicillin it is believed that the penicilloyl moiety of the penicillin molecule is responsible for the production of antibodies.

Occasionally the development of symptoms is delayed for some hours after the drug has been taken. It seems probable that antigen–antibody aggregates are involved which are capable of bringing about the release of histamine from mast cells. The antibody consists of IgG.

Type II reactions are due to antibodies of class IgG and IgM which on contact with antibodies on the surface of cells are able to fix complement. It is possible that some reactions due to quinidine, PAS and penicillin are of this type.

Type III (immune complex) reactions can produce several clinical allergic states including serum sickness and immune complex glomerulonephritis, and perhaps a syndrome resembling systemic lupus erythematosus. It has been shown to be responsible for some types of penicillin and sulphonamide allergy and may also be responsible for some forms of drug-induced pulmonary fibrosis (e.g. Furadantin lung).

Type IV (delayed hypersensitivity) reactions The classical example of this type of reaction is contact dermatitis: a drug applied to the skin may form an antigenic conjugate with the dermal proteins. This stimulates the formation of

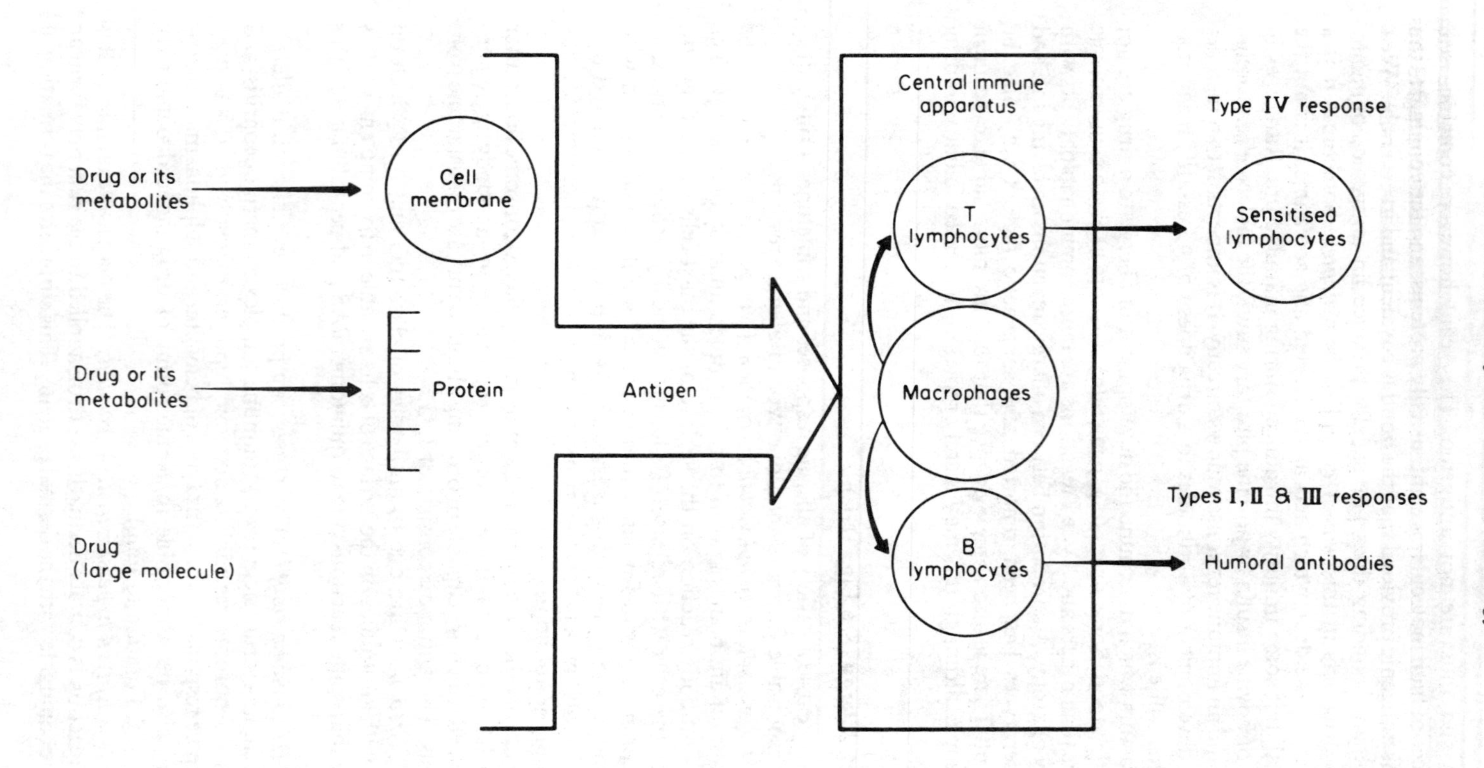

Fig. 21.1 The immune response to drugs.

sensitised T lymphocytes in the regional lymph nodes with a resultant rash if the drug is applied again. Delayed sensitivity can also result from the systemic administration of drugs.

Photosensitivity, when caused by drugs, is due to a photochemical combination between the drug and the dermal protein which acts as an antigen.

Some drug reactions in which allergy may play a part

Anaphylaxis See above.

Rashes are common manifestations of drug reaction. A number of immune mechanisms may be involved which produce many types of rash. In some cases (e.g. ampicillin) the rash is more commonly due to non-allergic factors; in others the cause is not known (see Table 21.3).

Serum sickness is caused by circulating immune complexes (Type III reaction). The onset is delayed for some days until the symptoms—fever, urticaria, arthropathy and lymphadenopathy—develop. Proteinuria occurs frequently. Recovery takes a few days. Among the causative agents are foreign serum, penicillin, sulphonamides, streptomycin and thiouracil.

Lymphadenopathy Lymph-node enlargement can result from taking drugs, commonly phenytoin. The reason for this is not known, but allergic factors may be involved. The importance of this reaction is that it may be confused with a lymphoma and inquiry about chronic drug taking is important in patients with lymphadenopathy of unknown cause.

Blood dyscrasias Thrombocytopenia, anaemia and agranulocytosis can all be produced by drugs, although immune mechanisms are not necessarily involved.

Thrombocytopenia can occur with many drugs and in many instances it is direct suppression of the megakarocytes rather than immune processes which is important. However, in sedormid thrombocytopenia it has been suggested that the platelet–drug complex acts as an antigen and similarly quinine thrombocytopenia may be an allergic phenomenon. The following are some of the drugs which most commonly cause thrombocytopenia although the mechanism varies:

phenylbutazone	thiazides	chloramphenicol
aspirin	quinidine	PAS
sulphonamides	quinine	gold
+ most cytotoxic agents		

Haemolytic anaemia can be caused by a number of drugs and sometimes immune mechanisms are responsible (but see also glucose 6-phosphate dehydrogenase deficiency). Some of these mechanisms are as follows.

Table 21.3 Skin reactions to some commonly used drugs

	Acne	*Alopecia*	*Bullous*	*Epidermo-necrolysis*	*Erythema multiforme*	*Erythema nodosa*	*Exfoliative dermatitis*	*Fixed*	*Lich-enoid*
Anticonvulsants				+		+	+		
Barbiturates			+	+		+	+	+	
β-blockers									+
Chlorpropamide					+		+		
Codeine						+			
Cytotoxics		+							
Gold							+	+	+
Griseofulvin									
Halides	+		+		+	+	+		
PAS							+	+	
Penicillins			+	+	+	+	+	+	
Phenolphthalein			+		+		+	+	
Phenothiazines					+		+		
Phenylbutazone				+			+	+	
Salicylates			+		+	+		+	
Steroids	+								
Streptomycin									
Sulphonamides				+	+	+	+	+	
Tetracyclines				+			+	+	
Thiazides					+	+			+
Thiouracils		+				+			

Table 21.3 (continued)

	Lupus erythe-matosus	*Morbil-liform*	*Nails*	*Photo-sensi-tivity*	*Porphyria*	*Purpura*	*Urticaria*	*Psoriasiform*
Anticonvulsants	+	+					+	
Barbiturates		+			+		+	
β-blockers	+							+
Chlorpropamide								
Codeine							+	
Cytotoxics		+	+			+		
Gold		+				+		
Griseofulvin	+			+	+			
Halides						+	+	
PAS		+						
Penicillins	+					+	+	
Phenolphthalein			+				+	
Phenothiazines	+	+		+		+		
Phenylbutazone	+							
Salicylates							+	
Steroids						+		
Streptomycin		+					+	
Sulphonamides	+			+		+	+	
Tetracyclines			+	+		+	+	
Thiazides		+		+		+		
Thiouracils		+					+	

(a) The drug can combine with the red-cell membrane and the conjugate acts as an antigen. This has been shown to occur with penicillin-induced haemolysis, and may also occur with chlorpromazine, chlorpropamide and sulphonamides.
(b) The drug can alter the red-cell membrane so that it becomes autoimmunogenic. This may happen with methyldopa, and a direct positive Coombs' test develops in about 20% of patients who have been treated with this drug for more than a year. In only a small proportion does haemolysis actually occur. Similar changes can take place with levodopa and mefenamic acid.
(c) Drugs can cause non-specific binding of plasma protein to red cells and thus cause haemolysis. This is believed to occur with cephalosporins.

Aplastic anaemia as an isolated entity is not common but may occur as part of a general depression of bone-marrow activity, particularly with chloramphenicol (see p. 724).

Agranulocytosis can be caused by a very large number of drugs. Several different mechanisms are probably involved and it is not known for certain whether allergy plays a part. Among the drugs most frequently implicated are:

phenylbutazone
phenothiazines
sulphonamides
anti-thyroid drugs
tolbutamide
antidepressants
+ most cytotoxic agents

Systemic lupus erythematosus A number of drugs produce a syndrome which resembles systemic lupus together with a positive antinuclear factor in the blood. The most usual drugs to cause this syndrome are:

procainamide
hydralazine
anticonvulsants
isoniazid
chlorpromazine

The development of this side effect is closely related to dose, and in the case of hydralazine also depends upon the rate of acetylation of the drug (see p. 105). There is some evidence that the drugs act as haptens combining with DNA and forming antigens. Symptoms usually disappear when the drug is stopped, but recovery may be slow.

Vasculitis Both acute and chronic vasculitis can result from taking drugs, and this may well have an allergic basis. Acute vasculitis with purpura and renal involvement occurs with penicillin and the sulphonamides. A more chronic form can occur with phenytoin.

Other reactions

Fever is a common manifestation of drug allergy and should be remembered in patients with PUO. *Liver involvement* as a side effect from drugs is not uncommon, but it is probable that immune mechanisms are rarely involved. *Gastrointestinal upsets* due to allergies are quite common.

Identification of the drug at fault

It may be difficult to decide whether a particular drug is responsible for an allergy, especially a rash, as frequently the patient is taking more than one drug. There are several ways of approaching the problem, though in practice none of them may give a clear answer.

(a) A careful drug history may be inconclusive, because although allergy to a drug implies previous exposure, the antigen may have occurred in foods (e.g. antibiotics are often fed to livestock and drug residues remain in the flesh), in drug mixtures or in some casual fashion.

(b) Provocative tests. This means giving a very small amount of the suspected drug and seeing if a reaction ensues. The commonest method is skin testing, where a drug is applied as a patch, or is pricked or scratched into the skin, or injected intradermally. Unfortunately prick and scratch testing are less useful for assessing the systemic reaction to drugs than they are for the more usual atopic antigens (e.g. pollens) and both false positives and false negatives can occur. Intradermal injection can provoke serious systemic anaphylaxis and fatalities have been recorded. Patch testing is safe and is useful for the diagnosis of contact sensitivity but does not reflect systemic reactions. It may also itself cause allergy.

Provocative tests can also involve giving small doses of the drug by inhalation, by mouth or parenterally. The initial dose should not exceed 1.0 μg by mouth or 1.0 ng by injection. The dose is increased at intervals until a therapeutic dose is reached or a reaction occurs. This type of testing should not be used when very serious reactions are involved (e.g. aplastic anaemia).

(c) Serological testing is rarely helpful as the demonstration of circulating antibodies does not mean that they are necessarily the cause of the symptoms.

(d) Sensitised lymphocytes. The demonstration of transformation occurring when lymphocytes are exposed to a drug suggests that they are T lymphocytes sensitised to the drug, but interpretation of results can be difficult in a clinical context. In this type of reaction the hapten itself will often provoke lymphocyte transformation as well as the conjugate.

(e) Often it is necessary to stop all the drugs which a patient is taking and reintroduce them one by one until the drug at fault is discovered. This should only be done if the reaction is not a serious one, otherwise any suspected drug should be banned for life. *The drug allergy should be recorded in the notes and the patient informed of the risks involved in taking the drug again.*

Prevention of allergic reactions

Although it is probably not possible to avoid allergic drug reactions completely, the following methods can decrease the incidence:

(a) Drug history is very important whenever drug treatment is anticipated, particularly with antibiotics and other drugs with a high allergy potential. A history of atopy, although not excluding the use of drugs, should put one on guard.

(b) Drugs given orally are less likely to cause severe allergic reactions.

(c) Prophylactic skin testing is not usually practicable and a negative test does not exclude the possibility of an allergic reaction.

(d) Desensitisation. This should only be used when continued use of the drug is essential. It consists of giving a very small dose of the drug and increasing the dose at regular intervals. It is often successful, though little is known of the mechanism by which it is achieved. Sometimes it may be necessary to control a drug allergy with antihistamines and/or steroids whilst giving the drug. This is not ideal but may allow essential treatment to be given.

Chapter 22
DRUG DEPENDENCE AND DRUG OVERDOSE

DEPENDENCE

The WHO definition (1969) of drug dependence is 'a state, psychic and sometimes physical, resulting from the interaction between a living organism and a drug, characterised by behavioural and other responses that always include a compulsion to take the drug on a continuous or periodic basis in order to experience its psychic effects, and sometimes to avoid the discomfort of its absence. Tolerance may or may not be present. A person may be dependent on more than one drug.' The term 'drug dependence' is now used instead of the terms 'drug addiction' and 'drug habituation'.

Dependence is always psychological and can in addition be physical. Psychological dependence is a condition in which a drug produces a feeling of satisfaction and in which there is a psychic need for periodic or continuous administration of the drug to produce pleasure or to avoid discomfort. Physical dependence is a state that manifests itself by intense physical disturbances when the administration of the drug is suspended.

In the management of drug dependence it is the psychological component that is most difficult to treat in the long term, even though on initial drug withdrawal the physical condition may endanger life. Initially it is the pleasure obtained from the drug or the ready escape from unpleasant pressures of living or acceptance in a group which maintains repeated drug taking. Later such positive conditioning may be followed by negative conditioning, in that the drug user has to remain on drugs in order to avoid unpleasant withdrawal phenomena.

Drug abuse has been defined as 'the consumption of a drug apart from medical need or in unnecessary quantities'. The harmful consequences of abuse include not only dependence but traffic accidents and antisocial behaviour. However, non-illicit drugs, such as alcohol and tobacco, may pose an even more important problem.

Up to 1961 most addicts to illicit drugs were middle-aged individuals who had initially experienced the drugs in a therapeutic situation or who handled drugs professionally. After this time the great increase in the number of addicts was due to the appearance of young, unstable, non-therapeutic (or epidemic) addicts who belonged to a subculture in which drug taking was the norm. The groups who are most at risk in epidemic addiction are mainly young, immature, adventurous and easily led. Those with school, social or work problems are vulnerable as are those who would otherwise find difficulty in being accepted in social cliques. These addicts initially obtain drugs from other addicts and do not make their first contact with drugs because of pain or psychological disturbances. Other forms of pleasure-seeking activity are often present, with early experience of smoking, alcohol and sex. There is often a history of truancy, poor work record, inability to stand frustration or to plan for distant goals and an increased incidence of criminal behaviour.

Even though addiction of the non-therapeutic (epidemic) type is usually a symptom of individual and social disturbances, once it is established, it becomes a self-perpetuating disease in its own right and not readily amenable to changes in environment or the individual.

The medical (therapeutic) addict differs from this picture. Table 22.1 summarises some of the points of difference.

Table 22.1 Differences between epidemic and medical addicts

Epidemic (non-medical) addict	*Medical (therapeutic) addict*
Dose of drug may escalate	Often on stable dosage
May stop taking drugs with increasing maturity	Age not a factor
Usually under 30 years	Usually over 30 years
6–8 males: 1 female	Equal sex incidence
Often delinquent	Not often delinquent, but may have an underlying psychiatric illness
Drug use in a group—seen as a mark of esteem	Solitary drug use—guilt about drug
Multiple drugs used	Usually single drug used—particularly narcotic analgesics, but amphetamine and barbiturates have been a problem

Opiates

Dependence on these drugs has become of increasing importance, particularly in the USA. In the UK the number of addicts to opioid drugs known to the Home Office in 1983 was 5864 but this figure is known to grossly underestimate the prevalence of the problem. Although some addicts receive their drugs from special clinics on a controlled basis there is a well-organised illicit distribution of opiates. Morphine, heroin, pethidine, methadone and less commonly pentazocine, dipipanone, propoxyphene, buprenorphine and diphenoxylate are abused. Heroin is, however, the drug of preference. It is known on the streets as H, white stuff, horse, smack, dope, scag, Lady Jane and so on, but is often adulterated with other indistinguishable white powders such as quinine (which is bitter like opiates), lactose and even starch and talc. The drug is taken intravenously, subcutaneously, orally and by inhalation ('chasing the dragon'). The latter method of abuse has become commoner recently, particularly among the 15–25 year age-group. To some extent this has resulted from a relative decrease in the price of street heroin over the past decade coinciding with greatly increased quantities of the drug reaching Europe and the USA from Asia and the Middle and Far East. In addition, younger drug abusers find that they can obtain the pleasurable effects of the drug without the need for unpleasant injections. It is not known if heroin inhalation over many years can produce respiratory damage. Thus the problems associated with acute and chronic opiate abuse discussed below apply to addicts administering heroin parenterally since it is not presently known whether they affect those taking heroin only by inhalation.

Acute overdose reaction

The medical hazards of chronic opiate abuse are summarised in Table 22.2. In addition the acute opiate overdose reaction may result in death. The acute reaction may take two main forms:

(a) Pulmonary oedema, which can be bilateral or unilateral and probably results from increased pulmonary capillary permeability.
(b) Hypoxic reaction (with cardiac arrhythmias in 25 %) which presents with severe bradypnoea, cyanosis, lethargy and coma. The pathophysiology is unknown but it could result from
  (i) anaphylaxis due to injected antigens;
  (ii) acute toxic reactions to adulterants;
  (iii) collapse due to injection of particles;
  (iv) excessive opiate effect due to loss of tolerance, irregular potency of supply or through a neophyte taking the dose used by a friend who has become tolerant.

The mortality in patients reaching hospital alive is about 5 % (which is much higher than in overdoses due to most other drugs—see below). Deaths on the street in New York City may amount to 1000/year, suggesting a mortality of 1 % per year amongst abusers there. About 25 % of overdose victims have taken another drug in addition, the commonest being alcohol, methadone, barbiturates and other sedatives.

Management of acute overdose (see also p. 868)

1. Ventilate with oxygen preferably via endotracheal tube to prevent aspiration.

2. Give naloxone 0.4 mg intravenously and wait for 3 min for effect; if no effect give a further 2.0 mg and wait for 3 min. At this time if there has been no increased ventilation, lightening of consciousness or dilatation of the pupils, it is unlikely that the patient has an opiate overdose. It should be remembered that the clinical $t_{1/2}$ of naloxone effect is short (about 10–20 min) compared to the $t_{1/2}$ of opiates, and when treating patients who have taken large amounts of opiate naloxone must be given by repeated bolus injections or as an infusion to avoid recurrence of respiratory depression. Since vomiting occurs in 80 % of patients with opiate overdose given naloxone and in some patients who have no opiate overdose it is important to prevent aspiration before this drug is given (aspiration pneumonia has a mortality of 30–40 %).

Gynaecological–neonatal problems Female addicts have a high rate of venereal disease because many earn money for drugs by prostitution; they may also transmit hepatitis by sexual intercourse. Pregnancy when it occurs is complicated by opiate abuse since the mother is often uncooperative with antenatal care. The newborns are frequently of low birth weight or premature (possibly because of the low oestriol levels in pregnant addicts). Neonatal

Table 22.2 Medical complications of opiate abuse

Complication	*Special features*
A. Infections	
1. Endocarditis	8 % of hospital admissions of opiate abusers. 50 % involve tricuspid valve (cf. 'usual' involvement of L side valves) *Staph. aureus* predominant organism but fungi not unusual.
2. Hepatitis	70 % of abusers with hepatitis have Australia antigen 5 % of abusers without hepatitis have Australia antigen i.e. similar to patients receiving multiple transfusions. 40 % of abusers have abnormal liver function tests and at autopsy at least 25 % of abusers have chronic active hepatitis.
3. HTLV III infection	50 % USA addicts positive
4. Osteomyelitis	Especially of vertebrae (*Pseudomonas*, *Staph.* and *Candida* common).
5. Skin infection	Associated with injection.
B. Immunological	
1. Raised IgM	False positive rheumatoid factor and syphilis tests
2. Nephropathy	Nephrotic syndrome with proliferative glomerulonephritis.
C. Neurological	
1. Transverse myelitis	Usually sudden shortly after injecting drugs. Paraplegia usual sequel.
2. Myopathy	? due to adulterants in drugs.
3. Postanoxic encephalopathy	Follows hypoxaemic episode; may result in prolonged coma.

addiction produces a withdrawal syndrome at birth which untreated has a mortality of 50%. The reaction begins within four days and consists of irritability and tremors (50 %), vomiting and diarrhoea (20 %), sneezing and yawning (10 %), respiratory depression (5 %) and convulsions (1–2 %). Death occurs from dehydration or circulatory collapse. Convulsions are not a complication of the adult withdrawal syndrome and may be a special feature of the electrolyte disturbance or prematurity. Treatment logically consists of methadone 0.1–0.5 mg/kg/day which is slowly reduced, but chlorpromazine 1 mg/kg 4 hourly is probably presently the drug of choice, this dose being reduced over 3–6 weeks.

Tolerance and physical dependence Chronic opiate abuse results in physical dependence and development of a tolerant state manifested by a decreased sensitivity to opiate agonists but an increased sensitivity to antagonists. Tolerance is cellular rather than metabolic and is defined as occurring when

Table 22.2 (continued)

Complication	*Special features*
D. Cardiovascular	
1. Arrhythmias	Supraventricular arrhythmias common in overdose reaction. Quinine (an adulterant) can produce heart block. Ventricular ectopics common with propoxyphene overdose.
2. Emboli	Multiple emboli (sometimes due to adulterants) into retinal and peripheral vessels. Gangrene common after intra-arterial injection.
E. Pulmonary	
1. Embolism by foreign particles	Pulmonary hypertension, cor pulmonale and granulomas may result.
2. Ventilation/perfusion defects	75% of abusers have abnormalities even when asymptomatic.
3. Aspiration pneumonia	Opiates block cough reflex and gastric emptying and provoke vomiting. Bronchiectasis may follow aspiration.
F. Gastrointestinal	
1. Constipation	Obstruction may follow swallowing condom filled with drugs by traffickers.
2. Biliary hypertension	Often causes transient increase in transaminases, amylase and alkaline phosphatase.
G. Skin	
1. Bullous eruptions	Seen in opiate overdose coma (like barbiturates and other drugs).
2. Localised oedema	Swelling of hands, feet, scalp, eyelids.
3. Urticaria	May be associated with serum sickness.
4. Needle tracks	

increasingly larger doses of drug must be administered to obtain the effects observed with the original dose. Tolerance affects the analgesic and euphoric effects of opiates so that the heroin addict requires more and more heroin for his 'buzz' although in the therapeutic setting patients with severe pain or addicts on maintenance opiate therapy do not appear to demonstrate large changes in tolerance. The increased 'habit' of street addicts may be one cause of their turning to crime to obtain money to buy increasing amounts of drug. Tolerance is less marked to the gastro-intestinal and miotic effects of opiates so that addicts remain constipated and have pin-point pupils. Withdrawal of opiates from or injection of an antagonist into an addict results in a physical withdrawal syndrome. This could be interpreted pharmacologically as the suppression of endogenous endorphin production due to opiate binding to brain receptors and to reduced sensitivity of brain opiate receptors. Withdrawal of opiates leads to the receptors being inadequately stimulated and therefore causes a temporary withdrawal syndrome. *Withdrawal symptoms* are unpleasant but the syndrome is never fatal in a healthy adult. They begin 8 h after the last dose and peak at 36–72 h. First yawning, rhinorrhoea, crying and sweating are seen, then at 20 h sweating, chills and gooseflesh ('cold turkey') appear. At 24–48 h nausea and vomiting, diarrhoea, hypertension and sometimes fever are seen and the patient complains of severe cramps which may last for up to a week. The reaction may be suppressed with methadone (20 mg in divided doses the first 3 days, then 10 mg for 3 days). Sleep disturbances (partly due to REM rebound) and anxiety may persist for weeks or months and require treatment with diazepam. Withdrawal from methadone, even if large doses are being taken, is mild and may be left untreated (except for diazepam).

Treatment of opiate dependence This may aim either for complete abstinence or for more effective functioning despite continued use of drugs. In the UK the 1967 Dangerous Drugs Act resulted in the establishment of clinics at which addicts continued to receive their drugs in a controlled way so that they cannot be sold or given to others. In selected cases a programme of dosage reduction with appropriate psychotherapy and social counselling is undertaken in an attempt to wean the patient off drugs.

An alternative approach, which has had widespread use in the USA, is *methadone maintenance*. Patients are given a gradually increasing dose of oral methadone as heroin is withdrawn (30 mg is usually a safe and effective dose even for hard-core addicts, but may cause somnolence in less addicted persons). Methadone maintenance results in tolerance to the effects of all opiates on the central nervous system. The dosage level can usually be stabilised at less than 100 mg daily when patients usually report no craving for other drugs and no psychological or physical effects even from large doses of other, self-administered opiates. Tolerance is not a problem under these circumstances. Dependence on methadone is a consequence of this treatment but the withdrawal syndrome is mild, although whether this is feasible in many patients remains to be determined. Methadone is usually given premixed in fruit juice (caution must be exercised to prevent children accidentally taking the patient's methadone mixture) or in non-injectable tablets. Partial opiate antagonists such as pentazocine and buprenorphine are contraindicated since they will precipitate a withdrawal syndrome. Heroin may cause temporary infertility in women and those who begin methadone maintenance treatment should be warned to take precautions if they wish to avoid pregnancy since there is often a restoration of normal menstrual cycles on methadone. The most important contraindication to methadone is the absence of physical dependence to heroin since in some communities 'street' heroin is so heavily adulterated that many patients are only psychologically dependent, so that methadone maintenance may convert them to physical dependence on opiates.

It should also be recognised that contrary to what was once believed, recent studies in the USA suggest that it may be possible to experiment with narcotics on an occasional basis without becoming addicted (although the practice is not recommended). The generally accepted view that there is a poor response to treatment and a high relapse rate among opiate users is based on statistics from prisons and hospitals where selected atypical groups, with poor prognoses, have been studied. There is evidence that a group of addicts exists in whom the condition remits in middle age when they become able to live without opiates. For many others methadone maintenance appears to lead to some improvement in terms of general stability of social life and functioning, although they remain dependent upon the prescribed drug.

Several new approaches to opiate withdrawal have been investigated recently. The administration of endogenous opioid peptides, e.g. β-endorphin, proved disappointing with no real evidence of clinical efficacy despite theoretical advantages. Acupuncture, which may release endogenous opioid peptides within the CNS is currently under investigation.

Clonidine (p. 442) a pre-synaptic α-agonist has short-term benefits in opiate withdrawal. In some patients it markedly reduces signs and symptoms of withdrawal, possibly by decreasing the increased brain noradrenaline concentrations which occur during opiate withdrawal. However, when clonidine itself is stopped a withdrawal syndrome may occur which limits the use of the drug.

Cocaine (see also p. 357)

This is the principal active alkaloid found in the leaves of the coca plant (*Erythroxylon coca*) and has been used for centuries by the Indians of Peru and Bolivia. Originally used for religious purposes it is now used as a recreational drug and to increase physical strength and endurance by workers who chew it with lime (alkali) to enhance extraction of cocaine from the leaf. The illicit use of cocaine has increased dramatically over the past 10 years, particularly in the USA. This may be attributed to increased availability and purity of the drug together with a marked reduction in street price. Cocaine is a white crystalline powder and is usually sold diluted with dried milk or talcum powder.

It is a CNS stimulant producing a euphoric 'rush' like amphetamine. With chronic administration it can produce a toxic psychosis associated with feelings of super strength and stamina, delusions of grandeur and convulsions. In addition to its psychological effects it may produce irregular respiration and anorexia. Cocaine blocks the re-uptake of catecholamines into nerve endings and this may account for various other somatic effects including peripheral vasoconstriction, dilation of the pupils, tachycardia and hypertension. Coronary artery vasoconstriction also occurs and may lead to infarction particularly in those with underlying ischaemic heart disease. Use of the drug has also been associated with ventricular arrhythmias and sudden death.

It is readily absorbed from the mouth but is often taken by sniffing ('snorting') since it is alleged to have a more rapid onset of action by this route. Unfortunately due to its potent vasoconstrictor action individuals who sniff the drug are prone to develop gangrene and/or perforation of the nasal septum. By contrast, cocaine is only poorly absorbed if swallowed since it is degraded in the stomach. The $t_{1/2}$ when given i.v. is 2–4 h. It is extensively metabolised to inactive metabolites by the mixed-function oxidase system of the liver.

Cocaine produces only psychological dependence; there is no physical dependence syndrome and withdrawal is less difficult than with opiates.

Cocaine is commonly taken with these drugs for it is believed by addicts to counteract opiate-induced impotence and lethargy (hence one of its street names 'love-affair': this mixture has also been called 'killer-stuff').

Barbiturates, Glutethimide, Methaqualone.

In Britain over the last 20 years there has been a marked increase in awareness of the existence of dependence upon these drugs which is both psychological and physical in type. Tolerance occurs and cross tolerance exists with alcohol. The withdrawal syndrome may include grand-mal seizures and can be fatal. The addict population includes many middle-aged females who are not in general regarded as likely addicts by those unfamiliar with the problem. Barbiturates are also taken with heroin, amphetamines, or alcohol as part of the pattern of multiple drug abuse which occurs in the younger age-group. More stringent voluntary controls on barbiturate prescription may result in a decreased availability of these drugs on the street and reduced incidence of new therapeutic addicts. The problem is further discussed in Chapter 9.

Benzodiazepines

Abuse of these drugs is still being evaluated and is presently somewhat uncommon considering their widespread use. Details are to be found on p. 219.

The hallucinogenic drugs

Even though the hallucinogens are of considerable research interest, they have no application in orthodox psychiatric practice. In clinical medicine their main importance is in their ability to produce psychiatric and physical illness when abused. The agents which are taken for their ability to alter perception include:

1. *Substances related to 5-hydroxytryptamine*

mescaline (from peyote cactus—*Lophophora williamsii*)
psilocybin psilocin (from mushrooms—*Psilocybe mexicanum* and *Stropharia cubensis*)
d-lysergic acid diethylamide (LSD) (from ergot—*Claviceps purpurea*)
dimethyltryptamine (DMT)
harmaline.

2. *Amphetamine derivatives*

amphetamine sulphate
dextroamphetamine sulphate
methamphetamine hydrochloride
dimethoxyamphetamine (methoxymethylamphetamine; STP; DOM)
3, 4-methylenedioxyamphetamine (MDA)

3. *Anticholinergics*

atropine
strammonium

4. *Cannabis preparations*

5. *Miscellaneous substances*
methylphenidate
phenmetrazine
phencyclidine HCl (PCP; constituent of 'angel dust')
petrol and other solvents
amyl nitrite
morning glory seeds.

The pharmacological properties of these substances vary considerably but the following are commonly seen:

1. The subjective effects are typically not true hallucinations, but are sensory illusions and distortions. These are accompanied by euphoria, excitement, sensations of watching while participating and feelings of tremendous insight. Unpleasant sensations include nausea and anxiety.
2. The EEG frequently shows an arousal pattern. This is associated with insomnia.
3. Sympathomimetic effects: dilatation of the pupil, peripheral vasoconstriction and raised systolic blood pressure.
4. Evidence of increased nervous activity: tremor, increased tendon jerks.
5. Deterioration in performance of tests involving motor coordination, reasoning and memory.
6. No evidence of physical dependence.
7. Dysphoric or psychotic reactions occur in about 20% of drug administrations. These are sometimes prolonged and can result in suicide.

Adverse reactions to hallucinogens

1. About 20% drug exposures ('trips') are unpleasant ('bummers'), but only a small proportion of victims present themselves for medical treatment. The commonest dysphoric reaction is fear and panic. The subjects experience loss of control of the drug effects ('freak out'). Other unpleasant presentations are paranoia, depression, illusions, visual hallucinations, delusions and feelings of going insane with resulting suicide.

Acute delusional states and hallucinations respond to chlorpromazine 100 mg intramuscularly or orally 3–4 hourly. The reactions to dimethoxyamphetamine last 4–12 days but chlorpromazine is contraindicated because of the danger of hypotensive reactions. Diazepam 50 mg orally daily (or more frequently) is often helpful. Strammonium can produce multifocal fits. With this type of drug gastric lavage is valuable up to 12 h after administration. Intravenous diazepam is used to control the fits.

2. 'Flashbacks' consist of episodes similar to the drug experience which recur whilst not taking the drug.

3. Chronic psychiatric states resembling dementia, schizophrenia or depression may persist for weeks or months following exposure to hallucinogens. It has never been established that chronic abuse of these drugs can result in cerebral atrophy.

Additional features of individual hallucinogens

LSD Adverse reactions can last 8–24 h after administration. Fits may occur.

Phencyclidine When sprinkled on to herbs and marijuanha, this is called 'angel dust'. Phencyclidine hydrochloride is related to ketamine and is used as an anaesthetic in veterinary practice. In man it can produce hypertension, stupor, coma and respiratory depression.

Amphetamines ('speed') are used for their euphoriant effects either as a spree drug, chronically or in a cocktail of drugs, often as a substitute for cocaine. They are taken orally or by injection. Originally there was a group of middle-aged women addicts who had initially received amphetamines either alone or in combination with barbiturates (Drinamyl or 'purple hearts'—a mixture of amphetamine and amylobarbitone). Following voluntary control of prescriptions this group has dwindled and the typically addicted person now is young and usually of unstable personality (qv opiate addicts). It is not necessarily true, however, that abusers of 'soft' drugs such as cannabis or amphetamines will progress to the abuse of 'hard' drugs like opiates. Tolerance to amphetamines occurs. The dependence produced is psychological and there is no withdrawal syndrome as such, although they may develop depressive reactions when the drug is stopped ('coming down' or 'the horrors') and a particular problem is the development of agitation, restlessness and schizophrenic-type psychoses, frequently with paranoid features.

Dimethoxyamphetamine (STP = serenity, tranquillity and peace). This can cause fatal respiratory failure. Treatment with chlorpromazine can precipitate circulatory collapse.

3,4 methylenedioxyamphetamine This drug can cause muscular rigidity, fever and cardiac arrhythmias.

Anticholinergics in large doses produce a dry flushed skin, dilated pupils and fits.

Cannabis

This term includes the various natural and derived products of *Cannabis sativa.* Two main forms exist which are called by a variety of local names:

(a) The resinous exudate of the flowering tops ('hashish')
(b) Chopped leaves and stalks (marijuana). Cannabis is usually smoked or taken orally and the various active substances probably vary according to the source of the plant and its mode of consumption and preparation.

The clinical effects of cannabis vary according to the individual, his mood, environment and expectations. Subjectively time may appear to be slowed down, sensory experiences may be heightened—and there may be a feeling of interchange between different modalities of sensation. The enjoyment of jokes, sex and music may be increased. Short-term memory is impaired. The subject feels relaxed, but a minority of subjects may feel restless and anxious. Auditory hallucinations may be experienced.

The physiological effects of cannabis are variable. The conjunctivae may become injected and there is a tachycardia and postural hypotension which may be due to its atropine-like actions. Antihypertensive effects have been demonstrated, possibly resulting from a reduction in sympathetic efferent outflow and suppression of inhibitory input into the sympathetic nervous system. Some attempts have been made to utilise these properties but so far the cannabis derivatives produced have either produced euphoria or shown rapidly increasing tolerance to their effects. Other properties which may show clinical potential are its sedative, antiepileptic, antiemetic, analgesic and appetite-enhancing effects. The blood sugar may be lowered or elevated by cannabis.

Pharmacokinetics The main active principles in cannabis are highly lipid soluble and therefore distribute widely in the body, their distribution and pattern of action being dependent upon the blood flow to tissues (cf. halothane, thiopentone). Tetrahydrocannabinol (THC) itself has a $t_{1/2}$ of 56 h. The major metabolite 11-hydroxy THC from microsomal oxidation is also psychoactive but continued cannabis administration has been demonstrated to inhibit microsomal function. Cumulation of cannabinols occurs with repeated administration.

Clinical uses A synthetic cannabinoid, nabilone (Cesemet), is now available for use as an antiemetic, principally for relief of nausea and vomiting associated with cytotoxic chemotherapy (see p. 563).

Adverse effects Occasional use of cannabis probably does no more harm to the individual than alcohol. Motor coordination is impaired in the majority of individuals and thus driving skills may be affected. Panic attacks occur both as 'bad trips' and 'flashbacks'. The effects of chronic consumption are hotly debated. Repeated use of cannabis does not appear to lead to physical dependence but psychological dependence is common. A phenomenon of 'reverse tolerance' is also described, i.e. habitués more easily experience subjective effects. This may relate to

(i) increased formation of active metabolites due to enzyme induction;
(ii) saturation of drug-binding sites in lipid;
(iii) increased awareness of nuances of the drug effect;
(iv) practice at inhaling drug.

Chronic toxicity may occur in various tissues:

(a) Respiratory system: pharyngitis, tracheitis, bronchitis, rhinitis.
(b) Nervous system: headache, memory loss, psychosis (acute and chronic). Dementia has been alleged but not proven.
(c) Chromosomal abnormalities and teratogenesis: unproven.

Solvent abuse The inhalation of volatile solvents has markedly increased over the past 10 years, particularly among adolescents. Glues, which contain toluene as the principal solvent, are the most popular but petrol, lighter fuel, paint thinners, hair lacquer and nail polish remover (acetone) are also abused.

These solvents are usually inhaled from a rag or plastic bag, often as a group activity.

The acute effects are predominantly on the central nervous system and commonly present as excitation with euphoria, hallucinations and behaviour change, followed by depression with ataxia, blurred vision and drowsiness. In occasional cases there are serious irreversible effects which have included toluene encephalopathy, optic atrophy, cerebellar ataxia and nephropathy. There have been deaths due to asphyxia during inhalation and occasionally sudden death possibly due to inhalation of fluorocarbons in aerosols which potentiate the effects of catecholamines on the heart.

Alcohol and Alcoholism

Ethyl alcohol (alcohol) has few clinical uses when given systemically, but is of great medical importance because of its pathological and psychological effects when used as a beverage. The alcohol content of drinks ranges from 3.5–6 % in beer, through 10 % in wine and 20 % in port to 40–55 % in spirits (100° proof is 57 % v/v). Most alcoholic beverages contain a number of congeneric substances formed as by-products during the fermentation or distilling processes. Many of these substances are pharmacologically active and include n-propyl, n-butyl and iso-amyl alcohols. They are collectively described as fusel oil and it has been suggested that different types of alcoholic beverage differ in their pharmacological effects due to the presence of fusel oil, large quantities of which have been shown to prolong the EEG changes produced in man by ethanol. These effects appear to be of little importance at the doses in which they are taken in alcoholic drinks. No evidence exists that these alter the pharmacokinetic or pharmacodynamic properties of coadministered ethanol and in these respects at least whisky is indistinguishable from an appropriate dilution of pure ethanol.

Alcohol is the most important drug of dependence, and in Western Europe and North America the incidence of alcoholism is about 5 % in the adult population. The maximum safe level of alcohol consumption is probably around 60 g pure ethanol daily for men and at least half this amount for women (10 g ethanol = 1 unit = 1/2 pint beer, one glass wine, 1 small glass port or sherry or 1 single measure of spirits).

Pharmacokinetics Ethyl alcohol is absorbed from the buccal, oesophageal, gastric and intestinal mucosae: approximately 80 % is absorbed from the small intestine. Alcohol delays gastric emptying and in high doses delays its own absorption by a negative feedback mediated via duodenal osmoreceptors. Large amounts of alcohol taken in dilute solution are also absorbed relatively slowly, possibly as a result of a volume effect on gastric emptying rate. Following oral administration alcohol can usually be detected in the blood within 5 min. Peak levels occur between $\frac{1}{2}$ and 2 h. Fats and carbohydrates delay absorption which follows zero-order kinetics. Individuals show great variation in speed of absorption and those habituated to alcohol often show a steeper rise and higher peak in blood level.

Alcohol is distributed throughout the body water (apparent volume of distribution is 55–60 % of body weight). Alcohol penetrates the CSF (1.1

× blood concentration) and urine (1.3 × blood concentration). 95% is metabolised (mainly in the liver) and the remainder is excreted unchanged in the breath, urine and sweat. Hepatic oxidation to acetaldehyde is catalysed by three parallel processes. The major pathway (Fig. 22.1) is rate limited by cytoplasmic alcohol dehydrogenase using NAD as coenzyme. This enzyme exhibits polymorphism, the less common variant (5–20% in Europeans) having a five-fold increase in specific activity. Despite this higher activity individuals possessing the atypical variant show no increase in alcohol oxidation rate in vivo. Less important is metabolism by microsomal enzymes using NADPH as cofactor. Another minor pathway involves catalase which oxidases ethanol in the presence of a hydrogen peroxide generating system. The importance of these minor pathways in vivo is undecided. The acetaldehyde formed is converted by acetaldehyde dehydrogenase to acetyl-coenzyme A, primarily in the mitochondria and then enters the tricarboxylic acid cycle. Large amounts of fructose (1–2 g/kg) accelerate alcohol metabolism but this has been found to be of relatively small clinical value.

Although nutritional defiencies may contribute to the toxicity of ethanol it is now believed that it is the altered intracellular redox balance caused by an increased NADH/NAD ratio which is responsible for the biochemical effects

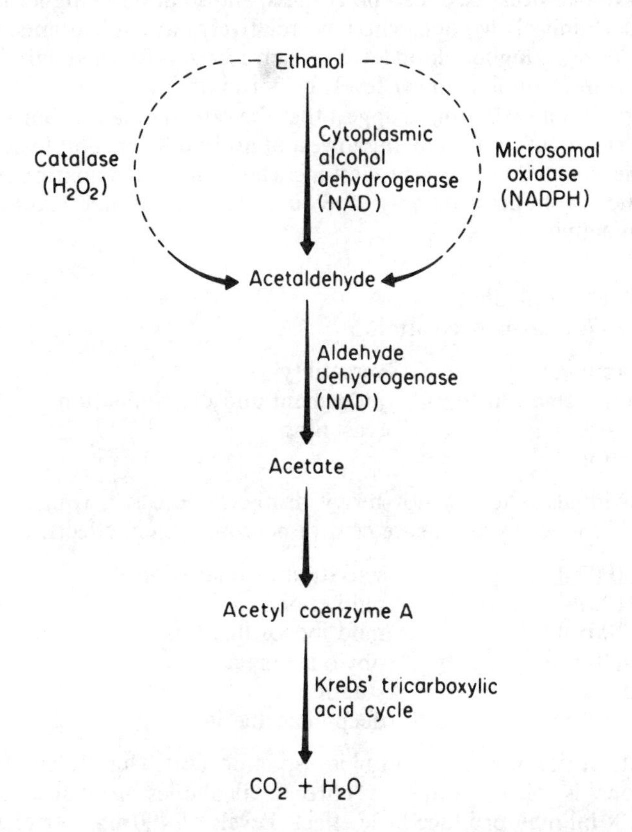

Fig. 22.1 Pathways of ethanol oxidation. (→ major pathway; → minor pathway).

of acute and chronic alcohol abuse. Increase in the relative concentration of NADH results in reduced metabolism and therefore accumulation of lactate, β-hydroxybutyrate, glutamate, malate, α-glycerophosphate and other substances requiring NAD for elimination. The net effect of such changes includes impaired gluconeogenesis resulting in alcohol-induced hypoglycaemia, and fatty infiltration of the liver due to impaired elimination of exogenous and endogenous fatty acids via the Krebs' cycle and enhanced triglyceride synthesis due to the increased levels of α-glycerophosphate. Originally it was postulated that alcohol elimination obeys zero-order kinetics, i.e. is independent of the blood concentration above about 0.1 mg/ml. There is substantial evidence now that Michaelis–Menten kinetics more accurately describe the situation. The V_m and K_m for the average man are approximately 25 mg/100 ml/h and 10.5 mg/100 ml respectively. It is, however, true to say that the average rate of alcohol elimination is approximately 10 ml/h so that once an intoxicated state is reached an intake of 10 ml each hour will suffice to maintain it. The rate of metabolism is much more nearly the same in identical twins than in fraternal twins and genetic factors rather than environmental differences appear to control the overall rate. The rate of metabolism is much the same in young and old subjects, although the aged have a smaller apparent volume of distribution, probably due to decreased lean body mass, and so develop higher levels for a given dose. Similarly women, who have relatively more subcutaneous fat than men, also develop higher blood levels, which accounts for their liability to toxic damage from alcohol at lower levels of consumption.

Some preliminary findings suggest that the rate of ethanol elimination may exhibit a circadian rhythm, being lowest at around 8 a.m. and faster at about 9 p.m. (the 'cocktail hour'). A modest increase in alcohol oxidation is observed in chronic alcoholics, possibly due to induction of microsomal ethanol oxidation activity.

Acute effects of alcohol

1. *Nervous system*: decrease in

learning ability,	versatility
association formation	judgement and discrimination
attention span	reasoning
concentration	

In individuals who are not heavy drinkers there is a rough correlation between blood levels and acute central nervous system effects:

20 mg/100 ml	sensation of relaxation
30 mg/100 ml	mild euphoria
50 mg/100 ml	mild incoordination
100 mg/100 ml	obvious ataxia
300 mg/100 ml	stupor
400 mg/100 ml	deep anaesthesia.

The rate of rise of concentration is also important. This table of blood level correlations is of no value in chronic alcoholics in whom a level of 200 mg/100 ml may produce little effect. Levels of 400 mg/100 ml and above can lead to death from respiratory depression. At high blood concentrations

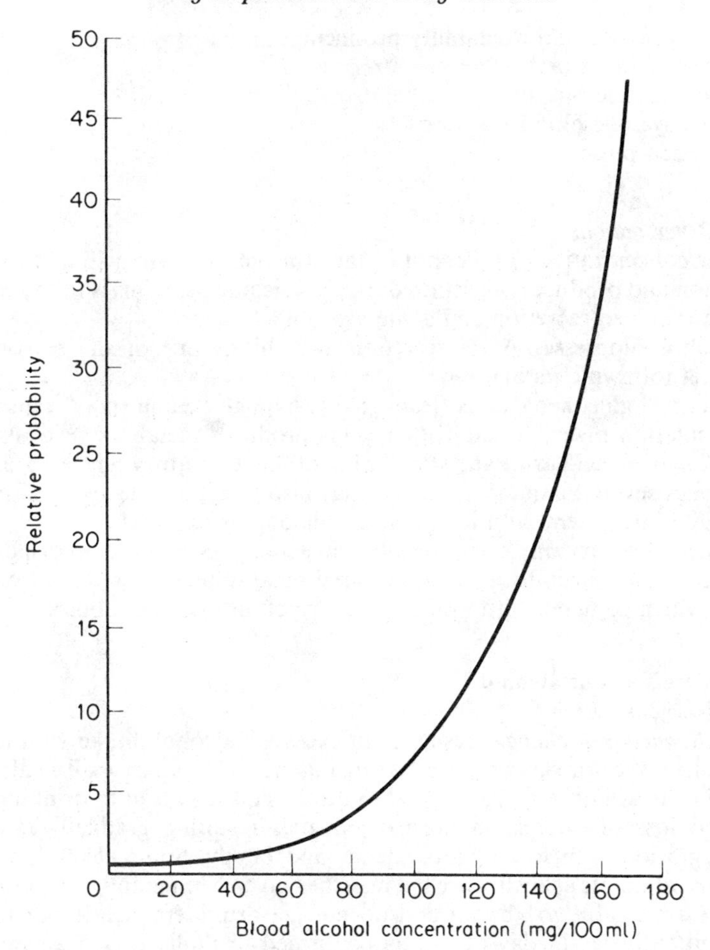

Fig. 22.2 Relative probability of causing a road traffic accident at various blood alcohol concentrations (From J. D. J. Havard, *Hospital Update*, **1**, 253 (1975)).

vomiting may occur and death may result from aspiration of gastric contents.

The importance of alcohol as a factor in road traffic accidents is well-known (Fig. 22.2). At present in the UK the legal limit for alcohol in the blood is 80 mg/100 ml. At this level of intoxication serious personal injuries or fatalities occur in some 10% of road accidents, which is more than double the rate occurring in accidents involving sober drivers.

The central depressant actions of alcohol greatly enhance the effects of other central depressant drugs.

In patients with organic brain damage alcohol may induce unusual aggression and destructiveness known as pathological intoxication.

2. *Circulatory system:*

Cutaneous vasodilatation, increased sweating (can produce hypothermia)
Splanchnic vasoconstriction

Increased myocardial excitability producing:
increased heart rate
raised cardiac output
raised systolic blood pressure
increased pulse pressure.

3. *Other actions*

Low concentrations of alcohol in the stomach increase acid and mucous secretion and produce congestion of the gastric mucosa. This is followed by a decrease in acid secretion and acute gastritis.

Alcohol suppresses ADH secretion and this is one of the reasons for polyuria following its ingestion:

Reduced gluconeogenesis leading to hypoglycaemia may cause fits. Accumulation of lactate and other acids produces metabolic acidosis with excretion of an acid urine and stimulation of the respiratory centre. In chronic alcoholics severe thiamine deficiency may also precipitate lactic acidosis and immediate treatment with intravenous thiamine is required.

Hyperuricaemia may occur, resulting in acute gout in those predisposed to this condition, partly because of increased renal tubular excretion of organic acids, which compete with uric acid for secretion into the tubules.

Chronic effects of alcohol

1. *Nervous system*

(a) *Behavioural changes* resulting in excessive alcohol intake with loss of control, i.e. the drinker can never be sure that he will be able to call a halt to his drinking at will once he has started to drink. This may lead to drinking with gradual loss of interest in normal activities resulting gradually in social disintegration with loss of job, friends and family. Some alcoholics make repeated attempts at abstinence but may then go on a binge and become drunk. Others are unable to abstain and do not get drunk frequently but top up intermittently day-in, day-out. In the confirmed alcoholic, periods of amnesia, emotional extremes (rage, depression, pathological jealousy), insomnia and seizures may occur. Acute withdrawal may result in:

tremor
convulsions
auditory hallucinations
paranoid reactions
delirium tremens (acute disorientation, autonomic hyperactivity, panic and unpleasant visual hallucinations), see below (p. 855).

Acute withdrawal symptoms reach a maximum 24–36 h after the last drink, but the anorexia, nausea, vomiting, tremor, anxiety, malaise and inability to concentrate may last for 1–2 weeks.

(b) *Wernicke's encephalopathy* (difficulty in concentrating, confusion, coma, nystagmus and ophthalmoplegia) and *Korsakov's psychosis* (gross memory defects with confabulation and disorientation in space and time) appear to be mainly due to the nutritional deficiency associated with alcoholism. There is usually a partial response to thiamine which should initially be given intravenously, e.g. 100 mg daily for 3 days. Recently it has been shown that some individuals inherit an abnormal form of the enzyme transketolase with reduced affinity for its coenzyme thiamine. Thus, if dietary thiamine intake falls, tissue transketolase activity is decreased which may result in neurological damage. This explains why only some alcoholics suffer these syndromes. The hypothesis demonstrates the general principle of a genetically determined variant being disclosed by an environmental stress or drug (cf. G6PD deficiency: p. 111). Similarly peripheral neuropathy and retrobulbar neuritis are due to thiamine lack. A pellagra-like state may develop from nicotinic acid deficiency.

(c) Chronic alcoholism can also produce:

Chronic cerebral degeneration (leading to dementia) with or without diffuse cerebral atrophy.

Marchiafava–Bignami syndrome (symmetrical demyelination of the corpus collasum leading to dementia, fits, paralysis and disturbance of motor skills).

Central pontine myelinosis (producing quadriplegia and pseudobulbar palsy).

2. *Alimentary system*

Morning nausea and vomiting. Abdominal pain, belching, gastritis.

Peptic ulceration, haematemesis (including the Mallory – Weiss syndrome which is haematemesis due to oesophageal tearing during forceful vomiting).

Enlargement of the liver due to fatty infiltration in 70–80 % alcoholics which is reversible.

Alcoholic hepatitis exhibits clinical features similar to other forms of toxic liver injury. The hypermetabolic state produced by alcohol produces maximal anoxia in the centrilobular hepatocytes which become necrotic. Lymphocytes may also cause cellular damage by becoming sensitive to alcoholic hyaline, a structureless material which accumulates in the liver poisoned by alcohol. This may be why the long-term prognosis of these patients is only modestly improved by abstinence.

How alcohol leads to *cirrhosis* has not been determined but poor dietary intake does not appear to be as important as was once believed. A direct hepatotoxic role for alcohol implies that dietary supplements cannot counteract its effects on the liver and that the only way to reduce its toxicity is complete abstinence. Approximately 10 % chronic alcoholics develop cirrhosis of variable severity. The level of alcohol intake at which the risk of liver disease becomes significant is contentious. Probably less than 60 g in men/day is innocuous but above this intake the risk of cirrhosis markedly increases. Predisposing factors for the development of cirrhosis include the female sex, histocompatibility antigens HLA B8, B13, B40 and the presence of hepatitis B markers. The rate of development of cirrhosis is independent of the duration of alcohol abuse and the amount consumed.

Pancreatitis (acute, subacute and chronic): alcohol stimulates secretin production which increases the flow of pancreatic enzymes. If these are retained in the pancreas due to oedema of the sphincter of Oddi, then autodigestion can lead to pancreatic destruction and inflammation.

3. Alcoholism is occasionally complicated by a *myopathy* affecting cardiac and/or skeletal muscle. A negative association between moderate alcohol intake and coronary disease has been demonstrated in several epidemiological

studies. There is now evidence of a positive correlation between chronic alcohol consumption and *hypertension*.

4. *Bone-marrow suppression* occurs, with consequent thrombocytopenia and inability to counter infections which are more common and serious in alcoholics. Macrocytic or hypochromic anaemias, probably nutritional in origin, may develop and occasionally a haemolytic or sideroblastic anaemia occurs.

5. Alcohol metabolism increases the intracellular NADH/NAD ratio which inhibits the pyruvate carboxylase step in gluconeogenesis thus allowing *hypoglycaemia* to occur if there is a substantial depletion of liver glycogen or in the fasting subject.

6. *Hypertriglyceridaemia* may occur in alcoholics with liver complications and also in those with normal liver function. *Zieve's syndrome* comprises jaundice, haemolytic anaemia and hyperlipaemia. Some patients with types III and IV hyperlipoproteinaemia develop more severe triglyceridaemia after alcohol.

7. *Hyperuricaemia*, sometimes associated with acute gout, occurs because alcohol oxidation increases hepatic uric acid synthesis and alcohol induced ketoacidosis decreases uric acid excretion by the kidneys.

The mortality of alcoholism is high, probably reducing life expectancy by around 10%. Furthermore, alcoholic mothers produce babies exhibiting features of intra-uterine growth retardation and mental deficiency, sometimes associated with motor deficits and failure to thrive. There are characteristic facial features which include microcephaly, micrognathia and a short upturned nose. This so-called *fetal-alcohol syndrome* is unlike that reported in severely undernourished women. Drinking in excess of 150 g alcohol daily carries substantial risks to the fetus, and most obstetricians now recommend either total abstinence or at the most 5 units per week during pregnancy.

Medical uses of alcohol

Apart from widespread use as a topical antiseptic and rubefacient systemic alcohol can be used:

1. As a night sedative in individuals who habitually take alcohol and are deprived of their drug in hospital.
2. Intravenous alcohol is occasionally used in obstetrics to suppress uterine contractions and delay premature labour. Given in moderate doses (30 ml/h for 2 h then 3 ml/h) it may induce drowsiness: higher intravenous doses may produce anaesthesia. Ethanol appears to be as effective as salbutamol in postponing pre-term labour.
3. In methanol poisoning, the administration of large amounts of ethanol compete for oxidation, slowing the rate of metabolism of methanol to toxic formaldehyde. An ethanol infusion is also useful in the management of ethylene glycol poisoning.
4. Alcohol included in oral opiate mixtures, e.g. of heroin and cocaine (Brompton mixture) for administration to the terminally ill patient. It may also improve appetite in such cases.
5. Vasodilator

Management of alcohol withdrawal

1. *Seizures* during alcohol withdrawal generally develop within 12–24 hours of withdrawal. They are usually generalised and status epilepticus is rare. They are managed with the usual agents. Development of features of the alcohol withdrawal syndrome, e.g. tremor, hallucinations, in a patient with a history of fits during previous withdrawal is an indication for the use of prophylactic anticonvulsants.

2. *Delirium tremens* is a medical emergency with a mortality of 5–10%. It occurs in less than 10% of patients withdrawing from alcohol. Management includes:

(a) careful nursing in a quiet evenly illuminated room, if possible by the same staff on each shift.
(b) sedation: either of the following agents are useful:
(i) Chlormethiazole. This is an effective sedative and anxiolytic but is potentially addictive. It may be given orally (2–4 capsules 8 hourly initially, reducing the dose to maintain light sedation) or as an intravenous infusion (0.8% solution, 40–100 ml initially over 10 minutes then reducing the rate to maintain sedation).
Chlormethiazole undergoes substantial pre-systemic metabolism when given orally and bioavailability is markedly increased in patients with cirrhosis in whom the oral dose must be reduced.
(ii) Benzodiazepines with a long half-life are suitable although cerebral sensitivity to these drugs is often decreased in alcoholics (cross-tolerance), so larger initial doses than usual are sometimes needed.
Note that deep sedation is undesirable as respiratory depression will predispose the patient to hypostatic pneumonia and pressure sores.
(c) Correction of fluid and electrolyte balance.
(d) Vitamin replacement with adequate thiamine (e.g. 100 mg parenterally, daily for 3 days).
(e) Psychiatric referral.

Long-term management of the alcoholic

1. Individual psychotherapy and group therapy may be appropriate. Many clinicians skilled in the management of such patients feel that they should never take alcohol again, while others feel that in certain cases alcohol can be allowed so long as consumption is carefully controlled.

2. Alcohol-sensitising drugs. These produce an unpleasant reaction when taken with alcohol.

(a) Disulfiram (Antabuse) inhibits aldehyde dehydrogenase leading to acetaldehyde accumulation if alcohol is taken which produces flushing, sweating, nausea, headache, tachycardia and hypotension. Cardiac arrhythmias may occur with large amounts of alcohol. The small amounts of alcohol included in many medicines may be sufficient to produce a reaction and it is advisable for the patient to carry a card warning of the danger of alcohol administration. The oral dose is 800 mg on the first day reducing over a week to 100–200 mg daily. Subcutaneous disulfiram implants are not recommended. It should be noted that disulfiram also inhibits phenytoin metabolism and can lead to phenytoin intoxication.

(b) Calcium carbimide (Abstem) acts similarly to disulfiram but usually produces a milder, more short-lived reaction with alcohol. It does not inhibit phenytoin metabolism. The dose is 50 mg twice daily.

Evidence for the efficacy of these agents in the routine treatment of alcoholism is lacking, but if the patient is motivated they may help during the first weeks of withdrawal when the craving for alcohol is strongest.

Interactions of alcohol with other drugs

1. Potentiation of effects of other CNS depressants, e.g. barbiturates, chloral, morphine, benzodiazepines.
2. Inhibition of metabolism of chloral via competition for alcohol dehydrogenase.
3. Acute alcohol ingestion may inhibit hepatic microsomal drug metabolising enzymes probably by binding to cytochrome P_{450}, thereby preventing cytochrome reduction by NADPH. Thus ethanol ingestion can retard the metabolism of some drugs, e.g. phenobarbitone.
4. Ethanol is a weak inducer of drug metabolism and its chronic administration results in increases in microsomal enzymes, cytochrome P_{450} and smooth endoplasmic reticulum. Increases in the rates of metabolism of warfarin, barbiturates, tolbutamide and phenytoin amongst others have been demonstrated. The evidence as to whether ethanol can induce its own metabolism is conflicting, probably most of the increased tolerance to ethanol seen in alcoholics is due to central adaptation, for they do not appear to metabolise ethanol very differently from non-drinkers.
5. Enhancement of gastric irritation of aspirin, indomethacin and other gastric irritants.
6. Alcohol apparently increases the rate of absorption of benzodiazepines but alcohol absorption is unchanged by codeine or cimetidine.
7. Alterations in ethanol metabolism by other drugs is relatively unusual, since unlike most drugs it is predominantly metabolised in the cytoplasm. Chlorpromazine inhibits ethanol metabolism by direct inhibition of the dehydrogenase whilst phenobarbitone, clofibrate and fructose enhance its elimination.
8. Disulphiram-type reactions (flushing of face, tachycardia, sweating, breathlessness, vomiting and hypotension) have been reported with metronidazole, procarbazine, sulphonylureas, latamoxef, cefamandole, cefoperazone and trichloroethylene (industrial exposure). There may be similar interactions with chloramphenicol and tolazoline. That these are caused by accumulation of acetaldehyde is not established.
9. Enhanced hypoglycaemia produced by insulin and oral hypoglycaemic agents.

Nicotine

Nicotine is an alkaloid present in the leaves of the tobacco plant, *Nicotiana tabacum.* There are no medical uses of nicotine but it is of very great importance in medicine because of its presence in tobacco.

Nicotine in low concentrations stimulates the nicotinic cholinergic receptors of autonomic ganglia, and in higher concentrations is a ganglion blocker. Thus smoking can accelerate the heart via sympathetic stimulation, or slow it due to sympathetic block or parasympathetic stimulation. There is usually cutaneous and splanchnic vasoconstriction with an increased peripheral vascular resistance. Respiration is stimulated, partly via stimulation of chemoreceptors in the carotid body. Adrenaline and noradrenaline are secreted from the adrenal medulla. The motor end-plate cholinergic receptors are initially stimulated and then blocked, producing a paralysis of voluntary muscle.

The results of extensive central stimulation include wakefulness, tremor, fits, anorexia, nausea, vomiting, tachypnoea and secretion of ADH. Nicotine is powerfully addicting, both psychologically and physically.

The percentage of nicotine in tobacco varies, but the smoke of a completely burned cigarette usually contains 1–6 mg and that of a cigar 15–40 mg. Acute administration of 60 mg of tobacco, (e.g. by ingestion) may be fatal.

Pharmacokinetics Large amounts of tobacco taken by mouth result in delayed gastric emptying and the nicotine may provoke vomiting. 90% of nicotine from inhaled smoke is absorbed, whilst smoke taken into the mouth results in only 25–50% absorption. As well as via the gastro-intestinal, buccal and respiratory epithelium, nicotine is also absorbed through the skin. A high concentration of nicotine may be present in the breast milk of smokers.

80–90% of circulating nicotine is metabolised in the liver, kidneys and lungs. Nicotine and its metabolites (cotinine, γ-(3-pyridyl)-γ-oxobutyric acid, 3-pyridylacetic acid and isomethylnicotinium ion) are excreted in the urine. Acidification of the urine accelerates excretion.

Each puff of cigarette smoke which is inhaled results in the absorption of 50–150 μg of nicotine. Smoking cigarette butts results in a much higher yield per inhalation. Thus each inhalation is equivalent to an intravenous injection of 1–2 μg/kg of nicotine. Smokers usually absorb 20–25% of the total nicotine in a cigarette. There is a rough correlation between the nicotine content of cigarettes and the peak plasma concentration of nicotine (see Table 22.3). The plasma elimination $t_{1/2}$ is 25–40 min.

Peak plasma levels after smoking cigarettes (1.2 mg nicotine) are similar to those after chewing gum containing 4 mg nicotine. However, the rate of rise is much slower after taking gum: peak nicotine levels were reached within 5 min after smoking a cigarette, whilst it took 15–30 min for the gum chewer to reach his peak. The use of such gums to wean smokers from cigarettes has therefore been of only limited success: perhaps because of this inability to mimic the

Table 22.3

Nicotine content of cigarette (mg)	*Peak plasma concentration (ng/ml)*
0.14	8.5
1.34	24.4
3.20	30.0

nicotine pharmacokinetics of smoking. However, some patients have found it useful, and nicotine chewing gum (Nicorette) in 2 mg and 4 mg pieces may now be prescribed. A high degree of motivation is always required if efforts to stop smoking are to be successful.

Adverse effects of smoking

1. In men under 70 years the ratio of death rate among cigarette smokers to non-smokers is 2 : 1. Above the age of 70 years this ratio is 1.5 : 1. The principal causes are heart disease, lung cancer, chronic obstructive lung disease and peripheral vascular diseases. Some of the specific causes of death which are positively related with smoking are:

ischaemic heart disease (strongest correlation);
cancers of lung, other respiratory sites and oesophagus, lip and tongue;
chronic bronchitis and emphysema, respiratory tuberculosis;
pulmonary heart disease;
non-syphilitic aortic aneurysm;
hernia.

There is a weak but positive association of smoking and death from the following:

cancers of rectum and pancreas;
pneumonia;
myocardial degeneration;
hypertension;
atherosclerotic disease;
cerebral thrombosis;
cirrhosis of liver and alcoholism;
peptic ulcer;
suicide and poisoning.

In several (but not all) surveys, cancer of the bladder is commoner in smokers compared with non-smokers. Naturally such statistical associations do not necessarily imply causal relationships. Smoking may, for example, be linked with some diseases because of personality factors, occupation or the association between smoking and alcohol consumption. One trial has shown a negative association between death from Parkinsonism and smoking.

2. Smoking is pleasurable for confirmed smokers, and once the habit is established it is very difficult to eradicate. Even though the rituals of smoking can enhance sociability and provide tactile, gustatory and oro-labial gratification, it is difficult to discount the role of nicotine or some other chemical agent in tobacco as being active as a drug of dependence. Both smoking and intravenous nicotine withdrawal can lead to an abstinence syndrome. This consists of craving, irritability, and sometimes physical features such as alimentary disturbances. The appetite for sugar is often increased during the withdrawal state.

3. Some of the metabolic disturbances of smoking, such as release of catecholamines and other amines from the adrenals, heart and platelets, rises in blood fatty acids and glucose, could predispose to cardiac arrhythmias, thrombosis and atherosclerosis. Further serious hazards from other products in smoke, in particular carbon monoxide, may also act as cardiotoxins and endanger ischaemic tissues.

4. Buerger's disease (thromboangiitis obliterans) is a disease of unknown aetiology, but it is severely aggravated by smoking. The coronary vessels may show other changes in addition to atherosclerosis: hyaline thickening in the arterioles occurs almost exclusively in heavy smokers; fibrous intimal thickening of the coronary arteries is also characteristic of 'smoker's heart'. Although smoking usually increases cardiac output, in patients with impaired cardiac function, a fall in cardiac output can result.

5. Smoking accelerates the ageing changes in the lungs. These processes include increased residual volume, decreased vital capacity, increase in the closing volume and a progressive fall in arterial oxygen tension. The underlying degenerative changes appear to be loss of lung elasticity and loss of compliance of the chest wall. In addition, chronic obstructive airways disease and bronchitis are associated with smoking. The development of emphysema can also be accelerated in cigarette smokers who have homozygous α_1 antitrypsin deficiency.

6. Smoking during pregnancy is associated with premature delivery, small babies and increased perinatal mortality. In households where the parents smoke, there is an increased risk of pneumonia and bronchitis in pre-school and school-children, most marked during the first year of life. This is presumably due to the effects of passive smoking by having to breathe in a polluted atmosphere.

Effect of smoking on drug disposition and effects

The commonest effect of tobacco smoking on drug disposition is an increase in elimination consistent with induction of drug-metabolising enzymes. Nicotine itself is metabolised more extensively by smokers than non-smokers and this is associated with an alteration in the rate of elimination of a number of other drugs. These effects are summarised in Table 22.4.

These changes in drug disposition may alter drug responses. Thus smokers require larger doses of pentazocine than non-smokers to achieve analgesia. The matter is complicated by the fact that smokers tend to have different sensory thresholds, psychosomatic characteristics and drug-consumption histories as compared to non-smokers. Thus whilst no effect on diazepam metabolism due to smoking has been observed, the Boston Collaborative Drug Surveillance Program (q.v.) has clearly demonstrated that heavy smokers

Table 22.4 Known effects of smoking on drug metabolism in man

Increased metabolism in smokers	*Unaffected by smoking*
Nicotine	Diazepam
Caffeine	Pethidine
Theophylline	Phenytoin
Phenacetin	Nortriptyline
Antipyrine	Ethanol
Imipramine	Warfarin
Pentazocine	

suffer less CNS depression after a standard dose of diazepam than non-smokers. Similar observations were also made for chlorpromazine and chlordiazepoxide. Whether these effects can be attributed to innate differences between smokers and non-smokers, to the presence of substances such as nicotine which exert their own pharmacological effects or to real pharmacokinetic differences has not yet been decided.

Xanthines

This group of compounds includes caffeine (present in the seeds of the coffee plant, *Coffea arabica*, tea leaves from *Thea sinensis*, cocoa from the seeds of *Theobroma cacao* and in soft drinks derived from the kola nut of the *Cola acuminata* tree.) Other members of the group are theobromine (in tea, coffee, cocoa and cola beverages) and theophylline (see p. 473). Caffeine is undoubtedly the most widely ingested alkaloid: in the USA the average intake from coffee alone is about 200 mg per day for persons over 10 years of age. In addition caffeine is included in a number of proprietary and prescription medicines, particularly occurring in analgesic combinations.

The major effects of these compounds are mediated by inhibition of phosphodiesterase, resulting in a raised intracellular cyclic AMP concentration.

1. *CNS effects* A very wide range of behaviour all the way from putting the shot to increased vigilance in boring tasks has been allegedly enhanced. These effects are less marked than with amphetamine and have been difficult to prove objectively. In large doses caffeine exerts an excitatory effect on the central nervous system manifested by tremor, anxiety, irritability and restlessness with interference with sleep. Such evidence as exists indicates that caffeine does not possess properties which lead to improved intellectual performance except perhaps when normal performance has been downgraded by fatigue or boredom. In animal experiments caffeine excites the CNS at all levels but the cerebral cortex is first affected, then the medulla, whilst the spinal cord is only affected by very large doses. The medullary respiratory, vagal and cardiovascular centres are all stimulated. Toxic doses result in convulsions but in man the toxic dose (over 10 g) is so large that human fatality is unlikely. Theophylline shares these actions but theobromine is virtually inactive in this respect.

2. *Circulatory effects* include direct myocardial stimulation producing tachycardia, increased cardiac output, ectopic beats and subjective feelings of palpitations. Direct effects on blood vessels result in dilatation of coronary, pulmonary and systemic vasculature but stimulation of the medullary vasomotor centre tends to counter this so that the effect on blood pressure is unpredictable. Recently it has been suggested that patients with hypertension may be susceptible to increased blood pressure following caffeine. The cerebral circulation responds differently by constriction, hence the use of caffeine in migraine.

3. *Bronchial smooth muscle* relaxes producing bronchodilatation. Respiration is also stimulated centrally.

4. *Mild diuresis* occurs due to an increased glomerular filtration rate subsequent to dilatation of the afferent arterioles. Theophylline is the most

powerful xanthine diuretic, theobromine has a more sustained effect but is less active whilst caffeine is the least powerful.

5. Caffeine increases *gastric acid secretion* via its action on cyclic AMP and xanthines in general may cause gastric irritation.

Pharmacokinetics Caffeine is rapidly and completely absorbed after oral administration. Xanthines undergo a complex series of hepatic metabolic transformations by demethylation and oxidation as well as eventual ring cleavage to produce a series of methylxanthines and methylurates. The plasma $t_{1/2}$ of caffeine is 2.5–12 h. There is some evidence that some of the enzymic steps in the metabolism of theophylline may obey Michaelis–Menten kinetics, resulting in overall dose-dependent kinetics. There is no evidence that this is true for caffeine. The plasma protein binding of caffeine is about 15% and there is significant salivary excretion of caffeine. Only 1–10% is excreted unchanged in the urine.

Caffeine dependence This is exceedingly common and doubtless benign since caffeine imparts a relaxed sense of social acceptance and mild stimulation. Tolerance is low grade but definitely exists, but does not appear to develop uniformly to all the effects of caffeine. Heavy users are allegedly less sensitive than light users to the nervousness and wakefulness caused by coffee but are more sensitive to the euphoriant and stimulant actions. A mild withdrawal syndrome manifested by headache (? due to withdrawal of caffeine's vasoconstrictor effect), lethargy, nervousness, irritability and inefficiency occurs 12–16 h after discontinuation. It is suggested that the breakfast cup of coffee wards off these dysphoric symptoms.

Adverse effects These are few. Much interest has recently been focused on the possibility that coffee drinking may be associated with an increased risk of myocardial infarction. Although known to cause extrasystoles this controversy has not yet been resolved.

Huge doses are teratogenic in rodents and other animal models: given the possibility of zero-order kinetics under such circumstances it is likely that this is of trivial interest to consumers.

DRUG OVERDOSE

Acute poisoning accounts for an increasing proportion of the work of medical units. In particular, self poisoning has become particularly common over the last 30 years and represents 10–30% of all acute admissions to medical hospital beds in the UK. A further 30% of patients with poisoning are treated at home by family doctors and an unknown proportion do not reach any medical aid.

The groups of drugs most commonly causing death from overdose have shown substantial changes over recent years. Whereas 15 years ago barbiturates were the commonest group to cause death their declining use has led to their being supplanted by other agents, particularly Distalgesic (dextropropoxyphene plus paracetamol), paracetamol alone and tricyclic antidepressants. Lithium, paraquat and salicylates continue to cause fatalities together with beta-adrenoceptor blockers, digoxin and aminophylline. However, the list of agents causing deaths from overdose does not reflect the incidence of overdose with individual compounds: in particular the benzodiazepines (often taken with alcohol) are the commonest group of drugs taken in overdose, but rarely lead to death. 80% of deaths from overdose occur out of hospital, with the mortality of those treated in hospital being less than 1%. The vast majority of cases of self-poisoning thus fall into the category of parasuicide (or a 'cry for help'), relatively few are serious suicide attempts.

The general principles of treatment of acute poisoning are:

(a) Diagnosis—clinical diagnosis; identification of drug (history, gastric aspiration, blood, urine); dose and blood concentration of drug; assessment of severity.
(b) Supportive therapy—maintenance of airways and respiration; treatment of circulatory failure; management of hypothermia; maintenance of fluid and electrolyte balance.
(c) Specific measures—prevention of further absorption; antidotes; forced diuresis; peritoneal dialysis and haemodialysis; haemoperfusion; exchange transfusion.
(d) Psychiatric assessment.

(a) **Diagnosis**

(i) The history from the patient or a companion should be taken whenever possible. A psychiatric history, particularly of depressive illness, previous suicide attempts and alcoholism or other drug dependence, is a most important clue of self-poisoning. Help in diagnosis may be given by clinical examination. Thus convulsions may be a feature of overdose with tricyclic antidepressants, antihistamines, narcotic analgesics, amphetamine, methaqualone and solvents (glue sniffing). The patient may present in coma with barbiturates, neuroleptics, alcohol, narcotic analgesics, glutethimide and tricyclic antidepressants. In early adult life acute poisoning is the commonest cause of coma in the absence of head injury. Extrapyramidal movements may indicate neuroleptic overdose whilst general motor restlessness could suggest salicylate or antihistamine poisoning. Pulmonary oedema may be a prominent feature of glutethimide and narcotic overdose. Although epidermal bullae are often thought to be a feature peculiar to barbiturate administration, this sign may appear in patients who are comatose due to a wide range of other causes: in particular poisoning with methaqualone, glutethimide, meprobamate, narcotics and tricyclics.

Glutethimide is the only drug which commonly causes papilloedema. Acute aspirin overdose may leave the patient alert, with flushing, pyrexia, overbreathing, tachycardia, tinnitus, deafness and sweating. Only in the most severe overdose is consciousness lost. The narcotic analgesics and anticholinesterases are unusual in producing small pupils. With both drugs, terminal respiratory failure leads to dilated pupils. However, dilated pupils (which react poorly to light) are also a feature of poisoning with tricyclic antidepressants, phenothiazines and other substances with anticholinergic activity, e.g. ingestion of the berries of the deadly nightshade, *Atropa belladonna*. Although patients are rarely comatose if these drugs alone have been taken, the clinical picture is confused if a CNS depressant, e.g. alcohol, has also been ingested. The patient may then present in coma with fixed dilated pupils. It is important to realise that full clinical recovery is usual if appropriate supportive care is provided.

It is important to look for skin puncture marks in addicts, although this may be made difficult in those who inject into tattoos or into the submucosal venous plexuses of the rectum or vagina. Necrosis and gangrene may follow injections of barbiturates and methaqualone. Depressed scars over veins may be left if these heal.

(ii) A history from the patient or his relatives or friends may reveal which drug has been taken and the likely dose. It is important to find out if alcohol or other drugs have been taken in addition. Mixtures of drugs are taken in approximately 30% of cases and alcohol has been taken in a further 30%. Although whenever possible the nature of the overdose should be elicited from the patient, in about 50% of instances the information given about the type and quantity of the drug taken is incorrect.

Analysis of gastric contents, blood and urine may be necessary in order to identify the drugs taken.

(iii) Even though the history often proves unreliable in assessing the severity of the overdose, in practice blood levels do not usually make much contribution to the patient's welfare. Clinical assessment and semiquantitative urine tests suffice for most patients.

(iv) The initial clinical assessment of the severity of poisoning is important because not only does this determine what treatment is required but it also provides a baseline from which to measure subsequent progress. The majority of drugs implicated in poisonings are central depressants and thus produce impairment of consciousness and depression of respiration and of the cardiovascular system.

A system of grading depression of consciousness is:

1. Patient is drowsy or asleep, but responds to vocal commands.
2. Patient is unconscious but responds to minimally painful stimuli.
3. Patient is unconscious and only responds to very painful stimuli.
4. Patient is unconscious and does not respond to any type of stimulus.

Respiratory function is assessed by monitoring respiratory minute volume. A Wright's respirometer may be used for this. If the minute volume is less than 4 l, then significant respiratory impairment is present, mechanical ventilation may be necessary and arterial blood pH, pCO_2, pO_2 and standard bicarbonate should be measured immediately. Respiratory depression may quickly progress to respiratory arrest followed by cardiac arrest. It is thus essential that intervention, with mechanical support of ventilation if necessary is begun as soon as possible. In addition, when respiratory depression is present the patient should always receive a test dose of intravenous naloxone (0.4–2.0 mg) which is a specific antagonist of opiates (see below). The action of naloxone is so specific and rapid (partial or complete reversal within 5 minutes) that it has a diagnostic as well as a therapeutic role in the management of acute opiate poisoning.

In addition to the CNS and respiratory depression, the cardiovascular system may also be depressed: either as a direct toxic effect of the drug or secondary to depression of these other two systems. Cardiovascular depression with hypotension may in turn lead to renal dysfunction and poor peripheral perfusion. Thus both blood pressure, urine output and central and peripheral temperature should be carefully monitored. Hypothermia (rectal temperature below 36°C) may also be due to hypothalamic depression.

In severely poisoned patients, baseline values of haematocrit, electrolytes, urea and creatinine should all be determined.

(b) Supportive therapy

(i) Maintenance of airway and respiration Once the airway has been cleared the patient should be nursed in a semiprone position. Even in the presence of respiratory failure analeptic drugs should never be given for hypnotic and psychotropic drug overdose. If the cough reflex is depressed in comatose patients a cuffed endotracheal tube should be inserted. However, in all unconscious patients accumulated oral, pharyngeal and tracheal secretions should be regularly aspirated. Intubation itself has complications, but the use of Portex tubes will allow tracheal intubation to last for 48–72 h. Tracheostomy is rarely required in acute poisoning.

When the pO_2 is reduced but above 8 kPa and pCO_2 between 5.2 and 6.6 kPa oxygen should be given by a Venturi mask, initially 24 % oxygen at a rate of 4 l oxygen/minute. If after 30 min the pCO_2 has not risen, then 28 % oxygen may be administered. If the pCO_2 rises above 6.6 kPa or pO_2 falls below 8 kPa, then assisted ventilation is required using a mechanical respirator.

(ii) Treatment of circulatory failure The restoration of respiration and acid–base balance may in themselves improve the circulation and therefore must have priority in order of treatment.

If hypotension persists, then active treatment should begin by raising the foot of the bed. This will be all that is required in 80 % of patients. In patients who do not respond to this measure, there is difference of opinion about the next step. Although plasma expanders such as blood, plasma or dextran may be initially effective, when the patient begins to recover they may develop acute circulatory overload due to the fact that many poisoned patients are not dehydrated and even though they may initially have a reduction in circulating fluid volume, they often have an increase in extravascular water. For this reason, it may be more sensible to use inotropic agents first to try and increase cardiac output and promote urine production, e.g. a combination of low dose dopamine and dobutamine. If these agents fail, then cautious infusion of plasma expanders may be indicated, with careful monitoring of central venous pressure.

(iii) Management of hypothermia Hypothermia increases the hazards of respiratory and circulatory failure. Severe hypothermia (30°C) in a young patient can be treated with rapid active rewarming in a bath of water at 40°C. In older patients and in those who have had prolonged severe hypothermia, rapid rewarming can produce cardiac arrhythmias or peripheral circulatory failure. Safer measures are warming the inspired air, by passing air through a Watter's cannister or by wrapping the patient in blankets and warming only one arm in a 43°C water bath.

(iv) Maintenance of fluid and electrolyte balance The importance of this has been mentioned in the management of peripheral circulatory failure. If the patient is conscious or recovers consciousness rapidly, fluids and electrolytes should be given by mouth. Patients who remain in coma for longer than 12 h are given intravenously alternate infusions of 0.5 l isotonic saline and 1 l of 5% glucose. From the start fluid balance charts are kept.

(c) Specific measures

(i) Prevention of further absorption The induction of vomiting in order to empty the stomach should only be attempted in conscious individuals. Mechanical stimulation of the pharynx (with a finger or other blunt instrument) is safer and usually more effective than drugs. Apomorphine can produce prolonged vomiting and shock. The effect of copper sulphate solution is uncertain and can be toxic. Ipecacuanha syrup (15 ml followed by a cup of water) may produce vomiting after about 15 min but the effect is not constant. Emetics do not completely empty the stomach and therefore gastric lavage is the treatment of choice, except in the case of children when a serious overdose is not suspected and when treating patients outside hospital (which should be avoided whenever possible). The most important danger of gastric lavage is vomiting followed by aspiration of gastric contents. The patient should be placed in the semi-prone position with the head lowered. If the cough reflex is absent, a cuffed endotracheal tube should be inserted. With most drugs the procedure is only of value if carried out within 4 h of ingestion. However, lavage may be of value when carried out up to 8 hours after a serious overdose with the following drugs which delay gastric emptying and are slowly absorbed: digoxin, β-adrenoceptor blockers, phenobarbitone, dextropropoxyphene, slow-release theophylline preparations, drugs with anticholinergic activity, e.g. tricyclic antidepressants, phenothiazines. In serious salicylate poisoning lavage is indicated up to 24 hours after the overdose.

A wide bore, lubricated tube is used, and in an adult a 30 gauge Jacques catheter is suitable. The stomach is aspirated and this first sample saved for future drug analysis if necessary. Lavage is then carried out with 300–600 ml aliquots of water at body temperature. Following an overdose of an iron preparation a solution of desferrioxamine is used, and desferrioxamine is left in the stomach at the end of the procedure.

Gastric lavage or induction of emesis are contraindicated if the patient has ingested corrosive agents, petroleum or related solvents like kerosene.

Activated charcoal is an oral adsorbant which is occasionally useful for prevention of further drug absorption. It is only of real benefit when present in a ratio of about 10 parts charcoal to 1 part drug, and when it is given within the first few hours of ingestion. It is thus likely to be useful when small amounts of a drug with the potential to cause substantial toxicity, e.g. a tricyclic antidepressant, have been taken. It is available both as 5 g sachets (Medicoal) which form an effervescent suspension in water or in powder form (Carbomix) for mixing with water. These liquid suspensions may be poured down a nasogastric tube if the patient is unable to drink.

(ii) Specific antidotes are available for a small number (about 2%) of poisons.

(iii) Forced diuresis as a method of accelerating excretion of a drug is only effective if the drug is normally substantially excreted by the kidney. In practice few drugs require this treatment. They are:

1. Salicylates; meprobamate (and other carbamates); barbitone and phenobarbitone—forced alkaline diuresis.
2. Amphetamine; fenfluramine; phencyclidine—forced acid diuresis.

NB. Contrary to previous belief, the elimination of quinine and quinidine does not seem to be substantially enhanced by forced acid diuresis.

Forced diuresis is discussed in more detail below (see p. 879).

(iv) Dialysis and haemoperfusion There are only a few patients who are so severely poisoned as to require the use of these techniques and there are relatively few drugs whose clearance is so substantially increased by them that they are removed in clinically useful amounts. It is obvious that to be successfully removed, a large proportion of the drug must either be present in plasma or be capable of rapid equilibration with it. Patients are considered for these techniques when they show signs of severe poisoning (e.g. Grade 4 coma) particularly if they deteriorate despite maximum supportive care, and they have high plasma levels of the toxic drug.

(*a*) *Peritoneal dialysis and haemodialysis* Although peritoneal dialysis requires no elaborate equipment and less medical supervision than haemodialysis, it is considerably less efficient than the former. In general, water-soluble drugs with relatively low molecular weight which are not extensively bound to protein or lipid are most readily dialysed. However, it is not always wise to act on theoretical considerations alone. For example, ethchlorvynol (Arvynol; Serenesil) is highly lipid soluble, yet is efficiently removed by dialysis. Also dialysis is of value in treating severe poisoning with phenobarbitone, salicylates and ethylene glycol. Lithium salts (as might be predicted) can be dialysed.

(*b*) *Haemoperfusion* through columns of ion-exchange resins or activated charcoal has been investigated because of the limitations of the older methods of removing drugs from the circulation. The use of charcoal is effective in severe barbiturate overdose, but several dangers complicate this. These include removal of electrolytes, platelets, leucocytes and fibrinogen. Fever and charcoal embolisation are other complications. The use of acrylic hydrogel-coated charcoal appears to be much safer and has been used to treat barbiturate and glutethimide overdose and may be of value in severe poisoning with methaqualone, salicylates, theophylline, ethchlorvynol, chloral and meprobamate.

(v) Exchange transfusion has been successfully used in the treatment of poisoning in young children and infants.

(d) Psychiatric assessment and treatment is of the utmost importance. The psychiatrist should not only be involved from the time the patient regains consciousness, but may have to diagnose and treat the family setting since the attempted suicide may be an expression of complex interpersonal problems.

ANTIDOTES TO POISONING

These are rarely of value since in many commonly encountered cases there is no specific antidote. A few examples are given below and others are discussed with the treatment of individual poisons (p. 868 et seq.)

1. Chelating agents

Chelating agents possess two or more electron donor groups in their molecule which can co-ordinate with a polyvalent metal. The resulting coordination metal complex has a ring structure.

For use in medicine the chelating agent and its metal complex must be non-toxic, soluble and readily excreted.

Dimercaprol (BAL) is effective in poisoning due to antimony, arsenic, copper, gold, lead and mercury. It is available as a 50 mg/ml solution in arachis oil and the dose is 2.5–5 mg/kg 4 hourly by deep intramuscular injection for 48 hours, reducing to 2.5 mg/kg, 12 hourly for 2 doses then once daily thereafter. Side effects include pain at the site of injection, nausea, vomiting, fever, salivation, discomfort in the mouth and throat, muscular aches and hypertension.

EDTA (ethylene diamine tetra acetic acid) is used as the trisodium salt (sodium versenate) or as the calcium disodium salt (calcium disodium versenate). The drug is given either intravenously or intramuscularly. If it is given by mouth it may enhance metal absorption. The main indication for its use is lead encephalopathy. However, Na_3EDTA can be given intravenously to remove calcium, plutonium, thorium and uranium. It is a toxic compound and the dose should not exceed 3 g/day. The immediate hazard is hypocalcaemia but it is also nephrotoxic.

Desferrioxamine mesylate (Desferal) is used in the treatment of iron salt poisoning (see below) and in the diagnosis of primary haemochromatosis.

Penicillamine (Distamine; Cuprimine) is dimethyl cysteine. It is rapidly absorbed from the gut and reaches peak levels in $\frac{1}{2}$–2 h. Clearance is almost complete in 24 h. Its main use in removing copper from patients with Wilson's disease and for the treatment of lead and mercury poisoning—although for the latter N-acetyl penicillamine may be preferable. In Wilson's disease 500–1000 mg penicillamine is given orally t.d.s. for life. The most serious toxic effect (usually seen with higher doses) is the nephrotic syndrome. Leucopenia is an indication to stop treatment. Pyridoxine deficiency can also occur.

Triethylene tetramine is an orally active chelating agent which may be suitable for patients with Wilson's disease who are intolerant to penicillamine.

2. Naloxone (Narcan) (see p. 330) is the alkyl derivative of oxymorphone. It is pure opiate antagonist with no intrinsic agonist activity—unlike nalorphine and levallorphan. Naloxone is an effective antagonist to a wide range of naturally occurring and synthetic narcotic analgesics—including morphine, diamorphine, pethidine, pentazocine, dextropropoxyphene, codeine and dipipanone.

Injected intravenously naloxone acts within 2 min and the plasma half-life is 1 hour, although the maximal clinical effect may last only 15 min. It is not itself sedating, does not depress respiration and does not affect pupil size. It may also be given intramuscularly. In a patient with suspected narcotic poisoning the initial dose is 1.2 mg intravenously. However, this usually has to be repeated since the $t_{1/2}$ of naloxone is much shorter than that of opiates and occasionally a naloxone infusion (2 mg in 500 ml of 0.9 % saline or 5 % dextrose) titrated to the patient's response is useful. Large doses of naloxone may be needed in cases of poisoning with long-acting narcotics, e.g. methadone, or the partial agonist buprenorphine.

The other principal uses of naloxone are reversal of narcotic depression of respiration in neonates and in anaesthesia. It can precipitate severe withdrawal reactions in narcotic addicts.

INDIVIDUAL POISONS

Opiates (see p. 839).

Paracetamol The patient remains conscious and yet as little as 10 g may produce fatal liver failure after a delay of 2–3 days. However, vomiting frequently occurs after swallowing large doses and this is sometimes sufficient to remove a dangerous overdose. The plasma level of paracetamol 4 h after ingestion gives an indication of prognosis (Fig. 22.3). In untreated patients, levels over 400 μg/ml are always followed by severe liver damage with a mortality of approximately 20 %. Four hour plasma levels of 150–300 μg/ml are followed by milder liver damage in 60–70 % of patients with a lower mortality. The mechanism of hepatocellular damage is not completely understood. Probably paracetamol itself is not toxic, but reactive metabolites produced by the action of hepatic cytochrome P_{450} are hepatotoxic and bind to the liver-cell proteins (see Fig. 22.4). This only occurs when hepatic glutathione stores have decreased to less than 30 % of normal and is promoted by pre-treatment with enzyme-inducing agents. After a paracetamol overdose it appears that the normal metabolic pathways (to glucuronide and sulphate) become saturated and in consequence an unstable reactive metabolite of unknown structure is formed. Normally this is detoxified by reaction with glutathione, but in the absence of the latter or if the capacity of this detoxication mechanism is exceeded it may react with liver cell proteins.

Substances which will substitute for or increase the level of glutathione have recently been used in treating paracetamol overdosage. They are protective

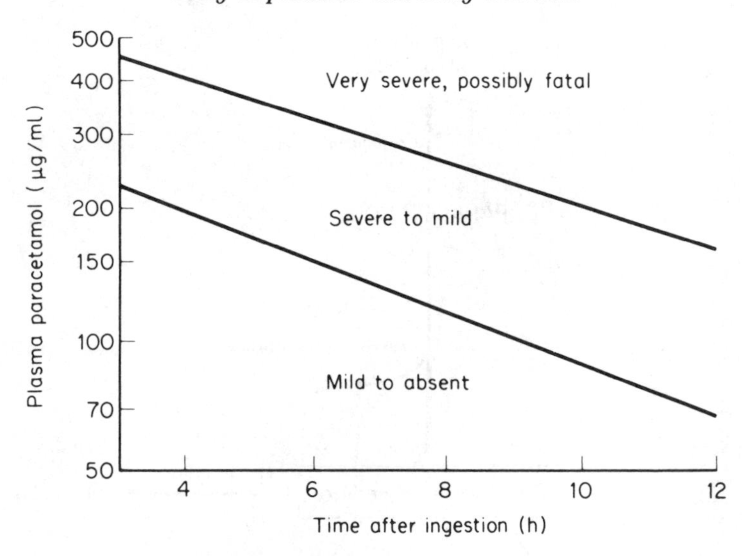

Fig. 22.3 Assessment of the probability of liver damage according to the plasma paracetamol concentration in relation to the time after ingestion (From L. F. Prescott *et al.*, *J. Int. Med. Res.*, **4**, Suppl. 4. 113 (1976))

agents rather than antidotes since they are ineffective once the reactive metabolite has become bound to the liver cells. At present it is not clear which of the following is the most effective treatment: our preference is for the least toxic, which is methionine. It is emphasised that all must be given as early as possible after overdosage:

1. Methionine (a precursor amino acid of glutathione)—2.5 g orally initially, followed by 2.5 g four hourly for 3 further doses (i.e. 10 g in 12 hours). There are usually no side effects from methionine, the only problem may be vomiting which can be controlled with an antiemetic. If the patient is unconscious (due to ingestion of other drugs) and cannot swallow, methionine tablets may be crushed and given via a stomach tube.
2. Acetylcysteine (Parvolex) (rapidly hydrolysed in the body to cysteine a precursor of glutathione)—150 mg/kg in 200 ml 5% dextrose over 15 minutes, then 50 mg/kg in 500 ml of 5% dextrose over 4 hours and 100 mg/kg in 1000 ml 5% dextrose over the next 16 hours. There have been several recent reports of adverse reactions to acetylcysteine both in therapeutic dose and following inadvertant overdose. These reactions are typically anaphylactoid in nature and commonly include flushing, rash, angioedema, hypotension and bronchospasm. They occur 20 to 60 min after commencing acetylcysteine and may be controlled by stopping the infusion and giving an antihistamine. Acetylcysteine should be used in preference to methionine if the patient is already vomiting, or in cases where a very large overdose has been taken.

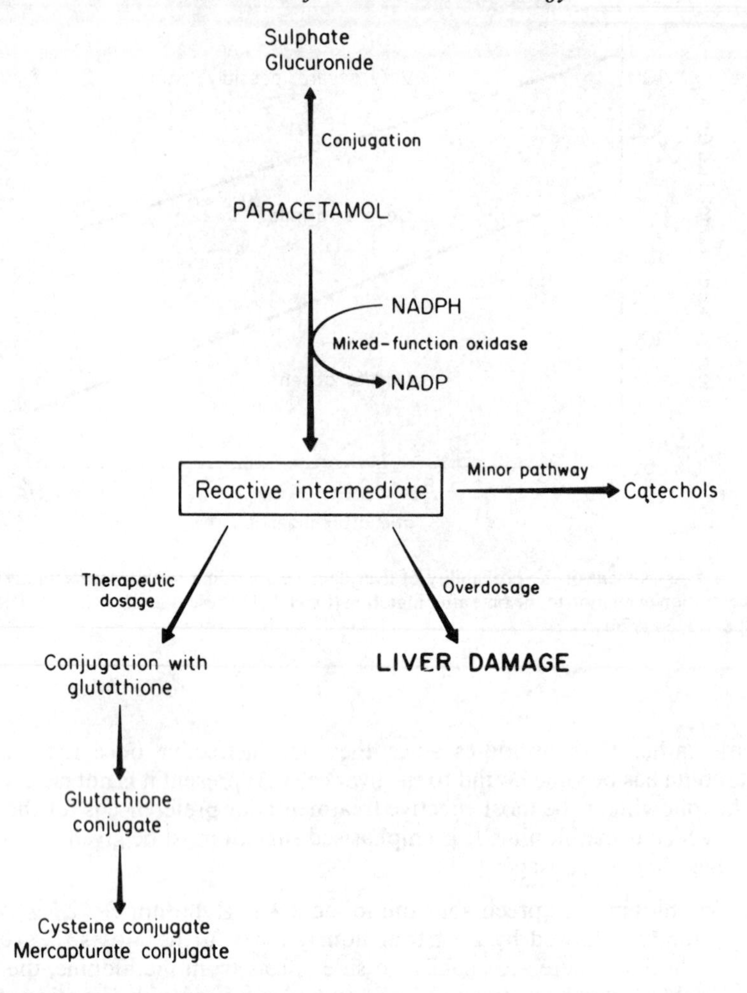

Fig. 22.4 Metabolic scheme for paracetamol in therapeutic and overdose.

As a rough guide, treatment should be given if the plasma paracetamol level exceeds the concentration line shown in Fig. 22.3 which joins 200 μg/ml at 4 h to 80 μg/ml at 12 h, since above this line there is a probability of mild to severe hepatoxicity. *The 'antidotes' should only be given if no more than* 10 *hours have elapsed since ingestion.* A kit is now available in many Casualty Departments which allows rapid estimation of plasma paracetamol concentration with reasonable accuracy which minimises the delay before appropriate management is instituted. If the plasma paracetamol level cannot be quickly estimated in this way, and there is a history of paracetamol overdose in the previous 12 hours a specific antidote should be started straight away. If the paracetamol level is subsequently found to be in the 'safe' range, treatment can then be stopped.

Cyanide at very low concentrations combines with ferric iron in cytochrome oxidase blocking tissue utilisation of oxygen. In treatment up to 50% of the patient's haemoglobin is converted to methaemoglobin by intravenous sodium nitrite (0.3 g in 10 ml) which preferentially combines with cyanide. Sodium thiosulphate (12.5 g in 50 ml) is then injected, which provides a sulphur donor for the conversion of cyanide to harmless thiocyanate by the tissue enzyme rhodanase. Hyperbaric oxygen is also used to bypass the tissue blockade of oxygen utilisation. An alternative and probably more effective treatment is intravenous *dicobalt edetate*. This chelates cyanide to form cobalticyanide, a stable and non-toxic compound. The dose is 600 mg as an intravenous bolus over 1 min, followed by a further 300 mg if there has been no response within one minute. The inhalation of amyl nitrite was previously popular as an antidote to cyanide poisoning but it can be regarded only as a short-term measure (as it yields inadequate levels of methaemoglobin) while a more definitive antidote is prepared.

Organophosphorus pesticides bind to cholinesterase, resulting in accumulation of acetylcholine at synapses and neuromuscular junctions. This produces initial stimulation followed by inhibition of transmission. Increased parasympathetic effects may be partially alleviated by atropine, but this has no effect on the neuromuscular effects which result from the nicotinic cholinergic receptors which are unaffected by atropine. *Pralidoxime* (30 mg/kg by i.v. or i.m. injection, 4 hourly for 24 h) reverses the toxic effects of organophosphorus compounds by attaching to cholinesterase-bound phosphate. This phosphate–pralidoxime complex then dissociates from the enzyme and so reactivates it.

Iron This initially produces a haemorrhagic gastroenteritis. After several hours headaches, confusion, fits and coma may be accompanied by shock. Patients may die from acute hepatic necrosis. *Desferrioxamine* treatment must be accompanied by appropriate supportive therapy. If the plasma iron is above 500 ng/ml in a child or 800 ng/ml in an adult then intravenous desferrioxamine should be given. Treatment often has to be started before the results of blood analysis are known. Gastric lavage is performed with a desferrioxamine solution (2 g/l) at the end of which 5 g desferrioxamine in 50 ml water is left in the stomach. The intravenous dose is 5 mg/kg/h but no more than 80 mg/kg/day should be given.

Digitalis A plasma digoxin level measured more than 6 hours after ingestion of the overdose provides an estimate of the severity of the overdose. The plasma potassium must also be measured: if low it may precipitate serious arrhythmias although hyperkalaemia often occurs in severe overdoses.

The patient should have continuous ECG monitoring and the plasma potassium must be normalised. Further absorption of digitoxin (but not digoxin) may be prevented by oral cholestyramine or colestipol. In seriously poisoned patients insertion of a temporary cardiac pacemaker is recommended. Ventricular arrhythmias are treated with conventional antiarrhythmic drugs although phenytoin (100 mg every 10 minutes up to a total dose of 1 g) has theoretical advantages because it speeds atrioventricular conduction. Quinidine and procainamide should be avoided. Magnesium sulphate (20 ml of 20% solution over 20 min) is useful to correct hypomagnesaemia and EDTA may be used to induce hypocalcaemia (which is antiarrhythmic). DC cardioversion should be avoided if possible. Recently a specific immunological antidote (Fab fragments of antidigoxin antibodies raised in sheep) has been used in severe digoxin poisoning with impressive results. This reagent is available from regional poisoning treatment centres.

β-adrenoceptor blockers Clinically patients usually present with hypotension and extreme bradycardia. The ECG may show intracardiac conduction defects or escape rhythms and seizures may occur.

Gastric lavage is worthwhile up to 8 hours after ingestion. Atropine should be given during lavage to prevent cardiac arrest due to vagal stimulation. For hypotension with severe reduction in cardiac output, the drug of choice is glucagon which has positive inotropic and chronotropic activity. It directly stimulates adenyl cyclase thus by-passing the β-receptors. An infusion of 5–15 mg glucagon/hour in 5% dextrose is often effective but if severe hypotension persists, other inotropes such as isoprenaline (providing β_2-receptor stimulation, but best avoided in ischaemic heart disease) or dobutamine (mainly β_1-receptor stimulation) may be used to compete for β-receptors and overcome the blockade. Severe bradycardia is treated with atropine and a pacing wire may be needed to manage conduction defects. Metabolic acidosis may develop and must be corrected as it exacerbates the arrhythmias.

Calcium blocking drugs Intravenous calcium gluconate (10–20 ml of 10% solution given slowly) may reverse both hypotension and arrhythmias although this is disputed. The blood pressure may be supported by infusion of appropriate amounts of saline.

Theophylline This is most commonly taken as a slow-release preparation, so gastric lavage followed by activated charcoal is useful up to 12 hours after the overdose. Oral activated charcoal may reduce absorption. Nausea, vomiting and gastritis are common. The major problems encountered are arrhythmias and fits but most patients respond to supportive measures. Hypokalaemia should be corrected and verapamil is probably the best drug for supraventricular tachycardia. Non-selective β-blockers may be useful in non-asthmatic patients but should be avoided in asthmatics because of the risk of bronchospasm. If the patient is severely poisoned as shown by the clinical picture and a high blood level, then haemoperfusion is indicated. However, drug levels must be closely monitored as a rebound increase may occur when haemoperfusion is discontinued.

Paraquat Large doses produce death in a few days by pulmonary oedema and haemorrhage, and by toxic effects on the kidney, liver, heart and adrenals. Smaller doses result in later mortality by progressive respiratory failure due to pulmonary fibrosis. Intermediate doses (10–20 ml of paraquat concentrate) initially produce only discomfort and ulceration of the mouth and pharynx, later progressive renal failure may develop.

Although blood levels give an indication of the severity of poisoning and of the likely outcome, in practice a strongly positive qualitative urine test is sufficient to predict a fatal outcome. The patient may feel initially well, but the lung progressively concentrates paraquat, and thus pulmonary deterioration is delayed. Treatment should therefore begin as early as possible and include gastric lavage, leaving adsorbents such as Fuller's Earth or bentonite in the stomach, purgation and haemoperfusion through charcoal. Forced diuresis may have a protective effect on the kidneys. The toxic effects of paraquat result from the oxidation of an unstable free radical formed by paraquat to form a superoxide (Fig. 22.5). The latter normally occurs in small amounts in the body and is detoxified by superoxide dysmutase. In paraquat overdose the capacity of the enzyme is exceeded and the superoxide produces cellular damage probably by peroxidation of membrane lipids and enzymes (this is probably how it acts as a weedkiller). At present no treatment can reverse these effects or absorb the superoxide to render it harmless, and antidotes such as superoxide dismutase, cyclophosphamide, steroids or vitamin E have not been of proven benefit.

Lomotil is an antidiarrhoeal preparation. Each tablet or 5 ml of liquid contains 2.5 mg of diphenoxylate hydrochloride (a narcotic analgesic) and 0.025 mg of atropine sulphate. The drug is dangerous in overdose and even apparently modest doses have produced dangerous respiratory depression in

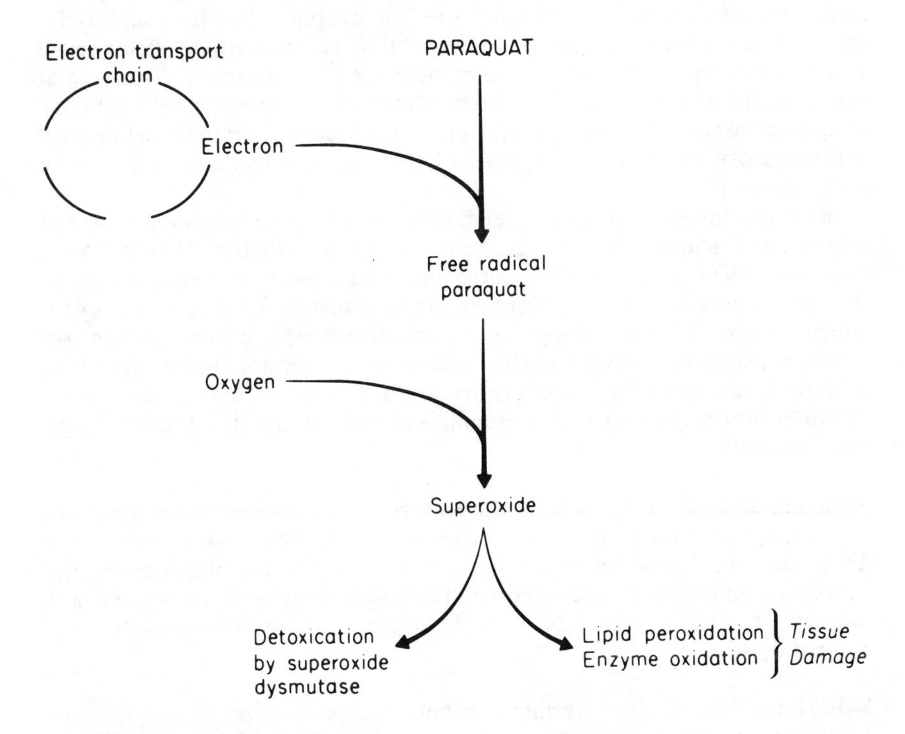

Fig. 22.5 Toxic activation of Paraquat.

young children. Atropine not only produces a dry mouth and skin, flushing and hallucinations, but delays gastric emptying so that the narcotic effects—coma and respiratory depression—may only begin after several hours. Even if gastric lavage is delayed, tablets may still be recovered from the stomach. Coma and respiratory depression is due to diphenoxylate and antagonised by naloxone.

Dextropropoxyphene This is available in the UK alone or in combination with paracetamol. Distalgesic tablets contain 32.5 mg dextropropoxyphene hydrochloride with 325 mg paracetamol and are becoming a common cause of drug overdose. Symptoms and signs appear within 30 min and are initially due to the dextropropoxyphene. These include nausea, vomiting, small pupils, drowsiness, generalised and focal fits and cardiovascular collapse. Serious respiratory depression, sometimes with pulmonary oedema, can develop in the first hour. Less commonly transient diabetes insipidus and cardiac conduction defects are also found. Toxicity can occur with ingestion of 10 mg/kg of dextropropoxyphene and respiratory arrest has occurred after 35 mg/kg. Serum and urine levels do not indicate the amount of drug ingested or severity of the poisoning. Naloxone is a specific antagonist, but general supportive measures must also be applied. The usual treatment for paracetamol overdosage is also necessary.

Tricyclic antidepressants in overdose may produce coma, seizures, hypotension, cardiac failure and arrhythmias as well as atropine-like effects such as dry mouth, dilated pupils, urinary retention and ileus. The cardiac effects result from a complex interaction between blockade of transmitter re-uptake at synapses and the anticholinergic effects. Metabolic acidosis may occur and is a dangerous complication as central depression of respiration reduces the usual compensatory response of hyperventilation. It also increases the risk of arrhythmias.

Management involves careful, repeated monitoring for the development of hypoxia and acidosis, which must be corrected immediately. If arrhythmias then occur, they should only be treated if they seriously impair cardiac output: the usual agents are used. Intravenous benzodiazepines should control any fits which occur. Physostigmine, an anticholinesterase which crosses the blood–brain barrier, was previously used to reverse the anticholinergic effects of these drugs. However, it has a short duration of action and the dose needs careful titration as it may itself cause fits and arrhythmias. It is thus no longer recommended.

Monoamine oxidase inhibitors The features of overdose include agitation, hallucinations, tachycardia, hyperreflexia, convulsions and hyperthermia. There may be hypertension or hypotension. A short-acting α-adrenergic blocking agent such as phentolamine (Rogitine) 5 mg with or without a β-blocker or alternatively labetalol (Trandate) 100 mg intravenously may control these effects.

Salicylates Except as a terminal event, the patient remains conscious. Vomiting is frequent even after relatively small amounts of salicylate. Plasma concentrations in the therapeutic range (200–350 mg/l) may result in deafness, tinnitus, headache, vertigo, nausea, irritability or other psychological disturbances. Hyperventilation usually occurs at levels of about 400 mg/l and this results in decreased pCO_2, and respiratory alkalosis can be severe enough to promote tetany. Metabolic acidosis is due to salicylate itself and tricarboxylic acid cycle intermediates (accumulating due to oxidative uncoupling by salicylate) acting as fixed acids and occurs above levels of 600 mg/l. In the range 700–900 mg/l coma, fever, hypothrombinaemia, cardiovascular collapse and renal failure may develop. Metabolic acidosis occurs sooner and at lower levels in children. Prognosis is related to the blood salicylate level, although in children it has been shown that with increasing overdosage the apparent volume of distribution is increased so that the plasma level measured is proportionately lower despite a higher salicylate body load. A nomogram relating plasma salicylate level and expected severity of intoxication at varying intervals following ingestion of a single dose of salicylate is shown in Fig. 22.6.

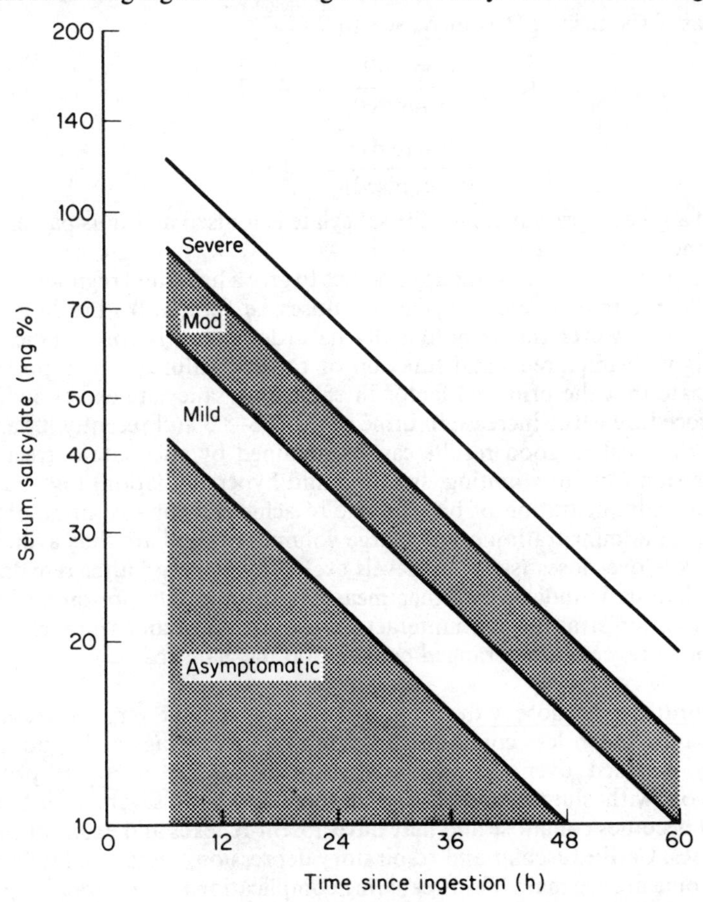

Fig. 22.6 Nomogram relating serum salicylate concentration and expected severity of intoxication at varying levels following ingestion of a single dose of salicylate (From A. K. Done, *Pediatrics*, **26**, 801 (1960). Copyright American Academy of Pediatrics (1960).)

A plasma level on admission of over 500 mg/l in adults or 300 mg/l in children warrants active treatment with alkalis. The underlying principle is that since the renal tubule acts as a lipid membrane an ionised molecule within the lumen cannot diffuse out into the peritubular space. From the Henderson–Hasselbalch equation,

$$\log_{10}\frac{\text{(ionised drug)}}{\text{(un-ionised drug)}} = \text{pH} - \text{pKa}.$$

Thus in urine at pH 5.4 for salicylate pKa 3.4

$$\log_{10}\frac{\text{(ionised)}}{\text{(un-ionised)}} = 5.4 - 3.4 = 2,$$

so

$$\frac{\text{(ionised)}}{\text{(un-ionised)}} = 100,$$

whereas if the urine pH is increased to 7.4

$$\log_{10}\frac{\text{(ionised)}}{\text{(un-ionised)}} = 7.4 - 3.4 = 4$$

and

$$\frac{\text{(ionised)}}{\text{(un-ionised)}} = 10\,000,$$

so that a greater proportion of the salicylate is ionised and thus passes out in the urine (see Fig. 22.7).

It has previously been standard practice to give a high fluid regimen together with alkali to treat severe salicylate overdoses, i.e. forced alkaline diuresis (see Fig. 22.8), however this is potentially hazardous, and is contraindicated in patients with impaired renal function or cardiac failure. It is important to appreciate that the principal factor in enhancing salicylate excretion during this procedure is the increase in urine pH to 7.5–8.5 and recently it has been found that just as good results can be obtained by adequate correction of dehydration (due to vomiting, sweating and hyperventilation) together with judicious administration of bicarbonate to achieve a suitable urine pH. The hazards of administration of very large volumes of fluid are thus avoided. In very severe overdoses (salicylate levels exceeding 800 mg/l after rehydration) haemodialysis is indicated. Other measures in salicylate poisoning include antacid administration to counteract gastric irritation and vitamin K in an attempt to reverse the deranged coagulation mechanisms.

Barbiturates Overdose with this group of drugs may be very dangerous but has become much less common as the use of these drugs as hypnotics has sharply declined over the past ten years. Moderate overdose produces confusion with slurred speech and nystagmus. With severe overdose the patient becomes comatose and may have absent reflexes and extensor plantar responses. Cardiovascular and respiratory depression, acute renal failure and pneumonia are the main life-threatening complications. In general, if a patient has taken 10 times the therapeutic dose then severe poisoning is likely.

Supportive measures are usually sufficient but in patients severely poisoned with barbitone or phenobarbitone, which are excreted by the kidneys, forced

Table 22.5 Drug levels in toxicology. NB The concentrations cited here are approximations and other factors may modify the patient's response. Interpretation may be complicated by multiple drug ingestion

Drug	Plasma concentration (mg/l) associated with severe toxicity	Approximate upper limit of therapeutic plasma concentration
Alcohols		
Ethanol	3.0 g/l	(0.8 g/l legal driving limit)
Methanol	0.2 g/l	
Anticonvulsants		
Phenobarbitone	100	30
Phenytoin	35	20
Hypnotics and anxiolytics		
Barbitone	100	15
Other barbiturates	50	5
Chloral (as trichlorethanol)	100	10
Chlordiazepoxide	5.5	1.5
Chlormethiazole	10	2
Diazepam	5	1
Desmethyldiazepam	5	1.5
Ethchlorvynol	100	20
Glutethimide	40	4
Meprobamate	40	20
Methaqualone	20	4
Antidepressants		
Amitriptyline + Nortriptyline	1	0.2
Nortriptyline	1	0.15
Phenothiazines		
Chlorpromazine	1.5	0.5
Analgesics		
Paracetamol	200–300 (4 h post ingestion) 100–150 (12 h post ingestion)	20
Pethidine	5	0.6
Salicylate	600	250
Miscellaneous		
Carbon monoxide	15–30%	—
Digoxin	5 μg/l (but variable)	2 μg/l
Iron	6	—
Lead	5 μmol/l (adult) 4 μmol/l (children)	2 μmol/l (adult) 1.5 μmol/l (children)

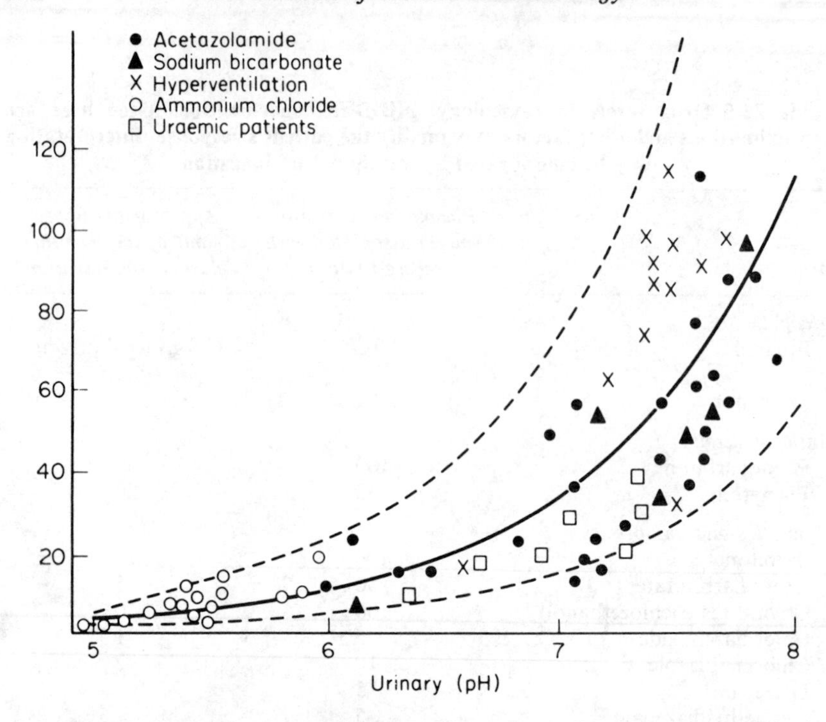

Fig. 22.7 Relationship between free salicylate clearance and urinary pH in normal subjects and patients with plasma salicylate levels of 15–18 mg/100 ml. Three alkalinising agents were used as shown but the effect on salicylate clearance was identical, i.e. urinary pH, not systemic acid-base balance, determines urinary salicylate clearance. The calculated regression line and the limits at twice the standard deviation (dotted lines) are shown. (From C. R. MacPherson *et al.*, *Brit. J. Pharmacol.*, **10**, 484 (1955). Reproduced by permission of the British Pharmacological Society.)

alkaline diuresis is effective. With other barbiturates (which are largely metabolised by the liver) haemoperfusion or haemodialysis should be considered if the patient is severely poisoned and has not responded to conservative measures.

Glutethimide Papilloedema can develop with fixed dilated pupils and episodes of apnoea. At the first sign of papilloedema, an intravenous infusion of 500 ml of 20% mannitol should be given over 20 min. This is followed by 500 ml of 5% glucose given over the next 4 h. It cannot be removed by haemodialysis because of its high lipophilicity, but haemoperfusion through charcoal columns is effective in lowering plasma levels.

Methaqualone Comatose patients may exhibit hyperreflexia, myoclonic jerks and fits. Papilloedema and pulmonary oedema may also develop.

Phenothiazines Comatose patients may also show Parkinsonism and dyskinesias which respond to benztropine 2 mg i.v. Fits are treated with diazepam.

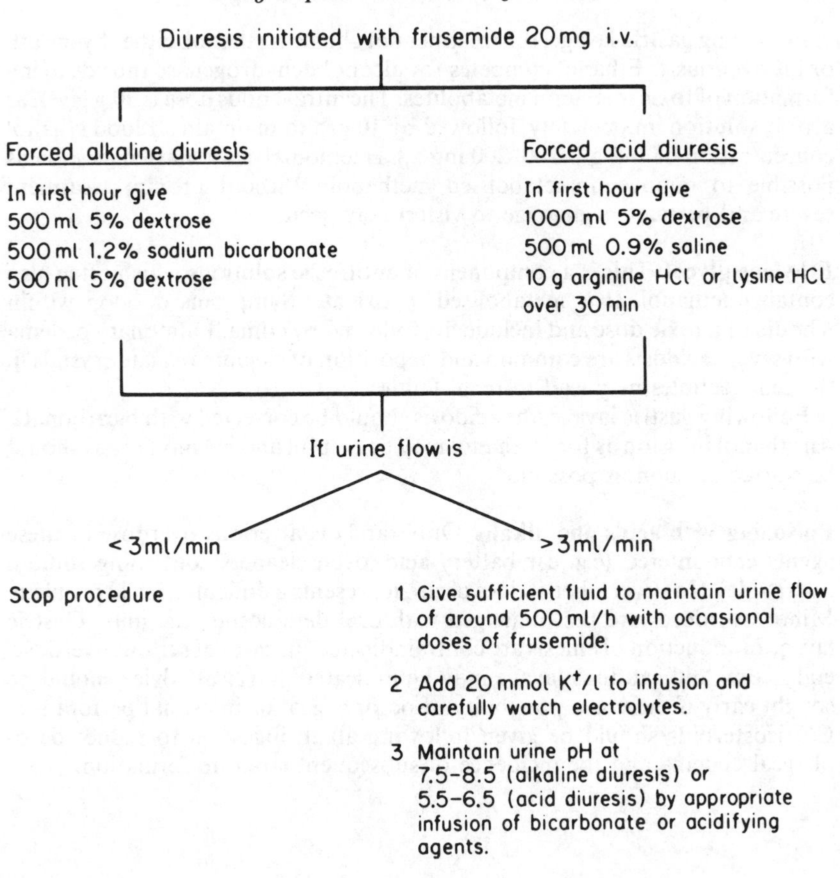

Fig. 22.8 Scheme for forced alkaline or acid diuresis.

Carbon monoxide binds to haemoglobin, forming carboxyhaemoglobin. Symptoms of headache begin at saturations of 10–20% of carboxyhaemoglobin and weakness, dizziness, nausea and failing vision occur at 40%. Syncope leading to coma with intermittent convulsions and death occur at 60–80%. The treatment consists of rest (to reduce oxygen demand) and administration of oxygen. Hyperbaric oxygen may be useful. Parkinsonism can follow damage to the basal ganglia by carbon monoxide and may be permanent. Some patients also suffer myocardial damage and care must be taken with infusions or too vigorous mobilisation.

Methanol Small amounts of methanol may cause severe toxicity, principally due to its metabolites, formaldehyde and formic acid, produced by alcohol dehydrogenase. Symptoms develop 10–48 hours after ingestion of an overdose and include confusion, visual disturbance and severe abdominal pain with nausea and vomiting. On examination the patient is typically hyperventilating due to metabolic acidosis, there is optic papillitis due to retinal toxicity and fits followed by coma may ensue.

Following gastric lavage, the treatment of choice is ethanol, either by mouth or intravenously. Ethanol competes for alcohol dehydrogenase thus delaying formation of toxic methanol metabolites. The intravenous dose is 30 g given as a 10 % solution immediately, followed by 10 g/h to maintain a blood ethanol concentration of 1–2 g/l (100–200 mg %). Haemodialysis is started as soon as possible to remove unmetabolised methanol. Without prompt treatment severe and permanent damage to vision may occur.

Ethylene glycol This is a component of antifreeze solutions which often also contain methanol. It is metabolised to oxalate. Symptoms develop within 6 hours of a toxic dose and include fits followed by coma. Pulmonary oedema with severe acidosis are common and deposition of calcium oxalate crystals in the renal tubules may lead to renal failure.

Following gastric lavage, the acidosis should be corrected with bicarbonate. An ethanol infusion as for methanol may be helpful and haemodialysis should be started as soon as possible.

Poisoning with acids and alkalis Only rarely is a serious overdose of these agents encountered (e.g. car battery acid, oven cleaners containing sodium hydroxide). However when it does occur, it presents a difficult clinical problem. Minor overdoses are best managed with oral demulcents, e.g. milk. Gastric lavage or induction of emesis are contraindicated. In cases of serious overdose, endoscopy and cautious lavage may be indicated. Surgical advice should be sought early if there is a possibility of oesophageal or intestinal perforation. Corticosteroids should be given following alkali ingestion to reduce oesophageal oedema and the incidence of subsequent stricture formation.

Appendix 1
LEGAL ASPECTS OF DRUG PRESCRIBING

The laws relating to the prescription and supply of drugs have recently undergone a major overhaul in the UK since previous regulations, which had grown up piecemeal, were manifestly unable to cope with the demands of modern medical practice. The laws chiefly affecting doctors are as follows.

1. Misuse of Drugs Act 1971

Drugs controlled under this Act are divided into three Classes, A, B and C, in decreasing order of harmfulness. This division is solely for the purpose of determining penalties under the Act. Thus some commonly encountered drugs in each category are:

Class A: Cannabinol and derivatives (except where contained in cannabis)
Cocaine
Dextromoramide (Palfium)
Diamorphine, Phenazocine, Pethidine
Fentanyl
Lysergide and its derivatives (LSD)
Mescaline
Methadone
Morphine and Opium

Class B: Amphetamine, Methylamphetamine, Methylphenidate and Phenmetrazine
Cannabis and Cannabis resin
Codeine, Dihydrocodeine and Pholcodeine

Class C: Benzphetamine, Chlorphentermine and Mephentermine
Methaqualone.

The Act gives powers to Ministers to combat changes in drug abuse by amending these lists as seems necessary on advice from the Advisory Council on the Misuse of Drugs. This consists of not less than 20 members, with wide experience of the medical and social effects of drug abuse, whose function is to keep the national drug-abuse situation under review. The Act prohibits import or export of controlled drugs without licence and makes it an offence to produce a controlled drug or to supply or offer to supply one to another person. It is therefore illegal to knowingly grow cannabis in the garden. Similarly unlawful possession of a controlled drug is an offence as is allowing the use of premises for illegally producing a controlled drug, for smoking cannabis or opium or for preparing opium for smoking.

Doctors acting in professional capacity may lawfully prescribe, administer, manufacture or supply a controlled drug but may be required to give information concerning quantities, number and frequency of occasions that the drug was prescribed, administered or supplied by him. It is an offence not to comply without reasonable excuse with this request or to give false information. There is no right of entry to a doctor's premises without a search warrant but the police may enter the premises and request the production of any documents relating to dealings with controlled drugs and inspect the stocks of such drugs.

2. Notification and Supply to Addicts Regulations 1973

These regulations imposed upon medical practitioners an obligation to notify addicts to the following drugs: cocaine, dextromoramide, diamorphine, dipipanone, hydrocodone, hydramorphone, levorphanol, methadone, morphine, opium, oxycodone, pethidine, phenazocine and piritramide. Notification must be made within 7 days to the Chief Medical Officer at the Home Office giving name, sex, date of birth, address and National Health Service number together with the drug involved and the date of attendance. Notification is not necessary if the doctor believes that the drug is medically necessary or if the doctor or his partner (or colleague in hospital) has notified the patient within the preceding 12 months. Notification should be confirmed in writing if the patient is still being treated by the doctor. Except for the treatment of organic disease or injury a doctor must not administer or supply heroin, cocaine or any of their salts to an addict unless he has a licence from the Secretary of State to do so. This regulation effectively gives the treatment of these addicts over to specially designated physicians.

The index of addicts at the Home Office may be consulted by any doctor for information about a person under his care. It is sensible to check (by telephone) all new cases of addiction or suspected addiction against the index before prescribing controlled drugs as a safeguard against addicts obtaining simultaneous prescriptions from two or more doctors.

Failure to notify an addict is an offence and can result in withdrawal of the doctor's authority to prescribe, administer, supply or authorise the supply of controlled drugs. Failure to comply with this direction is an offence and is treated in the same way as irresponsible prescribing of controlled drugs.

3. Misuse of Drugs Regulations 1973

Like the preceding regulations these amplify the provisions of the 1971 Act and control the use of a number of drugs specified into 4 schedules.

Schedule 1 This specifies preparations (excluding injections) of certain Controlled Drugs in which the drugs are in such small amounts or are combined with other substances so that they have no, or negligible, risk of abuse or so that the Controlled Drug cannot be recovered in a yield which would contribute a risk to public health. Of the many drugs in this schedule only the following are practically important:

(a) All commonly used preparations of codeine are exempt from the controls applying to codeine itself: thus codeine linctus and codeine phosphate tablets B.P. are not regarded as Controlled Drugs and so no record in the register of Controlled Drugs need be made when they are given.
(b) Pholcodeine and diphenoxylate preparations are exempt.
(c) Dihydrocodeine (DF118) tablets but not injection are exempt.
(d) Preparations containing not more than 0.2% morphine—thus kaolin and morphine mixture and similar proprietary mixtures—are exempt.
(e) Buprenorphine is not a controlled drug.

Schedules 2 *and* 3 These specify many drugs (some never marketed in the UK, but included because of international obligations under the United Nations Convention on Narcotic Drugs 1961). The opiates and the amphetamine group are included in this schedule, which details the controls required for the possession, supply and production of these drugs. From 1 January 1985 barbiturates (excluding hexobarbitone, methohexitone, thialbarbitone and thiopentone) and diethylpropion have been included in Schedule 3. Diethylpropion, but not the barbiturates must be securely stored (e.g. in a controlled drugs cabinet). The requirements for their prescription is therefore the same as for opiates (as specified below). It is allowable for an emergency supply of phenobarbitone to be given by a pharmacist to a patient for the treatment of epilepsy. Doctors have a general authority to possess these drugs and to administer or direct their administration to patients. A patient may possess these drugs only if they are supplied on prescription and commits an offence if he fails to disclose to the prescribing doctor that he is already being supplied with a controlled drug by another doctor. It is also illegal to make a false statement for the purpose of obtaining a prescription for a controlled drug. The purpose of these restrictions is to prevent addicts or traffickers in drugs from obtaining prescriptions for controlled drugs from several doctors. A prescription for a controlled drug in schedules 2 or 3 must conform to the following rules:

(a) In the doctor's own handwriting in ink or other indelible medium it must state:
    (i) name and address of patient
    (ii) the dose to be taken and the form (e.g. capsules, tablets) and, where appropriate, the concentration of the preparation.
    (iii) the total quantity of the preparation or the number of dosage units to be supplied, this to be written in both words and figures.
    (iv) the doctor's signature and date.
(b) The doctor's address need not be written but must appear on the prescription.

For the prescription to be dispensed the prescription must comply with the above format and in addition

(a) The prescriber's address must be within the UK.
(b) It must be presented within 13 weeks of the date on the prescription.
(c) The pharmacist must be assured that the signature of the prescriber is genuine.

Schedule 4 This contains substances such as cannabis, coca leaf and poppy straw which are not used in medicine and LSD and its derivatives. Possession of drugs in this schedule is limited to research or other special purposes and a licence from the Home Office is required.

Registers must be kept for all drugs specified in Schedules 2 and 4 and these can be examined by the authorities on demand. Entries must be chronological and must be indelible. No entry may be altered, cancelled or obliterated and any correction must be accompanied by an explanatory footnote.

4. Misuse of Drugs (Safe Custody) Regulations 1973

These regulations require that any controlled drug other than those in Schedule 1 must be kept in a locked receptacle which can only be opened by the doctor or somebody authorised by him to open it. A locked car or briefcase is not regarded as a locked receptacle for the purpose of the regulations.

5. Medicines Act 1968: Part III Medicines (Prescription Only) Order

These regulations became effective in February 1978, and replaced previous regulations restricting substances in Schedule 4 of the Poisons Rules and Part II of the Therapeutic Substances Act to prescription only. In place of these laws the Medicines Act categorises drugs into:

(a) General Sale List: these may be purchased in any kind of shop or even from an automatic machine.
(b) Prescription Only Medicines: for which a prescription is required.
(c) Pharmacy Only: drugs not in category (a) or (b) but which can be supplied to a patient directly by a pharmacist without prescription.

In some cases it is the dosage which determines whether a drug is in category (a) or (b). The pharmacist is also enabled to sell legally many ethical drugs previously limited to prescription provided the dosage is kept down. There is also provision made for the supply of emergency drugs at the request of a patient provided that only a small supply is given, that it has previously been prescribed by a doctor and that the substance requested is not in Schedule 2 of the Misuse of Drugs Act 1971 (see above) or one of a number of other substances like barbiturates (except for epilepsy) or poisons like cyanide or strychnine.

Note that provisionally registered doctors cannot write prescriptions for POMs for dispensing outside of hospital.

Appendix 2

GLOSSARY OF SYMBOLS

A	The ordinate (units of concentration) intercept obtained by extrapolating the secondary plot back to time zero when analysing a biexponential curve by the method of residuals
α	Apparent first-order rate constant of the distributive phase of a drug which confers upon the body the characteristics of a two-compartment model
AUC	Area under the plasma concentration–time curve
$(AUC)_{i.v.}$	Area under the plasma concentration–time curve following intravenous drug administration
$(AUC)_{oral}$	AUC for oral administration
B	The ordinate (units of concentration) intercept obtained by extrapolating the β-phase back to time zero on the log plasma concentration–time plot
β	Apparent first-order rate constant for elimination phase of a drug conferring upon the body the characteristics of a two-compartment model. The disposition rate constant
C	Drug concentration in plasma
$\frac{dC}{dt}$	Rate of change of drug concentration in plasma
$\int_0^\infty \bar{C}\,dt$	Total area under the plasma concentration–time curve
$\bar{C}$	'Average' plasma drug concentration at steady state after multiple dosing.
C_1	Drug concentration in the central compartment
C_2	Drug concentration in the peripheral compartment
C_{Cr}	Plasma creatinine concentration
C_{max}	Maximum plasma concentration attained
C_{min}	Minimum plasma concentration attained
C_{ss}	Steady-state plasma concentration
Cl	Total body clearance of drug
Cl_{cr}	Creatinine clearance
Cl_H	Hepatic clearance of drug
Cl_{int}	Intrinsic hepatic clearance of drug
Cl_r	Renal clearance of drug
D	Diffusion constant.
E	Hepatic extraction ratio
F	Fraction of dose available for absorption (bioavailability fraction)
$\underline{F}$	Fraction of administered dose available to the circulation: a more rigorously defined form of F
f_b	Fraction of unbound drug in the blood

f_t	Fraction of unbound drug in the tissues
K_a	Association constant
K_d	Dissociation constant
K_m	Apparent Michaelis constant
k	Apparent first-order elimination rate constant of a drug that confers upon the body the characteristics of a one-compartment model
k_a	Apparent first-order absorption rate constant
k_{nr}	First-order rate constant for non-renal elimination
k_o	Infusion rate of a drug, i.e. zero order input
k_r	First-order rate constant for renal elimination
k_{ij}	Apparent first-order intercompartment transfer rate constant where $i = 1, 2, \ldots$ and $j = 1, 2 \ldots$
L	Loading dose
P	Permeability constant
Q_L	Liver blood flow
R	Accumulation ratio for multiple dosing
T	Dosing interval
t	Time
t_{max}	Time after dosing at which maximum plasma concentration is reached
$t_{1/2}$	Half-life of drug
V_d	Apparent volume of distribution
$V_{d(area)}$, $V_{d(\beta)}$	Apparent volume of distribution during the β-phase.
$V_{d(ss)}$	Apparent volume of distribution at steady state
V_m	Theoretical maximum rate of a process described by Michaelis–Menten kinetics
V_1	Apparent volume of the central compartment
V_2	Apparent volume of the peripheral compartment
X_t or X_o	Amount of drug in the body at time t or zero time
$\frac{dX}{dt}$	Rate of change of drug amount in the body
X_u	Amount of free drug eliminated in the urine to time t
X_u^∞	Total amount of free drug eliminated in the urine

Appendix 3

FURTHER READING AND SOURCES OF INFORMATION ABOUT DRUGS

There are several sources of information about drugs, as follows.

A. Poisons Information Centres in the UK and Republic of Ireland may be consulted by doctors concerning the symptomatology and treatment of patients who have ingested toxic amounts of a wide variety of commercial and domestic products or drugs. Their addresses and telephone numbers are included for ready reference:

Belfast	Poisons Information Centre Royal Victoria Hospital, Belfast 0232 240503
Cardiff	Casualty Department, Royal Infirmary, Cardiff 0222 569200
Dublin	Poisons Information Centre, Jervis Street, Dublin 0001 745588
Edinburgh	The Scottish Poisons Information Bureau, Royal Infirmary, Edinburgh 031 229 2477 (Ask for Poisons Bureau)
Leeds	The Poisons Centre, Leeds General Infirmary, Leeds 0532 430715 or 432799
London	National Poisons Information Centre, Guy's Hospital, London 01 407 7600 (Ask for Poisons Enquiries) or 01 635 9191
Newcastle	Poisons Information Centre Royal Victoria Infirmary, Newcastle upon Tyne 0632 325131

B. Pharmacy-based drug information centres are now to be found in many district hospital pharmacies within the UK and are coordinated in most NHS regions by a Principal Pharmacist. The resources of such centres often include medical information-retrieval systems and a full-time drug information pharmacist able to deal with telephone enquiries, in some cases on a 24-h basis.

C. University departments of Clinical Pharmacology may in some cases be able to deal with specialist enquiries, especially if they relate to the interest of department members.

D. Libraries. In this rapidly expanding subject references are often outdated and the services of a medical librarian may be necessary for the newcomer to a subject to find the most recent and relevant information. We have not attempted to reference most of the statements made in this book but would refer the interested reader to the selection of reviews and original papers collected below under each chapter heading.

General Pharmacology and Therapeutics

AMA Drug Evaluations (1983) (5th edn.), Publishing Sciences Group, Littleton, Mass.
Avery, G. S. (1980) (ed.), (2nd edn.), *Drug Treatment*, ADIS Press, Sydney.
Crossland, J. (1980) (5th edn.) *Lewis's Pharamacology*, Churchill, Edinburgh.
Di Palma, J. R. (1971) (4th edn.), *Drill's Pharmacology in Medicine*, McGraw-Hill, New York.
Gilman, A. G., Goodman, L. S., T. W. Rall & F. Murad (1985) (eds.) (7th edn.), *The Pharmacological Basis of Therapeutics*, Macmillan, London.
Goldstein, A., Aronow, L. & Kalman, S. M. (1974) (2nd edn.), *The Principles of Drug Action*, Wiley, New York.
Goth, A. & Vesell, E. S. (1984) (11th edn.), *Medical Pharmacology*, Mosby, St Louis.
Rogers, H. J., Spector, R. G. & Trounce, J. R. (1976), *An Introduction to Mechanisms in Pharmacology and Therapeutics*, Heinemann, London.

Chapter 1 Introduction to Pharmacokinetics

Anton, A. H. & Solomon, H. M. (1976) (eds.), Drug–protein binding, *Ann. N. Y. Acad. Sci.*, **226,** 5.
Benet, L. Z., Massoud, N. & Gambertoglio, J. G. (1983) *Pharmacokinetic Basis for Drug Treatment*, Raven Press, New York.
Evans, W. E., Schentag, J. J. & Jusko, W. J. (1980) (eds.), *Applied Pharmacokinetics–Principles of Therapeutic Drug Monitoring*. Applied Therapeutics Inc., San Francisco.
Gerlowski, L. E. & Jain, R. K. (1983), Physiologically based pharmacokinetic modeling: principles and applications. *J. Pharm. Sci.*, **72,** 1103.
Gibaldi, M. & Perrier, D. (1982) (2nd edn.), *Pharmacokinetics*, M. Dekker, New York.
Greenblatt, D. J. & Koch-Weser, J. (1975), Clinical pharmacokinetics, *New Eng. J. Med.*, **293,** 707, 964.
Jeliffe; D. B. (1976), Plasma concentrations in the control of drug therapy, *Drugs*, **11,** 412.
Jusko, W. J. & Gretch, M. (1976), Plasma and tissue protein binding of drugs in pharmacokinetics, *Drug Metab. Rev.*, **5,** 43.
Koch-Weser, J. (1972), Serum drug concentrations as therapeutic guides, *New Eng. J. Med.*, **287,** 227.
Koch-Weser, J. & Sellers, E. M. (1976), Binding of drugs to serum albumin, *New Eng. J. Med.*, **294,** 311, 526.
MacKichan, J. J. (1984), Pharmacokinetic consequences of drug displacement from blood and tissue proteins. *Clin. Pharmacokin.*, **9** (Suppl. 1) 32.
Mungall, D. (1983) (ed), *Applied Clinical Pharmacokinetics*. Raven Press, New York.

Rossum, J. M. van (1977) (ed.), *Kinetics of Drug Action*, Vol. 47 of *Handbook of Experimental Pharmacology*, Springer-Verlag, Berlin.
Rowland, M. (1984) *Protein binding and drug clearance. Clin. Pharmacokin.*, **9** (Suppl. 1), 10.
Rowland, M., Benet, L. Z. & Graham, G. G. (1973), Clearance concepts in pharmacokinetics, *J. Pharmacokin. & Biopharm*, **1,** 123.
Rowland, M. & Tozer, T. N. (1980), *Clinical Pharmacokinetics: Concepts and Applications*. Lea & Febiger, Philadelphia.
Saunders, L. (1974), *The Absorption and Distribution of Drugs*, Ballière Tindall, London.
Sheiner, L. B., Rosenberg, B. & Melmon, K. L. (1972), Modelling of individual pharmacokinetics for computer-aided drug dosage, *Comp. Biomed. Res.*, 441.
Theorell, P., Dedrick, R. L. & Condliffe, P. G. (1974) (eds.), *Pharmacology and Pharmacokinetics*, Plenum Press, London.
Vallner, J. J. (1977), Binding of drugs by albumin and plasma protein, *J. Pharm. Sci.*, **66,** 447.
Wagner, J. G. (1971), *Biopharmaceutics and Relevant Pharmacokinetics*, Drug Intelligence Publications, Hamilton, Ill.
Wagner, J. G. (1973), Properties of the Michaelis–Menten equation and its integrated form which are useful in pharmacokinetics, *J. Pharmacokin. & Biopharm.*, **1,** 103, 337.
Wagner, J. G. (1975), Do you need a pharmacokinetic model and, if so, which one? *J. Pharmacokin. & Biopharm.*, **3,** 457.
Wagner, J. G. (1975), *Fundamentals of Clinical Pharmacokinetics*, Drug Intelligence Publications, Hamilton, Ill.

Chapter 2 Drug Absorption and Bioavailability

Azarnoff, D. L. & Huffmann, D. H. (1976), Therapeutic implications of bioavailability, *Ann. Rev. Pharmacol.*, **16,** 53.
Brodie, B. B. & Heller, W. H. (1972) (eds.), *Bioavailability of Drugs*, Karger, New York.
Cadwallader, D. E. (1983) (ed.), (3rd edn.), *Biopharmaceutics and Drug Interactions*, Raven Press, New York.
Chassaud, L. F. & Taylor, T. (1974), Bioavailability of drugs from formulations after oral administration, *Ann. Rev. Pharmacol.*, **14,** 35.
Goldman, P. (1982), Rate-controlled drug delivery. *New Eng. J. Med.*, **307,** 286.
Greenblatt, D. J. & Koch-Weser, J. (1976), Intramuscular injection of drugs, *New Eng. J. Med.*, **295,** 542.
Idson, B. (1975), Percutaneous absorption, *J. Pharm. Sci.*, **64,** 901.
Koch-Weser, J. (1974), Bioavailability of drugs, *New Eng. J. Med.*, **287,** 233, 503.
Lindenbaum, J. (1973), Bioavailability of digoxin tablets, *Pharmacol. Rev.*, **25,** 229.
Melander, A. (1978), Influence of food on the bioavailability of drugs, *Clin. Pharmacokin.*, **3,** 337.
Nimmo, W. S. (1976), Drugs, diseases and altered gastric emptying, *Clin. Pharmacokin.*, **1,** 189.
Riegelman, S. (1974), Pharmacokinetic factors affecting epidermal penetration and percutaneous absorption, *Clin. Pharm. Ther.*, **16,** 873.
Shanker, L. S. (1962), Passage of drugs across body membranes, *Pharmacol. Rev.*, **14,** 501.
Smolen, V. F. (1978), Bioavailability and pharmacokinetic analysis of drug responding systems, *Ann. Rev. Pharmacol.*, **18,** 495.
Thron, L. & Winne, D. (1971), Drug absorption, *Ann. Rev. Pharmacol.*, **11,** 56.

Welling, P. G. (1977), Influences of food and diet on gastrointestinal drug absorption: a review, *J. Pharmacokin. & Biopharm.*, **5,** 291.

Chapter 3 Drug Metabolism

Alvan, G. (1978), Individual differences in the disposition of drugs metabolised in the body, *Clin. Pharmacokin.,* **3,** 155.
Boobis, A. R. & Davies, D. S. (1984), Human cytochromes P–450. *Xenobiotica* **14,** 151.
Conney, A. H. (1967), Pharmacological implications of microsomal enzyme induction, *Pharmacol. Rev.*, **15,** 97.
Conney, A. H. & Burns, J. J. (1972), Metabolic interactions among environmental chemicals and drugs, *Science*, **173,** 756.
Conney, A. H., Pantuck, E. J., Kuntzman, R., Kappas, A., Anderson, K. E. & Alvares, A. P. (1978), Nutrition and chemical biotransformations in man, *Clin. Pharm. Ther.*, **22,** 707.
George, C. F., Shand, D. G. & Renwick, A. G. (1982) (eds.), *Presystemic Drug Elimination.* International Medical Reviews—Clinical Pharmacology and Therapeutics **1,** Butterworths, London.
Jusko, W. J. (1978), Role of tobacco smoking in pharmacokinetics, *J. Pharmacokin. & Biopharm.*, **6,** 7.
Kato, R. (1974), Sex-related differences in drug metabolism, *Drug Metab. Rev.*, **3,** 1.
Kuntzman, R. (1969), Drugs and enzyme induction, *Ann. Rev. Pharmacol.*, **9,** 21.
Miller, R. R. (1978), Effects of smoking on drug action, *Clin. Pharm. Ther.*, **22,** 749.
Nies, A. S., Shand, D. G. & Wilkinson, G. R. (1976), Altered hepatic blood flow in drug disposition, *Clin. Pharmacokin.*, **1,** 135.
Parke, D. V. (1968), *The Biochemistry of Foreign Compounds*, Pergamon Press.
Parke, D. V. (1975) (ed.), *Enzyme Induction*, Plenum Press, London.
Parke, D. V. & Smith, R. L. (1977) (eds.), *Drug Metabolism: from Microbe to Man*, Taylor & Francis, London.
Pond, S. M. & Tozer, T. N. (1984), First-pass Elimination—basic concepts and clinical consequences. *Clin. Pharmacokin.*, **9,** 1.
Reinberg, A. & Smolensky, M. H. (1982), Circadian changes of drug disposition in man. *Clin. Pharmacokin.*, **7,** 401.
Wilkinson, G. R. & Shand, D. G. (1975), A physiological approach to hepatic drug clearance, *Clin. Pharm. Ther.*, **18,** 377.
Wilson, K. (1984), Sex-related differences in drug disposition in man. *Clin. Pharmacokin.* **9,** 189.

Chapter 4 Pharmacogenetics

Drayer, D. E. & Reidenberg, M. M. (1977), Clinical consequences of polymorphic acetylation of basic drugs, *Clin. Pharm. Ther.*, **22,** 251.
Eichelbaum, M. (1982), Defective oxidation of drugs: pharmacokinetic and therapeutic implications. *Clin. Pharmacokin.*, **7,** 1.
Evans, D. A. P. (1965), Individual variations in drug metabolism as a factor in drug toxicity, *Ann. N. Y. Acad. Sci.*, **123,** 178.
Kalow, W. (1982), Ethnic differences in drug metabolism. *Clin. Pharmacokin.*, **7,** 373.
La Du, B. N. (1972), Pharmacogenetics: defective enzymes in relation to reactions to drugs, *Ann. Rev. Med.*, **23,** 453.
Motulsky, A. G. (1964), Pharmacogenetics, *Prog. Med. Genetics*, **3,** 49.
Vesell, E. S. (1974), Polygenic factors controlling drug response, *Med. Clin. N. America*, **58,** 951.

Vesell, E. S. (1978), Genetic and environmental factors affecting drug disposition in man, *Clin. Pharm. Ther.*, **22,** 659.
Wilding, G., Paigen, B. & Vesell, E. S. (1978), Genetic control of inter-individual variations in racemic warfarin binding to plasma and albumin of twins, *Clin. Pharm. Ther.*, **22,** 831.
Woosley, R. L., Drayer, D. E., Reidenberg, M. M., Nies, A. S., Carr, K. & Oates, J. A. (1978), Effect of acetylator phenotype on the rate at which procainamide induces antinuclear antibodies and the lupus syndrome, *New Eng. J. Med.*, **298,** 1157.

Chapter 5 Effects of Disease on Drug Kinetics

Benet, L. Z. (1976) (ed.), *The Effect of Disease States on Drug Pharmacokinetics*, American Pharmaceutical Association, Washington D.C.
Bennett, W. M., Bagley, S. P., McDonald, W. & Porter, G. A. (1979), *Drugs and Renal Disease*, Churchill Livingstone, Edinburgh.
Benowitz, N. L. & Meister, W. (1976), Pharmacokinetics in patients with cardiac failure, *Clin. Pharmacokin.*, **1,** 389.
Bessell, W. M., Singer, I., Golfer, T., Feig, P. & Coggins, C. J. (1977), Guidelines for drug therapy in renal failure, *Ann. Int. Med.*, **86,** 754.
Branch, R. A. & Shand, D. G. (1976), Propranolol disposition in chronic liver disease: a physiological approach, *Clin. Pharmacokin.*, **1,** 264.
Brater, D. C. (1982) *Drug Use in Renal Disease*, Wright, Bristol.
Doherty, J. E. & Perkins, W. H. (1966), Digoxin metabolism in patients with hypo- and hyperthyroidism, *Ann. Int. Med.*, **64,** 489.
Fabre, J. & Balant, L. (1976), Renal failure, drug pharmacokinetics and drug action, *Clin. Pharmacokin.*, **1,** 99.
Gibaldi, M. (1977), Drug distribution in renal failure, *Am. J. Med.*, **62,** 471.
Mawer, G. E. (1982), Dosage adjustment in renal insufficiency. *Brit. J. Clin. Pharmacol.*, **13,** 145.
Pagliaro, L. A. & Benet, L. Z. (1975), Critical compilation of half-lives, percent excreted unchanged and changes of half-life in renal and hepatic dysfunction for studies in humans, with references, *J. Pharmacokin. & Biopharm.*, **3,** 333.
Parsons, R. L. (1977), Drug absorption in gastrointestinal disease with particular reference to malabsorption syndromes, *Clin. Pharmacokin.*, **2,** 45.
Reidenberg, M. M. & Dreyer, D. E. (1984), Alteration of drug-protein binding in renal disease. *Clin. Pharmacokin.*, **9,** (Suppl. 1) 18.
Schenker, S., Hoyumpa, A. M. & Wilkinson, G. R. (1975), The effect of parenchymal liver disease on the disposition and elimination of sedatives and analgesics, *Med. Clin. N. America*, **59,** 887.
Shenfield, G. M. (1981), Influence of thyroid dysfunction on drug pharmacokinetics. *Clin. Pharmacokin*, **6,** 275.
Sotaniemi, E. R., Pelkonen, R. O., Mokka, R. E., Huttunen, R. & Viljakainen, E. (1977), Impairment of drug metabolism in patients with liver cancer, *Eur. J. Clin. Invest.*, **3,** 269.
Tillement, J. P., Lhoste, F. & Guidicelli, J. F. (1978), Diseases and drug protein binding, *Clin. Pharmacokin.*, **3,** 144.
Wilkinson, G. R. & Schenker, S. (1976), Effects of liver disease on drug disposition in man, *Biochem. Pharmacol.*, **25,** 2675.
Williams, R. L. & Mamelok, R. D. (1980), Hepatic disease and drug pharmacokinetics. *Clin. Pharmacokin.*, **5,** 528.

Chapter 6 Drugs at the Extremes of Age

Adamsons, K. & Joelsson, I. (1966), The effects of pharmacologic agents upon the fetus and newborn, *Am. J. Obs. Gyn.*, **96,** 437.

Boreus, L. O. (1982), *Principles of Paediatric Pharmacology*, Churchill Livingstone, Edinburgh.
Crooks, J., O'Malley, K. & Stevenson, I. H. (1976), Pharmacokinetics in the elderly, *Clin. Pharmacokin.*, **1,** 280.
Crooks, J. & Stevenson, I. H. (1979) (eds.), *Drugs and the Elderly—Perspectives in Geriatric Clinical Pharmacology*, Macmillan, London.
Done, A. K. (1966), Developmental pharmacology, *Ann. Rev. Pharmacol.*, **6,** 189.
Gosney, M. & Tallis, R. (1984), Prescription of contraindicated and interacting drugs in elderly patients admitted to hospital. *Lancet*, **2,** 564.
Greenblatt, D. J., Sellers, E. M. & Shader, R. I. (1982), Drug disposition in old age. *New Eng. J. Med.* **306,** 1081.
Jarvik, L. F., Greenblatt, D. J. & Harman, D. (1981), *Clinical Pharmacology and the Aged Patient*, Raven Press, New York.
Knowles, J. A. (1974), Breast milk: a source of more than nutrition for the neonate, *Clin. Toxicol.*, **7,** 69.
Krauer, B., Krauer, F. & Hytten, F. (1984), *Drug Prescribing in Pregnancy* (Current Reviews in Obstetrics and Gynaecology No. 7) Churchill Livingstone, Edinburgh.
Krasnor, J., Giacoia, P. & Yaffe, S. J. (1973), Drug protein binding in the newborn infant, *Ann. N.Y. Acad. Sci.*, **226,** 101.
Mirkin, B. L. (1976) (ed.), *Perinatal Pharmacology*, Academic Press, New York and London.
Mitenko, P. A., Comfort, A. & Crooks, J. (1983) (eds.), Drugs and the Elderly – A symposium. *J. Chronic Dis.*, **26,** 1.
Morselli, P. L., Garattini, S. & Sereni, F. (1975) (eds.), *Basic and Therapeutic Aspects of Perinatal Pharmacology*, Raven Press, New York.
Morselli, P. L. (1977) (ed.), *Drug Disposition during Development*, Spectrum Press, New York.
Palmisano, P. A. & Polhill, R. B. (1972), Fetal pharmacology, *Pediatric Clin. N. Amer.*, **19,** 3.
Richey, D. P. & Bender, A. D. (1977), Pharmacokinetic consequences of aging, *Ann. Rev. Pharmacol. Toxicol.*, **17,** 49.
Roberts, R. J. (1984), *Drug Therapy in Infants and Children*, Saunders, Philadelphia.
Royal College of Physicians (1984), Medication for the Elderly—A Report. *J. Roy. Coll. Phys. Lond.*, **18,** 7.
Shirkey, H. C. (1968), Clinical pharmacology in ambulatory children, *Clin. Pediatrics.*,**7,** 639.
Shirkey, H. C. (1970), Therapeutic orphans 1970, *J. Infect. Dis.*, **121,** 348.
Stern, L. (1984), *Drug Use in Pregnancy*, ADIS, Sydney.
Triggs, E. J. & Nation, R. L. (1975), Pharmacokinetics in the aged: a review, *J. Pharmacokin. & Biopharm.*, **3,** 387.
Tuchman-Duplessis, H. (1975), *Drug Effects on the Fetus*, ADIS Press, Sydney.
Wilson, J. T. *et al.* (1980), Drug excretion in human breast milk—Principles, pharmacokinetics and projected consequences. *Clin. Pharmacokin.*, **5,** 1.
Yaffe, S. J. & Juchan, M. R. (1974), Perinatal pharmacology, *Ann. Rev. Pharmacol.*, **14,** 219.

Chapter 7 Introduction of New Drugs, Clinical trials and Adverse-reaction Surveillance

Armitage, P. (1975), *Sequential Medical Trials*, Blackwell, Oxford.
Beyer, K. H. (1979), *Discovery, Development and Delivery of New Drugs*, Spectrum Press, London.
Blackwell, B. (1973), Patient compliance, *New Eng. J. Med.*, **289,** 249.

Borda, I. T., Slone, D. & Jick, H. (1968), Assessment of adverse reactions within a drug surveillance program, *J. Am. Med. Ass.*, **205,** 645.
Cluff, L. E., Caranasos, G. J. & Stewart, R. B. (1975), *Clinical Problems with Drugs*, Saunders, Philadelphia.
Davies, D. M. (1981), (ed) (2nd. edn.), *Textbook of Adverse Drug Reactions*, Oxford University Press, Oxford.
Dukes, M. N. G. (1977) (ed.), *Side Effects of Drugs*, Excerpta Medica, Amsterdam.
Folb, P. I. (1984), *Drug Safety in Clinical Practice*, Springer-Verlag, Berlin.
Freedman, L. M., Furburg, C. D. & DeMets, D. (1983), *Fundamentals of Clinical Trials*, Wright, Bristol.
Gross, F. H. & Inman, W. H. W. (1977) (eds.), *Drug Monitoring*, Academic Press, London.
Haynes, R. B., Taylor, D. W. & Sackett, D. (1979) (eds.), *Compliance in Health Care*, Johns Hopkins University Press, Baltimore.
Johnson, F. N. & Johnson, S. (1977) (eds.), *Clinical Trials*, Blackwell, Oxford.
Karch, F. E. & Lasagna, L. (1975), Adverse drug reactions—critical review, *J. Am. Med. Ass.*, **234,** 1236.
Koch-Weser, J., Sellers, E. M. & Zacest, R. (1977), The ambiguity of adverse drug reactions, *Eur. J. Clin. Pharmacol.*, **11,** 75.
Laurence, D. R. & Black, J. W. (1978), *The Medicines You Take*, Fontana Press, London.
Lawson, D. H. (1984) Pharmacoepidemiology: a new discipline, *Brit. Med. J.*, **289,** 940.
Miller, R. R. & Greenblatt, D. J. (1976) (eds.), *Drug Effects in Hospitalised Patients: Experiences of the Boston Collaborative Drug Surveillance Program 1966–1975*, Wiley, London.
Speirs, C. J., Griffin, J. P., Weber, J. C. P., *et al.* (1984), Demography of the U.K. adverse reaction register of spontaneous reports. *Health Trends*, **16,** 49.
Zarafonetis, C. J. D., Riley, P. A., Willis, P. W. *et al.* (1978), Clinically significant adverse effects in a phase I testing program, *Clin. Pharm. Ther.*, **24,** 127.

Chapter 8 Drug Interactions

Ariens, E. J. & Simonis, A. M. (1977), Pharmacodynamics of drug interactions, *Naunyn Schmiedebergs Arch. Pharmakol.*, **297,** 537.
Beeley, L. (1976), *Safer Prescribing*, Blackwell, Oxford.
Boston Collaborative Drug Surveillance Program (1972), Adverse drug interactions, *J. Am. Med. Ass.*, **220,** 1238.
Cluff, L. E. & Petrie, J. C. (1974) (eds.), *Clinical Effects of Interaction Between Drugs*, Excerpta Medica, Amsterdam.
Cohen, S. T. & Armstrong, M. F. (1974), *Drug Interactions: A Handbook for Clinical Use*, Williams & Wilkins, Baltimore.
Graham-Smith, D. G. (1977) (ed.), *Drug Interactions*, Macmillan, London.
Griffin, J. P. & D'Arcy, P. F. (1984) (2nd edn.), *A Manual of Adverse Drug Interactions*, Wright, Bristol.
Hansten, P. D. (1973), *Drug Interactions*, Lea & Febiger, Philadelphia.
Kabins, S. A. (1972), Interactions among antibiotics and other drugs, *J. Am. Med. Ass.*, **219,** 206.
Morselli, P. L. & Garattini, S. (1974) (eds.), *Drug Interactions*, Raven Press, New York.
Welling, P. G. (1984), Interactions affecting drug absorption. *Clin. Pharmacokin.*, **9,** 404.

Chapter 9 Nervous System

Amdisen, A. (1977), Serum level monitoring and clinical pharmacokinetics of lithium, *Clin. Pharmacokin.*, **2,** 73.
Baldessarini, R. J. & Lipinski, J. F. (1975), Lithium salts 1970–1975, *Ann. Int. Med.*, **83,** 527.
Baldessarini, R. J. (1977), *Chemotherapy in Psychiatry*, Harvard University Press, Cambridge.
Breimer, D. D. (1977), Clinical pharmacokinetics of hypnotics, *Clin. Pharmacokin.*, **2,** 93.
Burke, D. J. (1975), An approach to the treatment of spasticity, *Drugs*, **10,** 28.
Calne, D. B. & Reid, J. L. (1972), Anti-Parkinsonian drugs: pharmacological and therapeutic aspects, *Drugs*, **4,** 49.
Daniel, G. R. & Lader, M. H. (1976) (eds.), Symposium on the evaluation of psychotropic drugs, *Brit. J. Clin. Pharmacol.*, **3,** 1.
Drachman, D. B. (1978), Myasthenia gravis *New Eng. J. Med.*, **298,** 136, 186.
Eadie, M. J. & Tyrer, J. H. (1980) (2nd. edn), *Anticonvulsant Therapy: Pharmacological Basis and Practice*, Churchill Livingstone, Edinburgh.
Flacke, W. (1973), Treatment of myasthenia gravis, *New Eng. J. Med.*, **288,** 27.
Gottschalk, L. A. & Merlis, S. (1976) (eds.), *Pharmacokinetics of Psychoactive Drugs*, Spectrum Press, New York.
Grahame-Smith, D. G. & Orr, M. W. (1978), Clinical psychopharmacology, in P. Turner & D. G. Shand (eds.), *Recent Advances in Clinical Pharmacology* I, Churchill Livingstone, Edinburgh.
Hollister, L. H. (1978), *Clinical Pharmacology of Psychotherapeutic Drugs*, Churchill Livingstone, Edinburgh.
Hollister, L. H. (1978), Tricyclic antidepressants, *New Eng. J. Med.*, **299,** 1106, 1168.
Hvidberg, E. F. & Dam, M. (1976), Clinical pharmacokinetics of anticonvulsants, *Clin. Pharmacokin.*, **1,** 161.
Jefferson, J. (1977), *Primer of Lithium Therapy*, Williams & Wilkins, Baltimore.
Johns, M. W. (1975), Sleep and hypnotic drugs, *Drugs*, **9,** 448.
Laidlaw, J. & Richens, A. (1976) (eds.), *A Textbook of Epilepsy*, Churchill Livingstone, Edinburgh.
Nicholson, P. A. & Lader, M. H. (1976) (eds.), Symposium on the evaluation of psychotropic drugs, *Brit. J. Clin. Pharmacol.*, **3,** 1.
Nicholson, P. A. & Turner, P. (1977) (eds.), Symposium on Nomifensine, *Brit. J. Clin. Pharmacol.*, **4,** 535.
Peet, M. & Turner, P. (1978) (eds.), Symposium on Mianserin, *Brit. J. Clin. Pharmacol.*, **5,** 15.
Priest, R. G., Filho, U., Amrein, R. & Skreta, M. (1980), *Benzodiazepines Today and Tomorrow,* MTP Press, Lancaster.
Raskin, N. H. (1981), Pharmacology of migraine. *Ann. Rev. Pharmacol. Toxicol.*, **21,** 463.
Rose, F. C. & Capildeo, R. (1981) (eds), *Research progress in Parkinson's Disease.* Pitman, Tunbridge Wells.
Spector, R., Rogers, H. & Roy, D. (1984), *Psychiatry: Common Drug Treatments.* Martin Dunitz, London.
Tyrer, P. J. (1982) *Drugs in Psychiatric Practice*, Butterworth,
Woodbury, D. M., Penry, J. K. & Schmidt, R. P. (1972) (eds.), *Anti-epileptic Drugs*, Raven Press, New York.

Chapter 10 Analgesics and Antirheumatic Drugs

Beaver, W. I. (1965), Mild analgesics: a review of their clinical pharmacology, *Am. J. Med. Sci.*, **250,** 577.

Beecher, H. K. (1957), The measurement of pain, *Pharmacol. Rev.*, **9,** 59.
Clive, D. M. & Stoff, J. S. (1984) Renal syndromes associated with non-steroidal anti-inflammatory agents. *New Eng. J. Med.,* **310,** 563.
Dundee, J. W., Clarke, R. S. J. & Loan, W. B. (1967), Comparative toxicity of diamorphine, morphine and methadone, *Lancet*, **2,** 221.
Editorial (1977), Dangers of dextropropoxyphene, *Brit. Med. J.*, **1,** 668.
Editorial (1981) Aspirin and the stomach, *Brit. Med. J.*, **282,** 91.
Editorial (1981) Analgesic nephropathy, *Brit. Med. J.*, **282,** 339.
Flower, R. J. & Vane, J. R. (1974), Inhibition of prostaglandin biosynthesis, *Biochem. Pharmacol.*, **23,** 1439.
Hughes, J., Smith, T. W., Kosterlitz, H. W., Fothergill, L. A., Morgan, B. P. & Morris, H. R. (1975), Identification of two related pentapeptides from the brain with potent opiate agonist activity, *Nature*, **258,** 577.
Huskisson, E. C. (1974), Simple analgesics for arthritis, *Brit. Med. J.*, **2,** 196.
Huskisson, E. C. (1974), The measurement of pain, *Lancet*, **2,** 1127.
Ingelfinger, E. J. (1974), The side effects of aspirin, *New Eng. J. Med.*, **290,** 1196.
Lasagna, L. (1964), Clinical evaluation of morphine and its substitutes, *Pharmacol. Rev.*, **16,** 47.
Levy, G. & Tsuchiya, T. (1972), Salicylate accumulation kinetics in man, *New Eng. J. Med.*, **287,** 430.
Levy, G. & Giacomini, K. M. (1978), Rational aspirin dosage regiments, *Clin. Pharm. Ther.*, **23,** 247.
Lorber, A. (1977), Monitoring gold plasma levels in rheumatoid arthritis, *Clin. Pharmacokin.*, **2,** 127.
Macklan, W. F., Craft, A. W., Thompson, M. & Kerr, D. N. S. (1974), Aspirin and analgesic nephropathy, *Brit. Med. J.*, **1,** 597.
Mather, L. E. & Meffin, P. J. (1975), Clinical pharmacokinetics of pethidine, *Clin. Pharmacokin.*, **3,** 352.
Melzack, R. (1977), *The Mystery of Pain*, Pelican Books, London.
Mikkelsen, W. M. & Robinson, W. D. (1969), Physiologic and biochemical basis for the treatment of gout and hyperuricaemia, *Med. Clin. N. Amer.*, **53,** 1331.
Rundles, R. W., Metz, E. N. & Silberman, H. R. (1966), Allopurinol in the treatment of gout, *Ann. Int. Med.*, **64,** 229.
Simon, I. S. & Mills, J. A. (1980), Non-steroidal anti-inflammatory drugs. *New Eng. J. Med.*, **302,** 1237.
Thompson, J. W. (1984), Opioid peptides, *Brit. Med. J.*, **288,** 259.
Wallace, S. L. (1974), Colchicine, *Seminars in Arthritis and Rheumatism*, **3,** 369.
Willoughby, D. A., Wright, V. & Turner, P. (1977) (eds.), Symposium on diflunisal, *Brit. J. Clin. Pharmacol.*, **4,** 15.
Yu, T. F. (1974), Milestones in the treatment of gout, *Ann. Int. Med.*, **56,** 676.

Chapter 11 General and Local Anaesthetics; Muscle Relaxants

Cascorbi, H. F. (1973), Biotransformation of drugs used in anaesthesia, *Anaesthesiology*, **39,** 115.
Corino, B. G. (1972), Local anaesthesia, *New Eng. J. Med.*, **286,** 975, 1035.
Dundee, J. W. & Wyant, G. M. (1974), *Intravenous Anaesthesia*, Churchill Livingstone, Edinburgh,
Dyke, R. A. van & Chenoweth, M. R. (1965), Metabolism of volatile anaesthetics, *Anesthesiology*, **26,** 348.
Ghonesin, M. M. & Korltila, K. (1977), Pharmacokinetics of intravenous anaesthetics: implications for clinical use, *Clin. Pharmacokin.*, **2,** 344.
Greene, N. M. (1968), Halothane, *Clin. Anesthesia*, **1,** 1.
Hull, C. J. (1983), New drugs in anaesthesia. *Brit. J. Hosp. Med.*, **30,** 273.

Medical Research Council (1976), Conclusions of a working party on the effects of repeated exposure to anaesthetics, *Brit. J. Anaes.*, **48,** 1037.
Papper, E. M. & Kitz, R. J. (1963) (eds.), *Uptake and Distribution of Anaesthetic Agents*, McGraw-Hill, New York.
Roizen, M. F. & Feeley, T. W. (1978), Pancuronium bromide, *Ann. Int. Med.*, **88,** 64.
Sadove, M. S. & Wallace, V. E. (1962), *Halothane*, Blackwell, Oxford.
Smith, W. D. A. (1971), Pharmacology of nitrous oxide, *Int. Anesthesiology Clinics*, **9,** 91.
Thompson, M. A. (1980), Muscle relaxant drugs. *Brit. J. Hosp. Med.*, **23,** 153.
Vickers, M. D., Wood-Smith, F. G. & Stewart, H. C. (1978), *Drugs in Anaesthetic Practice* (5th edn.), Butterworths, London.

Chapter 12 Cardiovascular Drugs

Abrams, J. (1980), Nitroglycerine and long-acting nitrates. *New Eng. J. Med.*, **302,** 1234.
Antonaccio, M. J. (1982), Angiotensin converting enzyme (ACE) inhibitors. *Ann. Rev. Pharmacol. Toxicol.*, **22,** 57.
Aronson, J. K., Grahame-Smith, D. G. & Wigley, F. M. (1978), Monitoring digoxin therapy, *Quart. J. Med.*, **47,** 111.
Benowitz, N. L. & Meister, W. (1978), Clinical pharmacokinetics of lignocaine, *Clin. Pharmacokin.*, **3,** 177.
Breckenridge, A. (1982), Captopril—worldwide clinical experience. *Brit. J. Clin. Pharm.*, **14,** 65 S.
Breckenridge, A. (1983), Which beta blocker? *Brit. Med. J.*, **286,** 1085.
Chung, E. K. (1977), Tachyarrhythmias in Wolff–Parkinson–White syndrome—antiarrhythmic drug therapy, *J. Am. Med. Ass.*, **237,** 376.
Cohn, J. N. & Franciosa, J. A. (1977), Vasodilator therapy of cardiac failure, *New Eng. J. Med.*, **297,** 27, 254.
Cook, P. & James, I. (1981), Cerebral vasodilators. *New Eng. Med. J.*, **305,** 1508, 1560.
Dobbs, S. M. & Mawer, G. E. (1977), Prediction of digoxin dose requirements, *Clin. Pharmacokin.*, **2,** 281.
Ewy, G. A. & Bressler, R. (1984) (eds.), *Current Cardiovascular Therapy*. Raven Press, New York.
Frishman, W. H. (1981), β-Adrenoceptor antagonists: new drugs and new indications. *New Eng. J. Med.*, **305,** 500.
Frishman, W. H. (1982), Atenolol and timolol. *New Eng. J. Med.*, **306,** 1456.
Frishman, W. H. (1983), Pindolol. *New Eng. J. Med.*, **308,** 940.
Gillis, A. M. & Kates, R. E. (1984), Clinical pharmacokinetics of the newer antiarrhythmic agents. *Clin. Pharmacokin.*, **9,** 375.
Graham, R. M. & Pettinger, W. A. (1979), Prazosin, *New Eng. J. Med.*, **300,** 232.
Green, L. H. & Smith, T. W. (1977), The use of digitalis in patients with pulmonary disease, *Ann. Int. Med.*, **87,** 459.
Guz, A. & McHaffie, D. (1978), The use of digitalis glycosides in sinus rhythm, *Clin. Sci.*, **55,** 417.
Josephson, M. E. & Kastor, J. A. (1977), Supraventricular tachycardia: mechanisms and management, *Ann. Int. Med.*, **87,** 346.
Koch-Weser, J. (1976), Diazoxide, *New Eng. J. Med.*, **294,** 1271.
Koch-Weser, J. (1976), Hydralazine, *New Eng. J. Med.*, **295,** 321.
Kostis, J. B. & DeFelice E. A. (1983) (eds.), *Beta Blockers in the Treatment of Cardiovascular Diseases*. Raven Press, New York.
Krikler, D. M. (1974), A fresh look at arrhythmias, *Lancet*, **1,** 851, 913, 974, 1034.
Lawson, D. H. & Jick, H. (1977), Adverse reactions to procainamide, *Brit. J. Clin. Pharmacol.*, **4,** 507.

Leier, C. V. & Unverferth, D. V. (1983), Dobutamine. *Ann. Int. Med.*, **99,** 490.
Lewis, P. (1982) (ed.), Thirty years of drugs for hypertension. *Brit. J. Clin. Pharmacol.*, **13,** 1.
Lucchesi, B. R., Dingell, J. V. & Schwarz, R. P. (1984), *Clinical Pharmacology of Antiarrhythmic Therapy*. Raven Press, New York.
McDevitt, D. G. (1977), An assessment of beta adrenoceptor blocking drugs in man, *Brit. J. Clin. Pharmacol.*, **4,** 413.
McDevitt, D. G. (1978), β-adrenoceptor antagonists and respiratory function, *Brit. J. Clin. Pharmacol.*, **5,** 97.
Monady, F., Scheinman, M. M. & Desai, J. (1982), Disopyramide. *Ann. Int. Med.*, **96,** 337.
Mulrow, C. D., Feussner, J. R. & Velez, R. (1984), Re-evaluation of digitalis efficacy. *Ann. Int. Med.*, **101,** 113.
Opie, L. H. (1984), *Calcium Antagonists and Cardiovascular Disease*. Raven Press, New York.
Needleman, P. (1976), Organic nitrate metabolism, *Ann. Rev. Pharmacol.*, **16,** 81.
Parker, J. C. & Davidson, I. W. F. (1975), Organic nitrates in perspective, *Drug Metab. Rev.*, **4,** 135.
Prazosin Update (1983), *Drugs*, **5,** 339.
Pritchard, B. N. C. (1978), β-adrenergic blockade in hypertension, past, present and future, *Brit. J. Clin. Pharmacol.*, **5,** 379.
Reid, J. L. & Van Zwieten, P. A. (1983) (eds.), Round Table on Centrally Acting Antihypertensive drugs. *Brit. J. Clin. Pharmacol.*, **15,** 451S.
Richards, D. A. & Turner, P. (1976), Symposium on labetalol, *Brit. J. Clin. Pharmacol.*, **3,** 677.
Shaw, T. R. D. (1974), The digoxin affair, *Postgrad. Med. J.*, **50,** 98.
Singh, B. N., Ellrodt, G. & Peter, C. T. (1978), Verapamil: a review of its pharmacological properties and therapeutic use, *Drugs*, **15,** 169.
Smith, J. W. & Haber, E. (1973), Digitalis, *New Eng. J. Med.*, **289,** 945, 1010, 1063, 1125.
Sonnenblick, E. H., Frishman, W. H. & Le Jemtel, T. H. (1979), Dobutamine: a new synthetic cardioactive sympathetic amine, *New Eng. J. Med.*, **300,** 17.
Symposium on Digitalis (1977), *Federation Proceedings*, **36,** 2207.
Tinker, J. H. & Michenfelder, J. D. (1976), Sodium nitroprusside: pharmacology, toxicology, therapeutics, *Anaesthesiology*, **45,** 340.

Chapter 13 Respiratory System

Anthonisen, N. R. (1983), Long term oxygen therapy. *Ann. Int. Med.*, **99,** 519.
Arsdel, P. P. van & Paul, G. H. (1977), Drug therapy in management of asthma, *Ann. Int. Med.*, **87,** 68.
Bernstein, I. L., Johnson, C. L. & Tse, C. S. T. (1978), Therapy with cromolyn sodium, *Ann. Int. Med.*, **89,** 228.
Brogden, R. N., Speight, T. M. & Avery, G. S. (1974), Sodium cromoglycate: a review of its mode of action, pharmacology, therapeutic efficacy and use, *Drugs*, **7,** 164.
Collins, J. V., Clark, T. J. H., Brown, D. & Townsend, J. (1975), The use of corticosteroids in the treatment of acute asthma, *Quart. J. Med.*, **44,** 259.
Grant, I. W. B., Harris, D. M. & Turner, P. (1977), Symposium on Beclomethasone Dipropionate, *Brit. J. Clin. Pharmacol.*, **4,** 249S.
Hendeles, L., Laporte, P. & Weinberger, M. (1984), A clinical and pharmacokinetic basis for the selection and use of slow release theophylline. *Clin. Pharmacokin.*, **9,** 95.
Hoffbrand, B. I. (1975) (ed.), The place of parasympatholytic drugs in the management of chronic obstructive airways disease, *Postgrad. Med. J.*, **51,** suppl. 7.
Lieberman, J. (1970), The appropriate use of mucolytic agents, *Am. J. Med.*, **49,** 1.

Paterson, J. W. & Shenfield, G. M. (1974), Bronchodilators, *Brit. Thoracic & Tuberculosis Association Review* (supplement to *Tubercle*), **4,** 25.
Piafsky, K. M. & Ogilvie, R. I. (1975), Dosage of theophylline in bronchial asthma, *New Eng. J. Med.*, **292,** 1918.
Rebuck, A. S. (1974), Antiasthmatic drugs, *Drugs*, **7,** 344, 370.
Rees, J. (1984), Treatment of pulmonary hypertension in chronic bronchitis and emphysema. *Brit. Med. J.*, **289,** 1398.

Chapter 14 Diuretics and Drugs Acting on the Kidneys

Croxson, M. S., Neutze, J. M. & John, M. B. (1972), Exchangeable potassium in heart disease: long term effects of potassium supplements and amiloride, *Am. Heart J.*, **84,** 53.
Davies, D. L. & Wilson, G. M. (1975), Diuretics: mechanism of action and clinical application, *Drugs*, **9,** 178.
Frazier, H. S. & Yager, H. (1973), The clinical use of diuretics, *New Eng. J. Med.*, **288,** 246, 455.
Gennari, F. J. & Kassiver, J. P. (1974), Osmotic diuresis, *New Eng. J. Med.*, **29,** 714.
Goldberg, M. (1973), Renal physiology of diuretics in renal physiology, *Handbook of Physiology*, Section 8, American Physiology Society, Washington DC.
Hoffbrand, B. I. & Jones, G. (1975), Symposium on Bumetanide, *Postgrad. Med. J.*, **51,** suppl. 6.
Kleit, S. A., Hamburger, R. J., Martz, B. L. & Fisch, L. (1978), Diuretic therapy—current status, *Am. Heart J.*, **79,** 700.
Lawson, D. H. (1976), Potassium therapy, *Brit. J. Hosp. Med.*, **16,** 392.
Lindeman, R. D. & Papper, S. (1975), Therapy of fluid and electrolyte disorders, *Ann. Int. Med.*, **82,** 64.
Martinez-Maldomdo, M., Eknoyan, G. & Suki, W. N. (1973), Diuretics in non-oedematous states. Physiological basis for their clinical use, *Arch. Int. Med.*, **131,** 797.
Middler, S., Pak, C. Y. C., Murad, F. & Bartter, F. C. (1973), Thiazide diuretics and calcium metabolism, *Metabolism*, **22,** 139.
Milne, M. D., Schribner, B. H. & Crawford, M. A. (1958), Non-ionic diffusion and the excretion of weak acids and weak bases, *Am. J. Med.*, **243,** 709.
Odlind, B. (1984), Site and mechanism of the action of diuretics. *Acta Pharmacol. Toxiol.* **54,** (suppl 1), 5.
Pitts, R. F. (1974), *Physiology of the Kidney and Body Fluids: An Introductory Text* (3rd ed.), Year Book, Medical Publishers, Chicago.
Schedl, H. P. & Bartter, F. C. (1960), An explanation for and experimental correction of the abnormal water diuresis in cirrhosis, *J. Clin. Invest.*, **39,** 248.

Chapter 15 Alimentary System and Liver

Albibi, R. & McCalium, R. W. (1983), Metoclopramide—pharmacology and clinical application. *Ann. Int. Med.*, **98,** 86.
Avery, G. S., Davies, E. & Brogden, R. N. (1972), Lactulose, *Drugs*, **4,** 7.
Awouters, F., Niemegeers, C. J. E. & Janssen, P. A. J. (1983), Pharmacology of antidiarrhoeal drugs. *Ann. Rev. Pharmacol. Toxicol.*, **23,** 279.
Binder, H. J. & Donowitz, M. (1975), A new look at laxative action, *Gastroenterology*, **69,** 1001.
Das, K. M., Eastwood, M. A., McManus, J. P. A. & Sircus, W. (1973), Adverse reactions during salicylazosulphapyridine therapy and the relationship with drug metabolism and acetylator phenotype, *New Eng. J. Med.*, **289,** 491.
Fast, B., Wolfe, S. J., Stormont, J. & Davidson, C. S. (1968), Antibiotic therapy in the

management of hepatic coma, *Arch. Int. Med.*, **101,** 467.
Fordtran, J. S. & Collyns, J. A. H. (1966), Antacid pharmacology in duodenal ulcer, *New Eng. J. Med.*, **274,** 921.
Fordtran, J. S., Morawski, B. A. & Richardson, C. T. (1973), In vivo and in vitro evaluation of liquid antacids, *New Eng. J. Med.*, **288,** 923.
Fordtran, J. S. (1978), Placebos, antacids and cimetidine for duodenal ulcer, *New Eng. J. Med.*, **298,** 1081.
Freston, J. W. (1982), Cimetidine—developments, pharmacology, efficacy, adverse reactions, patterns of use. *Ann. Int. Med.*, **97,** 573, 728.
Goldman, P. & Peppercorn, M. A. (1975), Sulfasalazine, *New Eng. J. Med.*, **293,** 20.
Hermon-Taylor, J. (1977), An aetiological and therapeutic review of acute pancreatitis, *Brit. J. Hosp. Med.*, **19,** 546.
Homsky, J. (1973), The treatment of heartburn and oesophagitis, *Drugs*, **5,** 446.
Hurwitz, A. (1977), Antacid therapy and drug kinetics, *Clin. Pharmacokin.*, **2,** 269.
Iser, J. H., Dowling, R. H., Mok, H. Y. I. & Bell, G. D. (1975), Chenodeoxycholic acid treatment of gallstones: a follow-up report and analysis of factors influencing response to therapy, *New Eng. J. Med.*, **293,** 378.
Littmann, A. & Pine, B. H. (1975), Antacids and anticholinergic drugs, *Ann. Int. Med.*, **82,** 544.
Morrissey, J. F. & Barreras, R. F. (1974), Antacid therapy, *New Eng. J. Med.*, **290,** 550.
Palmer, R. H. & Carey, M. C. (1982), An optimistic view of the national cooperative gallstone study *New Eng. J. Med.*, **306,** 1171.
Roydhouse, N. (1973), Vertigo and its treatment, *Drugs*, **7,** 297.
Schroder, H., Lewkonia, R. M. & Price Evans, D. A. (1973), Metabolism of salicylazosulphapyridine in healthy subjects and in patients with ulcerative colitis, *Clin. Pharm. Ther.*, **14,** 802.
Sircus, W. (1972), Progress report: carbenoxolone sodium, *Gut.*, **13,** 816.
Symposium on Cimetidine (1978), *Gastroenterology*, **74,** Part 2.
Thistle, J. L. & Schoenfield, L. J. (1973), Efficacy, specificity and safety of chenodeoxycholic acid therapy for dissolving gallstones, *New Eng. J. Med.*, **289,** 655.

Chapter 16 Vitamins and Therapeutic Nutritional Drugs

Durrington, P. N. & Miller, J. P. (1984), Clinical aspects of hyperlipoproteinaemia. *Brit. J. Hosp. Med.*, **32,** 28.
Glueck, C. J. (1982), Cholestipol and Probucol: treatment of primary and familial hypercholesterolaemia and amelioration of atherosclerosis. *Ann. Int. Med.*, **96,** 475.
Goodman, DeW. S. (1984), Vitamin A and retinoids in health and disease. *New Eng. J. Med.*, **310,** 1023.
Innes, J. A., Watson, M. L., Ford, M. J., Munro, J. F., Stoddart, M. E. & Campbell, D. B. (1977), Plasma fenfluramine levels, weight loss and side effects, *Brit. Med. J.*, **2,** 1322.
Levy, R. I. & Rifkind, B. M. (1973), Lipid lowering drugs and hyperlipidaemia, *Drugs*, **6,** 12.
Northway, W. H. (1978), Bronchopulmonary dysplasia and vitamin E, *New Eng. J. Med.*, **299,** 599.
Oliver, M. F. (1978), Cholesterol, coronaries, clofibrate and death, *New Eng. J. Med.*, **209,** 1360.
Scott, P. J. (1975), Lipid lowering drugs and coronary heart disease, *Drugs*, **10,** 218.
Spivak, J. L. & Jackson, D. L. (1977), Pellagra: an analysis of 18 patients and a review of the literature, *Johns Hopkins Med. J.*, **140,** 295.
Yeshurun, D. & Gotto, A. M. (1976), Drug treatment of hyperlipidemia, *Am. J. Med.*, **60,** 379.

Chapter 17 Drugs Acting on the Blood

Babior, B. M. (1975), *Cobalamin. Biochemistry and Pathophysiology*, Wiley, New York.
Beal, R. W. (1971), Haematinics, *Drugs*, **2,** 190, 207.
Bjornsson, T. D. (1984), Clinical pharmacology of heparin in *Recent Advances in Clinical Pharmacology* (P. Turner & D. Shand, eds.) Churchill Livingstone, Edinburgh.
Canadian Cooperative Study Group (1978), A randomised trial of aspirin and sulphinpyrazone in threatened stroke, *New Eng. J. Med.*, **299,** 53.
Cederholm-Williams, S. A. (1983), Control of fibrinolysis. *Brit. J. Hosp. Med.*, **30,** 107.
Crosley, W. H. (1977), Who needs iron? *New Eng. J. Med.*, **297,** 543.
Gallop, P. M., Liam, J. B. and Hauschka, P. V. (1980), Carboxylated calcium-binding proteins and vitamin K. *New Eng. J. Med.*, **302,** 1460.
Hessler, S. & Gitel, S. N. (1984), Warfarin: from bedside to bench. *New Eng. J. Med.*, **311,** 654.
Jick, H., Slone, D., Borda, I. T. & Shapiro, S. (1968), Efficacy and toxicity of heparin in relation to age and sex, *New Eng. J. Med.*, **279,** 284.
Laffel, G. L. & Braunwald, E. (1984), Thrombolytic therapy: a new strategy for the treatment of acute myocardial infarction. *New Eng. J. Med.*, **311,** 710–770.
Lewis, R. L., Trager, W. F., Chan, K. K., *et al.* (1974), Warfarin. Stereochemical aspects of its metabolism and the interaction with phenylbutazone, *J. Clin. Invest.*, **53,** 1607.
McLean Baird, I., Walters, R. L. & Sutton, D. R. (1974), Absorption of slow-release iron and effects of ascorbic acid in normal subjects and after partial gastrectomy, *Brit. Med. J.*, **4,** 505.
Nagashima, R., O'Reilly, R. & Levy, G. (1969), Kinetics of pharmacologic effects in man; the anticoagulation of warfarin, *Clin. Pharm. Ther.*, **10,** 22.
O'Reilly, R. & Aggeler, P. (1968), Initiation of warfarin without a loading dose, *Circulation*, **23,** 169.
O'Reilly, R. A. & Aggeler, P. M. (1970), Determinants of the response to oral anticoagulants in man, *Pharmacol. Rev.*, **22,** 35.
Webster, J. (1983), Antiplatelet drugs. *Brit. J. Hosp. Med.*, **31,** 45.
Weiss, H. J. (1978), Antiplatelet therapy, *New Eng. J. Med.*, **298,** 1344, 1403.
Wessler, S. & Yin, E. T. (1973), Theory and practice of minidose heparin in surgical patients, *Circulation*, **47,** 671.

Chapter 18 Endocrine System

Chalmers, T. C. (1975), Settling the UGDP controversy, *J. Am. Med. Ass.*, **231,** 624.
Coburn, J. W., Brickman, A. S. & Massny, S. G. (1972), Medical treatment in primary and secondary hyperparathyroidism, *Seminars in Drug Treatment*, **2,** 117.
Cooper, D. S. (1984), Antithyroid drugs. *New Eng. J. Med.*, **311,** 1353.
Cope, C. L. (1972), *Adrenal Steroids and Disease* (2nd edn.), Pitman Medical, London.
Davis, J. O. & Freeman, R. H. (1976), Mechanisms regulating renin release, *Physiol. Rev.*, **56,** 1.
De Groot, L. J. (1977), Short-term antithyroid drug therapy, *New Eng. J. Med.*, **297,** 212.
De Rose, J., Avramides, A., Baker, R. K. & Wallach, S. (1972), Treatment of Paget's disease with calcitonin. *Seminars in Drug Treatment*, **2,** 1972.
Edwards, C. R. W., Kitau, M. J., Chand, T. & Besser, G. M. (1973), Vasopressin analogue DDAVP in diabetes insipidus: clinical and laboratory studies. *Brit. Med. J.*, **3,** 375.
Frantz, A. G. (1978), Prolactin, *New Eng. J. Med.*, **298,** 201.

Friedman, M. & Strang, L. B. (1966), Effect ot long-term corticosteroids and corticotrophin on the growth of children, *Lancet*, **2,** 568.
Hanssler, M. R. & McCain, T. A. (1977), Basic and clinical concepts related to vitamin D metabolism and action, *New Eng. J. Med.*, **297**, 974, 1041.
Hershman, J. M. (1974), Clinical application of thyrotropin-releasing hormone, *New Eng. J. Med.*, **290,** 886.
Karim, S. M. M. & Hillier, K. (1974), Prostaglandins: pharmacology and clinical application, *Drugs*, **8,** 176.
Kaye, R. (1975), Diabetic ketoacidosis—the bicarbonate controversy, *J. Pediatrics*, **87,** 156.
Krane, S. M. (1982), Etidronate disodium in the treatment of Paget's disease of bone. *Ann. Int. Med.*, **96,** 619.
Kreisberg, R. A. (1978), Diabetic ketoacidosis: new concepts and trends in pathogenesis and treatment, *Ann. Int. Med.*, **88,** 681.
Kurtzman, N. A. & Boojavern, S. (1975), Physiology of the antidiuretic hormone and the interrelationship between the hormone and the kidney, *Nephron*, **15,** 167.
Liao, S. (1975), Cellular receptors and mechanism of action of steroid hormones, *Int. Rev. Cytol.*, **41,** 87.
Liggins, G. C. (1974), Prostaglandins: current therapeutic status in obstetrics, *Drugs*, **8,** 161.
McEwan, J. (1977), Choosing which pill, *Brit. J. Hosp. Med.*, **19,** 364.
MacGregor, R. R., Sheagren, J. N., Lipsett, M. B. & Wolff, S. M. (1969), Alternate day prednisone therapy. Evaluation of delayed hypersensitivity responses, control of disease and steroid side effects, *New Eng. J. Med.*, **280,** 1427.
Mackin, J. F., Canary, J. J. & Pittman, C. S. (1974), Thyroid storm and its management, *New Eng. J. Med.*, **291,** 1396.
Marble, A. (1971), Glibenclamide, a new sulphonylurea, *Drugs*, **1,** 109.
Melby, J. (1974), Systemic corticosteroid therapy: pharmacology and endocrinologic considerations, *Ann. Int. Med.*, **81,** 505.
Peacock, M. (1977), Clinical uses of 1-α hydroxyvitamin D, *Clin. Endocrinol.*, **7,** supplement, 15.
Sterling, K. (1979), Thyroid hormone action at the cell level, *New Eng. J. Med.*, **300,** 117, 173.
Tomlinson, S. & O'Riordan, J. L. H. (1978), The parathyroids, *Brit. J. Hosp. Med.*, **20,** 40.
University Group Diabetes Program (1970), A study of the effects of hypoglycaemic agents in vascular complications in patients with adult onset diabetes, *Diabetes*, **19,** Suppl. 2, 747.
University Group Diabetes Program (1975), A study of the effects of hypoglycaemic agents on vascular complications in patients with adult onset diabetes, V. Evaluation of phenformin therapy, *Diabetes*, **24,** Suppl. 1, 65.
Utiger, R. D. (1978), Treatment of Graves' disease, *New Eng. J. Med.*, **298,** 681.
Vance, M. L., Evans, W. S. & Thorner, M. O. (1984), Bromocriptine. *Ann. Int. Med.*, **100,** 704.
Vaughan, N. J. A. & Oakley, N. (1983), The newer insulins. *Brit. J. Hosp. Med.*, **30,** 313.
Vessey, M. P., Wright, N. G., McPherson, K. & Wiggins, P. (1978), Fertility after stopping different methods of contraception, *Brit. Med. J.*, **1,** 265.
Woodhouse, N. J. Y. (1974), Clinical applications of calcitonin, *Brit. J. Hosp. Med.*, **16,** 677.

Chapter 19 Chemotherapy of Infections

Appel, G. B. & Neu, H. C. (1977), Nephrotoxicity of antimicrobial agents, *New Eng. J. Med.*, **296,** 663, 722, 784.

Appel, G. B. & Neu, H. C. (1978), Gentamicin in 1978, *Ann. Int. Med.*, **89,** 528.
Carne, P. E. (1984), *Interferons and Their Applications*, Springer-Verlag, Berlin.
Cook, F. V. & Farrow, W. E. (1978), Vancomycin revisited, *Ann. Int. Med.*, **89,** 813.
Craig, W. A. & Kunin, C. M. (1976), Significance of serum protein and tissue binding of antimicrobial agents, *Ann. Rev. Med.*, **27,** 287.
Editorial (1974), Tetracyclines after 25 years, *Brit. Med. J.*, **2,** 400.
Editorial (1975), Amikacin, *Lancet*, **2,** 804.
Editorial (1976), Mecillinam, *Lancet*, **2,** 503.
Eliopoulos, G. M. & Moellering, R. (1982), Azlocillin, Mezlocillin & Piperacillin: new broad spectrum penicillins. *Ann. Int. Med.*, **97,** 755.
Finland, M. & Hewitt, W. C. (1971), Second international symposium on gentamicin, *J. Infect. Dis.*, **124,** supplement.
Glassroth, J., Robins, A. G. & Snider, D. E. (1980), Tuberculosis in the 1980's. *New Eng. J. Med.*, **302,** 1441.
Garrod, L. P., James, D. G. & Lewis, A. A. G. (1969) (eds.), The synergy of Trimethoprim and Sulphonamides, *Postgrad. Med. J.*, **45,** supplement.
Garrod, L. P., Lambert, H. P. & O'Grady, F. (1981) (5th edn.), *Antibiotic and Chemotherapy*, Churchill Livingstone, Edinburgh.
Garrod, L. P. (1975), Chemoprophylaxis, *Brit. Med. J.*, **4,** 561.
Glover, S. C. (1983), Drug treatment of helminthic infections. *Brit. J. Hosp. Med.*, **30,** 169.
Holdiness, M. R. (1984), Clinical pharmacokinetics of the antituberculosis drugs. *Clin. Pharmacokin.*, **9,** 511.
Kucers, A. & Bennett, N. McK. (1979) (3rd edn.), *The Use of Antibiotics* (2nd edn.), Heinemann Medical, London.
McCormack, W. M. & Finland, M. (1976), Spectinomycin, *Ann. Int. Med.*, **84,** 72.
Kahlemeter, G. & Dahlajer, J. I. (1984), Aminoglycoside toxicity. *J. Antimicrobial Chemother.*, **13,** suppl. A, 9.
Laskin, O. L. (1984), Acyclovir. *Arch. Int. Med.*, **144,** 1241.
Medoff, G., Brajtburg, J. & Kobayashi, G. S. (1983), Antifungal agents useful in therapy of systemic fungal infections. *Ann. Rev. Pharmacol. Toxicol.*, **23,** 303.
Neu, H. C. (1975), New broad spectrum penicillins, *Drugs*, **9,** 81.
Neu, H. C. (1982), The new beta-lactamase-stable cephalosporins. *Ann. Int. Med.*, **97,** 408.
Nicholson, K. G. (1984), Properties of antiviral agents. *Lancet*, **ii,** 503, 562, & 617.
Nightingale, C. H., Green, D. S. & Quintiliani, R. (1975), Pharmacokinetics and clinical use of cephalosporin antibiotics, *J. Pharm. Sci.*, **64,** 1899.
Ory, E. M. (1970), The Tetracyclines, *Med. Clin. N. Amer.*, **54,** 1173.
Pearson, R. D. & Guerrant, R. L. (1983), Praziquantel—a major advance in anthelminthic therapy. *Ann. Int. Med.*, **99,** 195.
Rahal, J. J. (1978), Antibiotic combinations: the clinical relevance of synergy and antagonism, *Medicine*, **57,** 179.
Selwyn, S. (1980), *The β-lactam Antibiotics*, Hodder & Stoughton, London.
Trimethoprim–Sulphamethoxazole (1971), *Drugs*, **1,** 1.
Williams, J. D. (1974), The sulphonamides, *Brit. J. Hosp. Med.*, **16,** 722.
Willis, A. T. (1978), The treatment of anaerobic bacterial infections, *Brit. J. Hosp. Med.*, **20,** 579.
Youatt, J. (1969), A review of the action of isoniazid, *Am. Rev. Resp. Dis.*, **111,** 109.

Chapter 20 Cancer Chemotherapy

Balis, F. M., Holcenberg, J. S. & Bleyer, W. A. (1983), Clinical pharmacokinetics of commonly used anti-cancer drugs. *Clin. Pharmacokin.*, **8,** 202.

Bender, R. A., Zwelling, L. A., Doroshow, J. H., Locker, G. Y., Handel, K. R., Murinson, D. S., Cohen, M., Myers, C. E. & Chabner, B. A. (1978), Antineoplastic drugs—clinical pharmacology and therapeutic use, *Drugs,* **16,** 46.
Chabner, B. A., Myers, C. E., Coleman, C. H. & Johns, D. G. (1975), The clinical pharmacology of antineoplastic agents, *New Eng. J. Med.*, **292,** 1107, 1159.
De Vita, V. T., Young, R. C. & Canellos, G. P. (1975), Combination versus single chemotherapy: a review of the basis for selection of drug treatment in cancer, *Cancer*, **35,** 98.
Furr, B. J. A. & Jordan, V. C. (1984), The pharmacology and clinical use of tamoxifen. *Pharmacol. Ther.*, **25,** 127.
Golding, A. & Johnson, R. K. (1977), Resistance to antitumour agents, pp. 155 in *Recent Advances in Cancer Treatment*, Raven Press, New York.
Hellman, K. (1983) (ed.), Ifosfamide and mesna. *Cancer Treatment Rev.*, **10,** Suppl. A.
Jolivet, J., Cowan, K. H. *et al.* (1983), The pharmacology and clinical use of methotrexate. *New Eng. J. Med.*, **309,** 1094.
Lippman, M. E. & Allegra, J. C. (1978), Receptors in breast cancer, *New Eng. J. Med.*, **299,** 930.
Loehrer, P. J. & Einhorn, L. K. (1984), Cisplatin. *Ann. Int. Med.*, **100,** 704.
Powis, G. (1982), Effect of human renal and hepatic disease on the pharmacokinetics of anticancer drugs. *Cancer Treatment Rev.*, **9,** 85.
Salmon, S. E. & Jones, S. E. (1977) (eds.), *The Adjuvant Therapy of Cancer*, Elsevier–North Holland Press, Amsterdam.
Schein, P. S. & Winokur, S. H. (1975), Long term complications of immunosuppressive and cytotoxic chemotherapy, *Ann. Int. Med.*, **82,** 84.
Schornagel, J. H. & McVie, J. G. (1983), The clinical pharmacology of methotrexate. *Cancer Treatment Rev.*, **10,** 53.
Selby, P., Buick, R. N. & Tannock, I. (1983), A critical appraisal of the human tumor stem cell assay. *New. Eng. J. Med.*, **308,** 129.
Skipper, H. E. (1974), Combination therapy: some concepts and results, *Cancer Chemother. Rep.*, **4,** 137.
Spivack, S. (1974), Procarbazine, *Ann. Int. Med.*, **81,** 795.
Weinstein, G. D. (1977), Methotrexate, *Ann. Int. Med.*, **86,** 199.
Young, R. C., Lippman, M. & De Vita, V. T. (1977), Perspectives in the treatment of breast cancer, *Ann. Int. Med.*, **86,** 784.

Chapter 21 Allergy and Immunosuppression

Aisenberg, A. (1974), Inhibitors of immune reactions, *Life Sci.*, **15,** 1861.
Amos, H. E. (1976), *Allergic Drug Reactions* (Current Topics in Immunology No. 5), Edward Arnold, London.
Beaness, M. A. (1976), Histamine, *New Eng. J. Med.*, **294,** 30, 320.
Cohen, D. J., Loertscher, R. *et al.* (1984), Cyclosporine: a new immunosuppressive agent for organ transplantation. *Ann. Int. Med.*, **101,** 667.
Gerber, N. L. & Steinberg, A. D. (1976), Clinical use of immunosuppressive drugs, *Drugs*, **11,** 14, 90.
Heffner, G. H. & Calabresi, P. (1976), Selective suppression of humoral immunity by antineoplastic drugs, *Ann. Rev. Pharmacol.*, **16,** 367.
Hersh, E. M., Carbone, P. P., Wong, V. G. & Freirich, E. J. (1965), Inhibition of the primary immune response in man by antimetabolites, *Cancer Res.*, **25,** 997.
Liddle, G. W. (1961), Clinical pharmacology of the anti-inflammatory steroids, *Clin. Pharm. Ther.*, **2,** 615.
Pinofsky, B. J. & Bardana, E. J. (1977), Immunosuppressive therapy in rheumatic disease, *Med. Clin. N. Amer.*, **61,** 419.
Rozman, M. & Bertino, J. T. (1973), Azothioprine, *Ann. Int. Med.*, **79,** 694.

Skinner, M. D. & Schwartz, R. S. (1972), Immunosuppressive therapy, *New Eng. J. Med.*, **287,** 221, 281.

Chapter 22 Drug Dependence and Drug Overdose

Cherubin, C. E. (1967), The medical sequelae of narcotic addiction, *Ann. Int. Med.*, **67,** 23.
Graham, J. D. P. (1976) (ed.), *Cannabis and Health*, Academic Press, London.
Henderson, L. W. & Merrill, J. P. (1966), Treatment of barbiturate intoxication, *Ann. Int. Med.*, **64,** 876.
Hill, J. (1973), Salicylate intoxication, *New Eng. J. Med.*, **288,** 1110.
Hore, B. D. & Ritson, E. B. (1984), *Alcohol and Health—a Handbook for Medical Students*. Medical Council on Alcoholism, London.
Kaupman, R. E. & Levy, S. B. (1974), Overdose treatment: addict folklore and medical reality, *J. Am. Med. Ass.*, **227,** 411.
Louria, D. B. (1969), Medical complications of pleasure giving drugs, *Arch. Int. Med.*, **123,** 82.
Mezey, E. (1976), Ethanol metabolism and ethanol-drug interactions, *Biochem. Pharmacol.*, **25,** 869.
Mitchell, J. R., Thorgeirsson, S. S., Potter, W. Z., Jallow, D. J. & Keiser, H. (1974), Acetaminophen-induced hepatic injury: protective role of glutathione in man and rationale for therapy, *Clin. Pharm. Ther.*, **16,** 676.
Schachter, S. (1978), Pharmacological and psychological determinants of smoking. *Ann. Int. Med.*, **89,** 104.
Tashkin, D. P., Soares, J. R., Hepler, R. S., Shapiro, B. J. & Rachelepsky, G. E. (1978), Cannabis 1977, *Ann. Int. Med.*, **89,** 539.
Turner, T. B., Mezey, E. & Kimball, A. W. (1977), Measurement of alcohol-related effects in man: chronic effects in relation to levels of alcohol consumption, *Johns Hopkins Med. J.*, **141,** 235, 273.
Volans, G. V. & Henry, J. (1985) (eds.), *ABC of Poisoning*. British Medical Association, London.

INDEX

Page numbers in *italics* denote particularly important entries